D1558434

Vitamins in the prevention of human diseases

Edited by Wolfgang Herrmann and Rima Obeid

Vitamins in the prevention of human diseases

Edited by Wolfgang Herrmann and Rima Obeid

DE GRUYTER

Editors

Prof. Dr. Wolfgang Herrmann
Universitätsklinikum des Saarlandes
Klinische Chemie und
Laboratoriumsmedizin - Zentrallabor
Kirrberger Str.
Gebäude 57
66424 Homburg
kchwher@uniklinik-saarland.de

Dr. Rima Obeid
Universitätsklinikum des Saarlandes
Klinische Chemie und
Laboratoriumsmedizin - Zentrallabor
Kirrberger Str.
Gebäude 57
66424 Homburg
rima.obeid@uniklinik-saarland.de

This book contains num. figs. and tabs.

ISBN 978-3-11-021448-2 • e-ISBN 978-3-11-021449-9

Library of Congress Cataloging-in-Publication Data

Vitamins in the prevention of human diseases / edited by Wolfgang Herrmann, Rima Obeid.
   p. ; cm.
   ISBN 978-3-11-021448-2 (alk. paper)
   1. Vitamins.   2. Vitamin therapy.   I. Herrmann, Wolfgang, Prof.   II. Obeid, Rima.
   [DNLM: 1. Vitamins–pharmacology.   2. Vitamins–therapeutic use.   QU 160]

   QP801.V5V58 2010
   612.3'99–dc22   2010028998

Bibliographic information published by the Deutsche Nationalbibliothek
The Deutsche Nationalbibliothek lists this publication in the Deutsche Nationalbibliografie; detailed bibliographic data are available in the Internet at http://dnb.d-nb.de.

Project management: Dr. Petra Kowalski.
Production editor: Simone Pfitzner.
Production manager: Sabina Dabrowski.
Typesetting: Compuscript, Shanon – Ireland.
Cover image: Dr. Arthur Siegelman/Visuals Unlimited/gettyimages
Printing and binding: Druckhaus „Thomas Müntzer", Bad Langensalza.

Preface

This book provides an up-to-date knowledge on the role of the main water and fat soluble vitamins in the prevention of human diseases. The term vitamin originated from "vitamine", a word first used in 1911 by the Polish scientist Cashmir Funk to designate a group of compounds considered vital for life. Vitamins are essential food constituents with magnificent biological effects therefore, linking our biology to our lifestyle and environment. Our knowledge of the chemical composition of vitamins is much younger than the knowledge of the effect of vitamin deficiencies. Deficiency of essential vitamins has already been described in ancient Egypt.

One-sided nutrition, smoking, alcohol, genetic factors, and even geographical origin interfere with our dietary intake of the vitamins. Insufficient vitamin intake can impact our health and contribute significantly to the development of diseases. This book offers expert reviews and judgements on the role of vitamins in health and disease conditions at different stages of life. One classical example is the causal relationship between folate deficiency and neural tube defects and their prevention by folic acid supplementation. Furthermore, sufficient vitamin intake is considered essential for a healthy aging. Thus elderly people are a target group for vitamin-research aiming at prevention of age-related-diseases.

The significance of the vitamins as prevention factors has changed over the time. Vitamin research is still a modern field but one with great potential. Having knowledge about the association of vitamins and disease, as well as keeping track on the patients vitamin status has become increasingly important to physicians, clinical chemists, specialists in nutrition, and researchers. Recent development in laboratory methods has helped quantifying many vitamin biomarkers in biological materials.

A healthy well balanced diet has long been thought to be sufficient to prevent vitamin deficiency. However, vitamin deficiencies are found in affluent societies and may be very common in certain population groups like elderly people, pregnant women, or children. Vitamin deficiency may be due to a low intake, increased requirements, or turnover or impaired absorption in certain disease conditions. Food cultures, religion, ethical issues, and poverty are important factors that have impact on vitamin intake. Endemic deficiency of certain vitamins in some parts of the world has helped to understand the biological role of the vitamins.

The rapidly growing knowledge about the role of vitamins in human diseases and their relation to lifestyle factors has led to intensive scientific discussion. For example, in numerous secondary prevention trials the impact of supplementary vitamins on disease outcomes has been studied. Fortification of staple food with certain vitamins has been introduced in many countries as an effective way to reach all population groups. This book covers also vitamin supplementation recommendations and is therefore important updating the knowledge of a wide spectrum of health professionals. Furthermore, the book highlights controversial discussions in this area.

Wolfgang Herrmann and Rima Obeid
January 2011

Table of Contents

Authors Index

Emmanuel Andrés
Department of Internal Medicine
University Hospital of Strasbourg
1 Place de l'Hôpital
67000 Strasbourg Cedex
France
Emmanuel.andres@chru-strasbourg.fr

Arun B. Barua
4737 South Ellis Avenue
Chicago, IL 60615
USA
abbarua@gmail.com

Tapan K. Basu
University of Alberta
Dept. of Agricultural
Food and Nutritional Science
3-18B Agricultural Forestra Building
Edmonton, ALTA T6G 2P5
Canada

Elena Beltramo
Dept Internal Medicine
University of Turin
Corso Dogliotti 14
I-10126 Torino
Italy
elena.beltramo@unito.it

Peter C. Blumbergs
Hanson Institute/North Building
Institute of Medical and Veterinary Science
PO Box 14
Adelaide SA 5000
Australia

Jan Krzysztof Blusztajn
Department of Pathology and Laboratory
Medicine
Boston University School of Medicine
72 East Concord Street, L804
Boston MA 02118
USA
jbluszta@bu.edu

Mustafa Vakur Bor
Department of Clinical Biochemistry
Aarhus University Hospital
Norrebrogade 44
DK 8000 Aarhus
Denmark
vakbor@yahoo.com

Philip C. Calder
Institute of Human Nutrition
School of Medicine
University of Southampton
MP887 Southampton General Hospital
Tremona Road
Southampton SO16 6YD
UK
pcc@soton.ac.uk

Gabriella Calviello
Institute of General Pathology
School of Medicine
Catholic University
L. go f. Vito, 1
I-00168 Rome
Italy
g.calviello@rm.unicatt.it

Kanwaljit Chopra
UGC Centre of Advanced Study (UGC-CAS)
Panjab University
University Institute of Pharmaceutical Sciences
Chandigarh-160014
India
dr_chopra_k@yahoo.com

Karen E. Christensen
Departments of Human Genetics and
Pediatrics
McGill University and Montreal Children's
Hospital of the McGill University Health
Centre
Montreal Children's Hospital
2300 Tupper Street
Montreal, Quebec H3H 1P3
Canada

Robert Clarke
Clinical Trial Service Unit and Epidemiological
Studies Unit Richard Doll Building
University of Oxford
Old Road Campus
Roosevelt Drive Oxford
Oxford 3 7LF
UK
robert.clarke@ctsu.ox.ac.uk

Martin den Heijer
Department of Endocrinology
Radboud University Nijmegen
Medical Centre
PO-Box 9101
6500 HB Nijmegen
The Netherlands
m.denheijer@endo.umcn.nl

Jutta Dierkes
Institute of Agricultural and Nutritional
Sciences
Von-Danckelmann Platz 2
D-06120 Halle (Saale)
Germany
jutta.dierkes@landw.uni-halle.de
jutta.dierkes@med.ovgu.de

Victoria J. Drake
Linus Pauling Institute
Oregon State University
571 Weniger Hall
Corvallis
OR 97331-6512
USA

Gustavo Duque
Nepean Clinical School
Level 5, South Block
Nepean Hospital
12/81 Bertram Street
2137 Mortlake NSW
Australia
gduque@med.usyd.edu.au

Farah Esfandiari
Level 5, South Block
University of California Davis
Davis, CA 95616
USA

Richard H. Finnell
Nepean Hospital
Texas A&M Health Science Center
2121 W. Holcombe Blvd.
Houston
Texas 77030
USA
rfinnell@ibt.tmc.edu

Balz Frei
Linus Pauling Institute
Oregon State University
571 Weniger Hall
Corvallis
OR 97331-6512
USA
balz.frei@oregonstate.edu

Henriette Frikke-Schmidt
Section of Biomedicine, Department of
Disease Biology
Faculty of Life Sciences
University of Copenhagen
9 Ridebanevej
DK-1870 Frederiksberg C
Copenhagen
Denmark

Harold C. Furr
Department of Nutritional Sciences
University of Wisconsin – Madison
1415 Linden Dr.
Madison
WI 53706-1571
USA
hfurr581@yahoo.com

Claudia Glaser
Klinikum der Universität München
Dr. von Haunersches Kinderspital
Lindwurmstraße 4
D-80337 München
Germany

Elizabeth B. Gorman
Center for Environmental and Genetic
Medicine
Institute of Biosciences and Technology
Texas A&M Health Science Center
2121 W. Holcombe Blvd., Houston
Texas 77030
USA

Renata Gorska
Centre for Haemostasis & Thrombosis
St. Thomas' Hospital
1st Floor North Wing
London SE1 7EH
UK

Nils-Olof Hagnelius
Örebro University
School of Health and Medical Sciences
SE-701 82 Örebro
Sweden
nils-olof.hagnelius@oru.se

Charles H. Halsted
University of California Davis
Professor of Internal Medicine and Nutrition
Davis, CA 95616
USA
chhalsted@ucdavis.edu

Dominic J. Harrington
Centre for Haemostasis & Thrombosis
St. Thomas' Hospital
1st Floor North Wing
London SE1 7EH
UK

Judith Heinz
University Medical Center Hamburg-
Eppendorf
Center for Experimental Medicine
Department of Medical Biometry and
Epidemiology
Martinistraße 52
D-20246 Hamburg
Germany

Markus Herrmann
Nepean Clinical School
Level 5, South Block
Nepean Hospital
12/81 Bertram Street
2137 Mortlake NSW
Australia
markusherr@aol.com

Idanna Innocenti
Institute of General Pathology
School of Medicine
Catholic University
L.go f. Vito, 1
I-00168 Rome
Italy

Mario Klingler
Klinikum der Universität München
Dr. von Haunersches Kinderspital
Lindwurmstraße 4
D-80337 München
Germany

Berthold Koletzko
Klinikum der Universität München
Dr. von Haunersches Kinderspital
Lindwurmstraße 4
D-80337 München
Germany
office.koletzko@med.uni-muenchen.de

Anurag Kuhad
UGC Centre of Advanced Stduy
(UGC-CAS)
Panjab University
University Institute of Pharmaceutical
Sciences
Chandigarh-160014
India

J.S.E Laven
Erasmus Medical Center
Rotterdam
Department of Obstetrics &
Gynecology
Subdivision of Reproductive Medicine
Dr Molewaterplein 40
3015 GD Rotterdam
The Netherlands

Michael Lever
University of Canterbury
Canterbury Health Laboratories
Biochemistry Unit
PO Box 151
Christchurch 8140
New Zealand
michael.lever@otago.ac.nz

Jenny Libien
Department of Pathology
SUNY Downstate Medical Center
450 Clarkson Avenue
Box 25
Brooklyn
New York 11203
USA
jenny.libien@downstate.edu

Michael Linnebank
UniversitätsSpital Zürich
Neurologische Klinik
Frauenklinikstraße 26
CH-8091 Zürich
Switzerland
michael.linnebank@usz.ch

Jens Lykkesfeldt
Section of Biomedicine
Department of Disease Biology
Faculty of Life Sciences
University of Copenhagen
9 Ridebanevej
DK-1870 Frederiksberg C
Copenhagen
Denmark
jopl@life.ku.dk

Joel B. Mason
Friedman School of Nutritional Science &
Policy,
Vitamins & Carcinogenesis Laboratory
Jean Mayer U.S.D.A. Human Nutrition
Research Center on Aging at Tufts University
Tufts University School of Medicine
150 Harrison Avenue
Boston, MA 02111
USA

Patrizia Mecocci
Institute of Gerontology and Geriatrics
University of Perugia
Via Vanvitelli 1
06123 Perugia
Italy

Valentina Medici
Department of Internal Medicine
University of California Davis
Davis, CA 95616
USA

Joshua W. Miller
UC Davis Medical Center
University of California, Davis
Research 3, Room 3200A
4645 Second Avenue
Sacramento
CA 95817
USA
jwmiller@ucdavis.edu

Paul Newman
Epithelial Cell Biology Laboratory
Cancer Research UK
Cambridge Research Institute
Cambridge
UK

Ebba Nexo
Department of Clinical Biochemistry
Aarhus University Hospital
Norrebrogade 44
DK 8000 Aarhus
Denmark
e.nexo@dadlnet.dk

Torbjörn K. Nilsson
Kliniken för Laboratoriemedicin
Universitetssjukhuset
Dept of Laboratory Medicine
Örebro University Hospital
SE-70185 Örebro
Sweden
torbjorn.nilsson@orebroll.se

J.A. Petersen
UniversitätsSpital Zürich
Frauenklinikstr. 26
8091 Zürich
Switzerland
jens.petersen@usz.ch

Elisabetta Piccioni
Institute of General Pathology
School of Medicine
Catholic University
L.go f. Vito 1
I-00168 Rome
Italy

Maria Cristina Polidori
Department of Geriatrics
Marienhospital Herne
Ruhr University of Bochum
D- 44625 Herne
Germany

D. Pratico
Department of Pharmacology
Temple University
School of Medicine
MRB 706A
3420 North Broad Street
Philadelphia
PA 19140
USA
praticod@temple.edu

Jörg Reichrath
Klinik für Dermatologie
Venerologie und Allergologie
Universitätsklinikum des Saarlandes
Kirrberger Str.
D-66421 Homburg/Saar
Germany
hajrei@uniklinik-saarland.de

Natalie D. Riediger
University of Manitoba
St. Boniface Hospital Research
Centre
Taché Avenue 351
R2H 2A6 Winnipeg Manitoba
Canada
umriedin@cc.umanitoba.ca

Rima Rozen
McGill-Montreal Children's Hospital
James Administration Building
845 Sherbrooke Street West
Room 419, H3A 2T5 Montreal
Canada
rima.rozen@mcgill.ca

Leon J. Schurgers
Department of Biochemistry
University of Maastricht
P.O. Box 616
6200 MD Maastricht
The Netherlands

Robert Scragg
University of Auckland
School of Population Health
Biochemistry and Medical
Genetics
Private Bag 92019
Auckland 1142
New Zealand
r.scragg@auckland.ac.nz

Alexander Semmler
Neurologische Klinik
Universitätsspital Zürich
Frauenklinikstrasse 26
CH-8091 Zürich
Switzerland
alexander.semmler@usz.ch

Simona Serini
Catholic University
Institute of General Pathology
L. go F. Vito 1
I-00168 Rome
Italy

Martin J. Shearer
Centre for Haemostasis & Thrombosis
1st Floor North Wing
St Thomas' Hospital
London SE1 7EH
UK
martin.shearer@gstt.nhs.uk

Sandy Slow
Canterbury Health Laboratories
Biochemisty Unit
Corner Hagley Ave and Tuam Street,
P O Box 151,
Christchurch, 8140
New Zealand

Sally P. Stabler
University of Colorado
School of Medicine
Division of Hematology
University of Colorado
Sally.Stabler@ucdenver.edu

Maria Stacewicz-Sapuntzakis
University of Illinois at Chicago
College of Applied Health Sciences
Department of Kinesiology and
Nutrition
650 AHSB, MC 517
1919 W. Taylor Street
Chicago, IL 60612
USA
msapuntz@uic.edu

Regine P.M. Steegers-Theunissen
Departments of Obstetrics & Gynaecology,
Epidemiology, Paediatrics/Division
Paediatric Cardiology and Clinical
Genetics
Erasmus University Medical Center PO Box
2040
3000CA Rotterdam
The Netherlands
r.steegers@erasmusmc.nl

Patrick J. Stover
Division of Nutritional Sciences
Cornell University
127 Savage Hall
Ithaca NY 14850
USA
pjs13@cornell.edu

Peter Swaan
University of Maryland
Department of Pharmaceutical Sciences
School of Pharmacy
20 Penn Street, Rm 621
Baltimore MD 21201-1075
USA
pswaan@rx.umaryland.edu

Ya-Wen Teng
Nutrition Research Institute
University of North Carolina at Chapel Hill
Department of Nutrition – CB#7461
Chapel Hill
North Carolina 27599
USA
yteng@email.unc.edu

Vinod Tiwari
UGC Centre of Advanced Study (UGC-CAS)
Panjab University
University Institute of Pharmaceutical Sciences
Chandigarh-160014
India

Maret G. Traber
Linus Pauling Institute
Oregon State University
Department of Nutrition and Exercise Sciences
Corvallis
OR 97331
USA
maret.traber@oregonstate.edu

Pernille Tveden-Nyborg
Section of Biomedicine
Department of Disease Biology
Faculty of Life Sciences
University of Copenhagen
9 Ridebanevej
DK-1870 Frederiksberg C
Copenhagen
Denmark

J.M. Twigt
Erasmus Medical Center
Department of Obstetrics & Gynecology,
Ee2271
Dr. Molewaterplein 40
3015 GD Rotterdam
The Netherlands
j.twigt@erasmusmc.nl

Per M. Ueland
University of Bergen
Section for Pharmacology
Institute of Medicine
9th floor, New Laboratory Building
5021 Bergen
Norway
per.ueland@ikb.uib.no

Paul F. Williams
Medicine, Central Clinical School D06
Blackburn Building
The University of Sydney
NSW 2006
Australia
paul.williams@sydney.edu.au;
pwlms@med.usyd.edu.au"

Jayne V. Woodside
Centre for Public Health
School of Medicine, Dentistry and Biomedical
Sciences
Queen's University Belfast
First Floor ICS B Block
Royal Victoria Hospital
Grosvenor Road
Belfast BT12 6BJ
Northern Ireland

Ian S. Young
Centre for Public Health
School of Medicine, Dentistry and Biomedical
Sciences
Queen's University Belfast
First Floor ICS B Block
Royal Victoria Hospital
Grosvenor Road
Belfast BT12 6BJ
Northern Ireland
I.Young@qub.ac.uk

Steven H. Zeisel
Nutrition Research Institute
University of North Carolina at Chapel Hill
Department of Nutrition – CB#7461
500 Laureate Way
Kannapolis
North Carolina 28081
USA
steven_zeisel@unc.edu

Armin Zittermann
Clinic for Thoracic and Cardiovascular
Surgery
Heart Center North Rhine-Westphalia
Ruhr University Bochum
Georgstraße 11
D-32545 Bad Oeynhausen
Germany
azittermann@hdz-nrw.de

1 History of the vitamins

Discovery, syntheses, Nobel prizes, modern science

Rima Obeid; Wolfgang Herrmann

Deficiency of essential vitamins has been described in ancient Egypt. Our knowledge of the chemical composition of vitamins is much younger than the knowledge of the effect of vitamin deficiencies. The nature of specific deficiency of micronutrients began to emerge in the 19th century, when Magendie in 1816 fed dogs sugar and water for a long period. The animals developed severe starvation and corneal ulceration, which has been later shown to be related to vitamin A deficiency. It was not until the first 2 decades of the 20th century that research on a deprived diet fed to humans and laboratory animals began to identify essential food components, which came to be called 'vital amines'.

Scurvy was one of the first illnesses to be recognized as a nutritional deficiency disorder. In the 5th century BC, Hippocrates first described scurvy as bleeding gums, hemorrhaging and death. Outbreaks of scurvy were reported in 1500 BC in Egypt, during the winters. In 1250, during the Crusades, rampant scurvy forced the retreat and eventual capture of St. Louis and his knights. During the voyages of Christopher Columbus, some Portuguese sailors had come down with scurvy and asked to be dropped off at one of the nearby islands. On the return trip months later, they were found to be alive and healthy probably because of the fruits consumed. The island was named 'Curacao', meaning 'cure'.

Native Americans had concocted the first cure for scurvy. In 1593, during a voyage to the South Pacific, Sir Richard Hawkins recommended 'oranges and lemons' as treatment for scurvy.

Frederick Gowland Hopkins, an English biochemist, spent a major part of his life working on the hypothesis that food contains 'accessory factors' in addition to proteins, carbohydrates, fats, minerals and water. These factors were thought to be important to maintain life and health. Frederick Gowland Hopkins, Elmer Verner McCullum, Marguerite Davis, Thomas Burr Osborne and Lafayette Benedict Mendel described the importance of some fat-soluble food components for growth. Hopkins had established his methodology in an experiment whereby he fed mice 'an artificial diet consisting of pure carbohydrate, protein, fats and salts'. Hopkins observed that the animals failed to grow unless their diet was supplemented with milk, dairy products and cod liver oil. He concluded that the supplemented foods must contain small amounts of what he called 'additional food factors' for growth and the maintenance of health. Hopkins succeeded in isolating these factors what became known as 'vitamins A and D'.

The term vitamin originated from 'vitamine', a word first used in 1911 by the Polish scientist Cashmir Funk to designate a group of compounds considered vital for life. Vitamins were thought to have a nitrogen-containing component or an amine. Many of those compounds were found not to contain nitrogen, and therefore not to be amines. Thereafter, the final 'e' of vitamine was dropped.

Vitamin A (or retinol) deficiency has been related to visual disorders, particularly night blindness. Eber's Papyrus described night blindness in ancient Egypt. Vitamin A was discovered in 1909, isolated in 1931, crystallized in 1937 and synthesized in 1947. In 1955, Wald described the role of vitamin A in the formation of rhodopsin, which is responsible for retinal receptors and hence for dark adaptation. This disease was treated by squeezing the 'juices' of a grilled lambs's liver into the eyes of affected patients. In 1978, George Wolff speculated that these drops rich in retinol can reach the systemic circulation and thereby the retinal cells (Wolf, 1978). In 1978 Hussaini et al. reported on curing night blindness in an Indonesian child by applying goat juices into the eye (Hussaini et al., 1978). In order not to throw out foods, the remaining liver was fed to the child, but this was not considered a part of the treatment.

As early as 1913, the importance of feeding some lipids for growth has been recognized (Lanska, 2009). In 1913, Yale researchers, Thomas Osborne and Lafayette Mendel discovered that butter contained a fat-soluble nutrient soon known as vitamin A or at that time 'fat-soluble A factor'. In 1932, Ellison recognized the role of this factor in reducing the burden of measles. Almost 50 years later, studies performed on African children found that vitamin A can reduce the fatality of measles (Sommer and Emran, 1978). The 'fat-soluble A' which could cure xerophthalmia and rickets was believed to be one vitamin. In 1922, McCollum showed that the 'fat-soluble A' was indeed two vitamins, later identified as A and D, the latter effective against rickets.

Thiamine or vitamin B1 is the first vitamin to be discovered in 1897. It was the first vitamin to be isolated in the first years of the 20th century, while looking for an 'anti-beriberi' substance (Lonsdale, 2006), and it was crystallized from rice polishings in 1926 by Jansen and Donath. Almost 10 years after isolation of the vitamin, the structure of thiamine and its biochemical function were described by Peters in 1936 and Williams in 1938.

In the late 1800s a Dutch physician Christiaan Eijkman discovered that substituting unpolished rice for polished rice would prevent beriberi, a terrible disease which caused anemia and paralysis and was found mainly among the poor. However, it was not until 1911 that a Polish chemist Casimir Funk discovered the actual substance in unpolished rice that prevented the disease.

The effect of folate deficiency has been also documented in the early 1900s. In 1928, Lucy Wills was invited from London University to Bombay to investigate an anemia of pregnancy which was prevalent among certain population group in India (Bastian, 2008). The studies on Bombay women with anemia of pregnancy were published in 1929–1931 in the *Indian Journal of Medical Research*. In her works, Lucy performed surveys on dietary habits in different social classes. Liver extract has been found to cure anemia in women from Bombay. Later in 1943, folic acid was isolated.

A severe cobalamin deficiency form also called pernicious anemia could be cured by feeding patients with liver. For this elegant demonstration Minot won the 1937 Nobel Prize in Medicine. Cobalamin was isolated in 1948 only 5 years after folic acid. Two independent teams, one British and one American, isolated vitamin B12 in the same year, using two different procedures.

The Scottish naval surgeon James Lindin observed in 1747 that a nutrient in citrus foods, now known to be vitamin C, prevented scurvy. Ascorbic acid was the third substance found so it was given the third letter of the alphabet: C. An anti-scurvy (antiscorbutic) vitamin was postulated in 1911, just in time to be considered the third (or 'C') vitamin discovered. Because it was anti-scurvy or a-scorbutic, it received the name ascorbic acid. Vitamin C deficiency was produced in an animal model by Norwegians A. Hoist and T. Froelich in 1907 when they fed guinea pigs a cereal diet and eliminated fresh animal and vegetable foods. Vitamin C was the first vitamin to be artificially synthesized in 1935. In 1928, an Hungarian scientist, Albert Szent-Gyorgyi, isolated the substance that could treat scurvy. Already at that time, Szent-Gyorgyi recognized that there is a difference between the 'minimum daily doses' of vitamins needed to prevent deficiency diseases and optimal doses, which he referred to in Latin as the '*dosis optima quotidiana*'.

Our view of the vitamins has changed over the time. Vitamin research is still a modern science. Vitamins are essential food constitutes with magnificent biological effects therefore, linking our biology to our lifestyle and environment. Some investigators claim that people eating a healthy balanced diet are getting sufficient amount of the vitamins. Others reported on vitamin deficiencies particularly in relation to some diseases and even in affluent societies.

Food cultures, religion, ethical issues, diseases and poverty are factors that have been affecting our intake of the vitamins and therefore our health. Endemic deficiency of certain vitamins in some parts of the world has helped scientists learn about the functions of the vitamin. Today, it is well known that insufficient vitamin intake can impact our health and contribute significantly to the development of numerous diseases.

References

Bastian H, Lucy Wills (1888–1964), The life and research of an adventurous independent woman. J R Coll Physicians Edinb 2008;38: 89–91.

Hussaini G, Tarwotjo I, Sommer A, Cure for night blindness. Am J Clin Nutr 1978;31: 1489.

Lanska DJ, Chapter 29 Historical aspects of the major neurological vitamin deficiency disorders Overview and fat-soluble vitamin A. Handb Clin Neurol 2009;95: 435–44.

Lonsdale D, A review of the biochemistry, metabolism and clinical benefits of thiamin(e) and its derivatives. Evid Based Complement Alternat Med 2006;3: 49–59.

Sommer A, Emran N, Topical retinoic acid in the treatment of corneal xerophthalmia. Am J Ophthalmol 1978;86: 615–7.

Wolf G, A historical note on the mode of administration of vitamin A for the cure of night blindness. Am J Clin Nutr 1978;31: 290–2.

Vitamins

2 Vitamin A – Retinol

2.1 Vitamin A: sources, absorption, metabolism, functions and assessment of status

Arun B. Barua; Maria Stacewicz-Sapuntzakis; Harold C. Furr

2.1.1 Chemical structures

Vitamin A is a group name of several fat-soluble compounds consisting of four isoprenoid units [$H_2C=C(CH_3)–CH=CH_2$] joined in a head-to-tail manner (►Fig. 2.1). Each form of vitamin A has different and unique functions in the human body. Retinol is the transport form and circulates in the blood. Retinaldehyde and its *cis*-isomers are present in the eye and are required for vision. Retinyl esters are the storage form found in the liver and some other tissues. Retinoic acid, the active form in control of gene expression, is produced in very small amounts, but is essential for many biological functions of vitamin A apart from vision. There are two water-soluble forms of vitamin A, retinoyl glucuronide and retinyl glucuronide, which are carbohydrate derivatives of retinoic acid and retinol, respectively. They occur in small amounts, and are often regarded as excretory products (Barua and Sidell, 2004), although they have biological activity.

In several varieties of seawater and freshwater fish, another form of vitamin A, known as vitamin A2 (3,4-didehydroretinol) is present as the major form of vitamin A. Vitamin A2 differs from vitamin A in chemical structure in having an additional double bond in the cyclohexene ring at the 3,4 position (Embree and Shantz, 1943). Although its importance is not clear, vitamin A2 in various forms has been found in human skin (Vahlquist, 1994).

In an attempt to find compounds that are efficacious yet non-toxic, many new compounds related to vitamin A have been chemically synthesized and biologically tested. Compounds that can elicit specific biological responses by binding to and activating specific receptors or sets of receptors, with the resulting biological response of vitamin A compounds, are known as retinoids (Sporn and Roberts, 1994). The term 'retinoids' is now the group name for all of the naturally occurring vitamin A compounds as well as the synthetic compounds that possess some of the biological properties of vitamin A. Fenretinide, acitretin and TTNPB are examples of synthetic retinoids (►Fig. 2.2).

2.1.2 Dietary sources

Retinyl esters of fatty acids are the predominant dietary source of preformed vitamin A. Livers of all animals, birds and fish store vitamin A as retinyl esters and therefore liver is the richest food source of preformed vitamin A. When synthetic vitamin A was not available, cod liver oil was used as a source of vitamin A supplements. Other organs, such as kidney and heart, are good sources of vitamin A, as are eggs and fish. Vitamin A is also present in milk and other dairy products, such as cheese, butter and ice cream. In many countries, milk, margarine and breakfast cereals are often fortified with vitamin A (►Tab. 2.1).

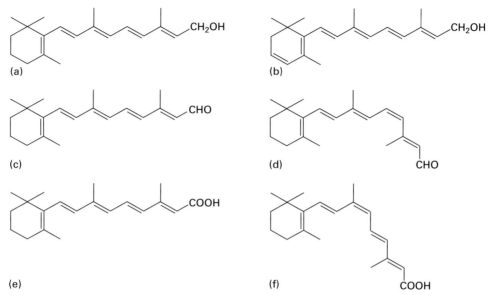

Fig. 2.1: Representative vitamin A compounds: (a) all-*trans* retinol (vitamin A alcohol); (b) all-*trans* 3,4-didehydroretinol (vitamin A2 alcohol); (c) all-*trans* retinaldehyde (all-*trans* retinal; vitamin A aldehyde); (d) 11-*cis* retinaldehyde (11-*cis* retinal); (e) all-*trans* retinoic acid (vitamin A acid; tretinoin); (f) 9-*cis* retinoic acid.

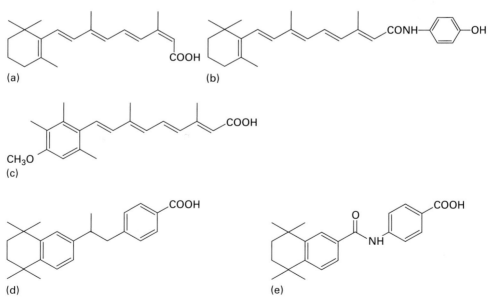

Fig. 2.2: Representative retinoid compounds of pharmacological interest: (a) 13-*cis* retinoic acid (isotretinoin; Accutane); (b) Fenretinide (4-hydroxyphenylretinamide; 4-HPR); (c) acitretin; (d) tetrahydrotetramethylnaphthalenylpropenylbenzoic acid (TTNPB); (e) AM-580.

Tab. 2.1: Food sources of vitamin A (per 100 g edible portion).

Provitamin A sources:	µg RAE/100 g
Fruits	
Apricots, dry	180
Cantaloupe, raw	169
Mango, raw	38
Papaya, raw	55
Tangerine, raw	42
Vegetables	
Broccoli, cooked	77
Carrots, raw	835
Carrots, cooked	852
Carrot juice	956
Collard greens, frozen, cooked	575
Mustard greens, cooked	316
Peppers, sweet, red, raw	157
Pumpkin, canned	778
Spinach, frozen, cooked	603
Squash, winter, baked	261
Sweet potato, baked	961
Turnip greens, cooked	381

Preformed vitamin A sources:	µg RAE/100 g
Dairy products	
Milk, whole	28
Milk, nonfat, added vitamin A	61
Butter	693
Margarine, added vitamin A	829
Cheddar cheese	268
Swiss cheese	221
Cream cheese	353
Cream, heavy, whipping	413
Ice cream, vanilla	105
Meat, poultry and fish products	
Beef liver	7744
Braunschweiger, pork	4198
Chicken liver	3900
Egg, large	140
Herring, pickled	258
Salmon, cooked, dry heat	63
Fortified cereals	
Kellogg's Complete Bran Flakes	1293
Cereals, fortified, oats, instant	186

Adapted from: USDA National Nutrient Database for Standard Reference, Release 20. Agricultural Research Service 2007. Nutrient Data Laboratory Home Page. http://www.ars.usda.gov/ba/bhnrc/ndl

For much of the population of the world, the major sources of vitamin A are the precursor compounds, the provitamin A carotenoids. Carotenoids are yellow to red fat-soluble pigments that give color to many fruits and vegetables. Many yellow and orange colored fruits, such as ripe mango, papaya, guava, orange, peach and apricot, and all green vegetables contain considerable amounts of carotenoids. Only a few carotenoids (beta-carotene, alpha-carotene, beta-cryptoxanthin) can be converted to vitamin A in the human body. Beta-carotene has the highest provitamin A activity and is the major carotene in carrots and many other fruits and vegetables (Ross, 2006).

In addition to provitamin A carotenoids, there are well over 600 known carotenoids in nature. Important carotenoids in the human diet and human tissues include lycopene (responsible for the red color of tomato and watermelon), lutein (present in all green vegetables and maize) and zeaxanthin (present in maize) (▶Fig. 2.3). Recent studies show that there might be a relation between the intake of lutein and zeaxanthin and prevention of macular disease (Loane et al., 2008). Lycopene is a very good antioxidant and might be protective against prostate cancer (Erdman et al., 2009).

2.1.3 Units of vitamin A activity

In the past it was common to use International Units to express vitamin A activity, but this is discouraged because of ambiguities in the definition regarding bioefficacy of carotenoids. One International Unit (IU) is equal to 0.3 µg of retinol, or 0.344 µg of retinyl acetate, or 0.54 µg of retinyl palmitate. Recent studies showed that provitamin A carotenoids are less well absorbed and less well converted to vitamin A than was previously thought, but the efficiency of intestinal absorption and extent of cleavage to vitamin A is still controversial (see discussion below on factors affecting absorption). The current international standard to measure vitamin A is retinol activity equivalents (RAE). One RAE is equal to 1 µg (3.5 nmol) of all-*trans* retinol or 12 µg of dietary beta-carotene. Therefore, the ratio of β-carotene to retinol is 12:1, whereas the ratio is 24:1 for α-carotene and other provitamin A carotenoids (Institute of Medicine, 2002). Previously it was believed that 6 µg of dietary β-carotene can provide 1 µg retinol or 1 retinol equivalent (RE), still used by FAO/WHO. However, β-carotene in supplements (oil or gelatin beadlets) is so efficiently absorbed that the conversion factor seems to be 2:1 (2 µg supplemental β-carotene = 1 RAE). In ▶Tab. 2.2, the conversion factors for RAE and IU for vitamin A and provitamin A carotenoids are shown.

2.1.4 Recommended dietary allowances

The recommended dietary allowance (RDA) for vitamin A in humans depends on the age and gender of the subject. Different national and international authorities have given somewhat different recommendations, depending on different interpretations of the data. However, it is agreed that a range of 300–1300 RAE of retinol is required daily. Current US and WHO/FAO recommended intakes are provided in ▶Tab. 2.3.

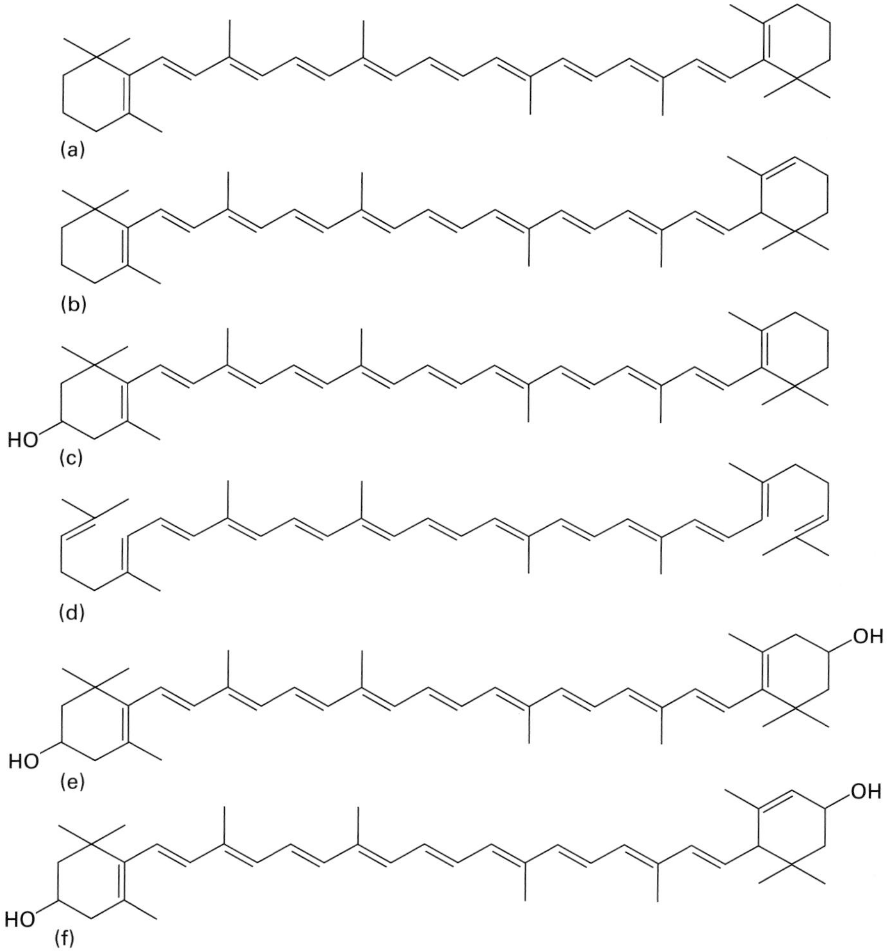

Fig. 2.3: Carotenoids of greatest interest in human foods and tissues: (a) beta-carotene; (b) alpha-carotene; (c) beta-cryptoxanthin; (d) lycopene; (e) zeaxanthin; (f) lutein. (Only the all-*trans* isomers are shown.)

US RDA is based on the estimated average requirement (EAR), which is designed to maintain minimal acceptable liver reserves. RDA exceeds EAR by 40% to supply the needs of 98% of targeted population (Institute of Medicine, 2002). FAO/WHO recommended safe intakes are similar to EAR, because they are set to prevent clinical signs of deficiency and allow normal growth, but are not sufficient for prolonged periods of infection or other stresses (WHO/FAO, 2002). The tolerable upper level (UL) of preformed vitamin A intake is set in the USA at 3000 μg of retinol per day, but it does not apply to provitamin A carotenoids because they do not evoke toxic symptoms.

Tab. 2.2: International Units (IU), Retinol Equivalents (RE) and Retinol Activity Equivalents (RAE).

Compound	µg/IU	IU/µg	RE/µg	µg/RE	RAE/µg	µg/RAE	µmol/µg	µg/µmol	µmol/IU	IU/µmol
Retinol (all-*trans*)	0.300	3.33	1.00	1.00	1.00	1.00	0.00350	286	0.00105	952
Retinyl acetate	0.344	2.91	0.873	1.15	0.873	1.15	0.00305	328	0.00105	954
Retinyl palmitate	0.549	1.82	0.546	1.83	0.546	1.83	0.00191	524	0.00105	954
β-Carotene (dietary sources, not supplements)	0.600	1.67	0.17	6	0.083	12.00	0.00187	536	0.00112	893
Other pro-vitamin A carotenoids	1.200	0.83	0.083	12	0.042	24.00	(not defined)	(not defined)	(not defined)	(not defined)

Adapted from Institute of Medicine (2002).

Tab. 2.3: Recommendations for vitamin A intake.

Life stage	Age	US RDA[a]		FAO/WHO Recommended Safe Intakes[b]	
		Males RAE/day	Females RAE/day	Males RE/day	Females RE/day
Infants	0–6 months	400	400	375	375
	7–12 months	500	500	400	400
Children	1–3 years	300	300	400	400
	4–6 years			450	450
	4–8 years	400	400		
	7–9 years			500	500
	9–13 years	600	600		
	10–18 years			600	600
	14–18 years	900	700		
Adults	>19 years	900	700	600	500
Pregnancy	<18 years		750		800
	>18 years		770		800
Breast feeding	<18 years		1200		850
	>18 years		1300		850

[a]Institute of Medicine, 2002.

[b]WHO/FAO (2002) http://www.fao.org/DOCREP/004/Y2809E/y2809e07.htm, accessed July 2009.

2.1.5 Absorption and metabolism

After foods are ingested, all preformed vitamin A and carotenoids present in foods are released from proteins by the action of digestive enzymes in the stomach and small intestine. The lipid molecules congregate in fatty globules and enter the duodenum. In the presence of bile salts, the globules are broken up into smaller lipid aggregates, which are digested by pancreatic lipase and retinyl ester hydrolase. The resulting mixed micelles, containing retinol and carotenoids, diffuse into the glycoprotein layer and make contact with the enterocyte membrane. Various components of the micelles are then readily absorbed into mucosal cells, mainly in the upper half of the intestine. The overall nutritional status of the individual and the integrity of the intestinal mucosa are very important (Olson, 1984).

Many factors influence the bioavailability and digestion of vitamin A and carotenoids (West and Castenmiller, 1998), including the preparation of the food (cooked or raw), the composition of the food (fat facilitates absorption), the health of the person (the presence of worms or diarrhea could decrease absorption), and possibly genetic differences. Some people cannot absorb carotenoids even though they consume lots of carotenoid-rich food. Owing to such differences in absorption, the amount of vitamin A available from carotenoids varies widely. By contrast, prolonged consumption of high amounts of carotenoids can result in hypercarotenemia (carotenemia), yellowish discoloration of the light-colored areas of the skin (carotenosis, carotenodermia). This condition is not dangerous, and readily reverses when consumption of carotenoids is decreased (Scientific Committee on Food, 2000).

After beta-carotene is absorbed in the mucosal cells of the small intestine, it can be cleaved to vitamin A aldehyde (retinal). Cleavage can occur at the central 15,15 double bond to produce two molecules of retinaldehyde and this is considered the major pathway for formation of vitamin A. Eccentric cleavage (i.e., at a position in the polyene chain other than at the 15,15' double bond) results in apo-carotenals which can be shortened to one molecule of retinaldehyde, and immediately reduced by a microsomal enzyme, retinal reductase, to retinol in the cytoplasm of intestinal cells. Retinol is then esterified to retinyl esters that are transported in the blood to the liver via chylomicrons. In periods of inadequate dietary intake of vitamin A, retinyl esters in tissues are hydrolyzed to retinol for mobilization and usage. This set of reactions occurs in many tissues, including the intestine, liver and adrenal gland. Retinaldehyde can also be irreversibly oxidized to retinoic acid. Several enzymes belonging to the reductase, hydrolase and esterase groups take part in these biochemical reactions. The possible pathways of the conversion of beta carotene to retinoids were described by Olson (1999) and an update on absorption and transport of vitamin A has been recently published (Wongsiriroj and Blaner, 2007).

2.1.6 Retinoid-binding proteins

Retinoids (with the exception of the glucuronides) have very low solubility in aqueous systems such as plasma and intracellular fluid, and so must have specific binding proteins as chaperones for transport and metabolism. Vitamin A-binding proteins can be extracellular or intracellular. Plasma retinol-binding protein (RBP) and interphotoreceptor retinol-binding protein (iRBP) are extracellular. RBP is the carrier of all-*trans* retinol and circulates in the blood in association with the protein transthyretin (TTR, also known as prealbumin). iRBP is involved in transferring retinoids between different cells in the retina of the eye. Cellular retinol-binding protein type I (CRBP-I) and type II (CRBP-II) are intracellular proteins required for metabolism (esterification or oxidation) within cells. Retinoic acid also binds to two specific intracellular proteins, CRABP-I and CRABP-II, which facilitate oxidative metabolism of retinoic acid and which deliver it to the cell nucleus. Retinaldehyde binds to a cellular retinal-binding protein (CRALBP), which participates in the formation of visual pigment. All these proteins are members of the protein family whose basic structural motif is a β-clam fold. The role of retinoid-binding proteins in metabolic channeling of retinoids and in pigment epithelium and their expression in adipose tissues, liver and cultured cell lines, and interaction with transthyretin have been reviewed (Livrea and Packer, 1993).

2.1.7 Biological functions of vitamin A

Vitamin A is necessary for growth, cell differentiation, cell proliferation, reproduction, immune function (resistance to infection) and vision (eyesight). Biochemically, the mechanism of action of vitamin A in vision is very different from that in other processes, where the mode of action is control of gene expression.

2.1.7.1 Vision

It is important to distinguish the two different functions of vitamin A in the eye. For vision *per se*, vitamin A (as retinaldehyde) forms part of the visual pigment needed for visual perception, and vitamin A deficiency results in night blindness (impaired ability to see in low levels of light); but this can be reversed by providing adequate vitamin A. By contrast, for maintenance of integrity of the cornea, retinoic acid is needed to sustain appropriate cell differentiation, and vitamin A deficiency results in hyperkeratinization of conjunctiva and disappearance of mucus-producing goblet cells. This, in turn, causes xerophthalmia, susceptibility to infection, eventual scarring of the cornea and permanent irreversible blindness.

Vitamin A alcohol (retinol) is transported in the blood by RBP to the retina of the eye. It accumulates in retinal pigment epithelial cells, and is esterified to form retinyl esters, which can be stored in a local pool. When needed, retinyl esters are hydrolyzed and isomerized to 11-*cis*-retinol and then oxidized to 11-*cis*-retinal. 11-*cis*-Retinal moves across the interphotoreceptor matrix (with the help of the binding protein iRBP) to the rod cells, where it binds to a protein called opsin to form the visual pigment, rhodopsin. Rod cells with rhodopsin can detect very small amounts of light, which is important for night vision. Absorption of a photon of light causes the isomerization of 11-*cis*-retinal to all-*trans*-retinal and results in its release from the opsin protein. This isomerization triggers a cascade of events, leading to the generation of an electrical signal to the optic nerve. The nerve impulse generated by the optic nerve is conveyed to the brain where it is interpreted as a visual event. Once released from opsin, all-*trans* retinal is converted to all-*trans*-retinol, which can be transported across the interphotoreceptor matrix (again via iRBP) to the retinal epithelial cell, thereby completing the visual cycle (Saari, 1994).

2.1.7.2 Retinoic acid receptors and control of gene expression

Experimental and clinical studies have shown that retinoic acid regulates a wide variety of biological processes. These include vertebrate embryonic morphogenesis and organogenesis, cell growth arrest, differentiation and apoptosis, and homeostasis, as well as their disorders. Retinoic acid exerts its pleiotropic effects through nuclear receptor proteins, the RAR (retinoic acid receptor) and RXR (retinoid X receptor) families. There are three RAR subtypes (RARα, RARβ and RARγ) and three RXR subtypes (RXRα, RXRβ and RXRγ), with isoforms for each subtype.

Upon binding of the appropriate isomer of retinoic acid (all-*trans* retinoic acid for RAR, either 9-*cis* or all-*trans* retinoic acid for RXR), the nuclear receptor protein-ligand complex translocates to the nucleus where it dimerizes (forming either a RAR-RAR or RXR-RXR homodimer or a RXR-RAR heterodimer or a heterodimer with another nuclear receptor protein) and binds to the promoter region (retinoic acid receptor response element, RARE) of an appropriate gene; the promoter region is usually in the 5′-regulatory region of the gene. Binding of the retinoic acid-nuclear receptor (as a homodimer or heterodimer) could result in either an increase or decrease in transcription, depending on the specific gene. The synthesis of the retinoic acid nuclear receptor proteins themselves is under transcriptional control by retinoic acid. Thus there are multiple control points for retinoid-responsive genes: provision of retinol and retinoic acid to the cell and synthesis of retinoic acid from retinol within the cell; synthesis of the individual retinoic acid nuclear receptor proteins; transfer of the retinoid-receptor protein complex to the nucleus; formation of a homodimer or heterodimer of nuclear receptor proteins; binding of the nuclear receptor proteins to the promoter region of the DNA; and interaction of several promoters/repressors of the gene (McGrane, 2007). Because retinoids function in a hormone-like manner, but can be converted to the active form (9-*cis* or all-*trans* retinoic acid) within the target tissues, they have been considered intracrine compounds (Reichrath et al., 2007).

2.1.7.3 Expression and functions of RARs

The expression of all three RARs has been demonstrated by *in situ* hybridization in mouse embryonic development. It has been shown that the three RARs have distinct physiological functions; individual RAR subtypes can have distinct activities even within the same cell line. Studies by Chambon's group using knockouts of the three RAR subtypes as well as the eight RAR isoforms through homologous recombination in embryonic stem cells have provided many valuable insights on the developmental functions of RARs (Mark et al., 2006). These studies provided the genetic evidence that RARs transduce retinoid signals *in vivo* and revealed that the various RAR subtypes have distinct functionalities during embryogenesis. Genetic studies revealed that retinoid signals are transduced by specific RXRα-RAR (α, β or γ) heterodimers during development (Germain et al., 2006).

2.1.8 Vitamin A deficiency

In the USA, only approximately 26% of vitamin A consumed by men and 34% of vitamin A consumed by women is in the form of provitamin A carotenoids (Institute of Medicine, 2002). In many developing countries where vitamin A is largely consumed in the form of fruits and vegetables, the daily intake is often insufficient to meet dietary requirements. The newborn child is particularly at risk of vitamin A deficiency because of very limited transfer of vitamin A across the placenta during embryonic development (perhaps to avoid teratogenesis), and because the maternal milk supply of vitamin A might be low. There is increased demand for the vitamin as children grow, but during periods of illness and common childhood infections the demand for vitamin A is even greater. As a result, vitamin A deficiency is prevalent in developing countries. From a global health point of view, vitamin A plays a major role in mortality and blindness of infants and children living in developing countries.

Xerophthalmia is a disease of the eye resulting from vitamin A deficiency, predominantly affecting young children (Heimburger et al., 2006). Lack of vitamin A initially affects rhodopsin formation in the eye, resulting in impaired dark adaptation and night blindness (XN) which is often the earliest sign of vitamin A deficiency. Progressing ocular surface changes are classified into conjunctival xerosis without Bitot's spot (X1A), with Bitot's spot (X1B) and corneal xerosis (X2). These ailments respond to vitamin A treatment (West, 1994; Heimburger et al., 2006; WHO, 2009). The next stage is corneal ulceration (keratomalacia) involving at first less than one-third of the corneal surface (X3A), and later more than one-third of the corneal surface (X3B). Ultimately, corneal scarring (XS) could result in complete blindness (Underwood, 1994a). Other symptoms of vitamin A deficiency include loss of appetite, follicular hyperkeratosis and skin dryness. The hyperkeratinization affects all epithelial tissues, including respiratory and urogenital tract. Because retinoic acid is required for correct differentiation and proliferation of cells, the impaired development of various white cell types decreases immunity and promotes susceptibility to infection (Semba, 1998).

It is now well known that there is a strong relation between infant mortality and vitamin A deficiency. Measles remains the most common precipitating cause of corneal xerophthalmia in Asia and Africa, and the cause of an estimated 1.5 million child deaths each year (West, 1994). Vitamin A deficiency increases the risk of dying from severe infection, such as enteric and respiratory diseases. Approximately 25 years ago the infant mortality rate in Nepal was 133 in every 1000 infants. Supplementation with vitamin A in 3.5 million children every year has resulted in cutting the mortality by half, and the prevalence of eye disease resulting from vitamin A deficiency plummeted from 23% to 3%. For deficient children, the periodic supply of high-dose vitamin A in swift, simple, low-cost, high-benefit interventions has also produced remarkable results, reducing mortality by 23% overall, and by up to 50% for acute measles sufferers.

2.1.9 Assessment of nutritional status

Vitamin A status is described as deficient, marginal, adequate, or excessive (▶Tab. 2.4), depending on liver reserves and circulating levels of retinol in plasma. Liver stores reflect total body vitamin A stores, and are the best measure of vitamin A status, but only indirect methods (such as isotope dilution) can usually be applied for this estimate (Furr et al., 2005). If the plasma level of retinol for a child falls below 0.7 µmol/l, the subject is considered vitamin A deficient; adults usually have higher plasma retinol concentrations, so 1.05 µmol/l (30 µg/dl) is often used as a cut-off (▶Tab. 2.3) (Underwood, 1994b; Ross, 2006; WHO, 2009). However, the plasma retinol range of 1–3 µmol/l (30–85 µg/dl) is maintained homeostatically over a wide range of liver concentrations of vitamin A and therefore is not a very specific marker of vitamin A status. In vitamin A deficiency, apo-RBP accumulates in hepatocytes, from where it can be released as holo-RBP when vitamin A becomes available again. This is the basis of the Relative Dose Response (RDR) and Modified Relative Dose Response (MRDR) techniques for assessing vitamin A status. Plasma response to an oral dose of vitamin A is employed in RDR (Underwood, 1990), whereas vitamin A2 is used in the MRDR (Tanumihardjo et al., 1996). In the marginal range of 0.7–1.05 µmol/l, no clinical signs are observed, but the liver reserves of vitamin A are low. In mild deficiency (0.35–0.7 µmol/l) there are still no apparent symptoms, but plasma levels are responsive to the supply of vitamin A. Therefore, to prevent xerophthalmia, it is appropriate to supplement subjects with suspected vitamin A deficiency before the plasma retinol level falls to a severely deficient level (below 0.35 µmol/l). Clinical assessments of vitamin A deficiency, including dark adaptation tests, scotometry or electroretinography, as well as evaluation of conjunctival impression cytology (counting mucin spots and goblet cells on an adhesive strip), have been used but have usually proven problematic in field applications. Dietary assessments are helpful but alone cannot determine vitamin A status.

Chemically, retinol and other vitamin A forms can be assessed in plasma or serum, breast milk and tissues (liver biopsy) by organic solvent extraction followed by high performance liquid chromatography (HPLC) with spectrophotometric or fluorometric

Tab. 2.4: Vitamin A (retinol) level in blood serum/plasma and clinical signs of deficiency or toxicity.

Category	Serum retinol concentration	Liver stores	Clinical signs
Deficient	<0.35 µmol/l (10 µg/dl)	Severely depleted (<5 µg/g)	Night blindness, ocular manifestations,
Marginal[a]	0.35–0.7 µmol/l (10–20 µg/dl)	Severely depleted	None (levels responsive to provision of vitamin A)
Adequate	1.05–3 µmol/l (30–85 µg/dl)	~20–300 µg/g	None
Excessive	High normal to >3 µmol/l (85 µg/dl)	High (>300 µg/g)	Not apparent or very mild; elevated liver enzymes in plasma
Toxic	Retinyl esters are elevated and might be higher than retinol	Very high in liver and increased in peripheral tissues	Headache, bone/joint pain, elevated liver enzymes in plasma, clinical signs of liver disease

Adapted from Ross (2006) and WHO (2009).

[a]The range 0.7–1.05 µmo/l is sometimes used to denote marginal status, and <0.7 µmol/l to indicate deficient status; these definitions might be more appropriate for adults, who typically have higher plasma retinol concentrations than do children. The reasons for differences in plasma retinol concentration with age have not been elucidated.

or mass spectrometric detection (Gunderson and Blomhoff, 2001). Most methods for analyzing retinoids and carotenoids depend on their sensitive absorption of light at 325 nm (retinol and retinyl esters), 350 nm (retinoic acid) or 375 nm (retinaldehyde) or approximately 450 nm (most carotenoids) (Barua et al., 2000).

2.1.10 Vitamin A toxicity (hypervitaminosis A)

Although vitamin A is an essential micronutrient, excessive intake could result in toxicity, which can be diagnosed by the high concentration of retinyl esters in plasma of fasting subjects. The acute poisoning causes a rise in intracranial pressure resulting in nausea, vomiting, headache, vertigo, irritability, stupor, fontanel bulging (in newborns), papilledema and pseudotumor cerebri (Heimburger et al., 2006), and could even result in death. Severe poisoning or fatal cases were documented among polar explorers after consumption of liver from polar bears, seals or husky dogs (Rodahl and Moore, 1943). Doses in excess of 30 mg/day ingested over a period of several months are sufficient to induce chronic toxicity, characterized by abdominal pain, headache, bone and joint pain, skin redness and peeling, loss of hair, irritability and lack of appetite (Rudman and Williams, 1983). Even doses of 4.5 mg/day could have teratogenic effects in the fetus although might not cause any toxicity symptoms in pregnant women. Excessive intake of vitamin A during the first trimester of pregnancy has been associated with increased incidence of cleft palate, harelip, macroglossia, developmental abnormalities in eyes, and hydrocephalus in newborns (Rothman et al., 1995) because of the role of retinoic acid in control of gene expression. Thus, although retinoids can be very effective pharmacological agents, particularly in dermatology, their use must be carefully monitored.

In older men and women, 1.5 mg/day of preformed vitamin A was associated with decreased bone mineral density and increased risk of hip fractures (Michaelsson et al., 2003). Increased risk of osteoporosis is correlated with plasma retinol levels above 80 µg/dl, which are common among older adults in developed countries. Life-long diets rich in animal sources of vitamin A and widespread use of supplements are characteristic for these countries (USA, Canada, Europe, Australia). Large intake of dietary provitamin A carotenoids does not cause vitamin A toxicity owing to limited absorption and conversion capability, but it is recommended that cigarette smokers not take supplements of beta-carotene. High doses of preformed vitamin A are ingested in the mistaken belief that it will improve vision and skin tone in old age. However, topical application of retinol or retinoic acid can reverse or retard many of the visible and histological changes of photodamaged skin. Retinoic acid treatment results in partial effacement of fine lines and wrinkles of the skin (Valquist, 1994).

Even though retinoids possess promising therapeutic value for the treatment of several forms of cancer and skin diseases, the systemic administration of retinoids must be cautious owing to their toxic side effects which include teratogenicity, increased serum triglycerides, headaches and bone toxicity. It is assumed that these toxic effects are all manifestations of imbalances in retinoid control of gene expression. All-*trans* retinoic acid (tretinoin) is more toxic than the 13-*cis* isomer (isotretinoin, Accutane). Accutane, taken orally as a prescription drug for the treatment of acute acne, must not be given to pregnant women or those who might become pregnant during therapy, as it significantly increases the risk of spontaneous abortion, premature delivery or developmental disabilities. Isotretinoin exposure causes a specific phenotype characterized by malformations of brain, heart and major arteries, craniofacies and thymus (Nau et al., 1994).

2.1.11 Current challenges in vitamin A research

A major challenge remains in elucidating the role of vitamin A in reducing the effects of chronic diseases, in particular measles. The interactions of zinc and vitamin A also remain to be explained at the molecular level. Most probably these effects will be explained by the functions of retinoids in the control of gene expression. At the public health level, there are still regional deficiencies of vitamin A in broad regions of the world, particularly in young children and their mothers. Solutions to those problems will require nutritional (changes in food habits, adoption of cultivars of food crops which are high in provitamin A content, as well as food fortification programs) and economic approaches. The concerns of aging populations in developed countries are very different, in fact opposite, stemming from the excess of preformed vitamin A. They also deserve the concern of medical research and practice.

References

Barua AB, Sidell N, Retinoyl beta-glucuronide: a biologically active interesting retinoid. J Nutr 2004;134: 286S–9S.

Barua AB, Olson JA, Furr HC, van Breemen RB, Vitamin A and carotenoids. In: De Leenheer AP, Lambert WE, van Bocxlaer JF, editors. Modern chromatographic analysis of vitamins. New York: Marcel Dekker; 2000. pp. 1–74.

Embree ND, Shantz EM, A possible new member of the vitamins A1 and A2 group. J Am Chem Soc 1943;65: 906–9.

Erdman JW Jr, Ford NA, Lindshield BL, Are the health attributes of lycopene related to its anti-oxidant function? Arch Biochem Biophys 2009;483: 229–35.

Furr HC, Green MH, Haskell M, Mokhtar N, Nestel P, Newton S, Ribaya-Mercado JD, Tang G, Tanumihardjo S, Wasantwisut E, Stable isotope dilution techniques for assessing vitamin A status and bioefficacy of provitamin A carotenoids in humans. Public Health Nutr 2005;8: 596–607.

Germain P, Chambon P, Eichele G, Evans RM, Lazar MA, Leid M, De Lera AR, Lotan R, Mangelsdorf DJ, Gronemeyer H, International union of pharmacology. LX. Retinoic acid receptors. Pharmacol Rev 2006;58: 712–25.

Gunderson TE, Blomhoff R, Qualitative and quantitative liquid chromatographic determination of natural retinoids in biological samples. J Chromatogr A 2001;935: 13–43.

Heimburger DC, McLaren DS, Shils ME, Clinical manifestations of nutrient deficiencies and toxicities: a resume. In: Shils ME, Shike M, Ross AC, Caballero B, Cousins RJ, editors. Modern nutrition in health and disease. Philadelphia: Lippincott Williams & Wilkins; 2006. pp. 595–612.

Institute of Medicine, Dietary reference intakes for vitamin A, vitamin K, arsenic, boron, chromium, copper, iodine, iron, manganese, molybdenum, nickel, silicon, vanadium, and zinc. A report of the panel on micronutrients, subcommittees on upper reference levels of nutrients and of interpretation and uses of Dietary Reference Intakes, and the standing committee on the scientific evaluation of Dietary Reference Intakes. Washington, DC: National Academy Press; 2002. 728 pp.

Livrea MA, Packer L, Retinoids: progress in research and clinical applications. New York: Marcel Dekker; 1993. 634 pp.

Loane E, Kelliher C, Beatty S, Nolan JM, The rationale and evidence base for a protective role of macular pigment in age-related maculopathy. Br J Ophthalmol 2008;92: 1163–8.

Mark M, Ghyselinck NB, Chambon P, Function of retinoid nuclear receptors: lessons from genetic and pharmacological dissections of the retinoic acid signaling pathway during mouse embryogenesis. Ann Rev Pharmacol Toxicol 2006;46: 451–80.

McGrane MM, Vitamin A regulation of gene expression: molecular mechanism of a prototype gene. J Nutr Biochem 2007;18: 497–508.

Michaelsson K, Lithell H, Vessby B, Melhus H, Serum retinol levels and the risk of fractures. N Engl J Med 2003;348: 287–94.

Nau H, Chahoud I, Dencker L, Lammer EJ, Scott WJ, Teratogenicity of vitamin A and retinoids. In:Blomhoff R, editor. Vitamin A in health and disease. New York, NY: Marcel Dekker; 1994. pp. 615–63.

Olson JA, Vitamin A. In: Machlin LJ, editor. Handbook of vitamins. New York, NY: Marcel Dekker; 1984. pp. 1–43.

Olson JA, Carotenoids. In: Shils ME, Olson JA, Shike M, Ross AC, editors. Modern nutrition in health and disease. Philadelphia: Lippincott Williams & Wilkins; 1999. pp. 525–41.

Reichrath J, Lehmann B, Carlberg C, Varani J, Zouboulis CC, Vitamins as hormones. Horm Metab Res 2007;39: 71–84.

Rodahl K, Moore T, The vitamin A content and toxicity of bear and seal liver. Biochem J 1943;37: 166–8.

Ross AC, Vitamin A and carotenoids. In: Shils ME, Shike M, Ross AC, Caballero B, Cousins RJ, editors. Modern nutrition in health and disease. Philadelphia: Lippincott Willams & Wilkins; 2006. pp. 351–75.

Rothman KJ, Moore LL, Singer MR, Nguyen US, Mannino S, Milunsky A, Teratogenicity of high vitamin A intake. N Engl J Med 1995;21: 1369–77.

Rudman D, Williams PJ, Megadose vitamins. Use and misuse. N Engl J Med 1983;309: 488–90.

Saari JC, Retinoids in photosensitive systems. In: Sporn MB, Roberts AB, Goodman DS, editors. The retinoids: biology, chemistry and medicine. 2nd ed. New York: Raven Press; 1994. pp. 351–85.

Scientific Committee on Food, Opinion of the scientific committee on food on the tolerable upper intake level of beta-carotene. Brussels: European Commission, Health & Consumer Protection Directorate-General; 2000. 21 pp.

Semba RD, The role of vitamin A and related retinoids in immune function. Nutr Rev 1998;56: S38–48.

Sporn MB, Roberts AB, In: Sporn MB, Roberts AB, Goodman DS, editors. The retinoids, 2nd ed. New York, NY: Raven Press; 1994. pp. 1–3.

Tanumihardjo SA, Cheng JC, Permaesih D, Muherdiyantiningsih, Rustan E, Muhilal, Karyadi D, Olson JA, Refinement of the modified-relative dose response test as a method for assessing vitamin A status in a field setting: experience with Indonesian children. Am J Clin Nutr 1996;64, 966–71.

Underwood BA, Methods for assessment of nutritional status. J Nutr 1990;120: 1459–63.

Underwood BA, Vitamin A in human nutrition: Public health considerations. In: Sporn MB, Roberts AB, Goodman DS, editors. The retinoids: biology, chemistry and medicine. 2nd ed. New York: Raven Press; 1994a. pp. 211–27.

Underwood BA, Hypovitaminosis A: international programmatic issues, J Nutr 1994b;124: 1467S–72S.

USDA National Nutrient Database for Standard Reference, Release 20. Agricultural Research Service 2007. Nutrient Data Laboratory Home Page.

Valquist A, Role of retinoids in normal and diseased skin. In: Blomhoff R, editor. Vitamin A in health and disease. New York: Marcel Dekker; 1994. pp. 365–424.

West KP, Vitamin A deficiency: its epidemiology and relation to child mortality and morbidity. In: Blomhoff R, editor. Vitamin A in health and disease. New York: Marcel Dekker; 1994. pp. 585–614.

West CE, Castenmiller JJ, Quantification of the 'SLAMENGHI' factors for carotenoid bioavailability and bioconversion. Int J Vitam Nutr Res 1998;68: 371–7.

Wongsiriroj N, Blaner W, Recent advances in vitamin A absorption and transport. Sight Life 2007;3: 32–7.

WHO, Global prevalence of vitamin A deficiency in populations at risk 1995–2005. WHO Global Database on Vitamin A Deficiency. Geneva: World Health Organization; 2009.

WHO/FAO, Human vitamin and mineral requirements: report of a joint FAO/WHO expert consultation, Bangkok, Thailand. Rome: World Health Organization and Food and Agriculture Organization of the United Nations; 2002.

2.2 Vitamin A in human diseases

Jenny Libien; Wei-ping Chen

2.2.1 Introduction

The role of vitamin A in maintaining human health and preventing disease has been recognized for almost a century but is still intensely investigated owing to the complexities of retinoid signaling in the human body. Vitamin A in human disease encompasses vitamin A deficiency (VAD) and toxicity related signs and symptoms, vitamin A and beta-carotene supplementation for prevention of morbidity and mortality, synthetic and natural retinoid-based therapies for treatment of cancer and dermatologic diseases, and retinoid signaling in the pathogenesis of various diseases. This chapter will primarily focus on the role of beta-carotene and vitamin A in disease prevention.

Numerous clinical trials have now investigated the influence of vitamin A and beta-carotene supplementation on human diseases. In populations in which deficiency is common, the supplementation studies have primarily examined mortality and infectious disease in infants, children and lactating women, the groups most susceptible to the harmful consequences of deficiencies (WHO, 2009). In populations in which clinical deficiency is rare, studies have examined whether inadequate intake leading to a subtle deficiency is associated with cancer, diabetes, cardiovascular disease, Alzheimer's disease, or other diseases associated with aging. Clinical trials indicate that factors such as age, sex, smoking history, alcohol use, geographic location, nutritional status and vitamin A status help to determine whether provitamin A carotenoid or retinoid supplementation improves health and survival or leads to greater morbidity and mortality. Often, the results of large scale randomized clinical trials have been surprising and contradict hypotheses formulated from observational, epidemiologic studies.

2.2.2 Child mortality

A higher risk of death was observed in young Indonesian children with signs of VAD, xeropthalmia, Bitot's spots, and night blindness (Sommer, 1983). This recognition led to several randomized field trials investigating the impact of vitamin A supplementation on child mortality. The first field trial showed that supplementation with 200 000 IU vitamin A (60 mg) every 6 months reduced mortality by 34% among Indonesian children aged 1–5 years (Sommer et al., 1986; Sommer, 2008). Multiple studies in Asia and Africa subsequently showed that periodic large doses of vitamin A resulted in a decrease in mortality of 29–54% in children aged 6 months to 5 years. The supplementation reduced the severity but not the incidence of diarrheal disease and measles (Sommer, 2008). Vitamin A fortified foods such as monosodium glutamate (Muhilal et al., 1988) and sugar (Krause et al., 1998) also reduce childhood mortality in populations with high rates of VAD. The WHO recommends universal vitamin A supplementation of children aged 6–60 months, in countries with evidence of VAD and this has been adopted as government policy in many countries (WHO, 2009), additional reference (Prentice, 2010).

2.2.3 Neonatal and infant morbidity and mortality

Vitamin A supplementation of neonates is not currently recommended by the WHO. Clinical trials examining vitamin A supplementation in neonates have shown a geographic and a sex difference in the mortality rate. Studies in India (Tielsch et al., 2007), Bangladesh (Klemm et al., 2008) and Indonesia (Humphrey et al., 1996) reported an approximately 20% reduction in infant mortality with 48 000–50 000 IU of vitamin A administered within the first several days after delivery. By contrast, there was no overall improvement in survival with vitamin A supplementation in two studies which took place in Africa (Benn et al., 2008, 2010). In the most recent study, a two-by-two factorial randomized controlled trial of 1717 low birthweight neonates in Guinea Bissau, 25 000 IU vitamin A resulted in lower mortality in boys but in greater mortality in girls (mortality rate ratio of 1.42) (Benn et al., 2010; Prentice, 2010). Differences in vitamin A metabolism and actions in boys and girls and men and women are not yet well understood.

In the developed world, intramuscular administration of vitamin A (5000 IU, 3 times per week for 4 weeks) has been used to reduce chronic lung disease in extremely-low-birthweight infants weighing less than 1000 g (Tyson et al., 1999). A meta-analysis of eight studies showed a slight reduction in mortality or oxygen requirement at 1 month of age and of oxygen requirement at 36 weeks' postmenstrual age (Darlow and Graham, 2007). In the largest study, one additional infant was not affected by chronic lung disease for every 14–15 infants supplemented with vitamin A (Tyson et al., 1999). The outcome at 18–22 months of age showed no significant difference between the vitamin A supplemented group and the control group; both groups had approximately the same number of rehospitalizations and pulmonary problems after initial discharge (Ambalavanan et al., 2005). Perhaps, because of this lack of long-term effect, vitamin A supplementation of extremely-low-birthweight infants is not common practice in neonatal intensive care units.

2.2.4 Vitamin A and beta-carotene supplementation during pregnancy

Vitamin A or beta-carotene supplementation in women of reproductive age has yielded different outcomes in Asia versus Africa, as was seen with neonatal supplementation. Weekly Vitamin A (7000 µg retinol equivalents) or beta-carotene (42 mg, or 7000 µg retinol equivalents) supplementation reduced pregnancy-related mortality by 44% in Nepal (West et al., 1999), but had no significant impact on all-cause mortality or pregnancy-related mortality in a randomized, double-blind, placebo-controlled trial in Ghana (Kirkwood et al., 2010). Although there was no improvement in survival, the weekly doses of 25 000 IU of vitamin A administered to women 15–45 years of age were not harmful in this population (Kirkwood et al., 2010). In Nepal, in which chronic vitamin A deficiency is common, vitamin A supplementation before, during and after pregnancy resulted in improved lung function in offspring (Checkley et al., 2010). In developed countries, vitamin A supplementation is contraindicated in pregnant women owing to the well-established teratogenic effects of retinoids.

2.2.5 Adult mortality

Increased adult mortality has been seen in several cancer prevention trials in which vitamin A or beta-carotene supplements were administered (Qiao et al., 2009). Daily vitamin A supplementation (5000 IU as retinol palmitate) was associated with increased stroke mortality and total mortality in The General Population Nutrition Intervention Trial, a randomized primary esophageal and gastric cancer prevention trial conducted in Linxian, China from 1985 to 1991 and followed for 10 years after active intervention (Qiao et al., 2009). In the same study, beta-carotene (15 mg) in combination with selenium (50 µg) and vitamin E (30 mg) resulted in reduced mortality from gastric cancer, cancer overall, and from all causes (Qiao et al., 2009). Surprisingly, a topical retinoid (tretinoin, 0.1%, twice daily) also increased mortality in the Veterans Affairs Topical Tretinoin Chemoprevention Trial (Weinstock et al., 2009). In a meta-analysis of 47 randomized clinical trials of antioxidant supplements used for primary or secondary prevention of several diseases, beta-carotene and vitamin A supplementation increased the risk of mortality by 7% and 16%, respectively (Bjelakovic et al., 2007). These findings suggest that both beta-carotene and vitamin A supplementation should be used with caution. The impact of beta-carotene supplementation on cancer mortality is discussed further in Section 2.2.7.1.

2.2.6 Infectious disease/immunity

Vitamin A supplementation was first used to prevent infectious disease in the late 1920s as a prophylactic against puerperal infection. Evidence that vitamin A can favorably influence the course of a disease already in progress was first published in 1932 (Ellison, 1932). Measles mortality was reduced by more than half and pulmonary complications were less severe in the group of young children treated with daily cod liver oil with 300 units of vitamin A than in control patients. Vitamin A supplements are still recommended in the treatment of measles in populations with a high prevalence of VAD.

Maintenance of epithelial cell integrity was proposed to be the major mechanism by which vitamin A limited the severity of measles (Ellison, 1932). VAD-associated squamous metaplasia was hypothesized to make tissues more susceptible to infection or to superinfection. Numerous studies have since shown that although vitamin A lessens the severity of certain infectious diseases, most notably of measles and diarrhea, the overall incidence of disease is the same with or without vitamin A supplementation (Grotto et al., 2003). There is some evidence that incidence of infectious disease might change with vitamin A supplementation in some study participants but not in others. A randomized clinical trial in Mexico City found that vitamin A supplementation reduced the overall risk of diarrheal disease only among children with better socioeconomic measures. Vitamin A supplementation also reduced the incidence of mild watery diarrhea and cough with fever in all children (Long et al., 2007). No impact on other acute respiratory infections or on overall diarrheal disease was seen with supplementation. The investigators suggest that vitamin A could be protective against only a specific group of pathogens. Characteristics of the host, such as socioeconomic status, overall nutritional status, and vitamin A status, might influence whether vitamin A can act to prevent infectious disease via influencing the pathogen-specific immune response of the host.

Animal models have contributed much to our understanding of the influence of vitamin A on immune response. Vitamin A supplementation and retinoic acid treatment have been shown to augment antibody responses in animals (Ross et al., 2009). Retinoic acid has also been shown to influence the differentiation or function of various immune cells, including CD4+ T cells, natural killer cells, dendritic cells and antigen-activated B-cells (Ross et al., 2009). Human studies confirm the influence of vitamin A on immune function. In a study of 80 preschool children in Venezuela, the phagocytic capacity of neutrophils increased 30 days after a single 200 000 IU dose of vitamin A (Jimenez et al., 2010).

2.2.7 Cancer

2.2.7.1 Overall cancer prevention and mortality

Support for a role of retinoids and carotenoids in cancer prevention initially came from observational epidemiologic studies in which individuals with diets rich in carotenoids had a reduced risk of cancer (Peto et al., 1981). The carotenoids were thought to act in cancer prevention by acting as antioxidants. *In vitro*, beta-carotene and other carotenoids are antioxidants, although pro-oxidant activity has also been shown (Rao and Rao, 2007). It was hypothesized that beta-carotene would prevent the oxidative damage to cells caused by reactive oxygen species and inhibit carcinogenesis. It was also proposed that carotenoids and retinoids might inhibit aberrant cellular proliferation and prevent cancers from forming. Beta-carotene, as a pro-vitamin A carotenoid, is metabolized to retinoic acid and acts as a regulator of cellular proliferation and differentiation via activation of nuclear retinoic acid receptors.

Multiple randomized clinical trials have explored whether vitamin A and beta-carotene supplementation can prevent cancer. The results have mostly been negative. In a meta-analysis of 12 randomized clinical trials of antioxidants and primary prevention of cancer, there was a slight increase (6%) in cancer incidence and no reduction in cancer mortality with beta-carotene supplementation (Bardia et al., 2008). For smokers, beta-carotene supplementation was associated with a 10% increase in the incidence of cancer but only a trend toward increased cancer mortality (Bardia et al., 2008). In the Women's Antioxidant Cardiovascular Study, beta-carotene supplementation (50 mg, every other day) did not impact cancer incidence or mortality (Lin et al., 2009), although the women in this study already had dietary intakes of vitamin A and of antioxidants above the recommended daily allowance. The Physicians' Health Study similarly showed no overall effect of beta-carotene supplementation (50 mg, every other day) on total cancer incidence, but did show a 20% reduction in cancer incidence in men over 70 years of age, a 10% reduction among daily drinkers of alcohol and among men with the highest body mass index (Cook et al., 2000). Clearly, the studies indicate that it is not possible to make a general recommendation about beta-carotene and cancer.

2.2.7.2 Lung cancer

The strongest data against beta-carotene and vitamin A supplementation for the primary prevention of cancer come from randomized clinical trials examining the risk for lung cancer. Observational epidemiologic studies found that people consuming a diet rich in carotenoids had a lower risk of lung cancer (Mettlin et al., 1979) at all levels of cigarette smoking (Shekelle et al., 1981). Serum levels of beta-carotene were also inversely related to lung cancer risk. However, the Finnish Alpha-Tocopherol Beta-Carotene (ATBC) trial, a large-scale randomized clinical trial, found that beta-carotene (20 mg) supplementation increased lung cancer incidence by 16–35%, with the greatest risk seen among the heaviest smokers and regular alcohol users (Albanes et al., 1996; Fairfield and Fletcher, 2002; Bowen et al., 2003; Rao and Rao, 2007). The Beta-Carotene and Retinol Efficacy Trial (CARET) found a 28% increase in the incidence of lung cancer and a 17% increase in incidence of death with daily supplementation with beta-carotene (30 mg) and retinyl palmitate (25 000 IU) (Omenn, 1996). It is important to note that all of the participants in CARET had a history of smoking or asbestos exposure and were at high risk for lung cancer. Although the active intervention arm of the study was stopped early owing to the increased risk, the participants continued to be followed and the increased risk of mortality persisted, particularly in women. Analysis of post-intervention data at 6 years showed women who received the beta-carotene and retinyl ester supplementation had a 33% increase in risk in lung cancer mortality, 37% increase in all-cause mortality, and 44% increase in cardiovascular mortality (Goodman et al., 2004). Several other randomized clinical trials found no increase in mortality but also no benefit with beta-carotene supplementation (Blot et al., 1993; Hennekens et al., 1996; Lin et al., 2009). As a result of these studies, beta-carotene supplementation is not recommended in smokers. Carotenoids other than beta-carotene, such as alpha-carotene or lycopene, might play a role in cancer prevention and account for the contrasting results of the epidemiologic studies and randomized clinical trials (Rao and Rao, 2007).

2.2.7.3 Colon cancer

Beta-carotene supplementation could be beneficial for certain cancers and for subsets of the population. For colon cancer, beta-carotene supplementation decreased colon cancer risk among regular alcohol users but not among other participants in the Physicians' Health Study in the USA (Cook et al., 2000) and in the ATBC study in Finland (Glynn et al., 1996; Fairfield and Fletcher, 2002). A 50% decrease in colon cancer risk was seen in regular alcohol drinkers who took a 50 mg dose of beta-carotene on alternate days for multiple years (Cook et al., 2000). A possible reason for a benefit in the alcohol users is that they might have lower baseline levels of beta-carotene and the supplementation corrects a subtle deficiency (Fairfield and Fletcher, 2002).

2.2.7.4 Prostate cancer

Diet is thought to contribute significantly to prostate cancer risk and there is evidence that carotenoids such as lycopene offer protection (Rao and Rao, 2007). However, it is unclear whether beta-carotene and retinol play a beneficial or harmful role (or any role) in prostate cancer risk and survival. Serum levels of beta-carotene and retinol are not associated with prostate cancer risk or with prostate cancer survival (Goodman et al., 2003; Key et al., 2007). An increased risk of fatal or aggressive prostate cancer was reported in the ATBC trial during beta-carotene supplementation (20 mg/day) (Watters et al., 2009) and with 30 mg beta-carotene + 25 000 IU retinyl palmitate + other dietary supplement in CARET (Neuhouser et al., 2009). After discontinuation of the supplementation, the risk of aggressive prostate cancer returned to baseline. Interestingly, CARET also found a significant decrease in the risk of non-aggressive prostate cancer (Gleason score <7, Stage 1 and 2) with beta-carotene supplementation (Neuhouser et al., 2009). A reduced risk of prostate cancer with beta-carotene supplementation (50 mg every other day) was also seen in men with low baseline serum beta-carotene levels, but not in participants overall, in the Physicians' Health Study (Cook et al., 1999). Overall, the evidence does not support beta-carotene supplementation for prostate cancer prevention.

2.2.7.5 Breast cancer

The association of dietary carotenoid and vitamin A intake and breast cancer risk has been inconsistent (Zhang et al., 1999), with most studies showing no impact (Jarvinen et al., 1997; Verhoeven et al., 1997; Michels et al., 2001; Fairfield and Fletcher, 2002). In one study, the inverse association of vitamin A, beta-carotene and alpha-carotene intake and breast cancer was seen only in premenopausal women who had a smoking history (Mignone et al., 2009). An inverse association of serum alpha-carotene and beta-carotene levels and breast cancer was also recently reported (Kabat et al., 2009). There have been no prospective trials examining vitamin A supplementation and breast cancer risk.

2.2.7.6 Retinoid-based therapies to prevent or treat cancer

Retinoids have been used as chemopreventive agents in survivors of breast cancer (Fairfield and Fletcher, 2002; Veronesi et al., 2006), of head and neck cancers (Armstrong and Meyskens, 2000; Dragnev et al., 2000; Dragnev et al., 2003), and in individuals with *xeroderma pigmentosum* and nevoid basal cell carcinoma syndrome who are at high risk of developing skin cancers. Retinoids have also been used in preventing premalignant lesions such as oral leukoplakia from progressing to invasive cancer (Epstein and Gorsky, 1999; Gorsky and Epstein, 2002; Lippman et al., 2006), and for the treatment of various malignant neoplasms including acute promyelocytic leukemia, neuroblastoma, medulloblastoma and glioblastoma (Dragnev et al 2003). The major use for retinoic acid in cancer is in the treatment of acute promyelocytic leukemia, a disease in which a (15:17) translocation results in the fusion of a truncated retinoic acid receptor α on chromosome 17 with the PML gene on chromosome 15 (de The et al., 1990; Tallman et al., 1997). The abnormal retinoic acid receptor encoded by the fusion gene prevents myeloid cells from differentiating. All-*trans* retinoic acid induces the acute promyelocytic leukemia cells to differentiate into mature granulocytes. This differentiation therapy often leads to remission (de The et al., 1990), and improves disease-free and overall survival (Tallman et al., 1997).

2.2.8 Retinoids in the treatment of dermatologic disease

The efficacy of retinoids is best illustrated by their use in the treatment of acne and other dermatologic diseases. In addition to acne, oral and/or topical retinoids are effective in treating disorders of cornification, psoriasis, pigmentary disorders, cutaneous T cell lymphoma, and in chemoprevention of basal cell carcinoma and squamous cell carcinoma in high-risk individuals (Zouboulis, 2001; Goldsmith et al., 2004). Use of oral retinoids is limited by toxicity. Toxicities include teratogenesis, elevations in triglycerides and liver enzymes, decreased bone mineral density, and elevated intracranial pressure (Goldsmith et al., 2004). In addition, an association of 13-*cis* retinoic acid with depression and suicide has been reported but is not supported by evidence in the current literature (Marqueling and Zane, 2007). Detailed description of the use of retinoids in dermatologic disease is reviewed in the literature (Shalita, 2001; Ghali et al., 2009; Kang et al., 2009a; Thiboutot et al., 2009) and beyond the scope of the focus of this chapter.

2.2.9 Idiopathic intracranial hypertension

Vitamin A toxicity is a well-recognized cause of intracranial hypertension (Morrice et al., 1960; Corbett, 2004) and recent data suggest that abnormal retinoid transport and metabolism could be involved in the pathogenesis of idiopathic intracranial hypertension (Libien and Blaner, 2007; Warner et al., 2007). There are numerous case reports and series documenting elevated intracranial pressure following overconsumption of vitamin A-rich foods (usually liver) (Selhorst et al., 1984; Fishman, 2002; O'Donnell, 2004) and after administration of therapeutic doses of the synthetic vitamin A derivative, 13-*cis*-retinoic acid (Isotretinoin) (Visani et al., 1996; Fraunfelder and Fraunfelder, 2004). The elevated intracranial pressure resolves after removing the vitamin A-rich food from the diet or after stopping retinoic acid administration. In several clinical studies of patients with idiopathic intracranial hypertension, high serum or CSF vitamin A levels and altered levels of RBP were reported (Jacobson et al., 1999; Sass et al., 2000; Selhorst et al., 2000; Warner et al., 2002; Tabassi et al., 2005; Warner et al., 2007). The mechanism by which vitamin A leads to elevated intracranial pressure is not yet known.

2.2.10 Osteoporosis and hip fracture

Bone resorption and fracture are known consequences of vitamin A toxicity (Penniston and Tanumihardjo, 2006). According to animal and *in vitro* studies, the actions of vitamin A on bone are mediated via retinoic acid induced stimulation of osteoclast formation and inhibition of osteoblast activity (Scheven and Hamilton, 1990; Togari et al., 1991). In humans, epidemiologic studies have found that higher levels of dietary vitamin A intake are associated with lower bone mineral density and greater risk of hip fracture (Melhus et al., 1998; Feskanich et al., 2002; Promislow et al., 2002). Beta-carotene intake did not contribute significantly to fracture risk (Feskanich et al., 2002). In addition to vitamin A intake from diet and supplements, serum retinol is also associated with risk of fracture (Michaelsson et al., 2003).

In a study from Sweden, where there are high rates of hip fracture and of dietary vitamin A intake, the risk for hip fracture increased by 68% for every 1 mg increase in daily intake of retinol. In addition, there was a 10% decrease in bone mineral density at the femoral head and 14% at the lumbar spine with vitamin A intake greater than 1.5 mg/day compared with intake less than 0.5 mg/day (Melhus et al., 1998). The Women's Health Initiative Observational Study of postmenopausal women had partly conflicting results and reported that a modest increase in fracture risk with high vitamin A intake was only seen in women with low vitamin D intake (Caire-Juvera, 2009). In a cohort of men and women aged 55 years and older, consumption of vitamin A in amounts approximating the recommended daily allowance (700 µg or 2330 IU for women and 900 µg or 3000 IU for men) was associated with peak bone mineral density and bone maintenance. Individuals with the lowest and highest vitamin A intake had reduced bone density (Promislow et al., 2002). The investigators conclude that it is important for skeletal health to ensure adequate but not excessive vitamin A intake (Promislow et al., 2002).

2.2.11 Diabetes

The main transport protein for vitamin A in blood, retinol binding protein (RBP; also known as RBP4), has received much attention after its identification as an adipokine in 2005. In animal studies, adipose-derived RBP was linked to (and suggested to cause) insulin resistance (Yang et al., 2005). Multiple human studies investigating the association of RBP with insulin resistance, diabetes, metabolic syndrome, and obesity have since been published. The initial human study found a correlation of serum RBP levels with the magnitude of insulin resistance in subjects with obesity, impaired glucose tolerance, and type 2 diabetes and in non-obese, non-diabetic subjects with strong family histories of type 2 diabetes. Serum RBP levels correlated with body-mass index and with fasting insulin level (Graham et al., 2006). The investigators did not measure vitamin A levels. Subsequent studies have had conflicting results; some investigators report a correlation of RBP levels with insulin resistance (Aeberli et al., 2007; Mills et al., 2008) and others report a lack of association between RBP levels and insulin resistance (von Eynatten et al., 2007; Lewis et al., 2008a, b; Shim et al., 2010) or insulin sensitivity (Janke et al., 2006; Pfutzner et al., 2009).

Serum retinol (vitamin A) has been measured by several investigators who found that the ratio of RBP to retinol, but not the level of RBP itself, was higher in subjects with type 2 diabetes mellitus than in subjects with normal glucose tolerance (Erikstrup et al., 2009) and correlated with fasting insulin levels (Aeberli et al., 2007). This suggests that apo-RBP (RBP not bound to retinol) is the key player in insulin resistance (Mills et al., 2008). This could also suggest that serum vitamin A levels are low or relatively low in diabetes. However, serum retinol levels are tightly controlled and do not necessarily reflect tissue levels. It is possible that high levels of RBP lead to greater tissue delivery of retinol and activation of retinoid responsive or PPAR-gamma activated genes.

There has not been a consistent association between serum retinol or beta-carotene levels and diabetes mellitus. Beta-carotene serum levels were higher in control subjects than in subjects with type 2 diabetes mellitus, whereas retinol and alpha-carotene were the same for both groups (Abahusain et al., 1999). Men with higher serum beta-carotene were also less likely to develop diabetes than men with lower serum beta-carotene in the Uppsala Longitudinal Study of Adult Men (Arnlov et al., 2009). However, beta-carotene supplementation did not impact the risk of subsequent type 2 diabetes mellitus in men in the Physicians' Health Study (Liu, 1999) or in male smokers in the ATBC study (Kataja-Tuomola et al., 2008). Dietary vitamin A intake also was not associated with blood glucose or insulin levels (Zulet et al., 2008). Clinical trial results could help to define the connection between RBP and retinol with insulin resistance and diabetes. Fenretininde, a synthetic retinoid that reduces serum RBP and total body retinol levels, is in Phase 2 clinical trials for assessment of insulin sensitizing activity in subjects with insulin resistance and obesity.

2.2.12 Obesity

The association of RBP with body mass index and adiposity has also been confirmed by some investigators (Aeberli et al., 2007; Haider et al., 2007) and disputed by others (Janke et al., 2006; Takashima et al., 2006; Yoshida et al., 2006; Lewis et al., 2008b). In one study, dietary vitamin A intake was inversely correlated with body weight, BMI, waist circumference and waist-to-hip ratio (Zuletet al., 2008). Evidence from animal studies suggests that vitamin A is involved in regulating energy balance and that retinoic acid administration leads to weight loss via activation of PPAR β/δ receptors (Berry and Noy, 2009). Randomized clinical trials examining the role of retinoids in energy balance and control of adiposity are needed to determine whether the animal studies translate to humans.

2.2.13 Cardiovascular and cerebrovascular disease

Large-scale randomized clinical trials have largely found no association between beta-carotene and cardiovascular disease (Hennekens et al., 1996; Omenn et al., 1996). However, in women smokers in CARET, beta-carotene (30 mg) and retinyl palmitate (25 000 IU) supplementation were detrimental and lead to a 44% increase in cardiovascular mortality (Goodman et al., 2004).

A link between RBP and cardiovascular disease has also been proposed. RBP levels are associated with a proatherogenic lipid profile with increased triglyceride levels and/or low HDL cholesterol (Graham et al., 2006; Janke et al., 2006; Kloting et al., 2007; von Eynatten et al., 2007; Ingelsson and Lind, 2009; von Eynatten and Humpert, 2009). However, there is little evidence that RBP is associated with cardiovascular disease directly. In the Uppsala Longitudinal Study of Adult Men, RBP was associated with prior cerebrovascular disease in men but not with prior myocardial infarction (Ingelsson et al., 2009). Because stroke mortality was associated with vitamin A supplementation in The General Population Nutrition Intervention Trial in China (Qiao et al., 2009), the association of RBP and stroke might be via retinoid actions on the cerebral blood vessels. More studies are needed to define the association of RBP and vitamin A with stroke.

2.2.14 Age-related macular degeneration

The Age-Related Eye Disease Study (AREDS) is a large-scale, randomized, controlled clinical trial examining the effect of nutritional supplementation on progression of age-related macular degeneration (AMD), the major cause of visual loss in older adults in developed countries. The AREDS supplements, consisting of 15 mg of beta-carotene, 500 mg of vitamin C, 400 IU of vitamin E, 80 mg of zinc oxide and 2 mg cupric oxide, lead to a 25% risk reduction in progression to advanced AMD over 5 years. Only patients with intermediate AMD or advanced AMD in one eye were included in the study. There is not yet evidence that nutritional supplementation can be used for primary prevention of AMD (Krishnadev et al., 2010).

2.2.15 Mild cognitive impairment and Alzheimer's disease

Oxidative damage leading to impaired neuronal function is thought be an early event in Alzheimer's disease. It has been hypothesized that antioxidants such as beta-carotene might prevent neuronal damage and help to maintain cognitive function during aging. There is also significant data from animal studies that retinoic acid influences learning and memory formation and that memory formation is impaired in vitamin A deficiency (Chiang et al., 1998; Etchamendy et al., 2001; Cocco et al., 2002; Etchamendy et al., 2003; Lane and Bailey, 2005; McCaffery et al., 2006; Mingaud et al., 2008; Olson and Mello, 2010).

Data on the influence of antioxidative vitamins on cognitive function are inconsistent. Intake of antioxidant vitamins was not associated with cognitive performance in more than 12 000 middle-aged participants of The Atherosclerosis Risk in Communities (ARIC) Study (Peacock et al., 2000), but these subjects might have been too young (age 48–67 years) to show an effect. In subjects aged 65–94 years, a positive correlation was found between the plasma levels of beta-carotene and cognitive performance in tests of free recall, recognition and vocabulary but not in tests of priming or working memory (Perrig et al., 1997). Several studies have found lower serum levels of beta-carotene and/or vitamin A in Alzheimer's disease patients than in control subjects (Zaman et al., 1992; Jimenez-Jimenez et al., 1999; Rinaldi et al., 2003; Wang et al., 2008) and one study found lower levels of beta-carotene and lutein in patients with moderately severe Alzheimer's disease than in patients with mild Alzheimer's disease (Wang et al., 2008). However, there is not a direct correlation of plasma levels of carotenoids with cognitive performance (Kang and Grodstein, 2008) or with degree of memory impairment (Rinaldi et al., 2003). Significantly decreased plasma levels of vitamin A, alpha and beta-carotene, and other carotenoids were present both in subjects with mild cognitive impairment and in patients with Alzheimer's disease as compared with controls (Rinaldi et al., 2003). Vitamin A and carotenoids have also been measured in postmortem brain samples and show an age-related decline in the frontal lobe, a region frequently involved in Alzheimer's disease, but not in the occipital lobe, a region rarely involved in Alzheimer's disease (Craft et al., 2004).

Randomized, placebo-controlled double-blind clinical trials examining the impact of beta-carotene supplementation on cognitive performance indicate that the effect, if any, is subtle (Yaffe, 2007). Very long-term supplementation could be necessary to see improvement in cognitive performance. In the Physicians' Health Study II (PHSII) cognitive ancillary study, subjects who had been supplemented with beta-carotene (50 mg on alternate days) for an average of 18 years performed better on cognitive tests overall and on verbal memory tests than subjects who had received a placebo, whereas subjects who received beta-carotene supplementation for only 1 year performed the same as those receiving placebo (Grodstein et al., 2007). In a study in Germany, 6 months of multivitamin supplements, which included beta-carotene, did not improve cognitive performance in well-educated women without dementia, aged 60–91 years (Wolters et al., 2005). Similarly, there was no impact of supplementation on cognitive performance with a combination of beta-carotene, vitamin E and vitamin C after approximately 5–7 years in the Age-Related Eye Disease Study (Yaffe et al., 2004) or the Women's Antioxidant Cardiovascular Study (Kang et al., 2009b). The influence of vitamin A or retinoic acid on human cognitive performance has not been studied in prospective clinical trials. In a transgenic mouse model of Alzheimer's disease, all-*trans* retinoic acid treatment for 8 weeks decreased Alzheimer's disease type pathology and improved spatial learning and memory (Ding et al., 2008).

2.2.16 Conclusions and future directions

There is no uniform consensus statement for the use of beta-carotene and vitamin A supplementation in human disease. Clinical outcomes vary by age, sex, smoking history, alcohol use, geographic location, nutritional status and vitamin A status. Where is there consensus? Vitamin A supplementation is recommended for children aged 6 months to 5 years to decrease mortality and severity of infectious disease in populations at risk of VAD (Sommer, 2008; WHO, 2009). Beta-carotene supplementation is contraindicated in smokers owing to the increased risk of cancer, lung cancer and mortality (Albanes et al., 1996; Omenn et al., 1996a; Goodman et al., 2004). Although a meta-analysis of 47 studies showed increased mortality with both beta-carotene and with vitamin A supplementation (Bjelakovic et al., 2007), there is evidence that supplementation could be beneficial for older individuals. For example, men over 70 years of age had a 20% reduction in cancer incidence with beta-carotene supplementation (Cook et al., 2000). For most people, vitamin A intake should not exceed the recommended dietary allowance because even small excesses lead to reduced bone density and increased risk of hip fracture (Melhus et al., 1998). Low levels of vitamin A could also lead to reduced bone density (Promislow et al., 2002). This highlights the concept of maintaining adequate but not excessive vitamin A levels for good health. Randomized clinical trials examining vitamin A and/or beta-carotene supplementation for prevention of diabetes, obesity, mild cognitive impairment and Alzheimer's disease are needed. Our understanding of RBP and retinol in insulin resistance and energy balance is rapidly evolving and there is considerable enthusiasm for the potential of new retinoid-based therapies for diabetes and obesity. The Finnish Alpha-Tocopherol Beta-Carotene trial and The Beta-Carotene and Retinol Efficacy Trial (CARET) have hopefully taught us that epidemiologic, observational studies are not able to predict the results of prospective clinical trials. Therefore, the results of future trials are eagerly anticipated. Finally, there is general agreement that a diet rich in a variety of fruits and vegetables could offer the best protection against chronic diseases.

References

Abahusain MA, Wright J, Dickerson JW, de Vol EB, Retinol, alpha-tocopherol and carotenoids in diabetes. Eur J Clin Nutr 1999;53: 630–5.

Aeberli I, Biebinger R, Lehmann R, L'Allemand D, Spinas GA, Zimmermann MB, Serum retinol-binding protein 4 concentration and its ratio to serum retinol are associated with obesity and metabolic syndrome components in children. J Clin Endocrinol Metab 2007;92: 4359–65.

Albanes D, Heinonen OP, Taylor PR, Virtamo J, Edwards BK, Rautalahti M, Hartman AM, Palmgren J, Freedman LS, Haapakoski J, Barrett MJ, Pietinen P, Malila N, Tala E, Liippo K, Salomaa ER, Tangrea JA, Teppo L, Askin FB, Taskinen E, Erozan Y, Greenwald P, Huttunen JK, Alpha-tocopherol and beta-carotene supplements and lung cancer incidence in the alpha-tocopherol, beta-carotene cancer prevention study: effects of base-line characteristics and study compliance. J Natl Cancer Inst 1996;88: 1560–70.

Ambalavanan N, Tyson JE, Kennedy KA, Hansen NI, Vohr BR, Wright LL, Carlo WA, Vitamin A supplementation for extremely low birth weight infants: outcome at 18 to 22 months. Pediatrics 2005;115: e249–54.

Armstrong WB, Meyskens FL Jr, Chemoprevention of head and neck cancer. Otolaryngol Head Neck Surg 2000;122: 728–35.

Arnlov J, Zethelius B, Riserus U, Basu S, Berne C, Vessby B, Alfthan G, Helmersson J, Serum and dietary beta-carotene and alpha-tocopherol and incidence of type 2 diabetes mellitus in a community-based study of Swedish men: report from the Uppsala Longitudinal Study of Adult Men (ULSAM) study. Diabetologia 2009;52: 97–105.

Bardia A, Tleyjeh IM, Cerhan JR, Sood AK, Limburg PJ, Erwin PJ, Montori VM, Efficacy of antioxidant supplementation in reducing primary cancer incidence and mortality: systematic review and meta-analysis. Mayo Clin Proc 2008;83: 23–34.

Benn CS, Diness BR, Roth A, Nante E, Fisker AB, Lisse IM, Yazdanbakhsh M, Whittle H, Rodrigues A, Aaby P, Effect of 50,000 IU vitamin A given with BCG vaccine on mortality in infants in Guinea-Bissau: randomised placebo controlled trial. Br Med J 2008;336: 1416–20.

Benn CS, Fisker AB, Napirna BM, Roth A, Diness BR, Lausch KR, Ravn H, Yazdanbakhsh M, Rodrigues A, Whittle H, Aaby P, Vitamin A supplementation and BCG vaccination at birth in low birthweight neonates: two by two factorial randomised controlled trial. Br Med J 2010;340: c1101.

Berry DC, Noy N, All-trans-retinoic acid represses obesity and insulin resistance by activating both peroxisome proliferation-activated receptor beta/delta and retinoic acid receptor. Mol Cell Biol 2009;29: 3286–96.

Bjelakovic G, Nikolova D, Gluud LL, Simonetti RG, Gluud C, Mortality in randomized trials of antioxidant supplements for primary and secondary prevention: systematic review and meta-analysis. J Am Med Assoc 2007;297: 842–57.

Blot WJ, Li JY, Taylor PR, Guo W, Dawsey S, Wang GQ, Yang CS, Zheng SF, Gail M, Li GY, et al., Nutrition intervention trials in Linxian, China: supplementation with specific vitamin/mineral combinations, cancer incidence, and disease-specific mortality in the general population. J Natl Cancer Inst 1993;85: 1483–92.

Bowen DJ, Thornquist M, Anderson K, Barnett M, Powell C, Goodman G, Omenn G, Stopping the active intervention: CARET. Control Clin Trials 2003;24: 39–50.

Caire-Juvera G, Ritenbaugh C, Wactawski-Wende J, Snetselaar LG, Chen Z. Vitamin A and retionl intakes and the risk of fractures among participants of the Women's Health Initiative Observational Study. Am J Clin. Nutr. 2009 Jan;89(1): 323–30.

Checkley W, West KP Jr., Wise RA, Baldwin MR, Wu L, LeClerq SC, Christian P, Katz J, Tielsch JM, Khatry S, Sommer A, Maternal vitamin A supplementation and lung function in offspring. N Engl J Med 2010;362: 1784–94.

Chiang MY, Misner D, Kempermann G, Schikorski T, Giguere V, Sucov HM, Gage FH, Stevens CF, Evans RM, An essential role for retinoid receptors RARbeta and RXRgamma in long-term potentiation and depression. Neuron 1998;21: 1353–61.

Cocco S, Diaz G, Stancampiano R, Diana A, Carta M, Curreli R, Sarais L, Fadda F, Vitamin A deficiency produces spatial learning and memory impairment in rats. Neuroscience 2002;115: 475–82.

Cook NR, Stampfer MJ, Ma J, Manson JE, Sacks FM, Buring JE, Hennekens CH, Beta-carotene supplementation for patients with low baseline levels and decreased risks of total and prostate carcinoma. Cancer 1999;86: 1783–92.

Cook NR, Le IM, Manson JE, Buring JE, Hennekens CH, Effects of beta-carotene supplementation on cancer incidence by baseline characteristics in the Physicians' Health Study (United States). Cancer Causes Control 2000;11: 617–26.

Corbett JJ, Increased intracranial pressure: idiopathic and otherwise. J Neuroophthalmol 2004;24: 103–5.

Craft NE, Haitema TB, Garnett KM, Fitch KA, Dorey CK, Carotenoid, tocopherol, and retinol concentrations in elderly human brain. J Nutr Health Aging 2004;8: 156–62.

Darlow BA, Graham PJ, Vitamin A supplementation to prevent mortality and short and long-term morbidity in very low birthweight infants. Cochrane Database Syst Rev 2007;CD000501.

de The H, Chomienne C, Lanotte M, Degos L, Dejean A, The t(15;17) translocation of acute promyelocytic leukaemia fuses the retinoic acid receptor alpha gene to a novel transcribed locus. Nature 1990;347: 558–61.

Ding Y, Qiao A, Wang Z, Goodwin JS, Lee ES, Block ML, Allsbrook M, McDonald MP, Fan GH, Retinoic acid attenuates beta-amyloid deposition and rescues memory deficits in an Alzheimer's disease transgenic mouse model. J Neurosci 2008;28: 11622–34.

Dragnev KH, Rigas JR, Dmitrovsky E, The retinoids and cancer prevention mechanisms. Oncologist 2000;5: 361–8.

Dragnev KH, Petty WJ, Dmitrovsky E, Retinoid targets in cancer therapy and chemoprevention. Cancer Biol Ther 2003;2: S150–6.

Ellison JB, Intensive vitamin therapy in measles. Br Med J 1932;2: 708–11.

Epstein JB, Gorsky M, Topical application of vitamin A to oral leukoplakia: a clinical case series. Cancer 1999;86: 921–7.

Erikstrup C, Mortensen OH, Nielsen AR, Fischer CP, Plomgaard P, Petersen AM, Krogh-Madsen R, Lindegaard B, Erhardt JG, Ullum H, Benn CS, Pedersen BK, RBP-to-retinol ratio, but not total RBP, is elevated in patients with type 2 diabetes. Diabetes Obes Metab 2009;11: 204–12.

Etchamendy N, Enderlin V, Marighetto A, Vouimba RM, Pallet V, Jaffard R, Higueret P, Alleviation of a selective age-related relational memory deficit in mice by pharmacologically induced normalization of brain retinoid signaling. J Neurosci 2001;21: 6423–9.

Etchamendy N, Enderlin V, Marighetto A, Pallet V, Higueret P, Jaffard R, Vitamin A deficiency and relational memory deficit in adult mice: relationships with changes in brain retinoid signalling. Behav Brain Res 2003;145: 37–49.

Fairfield KM, Fletcher RH, Vitamins for chronic disease prevention in adults: scientific review. J Am Med Assoc 2002;287: 3116–26.

Feskanich D, Singh V, Willett WC, Colditz GA, Vitamin A intake and hip fractures among postmenopausal women. J Am Med Assoc 2002;287:47–54.

Fishman RA, Polar bear liver, vitamin A, aquaporins, and pseudotumor cerebri. Ann Neurol 2002;52: 531–3.

Fraunfelder FW, Fraunfelder FT, Evidence for a probable causal relationship between tretinoin, acitretin, and etretinate and intracranial hypertension. J Neuroophthalmol 2004;24: 214–6.

Ghali F, Kang S, Leyden J, Shalita AR, Thiboutot DM, Changing the face of acne therapy. Cutis 2009;83: 4–15.

Glynn SA, Albanes D, Pietinen P, Brown CC, Rautalahti M, Tangrea JA, Taylor PR, Virtamo J, Alcohol consumption and risk of colorectal cancer in a cohort of Finnish men. Cancer Causes Control 1996;7: 214–23.

Goldsmith LA, Bolognia JL, Callen JP, Chen SC, Feldman SR, Lim HW, Lucky AW, Reed BR, Siegfried EC, Thiboutot DM, Wheeland RG, American Academy of Dermatology Consensus Conference on the safe and optimal use of isotretinoin: summary and recommendations. J Am Acad Dermatol 2004;50: 900–6.

Goodman GE, Schaffer S, Omenn GS, Chen C, King I, The association between lung and prostate cancer risk, and serum micronutrients: results and lessons learned from beta-carotene and retinol efficacy trial. Cancer Epidemiol Biomarkers Prev 2003;12: 518–26.

Goodman GE, Thornquist MD, Balmes J, Cullen MR, Meyskens FL Jr, Omenn GS, Valanis B, Williams JH Jr, The Beta-Carotene and Retinol Efficacy Trial: incidence of lung cancer and cardiovascular disease mortality during 6-year follow-up after stopping beta-carotene and retinol supplements. J Natl Cancer Inst 2004;96: 1743–50.

Gorsky M, Epstein JB, The effect of retinoids on premalignant oral lesions: focus on topical therapy. Cancer 2002;95: 1258–64.

Graham TE, Yang Q, Bluher M, Hammarstedt A, Ciaraldi TP, Henry RR, Wason CJ, Oberbach A, Jansson PA, Smith U, Kahn BB, Retinol-binding protein 4 and insulin resistance in lean, obese, and diabetic subjects. N Engl J Med 2006;354: 2552–63.

Grodstein F, Kang JH, Glynn RJ, Cook NR, Gaziano JM, A randomized trial of beta carotene supplementation and cognitive function in men: the Physicians' Health Study II. Arch Intern Med 2007;167: 2184–90.

Grotto I, Mimouni M, Gdalevich M, Mimouni D, Vitamin A supplementation and childhood morbidity from diarrhea and respiratory infections: a meta-analysis. J Pediatr 2003;142: 297–304.

Haider DG, Schindler K, Prager G, Bohdjalian A, Luger A, Wolzt M, Ludvik B, Serum retinol-binding protein 4 is reduced after weight loss in morbidly obese subjects. J Clin Endocrinol Metab 2007;92: 1168–71.

Hennekens CH, Buring JE, Manson JE, Stampfer M, Rosner B, Cook NR, Belanger C, LaMotte F, Gaziano JM, Ridker PM, Willett W, Peto R, Lack of effect of long-term supplementation with beta carotene on the incidence of malignant neoplasms and cardiovascular disease. N Engl J Med 1996;334: 1145–9.

Humphrey JH, Agoestina T, Wu L, Usman A, Nurachim M, Subardja D, Hidayat S, Tielsch J, West KP Jr, Sommer A, Impact of neonatal vitamin A supplementation on infant morbidity and mortality. J Pediatr 1996;128: 489–96.

Ingelsson E, Lind L, Circulating retinol-binding protein 4 and subclinical cardiovascular disease in the elderly. Diabetes Care 2009;32: 733–5.

Ingelsson E, Sundstrom J, Melhus H, Michaelsson K, Berne C, Vasan RS, Riserus U, Blomhoff R, Lind L, Arnlov J, Circulating retinol-binding protein 4, cardiovascular risk factors and prevalent cardiovascular disease in elderly. Atherosclerosis 2009;206: 239–44.

Jacobson DM, Berg R, Wall M, Digre KB, Corbett JJ, Ellefson RD, Serum vitamin A concentration is elevated in idiopathic intracranial hypertension. Neurology 1999;53: 1114–8.

Janke J, Engeli S, Boschmann M, Adams F, Bohnke J, Luft FC, Sharma AM, Jordan J, Retinol-binding protein 4 in human obesity. Diabetes 2006;55: 2805–10.

Jarvinen R, Knekt P, Seppanen R, Teppo L, Diet and breast cancer risk in a cohort of Finnish women. Cancer Lett 1997;114: 251–3.

Jimenez C, Leets I, Puche R, Anzola E, Montilla R, Parra C, Aguilera A, Garcia-Casal MN, A single dose of vitamin A improves haemoglobin concentration, retinol status and phagocytic function of neutrophils in preschool children. Br J Nutr 2010;103: 798–802.

Jiménez-Jiménez FJ, Molina JA, de Bustos F, Ortf-Pareja M, Benito-León J, Tallón-Barranco A, Gasalla T, Porta J, Arenas J. Serum levels of beta-carotene, alpha-carotene and vitamin A in patients with Alzheimer's disease. Eur J Neurol. 1999 Jul;6(4): 495–7.

Kabat GC, Kim M, Adams-Campbell LL, Caan BJ, Chlebowski RT, Neuhouser ML, Shikany JM, Rohan TE, Longitudinal study of serum carotenoid, retinol, and tocopherol concentrations in relation to breast cancer risk among postmenopausal women. Am J Clin Nutr 2009;90: 162–9.

Kang HY, Valerio L, Bahadoran P, Ortonne JP, The role of topical retinoids in the treatment of pigmentary disorders: an evidence-based review. Am J Clin Dermatol 2009a;10: 251–60.

Kang JH, Cook NR, Manson JE, Buring JE, Albert CM, Grodstein F, Vitamin E, vitamin C, beta carotene, and cognitive function among women with or at risk of cardiovascular disease: The Women's Antioxidant and Cardiovascular Study. Circulation 2009b;119: 2772–80.

Kang JH, Grodstein F, Plasma carotenoids and tocopherols and cognitive function: a prospective study. Neurobiol Aging 2008;29: 1394–403.

Kataja-Tuomola M, Sundell JR, Mannisto S, Virtanen MJ, Kontto J, Albanes D, Virtamo J, Effect of alpha-tocopherol and beta-carotene supplementation on the incidence of type 2 diabetes. Diabetologia 2008;51: 47–53.

Key TJ, Appleby PN, Allen NE, Travis RC, Roddam AW, Jenab M, Egevad L, Tjonneland A, Johnsen NF, Overvad K, Linseisen J, Rohrmann S, Boeing H, Pischon T, Psaltopoulou T, Trichopoulou A, Trichopoulos D, Palli D, Vineis P, Tumino R, Berrino F, Kiemeney L, Bueno-de-Mesquita HB, Quiros JR, Gonzalez CA, Martinez C, Larranaga N, Chirlaque MD, Ardanaz E, Stattin P, Hallmans G, Khaw KT, Bingham S, Slimani N, Ferrari P, Rinaldi S, Riboli E, Plasma carotenoids, retinol, and tocopherols and the risk of prostate cancer in the European Prospective Investigation into Cancer and Nutrition study. Am J Clin Nutr 2007;86: 672–81.

Kirkwood BR, Hurt L, Amenga-Etego S, Tawiah C, Zandoh C, Danso S, Hurt C, Edmond K, Hill Z, Ten Asbroek G, Fenty J, Owusu-Agyei S, Campbell O, Arthur P, Effect of vitamin A supplementation in women of reproductive age on maternal survival in Ghana (ObaapaVitA): a cluster-randomised, placebo-controlled trial. Lancet 2010;375: 1640–9.

Klemm RD, Labrique AB, Christian P, Rashid M, Shamim AA, Katz J, Sommer A, West KP Jr, Newborn vitamin A supplementation reduced infant mortality in rural Bangladesh. Pediatrics 2008;122: e242–50.

Kloting N, Graham TE, Berndt J, Kralisch S, Kovacs P, Wason CJ, Fasshauer M, Schon MR, Stumvoll M, Bluher M, Kahn BB, Serum retinol-binding protein is more highly expressed in visceral than in subcutaneous adipose tissue and is a marker of intra-abdominal fat mass. Cell Metab 2007;6: 79–87.

Krause VM, Delisle H, Solomons NW, Fortified foods contribute one half of recommended vitamin A intake in poor urban Guatemalan toddlers. J Nutr 1998;128: 860–4.

Krishnadev N, Meleth AD, Chew EY, Nutritional supplements for age-related macular degeneration. Curr Opin Ophthalmol 2010;21: 184–9.

Lane MA, Bailey SJ, Role of retinoid signalling in the adult brain. Prog Neurobiol 2005;75: 275–93.

Lewis JG, Shand BI, Elder PA, Scott RS, Plasma retinol-binding protein is unlikely to be a useful marker of insulin resistance. Diabetes Res Clin Pract 2008a;80: e13–5.

Lewis JG, Shand BI, Frampton CM, Elder PA, Scott RS, Plasma retinol-binding protein is not a marker of insulin resistance in overweight subjects: a three year longitudinal study. Clin Biochem 2008b;41: 1034–8.

Libien J, Blaner WS, Retinol and retinol-binding protein in cerebrospinal fluid: can vitamin A take the 'idiopathic' out of idiopathic intracranial hypertension? J Neuroophthalmol 2007;27: 253–7.

Lin J, Cook NR, Albert C, Zaharris E, Gaziano JM, Van Denburgh M, Buring JE, Manson JE, Vitamins C and E and beta carotene supplementation and cancer risk: a randomized controlled trial. J Natl Cancer Inst 2009;101: 14–23.

Lippman SM, Lee JJ, Martin JW, El-Naggar AK, Xu X, Shin DM, Thomas M, Mao L, Fritsche HA Jr, Zhou X, Papadimitrakopoulou V, Khuri FR, Tran H, Clayman GL, Hittelman WN, Hong WK, Lotan R, Fenretinide activity in retinoid-resistant oral leukoplakia. Clin Cancer Res 2006;12: 3109–14.

Liu S, Ajanl U, Chae C, Hennekens C, Buring JE, Manson JE. Long-term beta-carotene supplementation and risk of type 2 diabetes mellitus a randomized controlled trial. JAMA. 1999 Sep 15; 282(11): 1073–5.

Long KZ, Rosado JL, DuPont HL, Hertzmark E, Santos JI, Supplementation with vitamin A reduces watery diarrhoea and respiratory infections in Mexican children. Br J Nutr 2007;97: 337–43.

Marqueling AL, Zane LT, Depression and suicidal behavior in acne patients treated with isotretinoin: a systematic review. Semin Cutan Med Surg 2007;26: 210–20.

McCaffery P, Zhang J, Crandall JE, Retinoic acid signaling and function in the adult hippocampus. J Neurobiol 2006;66: 780–91.

Melhus H, Michaelsson K, Kindmark A, Bergstrom R, Holmberg L, Mallmin H, Wolk A, Ljunghall S, Excessive dietary intake of vitamin A is associated with reduced bone mineral density and increased risk for hip fracture. Ann Intern Med 1998;129: 770–8.

Mettlin C, Graham S, Swanson M, Vitamin A and lung cancer. J Natl Cancer Inst 1979;62: 1435–8.

Michaelsson K, Lithell H, Vessby B, Melhus H, Serum retinol levels and the risk of fracture. N Engl J Med 2003;348: 287–94.

Michels KB, Holmberg L, Bergkvist L, Ljung H, Bruce A, Wolk A, Dietary antioxidant vitamins, retinol, and breast cancer incidence in a cohort of Swedish women. Int J Cancer 2001;91: 563–7.

Mignone LI, Giovannucci E, Newcomb PA, Titus-Ernstoff L, Trentham-Dietz A, Hampton JM, Willett WC, Egan KM, Dietary carotenoids and the risk of invasive breast cancer. Int J Cancer 2009;124: 2929–37.

Mills JP, Furr HC, Tanumihardjo SA, Retinol to retinol-binding protein (RBP) is low in obese adults due to elevated apo-RBP. Exp Biol Med (Maywood) 2008;233: 1255–61.

Mingaud F, Mormede C, Etchamendy N, Mons N, Niedergang B, Wietrzych M, Pallet V, Jaffard R, Krezel W, Higueret P, Marighetto A, Retinoid hyposignaling contributes to aging-related decline in hippocampal function in short-term/working memory organization and long-term declarative memory encoding in mice. J Neurosci 2008;28: 279–91.

Morrice G Jr, Havener WH, Kapetansky F, Vitamin A intoxication as a cause of pseudotumor cerebri. J Am Med Assoc 1960;173: 1802–5.

Muhilal, Permeisih D, Idjradinata YR, Muherdiyantiningsih, Karyadi D, Vitamin A-fortified monosodium glutamate and health, growth, and survival of children: a controlled field trial. Am J Clin Nutr 1988;48: 1271–6.

Neuhouser ML, Barnett MJ, Kristal AR, Ambrosone CB, King IB, Thornquist M, Goodman GG, Dietary supplement use and prostate cancer risk in the Carotene and Retinol Efficacy Trial. Cancer Epidemiol Biomarkers Prev 2009;18: 2202–6.

O'Donnell J, Polar hysteria: an expression of hypervitaminosis A. Am J Ther 2004;11: 507–16.

Olson CR, Mello CV. Significance of vitamin A to brain function, behavior and learning. Mol Nutr Food Res 2010;54: 489–95.

Omenn GS, Goodman GE, Thornquist MD, Balmes J, Cullen MR, Glass A, Keogh JP, Meyskens FL, Valanis B, Williams JH, Barnhart S, Hammar S, Effects of a combination of beta carotene and vitamin A on lung cancer and cardiovascular disease. N Engl J Med 1996;334: 1150–5.

Peacock JM, Folsom AR, Knopman DS, Mosley TH, Goff DC Jr, Szklo M, Dietary antioxidant intake and cognitive performance in middle-aged adults. The Atherosclerosis Risk in Communities (ARIC) Study investigators. Public Health Nutr 2000;3: 337–43.

Penniston KL, Tanumihardjo SA, The acute and chronic toxic effects of vitamin A. Am J Clin Nutr 2006;83: 191–201.

Perrig WJ, Perrig P, Stahelin HB. The relation between antioxidants and memory performance in the old and very old. J Am Geriatr Soc 1997;45: 718–24.

Peto R, Doll R, Buckley JD, Sporn MB, Can dietary beta-carotene materially reduce human cancer rates? Nature 1981;290: 201–8.

Pfutzner A, Schondorf T, Hanefeld M, Lubben G, Kann PH, Karagiannis E, Wilhelm B, Forst T, Changes in insulin resistance and cardiovascular risk induced by PPARgamma activation have no impact on RBP4 plasma concentrations in nondiabetic patients. Horm Metab Res 2009;41: 202–6.

Prentice AM, Vitamin A supplements and survival in children. Br Med J 2010;340: c977.

Promislow JH, Goodman-Gruen D, Slymen DJ, Barrett-Connor E, Retinol intake and bone mineral density in the elderly: the Rancho Bernardo Study. J Bone Miner Res 2002;17: 1349–58.

Qiao YL, Dawsey SM, Kamangar F, Fan JH, Abnet CC, Sun XD, Johnson LL, Gail MH, Dong ZW, Yu B, Mark SD, Taylor PR, Total and cancer mortality after supplementation with vitamins and minerals: follow-up of the Linxian General Population Nutrition Intervention Trial. J Natl Cancer Inst 2009;101: 507–18.

Rao AV, Rao LG, Carotenoids and human health. Pharmacol Res 2007;55: 207–16.

Rinaldi P, Polidori MC, Metastasio A, Mariani E, Mattioli P, Cherubini A, Catani M, Cecchetti R, Senin U, Mecocci P, Plasma antioxidants are similarly depleted in mild cognitive impairment and in Alzheimer's disease. Neurobiol Aging 2003;24: 915–9.

Ross AC, Chen Q, Ma Y, Augmentation of antibody responses by retinoic acid and costimulatory molecules. Semin Immunol 2009;21: 42–50.

Sass JO, Arnhold T, Tzimas G, Jacobson DM, Serum vitamin A is elevated in idiopathic intracranial hypertension. Neurology 2000;54: 2192–93.

Scheven BA, Hamilton NJ, Retinoic acid and 1,25-dihydroxyvitamin D3 stimulate osteoclast formation by different mechanisms. Bone 1990;11: 53–9.

Selhorst JB, Waybright EA, Jennings S, Corbett JJ, Liver lover's headache: pseudotumor cerebri and vitamin A intoxication. J Am Med Assoc 1984;252: 3365.

Selhorst JB, Kulkantrakorn K, Corbett JJ, Leira EC, Chung SM, Retinol-binding protein in idiopathic intracranial hypertension (IIH). J Neuroophthalmol 2000;20: 250–2.

Shalita A, The integral role of topical and oral retinoids in the early treatment of acne. J Eur Acad Dermatol Venereol 2001;15(Suppl 3): 43–9.

Shekelle RB, Lepper M, Liu S, Maliza C, Raynor WJ Jr, Rossof AH, Paul O, Shryock AM, Stamler J, Dietary vitamin A and risk of cancer in the Western Electric study. Lancet 1981;ii: 1185–90.

Shim CY, Park S, Kim JS, Shin DJ, Ko YG, Kang SM, Choi D, Ha JW, Jang Y, Chung N, Association of plasma retinol-binding protein 4, adiponectin, and high molecular weight adiponectin with insulin resistance in non-diabetic hypertensive patients. Yonsei Med J 2010;51: 375–84.

Sommer A, Mortality associated with mild, untreated xerophthalmia. Trans Am Ophthalmol Soc 1983;81: 825–53.

Sommer A, Vitamin A deficiency and clinical disease: an historical overview. J Nutr 2008;138: 1835–9.

Sommer A, Tarwotjo I, Djunaedi E, West KP Jr, Loeden AA, Tilden R, Mele L, Impact of vitamin A supplementation on childhood mortality. A randomised controlled community trial. Lancet 1986;i: 1169–73.

Tabassi A, Salmasi AH, Jalali M, Serum and CSF vitamin A concentrations in idiopathic intracranial hypertension. Neurology 2005;64: 1893–6.

Takashima N, Tomoike H, Iwai N, Retinol-binding protein 4 and insulin resistance. N Engl J Med 2006;355: 1392; author reply 1394–5.

Tallman MS, Andersen JW, Schiffer CA, Appelbaum FR, Feusner JH, Ogden A, Shepherd L, Willman C, Bloomfield CD, Rowe JM, Wiernik PH, All-trans-retinoic acid in acute promyelocytic leukemia. N Engl J Med 1997;337: 1021–8.

Thiboutot D, Gollnick H, Bettoli V, Dreno B, Kang S, Leyden JJ, Shalita AR, Lozada VT, Berson D, Finlay A, Goh CL, Herane MI, Kaminsky A, Kubba R, Layton A, Miyachi Y, Perez M, Martin JP, Ramos ESM, See JA, Shear N, Wolf J Jr, New insights into the management of acne: an update from the Global Alliance to Improve Outcomes in Acne group. J Am Acad Dermatol 2009;60: S1–50.

Tielsch JM, Rahmathullah L, Thulasiraj RD, Katz J, Coles C, Sheeladevi S, John R, Prakash K, Newborn vitamin A dosing reduces the case fatality but not incidence of common childhood morbidities in South India. J Nutr 2007;137: 2470–4.

Togari A, Kondo M, Arai M, Matsumoto S (Effects of retinoic acid on bone formation and resorption in cultured mouse calvaria. Gen Pharmacol 1991;22: 287–92.

Tyson JE, Wright LL, Oh W, Kennedy KA, Mele L, Ehrenkranz RA, Stoll BJ, Lemons JA, Stevenson DK, Bauer CR, Korones SB, Fanaroff AA, Vitamin A supplementation for extremely-low-birth-weight infants. National Institute of Child Health and Human Development Neonatal Research Network. N Engl J Med 1999;340: 1962–8.

Verhoeven DT, Assen N, Goldbohm RA, Dorant E, van 't Veer P, Sturmans F, Hermus RJ, van den Brandt PA, Vitamins C and E, retinol, beta-carotene and dietary fibre in relation to breast cancer risk: a prospective cohort study. Br J Cancer 1997;75: 149–55.

Veronesi U, Mariani L, Decensi A, Formelli F, Camerini T, Miceli R, Di Mauro MG, Costa A, Marubini E, Sporn MB, De Palo G, Fifteen-year results of a randomized phase III trial of fenretinide to prevent second breast cancer. Ann Oncol 2006;17: 1065–71.

Visani G, Manfroi S, Tosi P, Martinelli G. All-trans-retinoic acid and pseudotumor cerebri. Leuk Lymphoma 1996;23: 437–42.

von Eynatten M, Humpert PM, Retinol-binding protein 4 & atherosclerosis: risk factor or innocent bystander? Atherosclerosis 2009;206: 38–9.

von Eynatten M, Lepper PM, Liu D, Lang K, Baumann M, Nawroth PP, Bierhaus A, Dugi KA, Heemann U, Allolio B, Humpert PM, Retinol-binding protein 4 is associated with components of the metabolic syndrome, but not with insulin resistance, in men with type 2 diabetes or coronary artery disease. Diabetologia 2007;50: 1930–7.

Wang W, Shinto L, Connor WE, Quinn JF, Nutritional biomarkers in Alzheimer's disease: the association between carotenoids, n-3 fatty acids, and dementia severity. J Alzheimers Dis 2008;13: 31–8.

Warner JE, Bernstein PS, Yemelyanov A, Alder SC, Farnsworth ST, Digre KB, Vitamin A in the cerebrospinal fluid of patients with and without idiopathic intracranial hypertension. Ann Neurol 2002;52: 647–50.

Warner JE, Larson AJ, Bhosale P, Digre KB, Henley C, Alder SC, Katz BJ, Bernstein PS, Retinol-binding protein and retinol analysis in cerebrospinal fluid and serum of patients with and without idiopathic intracranial hypertension. J Neuroophthalmol 2007;27: 258–62.

Watters JL, Gail MH, Weinstein SJ, Virtamo J, Albanes D, Associations between alpha-tocopherol, beta-carotene, and retinol and prostate cancer survival. Cancer Res 2009;69: 3833–41.

Weinstock MA, Bingham SF, Lew RA, Hall R, Eilers D, Kirsner R, Naylor M, Kalivas J, Cole G, Marcolivio K, Collins J, Digiovanna JJ, Vertrees JE, Topical tretinoin therapy and all-cause mortality. Arch Dermatol 2009;145: 18–24.

West KP Jr, Katz J, Khatry SK, LeClerq SC, Pradhan EK, Shrestha SR, Connor PB, Dali SM, Christian P, Pokhrel RP, Sommer A, Double blind, cluster randomised trial of low dose supplementation with vitamin A or beta carotene on mortality related to pregnancy in Nepal. The NNIPS-2 Study Group. Br Med J 1999;318: 570–5.

WHO (2009) Global prevalence of vitamin A deficiency in populations at risk 1995–2005. In: Deficiency. WGDoVA, editor. Geneva: World Health Organization.

Wolters M, Hickstein M, Flintermann A, Tewes U, Hahn A, Cognitive performance in relation to vitamin status in healthy elderly German women-the effect of 6-month multivitamin supplementation. Prev Med 2005;41: 253–9.

Yaffe K, Antioxidants and prevention of cognitive decline: does duration of use matter? Arch Intern Med 2007;167: 2167–8.

Yaffe K, Clemons TE, McBee WL, Lindblad AS, Impact of antioxidants, zinc, and copper on cognition in the elderly: a randomized, controlled trial. Neurology 2004;63: 1705–7.

Yang Q, Graham TE, Mody N, Preitner F, Peroni OD, Zabolotny JM, Kotani K, Quadro L, Kahn BB, Serum retinol binding protein 4 contributes to insulin resistance in obesity and type 2 diabetes. Nature 2005;436: 356–62.

Yoshida A, Matsutani Y, Fukuchi Y, Saito K, Naito M, Analysis of the factors contributing to serum retinol binding protein and transthyretin levels in Japanese adults. J Atheroscler Thromb 2006;13: 209–15.

Zaman Z, Roche S, Fielden P, Frost PG, Niriella DC, Cayley AC. Plasma concentrations of vitamins A and E and carotenoids in Alzheimer's disease. Age Ageing. 1992;21(2): 91–4.

Zhang S, Hunter DJ, Forman MR, Rosner BA, Speizer FE, Colditz GA, Manson JE, Hankinson SE, Willett WC, Dietary carotenoids and vitamins A, C, and E and risk of breast cancer. J Natl Cancer Inst 1999;91: 547–56.

Zouboulis CC, Retinoids – which dermatological indications will benefit in the near future? Skin Pharmacol Appl Skin Physiol 2001;14: 303–15.

Zulet MA, Puchau B, Hermsdorff HH, Navarro C, Martinez JA, Vitamin A intake is inversely related with adiposity in healthy young adults. J Nutr Sci Vitaminol (Tokyo) 2008;54: 347–52.

3 Vitamin B1 – Thiamine

3.1 Nutritional and biological aspects of vitamin B1

Elena Beltramo

3.1.1 Introduction

Thiamine, or vitamin B1, is a water-soluble, B-complex vitamin, necessary for the metabolism of carbohydrates, fats and proteins in most organisms (Stryer, 1988), which probably played a role in the earliest phases of the evolution of life (Frank et al., 2007). It was the first vitamin to be isolated in the first years of the 20th century, while looking for an 'anti-beriberi' substance (Lonsdale, 2006), and it was crystallized from rice polishings in 1926 by Jansen and Donath. The structure and synthesis of thiamine and its biochemical function were described by Peters in 1936 and Williams in 1938.

The active form of thiamine, thiamine-diphosphate (TDP), works as a co-factor for more than 24 enzymes and it is required at several stages of anabolic and catabolic intermediary metabolism, such as intracellular glucose metabolism (glycolysis, Krebs cycle, pentose-phosphate cycle) (Frank et al., 2007). TDP is essential for ATP production through the Krebs cycle within each cell and is also a modulator of neuronal and neuro-muscular transmission, probably through activation of an ionic channel for chlorine (Bender, 1999; Beltramo et al., 2008). Thiamine has also been reported to mimic acetylcholine in the brain, possibly exerting a function in Alzheimer's disease and other dementias (Meador et al., 1993a,b).

3.1.2 Biochemistry

Thiamine is chemically structured as a five-membered thiazolium ring and a six-membered aminopyrimidine ring joined together by a methyl group (▶Fig. 3.1a). The active form (TDP) has a diphosphate-terminated side-chain (▶Fig. 3.1b).

In intestinal lumen, thiamine is present in a free form and in very low concentrations; it is absorbed mainly in the proximal part of the small intestine, by passive diffusion at higher concentrations (>1 µmol/l), whereas at lower concentrations, an active, carrier-mediated system, involving the phosphorylation of the vitamin, is needed (Hoyumpa et al., 1982; Rindi and Ferrari, 1997). Thiamine deficiency enhances thiamine uptake (Laforenza et al., 1997), which can instead be reduced by thyroid hormone and insulin (Rindi and Laforenza, 2000).

Lipid-soluble thiamine derivatives (allithiamines) have much higher absorption and bioavailability than water-soluble thiamine salts, reaching higher concentrations in the blood and tissues and maintaining them longer (Baker and Frank, 1976; Fujimara, 1976). In particular, benfotiamine, a compound which contains an open thiazole

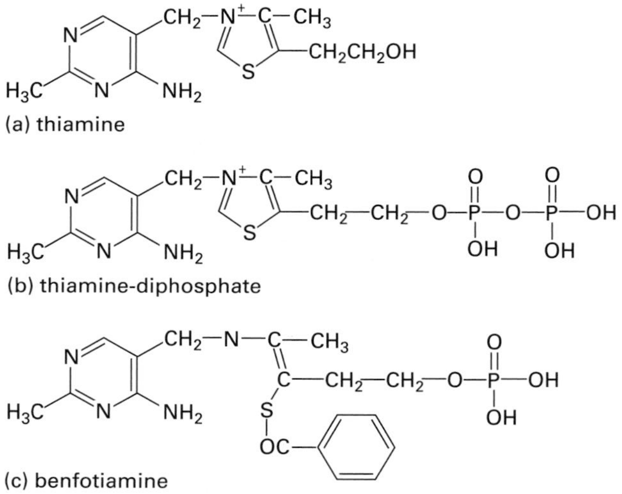

Fig. 3.1: Chemical structures of (a) thiamine, (b) its activated form, thiamine diphosphate (TDP), and (c) its lipophilic-analogue, benfotiamine.

ring (▶Fig. 3.1c) and was developed to improve bioavailability for pharmacological administration (Schreeb et al., 1997; Greb and Bitsch, 1998), seems to be the most effective (Loew, 1996). Lipid-soluble compounds are converted to biologically-active thiamine after the passage through the mucous membranes and, subsequently, to the active form, TDP.

TDP acts as a cofactor for enzymatic reactions that cleave alpha-keto acids, producing energy from glucose or converting glucose to fat for storage inside the tissues: among them, transketolase (TK), the pyruvate dehydrogenase and α-ketoglutarate dehydrogenase complexes, and the macromolecular aggregation in charge to decarboxylate the keto acids deriving from the branched chain amino acids (valine, leucine and isoleucine) are the most important (▶Fig. 3.2).

TK, which contains a tightly bound TDP as its prosthetic group, is able to shift excess fructose-6-phosphate and glycerhaldeyde-3-phosphate (G3P) from glycolysis into the pentose-phosphate shunt. G3P is one of the most effective agents of advanced-glycation end-products (AGE) formation into the cytoplasm (Brownlee, 1994) and also an end-product of the non-oxidative branch of the pentose phosphate pathway, the function of which is to provide pentose phosphate for nucleotide synthesis and reduced NADP for several metabolic pathways (Lonsdale, 2006). TK activity in erythrocytes is often used as a marker of thiamine deficiency (Nixon et al., 1990).

Because the pyruvate dehydrogenase complex is responsible for the oxidative decarboxylation of pyruvate, the final product of glycolysis, and the subsequent synthesis of acetyl-CoA, which then enters the Krebs' cycle, a deficit in thiamine is responsible for an accumulation of pyruvate and lactate (Horwitt and Kreisler, 1949). Similarly, the α-ketoglutarate dehydrogenase complex is responsible for the oxidative decarboxylation of α-ketoglutarate into succinyl-CoA inside the Krebs' cycle.

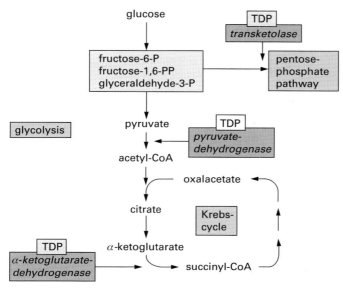

Fig. 3.2: Thiamine-diphosphate (TDP) works as a cofactor for several enzymes, the most important of which, playing a fundamental role in the intracellular glucose metabolism, are transketolase and the pyruvate dehydrogenase and α-ketoglutarate dehydrogenase complexes.

3.1.3 Natural sources, interactions, dosage, recommended intake

Natural sources of thiamine are meats (particularly lean pork), liver, poultry, eggs, fish, beans, peas, nuts and whole grains, whereas little thiamine is present in fruit, vegetables and dairy products (Flodin, 1988). Cooking and other heat-processing of food causes a considerable loss of this vitamin.

Lack of thiamine can be caused by several factors in diet. Sulphites, largely used as preservatives, attack thiamine at the methylene bridge, cleaving the pyrimidine ring from the thiazole ring (Combs, 2008). Thiamine is also degraded by thermolabile thiaminases, present in milled rice, raw freshwater fish, raw shellfish, and ferns. Heat-stable poly-phenolic plant thiamine antagonists, such as caffeic acid, chlorogenic acid and tannic acid, present in tea, coffee and betel nuts, impair thiamine absorption by oxidizing the thiazole ring. Approximately two times the RDA of thiamine can be destroyed and degraded by the consumption of 100 g tea or coffee over a period of 3 h. This effect can be partially inhibited and reversed by vitamin C.

Heavy alcohol consumption is a major cause of thiamine deficiency, for several reasons: alcoholics tend to assume little thiamine in their diet, the active transport of thiamine from the gastrointestinal tract is impaired by acute ethanol intoxication, which also blocks the phosphorylation of thiamine to its active form (TDP), liver storage is reduced by hepatic steatosis or fibrosis, and thiamine utilization is impaired by magnesium deficiency owing to alcohol consumption (Leevy, 1982; Rindi et al., 1986; Butterworth et al., 1993).

Phenytoin, penicillins, cephalosporins, tetracycline derivatives, aminoglycosides, loop diuretics, fluoroquinolones, sulphonamide derivatives and trimethoprim can deplete thiamine, as well as long-term use of oral contraceptives (Pelton et al., 1999).

Approximately 25–30 mg of thiamine are stored into the body, mainly in organs with high metabolic needs, such as skeletal muscle, heart, brain, liver and kidneys. Two to 3 weeks of depletion are sufficient to fully consume body storage (Velez et al., 1985), but after 1 week only, the blood-brain barrier is disrupted, with local cerebral hypoperfusion and onset of the classic symptoms of Wernicke's encephalopathy (Heye et al., 1994).

The recommended thiamine intake for healthy individuals is 0.2–0.9 mg/day in infants/children, 1.1–1.2 mg/day in adolescents and adults and 1.4–1.5 mg/day during pregnancy and lactation (FAO/WHO, 2004). The recommended intake for elderly people is the same as for adults. In fact, although some reports suggested that requirements might be higher in the elderly, there is also a concomitant decrease in their energy utilisation (IOM, 1998).

Fortification of white flour, cereals, pasta and rice with thiamine began in the USA during the World War and other countries quickly followed. Fortification of staple foods has virtually eradicated the thiamine deficiency owing to the low vitamin intake in developed nations. Nowadays, thiamine fortification of white flour is mandatory in Australia and is common practice in other industrialized countries (such as the UK, USA and Canada) to restore losses from wheat during milling. Fortification of rice, however, is much more difficult and this is a problem in those countries where rice constitutes the main food. Experiments of beer and wine fortification have been made in Australia (because alcoholics are commonly thiamine-deficient), but the project has been left behind owing to the opposition of nutritionists, brewers and anti-alcohol groups.

3.1.4 Thiamine deficiency

Thiamine deficiency has long been considered a problem only in non-developed countries and in advanced alcoholics. However, it has been shown that lack of thiamine or defects in its intracellular transport can cause several severe disorders and can occur in a variety of situations.

The best known manifestation of thiamine deficiency is beriberi, a neurological and cardiovascular disease, known since antiquity (the first document describing it as 'Kakke' dates back to 808 AD) (Lonsdale, 2006) and so-called in 1630 by a Dutch physician who worked in Java because its symptoms cause walking like sheep (*beri-beri* in the local dialect) (Beltramo et al., 2008).

In adults, beriberi can occur in different forms: wet beriberi, which affects heart and circulation, and dry beriberi, affecting the nervous system. Recently, this classical division has been overcome by the evidence that symptoms can co-exist in the same individual, might or might not be associated with oedema, and vary according to age (Lonsdale, 2006). In cardiovascular beriberi, the heart could be enlarged and cardiac output inadequate (Stryer, 1988); a severe, although less common, cardiovascular form is *shoshin*, in which acute heart failure occurs rapidly, and frequently the consequence is sudden death (within hours or days) (Jansen and Donath, 1926; Kawano et al., 2005). Neuronal symptoms (dry beriberi) consist of damage of the peripheral nervous system, with pain in the limbs, weakness of the musculature and distorted skin sensation, owing to degeneration of myelin in the muscular sheaths without inflammation (Karuppagounder et al., 2008). Absence or severe lack of thiamine in the diet can cause the *Wernicke-Korsakoff syndrome*, (also known as 'cerebral beriberi'), a striking neuropsychiatric disorder characterized by paralysis of eye movements, horizontal nystagmus, fever, ataxia, abnormal stance and gait, and finally markedly deranged mental function (Harper, 1979; Stryer, 1988). Infantile beriberi can occur in breast-fed infants, whose mothers are thiamine-deficient.

Beriberi is particularly common in Far Eastern countries, because of the low content of thiamine in rice, particularly polished rice, because only the outer layer contains an appreciable amount of the vitamin. In western countries, it can occur, mainly in the form of Wernicke's encephalopathy, in severely-malnourished alcoholics (Cook et al., 1998), but it has been also described in cases of total parental nutrition (Kitamura et al., 1996), diets high in simple carbohydrates deriving from processed food (Lonsdale, 1987), gastrointestinal surgery (Seehra et al., 1996), chronic renal dialysis (Reuler et al., 1985), hyperemesis gravidarum (Togay-Isikay et al., 2001), severe infections (Lindoe and Loberg, 1989), cancer (particularly after chemotherapy) (Kuo et al., 2009) and AIDS (Butterworth et al., 1991).

Thiamine levels are often reduced in alcoholics, mainly owing to their diet rich in carbohydrates, the impairment of thiamine absorption for the effects of chronic alcohol intake on the absorptive mechanisms of the gut and the accumulation of acetaldehyde, which interferes with thiamine utilization. Thiamine deficiency in alcoholics often is not resolved by thiamine supplementation (Thomson, 2000). A deficit in thiamine is described also in pregnancy, particularly in women with gestational diabetes (Bakker et al., 2000) and hyperemesis gravidarum (Togay-Isikay et al., 2001), and in diabetic patients (Thornalley et al., 2007), particularly in those with diabetic neuropathy (Abbas and Swai, 1997; Wu and Ren, 2006).

Finally, an inborn defect in the intracellular transport of thiamine could be the cause of TRMA syndrome (thiamine-responsive megaloblastic anaemia), an autosomal recessive disorder characterized by megaloblastic anaemia with ringed sideroblasts, diabetes and progressive sensorineural deafness. The TRMA gene, a member of the solute carrier gene superfamily, whose product is a membrane protein which transports thiamine with sub-micromolar affinity, is mutated in all patients with TRMA. Cells from TRMA patients are uniquely sensitive to thiamine depletion to the nanomolar range, whereas pharmacologic doses of thiamine relieve the symptoms of anaemia and diabetes (Neufeld et al., 2001).

Symptoms of thiamine deficiency vary according to the severity of the deficiency itself and can include weakness, dizziness, insomnia, myalgia, back pain, muscular atrophy, depression, nausea, vomit, weight loss, hypotension, hypothermia, bradycardia at rest, tachycardia with sinus arrhythmia on exertion, constipation, digestive disturbances, memory loss, peripheral neuropathy, pain sensitivity, dyspnoea and sonophobia (Williams et al., 1943). Emotional instability, mood lability, uncooperative behaviour and fearfulness with agitation have also been seen in adolescents with documented thiamine deficiency (Lonsdale and Schamberger, 1980).

3.1.5 Biochemical indicators

Thiamine status is usually estimated as urinary excretion of thiamine and its metabolites, under basal conditions or after thiamine loading, or blood concentrations of thiamine itself, free or phosphorylated, pyruvate, alpha-ketoglutarate, lactate and glyoxylate (Lu et al., 2008). Erythrocyte tranketolase activity is a marker of TDP levels and could indicate genetic defects (FAO/WHO, 2004). Erythrocyte thiamine is used as a direct measure of TDP, but it is possible to discriminate among thiamine, TDP and thiamine monophosphate by high liquid chromatography separation (Gerrits et al., 1997). The erythrocyte tranketolase activity assay continues to be a main functional indicator, but sometimes it could appear to be normal after prolonged deficiency and in a study was found to scarcely correlate with dietary intake in a group of English adolescents (Bailey et al., 1994). Moreover, inter-individual and genetic factors might affect the transketolase (Singleton et al., 1995). The direct determination of erythrocyte TDP (Baines and Davies, 1988) or whole blood thiamine and its phosphate esters (Gerrits et al., 1997) seems to be more useful, because the coenzyme is less susceptible to factors affecting enzyme activity.

3.1.6 Toxicity

Thiamine toxicity is very uncommon because renal clearance is rapid (FAO/WHO, 2004). Most reports of adverse effects follow parenteral nutrition. High oral doses of thiamine hydrochloride (>7000 mg) can cause headache, nausea, irritability, insomnia, rapid pulse and weakness, symptoms relieved upon cessation of treatment or dose reduction.

3.1.7 Thiamine and diabetes

Diabetes is known to strongly affect large vessels, accelerating atherosclerosis and increasing the risk of myocardial infarction, stroke and limb amputation, whereas diabetic microangiopathy is a major cause of blindness, renal failure and nerve damage. Two large prospective clinical trials have closely linked the severity of vascular complications in both type 1 and 2 diabetes with the duration and degree of hyperglycaemia (DCCT, 1993; UKPDS, 1998).

Vascular cells are highly sensible to the direct exposure to high glucose concentrations, which cause several pathological changes in small and large vessels (Brignardello et al., 1998; Podestà et al., 2000; Beltramo et al., 2004). Among the possible mechanisms of glucose-induced vascular damage, four hypotheses gained major credit: (1) increased flux through the polyol pathway; (2) increased formation of AGE; (3) protein kinase C (PKC) activation; (4) increased flux through the hexosamine pathway. It has been hypothesized that the possible common denominator ('unifying mechanism') of these apparently independent biochemical pathways is high glucose-induced excess production of reactive oxygen species by the mitochondrial electron transport chain, as a result of increased flux through the Krebs' cycle (Nishikawa et al., 2000). Thus, potentially, thiamine can prevent cell damage induced by hyperglycaemia, by removing excess glycating metabolites from the cytoplasm, as described above (see Section 3.1.2) and, through activation of α-ketoglutarate dehydrogenase, by facilitating the utilization, in the Krebs' cycle, of acetyl-CoA derived from accelerated glycolysis (La Selva et al., 1996).

Several reports in the literature show that thiamine and benfotiamine act as protective agents against the metabolic damage induced by high glucose in vascular cells (reviewed in Thornalley, 2005; Beltramo et al., 2008). One possible mechanism is by reducing excess ROS production through the normalization of the four branches of the 'unifying mechanism' proposed to be at the basis of the pathogenesis of diabetic vascular complications (Hammes et al., 2003; Berrone et al., 2006).

Studies on thiamine-deficient streptozotocin (STZ)-induced diabetic rats or mice reported that thiamine and/or benfotiamine can prevent incipient diabetic nephropathy (Babaei-Jadidi et al., 2003) and ischemia-induced toe necrosis, improve hind-limb perfusion and oxygenation, restore endothelium-dependent vasodilatation (Gadau et al., 2006), have beneficial effects on detrusor contractility, progression of diabetic cystopathy (Yenilmez et al., 2006), peripheral nerve function (motor nerve conduction velocity) and the formation of glycation products in nervous tissue (Stracke et al., 2001), alleviate oxidative stress both in cerebral cortex tissue (Wu and Ren, 2006) and cardiomyocytes (Ceylan-Isik et al., 2006). Moreover, high-dose thiamine therapy (70 mg/kg) in STZ-induced diabetic rats normalizes food intake, which was increased by more than 60% in comparison with non-diabetics, decreases diuresis and glicosuria, and prevents diabetic-induced increases in plasma cholesterol and triglycerides, thus counteracting dyslipidaemia (Babaei-Jadidi et al., 2004).

As regards human studies, diabetic patients seem to have lower blood thiamine concentrations than healthy subjects, together with a reduced erythrocyte transketolase activity (Saito et al., 1987; Valerio et al., 1999; Jermendy, 2006), an increased thiamine renal clearance (Thornalley et al., 2007), and a decreased intestinal absorption and membrane transport (Laforenza et al., 1997). However, diabetic subjects usually do not manifest the typical clinical markers of thiamine deficiency, probably because their low thiamine levels are owing to a specific pattern of vascular cells, which are unable to regulate glucose transport, reaching high levels of intracellular glucose concentrations (Kaiser et al., 1993), in the presence of hyperglycaemia. Such high levels of glucose determine high production of ROS, which could oxidize thiamine, with the production of inactive compounds (Stepuro et al., 1997).

The possible positive effects of thiamine supplementation in diabetic patients, however, have not been fully investigated. An amelioration in neuropathy symptoms (nerve conduction velocity and vibration perception threshold) and decrease in pain, together with the patients' sensation of improved clinical conditions, were signalled in diabetic subjects with polyneuropathy treated with either thiamine (Abbas and Swai, 1997) or benfotiamine (Stracke et al., 1996; Haupt et al., 2005; Stracke et al., 2008).

Macro- and microvascular endothelial dysfunction and oxidative stress, as assessed by measurement of flow-mediated dilatation and hyperaemia, following an AGE-rich meal in type 2 diabetic patients, were prevented by benfotiamine, possibly through reduction of endogenous AGE and dycarbonyl (methyl-glyoxal) production, suggesting a role for benfotiamine in atherosclerosis prevention in diabetic patients (Stirban et al., 2006). The intravenous administration of 100 mg of thiamine improved endothelium-dependent vasodilatation in the presence of hyperglycaemia (Arora et al., 2006). Both studies showed that thiamine/benfotiamine effects were not owing to a glucose-lowering mechanism because either compound had no effects in normoglycaemic conditions.

In a recent pilot study, high-dose thiamine therapy produced regression of urinary albumin excretion in type 2 diabetic patients with microalbuminuria, showing that thiamine supplementation at high doses could provide improved therapy for early-stage diabetic nephropathy (Rabbani et al., 2009).

3.1.8 Summary

Thiamine, or vitamin B1, is an essential coenzyme, required at several stages of anabolic and catabolic metabolism. Natural sources of thiamine are meats, eggs, fish, legumes, nuts and whole grains, whereas little is present in fruit, vegetables and dairy products. Lack of thiamine in the diet can be caused by addition of sulphites as preservatives, degradation by thiaminases present in milled rice, raw fish and ferns, excess use of tea and coffee, and, particularly, heavy alcohol consumption. Thiamine deficiency can cause several severe disorders, the best known of which is beriberi, a neurological and cardiovascular disease, particularly common in Far Eastern countries, because of the low content of thiamine in rice. In Western countries, it can occur, mainly in form of Wernicke's encephalopathy, in severely-malnourished alcoholics, but also in cases of total parental nutrition, diets high in simple carbohydrates, gastrointestinal surgery, chronic renal dialysis, hyperemesis gravidarum, severe infections, cancer, AIDS and diabetes, in particular in patients with diabetic neuropathy. An inborn defect in the intracellular transport of thiamine can cause the TRMA syndrome, characterized by megaloblastic anaemia, diabetes and progressive sensorineural deafness. Symptoms of thiamine deficiency vary according to the severity of the deficiency itself. Thiamine status can be estimated as blood concentration or urinary excretion of thiamine itself and its metabolites. Erythrocyte tranketolase activity might indicate genetic defects. Thiamine toxicity is very uncommon because of its rapid renal clearance.

In recent years, there has been an increasing interest in the role of thiamine in the prevention of diabetic complications. Several studies have demonstrated beneficial effects of thiamine and its lipophilic derivatives in counteracting excess glucose-induced damage in vascular cells.

References

Abbas ZG, Swai AB, Evaluation of the efficacy of thiamine and pyridoxine in the treatment of symptomatic diabetic peripheral neuropathy. East Afr Med J 1997;74: 803–8.

Arora S, Lidor A, Abularrage CJ, Weiswasser JM, Nylen E, Kellicut D, Sidawy AN, Thiamine (vitamin B1) improves endothelium-dependent vasodilatation in the presence of hyperglycemia. Ann Vasc Surg 2006;20: 653–8.

Babaei-Jadidi R, Karachalias N, Ahmed N, Battah S, Thornalley PJ, Prevention of incipient diabetic nephropathy by high-dose thiamine and benfotiamine. Diabetes 2003;52: 2110–20.

Babaei-Jadidi R, Karachalias N, Kupich C, Ahmed N, Thornalley PJ, High-dose thiamine therapy counters dyslipidaemia in streptozotocin-induced diabetic rats. Diabetologia 2004;47: 2235–46.

Baker H, Frank O, Absorption, utilization and clinical effectiveness of allithiamines compared to water-soluble thiamines. J Nutr Sci Vitaminol (Tokyo) 1976;22(Suppl): 63–8.

Bakker SJ, ter Maaten JC, Gans RO, Thiamine supplementation to prevent induction of low birth weight by conventional therapy for gestational diabetes mellitus. Med Hypotheses 2000;55: 88–90.

Bailey AL, Finglas PM, Wright AJ, Southon S, Thiamin intake, erythrocyte transketolase (EC 2.2.1.1) activity and total erythrocyte thiamin in adolescents. Br J Nutr 1994;72: 111–25.

Baines M, Davies G, The evaluation of erythrocyte thiamin diphosphate as an indicator of thiamin status in man, and its comparison with erythrocyte transketolase activity measurements. Ann Clin Biochem 1988;25(Part 6): 698–705.

Beltramo E, Berrone E, Buttiglieri S, Porta M, Thiamine and benfotiamine prevent increased apoptosis in endothelial cells and pericytes cultured in high glucose. Diabetes Metab Res Rev 2004;20: 330–6.

Beltramo E, Berrone E, Tarallo S, Porta M, Effects of thiamine and benfotiamine on intracellular glucose metabolism and relevance in the prevention of diabetic complications. Acta Diabetol 2008;45: 131–41.

Bender DA, Optimum nutrition: thiamin, biotin and pantothenate. Proc Nutr Soc 1999;58: 427–33.

Berrone E, Beltramo E, Solimine C, Ape AU, Porta M, Regulation of intracellular glucose and polyol pathway by thiamine and benfotiamine in vascular cells cultured in high glucose. J Biol Chem 2006;281: 9307–13.

Brignardello E, Beltramo E, Molinatti PA, Aragno M, Gatto V, Tamagno E, Danni O, Porta M, Boccuzzi G, Dehydroepiandrosterone protects bovine retinal capillary pericytes against glucose toxicity. J Endocrinol 1998;158: 21–6.

Brownlee M, Glycation and diabetic complications. Diabetes 1994;43: 836–41.

Butterworth RF, Pathophysiologic mechanisms responsible for the reversible (thiamine-responsive) and irreversible (thiamine non-responsive) neurological symptoms of Wernicke's encephalopathy. Drug Alcohol Rev 1993;12: 315–22.

Butterworth RF, Gaudreau C, Vincelette J, Bourgault AM, Lamothe F, Nutini AM, Thiamine deficiency and Wernicke's encephalopathy in AIDS. Metab Brain Dis 1991;6: 207–12.

Ceylan-Isik AF, Wu S, Li Q, Li SY, Ren J, High-dose benfotiamine rescues cardiomyocyte contractile dysfunction in streptozotocin-induced diabetes mellitus. J Appl Physiol 2006;100: 150–6.

Combs GF Jr, The vitamins: fundamental aspects in nutrition and health. 3rd ed. Ithaca: Elsevier Academic Press; 2008.

Cook C, Hallwood PM, Thomson AD, B vitamin deficiency and neuropsychiatric syndromes in alcohol misuse. Alcohol Alcohol 1998;33: 317–36.

DCCT: The Diabetes Control and Complications Trial Research Group, The effect of intensive treatment of diabetes on the development and progression of long-term complications in insulin-dependent diabetes mellitus. N Engl J Med 1993;329: 977–86.

FAO/WHO expert consultation on human vitamin and mineral requirements, Thiamine, riboflavin, niacin, vitamin B6, pantothenic acid, and biotin. In: Vitamin and mineral requirements in human nutrition. 2nd ed. 2004. pp. 164–8.

Flodin NW, Thiamine (vitamin B1). In: Alan R, editor. Current topics in nutrition and disease. New York: Liss Inc; 1988. pp. 103–16.

Frank RAW, Leeper FJ, Luisi BF, Structure, mechanism and catalytic duality of thiamine-dependent enzymes. Cell Mol Life Sci 2007;64: 892–905.

Fujimara M, Allithiamine and its properties. J Nutr Sci Vitaminol (Tokyo) 1976;22(Suppl): 57–62.

Gadau S, Emanueli C, Van Linthout S, Graiani G, Todaro M, Meloni M, Campesi I, Invernici G, Spillmann F, Ward K, Madeddu P, Benfotiamine accelerates the healing of ischaemic diabetic limbs in mice through protein kinase B/Akt-mediated potentiation of angiogenesis and inhibition of apoptosis. Diabetologia 2006;49: 405–20.

Gerrits J, Eidhof H, Brunnekreeft JW, Hessels J, Determination of thiamin and thiamin phosphates in whole blood by reversed-phase liquid chromatography with precolumn derivatization. In: McCormick DB, Suttie JW, Wagner C, editors. Methods in enzymology, vol. 279. Vitamins and co-enzymes. San Diego: Academic Press; 1997. pp. 74–82.

Greb A, Bitsch R, Comparative bioavailability of various thiamine derivatives after oral administration. Int J Clin Pharmacol Ther 1998;36: 216–21.

Hammes HP, Du X, Edelstein D Taguchi T, Matsumura T, Ju Q, Lin J, Bierhaus A, Nawroth P, Hannak D, Neumaier M, Bergfeld R, Giardino I, Brownlee M, Benfotiamine blocks three major pathways of hyperglycemic damage and prevents experimental diabetic retinopathy. Nat Med 2003;9: 294–9.

Harper C, Wernicke's encephalopathy, a more common disease than realised (a neuropathological study of 51 cases). J Neurol Neurosurg Psych 1979;42: 226–31.

Haupt E, Ledermann H, Kopcke W, Benfotiamine in the treatment of diabetic polyneuropathy – a three-week randomized, controlled pilot study (BEDIP study). Int J Clin Pharmacol Ther 2005;43: 71–7.

Heye N, Terstegge K, Sirtl C, McMonagle U, Schreiber K, Meyer-Gessner M, Wernicke's encephalopathy – causes to consider. Intensive Care Med 1994;20: 282–6.

Horwitt MK, Kreisler O, The determination of early thiamine deficient states by estimation of blood lactate and pyruvate after glucose administration and exercise. J Nutr 1949;37: 411–27.

Hoyumpa AM Jr, Strickland R, Sheehan JJ, Yarborough G, Nichols S, Dual system of intestinal thiamine transport in humans. J Lab Clin Med 1982;99: 701–8.

IOM (Institute of Medicine, USA), Thiamin. In: Dietary references intakes for thiamine, riboflavin, niacin, vitamin B6, folate, vitamin B12, pantothenic acid, biotin and choline, ch. 4. Food and Nutrition Board, Institute of Medicine. Washington DC: National Academy Press, 1998. pp. 58–86.

Jansen BCT, Donath WF, On the isolation of the anti-beriberi vitamin. Proc K Acad Wet Amsterdam 1926;29: 1390.

Jermendy G, Evaluating thiamine deficiency in patients with diabetes. Diab Vasc Dis Res 2006;3: 120–1.

Kaiser N, Sasson S, Feener EP, Boukobza-Vardi N, Higashi S, Moller DE, Davidheiser S, Przybylski RJ, King GL, Differential regulation of glucose transport and transporters by glucose in vascular endothelial and smooth muscle cells. Diabetes 1993;42: 80–9.

Karuppagounder SS, Xu H, Pechman D, Chen LH, DeGiorgio LA, Gibson GE, Translocation of amyloid precursor protein C-terminal fragment(s) to the nucleus precedes neuronal death due to thiamine deficiency-induced mild impairment of oxidative metabolism. Neurochem Res 2008;33: 1365–72.

Kawano H, Hayashi T, Koide Y, Toda G, Yano K, Histopathological changes of biopsied myocardium in Shoshin beriberi. Int Heart J 2005;46: 751–9.

Kitamura K, Yamaguchi T, Tanaka H, Hashimoto S, Yang M, Takahashi T, TPN-induced fulminant beriberi: a report on our experience and a review of the literature. Surg Today 1996;26: 769–76.

Kuo SH, Debnam JM, Fuller GN, de Groot J, Wernicke's encephalopathy: an underrecognized and reversible cause of confusional state in cancer patients. Oncology 2009;76: 10–8.

La Selva M, Beltramo E, Pagnozzi F, Bena E, Molinatti PA, Molinatti GM, Porta M, Thiamine corrects delayed replication and decreases production of lactate and advanced glycation end-products in bovine retinal and umbilical vein endothelial cells cultured under high glucose conditions. Diabetologia 1996;39: 1263–8.

Laforenza U, Patrini C, Alvisi C, Faelli A, Licandro A, Rindi G, Thiamine uptake in human intestinal biopsy specimen, including observations from a patient with acute thiamine deficiency. Am J Clin Nutr 1997;66: 320–6.

Leevy CM, Thiamin deficiency and alcoholism. Ann NY Acad Sci 1982;378: 316–26.

Lindboe CF, Loberg EM, Wernicke's encephalopathy in non-alcoholics. An autopsy study. J Neurol Sci 1989;90: 125–9.

Loew D, Pharmacokinetics of thiamine derivatives especially of benfotiamine. Int J Clin Pharmacol Ther 1996;34: 47–50.

Lonsdale D, Schamberger RJ, Red cell transketolase as indicator of nutritional deficiency. Am J Clin Nutr 1980;33: 205–11.

Lonsdale D, The nutritionist's guide to the clinical use of vitamin B-1. Tacoma: Life Sciences Press; 1987.

Lonsdale D, A review of the biochemistry, metabolism and clinical benefits of thiamin(e) and its derivatives. Evid Based Complement Alternat Med 2006;3: 49–59.

Lu J, Frank EL, Rapid HPLC measurement of thiamine and its phosphate esters in whole blood. Clin Chem 2008;54: 901–6.

Meador KJ, Loring D, Nichols M, Zamrini E, Rivner M, Posas H, Thompson E, Moore E, Preliminary findings of high-dose thiamine in dementia of Alzheimer's type. J Geriatr Psychiatry Neurol 1993;6: 222–9.

Meador KJ, Nichols ME, Franke P, Durkin MW, Oberzan RL, Moore EE, Loring DW, Evidence for a central cholinergic effect of high-dose thiamine. Ann Neurol 1993;34: 724–6.

Neufeld EJ, Fleming JC, Tartaglini E, Steinkamp MP, Thiamine-Responsive Megaloblastic Anemia syndrome: a disorder of high-affinity thiamine transport. Blood Cells Mol Dis 2001;27: 135–8.

Nishikawa T, Edelstein D, Du XL, Yamagishi S, Matsumura T, Kaneda Y, Yorek MA, Beebe D, Oates PJ, Hammes HP, Giardino I, Brownlee M, Normalizing mitochondrial superoxide production blocks three pathways of hyperglycaemic damage. Nature 2000;404: 787–90.

Nixon PF, Price J, Norman-Hick M, Williams GM, Kerr RA, The relationship between erythrocyte transketolase activity and the 'TPP effect' in Wernicke's encephalopathy and other thiamine deficiency states. Clin Chim Acta 1990;192: 89–98.

Pelton R, LaValle JB, Hawkins E, Krinsky DL, editors. Drug-induced nutrient depletion handbook. Hudson: Lexi-Comp; 1999. p. 258.

Peters RA, The biochemical lesion in vitamin B1 deficiency. Lancet 1936;i: 1162–5.

Podestà F, Romeo G, Liu WH, Krajewski S, Reed JC, Gerhardinger C, Lorenzi M, Bax is increased in the retina of diabetic subjects and is associated with pericyte apoptosis in vivo and in vitro. Am J Pathol 2000;156: 1025–32.

Rabbani N, Alam SS, Riaz S, Larkin JR, Akhtar MW, Shafi T, Thornalley PJ, High-dose thiamine therapy for patients with type 2 diabetes and microalbuminuria: a randomised, double-blind placebo-controlled pilot study. Diabetologia 2009;52: 208–12.

Reuler JB, Girard DE, Cooney TG, Wernicke's encephalopathy. N Engl J Med 1985;312: 1035–9.

Rindi G, Imarisio L, Patrini C, Effects of acute and chronic ethanol administration on regional thiamin pyrophosphokinase activity of the rat brain. Biochem Pharmacol 1986;35: 3903–8.

Rindi G, Ferrari G, Thiamine transport by human intestine in vitro. Experientia 1997;33: 211–3.

Rindi G, Laforenza U, Thiamine intestinal transport and related issues: recent aspects. Proc Soc Exp Biol Med 2000;224: 246–255.

Saito N, Kimura M, Kuchiba A, Itokawa Y, Blood thiamine levels in outpatients with diabetes mellitus. J Nutr Sci Vitaminol 1987;33: 421–30.

Schreeb KH, Freudenthaler S, Vormfelde SV, Gundert-Remy U, Gleiter CH, Comparative bioavailability of two vitamin B1 preparations: benfotiamine and thiamine mononitrate. Eur J Pharmacol 1997;52: 319–20.

Seehra H, MacDermott N, Lascelles RG, Taylor TV, Wernicke's encephalopathy after vertical banded gastroplasty for morbid obesity. Br Med J 1996;312: 434.

Singleton CK, Pekovich SR, McCool BA, Martin PR, The thiamine dependent hysteretic behavior of Human transketolase: implications for thiamine deficiency. J Nutr 1995;125: 189–94.

Stepuro II, Piletskaya TP, Stepuro VI, Maskevich SA, Thiamine oxidative transformations catalyzed by copper ions and ascorbic acid. Biochemistry 1997;62: 1409–14.

Stirban A, Negrean M, Stratmann B Gawlowski T, Horstmann T, Götting C, Kleesiek K, Mueller-Roesel M, Koschinsky T, Uribarri J, Vlassara H, Tschoepe D, Benfotiamine prevents macro- and microvascular endothelial dysfunction and oxidative stress following a meal rich in advanced glycation end products in individuals with type 2 diabetes. Diabetes Care 2006;29: 2064–71.

Stracke H, Lindemann A, Federlin K, A benfotiamine-vitamin B combination in treatment of diabetic polyneuropathy. Exp Clin Endocrinol Diabetes 1996;104: 311–6.

Stracke H, Hammes HP, Werkmann D, Mavrakis K, Bitsch I, Netzel M, Geyer J, Köpcke W, Sauerland C, Bretzel RG, Federlin KF, Efficacy of benfotiamine versus thiamine on function and glycation products of peripheral nerves in diabetic rats. Exp Clin Endocrinol Diabetes 2001;109: 330–6.

Stracke H, Gaus W, Achenbach U, Federlin K, Bretzel RG, Benfotiamine in diabetic polyneuropathy (BENDIP): results of a randomised, double blind, placebo-controlled clinical study. Exp Clin Endocrinol Diabetes 2008;116: 600–5.

Stryer L, Biochemistry. New York: Freeman WH and Co; 1988.

Thomson AD, Mechanisms of vitamin deficiency in chronic alcohol misusers and the development of the Wernicke-Korsakoff syndrome. Alcohol Alcohol 2000;35(Suppl): 2–7.

Thornalley PJ, The potential role of thiamine (vitamin B1) in diabetic complications. Curr Diabetes Rev 2005;1: 287–98.

Thornalley PJ, Babaei-Jadidi R, Al Ali H, Rabbani N, Antonysunil A, Larkin J, Ahmed A, Rayman G, Bodmer CW, High prevalence of low plasma thiamine concentration in diabetes linked to a marker of vascular disease. Diabetologia 2007;50: 2164–70.

Togay-Isikay C, Yigit A, Mutluer N, Wernicke's encephalopathy due to hyperemesis gravidarum: and under-recognised condition. Aust N Z J Obstet Gynaecol 2001;41: 453–6.

UK Prospective Diabetes Study Group, Intensive blood-glucose control with sulphonylureas or insulin compared with conventional treatment and risk of complications in patients with type 2 diabetes (UKPDS 33). Lancet 1998;352: 837–53.

Valerio G, Franzese A, Poggi V, Patrini C, Laforenza U, Tenore A, Lipophilic thiamine treatment in long-standing insulin-dependent diabetes mellitus. Acta Diabetol 1999;36: 73–6.

Velez RJ, Myers B, Guber MS, Severe acute metabolic acidosis (acute beriberi): an avoidable complication of total parenteral nutrition. J Parenter Enteral Nutr 1985;9: 216–9.

Williams RD, Mason HL, Power MH, Induced thiamine deficiency in man; relation of depletion of thiamine to development of biochemical defect and of polyneuropathy. Arch Int Med 1943;71: 2176–7.

Williams RR, Chemistry of thiamine (vitamin B1). J Am Med Assoc 1938; 110: 727–31.

Wu S, Ren J. Benfotiamine alleviates diabetes-induced cerebral oxidative damage independent of advanced glycation end-product, tissue factor and TNF-alpha. Neurosci Lett 2006; 394: 158–62.

Yenilmez A, Ozçifçi M, Aydin Y, Turgut M, Uzuner K, Erkul A, Protective effect of high-dose thiamine (B1) on rat detrusor contractility in streptozotocin-induced diabetes mellitus. Acta Diabetol 2006;43: 103–8.

3.2 Clinical and biological aspects of thiamine deficiency

Jens A. Petersen; Michael Linnebank

3.2.1 Physiology

Heat-labile thiamine (thiamine monophosphate, thiamine diphosphate, thiamine triphosphate, adenosine thiamine triphosphate, adenosine thiamine diphosphate) is a water-soluble B-complex vitamin also known as vitamin B1 or aneurine. In the 1920s, thiamine was one of the first organic compounds to be recognized as a vitamin. It acts as a cofactor for numerous enzymes such as the α-ketoglutarate-dehydrogenase complex and the pyruvate-dehydrogenase complex in the tricarboxylic acid cycle, and transketolase in the pentose-phosphate pathway. In neuronal and glial cells, the enzyme thiamine pyrophosphokinase converts thiamine into thiamine pyrophosphate (Voskoboyev and Ostrovsky, 1982) which is necessary in several biochemical pathways such as carbohydrate metabolism (for energy production), lipid metabolism (for myelin production) and synthesis of amino acids and neurotransmitters such as GABA and glutamic acid. Thiamine has been shown to mimic acetylcholine in the brain which might explain its possible action in Alzheimer's disease and other dementias (Meador et al., 1993). Thiamine deficiency results in decreased ATP production and increased cellular acidosis (Pannunzio et al., 2000).

3.2.2 Thiamine deficiency

Thiamine deficiency can cause severe neurological deficits and end lethally. The stores of thiamine in the body last for up to 3 weeks. Then, in the case of thiamine depletion, enzymes requiring thiamine pyrophosphate as a coenzyme become impaired (Schenker et al., 1980). Alcoholism, particularly along with malnutrition, is the most common reason for thiamine deficiency in western countries (Baines, 1978; Thomson et al., 1987;

Cook et al., 1998). Ethanol inhibits the resorption of thiamine, but thiamine deficiency has even been observed in adolescents eating an average American diet (Lonsdale and Shamberger, 1980), in psychiatric (Schwartz et al., 1979) and in geriatric patients (Chen et al., 1996). In non-developed countries, thiamine deficiency is most prevalent where polished rice is a major source of food but it can also be owing to consumption of food containing antithiamin factors such as betel nuts and raw fermented fish (Vimokesant et al., 1975). Furthermore, thiamine deficiency occurs in a variety of situations, including parenteral nutrition (Kitamura et al., 1996), gastrointestinal/bariatric surgery (Seehra et al., 1996; Sechi, 2008), pregnancy, long-term use of diuretics (Wilcox, 1999), breast feeding (Soukaloun et al., 2003), diarrhea, (Boonsiri et al., 2007), severe infections (Lindboe and Loberg, 1989), a diet high in carbohydrates, eating disorders (Winston et al., 2000), cancer (Bleggi-Torres et al., 1997), an elevated need as in alcoholism and diabetes mellitus (Beltramo et al., 2008), hyperemesis gravidarum (Togay-Isikay et al., 2001) and renal dialysis (Reuler et al., 1985; Hung et al., 2001). In HIV/AIDS patients, an encephalopathy owing to thiamine deficiency has been described even though they did not abuse alcohol (Lindboe and Loberg, 1989). Moderate to severe thiamine deficiency has been described in approximately one-fourth of HIV- or AIDS-diagnosed individuals (Butterworth et al., 1991). Formaldehyde exposure, aminoglycosides, fluoroquinolones, trimethoprin, tetracycline derivates, phenytoin, penicilline, cephalosporins and sulfonamide derivates could also lead to a reduced availability of thiamine (Zenuk et al., 2003).

A broad spectrum of symptoms has been associated with thiamine deficiency, including memory loss, vomiting, hypotension, constipation, weakness, depression, insomnia, dizziness, back pain, dyspnea and sonophobia, myalgia, palpitations, nausea, anorexia, bradycardia, digestive disturbances, muscular atrophy, weight loss, peripheral neuropathy, and pain sensitivity. In Wernicke's encephalopathy, ophthalmoplegia, ataxia, nystagmus and delirium are frequently observed (Liang, 1977; Cook et al., 1998).

3.2.2.1 Beriberi

Beriberi mainly occurs in non-developed countries in East Asia where polished rice is the major source of food. Because thiamine is contained in the outer coat of rice, polishing destroys it. In Indonesia, the prevalence of thiamine deficiency among low-income families is thought to be as high as 66% (Djoenaidi et al., 1996).

Biventricular heart failure is known as 'wet (cardiac) beriberi': thiamine deficiency causes impaired oxidative metabolism and thereby induces an increase of pyruvate and lactate levels, leading to acidosis, peripheral vasodilation, and retention of water and sodium by activation of the renin-angiotensin system (Soukoulis et al., 2009). The consequence is edema and high-output heart failure. Sudden thiamine supplementation can reverse these symptoms. Cardiac beriberi could be missed in clinical practice owing to the absence of pedal edema/anasarca and therefore, in developing countries, thiamine therapy is recommended for infants from a precarious socioeconomic background with unexplained congestive heart failure or acute respiratory failure because it might be life-saving (Rao and Chandak, 2009).

In the western world, the incidence of beriberi is not known, but 'wet' beriberi is rarely encountered and the concern focuses on patients with moderate thiamine deficiency. The so-called 'dry' form of beriberi occurs mostly in first-world countries in subjects with disposition and includes mild symptoms, in particular, a symmetric sensimotor polyneuropathy (in severe cases including the brain nerves) and dilative cardiomyopathy.

In patients with heart failure, thiamine deficiency is common (Pfitzenmeyer et al., 1994; Zenuk et al., 2003; Hanninen et al., 2006) and seems to correlate with its functional severity. Animal models have shown that thiamine deficiency can lead to cardiac dysfunction, hypertrophy, and arrhythmias without the presence of beriberi (Yoshitoshi et al., 1961; Boullin, 1963; Davies and Jennings, 1970). In patients with heart failure, average nutritional amounts of thiamine might be too low (Hanninen et al., 2006).

3.2.2.2 Wernicke's encephalopathy

In developed countries, Wernicke-Korsakoff syndrome mostly occurs in advanced alcoholics. Wernicke's encephalopathy, the acute course of vitamin B1-deficiency, can also develop in non-alcoholic conditions (Shah and Wolff, 1973; Ebels, 1978; Butterworth et al., 1991). It is a rare but known complication of severe hyperemesis gravidarum, diets with polished rice, gastrointestinal surgical procedures, chronic diarrhea, cancer and chemotherapeutic treatments, systemic diseases, magnesium depletion, the use of chemical compounds and drugs and unbalanced nutrition (Sechi and Serra, 2007). Its prevalence and incidence vary throughout the world. In adults, the prevalence was found to be higher than predicted by clinical studies, ranging from 0.8% to 2.8% (Victor et al., 1971; Harper et al., 1986; Vasconcelos et al., 1999). Particularly in adult patients with AIDS and in those who misused alcohol, Wernicke's encephalopathy had been missed by routine clinical examination in 75–80% of cases.

In alcoholism, thiamine deficiency stems from a variety of causes. In addition to low intake, absorption is inhibited, hepatic activation of thiamine coenzymes is decreased, and thiamine is consumed by the metabolism of ethanol (Leevy, 1982). Thiamine deficiency is discussed to be involved in the etiology of psychotic symptoms associated with chronic alcohol abuse. Its pathological features are symmetrical areas of profound neuronal loss and accompanying gliosis, occurring most frequently in diencephalic regions such as the thalamus, on the ground of the fourth ventricle, in the cerebellum and in the hypothalamus close to the aqueduct. Lesions can include the vestibular nuclei and the inferior olivary complex and in some cases, the mamillary bodies are affected (▶Fig. 3.3).

Although Wernicke's encephalopathy is thought to be a primary consequence of thiamine deficiency (Lishman, 1981), the precise mechanisms that lead to the selective histological lesions characteristic of this disorder remains unknown. As early as 1 week after thiamine stores are depleted, the blood-brain barrier is disrupted, leading to local hypoperfusion in the brain followed by the classic symptoms of Wernicke's encephalopathy. These are nystagmus, acute oculomotor palsy, papillary motor affection, ataxia, vegetative dysregulation (hypotension, hypothermia, heart rhythm disturbance), grand-mal seizures and mental symptoms with impairment of conscience, loss of orientation and impulse control as well as psychotic symptoms and aphasia.

In the course of Wernicke's encephalopathy, Korsakoff's psychosis and Korsakoff's syndrome can occur owing to irreversible damage of the thalamus and the hypothalamus. Korsakoff's syndrome contains a chronic disturbance of anterograde memory, whereas retrograde memory is mostly intact.

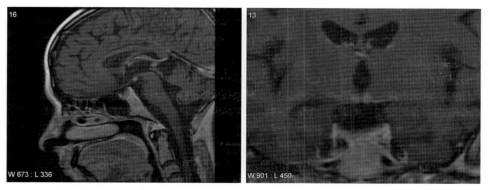

Fig. 3.3: MRI in Wernicke's Encephalopathy. An enhancement of the mamillary bodies appear after application of contrast agent.

3.2.2.3 Strachan's syndrome

Thiamine deficiency, possibly only in combination with a lack of further vitamins and proteins and the effects of toxic ingredients of the manioc fruit, also seems to be involved in the etiology of Strachan's syndrome presenting with bilateral optic neuropathy with cecocentral scotomata or a distal predominantly sensory neuropathy sometimes associated with deafness, or a combination of both optic and peripheral sensory neuropathy (Thomas et al., 1995).

3.2.2.4 Thiamine-responsive megaloblastic anemia

Thiamine-responsive megaloblastic anemia syndrome is an autosomal recessive disorder so far diagnosed in less than 30 families throughout the world. It features diabetes mellitus, megaloblastic anemia and sensorineural hearing loss. Other manifestations include optic atrophy, cardiomyopathy and stroke-like episodes. The causes are mutations in the SLC19A2 gene, encoding a high-affinity thiamine transporter protein, THTR-1. To date, more than 20 distinct mutations have been reported (Bergmann et al., 2009). Animal models showed defects in insulin secretion and selective loss of inner hair cells in the cochlea (Oishi et al., 2002; Liberman et al., 2006) but the exact pathophysiological mechanisms are not known. Also, the role of thiamine in normal hematopoiesis is unclear, and so are the biochemical mechanisms of megaloblastic anemia.

Progressive hearing loss can be detected in toddlers whereas diabetes mellitus is non-type 1 in nature, with age of onset from infancy to adolescence.

3.2.3 Differential diagnosis

Differential diagnoses of acute thiamine deficiency include acute intoxication with alcohol or other substances, hepatic encephalopathy, chronic subdural hematoma (in alcoholism, impaired blood coagulation and downfalls are frequent), and central pontine myelinolysis. Owing to its variety of symptoms, several differential diagnoses could lead to symptoms very similar to thiamine deficiency. Dry beriberi might even mimic Guillain-Barré syndrome (Murphy et al., 2009). In patients with predisposition, thiamine deficiency should be taken into account if symptoms of central or peripheral nervous disturbances or of impairment of neuromuscular transmission occur.

3.2.4 Thiamine deficiency during pregnancy

In pregnancy, thiamine deficiency is common. Owing to accumulation of thiamine in fetal tissue, thiamine requirements are much higher than normal (Butterworth, 1993). In one study, 25–30% of pregnant women were found to be thiamine-depleted (Heller et al., 1974). Causes of thiamine deficiency during pregnancy include the following: inadequate dietary intake, increased dietary requirements, hyperemesis gravidarum, malabsorption of the vitamin owing to gestational disorders, alcohol abuse, infections including HIV, effects of various drugs and genetic factors. Psychomotor abnormalities and intrauterine growth retardation are attributed to maternal thiamine deficiency. Brain tissue is particularly vulnerable to thiamine deprivation during ontogenesis (Ba et al., 2005) and thiamine deficiency during pregnancy is a risk factor for stillbirths (Ba, 2009). Infantile beriberi might occur in infants breast-fed by mothers who themselves are thiamine-deficient but asymptomatic.

In mothers with gestational diabetes mellitus, thiamine hypovitaminemia was found in almost 20% of cases despite vitamin supplementation and treatment for gestational diabetes; neonates born to mothers with hypovitaminemia were also thiamine hypovitaminemic (Baker et al., 2000). Thiamine supplementation in gestational diabetic mothers is thought not only to improve the glucose tolerance but also to stimulate the intrauterine growth, thereby preventing a low birthweight (Bakker et al., 2000).

Wernicke's encephalopathy can be a rare complication caused by thiamine deficiency owing to severe hyperemesis gravidarum. The overall pregnancy loss rate owing to Wernicke's encephalopathy was found to be as high as 48% (Chiossi et al., 2006).

3.2.5 Treatment

3.2.5.1 Beriberi

The presumptive diagnosis of thiamine deficiency can be confirmed either by directly measuring the concentration of the vitamin in the serum or indirectly by estimating the red blood cell transketolase activity (Dreyfus, 1962). Recently, reproducibility, practicability and performance have been improved by high-performance liquid chromatography which is suitable for clinical as well as for research purposes. As a therapy, 100 mg vitamin B1 per day can be substituted intravenously for 1 day, followed by 100 mg intramuscularly each day for 5 days, and then permanent oral maintenance of 50–100 mg daily (Matrana and Davis, 2009). Symptoms of dry beriberi can persist for weeks to months following the replacement of thiamine, but wet beriberi typically responds quickly to treatment.

3.2.5.2 Wernicke's encephalopathy

Acute Wernicke's syndrome is a neurological emergency. Its appearance is heterogeneous: in the case of anamnestical, clinical or laboratory-supported suspicion of chronic abuse of alcohol or other possible causes of thiamine deficiency in combination with the symptoms described (psychosyndrome, ataxia, double-vision), the therapy has to be initiated urgently. Depending on the clinical course (vegetative involvement), treatment in the intensive care unit might be necessary.

Patients suspected of having Wernicke-Korsakoff syndrome should promptly receive parenteral thiamine hydrochloride. Rare adverse effects include pruritus, local irritation or, rarely, anaphylaxis. If treated inadequately with thiamine (given by the wrong route, in too small a dose or too late), Wernicke's encephalopathy can lead to irreversible structural changes producing loss of short-term memory and an impaired ability to acquire new information. The estimated mortality rate is approximately 20%, whereas 85% of survivors develop chronic and irreversible Korsakoff's syndrome (Thomson et al., 2002). Thiamine for parenteral use should be diluted in 100 ml of normal saline and 5% glucose and be infused over 30 min (Cook et al., 1998). The solution should be fresh because thiamine hydrochloride can be inactivated by heat (Sechi and Serra, 2007). Several different regimens for patients with the disorder and those at risk for developing it have been proposed, but there is insufficient evidence from randomized controlled clinical trials to guide clinicians in the dose, frequency, route or duration of thiamine treatment for prophylaxis against or treatment of Wernicke-Korsakoff syndrome owing to alcohol abuse (Day et al., 2004). In some studies, a common thiamine replacement regimen is 100 mg every 8 h (Foster et al., 2005) but this might not be sufficient to ameliorate clinical signs (Tallaksen et al., 1993) or prevent death (Cook, 2000). In the setting of Wernicke's encephalopathy owing to alcoholism, it was proposed to initiate treatment with a minimum of 500 mg thiamine hydrochloride (dissolved in 100 ml of normal saline) three times per day for 2–3 days (Sechi and Serra, 2007). Treatment should be continued with 250 mg thiamine given intravenously or intramuscularly daily for 3–5 days, or until clinical improvement ceases. Usually, the recovery from Wernicke's encephalopathy starts as soon as a few hours after the therapy has been initiated. The mental status improves 2–3 weeks after therapy. Oral thiamine supplementation should be continued at a dose of 30 mg twice daily for several months (Sechi and Serra, 2007).

In alcohol-dependent patients without clinically apparent Wernicke's encephalopathy, the parenteral administration of at least 200 mg thiamine might ameliorate neurologic symptoms (Ambrose et al., 2001). People with alcohol withdrawal, poorly nourished patients and those with poor diet and signs of malnutrition, should receive 250 mg of intramuscular thiamine for 3–5 consecutive days (Cook et al., 1998; Cook, 2000; Thomson et al., 2002). In patients with Wernicke's encephalopathy or otherwise suspected thiamine deficiency, other B-vitamins could be additionally substituted owing to possible co-incidences of deficiency (Cook et al., 1998). To avoid the risk of Wernicke's encephalopathy, hypoglycemic patients who are treated with glucose i.v. must be given i.v. thiamine at the same time (Thomson et al., 2002).

3.2.5.3 Thiamine-responsive megaloblastic anemia

Treatment with pharmacological doses of thiamine (25–75 mg/day) can often correct the megaloblastic anemia and diabetes mellitus (Diaz et al., 1999). Theses symptoms can reappear when thiamine is withdrawn. It is unclear whether hearing can be improved, or hearing loss delayed by high-dose thiamine.

3.2.5.4 Pregnancy

Thiamine requirements of pregnant women are much higher than normal (Butterworth, 2001). The US National Academy of Sciences' recommended dietary allowance for thiamine in pregnancy is 1.5 mg (non-pregnant adult women: 1.1 mg). Supplementation with multivitamin products does not sufficiently reduce thiamine hypovitaminemia (Baker et al., 1975). Wernicke's encephalopathy is a rare but known complication in hyperemesis gravidarum resulting from poor nutritional intake, frequent vomiting, and increased metabolic demands of pregnancy. Body stores of B1 can be depleted in only 3 weeks. Therefore, pregnant women who present with vomiting and feeding difficulties for more than 3 weeks should receive oral or intramuscular thiamine supplement (100 mg per day), and intravenous thiamine supplements should be administered when a patient with hyperemesis gravidarum of longstanding duration receives parenteral carbohydrate-containing nutrition (Chiossi et al., 2006).

3.2.6 Course and prognosis

The symptoms of chronic vitamin B1-deficiency (beriberi) can be stabilized by substitution and are often reversible.

Wernicke's syndrome can be lethal but can be fully reversible if an adequate therapy is administered in the early course. As a residual state, chronic Korsakoff's syndrome can occur (see above).

3.2.7 Vitamin B1-hypervitaminosis

The therapeutic spectrum of vitamin B1 is broad. Presently, cases of thiamine toxicity from oral dosage are not known. Is has been discussed if the intake of high doses of vitamin B1 ameliorates mental capability. One controlled trial with 127 young adults given 15 mg of thiamine along with other B vitamins found the most significant association between enhanced cognitive function and improved thiamine status in females (Benton et al., 1995). In another trial, 80 elderly females were given 10 mg thiamine daily for 10 weeks (Smidt et al., 1991). The women experienced increases in appetite, body weight, energy intake, general well-being, reduced daytime sleep, improved sleep patterns, decreased fatigue and increased activity levels.

References

Ambrose ML, Bowden SC, Whelan G, Thiamin treatment and working memory function of alcohol-dependent people: preliminary findings. Alcohol Clin Exp Res 2001;25: 112–6.

Ba A, Alcohol and B1 vitamin deficiency-related stillbirths. J Matern Fetal Neonatal Med 2009;22: 452–7.

Ba A, N'Douba V, D'Almeida MA, Seri BV, Effects of maternal thiamine deficiencies on the pyramidal and granule cells of the hippocampus of rat pups. Acta Neurobiol Exp (Wars) 2005;65: 387–98.

Baines M, Detection and incidence of B and C vitamin deficiency in alcohol-related illness. Ann Clin Biochem 1978;15: 307–12.

Baker H, Frank O, Thomson AD, Langer A, Munves ED, De Angelis B, et al., Vitamin profile of 174 mothers and newborns at parturition. Am J Clin Nutr 1975;28: 59–65.

Baker H, Hockstein S, DeAngelis B, Holland BK, Thiamin status of gravidas treated for gestational diabetes mellitus compared to their neonates at parturition. Int J Vitam Nutr Res 2000;70: 317–20.

Bakker SJ, ter Maaten JC, Gans RO, Thiamine supplementation to prevent induction of low birth weight by conventional therapy for gestational diabetes mellitus. Med Hypotheses 2000;55: 88–90.

Beltramo E, Berrone E, Tarallo S, Porta M, Effects of thiamine and benfotiamine on intracellular glucose metabolism and relevance in the prevention of diabetic complications. Acta Diabetol 2008;45: 131–41.

Benton D, Fordy J, Haller J, The impact of long-term vitamin supplementation on cognitive functioning. Psychopharmacology (Berl) 1995;117: 298–305.

Bergmann AK, Sahai I, Falcone JF, Fleming J, Bagg A, Borgna-Pignati C, et al., Thiamine-responsive megaloblastic anemia: identification of novel compound heterozygotes and mutation update. J Pediatr 2009;155: 888–92.

Bleggi-Torres LF, de Medeiros BC, Ogasawara VS, Loddo G, Zanis Neto J, Pasquini R, et al., Iatrogenic Wernicke's encephalopathy in allogeneic bone marrow transplantation: a study of eight cases. Bone Marrow Transplant 1997;20: 391–5.

Boonsiri P, Tangrassameeprasert R, Panthongviriyakul C, Yongvanit P, A preliminary study of thiamine status in northeastern Thai children with acute diarrhea. Southeast Asian J Trop Med Public Health 2007;38: 1120–5.

Boullin DJ, Pharmacological responses of thiamine-deficient rat tissues. Br J Pharmacol Chemother 1963;20: 190–203.

Butterworth RF, Maternal thiamine deficiency. A factor in intrauterine growth retardation. Ann N Y Acad Sci 1993;678: 325–9.

Butterworth RF, Maternal thiamine deficiency: still a problem in some world communities. Am J Clin Nutr 2001;74: 712–3.

Butterworth RF, Gaudreau C, Vincelette J, Bourgault AM, Lamothe F, Nutini AM, Thiamine deficiency and Wernicke's encephalopathy in AIDS. Metab Brain Dis 1991;6: 207–12.

Chen MF, Chen LT, Gold M, Boyce HW Jr, Plasma and erythrocyte thiamin concentrations in geriatric outpatients. J Am Coll Nutr 1996;15: 231–6.

Chiossi G, Neri I, Cavazzuti M, Basso G, Facchinetti F, Hyperemesis gravidarum complicated by Wernicke encephalopathy: background, case report, and review of the literature. Obstet Gynecol Surv 2006;61: 255–68.

Cook CC, Prevention and treatment of Wernicke-Korsakoff syndrome. Alcohol Alcohol 2000;35(Suppl): 19–20.

Cook CC, Hallwood PM, Thomson AD, B Vitamin deficiency and neuropsychiatric syndromes in alcohol misuse. Alcohol Alcohol 1998;33: 317–36.

Davies MJ, Jennings RB, The ultrastructure of the myocardium in the thiamine-deficient rat. J Pathol 1970;102: 87–95.

Day E, Bentham P, Callaghan R, Kuruvilla T, George S, Thiamine for Wernicke-Korsakoff Syndrome in people at risk from alcohol abuse. Cochrane Database Syst Rev 2004;1: CD004033.

Diaz GA, Banikazemi M, Oishi K, Desnick RJ, Gelb BD, Mutations in a new gene encoding a thiamine transporter cause thiamine-responsive megaloblastic anaemia syndrome. Nat Genet 1999;22: 309–12.

Djoenaidi W, Notermans SL, Verbeek AL, Subclinical beriberi polyneuropathy in the low income group: an investigation with special tools on possible patients with suspected complaints. Eur J Clin Nutr 1996;50: 549–55.

Dreyfus PM, Clinical application of blood transketolase determinations. N Engl J Med 1962;267: 596–8.

Ebels EJ, How common is Wernicke-Korsakoff syndrome? Lancet 1978;ii: 781–2.

Foster D, Falah M, Kadom N, Mandler R, Wernicke encephalopathy after bariatric surgery: losing more than just weight. Neurology 2005;65: 1987; discussion 847.

Hanninen SA, Darling PB, Sole MJ, Barr A, Keith ME, The prevalence of thiamin deficiency in hospitalized patients with congestive heart failure. J Am Coll Cardiol 2006;47: 354–61.

Harper CG, Giles M, Finlay-Jones R, Clinical signs in the Wernicke-Korsakoff complex: a retrospective analysis of 131 cases diagnosed at necropsy. J Neurol Neurosurg Psychiatry 1986;49: 341–5.

Heller S, Salkeld RM, Korner WF, Vitamin B1 status in pregnancy. Am J Clin Nutr 1974;27: 1221–4.

Hung SC, Hung SH, Tarng DC, Yang WC, Huang TP, Chorea induced by thiamine deficiency in hemodialysis patients. Am J Kidney Dis 2001;37: 427–30.

Kitamura K, Yamaguchi T, Tanaka H, Hashimoto S, Yang M, Takahashi T, TPN-induced fulminant beriberi: a report on our experience and a review of the literature. Surg Today 1996;26: 769–76.

Leevy CM, Thiamin deficiency and alcoholism. Ann N Y Acad Sci 1982;378: 316–26.

Liang CC, Bradycardia in thiamin deficiency and the role of glyoxylate. J Nutr Sci Vitaminol (Tokyo) 1977;23: 1–6.

Liberman MC, Tartaglini E, Fleming JC, Neufeld EJ, Deletion of SLC19A2, the high affinity thiamine transporter, causes selective inner hair cell loss and an auditory neuropathy phenotype. J Assoc Res Otolaryngol 2006;7: 211–7.

Lindboe CF, Loberg EM, Wernicke's encephalopathy in non-alcoholics. An autopsy study. J Neurol Sci 1989;90: 125–9.

Lishman WA, Cerebral disorder in alcoholism: syndromes of impairment. Brain 1981;104: 1–20.

Lonsdale D, Shamberger RJ, Red cell transketolase as an indicator of nutritional deficiency. Am J Clin Nutr 1980;33: 205–11.

Matrana MR, Davis WE, Vitamin deficiency after gastric bypass surgery: a review. South Med J 2009;102: 1025–31.

Meador KJ, Nichols ME, Franke P, Durkin MW, Oberzan RL, Moore EE, et al., Evidence for a central cholinergic effect of high-dose thiamine. Ann Neurol 1993;34: 724–6.

Murphy C, Bangash IH, Varma A, Dry beriberi mimicking the Guillain-Barre syndrome. Pract Neurol 2009;9: 221–4.

Oishi K, Hofmann S, Diaz GA, Brown T, Manwani D, Ng L, et al., Targeted disruption of Slc19a2, the gene encoding the high-affinity thiamin transporter Thtr-1, causes diabetes mellitus, sensorineural deafness and megaloblastosis in mice. Hum Mol Genet 2002;11: 2951–60.

Pannunzio P, Hazell AS, Pannunzio M, Rao KV, Butterworth RF, Thiamine deficiency results in metabolic acidosis and energy failure in cerebellar granule cells: an in vitro model for the study of cell death mechanisms in Wernicke's encephalopathy. J Neurosci Res 2000;62: 286–92.

Pfitzenmeyer P, Guilland JC, d'Athis P, Petit-Marnier C, Gaudet M, Thiamine status of elderly patients with cardiac failure including the effects of supplementation. Int J Vitam Nutr Res 1994;64: 113–8.

Rao SN, Chandak GR, Cardiac beriberi: often a missed diagnosis. J Trop Pediatr 2009; 24 [E-pub].

Reuler JB, Girard DE, Cooney TG, Current concepts. Wernicke's encephalopathy. N Engl J Med 1985;312: 1035–9.

Schenker S, Henderson GI, Hoyumpa AM Jr, McCandless DW, Hepatic and Wernicke's encephalopathies: current concepts of pathogenesis. Am J Clin Nutr 1980;33: 2719–26.

Schwartz RA, Gross M, Lonsdale D, Shamberger R, Transketolase activity in psychiatric patients. J Clin Psychiatry 1979;40: 427–9.

Sechi G, Prognosis and therapy of Wernicke's encephalopathy after obesity surgery. Am J Gastroenterol 2008;103: 3219.

Sechi G, Serra A, Wernicke's encephalopathy: new clinical settings and recent advances in diagnosis and management. Lancet Neurol 2007;6: 442–55.

Seehra H, MacDermott N, Lascelles RG, Taylor TV. Wernicke's encephalopathy after vertical banded gastroplasty for morbid obesity. Br Med J 1996;312: 434.

Shah N, Wolff JA, Thiamine deficiency: probable Wernicke's encephalopathy successfully treated in a child with acute lymphocytic leukemia. Pediatrics 1973;51: 750–1.

Smidt LJ, Cremin FM, Grivetti LE, Clifford AJ, Influence of thiamin supplementation on the health and general well-being of an elderly Irish population with marginal thiamin deficiency. J Gerontol 1991;46: M16–22.

Soukaloun D, Kounnavong S, Pengdy B, Boupha B, Durondej S, Olness K, et al., Dietary and socio-economic factors associated with beriberi in breastfed Lao infants. Ann Trop Paediatr 2003;23: 181–6.

Soukoulis V, Dihu JB, Sole M, Anker SD, Cleland J, Fonarow GC, et al., Micronutrient deficiencies an unmet need in heart failure. J Am Coll Cardiol 2009;54: 1660–73.

Tallaksen CM, Bell H, Bohmer T, Thiamin and thiamin phosphate ester deficiency assessed by high performance liquid chromatography in four clinical cases of Wernicke encephalopathy. Alcohol Clin Exp Res 1993;17: 712–6.

Thomas PK, Plant GT, Baxter P, Bates C, Santiago Luis R, An epidemic of optic neuropathy and painful sensory neuropathy in Cuba: clinical aspects. J Neurol 1995;242: 629–38.

Thomson AD, Jeyasingham MD, Pratt OE, Shaw GK, Nutrition and alcoholic encephalopathies. Acta Med Scand Suppl 1987;717: 55–65.

Thomson AD, Cook CC, Touquet R, Henry JA, The Royal College of Physicians report on alcohol: guidelines for managing Wernicke's encephalopathy in the accident and Emergency Department. Alcohol Alcohol 2002;37: 513–21.

Togay-Isikay C, Yigit A, Mutluer N, Wernicke's encephalopathy due to hyperemesis gravidarum: an under-recognised condition. Aust NZ J Obstet Gynaecol 2001;41: 453–6.

Vasconcelos MM, Silva KP, Vidal G, Silva AF, Domingues RC, Berditchevsky CR, Early diagnosis of pediatric Wernicke's encephalopathy. Pediatr Neurol 1999;20: 289–94.

Victor M, Adams RD, Collins GH, The Wernicke-Korsakoff syndrome. A clinical and pathological study of 245 patients, 82 with post-mortem examinations. Contemp Neurol Ser 1971;7: 1–206.

Vimokesant SL, Hilker DM, Nakornchai S, Rungruangsak K, Dhanamitta S, Effects of betel nut and fermented fish on the thiamin status of northeastern Thais. Am J Clin Nutr 1975;28: 1458–63.

Voskoboyev AI, Ostrovsky YM, Thiamin pyrophosphokinase: structure, properties, and role in thiamin metabolism. Ann NY Acad Sci 1982;378: 161–76.

Wilcox CS, Do diuretics cause thiamine deficiency? J Lab Clin Med. 1999;134: 192–3.

Winston AP, Jamieson CP, Madira W, Gatward NM, Palmer RL, Prevalence of thiamin deficiency in anorexia nervosa. Int J Eat Disord 2000;28: 451–4.

Yoshitoshi Y, Shibata N, Yamashita S, Experimental studies on the beriberi heart. I. Cardiac lesions in thiamine deficient rats. Jpn Heart J 1961;2: 42–64.

Zenuk C, Healey J, Donnelly J, Vaillancourt R, Almalki Y, Smith S, Thiamine deficiency in congestive heart failure patients receiving long term furosemide therapy. Can J Clin Pharmacol 2003;10: 184–8.

4 Vitamin B2 – Riboflavin

Riboflavin in human nutrition, biological function, acquired deficiency and the significance of riboflavin deficiency

Peter W. Swaan

4.1 Introduction

Since its discovery in 1920s, riboflavin, also known as vitamin B2, has been one of the main focuses in vitamin research. Numerous studies have contributed to substantial information in the chemistry, physiology and medical significance of this essential vitamin (Rivlin, 1979). Cellular homeostasis of vitamins is tightly controlled in the body owing to their unique and indispensable roles in normal cellular function, growth and development. Riboflavin is a water-soluble vitamin essential for normal cellular functions, growth and development. In its coenzyme forms of flavin adenine dinucleotide (FAD) and flavin mononucleotide (FMN), riboflavin performs key metabolic functions as an intermediary in the transfer of electrons in biological oxidation-reduction reactions. During periods of dietary deprivation or physiological and pathological stress, humans are vulnerable to developing riboflavin deficiency. This could lead to a variety of clinical abnormalities, including growth retardation, anemia, skin lesions and degenerative changes in the nervous system (Cooperman and Lopez, 1991). Humans cannot synthesize riboflavin and, thus, must obtain the vitamin from their diet through absorption in the small intestine. Alternatively, riboflavin is also obtained from indigenous bacteria that colonize the large intestine, which naturally synthesize this vitamin. Although many studies have focused on the mechanism of riboflavin uptake using various tissues and cell lines, transepithelial absorption is controversial and its exact mechanism(s) remains to be defined further. Intracellular processes in riboflavin absorption, such as cellular homoeostasis, and riboflavin function and regulation are also poorly understood. The purpose of this review is to illustrate current *in vitro* and *in vivo* data defining riboflavin uptake mechanisms noted in different studies and to compare and contrast the various implicated parameters defining this (these) absorption mechanism(s). In addition, riboflavin subcellular trafficking events involving receptor-mediated endocytosis and cytoskeletal elements will be discussed. The involvement of a soluble riboflavin binding/carrier protein (RfBP, RCP) in riboflavin uptake and trafficking is currently elusive. Although several studies have reported its existence (Natraj et al., 1988; Prasad et al., 1992), it has not been characterized in detail. The majority of the work on RfBP has been focused on oviparous species and has shown a crucial role in embryo development. Few studies have been conducted on mammalian RfBP analogs despite its promising therapeutic applications.

4.2 Biochemical function

4.2.1 Biochemical function and clinical significance of riboflavin

In its coenzyme forms of FAD and riboflavin 5'-phosphate (FMN), riboflavin performs as an electron transfer intermediary in biological oxidation-reduction reactions. Flavoproteins, enzymes containing FMN or FAD as cofactors, catalyze a remarkable spectrum of biological processes in both prokaryotic and eukaryotic cells. They are not only essential for biosynthesis and metabolism of carbohydrate, lipid, and amino acid, but also crucially involved in activation of other vitamins such as pyridoxine and folic acid (Cooperman et al., 1973). Riboflavin is present in many food substances, mainly in eggs, dairy products such as cheese, meats (particularly liver), cereals (usually fortified) and certain vegetables (broccoli, asparagus). In food products, it is almost exclusively bound to proteins, mainly in the form of FMN and FAD. Riboflavin is extremely stable to heat and most food preparations (cooking, sterilizing), do not affect the riboflavin contents of foods. However, it is very sensitive to light which can lead to rapid degradation if exposure to sunlight is combined with cooking.

In animals, riboflavin deficiency results in lack of growth, failure to thrive, and eventual death (Cooperman and Lopez, 1991). Experimental riboflavin deficiency in dogs results in growth failure, weakness, ataxia and inability to stand. The animals collapse, become comatose and die (Cooperman and Lopez, 1991). During the deficiency state, dermatitis develops together with hair-loss. Other signs include corneal opacity, lenticular cataracts, hemorrhagic adrenals, fatty degeneration of the kidney and liver, and inflammation of the mucus membrane of the gastrointestinal tract (Horwitt, 1972). Post-mortem studies in rhesus monkeys fed a riboflavin-deficient diet revealed that approximately one-third the normal amount of riboflavin was present in the liver (Foy and Mbaya, 1977), which is the main storage organ for riboflavin.

In humans, riboflavin deficiency results in dermatitis, angular stomatitis, cheilosis and neuropathy (Cooperman and Lopez, 1991). Despite its important involvement in metabolic pathways, these overt clinical signs of riboflavin deficiency are rare among inhabitants of the developed countries. However, approximately 28 million Americans exhibit a common 'subclinical' deficiency stage, characterized by a change in biochemical indices (e.g., erythrocyte glutathione reductase) (Lemoine et al., 1991). In this stage, such a person's dietary uptake is sufficient to prevent clinical manifestations but inadequate to sustain flavoproteins for their optimal activities. Although the long-term effects of this subclinical deficiency are unknown in adults, this deficiency results in growth retardation in children (Goldsmith, 1975). Moreover, a severe primary riboflavin deficiency is often followed by secondary deficiencies of other B vitamins (Pinto and Rivlin, 1987). Subclinical riboflavin deficiency has also been observed in women taking oral contraceptives (Wynn, 1975), in the elderly, eating disorders, and in disease states such as HIV (Beach et al., 1992), inflammatory bowel disease (Fernandez-Banares et al., 1989), diabetes and chronic heart disease (Cooperman and Lopez, 1991). The fact that riboflavin-deficiency does not immediately lead to gross clinical manifestations indicates that the systemic levels of this essential vitamin are tightly regulated.

Breast cancer remains the highest cause of malignancy-related death for women in the USA (Castrellon and Gluck, 2008). The first specific soluble plasma protein marker for breast cancer was recently identified as riboflavin carrier protein (RCP) following clinical studies that revealed a significant elevation in RCP serum levels (Karande et al., 2001) and simultaneous decrease in riboflavin levels (Vaidya et al., 1998) in breast cancer patients. This effect is suggested to be the result of an up-regulation in riboflavin-specific cell surface receptors and riboflavin internalization similar to other vitamin systems (Russell-Jones, 2004). Riboflavin, or vitamin B2, is the sole absorptive species of flavin and is necessary for mitochondrial energy production through the metabolism of its cofactors FMN and FAD. Kinetic analysis of riboflavin internalization in a variety of cell lines revealed a high-affinity, saturable mechanism that is Na^+-, potential-, and pH-independent, suggesting an riboflavin-specific carrier-mediated system (Yonezawa et al., 2008). Further characterization in human breast cancer cells (MCF-7 and SKBR-3) demonstrated riboflavin absorption to occur predominantly via receptor-mediated endocytosis (RME) at physiological concentrations (~12 nM) (Bareford et al., 2008) before its vesicular trafficking to subcellular organelle compartments (D'Souza et al., 2006). These data suggest an encouraging clinical application for riboflavin as a novel targeting agent for breast cancer-directed chemotherapeutics.

Additionally, riboflavin has gained renewed therapeutic interest after it was shown to protect vital tissues from ischemia-induced oxidative injury resulting from heart attack or stroke (Hultquist et al., 1993; Betz et al., 1994).

4.2.2 Absorption and disposition of riboflavin

Unlike microorganisms, mammals cannot biosynthesize riboflavin. The only way to obtain this essential vitamin is from diet via intestinal absorption or in the case of a fetus, through maternal sources. Most dietary riboflavin is in the form of flavoproteins or its coenzyme forms, which must first be hydrolyzed to riboflavin before absorption can occur (▶Fig. 4.1). Digestion of flavoproteins, FAD, FMN occurs by both non-specific and specific enzymes in the intestine, suggesting a physiologic preference of riboflavin as the absorptive species of dietary flavins.

Upon entry into the cell, most of the water-soluble vitamins are metabolically altered, and, as a consequence, become trapped within the cell (McCormick and Zhang, 1993). Much evidence indicates that a two-step phosphorylation process is involved in metabolic trapping of riboflavin (Jusko and Levy, 1975; Okuda et al., 1978). Two cytosolic enzymes, flavokinase and FAD synthetase (also known as FAD-pyrophosphorylase), have been identified in enterocytes and hepatocytes to catalyze these specific conversions of riboflavin into its anionic coenzyme forms (Merrill et al., 1978). Some studies also further suggest this phosphorylation process is closely coupled to an absorption mechanism of riboflavin and is necessary for its intestinal absorption (Kasai et al., 1972), although direct proof of this mechanism remains elusive. Excessive riboflavin and catabolic metabolites of intracellular flavoenzymes could exit the enterocytes via a basolateral-located transporter.

In humans, approximately 50% of total riboflavin in plasma is non-covalently protein-bound. Circulatory transport of riboflavin is known to involve both weak associations with albumin and tight binding to a subclass of immunoglobulins (McCormick, 1972). In oviparous vertebrates, a class of pregnancy specific, estrogen-induced riboflavin-carrier proteins is found, that transport riboflavin to the embryonic tissue. Recently, a similar protein has also been identified in mammals, including humans. A more detailed review of this protein will be discussed below.

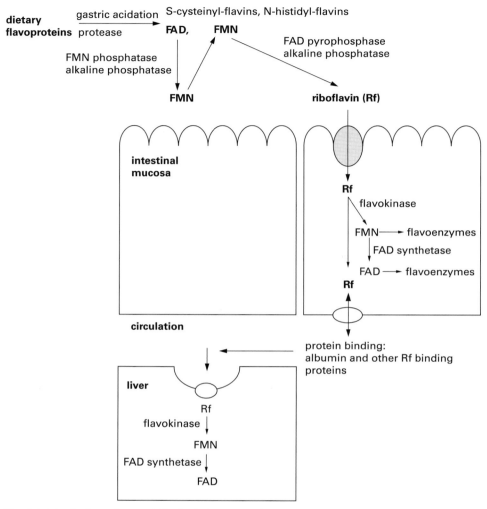

Fig. 4.1: Metabolic pathway of riboflavin in mammalian tissue.

After reaching systemic circulation, riboflavin is imported and converted into FMN and FAD inside the tissues. The liver is the major storage site, containing approximately one-third of total body flavins. Excessive amounts of riboflavin are excreted primarily in the urine, mostly in its intact form. Both *in vitro* and *in vivo* studies have demonstrated that after glomerular filtration, riboflavin is secreted and reabsorbed by the renal tubules via saturable processes (Yanagawa et al., 1997).

4.2.2.1 Effect of drugs on disposition of riboflavin

The structure of riboflavin consists of two main parts: an isoalloxazine ring and a D-ribose side chain. Interestingly, several groups of therapeutic compounds are

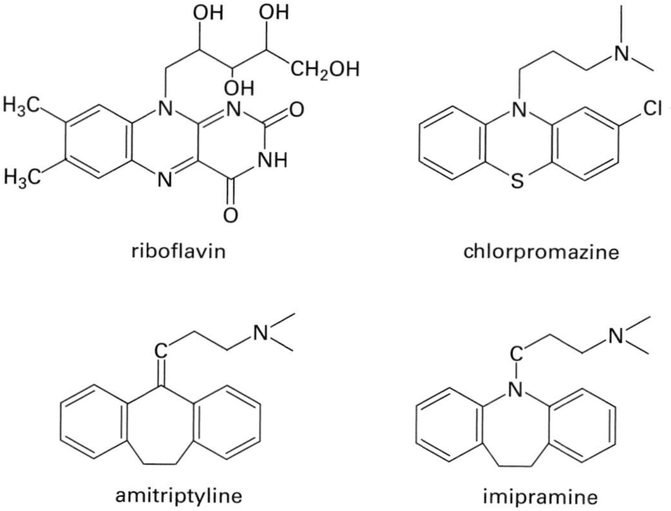

Fig. 4.2: Chemical structures of riboflavin and its phenothiazine drug derivatives.

structurally related to riboflavin, e.g., phenothiazine derivatives such as chlorproma-zine and tricyclic antidepressant agents (TCAs) such as imipramine and amitriptyline (►Fig. 4.2). Co-administration of these agents has been shown to enhance urinary excretion of riboflavin and to accelerate tissue depletion of FAD levels in liver (Pelliccione et al., 1983; Rivlin, 1986). Because psychoactive drugs that are structurally unrelated to riboflavin fail to produce comparable outcome, these studies suggested that the phe-nothiazines and TCAs might exert their inhibitory effects on the cellular disposition of riboflavin. Although the exact mechanism of these drugs remains unclear, it is probable that these metabolic changes are caused by modulation of riboflavin-specific enzymes and/or membrane translocating systems.

4.3 Riboflavin carrier protein

During pregnancy, rapid embryonic development demands a continuous supply of nutrients including riboflavin from the maternal system. However, as with most epithe-lium, the placental/vitelline membrane prevents the transit of free riboflavin into the fetus/egg. In oviparous vertebrates, a specific riboflavin carrier protein (RCP) is involved in transport of riboflavin from plasma to oocytes. The best characterized of the RCPs, chicken RCP (cRCP), is a 37-kDa phosphoglycoprotein synthesized in the liver and oviduct. RCP is unique among flavoproteins because it preferentially binds to riboflavin (in 1:1 molar ratio) over its coenzyme forms (Adiga and Murty, 1983). Although attempts to locate the cRCP-specific receptors have been inconclusive, cRCP-mediated delivery of riboflavin in eggs has been shown to occur via endocytosis of the cRCP-riboflavin complexes through the lipoprotein receptor (Mac Lachlan et al., 1994).

Using antibodies raised against cRCP, Adiga and coworkers are able to identify RCP in the plasma of pregnant mice, rats, monkeys and women. Although these carriers have not been characterized thoroughly, the rodent and primate RCP display marked similarities to cRCP with regard to size, affinity, isoelectric point and immunological cross-reactivity. In humans, the distribution and role of an RCP is more elusive. One study reports the presence of a binding protein in the amniotic fluid of pregnant women. RCPs have also been detected in plasma of male monkeys as well as rat testicular Leydig and Sertoli cells. Similar to their female counterparts, RCP production in male rats and monkeys was sensitive to estradiol-17 and follicle-stimulating hormone.

Recently, two separate groups have independently shown elevated serum RCP levels in breast cancer patients (Karande et al., 2001). The rising serum RCP seems to correlate with the progression of the breast cancer. Advanced breast cancer patients harbor the highest RCP levels compared with early breast cancer patients or normal disease-free women (Karande et al., 2001). Immunohistochemical analysis in breast cancer biopsy specimens also detected the presence of RCP in the cytoplasma of neoplastic cells. Although it remains to be verified whether the elevated patient RCP resulted from overexpression of RCP in breast cancer cells, these studies suggest that circulatory RCP could present as a promising marker for breast cancer diagnosis and prognosis.

In summary, although RCP has been identified in plasma and reproductive organs of either sex, its function in mammalian riboflavin transport remains to be defined. Nevertheless, based on the remarkably conserved features between cRCP and mammalian RCPs, it is proposed that a similar RCP-mediated mechanism could also exist in maternal-fetal transport of riboflavin (Adiga et al., 1997).

4.4 Cellular transport mechanisms of riboflavin

Riboflavin is the preferred absorption species among all flavins, but its low partition coefficient (log $P_{octanol}$ = –1.46) prevents its permeation across cell membrane by simple passive diffusion. By contrast, when riboflavin is given orally in human subjects, maximal plasma concentration and urinary excretion are observed within the first 1.5 h, indicating a rapid absorption and/or elimination process (Jusko and Levy, 1967; Zempleni et al., 1996). The efficient disposition together with a dose-dependent absorption strongly suggests the involvement of a specialized pathway in cellular translocation of riboflavin.

Several *in vitro* techniques such as everted sacs, membrane vesicles, and isolated cell preparations have been applied to directly investigate the specialized transport process of riboflavin. An active transport mechanism has been observed in uptake of riboflavin in intestine, liver, kidney, choroid plexus of species rat, rabbit and human.

4.4.1 Intestine

Because of its pivotal role in absorption of riboflavin, the intestinal uptake mechanism of riboflavin is the most extensively studied among all tissues (▶Tab. 4.1). Taken together, these results suggest that riboflavin is taken up by enterocytes via an active, saturable, temperature-dependent carrier-mediated mechanism.

Tab. 4.1: Intestinal uptake of riboflavin.

Species	Techniques	K_m	J_{max}	Properties
Rat	BBMV	0.12 M	0.36 pmol/5 s per mg protein	Na$^+$-independent
	BBMV (jejunum)	0.38 M	0.9 pmol/5 s per mg protein	Na$^+$-dependent, pH-dependent
	Everted sacs	0.177 M	25.8 pmol/min per 100 mg tissue	Na$^+$-dependent
	Everted sacs	0.54 M	0.182 pmol/min per cm^2	Na$^+$-dependent, ouabain sensitive
	Single pass perfusion	0.38 M	12 pmol/min per g tissue	
Rabbit	BBMV (jejunum)	7.24 M	24.3 pmol/5 s per mg protein	Na$^+$-independent, pH-independent
	BBMV (ileum)	8.88 M	32.2 pmol/5 s per mg protein	Probenecid, PAH insensitive
	BLMV (jejunum)	5 M	91.6 pmol/5 s per mg protein	Na$^+$-independent, pH-independent
	BLMV (ileum)	4.4 M	60.8 pmol/5 s per mg protein	Probenecid, PAH insensitive
Human	BBMV (jejunum)	7.26 M	0.48 pmol/5 s per mg protein	Partial Na$^+$ dependent, electrogenic uptake
	Caco-2 cell line	0.3 M	210 pmol/3 min per mg protein	Na$^+$-independent, ouabain insensitive, pH-independent, probenecid, PAH insensitive
Frog	*Xenopus* oocytes	0.41 M	2.86 fmol/h per oocyte	Na$^+$-independent ouabain insensitive, probenecid, PAH insensitive

Abbreviations: BBMV, brush border membrane vesicle; BLMV, basolateral membrane vesicle; PAH, *p*-aminohippurate.

4.4.1.1 Affinity

The high affinity specialized intestinal uptake process has a K_m value within a lower M range (<10 M). The riboflavin transporter system in rat intestine exhibits a lower capacity but an approximately 10-fold higher affinity compared with that in rabbit intestine.

4.4.1.2 Site specificity and distribution

Early pharmacokinetics studies suggest riboflavin is absorbed more rapidly in the proximal small intestine (Jusko and Levy, 1975). However, several recent studies showed a similar level of uptake activity in both the jejunum and ileum (Said and Mohammadkhani, 1993).

Intestinal absorption of riboflavin involves vectorial transport across both apical and basolateral cell membrane. Using rabbit intestinal membrane vesicles, Said and co-workers reported the existence of a specialized carrier-mediated process on basolateral membrane of enterocytes (Said et al., 1993).

4.4.1.3 Co-transporter properties

The influence of Na^+ on riboflavin uptake in intestine remains controversial: although some studies report Na^+ dependency, most reports indicate riboflavin transport to be Na^+-independent. Furthermore, riboflavin uptake is mostly insensitive to ouabain, which confirms the apparent Na^+-independent behavior of this transport system.

4.4.1.4 Regulation

In both rat intestine and Caco-2 cells, Said and co-workers have shown that intestinal uptake of riboflavin is closely regulated by its dietary level (Said et al., 1993; Said and Ma, 1994). Riboflavin uptake in riboflavin-deficient intestine and Caco-2 cells is up-regulated with significant increase in their J_{max} values without affecting K_m of the systems.

In Caco-2 cells, treatment of intracellular cAMP modulators results in significant inhibition of riboflavin uptake, suggesting possible involvement of a protein kinase A (PKA)-mediated pathway(s) in regulation of the transporter activity (Said et al., 1994).

4.4.2 Kidney

In renal tubules, riboflavin is imported bi-directionally via a carrier-mediated process (▶Tab. 4.2). In term of Na^+ and pH dependency, these two systems exhibit different co-transporter properties (Yanagawa et al., 1998). Compared with that of intestine, the renal riboflavin transporter systems have relatively lower affinity but higher capacity.

Tab. 4.2: Kidney uptake of riboflavin.

Species	Techniques	K_m	J_{max}	Properties
Rat	Isolated cells	8.4 M	7 pmol/30 s per 10^6 cells	Na^+-dependent, ouabain insensitive, PAH insensitive
Rabbit	BBMV	25.7 M	76 pmol/10 s per mg protein	Partial Na^+-dependent, pH-independent, probenecid, PAH sensitive
	BLMV	8.3 M	14.3 pmol/10 s per mg protein	Na^+-independent, pH-dependent, Probenecid, PAH sensitive
Human	HK-2 cell line	0.67 M	10 pmol/3 min per mg protein	Na^+-independent, ouabain insensitive, probenecid, PAH sensitive

Abbreviation: PAH, *p*-aminohippurate.

In early *in vivo* studies in human, probenecid, a substrate of organic anion transporter, was shown to inhibit renal excretion in a dose-dependent fashion. Consistent with this result, renal uptake in most *in vitro* studies are found to be inhibited by probenecid and other organic acids such as *p*-aminohippurate.

Using HK-2 cells, a human renal proximal tubule epithelial cell line, Kumar and colleagues demonstrated renal uptake of riboflavin is also adaptively regulated according to riboflavin supplement (Kumar, 1998). However, up-regulation of riboflavin uptake in riboflavin-deficient HK-2 cells is accompanied by an increase of both the apparent K_m and J_{max} values. Moreover, unlike Caco-2 cells, riboflavin uptake in HK-2 is under the regulation of a Ca^{2+}/calmodulin-mediated pathway(s).

4.4.3 Liver

The liver is the major storage site of riboflavin and plays an important role in riboflavin homeostasis. Hepatic uptake of riboflavin proceeds by a carrier-mediated process (►Tab. 4.3). Riboflavin import in Hep G2 cells, a human-derived liver cell line, is regulated by riboflavin levels in the growth medium and a Ca^{2+}/calmodulin-mediated pathway (Said, 1998).

4.4.4 Choroid plexus and brain

Unlike in other tissues, the concentration of riboflavin in brain is maintained relatively constant. Because this essential factor is not biosynthesized in brain cells, it must enter the brain and cerebrospinal fluid (CSF) from the blood. Choroid plexuses, which comprise the blood and CSF barrier, together with the blood-brain barrier, are responsible for controlling the nutrient homeostasis in the brain. A saturable, Na^+-dependent, ouabain-, probenecid-sensitive carrier-mediated uptake process has been reported by Spector and colleagues (K_m: 78 M; J_{max}: 1.66 mmol/kg per 15 min) (Spector, 1979, 1980).

4.5 What transport mechanisms govern cellular riboflavin homeostasis?

Until recently, it was generally accepted that riboflavin translocation followed an active, carrier-mediated pathway. However, the criteria used to define active transport, i.e., energy dependency and saturation transport kinetics, do not effectively distinguish

Tab. 4.3: Hepatic uptake of riboflavin.

Species	Techniques	K_m	J_{max}	Properties
Rat	BLMV	3.55 M	39.9 pmol/5 s per mg protein	Na^+-independent, pH-independent, probenecid, PAH insensitive
	Isolated hepatocytes	11.8 M	81.7 pmol/min per 10^6 cells	
Human	Hep G2 cell line	0.41 M	3.6 pmol/3min per mg protein	Na^+-independent

carrier-mediated transport from receptor-mediated endocytosis (RME). Receptor-mediated events typically involve endocytosis followed by microtubule-driven vesicular sorting to various cellular organelles (Mukherjee et al., 1997). In an effort to determine whether a receptor-mediated component is involved in riboflavin transport, our laboratory treated Caco-2 cells with either brefeldin A (BFA), which induces mis-sorting of vesicles at the trans-Golgi network, or nocodazole, a microtubule depolymerizing agent (Huang and Swaan, 2000). Our data revealed nocodazole to significantly inhibit the basolateral to apical flux of riboflavin as well as fluorescently labeled transferrin (56.7% and 31.8% of control, respectively), an iron transport protein that has been extensively established to be internalized by a transferrin-specific receptor via a receptor-mediated endocytosis mechanism. In addition, the apical to basolateral transport of both riboflavin and transferrin was significantly increased (37.1% increase compared with controls for riboflavin) upon treatment with nocodazole. BFA led to a significant increase in transport in both directions for transferrin (13-fold higher in apical to basolateral, and 5-fold increase in basolateral to apical). BFA caused a slight, although not significant, increase in basolateral to apical riboflavin transport, and a significant increase was observed for the apical to basolateral flux. The effects of BFA to induce increased concentrations of membrane receptor on the apical membrane as opposed to the basolateral membrane are comparable with similar studies on transferrin by Shah and colleagues (Shah and Shen, 1994).

More recently, the subcellular localization of riboflavin in BeWo cells was studied (Huang et al., 2003). Rhodamine-labeled riboflavin and FITC-labeled transferrin (FITC-Tf) were used to trace subcellular distribution patterns of both compounds upon cellular uptake. Specifically, various RME markers such as fluorescently labeled antibodies specific for human clathrin heavy chain and LAMP-1, a late endosomal marker, were implemented. Using fluorescence microscopy, a distinct perinuclear punctate staining pattern was observed for rhodamine-riboflavin, which colocalized with FITC-Tf. Furthermore, a membrane diffusible probe specific for acidic organelles (e.g., late endosomes), LysoTracker Blue-white DPX, did not colocalize with Rhodamine-riboflavin. Colocalization of riboflavin was also observed with Rab-5, a small GTPase that specifically resides with the clathrin coat, and LAMP-1. All these findings suggest riboflavin transport involves RME in BeWo cells (Huang et al., 2003).

4.6 Conclusion

Understanding the cellular kinetics and mechanisms regulating riboflavin absorption, intracellular trafficking, and recycling, is crucial in facilitating future studies aimed at utilizing this important vitamin for applications in food science or drug delivery. Identifying riboflavin regulatory processes will also allow the characterization of intracellular events which can be manipulated in riboflavin-responsive diseased tissue, such as cancer and ischemia. An abundance of clinical evidence has proposed a role of riboflavin-molecular sensors in breast and liver cancer progression rendering the riboflavin cellular pathway of high interest in targeting these tissue types. Targeting drug delivery vehicles with high affinity ligands, such as riboflavin, would theoretically allow for a more efficient means of therapy.

References

Adiga PR, Murty CV, Vitamin carrier proteins during embryonic development in birds and mammals. Ciba Found Symp 1983;98: 111–36.

Adiga PR, Subramanian S, Rao J, Kumar M, Prospects of riboflavin carrier protein (RCP) as an antifertility vaccine in male and female mammals. Hum Reprod Update 1997;3: 325–34.

Bareford LM, Phelps MA, Foraker AB, Swaan PW, Intracellular processing of riboflavin in human breast cancer cells. Mol Pharm 2008;5: 839–48.

Beach RS, Mantero-Atienza E, Shor-Posner G, Javier JJ, Szapocznik J, Morgan R, Sauberlich HE, Cornwell PE, Eisdorfer C, Baum MK, Specific nutrient abnormalities in asymptomatic HIV-1 infection. Aids 1992;6: 701–8.

Betz AL, Ren XD, Ennis SR, Hultquist DE, Riboflavin reduces edema in focal cerebral ischemia. Acta Neurochir Suppl (Wien) 1994;60: 314–7.

Castrellon AB, Gluck S. Chemoprevention of breast cancer. Expert Rev Anticancer Ther 2008;8: 443–52.

Cooperman JM, Cole HS, Gordon M, Lopez R, Erythrocyte glutathione reductase as a measure of riboflavin nutritional status of pregnant women and newborns. Proc Soc Exp Biol Med 1973;143: 326–8.

Cooperman JM, Lopez, R, Riboflavin. Handbook of vitamins. New York: Marcel Dekker; 1991. pp. 283–310.

D'Souza VM, Foraker AB, Free RB, Ray A, Shapiro PS, Swaan PW, cAMP-Coupled riboflavin trafficking in placental trophoblasts: a dynamic and ordered process. Biochemistry 2006;45: 6095–104.

Fernandez-Banares F, Abad-Lacruz A, Xiol X, Gine JJ, Dolz C, Cabre E, Esteve M, Gonzalez-Huix F, Gassull MA, Vitamin status in patients with inflammatory bowel disease. Am J Gastroenterol 1989;84: 744–8.

Foy H, Mbaya V, Riboflavin. Prog Food Nutr Sci 1977;2: 357–94.

Goldsmith GA, Vitamin B complex. Thiamine, riboflavin, niacin, folic acid (folacin), vitamin B12, biotin. Progr Food Nutr Sci 1975;1: 559–609.

Horwitt MK, In: Sebrell WH, Harris RS, editors. The vitamins, vol. 5. New York: Academic Press; 1972. p. 73.

Huang SN, Swaan, PW, Involvement of a receptor-mediated component in cellular translocation of riboflavin. J Pharmacol Exp Ther 2000;294: 117–25.

Huang SN, Phelps, MA, Swaan, PW, Involvement of endocytic organelles in the subcellular trafficking and localization of riboflavin. J Pharmacol Exp Ther 2003;306: 681–7.

Hultquist DE, Xu F, Quandt KS, Shlafer M, Mack CP, Evidence that NADPH-dependent methaemoglobin reductase and administered riboflavin protect tissue from oxidative injury. Am J Hematol 1993;42: 13–8.

Jusko WJ, Levy G, Absorption, metabolism, and excretion of riboflavin-5'-phosphate in man. J Pharm Sci 1967;56: 58–62.

Jusko WJ, Levy G, Effect of probenecid on riboflavin absorption and excretion in man. J Pharm Sci 1967;56: 1145–9.

Jusko WJ, Levy G. Absorption, protein binding, and elimination of riboflavin. In: Rivlin RS, editor. Riboflavin. New York: Plenum Press; 1975. pp. 99–152.

Karande AA, Sridhar L, Gopinath KS, Adiga PR, Riboflavin carrier protein: a serum and tissue marker for breast carcinoma. Int J Cancer 2001;95: 277–81.

Kasai S, Isemura S, Masuoka M, Matsui K. Identification of riboflavinyl-D-glucoside in cat liver. J Vitaminol 1972;18: 17–23.

Kumar CK, Yanagawa N, Ortiz A, Said HM, Mechanism and regulation of riboflavin uptake by human renal proximal tubule epithelial cell line HK-2. Am J Physiol 1998;274: F104–110.

Lemoine A, Williams DE, Cresteil T, Leroux JP, Hormonal regulation of microsomal flavin-containing monooxygenase: tissue-dependent expression and substrate specificity. Mol Pharmacol 1991;40: 211–7.

Mac Lachlan I, Nimpf J, Schneider WJ, Avian riboflavin binding protein binds to lipoprotein receptors in association with vitellogenin. J Biol Chem 1994;269: 24127–32.

McCormick DB, The fate of riboflavin in the mammal. Nutr Rev 1972;30: 75–9.

Merrill AH, Addison R, McCormick DB, Induction of hepatic and intestinal flavokinase after oral administration of riboflavin to riboflavin-deficient rats. Proc Soc Exp Biol Med 1978;158: 572–4.

Mukherjee S, Ghosh RN, Maxfield FR, Endocytosis. Physiol Rev 1997;77: 759–803.

Natraj U, George S, Kadam P, Isolation and partial characterisation of human riboflavin carrier protein and the estimation of its levels during human pregnancy. J Reprod Immunol 1988;13: 1–16.

Okuda J, Nagamine J, Okumura M, Yagi K, Metabolism of injected flavins studied by using double-labeled [14C]flavin adenine dinucleotide and [14C, 32P]flavin mononucleotide. J Nutr Sci Vitaminol 1978;24: 505–10.

Pelliccione N, Pinto J, Huang YP, Rivlin RS, Accelerated development of riboflavin deficiency by treatment with chlorpromazine. Biochem Pharmacol 1983;32:2949–53.

Pinto JT, Rivlin RS, Drugs that promote renal excretion of riboflavin. Drug-Nutr Interact 1987;5: 143–51.

Prasad PD, Malhotra P, Karande AA, Adiga PR, Isolation and characterization of riboflavin carrier protein from human amniotic fluid. Biochem Int 1992;27: 385–95.

Rivlin RS, Hormones, drugs and riboflavin. Nutr Rev 1979;37: 241–5.

Rivlin RS, Riboflavin. Adv Exp Med Biol 1986;206: 349–55.

Russell-Jones GJ, Use of targeting agents to increase uptake and localization of drugs to the intestinal epithelium. J Drug Target 2004;12: 113–23.

Said HM, Ma TY, Mechanism of riboflavine uptake by Caco-2 human intestinal epithelial cells. Am J Physiol 1994;266: G15-21.

Said HM, Mohammadkhani R, Uptake of riboflavin across the brush border membrane of rat intestine: regulation by dietary vitamin levels. Gastroenterology 1993;105: 1294–8.

Said HM, Hollander D, Mohammadkhani R. Uptake of riboflavin by intestinal basolateral membrane vesicles: a specialized carrier-mediated process. Biochim Biophys Acta 1993;1148: 263–8.

Said HM, Ma TY, Grant K, Regulation of riboflavin intestinal uptake by protein kinase A: studies with Caco-2 cells. Am J Physiol 1994;267: G955-9.

Said HM, Ortiz A, Ma TY, McCloud E, Riboflavin uptake by the human-derived liver cells Hep G2: mechanism and regulation. J Cell Physiol 1998;176: 588–594.

Shah D, Shen, WC, The establishment of polarity and enhanced transcytosis of transferrin receptors in enterocyte-like Caco-2 cells. J Drug Target 1994;2:93–9.

Spector R, Riboflavin homeostasis in the central nervous system. J Neurochem. 1980;35: 202–209.

Spector R, Boose B, Active transport of riboflavin by the isolated choroid plexus in vitro. J Biol Chem. 1979;254:10286–10289.

Vaidya SM, Kamlakar PL, Kamble SM, Molybdenum, xanthine oxidase and riboflavin levels in tamoxifen treated postmenopausal women with breast cancer. Indian J Med Sci 1998;52: 244–7.

Wynn V, Vitamins and oral contraceptive use. Lancet 1975;i: 561–4.

Yanagawa N, Jo OD, Said HM, Riboflavin transport by rabbit renal brush border membrane vesicles. Biochim Biophys Acta 1997;1330: 172–8.

Yanagawa N, Jo OD, Said HM, Riboflavin transport by rabbit renal basolateral membrane vesicles. Biochim Biophys Acta 1998;1415: 56–62.

Yonezawa A, Masuda S, Katsura T, Inui K, Identification and functional characterization of a novel human and rat riboflavin transporter, RFT1. Am J Physiol Cell Physiol. 2008;295: C632–41.

Zempleni J, Galloway JR, McCormick DB, Pharmacokinetics of orally and intravenously administered riboflavin in healthy humans. Am J Clin Nutr 1996;63: 54–66.

5 Vitamin B6 – Pyridoxine

Nutritional and biological aspects and relation to cardiovascular disease

Martin den Heijer

5.1 Introduction

Vitamin B6 is a water-soluble vitamin which is involved in many metabolic processes. The relation between vitamin B6 deficiency and vascular disease attracted most attention in relation to the concept of hyperhomocysteinemia and vascular disease, but several studies suggested that it has an independent role. In this chapter we describe first the biochemistry of vitamin B6, its metabolic functions and the nutritional aspects. Furthermore, we review the data about vitamin B6 deficiency and the risk for vascular disease.

5.2 Biochemistry of vitamin B6

Vitamin B6 was discovered in 1934 by György as a B-vitamin distinct from riboflavin (vitamin B2) (György, 1934). He defined vitamin B6 activity as "that part of the vitamin B-complex responsible for the cure of a specific dermatitis developed by rats on a vitamin-free diet supplemented with vitamin B1 and lactoflavin". In 1938 the vitamin was purified and called pyridoxine (Combs, 2008).

Vitamin B6 is the generic name of all the 3-hydroxy-2-methylpyridine derivates that have a comparable biological activity to 3-hydroxy-4,5bis(hydroxymethyl)-2-methylpyridine (i.e., pyridoxine). ▶Fig. 5.1 shows the different vitamers and their inter-relations. The interconversion of these vitamers is regulated by several enzymes: pyridox(am)ine phosphatase oxidase (PNPO, EC 1.4.3.5), pyridoxal kinase (PDXK, EC 2.7.1.35), pyridoxal phosphatase (PDXP, EC 3.1.3.74) and other phosphatases (alkaline phosphatase (ALP, EC 3.1.3.1) and acid phosphatase (ACP, EC 3.1.3.2). Pyridoxal is eliminated by conversion to 4-pyridoxate by aldehyde oxidase 1 (AOX1, EC 1.2.3.1).

Pyridoxal phosphate (PLP) is the most active B6-vitamer and acts as a coenzyme in more than 180 enzymatic reactions, related to amino acid metabolism and sugar and fatty acid metabolism. Enzymatic reactions include transaminations, aldol cleavages, α-decarboxylations, racemizations, β- and γ-eliminations and replacement reactions (Percudani and Peracchi, 2009; Hellmann and Mooney, 2010). These enzymes can be found at the online B6 database (http://bioinformatics.unipr.it/B6db) (Percudani and Peracchi, 2009).

In addition to be the most active vitamer, pyridoxal phosphate is also the principal form of vitamin B6 in the blood. Several assays have been developed to measure vitamin B6 (Rybak et al., 2005). These include enzymatic assays that make use of a PLP-dependent enzyme such as apo-tyrosine decarboxylase, erythrocyte aspartate amino transferase or apo-homocysteine-lyase (Edwards et al., 1989; Han and Hoffman, 2008).

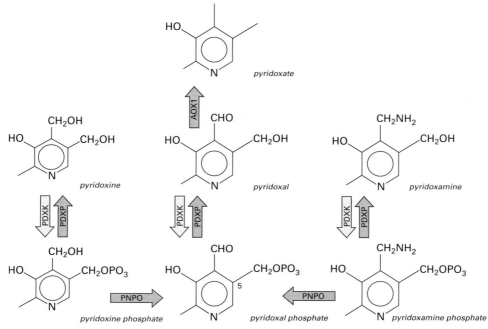

Fig. 5.1: Interconversion of B6 vitamers. Pyridoxal phosphate (PLP) is formed primarily of pyridoxine and pyridoxamine by the enzymes pyridoxal kinase (PDXK) and pyridox(am)ine phosphatase oxidase (PNPO). PLP is dephosphorylated by pyridoxal phosphatase (PDXP) or alkaline phosphatase (ALP). Pyridoxal is eliminated by conversion to 4-pyridoxate by aldehyde oxidase 1 (AOX1).

The product of these enzymes can be measured radioactively or chromogenically. These assays give one summary estimate of all B6-vitamers that have PLP activity. More recently HPLC and mass-spectrometric assays allow the concomitant measurement of the distinct vitamers (pyridoxal 5′-phosphate, pyridoxal, 4-pyridoxic acid, pyridoxine and pyridoxamine) (Bisp et al., 2002; Midttun et al., 2005).

Next to measure the B6 vitamers directly, several other tests could be used to assess the functional B6 activity. Most of these tests measure metabolites that are related to vitamin B6-dependent pathways. Homocysteine (particularly after methionine loading) is elevated in B6 deficiency. Also, tryptophan metabolites could be used as functional indicators of vitamin B6 status (Food and Nutrition Board, Institute of Medicine, 1998; Midttun et al., 2007). Other vitamin B6 status indicators are erythrocyte alanine aminotransferase activity coefficient (EALT-AC), aspartate aminotransferase activity coefficient (EAST-AC) and urinary 4-pyridoxic acid (4-PA).

5.3 Nutritional aspects

In contrast to bacteria, humans cannot synthesize vitamin B6 and therefore they need to have adequate intake of vitamin B6 through food. Important sources of vitamin B6 are meat, whole-grain products and vegetables. In food derived from plant tissue, pyridoxine is the predominant form, whereas in animal-derived food, pyridoxal and pyridoxamine are the predominant forms. Because pyridoxine is more stable than pyridoxal and pyridoxamine, the loss of vitamin B6 by cooking is much higher in animal-derived food than in plant-derived food (Combs, 2008).

The bioavailability of vitamin B6 is approximately 70–80%. Most of the vitamin B6 is absorbed via passive diffusion in the jejunum and ileum. Before entering the gut the vitamers must be dephosphorylated, which is catalyzed by the enzyme ALP. In the liver the vitamers are converted to pyridoxal phosphate (▶Fig. 5.2).The total body pools of vitamin B6 in the human adult is approximately 40–150 mg. Most of the vitamin B6 in the body is found in muscles, where it is bound to glycogen phosphorylase (Combs, 2008).

The Recommended Dietary Allowance (RDA) of vitamin B6 varies from 1.3 to 1.7 mg/day in the US (Food and Nutrition Board, Institute of Medicine, 1998) and is 1.4 in Europe (Commission Directive, 2008). The mean intake in the US population in 2003–2004 was 1.86 ± 0.02 mg/day in non-users of supplements containing vitamin B6 and 1.92 ± 0.02 mg/day in supplement users (36% of the population) (Morris et al., 2008). Plasma PLP concentrations were linearly correlated with vitamin B6 intake. Geometric means of plasma PLP was 41 nmol/l in men and 29 nmol/l in women not using

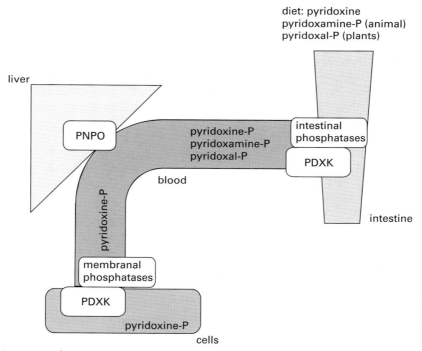

Fig. 5.2: Vitamin B6 absorption and metabolism in the body. Vitamin B6 in the diet is primarily in the form of pyridoxine (plant food) or pyridoamine (animal food) or its phosphate-esters. To be absorbed it should be dephosphorylated by intestinal phosphatases. Pridoxine and pyridoxamine are converted to pyridoxal-phosphate (PLP). PLP has to be dephosphorylated before it can enter the cell.

supplements with vitamin B6. However, in the group with a vitamin intake between 2 and 2.9 mg/day (above the RDA) 10% of the men and 20% of the women had plasma PLP levels below 20 nmol/l (Morris et al., 2008). Comparable intake data are found in Europe (Olsen et al., 2009).

5.4 Determinants of vitamin B6

The plasma PLP levels are lower in smokers, coffee drinkers and oral contraceptive users. Coffee consumption of four cups a day is associated with a 14% lower PLP (Ulvik et al., 2008). However, this effect is absent at lower concentrations and increases to 40% at high levels of PLP. This might be explained by effect of caffeine on the excretion of PLP in the urine. PLP concentrations were 20–25% lower in active smokers compared with never smokers (Morris et al., 2008; Ulvik et al., 2010). One of the explanations for the effect of smoking is a higher demand and turnover of PLP as an antioxidant because of the oxidative stress induced by smoking. Vitamin B6 levels are also lower in oral contraceptive users although their homocysteine levels do not differ (Massé et al., 1996b; Lussana et al., 2003).

An important determinant of plasma PLP is inflammation. This was observed in patients with rheumatoid arthritis (Roubenoff et al., 1995). Several other studies have demonstrated a clear inverse relation between plasma PLP levels and C-reactive protein as a marker of inflammation (Friso et al., 2001; Saibeni et al., 2003; Shen et al., 2010). In the Framingham Heart Study plasma PLP was 35% lower in subjects with CRP 6 mg/l compared with those with CRP <6 mg/l (Friso et al., 2001). A possible explanation could be increased consumption of vitamin B6 in the production of cytokines and other mediators of the inflammatory process. Another explanation could also be redistribution of PLP from circulation to tissues with high demand. This is supported by the observation that red cell PLP is higher in critically ill patients (Talwar et al., 2003; Vasilaki et al., 2008). In the study of Friso et al. (2001) the lower PLP levels at higher CRP levels could not be explained by changes in vitamin B6 intake. However, another study showed also a decreased intake of vitamin B6 in subjects with higher CRP levels (Morris et al., 2010). Moreover, Cheng et al. (2006) found a decrease in inflammation after supplementation with vitamin B6.

5.5 Genetics of vitamin B6

The vitamin B6 metabolism in humans consist essentially of four enzymes: PNPO, PDXK, PDXP and AOX. Mutations in PNPO have been associated with neonatal seizures (Mills et al., 2005; Khayat et al., 2008). However, these mutations or polymorphisms have not been associated with vitamin B6 levels in population studies. Two genome-wide studies on homocysteine and folate, vitamin B6 and vitamin B12 revealed genome-wide significant association for PLP with variants on chromosome 1p36 (Hazra et al., 2009; Tanaka et al., 2009). This region harbors the *ALP* gene which codes for alkaline phosphatase. Mutations in the *ALP* gene are associated with hypophosphatasia and increased PLP levels have been observed in all clinical forms of hypoplasia (Whyte et al., 1985).

5.6 Vitamin B6 and disease

Vitamin B6 has implications for health and disease in several ways: (1) through vitamin B6 deficient diet, (2) through disturbed vitamin B6 metabolism, and (3) through impaired B6-dependent enzymes that could be restored by a high amount of vitamin B6. Certainly, these three possibilities can occur simultaneously.

- Historically vitamin B6 deficiency has been related to pellagra and anemia which occurs in severe vitamin B6 deficiency. Mild deficiencies are related to many diseases including premenstrual syndrome (Wyatt et al., 2000), carpal tunnel syndrome (Piazzini et al., 2007) and psychiatric diseases (Merete et al., 2008; Rossignol, 2009). However, none of these relations have been proven.
- An important disease caused by disturbed vitamin B6 metabolism is the neonatal seizures caused by PNPO deficiency (Clayton et al., 2003; Mills et al., 2005; Khayat et al., 2008; Plecko and Stöckler, 2009). For a long time neonatal seizures have been found to respond sometimes to high doses of folate and pyridoxine or PLP. The fact that sometimes the seizures respond to PLP but not to pyridoxine suggested that the conversion to the active form could be the cause of the disease (Mills et al., 2005; Khayat et al., 2008). This has been shown in several but not all cases. Recently, another cause of neonatal seizures has been found that induce a secondary form of PLP deficiency (Salomons et al., 2007).
- PLP as the active B6 vitamer acts as a cofactor in approximately 180 enzymatic reactions (Percudani and Peracchi, 2009). Most of them are associated with amino acid metabolism and include transamination, decarboxylation, racemization and elimination or replacements at the beta- or gamma-carbons (see for some examples ►Tab. 5.1). Vitamin B6 has been prescribed for several conditions (some of them listed in ►Tab. 5.1). In the case of impaired enzyme function, high doses of pyridoxine (up to 750 mg/day) are given to restore enzyme function. However, high doses of vitamin B6 can lead to peripheral sensory neuropathy and nerve degeneration (Parry and Bredesen, 1985; Gdynia et al., 2008).

Tab. 5.1: Vitamin B6-dependent enzymes. Some examples of more than 180 vitamin B6-dependent enzymes and their function or associated disease are listed.

Enzyme	Associated disease/function
Cystathionine β-synthase	Homocystinuria
Cystathionine γ-lyase	Cystathioninuria
Ornithine aminotransferase	Hyperornithinemia/gyrate atrophy
Glycogen phosphorylase	McArdle disease
Kynureninase	Xanthurenic aciduria
Tryptophan decarboxylase	Biosynthesis of serotonin
Tyrosine carboxylase	Biosynthesis of catecholamines
Glutamate decarboxylase	Biosynthesis of GABA

Much research interest has been devoted to the relation between nutrition and cancer. Regarding vitamin B6 the strongest relation was found with colon cancer. Recently a meta-analysis was conducted of nine studies on vitamin B6 intake and four studies on blood PLP levels. The pooled RRs of colorectal cancer for the highest versus lowest category of vitamin B6 intake and blood PLP levels were 0.90 (95% CI, 0.75–1.07) and 0.52 (95% CI, 0.38–0.71), respectively. After omitting one study which contributed substantially to the heterogeneity among studies of vitamin B6 intake the pooled RR was 0.80 (95% CI, 0.69–0.92). Also, gastric cancer has been associated with plasma vitamin B6 levels (Eussen et al., 2010). No relation was found for breast cancer (Lin et al., 2008; Ma et al., 2009) or prostate cancer (Johansson et al., 2009).

5.6.1 Vitamin B6 and vascular disease

The relation between vitamin B6 and vascular disease has been studied first by Rinehart and Greenberg (1949) who described arteriosclerotic lesions in pyridoxine-deficient monkeys.

The first case-control study on PLP in the coronary artery was published in 1985 showing lower PLP levels in patients compared with controls (Serfontein et al., 1985). ▶Tab. 5.2 shows all the studies published with risk estimates for low PLP and cardiovascular disease (Verhoef et al., 1996; Folsom et al., 1998; Robinson et al., 1998; Kelly et al., 2003; Friso et al., 2004; Dierkes et al., 2005, 2007; Vanuzzo et al., 2007; Cheng et al., 2008; Page et al., 2009). Both the retrospective and prospective studies show a clearly elevated risk for crude estimates (or adjusted for age and sex). However, as mentioned above, plasma PLP is influenced by several factors such as smoking and inflammation which are directly related to cardiovascular disease. Moreover, plasma PLP is an important factor of homocysteine which might explain the relation with cardiovascular disease.

In two studies, Dierkes and colleagues showed that the effect of PLP diminished strongly after adjustment for hs-CRP (Dierkes et al., 2005, 2007). However, in some other studies the effect of PLP remained after adjustment for hs-CRP. Therefore, the current debate as to whether plasma PLP is indeed a causal and independent risk factor is still not closed.

Other sources of evidence resulted from studies on the relation of B6 intake and cardiovascular disease. In the Nurses' Health Study vitamin intake in the highest quintile was associated with a decreased risk of coronary heart disease (Rimm et al., 1998). Similar results were found in the Physician Health Study (Chasan-Taber et al., 1996). Although these intake data might be less sensitive to influences by inflammation, it remains difficult to exclude other possible confounders as lifestyle and nutritional habits.

As in the case of homocysteine, the final answer on causality has to come from clinical trials. In fact, a lot of homocysteine-lowering trials (that are discussed elsewhere in this book) use vitamin B6 – next to folate and vitamin B12 – as homocysteine-lowering agent. These trials did not show any effect, but one should take into account that these trials are not performed in vitamin B6 deficient subjects.

Very recently two trials with pyridoxal phosphate (under the name MC-1) in patients undergoing coronary artery bypass surgery were published. Although the first study shows a preventive effect (Tardif et al., 2007), this could not be confirmed in the second study (MEND-CABG II Investigators, 2008).

Tab. 5.2: Vitamin B6 and arterial vascular disease.

Reference	Type of study	Disease	Cases	Controls	Comparison	Adjustment	Risk estimate
Verhoef et al. (1996)	CC	MI	130	118	Bottom/top quintile	Age, sex	3.13
						+CVD risk	1.96 (0.74–5.26)
Robinson et al. (1998)	CC	VD	750	800	<23.3 nmol/l (20th percentile)	Age, sex, CVD risk	1.84 (1.39–2.42)
Kelly et al. (2003)	CC	CVA/TIA	180	140	<20 nmol/l	Age, sex	7.1 (3.13–15.86)
						+CVD risk	4.58 (1.39–15.12)
Friso et al. (2004)	CC	CAD	475	267	<36.3 nmol/l (50th percentile)	Crude	1.71 (1.26–2.32)
						+Age, sex, CVD risk	1.61 (1.05–2.45)
						+hs-CRP	1.73 (1.11–2.72)
Dierkes et al. (2005)	CC women	CAD	200	225	Bottom/top quintile	Crude	5.88 (2.70–12.5)
						+Age, sex, CVD risk	7.14 (1.96–25.0)
						+hs-CRP	1.23 (0.22–7.14)
Cheng et al. (2008)	CC	CAD (>70% stenosis)	184	516	<20 nmol/l	Crude	5.07 (3.31–7.78)
						+Age, sex , CVD risk	2.39 (1.24–4.60)
						+hs-CRP<0.6 mg/dl	2.34 (1.12–4.92)

(Continued)

Tab. 5.2 (Continued)

Reference	Type of study	Disease	Cases	Controls	Comparison	Adjustment	Risk estimate
Folsom et al. (1998)	NCC	CAD	232	537	Bottom/top quintile	Age and sex	2.38 (0.98–6.67)
						+CVD risk	3.57 (1.43–10.0)
Dierkes et al. (2007)	NCC	MI	148	810	Bottom/top quintile	Age and sex	2.00 (1.20–3.45)
						+hrCRP, CVD risk	1.14 (0.65–1.96)
Vanuzzo et al. (2007)	NCC	CAD, CVD	109	109	Bottom/top quintile	Age and sex (matched)	1.43 (1.03–1.96)
						+CVD risk+CRP	1.45 (1.02–2.04)
Page et al. (2009)	NCC	MI	144	258	Bottom/top quintile	Age and sex	4.17 (2.08–8.33)
						+CVD risk	4.55 (1.82–11.1)
						+hs-CRP	5.56 (1.92–16.7)

CC, case control study; NCC, nested case control study; MI, myocardial infarction; VD, vascular disease; CVA, cerebrovascular accident; TIA, transient ischemic attack; CAD, coronary artery disease; CVD, cerebrovascular disease. CVD risk, adjusted for cardiovascular risk factors. Hs-CRP, high-sensitivity C-reactive protein. For the studies that provide risk estimates for top versus bottom quintiles these estimates have been converted to bottom versus top comparisons for reasons of comparability with other studies.

5.6.2 Venous thrombosis and other vascular diseases

Next to studies on the relation with cardiovascular disease, several studies evaluated the relation with venous thrombosis (▶Tab. 5.3). In 2001 it was reported that low plasma levels of vitamin B6 are independently associated with a heightened risk of deep-vein thrombosis (Cattaneo et al., 2001). Also, in a prospective study with recurrent venous thrombosis low plasma PLP was associated with an increased risk (Hron et al., 2007). In a prospective study on vitamin B6 intake and thrombosis, a low intake of vitamin B6 was associated with an increased risk (Steffen et al., 2007), but this could not be confirmed in another study (Lutsey et al., 2009).

Two homocysteine lowering trials did not show a beneficial effect (den Heijer et al., 2007; Ray et al., 2007), although in one study there was a trend of such an effect, particularly in patients with low PLP levels at baseline (Cattaneo et al., 2005). In none of these studies has the CRP levels been taken into account.

Other studies focused on the relation between abdominal aneurysm (Peeters et al., 2007) and central retinal vein obstruction (Sofi et al., 2008). Also, in these studies the CRP has not been taken into account.

5.6.3 Pathophysiology

A possible relation between vitamin B6 deficiency and vascular disease requires a pathophysiological explanation. Several animal and cell culture studies have shown effects of both experimentally induced vitamin B6 deficiency on the one hand, and vitamin B6 supplementation on the other hand, in relation to vascular and thrombotic changes.

The first study in the literature is from Rinehart and Greenberg (1949). They reported arteriosclerotic lesions in pyridoxine-deficient monkeys. However, most published studies on effects of pyridoxine relate to platelets. Several studies have shown inhibitory effects of pyridoxine in platelets. For instance, Chang et al. (2002) found B-6 vitamers inhibiting platelet aggregation *in vitro* through occupancy of glycoprotein IIb/IIIa receptors. Earlier studies showed platelet inhibitory effects of vitamin B6 using different stimuli (Anonymous, 1981; Nolan et al., 1996; Wu et al., 2009).

Two small trials with supplementation of vitamin B6 in humans showed conflicting results. Schoene and colleagues performed a trial in 12 healthy volunteers with a dose of vitamin B6 (100 mg/day) for 6 weeks and did not find any effects on platelet aggregation (Schoene et al., 1986). However, Van Wyk and colleagues assessed the *in vivo* effect of vitamin B6 by measuring the effect of long-term administration of vitamin B6 (100 mg twice daily p.o. for 15 days) on platelet function and blood coagulation in ten healthy volunteers (van Wyk et al., 1992). Platelet aggregation induced with the agonists ADP or epinephrine was significantly inhibited by vitamin B6, and the platelets tended to aggregate at a slightly decreased rate. Vitamin B6 had no effect on the sensitivity of platelets to prostacyclin, or on the coagulation system.

Regarding a possible relation between vitamin B6 deficiency and abdominal aneurysm, collagen and elastin are major components of the vascular wall. In aneurysms, the elastic lamellae of the vascular wall are degraded, and collagen production is enhanced. Pyridoxal 5-phosphate is an important cofactor for lysyl oxidase, an enzyme responsible for cross-linking collagen and elastin. Animal studies have reported that pyridoxal

Tab. 5.3: Vitamin B6 and venous thrombosis, abdominal aneurysm and central retinal vein thrombosis.

First author	Type of study	Disease	Cases	Controls	Comparison	Adjustment	Risk estimate
Cattaneo et al. (2001)	CC	VT	397	585	Bottom/top quartile	Crude	1.5 (1.0–2.1)
						+Age, sex, risk VT, hcy	1.7 (1.1–2.4)
Hron et al. (2007)	Cohort	RVT	130	757	<15th vs. >75th perc	Crude	1.79 (1.05–2.08)
						+Age, sex, risk VT, hcy	1.72 (1.00–3.00)
Peeters et al. (2007)	CC	AAA	88	88	Bottom/top quartile	Age, sex	3.75 (1.22–11.54)
						+Creatinine	6.92 (1.63–29.3)
Sofi et al. (2008)	CC	CRVO	262	262	Bottom/top tertile	Age sex	4.03 (2.58–6.31)
						+risk CVD+hcy	3.29 (1.89–5.70)

VT, venous thrombosis; RVT, recurrent venous thrombosis; AAA, aortic abdominal aneurysm; CRVO, central retinal vein occlusion.

5-phosphate depletion inhibits lysyl oxidase (Carrington et al., 1984; Levene et al., 1992). Pyridoxine deficiency was also responsible for alterations in bone collagen (Massé et al., 1996a) and for loss of connective tissue integrity (Massé et al., 1995).

5.7 Conclusion

In this chapter we summarized the nutritional and biochemical aspects of vitamin B6. Although many possible relations between different diseases and vitamin B6 deficiency have been postulated, none has been proven yet. This is also true for the relation between vitamin B6 deficiency and vascular disease. However, such relation could not be ruled out. Further evidence should come from genetic studies that could evaluate the role of vitamin B6 related genes on cardiovascular disease (based on the concept of Mendelian randomization) and from meta-analyses on sub-group effects in vitamin B6-deficient participants.

References

Anonymous, Is vitamin B6 an antithrombotic agent? Lancet 1981;1: 1299–300.

Bisp MR, Bor MV, Heinsvig EM, Kall MA, Nexø E, Determination of vitamin B6 vitamers and pyridoxic acid in plasma: development and evaluation of a high-performance liquid chromatographic assay. Anal Biochem 2002;305: 82–9.

Carrington MJ, Bird TA, Levene CI, The inhibition of lysyl oxidase in vivo by isoniazid and its reversal by pyridoxal: Effect on collagen cross-linking in the chick embryo. Biochem J 1984;221: 837–43.

Cattaneo M, Lombardi R, Lecchi A, Bucciarelli P, Mannucci PM, Low plasma levels of vitamin B(6) are independently associated with a heightened risk of deep-vein thrombosis. Circulation 2001;104: 2442–6.

Cattaneo M, Lombardi R, Lecchi A, Bos G, Blom H, Rosendaal F, den Heijer M, Low plasma levels of vitamin B6 and recurrent venous thrombosis: risk assessment and effect of combined vitamin supplementation in the VITRO-trial. J Thromb Haemost 2005;3: P1079.

Chang SJ, Chang CN, Chen CW, Occupancy of glycoprotein IIb/IIIa by B-6 vitamers inhibits human platelet aggregation. J Nutr 2002;132: 3603–6.

Chasan-Taber L, Selhub J, Rosenberg IH, Malinow MR, Terry P, Tishler PV, Willett W, Hennekens CH, Stampfer MJ, A prospective study of folate and vitamin B6 and risk of myocardial infarction in US physicians. J Am Coll Nutr 1996;15: 136–43.

Cheng CH, Chang SJ, Lee BJ, Lin KL, Huang YC, Vitamin B6 supplementation increases immune responses in critically ill patients. Eur J Clin Nutr 2006;60: 1207–13.

Cheng CH, Lin PT, Liaw YP, Ho CC, Tsai TP, Chou MC, Huang YC, Plasma pyridoxal 5′-phosphate and high-sensitivity C-reactive protein are independently associated with an increased risk of coronary artery disease. Nutrition 2008;24: 239–44.

Clayton PT, Surtees RA, DeVile C, Hyland K, Heales SJ, Neonatal epileptic encephalopathy. Lancet 2003;361: 1614.

Combs GF, The vitamins – fundamental aspects of nutrition and health. 3rd ed. Amsterdam: Elsevier; 2008.

Commission Directive 2008/100/EC.

den Heijer M, Willems HP, Blom HJ, Gerrits WB, Cattaneo M, Eichinger S, Rosendaal FR, Bos GM, Homocysteine lowering by B vitamins and the secondary prevention of deep vein thrombosis and pulmonary embolism: A randomized, placebo-controlled, double-blind trial. Blood 2007;109: 139–44.

Dierkes J, Hoffmann K, Klipstein-Grobusch K, et al., Low plasma pyridoxal-5-phosphate and cardiovascular disease risk in women: results from the Coronary Risk Factors for Atherosclerosis in Women Study. Am J Clin Nutr 2005;81: 725–7.

Dierkes J, Weikert C, Klipstein-Grobusch K, Westphal S, Luley C, Möhlig M, Spranger J, Boeing H, Plasma pyridoxal-5-phosphate and future risk of myocardial infarction in the European Prospective Investigation into Cancer and Nutrition Potsdam cohort. Am J Clin Nutr 2007;86: 214–20.

Edwards P, Liu PK, Rose GA, Determination of plasma pyridoxal phosphate levels using a modified apotryptophanase assay. Ann Clin Biochem 1989;26: 158–63.

Eussen SJ, Vollset SE, Hustad S, Midttun Ø, Meyer K, Fredriksen A, Ueland PM, Jenab M, Slimani N, Ferrari P, Agudo A, Sala N, Capellá G, Del Giudice G, Palli D, Boeing H, Weikert C, Bueno-de-Mesquita HB, Büchner FL, Carneiro F, Berrino F, Vineis P, Tumino R, Panico S, Berglund G, Manjer J, Stenling R, Hallmans G, Martínez C, Arrizola L, Barricarte A, Navarro C, Rodriguez L, Bingham S, Linseisen J, Kaaks R, Overvad K, Tjønneland A, Peeters PH, Numans ME, Clavel-Chapelon F, Boutron-Ruault MC, Morois S, Trichopoulou A, Lund E, Plebani M, Riboli E, González CA, Vitamins B2 and B6 and genetic polymorphisms related to one-carbon metabolism as risk factors for gastric adenocarcinoma in the European prospective investigation into cancer and nutrition. Cancer Epidemiol Biomarkers Prev 2010;19: 28–38.

Folsom AR, Nieto FJ, McGovern PG, et al., Prospective study of coronary heart disease incidence in relation to fasting total homocysteine, related genetic polymorphisms, and B vitamins: the Atherosclerosis Risk in Communities (ARIC) study. Circulation 1998;98: 204–10.

Food and Nutrition Board, Institute of Medicine. Vitamin B_6. Dietary reference intakes for thiamin, riboflavin, niacin, vitamin B_6, folate, vitamin B_{12}, pantothenic acid, biotin, and choline. Washington DC: National Academies Press; 1998. pp. 150–95.

Friso S, Jacques PF, Wilson PW, Rosenberg IH, Selhub J, Low circulating vitamin B(6) is associated with elevation of the inflammation marker C-reactive protein independently of plasma homocysteine levels. Circulation 2001;103: 2788–91.

Friso S, Girelli D, Martinelli N, et al., Low plasma vitamin B-6 concentrations and modulation of coronary artery disease risk. Am J Clin Nutr 2004;79: 992–8.

Gdynia HJ, Müller T, Sperfeld AD, Kühnlein P, Otto M, Kassubek J, Ludolph AC, Severe sensorimotor neuropathy after intake of highest dosages of vitamin B6. Neuromuscul Disord 2008;18: 156–8.

György P, Vitamin B2 and the pellagra-like dermatitis in rats. Nature 1934;133: 498–9.

Han Q, Hoffman RM, Nonradioactive enzymatic assay for plasma and serum vitamin B(6). Nat Protoc 2008;3: 1815–9.

Hazra A, Kraft P, Lazarus R, Chen C, Chanock SJ, Jacques P, Selhub J, Hunter DJ, Genome-wide significant predictors of metabolites in the one-carbon metabolism pathway. Hum Mol Genet 2009;18: 4677–87.

Hellmann H, Mooney S, Vitamin B6: a molecule for human health? Molecules 2010;15: 442–59.

Hron G, Lombardi R, Eichinger S, Lecchi A, Kyrle PA, Cattaneo M, Low vitamin B6 levels and the risk of recurrent venous thromboembolism. Haematologica 2007;92: 1250–3.

Johansson M, Van Guelpen B, Vollset SE, Hultdin J, Bergh A, Key T, Midttun O, Hallmans G, Ueland PM, Stattin P, One-carbon metabolism and prostate cancer risk: prospective investigation of seven circulating B vitamins and metabolites. Cancer Epidemiol Biomarkers Prev 2009;18: 1538–43.

Kelly PJ, Shih VE, Kistler JP, et al., Low vitamin B6 but not homocyst(e)ine is associated with increased risk of stroke and transient ischemic attack in the era of folic acid grain fortification. Stroke 2003;34: e51–4.

Khayat M, Korman SH, Frankel P, Weintraub Z, Hershkowitz S, Sheffer VF, Ben Elisha M, Wevers RA, Falik-Zaccai TC, PNPO deficiency: an under diagnosed inborn error of pyridoxine metabolism. Mol Genet Metab 2008;94: 431–4.

Larsson SC, Orsini N, Wolk A, Vitamin B6 and risk of colorectal cancer: a meta-analysis of prospective studies. J Am Med Assoc 2010;303: 1077–83.

Levene CI, Sharman DF, Callingham BA, Inhibition of chick embryo lysyl oxidase by various lathyrogens and the antagonistic effect of pyridoxal. Int J Exp Pathol 1992;73: 613–24.

Lin J, Lee IM, Cook NR, Selhub J, Manson JE, Buring JE, Zhang SM, Plasma folate, vitamin B-6, vitamin B-12, and risk of breast cancer in women. Am J Clin Nutr 2008;87: 734–43.

Lussana F, Zighetti ML, Bucciarelli P, Cugno M, Cattaneo M, Blood levels of homocysteine, folate, vitamin B6 and B12 in women using oral contraceptives compared to non-users. Thromb Res 2003;112: 37–41.

Lutsey PL, Steffen LM, Virnig BA, Folsom AR, Diet and incident venous thromboembolism: the Iowa Women's Health Study. Am Heart J 2009;157: 1081–7.

Ma E, Iwasaki M, Kobayashi M, Kasuga Y, Yokoyama S, Onuma H, Nishimura H, Kusama R, Tsugane S, Dietary intake of folate, vitamin B2, vitamin B6, vitamin B12, genetic polymorphism of related enzymes, and risk of breast cancer: a case-control study in Japan. Nutr Cancer 2009;61: 447–56.

Massé PG, Yamauchi M, Mahuren JD, Coburn SP, Muniz OE, Howell DS, Connective tissue integrity is lost in vitamin B6 deficient chicks. J Nutr 1995;125: 26–34.

Massé PG, Rimnac CM, Yamauchi M, Coburn SP, Rucker RB, Howell DS et al., Pyridoxine deficiency affects biomechanical properties of chick tibial bone. Bone 1996a;18: 567–74.

Massé PG, van den Berg H, Duguay C, Beaulieu G, Simard JM, Early effect of a low dose (30 micrograms) ethinyl estradiol-containing Triphasil on vitamin B6 status. A follow-up study on six menstrual cycles. Int J Vitam Nutr Res 1996b;66: 46–54.

MEND-CABG II Investigators, Alexander JH, Emery RW Jr, Carrier M, Ellis SJ, Mehta RH, Hasselblad V, Menasche P, Khalil A, Cote R, Bennett-Guerrero E, Mack MJ, Schuler G, Harrington RA, Tardif JC, Efficacy and safety of pyridoxal 5'-phosphate (MC-1) in high-risk patients undergoing coronary artery bypass graft surgery: the MEND-CABG II randomized clinical trial. J Am Med Assoc 2008;299: 1777–87.

Merete C, Falcon LM, Tucker KL, Vitamin B6 is associated with depressive symptomatology in Massachusetts elders. J Am Coll Nutr 2008;27: 421–7.

Midttun O, Hustad S, Solheim E, Schneede J, Ueland PM, Multianalyte quantification of vitamin B6 and B2 species in the nanomolar range in human plasma by liquid chromatography-tandem mass spectrometry. Clin Chem 2005;51: 1206–16.

Midttun Ø, Hustad S, Schneede J, Vollset SE, Ueland PM, Plasma vitamin B-6 forms and their relation to transsulfuration metabolites in a large, population-based study. Am J Clin Nutr 2007;86: 131–8.

Midttun Ø, Hustad S, Ueland PM, Quantitative profiling of biomarkers related to B-vitamin status, tryptophan metabolism and inflammation in human plasma by liquid chromatography/tandem mass spectrometry. Rapid Commun Mass Spectrom 2009;23: 1371–9.

Mills PB, Surtees RA, Champion MP, Beesley CE, Dalton N, Scambler PJ, Heales SJ, Briddon A, Scheimberg I, Hoffmann GF, Zschocke J, Clayton PT, Neonatal epileptic encephalopathy caused by mutations in the PNPO gene encoding pyridox(am)ine 5'-phosphate oxidase. Hum Mol Genet 2005;14: 1077–86.

Morris MS, Picciano MF, Jacques PF, Selhub J, Plasma pyridoxal 5'-phosphate in the US population: the National Health and Nutrition Examination Survey, 2003–2004. Am J Clin Nutr 2008;87: 1446–54.

Morris MS, Sakakeeny L, Jacques PF, Picciano MF, Selhub J, Vitamin B-6 intake is inversely related to, and the requirement is affected by, inflammation status. J Nutr 2010;140: 103–10.

Nolan ML, Harrington MG, Eljamil A, Effect of pyridoxal-5'-phosphate on aggregation of platelets from stored human concentrates induced by arachidonic acid. Biochem Soc Trans 1996;24: 95S.

Olsen A, Halkjaer J, van Gils CH, Buijsse B, Verhagen H, Jenab M, Boutron-Ruault MC, Ericson U, Ocké MC, Peeters PH, Touvier M, Niravong M, Waaseth M, Skeie G, Khaw KT, Travis R, Ferrari P, Sanchez MJ, Agudo A, Overvad K, Linseisen J, Weikert C, Sacerdote C, Evangelista A, Zylis D, Tsiotas K, Manjer J, van Guelpen B, Riboli E, Slimani N, Bingham S,

Dietary intake of the water-soluble vitamins B1, B2, B6, B12 and C in 10 countries in the European Prospective Investigation into Cancer and Nutrition. Eur J Clin Nutr 2009;63(Suppl 4): S122–49.

Page JH, Ma J, Chiuve SE, Stampfer MJ, Selhub J, Manson JE, Rimm EB, Plasma vitamin B(6) and risk of myocardial infarction in women. Circulation 2009;120: 649–55.

Parry GJ, Bredesen DE, Sensory neuropathy with low-dose pyridoxine. Neurology 1985;35: 1466–8.

Peeters AC, van Landeghem BA, Graafsma SJ, Kranendonk SE, Hermus AR, Blom HJ, den Heijer M, Low vitamin B6, and not plasma homocysteine concentration, as risk factor for abdominal aortic aneurysm: a retrospective case-control study. J Vasc Surg 2007;45: 701–5.

Percudani R, Peracchi A, The B6 database: a tool for the description and classification of vitamin B6-dependent enzymatic activities and of the corresponding protein families. BMC Bioinformatics 2009;10: 273.

Piazzini DB, Aprile I, Ferrara PE, Bertolini C, Tonali P, Maggi L, Rabini A, Piantelli S, Padua L, A systematic review of conservative treatment of carpal tunnel syndrome. Clin Rehabil 2007;214: 299–314.

Plecko B, Stöckler S, Vitamin B6 dependent seizures. Can J Neurol Sci 2009;36(Suppl 2): S73–7.

Ray JG, Kearon C, Yi Q, Sheridan P, Lonn E; Heart Outcomes Prevention Evaluation 2 (HOPE-2) Investigators, Homocysteine-lowering therapy and risk for venous thromboembolism: a randomized trial. Ann Intern Med 2007;146: 761–7.

Rimm EB, Willett WC, Hu FB, Sampson L, Colditz GA, Manson JE, Hennekens C, Stampfer MJ, Folate and vitamin B6 from diet and supplements in relation to risk of coronary heart disease among women. J Am Med Assoc 1998;279: 359–64.

Rinehart JF, Greenberg LD, Arteriosclerotic lesions in pyridoxine-deficient monkeys. Am J Pathol 1949;25: 481–91.

Robinson K, Arheart K, Refsum H, et al., Low circulating folate and vitamin B6 concentrations: risk factors for stroke, peripheral vascular disease, and coronary artery disease. European COMAC Group. Circulation 1998;97: 437–43.

Rossignol DA, Novel and emerging treatments for autism spectrum disorders: a systematic review. Ann Clin Psychiatry 2009;21: 213–36.

Roubenoff R, Roubenoff RA, Selhub J, Nadeau MR, Cannon JG, Freeman LM, Dinarello CA, Rosenberg IH, Abnormal vitamin B6 status in rheumatoid cachexia. Association with spontaneous tumor necrosis factor alpha production and markers of inflammation. Arthritis Rheum 1995;38: 105–9.

Rybak ME, Jain RB, Pfeiffer CM, Clinical vitamin B6 analysis: an interlaboratory comparison of pyridoxal 5′-phosphate measurements in serum. Clin Chem 2005;51: 1223–31.

Saibeni S, Cattaneo M, Vecchi M, Zighetti ML, Lecchi A, Lombardi R, Meucci G, Spina L, de Franchis R, Low vitamin B(6) plasma levels, a risk factor for thrombosis, in inflammatory bowel disease: role of inflammation and correlation with acute phase reactants. Am J Gastroenterol 2003;98: 112–7.

Salomons GS, Bok LA, Struys EA, Pope LL, Darmin PS, Mills PB, Clayton PT, Willemsen MA, Jakobs C, An intriguing 'silent' mutation and a founder effect in antiquitin (ALDH7A1). Ann Neurol 2007;62: 414–8.

Schoene NW, Chanmugam P, Reynolds RD, Effect of oral vitamin B6 supplementation on in vitro platelet aggregation. Am J Clin Nutr 1986;43: 825–30.

Serfontein WJ, Ubbink JB, De Villiers LS, Rapley CH, Becker PJ, Plasma pyridoxal-5-phosphate level as risk index for coronary artery disease. Atherosclerosis 1985;55: 357–61.

Shen J, Lai CQ, Mattei J, Ordovas JM, Tucker KL, Association of vitamin B-6 status with inflammation, oxidative stress, and chronic inflammatory conditions: the Boston Puerto Rican Health Study. Am J Clin Nutr 2010;91: 337–42.

Sofi F, Marcucci R, Bolli P, Giambene B, Sodi A, Fedi S, Menchini U, Gensini GF, Abbate R, Prisco D, Low vitamin B6 and folic acid levels are associated with retinal vein occlusion independently of homocysteine levels. Atherosclerosis 2008;198: 223–7.

Steffen LM, Folsom AR, Cushman M, Jacobs DR Jr, Rosamond WD, Greater fish, fruit, and vegetable intakes are related to lower incidence of venous thromboembolism: the Longitudinal Investigation of Thromboembolism Etiology. Circulation 2007;115: 188–95.

Talwar D, Quasim T, McMillan DC, Kinsella J, Williamson C, O'Reilly DS, Pyridoxal phosphate decreases in plasma but not erythrocytes during systemic inflammatory response. Clin Chem 2003;49: 515–8.

Tanaka T, Scheet P, Giusti B, Bandinelli S, Piras MG, Usala G, Lai S, Mulas A, Corsi AM, Vestrini A, Sofi F, Gori AM, Abbate R, Guralnik J, Singleton A, Abecasis GR, Schlessinger D, Uda M, Ferrucci L, Genome-wide association study of vitamin B6, vitamin B12, folate, and homocysteine blood concentrations. Am J Hum Genet 2009;84: 477–82.

Tardif JC, Carrier M, Kandzari DE, Emery R, Cote R, Heinonen T, Zettler M, Hasselblad V, Guertin MC, Harrington RA; MEND-CABG Investigators, Effects of pyridoxal-5'-phosphate (MC-1) in patients undergoing high-risk coronary artery bypass surgery: results of the MEND-CABG randomized study. J Thorac Cardiovasc Surg 2007;133: 1604–11.

Ulvik A, Vollset SE, Hoff G, Ueland PM, Coffee consumption and circulating B-vitamins in healthy middle-aged men and women. Clin Chem 2008;54: 1489–96.

Ulvik A, Ebbing M, Hustad S, Midttun O, Nygård O, Vollset SE, Bønaa KH, Nordrehaug JE, Nilsen DW, Schirmer H, Ueland PM, Long- and short-term effects of tobacco smoking on circulating concentrations of B vitamins. Clin Chem 2010;56: 755–63.

Vanuzzo D, Pilotto L, Lombardi R, Lazzerini G, Carluccio M, Diviacco S, Quadrifoglio F, Danek G, Gregori D, Fioretti P, Cattaneo M, De Caterina R, Both vitamin B6 and total homocysteine plasma levels predict long-term atherothrombotic events in healthy subjects. Eur Heart J 2007;28: 484–91.

van Wyk V, Luus HG, Heyns AD, The in vivo effect in humans of pyridoxal-5'-phosphate on platelet function and blood coagulation. Thromb Res 1992;66: 657–68.

Vasilaki AT, McMillan DC, Kinsella J, Duncan A, O'Reilly DS, Talwar D, Relation between pyridoxal and pyridoxal phosphate concentrations in plasma, red cells, and white cells in patients with critical illness. Am J Clin Nutr 2008;88: 140–6.

Verhoef P, Stampfer MJ, Buring JE, et al., Homocysteine metabolism and risk of myocardial infarction: relation with vitamins B6, B12, and folate. Am J Epidemiol 1996;143: 845–59.

Whyte MP, Mahuren JD, Vrabel LA, Coburn SP, Markedly increased circulating pyridoxal-5'-phosphate levels in hypophosphatasia. Alkaline phosphatase acts in vitamin B6 metabolism. J Clin Invest 1985;76: 752–6.

Wu Y, Liu Y, Han Y, Cui B, Mi Q, Huang Y, Wang L, Jiang Q, Chen Q, Liu N, Ferro A, Ji Y, Pyridoxine increases nitric oxide biosynthesis in human platelets. Int J Vitam Nutr Res 2009;79: 95–103.

Wyatt K, Dimmock P, Jones P, Poor-quality studies suggest that vitamin B(6) use is beneficial in premenstrual syndrome. West J Med 2000;172: 245.

6 Vitamin B9 – Folate

6.1 Folate in human nutrition

Patrick J. Stover

6.1.1 Folate

Folate is a generic term that refers to a family of water-soluble B-vitamins that are found in food and function as enzyme cofactors by carrying and chemically activating single carbons (1Cs) for biosynthetic reactions (▶Fig. 6.1a). Folate is required for the synthesis of DNA and regulation of gene expression, and therefore is found in virtually all forms of life. Tetrahydrofolate (THF), which is the fully reduced form of the vitamin, carries 1Cs at one of three different oxidation levels ranging from methanol to formate (Appling 1991; Fox and Stover, 2008). The 1Cs are covalently bound to the N-5 and/or N-10 position of THF. In the cell, there are five different 1C-substituted forms of THF: 10-formyl-THF, 5-formyl-THF, 5,10-methenyl-THF, 5,10-methylene-THF and 5-methyl-THF, and each of these THF 1C forms are interconverted in the cell through enzyme-mediated catalysis (▶Fig. 6.2). Folates are also modified through the addition of a glutamate polypeptide that is polymerized through unusual γ-linked peptide bonds (Shane, 1995; Moran, 1999). During digestion, the γ-glutamyl polypeptide is hydrolyzed from natural food folate to generate folate monoglutamate forms, through a reaction catalyzed by the enzyme γ-glutamyl hydrolase. Only folate monoglutamates are absorbed across the intestinal epithelium by the proton-coupled folate transporter (Zhao et al., 2009), and circulate in serum as monoglutamate derivatives. Upon transport into cells, folate monoglutamate derivatives are reconverted to their polyglutamate forms by the addition of a γ-glutamyl polypeptide usually consisting of five to eight glutamate residues. The glutamate polypeptide serves to retain the vitamin within cells and to increase its affinity for folate-dependent enzymes.

6.1.2 Biological roles of folate

THF polyglutamates function as coenzymes that donate or accept 1Cs in a network of reactions involved in nucleotide and amino acid biosynthesis and catabolism, known as 1C metabolism. Folate-mediated 1C metabolism occurs in the cytoplasm, mitochondria and nucleus, and each of these intracellular compartments is associated with specific metabolic pathways (▶Fig. 6.2) (Appling, 1991; Stover, 2004).

6.1.2.1 Cytoplasm

1C metabolism in the cytoplasm involves all of the 1C-substituted forms of THF, which function in the synthesis of purines, thymidylate and remethylation of homocysteine to methionine (Fox and Stover, 2008). Formate serves as the primary source of 1C units for 1C metabolism in the cytoplasm, and is derived from 1C metabolism in

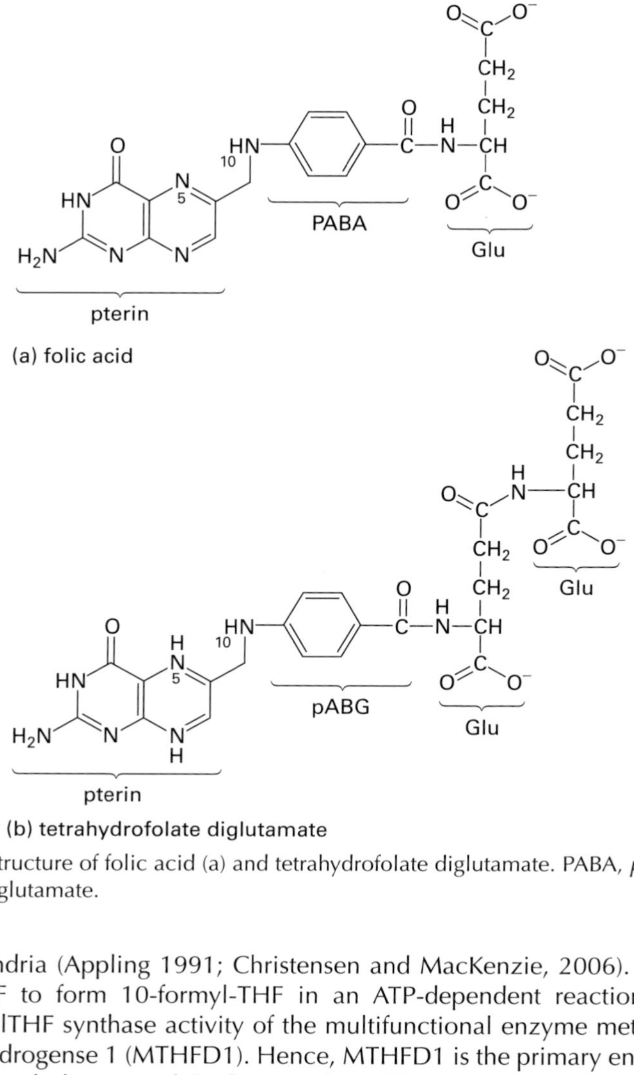

Fig. 6.1: Structure of folic acid (a) and tetrahydrofolate diglutamate. PABA, *para*-aminobenzoic acid; glu, glutamate.

mitochondria (Appling 1991; Christensen and MacKenzie, 2006). Formate condenses with THF to form 10-formyl-THF in an ATP-dependent reaction catalyzed by the 10-formylTHF synthase activity of the multifunctional enzyme methylenetetrahydrofolate dehydrogense 1 (MTHFD1). Hence, MTHFD1 is the primary entry point of 1Cs into the 1C metabolic network in the cytoplasm. The folate-dependent *de novo* synthesis of purines occurs in the cytoplasm through a multi-enzyme complex termed a purineosome, which assembles when exogenous sources of purines are not available (An et al., 2008). The activated formyl moiety of 10-formyl-THF is incorporated directly into the #2 and #8 positions of the purine ring. Alternatively, the 1C of 10-formyl-THF can be reduced to 5,10-methylene-THF through the cyclohydrolase and NADPH-dependent dehydrogenase activities of MTHFD1.

The *de novo* synthesis of thymidylate requires 5,10-methylene-THF as the 1C donor. In a reaction catalyzed by the enzyme thymidylate synthase (TYMS), 5,10-methylene-THF and uridylate are converted to thymidylate and dihydrofolate. In this reaction, the 5,10-methylene-THF cofactor serves both as a donor of a 1C unit, and also as a

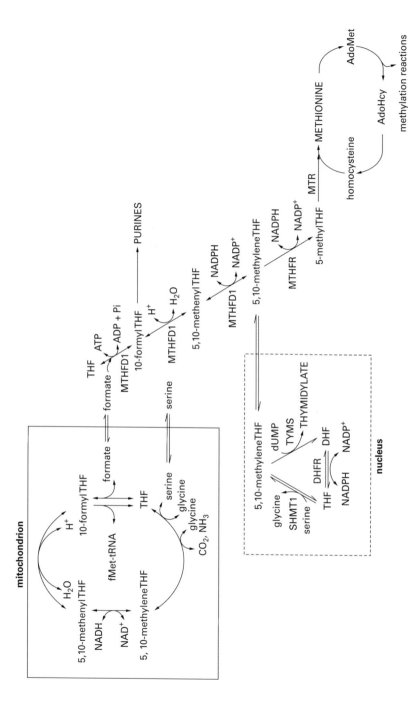

Fig. 6.2: Compartmentation of folate-mediated 1C metabolism in the cytoplasm, mitochondria and nucleus. 1C metabolism in the cytoplasm is required for the *de novo* synthesis of purines and thymidylate, and for the remethylation of homocysteine to methionine. 1C metabolism in the mitochondria is required to generate formate for 1C metabolism in the cytoplasm. 1C metabolism in the nucleus synthesizes thymidylate from uridylate and serine. MTHFD1, methylenetetrahydrofolate dehydrogenase; MTHFR, methylenetetrahydrofolate reductase; SHMT1, cytoplasmic serine hydroxymethyltransferase; TYMS, thymidylate synthase; DHFR, dihydrofolate reductase; MTR, methionine synthase; THF, tetrahydrofolate; DHF, dihydrofolate.

source of two electrons through the oxidation of THF to dihydrofolate (DHF). THF is regenerated from DHF in a reaction catalyzed by the NADPH-dependent enzyme dihydrofolate reductase (DHFR). To complete the *de novo* thymidylate synthesis cycle in the cytoplasm, THF is converted to 5,10-methylene-THF by MTHFD1 as described above, or alternatively by the vitamin B6-(pyridoxal-phosphate) requiring enzyme serine hydroxymethyltransferase (SHMT1 and SHMT2α). The SHMT isozymes catalyze the conversion of serine to glycine to generate 5,10-methylene-THF from THF (▶Fig. 6.2) (Anderson and Stover, 2009). 5,10-Methylene-THF can also be reduced to 5-methyl-THF for methionine biosynthesis in a reaction catalyzed by the NADPH- and FAD-dependent enzyme methylenetetrahydrofolate reductase (MTHFR).

The remethylation of homocysteine to methionine occurs through folate-dependent and folate-independent pathways. Homocysteine can be converted to methionine in a folate-independent reaction catalyzed by the enzyme betaine homocysteine methyltransferase, a reaction in which betaine serves as the 1C donor. Folate-dependent homocysteine remethylation, which is catalyzed by methionine synthase, requires vitamin B12 in the form of cobalamin to convert 5-methyl-THF and homocysteine to methionine and THF. Because the MTHFR-catalyzed generation of 5-methyl-THF is essentially irreversible *in vivo*, accumulation of 5-methyl-THF can impair purine and thymidylate *de novo* biosynthesis, which occurs in severe vitamin B12 deficiency (Scott, 1999). Once formed, methionine can be adenosylated to form *S*-adenosylmethionine (AdoMet), which is a cofactor and 1C donor for numerous other methylation reactions (Finkelstein, 2000, 2007). S-Adenosylhomocysteine (AdoHcy) is a product of AdoMet-dependent transmethylation reactions, and is cleaved to form adenosine and homocysteine, which completes the homocysteine remethylation pathway.

6.1.2.2 Mitochondria

Mitochondria contain as much as 40% of total cellular folate, and folate polyglutamates in mitochondria are a distinct pool that does not exchange with folate polyglutamates in the cytoplasm. In this compartment, 1C metabolism is necessary to formylate Met-tRNA to form fMet-tRNA, for the initiation of mitochondrial protein synthesis, and to generate formate for 1C metabolism in the cytoplasm; both of these pathways require 10-formyl-THF. These 1Cs that support these pathways are generated from the THF-dependent catabolism of the amino acids glycine, serine, dimethylglycine and sarcosine, which donate a 1C to THF generating 5,10-methylene-THF, which is subsequently oxidized to form 10-formyl-THF through the activities of MTHFD2 and MTHFD1L (Christensen and MacKenzie, 2006). Formate derived in mitochondria traverses to the cytoplasm (Appling, 1991).

6.1.2.3 Nucleus

Approximately 10% of total liver folate resides in the nuclear compartment (Shin et al., 1976). 1C metabolism in the nucleus functions to generate thymidylate from uridylate (Anderson and Stover, 2009). During S-phase of the cell cycle, the enzymes that constitute the entire thymidylate synthesis pathway in the cytoplasm, which includes the enzymes SHMT1, SHMT2, TYMS and dihydrofolate reductase (DHFR), are modified by the Small Ubiquitin-like Modifier (SUMO), which facilitates the nuclear translocation of the entire pathway. SHMT is the only known source of 1Cs for nuclear thymidylate synthesis; mice lacking SHMT1 exhibit impaired thymidylate synthesis (MacFarlane et al., 2008). The necessity for redundancy in the compartmentation of *de novo* thymidylate synthesis in the cytoplasm and nucleus is not known.

6.1.3 Laboratory diagnosis and biomarkers of impaired 1C metabolism

Impairments in the folate-dependent 1C metabolic network can result from a primary dietary folate deficiencies, from secondary deficiencies of nutrients that function in 1C metabolism including vitamin B6, vitamin B12, and riboflavin and/or from genetic variation that influences the activity or expression of folate-dependent enzymes (Stover, 2004). Folate-dependent enzymes bind folate polyglutamate cofactors tightly with binding constants in the low micromolar or nanomolar range. Furthermore, the cellular concentration of folate-binding proteins exceeds that of folate derivatives (which are present at 25–35 μM), and therefore the concentration of free folate in the cell is negligible (Schirch and Strong, 1989; Strong et al., 1990; Suh et al., 2001). Therefore, independent or origin, metabolic impairments of 1C metabolism rarely impact a single pathway, but rather influence the entire network. This primarily occurs because the folate dependent pathways compete for a limiting pool of folate cofactors in the cytoplasm (Scott et al., 1981; Suh et al., 2001).

Two of the most sensitive biomarkers of impaired folate metabolism are uracil content in nuclear DNA (Blount et al., 1997) and elevations in homocysteine concentrations in serum and tissue. Decreased rates of folate-dependent methionine synthesis result in elevations of cellular and plasma homocysteine (Finkelstein, 2007). This leads to elevations in *S*-adenosylhomocysteine (AdoHcy) concentrations, because the equilibrium for the hydrolysis AdoHcy to adenosine and homocysteine favors AdoHcy synthesis (Finkelstein, 2007). AdoHcy is a potent inhibitor of AdoMet-dependent methylation reactions including DNA and protein methyltransferases (Clarke and Banfield, 2001), leading to hypomethylated DNA and protein (including histones) (Friso et al., 2002a,b; Huang et al., 2003; Jaenisch and Bird, 2003). Decreased rates of deoxythymidine triphosphate (dTTP) synthesis (Blount et al., 1997) results in incorporation of deoxyuridine triphosphate (dUTP) into DNA, because DNA polymerases do not discriminate between dUTP and dTTP (Blount et al., 1997; Ames, 1999). Other biomarkers of whole-body folate deficiency include low serum and/or red blood cell folate concentrations, DNA hypomethylation, elevated formiminoglutamate in urine (an intermediate in folate-dependent histidine catabolism), megaloblastic anemia and neutrophil hypersegmentation (O'Connor, 1991; Lindenbaum and Allen, 1995). More recently, there has been interest in quantifying the distribution of the 1C forms of folate in serum or erythrocytes as markers of folate status and/or impaired 1C metabolism (Huang et al., 2008).

6.1.4 Folate nutritional requirements and acquired causes of deficiency

Folate nutritional status is supported by the intake of the vitamin found in natural food, as well as dietary supplements and fortified foods. Good dietary sources of natural folate include fresh fruits, leafy green vegetables and legumes (Allen, 2008). Natural food folates are chemically unstable and readily undergo irreversible oxidative degradation during food preparation and cooking. Folic acid, which is a synthetic, fully oxidized and stable provitamin, is commonly found in dietary supplements and fortified food (▶Fig. 6.1a). Because of its chemical stability and lack of a polyglutamate moiety, it has greater bioavailability than natural folate, but once transported into the cell is reduced to DHF and subsequently THF by the enzyme DHFR. Low levels of DHFR expression could result in the appearance of folic acid in the serum of individuals with high levels of folic acid intake (Yang et al., 2009), and there is evidence that total DHFR activity is highly variable among individuals (Bailey and Ayling, 2009). Dietary folate requirements are expressed as Dietary Folate Equivalents (DFEs) to adjust for the increased bioavailability of folic acid compared with natural food folate (Bailey, 1998). The Recommended Dietary Allowance (RDA) for adults is 400 µg/day of dietary folate equivalents.

Biomarkers of folate nutritional status are responsive to inadequate dietary intake of folate, although secondary nutrient deficiencies and genetics can influence metabolic biomarkers that are used to assess whole-body folate status (Bailey and Gregory, 1999). The biomarkers that were used to determine the RDA for dietary folate intake by the Institute of Medicine include serum and erythrocyte folate concentrations and plasma homocysteine concentrations. However, it should be noted that plasma homocysteine levels do not report exclusively on folate status. Normal plasma homocysteine levels range from 10 to 12 µM during folate sufficiency, but are elevated by vitamin B6 and B12 deficiency. Erythrocyte folate concentrations less than 140 ng/ml indicate folate deficiency, but are also influenced by genetic variation, including the common 677 C→T polymorphism in the MTHFR gene (Friso et al., 2002), and there is increasing evidence that dietary folate requirements may differ by MTHFR genotype (Solis et al., 2008).

6.1.4.1 Folate and neural tube defects

Neural tube defects (NTDs) refer to neurodevelopmental anomalies resulting from the failure of the neural tube to close during early embryonic development (Beaudin and Stover, 2009). These are among the most common congenital birth defects, with worldwide prevalence ranging from 0.5 to 60 per 10 000 births (ICBDMS, 2000). The most common and severe NTDs include spina bifida, which results from a failure of the posterior neural tube to close resulting in exposure of the spinal cord, and anencephaly, which is defined by absence of the cranial vault and brain owing to failure of the anterior neural tube to close. Maternal folic acid supplementation is the most effective intervention known to prevent NTDs, and can prevent up to 70% of NTDs (Czeizel and Dudas, 1992). Despite the unambiguous impact of folate status on NTD risk reduction, the mechanism for this protective effect has yet to be established. In the USA and Canada, folic acid fortification of enriched flour was initiated in 1998 to lower the incidence of NTDs and has been effective (Ray, 2008). The Institute of Medicine recommends that women of child-bearing age consume a total of 400 µg of folic acid/day from fortified foods and/or dietary supplements in addition to food folate from a varied diet (Bailey and Gregory, 1999). Human genetic variation that contributes to the risk of having an NTD-affected pregnancy includes genes that encode the folate-dependent enzymes MTHFR (Botto and Yang, 2000; van der Put and Blom, 2000; Blom et al., 2006) and MTHFD1 (Brody et al., 2002). Both maternal and fetal MTHFR variants contribute to risk, whereas MTHFD1 risk is exclusively maternal.

The metabolic pathway responsible for failure of neural tube closure has not been established. Homocysteine is cytotoxic at high levels and induces oxidative stress, but several mouse models of inborn errors of metabolism that exhibit severe hyperhomo-cysteinemia, including MTHFR deletion, do not develop NTDs. Furthermore, elevated homocysteine in fetal culture medium does not induce NTDs in developing embryos (Watanabe et al., 1995). Impairments in AdoMet-dependent methylation reactions, including genomic methylation, have also been suggested to underlie NTD etiology. Depressed chromatin methylation might affect neural tube closure by affecting cellular differentiation (Kobayakawa et al., 2007) and/or cellular migration processes (Rahnama et al., 2006; Issaeva et al., 2007), both of which are crucial for neurulation. Mice with targeted deletion of the *de novo* methyltransferase enzyme Dnmt3b exhibit altered differentiation capacity in embryonic stem (ES) cells (Jackson et al., 2004), and embryos exhibit NTDs, confirming the essentiality of *de novo* methylation and cell differentiation in neural tube closure. Targeted deletion of genes that mediate methylation-mediated suppression of gene expression also resulted in NTDs (Kim et al., 2001). However, the relevance of these mouse models to human NTDs is unknown, nor it is known if these NTDs can be prevented with folic acid.

Human embryos with NTDs have been shown to exhibit impaired *de novo* thymi-dylate synthesis (Dunlevy et al., 2007), indicating a potential causal relationship between impaired thymidylate biosynthesis and NTDs. The rapid growth of the neuroepithelium during neural tube closure requires robust *de novo* nucleotide biosynthesis to sustain rates of cell division and limit uracil accumulation in DNA. Impairments in nucleotide biosynthesis for DNA replication and repair decrease rates of cell division during the crucial period of neural tube closure (Keller-Peck and Mullen, 1997). Mouse models of genomic instability exhibit NTDs, although genomic instability resulting from increased uracil accumulation in DNA has not been investigated (Herrera et al., 1999; Hollander et al., 1999; Wang et al., 2004). Disruption of the *Pax3* locus in mice, which encodes a homeobox transcription factor, results in 100% penetrant spina bifida and impaired *de novo* thymidylate biosynthesis (Fleming and Copp, 1998; Wlodarczyk et al., 2005). Maternal *in utero* supplementation or supplementation of culture media with either thymidine or folic acid prevented NTDs in homozygous *Pax3* null embryos whereas methionine supplementation exacerbated the NTD phenotype. Collectively, these data indicate that thymidylate biosynthesis is a strong candidate for the causal biosynthetic pathway involved in folate-responsive NTD pathogenesis. However, human epidemiological and murine fetal culture models have also identified choline as a modifier of NTD risk (Zeisel, 2006). Choline interacts with folate-mediated 1C metabolism by two distinct mechanisms. Choline degradation can be a source of 1C units for 1C metabolism in the cytoplasm; choline biosynthesis from glycine requires three equivalents of AdoMet. Clearly, more research is required to conclusively demonstrate which disruptions in 1C metabolism are causal and which are bystanders in the etiology of folate-responsive developmental anomalies.

6.1.4.2 Folate and chronic disease

Deleterious gene-diet interactions are fundamental to the etiologies of virtually all folate-associated chronic disease, although underlying mechanisms have yet to be established. Impairments in folate metabolism have been associated with cardiovascular disease (McNulty et al., 2008; Bazzano, 2009), cancers (Martinez et al., 2008), and cognitive decline (Vogel et al., 2009), although randomized, placebo-controlled clinical trials have not conclusively validated observation studies that suggested these associations. Impairments in folate-dependent methylation and/or nucleotide biosynthesis are the probable molecular antecedents of these pathologies. Proposed roles of low folate status in carcinogenesis have been the subject of several excellent reviews (Martinez et al., 2008; Hubner and Houlston, 2009). Low folate status increases DNA mutation rates and uracil content in DNA, which can lead to double strand breaks and altered DNA methylation patterns, all of which are involved in cellular transformation. However, randomized clinical trials do not support a role for folic acid supplementation in the prevention of colon cancer, indicating that cancer risk might only be associated with overt folate deficiency. Genetic variation in the 1C metabolic network has also been shown to influence cancer risk; the MTHFR 677C→T polymorphism is associated with an increased risk of NTDs but a decreased risk of colon cancer (Ma et al., 1997). Given the role of folate in nucleotide biosynthesis, it has been suggested that elevated folate status could accelerate cellular transformation and/or tumor growth in colon cancer, but definitive evidence from randomized controlled trails have not supported this hypothesis to date (Ebbing et al., 2009).

1C metabolism remains an attractive target for nutritional intervention to prevent and/or manage chronic disease, but a deeper understanding of the causal pathways, their regulation and mechanism of pathogenesis is required. Recent genome-wide association studies are indicating a role for 1C metabolism in mitochondria in vascular disease (Samani et al., 2007), and virtually nothing is known about the regulation of 1C metabolism in this compartment, including if formate production is limiting in the 1C network in the cytoplasm. As causal pathways are identified, new approaches to nutrition intervention could be developed and tested that supply the end products of 1C metabolism (purines, thymidylate, methionine, formate, etc.), which might be more efficacious than improving folate status with folic acid.

References

Allen LH, Causes of vitamin B12 and folate deficiency. Food Nutr Bull 2008;29(2 Suppl): S20–34; discussion S35–7.
Ames BN, Micronutrient deficiencies. A major cause of DNA damage. Ann N Y Acad Sci 1999;889: 87–106.
An S, Kumar R, et al., Reversible compartmentalization of de novo purine biosynthetic complexes in living cells. Science 2008;320: 103–6.
Anderson DD, Stover PJ, SHMT1 and SHMT2 are functionally redundant in nuclear De novo thymidylate biosynthesis. PLoS One 2009;4: e5839.
Appling DR, Compartmentation of folate-mediated one-carbon metabolism in eukaryotes. FASEB J 1991;5: 2645–51.
Bailey LB, Dietary reference intakes for folate: the debut of dietary folate equivalents. Nutr Rev 1998;56: 294–9.
Bailey SW, Ayling JE, The extremely slow and variable activity of dihydrofolate reductase in human liver and its implications for high folic acid intake. Proc Natl Acad Sci USA 2009;106: 15424–9.
Bailey LB, Gregory JF 3rd, Folate metabolism and requirements. J Nutr 1999;129: 779–82.
Bazzano LA, Folic acid supplementation and cardiovascular disease: the state of the art. Am J Med Sci 2009;338: 48–9.

Beaudin AE, Stover PJ, Insights into metabolic mechanisms underlying folate-responsive neural tube defects: a minireview. Birth Defects Res A Clin Mol Teratol 2009;85: 274–84.

Blom HJ, Shaw GM, et al., Neural tube defects and folate: case far from closed. Nat Rev Neurosci 2006;7: 724–31.

Blount BC, Mack MM, et al., Folate deficiency causes uracil misincorporation into human DNA and chromosome breakage: implications for cancer and neuronal damage. Proc Natl Acad Sci USA 1997;94: 3290–5.

Botto LD, Yang Q, 5,10-Methylenetetrahydrofolate reductase gene variants and congenital anomalies: a HuGE review. Am J Epidemiol 2000;151: 862–77.

Brody LC, Conley M, et al., A polymorphism, R653Q, in the trifunctional enzyme methylene-tetrahydrofolate dehydrogenase/methenyltetrahydrofolate cyclohydrolase/formyltetrahydrofolate synthetase is a maternal genetic risk factor for neural tube defects: report of the Birth Defects Research Group. Am J Hum Genet 2002;71: 1207–15.

Christensen KE, MacKenzie RE, Mitochondrial one-carbon metabolism is adapted to the specific needs of yeast, plants and mammals. Bioessays 2006;28: 595–605.

Clarke S, Banfield K, S-Adenosylmethionine-dependent methyltransferases. In: Carmel R, Jacobson DW. Homocysteine in health and disease. Cambridge: Cambridge Press; 2001.

Czeizel AE, Dudas I, Prevention of the first occurrence of neural-tube defects by periconceptional vitamin supplementation. N Engl J Med 1992;327: 1832–5.

Dunlevy LP, Chitty LS, et al., Abnormal folate metabolism in foetuses affected by neural tube defects. Brain 2007;130: 1043–9.

Ebbing M, Bonaa KH, et al., Cancer incidence and mortality after treatment with folic acid and vitamin B12. J Am Med Assoc 2009;302: 2119–26.

Finkelstein JD, Pathways and regulation of homocysteine metabolism in mammals. Semin Thromb Hemost 2000;26: 219–25.

Finkelstein JD, Metabolic regulatory properties of S-adenosylmethionine and S-adenosylhomocys-teine. Clin Chem Lab Med 2007;45: 1694–9.

Fleming A, Copp AJ, Embryonic folate metabolism and mouse neural tube defects. Science 1998; 280: 2107–9.

Fox JT, Stover PJ, Folate-mediated one-carbon metabolism. Vitam Horm 2008;79: 1–44.

Friso S, Choi SW, et al., A method to assess genomic DNA methylation using high-performance liq-uid chromatography/electrospray ionization mass spectrometry. Anal Chem 2002a;74:4526–31.

Friso S, Choi SW, et al., A common mutation in the 5,10-methylenetetrahydrofolate reductase gene affects genomic DNA methylation through an interaction with folate status. Proc Natl Acad Sci USA 2002b;99: 5606–11.

Herrera E, Samper E, et al., Telomere shortening in mTR-/- embryos is associated with failure to close the neural tube. EMBO J 1999;18: 1172–81.

Hollander MC, Sheikh MS, et al., Genomic instability in Gadd45a-deficient mice. Nat Genet 1999;23: 176–84.

Huang C, Sloan EA, et al., Chromatin remodeling and human disease. Curr Opin Genet Dev 2003;13: 246–52.

Huang Y, Khartulyari S, et al., Quantification of key red blood cell folates from subjects with defined MTHFR 677C>T genotypes using stable isotope dilution liquid chromatography/mass spectrometry. Rapid Commun Mass Spectrom 2008;22: 2403–12.

Hubner RA, Houlston RS, Folate and colorectal cancer prevention. Br J Cancer 2009;100: 233–9.

ICBDMS Birth Defects Annual Report, 2000.

Issaeva I, Zonis Y, et al., Knockdown of ALR (MLL2) reveals ALR target genes and leads to altera-tions in cell adhesion and growth. Mol Cell Biol 2007;27: 1889–903.

Jackson M, Krassowska A, et al., Severe global DNA hypomethylation blocks differentiation and induces histone hyperacetylation in embryonic stem cells. Mol Cell Biol 2004;24: 8862–71.

Jaenisch R, Bird A, Epigenetic regulation of gene expression: how the genome integrates intrinsic and environmental signals. Nat Genet 2003;33 Suppl: 245–54.

Keller-Peck CR, Mullen RJ, Altered cell proliferation in the spinal cord of mouse neural tube mutants curly tail and Pax3 splotch-delayed. Brain Res Dev Brain Res 1997;102: 177–88.

Kim JK, Huh SO, et al., Srg3, a mouse homolog of yeast SWI3, is essential for early embryogenesis and involved in brain development. Mol Cell Biol 2001;21: 7787–95.

Kobayakawa S, Miike K, et al., Dynamic changes in the epigenomic state and nuclear organization of differentiating mouse embryonic stem cells. Genes Cells 2007;12: 447–60.

Lindenbaum J, Allen RH, Clinical spectrum and diagnosis of folate deficiency. In: Bailey LB, editor. Folate in health and disease. New York: Marcel Dekker Inc.; 1995.

Ma J, Stampfer MJ, et al., Methylenetetrahydrofolate reductase polymorphism, dietary interactions, and risk of colorectal cancer. Cancer Res 1997;57: 1098–102.

MacFarlane AJ, Liu X, et al., Cytoplasmic serine hydroxymethyltransferase regulates the metabolic partitioning of methylenetetrahydrofolate but is not essential in mice. J Biol Chem 2008;283: 25846–53.

Martinez ME, Marshall JR, et al., Diet and cancer prevention: the roles of observation and experimentation. Nat Rev Cancer 2008;8: 694–703.

McNulty H, Pentieva K, et al., Homocysteine, B-vitamins and CVD. Proc Nutr Soc 2008;67: 232–7.

Moran RG, Roles of folylpoly-gamma-glutamate synthetase in therapeutics with tetrahydrofolate antimetabolites: an overview. Semin Oncol 1999;26(2 Suppl 6): 24–32.

O'Connor DL, Interaction of iron and folate during reproduction. Prog Food Nutr Sci 1991;15: 231–54.

Rahnama F, Shafiei F, et al., Epigenetic regulation of human trophoblastic cell migration and invasion. Endocrinology 2006;147: 5275–83.

Ray JG, Efficacy of Canadian folic acid food fortification. Food Nutr Bull 2008;29(2 Suppl): S225–30.

Samani NJ, Erdmann J, et al., Genomewide association analysis of coronary artery disease. N Engl J Med 2007;357: 443–53.

Schirch V, Strong WB, Interaction of folylpolyglutamates with enzymes in one-carbon metabolism. Arch Biochem Biophys 1989;269: 371–80.

Scott JM, Folate and vitamin B12. Proc Nutr Soc 1999;58: 441–8.

Scott JM, Dinn JJ, et al., Pathogenesis of subacute combined degeneration: a result of methyl group deficiency. Lancet 1981;2(8242): 334–7.

Shane B, Folate chemistry and metabolism. In: Bailey LB, editor. Folate in health and disease. New York: Marcel Dekker Inc; 1995. pp. 1–22.

Shin YS, Chan C, et al., Subcellular localization of gamma-glutamyl carboxypeptidase and of folates. Biochim Biophys Acta 1976;444: 794–801.

Solis C, Veenema K, et al., Folate intake at RDA levels is inadequate for Mexican American men with the methylenetetrahydrofolate reductase 677TT genotype. J Nutr 2008;138: 67–72.

Stover PJ, Physiology of folate and vitamin B12 in health and disease. Nutr Rev 2004;62(6 Pt 2): S3–12; discussion S13.

Strong WB, Tendler SJ, et al., Purification and properties of serine hydroxymethyltransferase and C1-tetrahydrofolate synthase from L1210 cells. J Biol Chem 1990;265: 12149–55.

Suh JR, Herbig AK, et al., New perspectives on folate catabolism. Annu Rev Nutr 2001;21: 255–82.

van der Put NM, Blom HJ, Neural tube defects and a disturbed folate dependent homocysteine metabolism. Eur J Obstet Gynecol Reprod Biol 2000;92: 57–61.

Vogel T, Dali-Youcef N, et al., Homocysteine, vitamin B12, folate and cognitive functions: a systematic and critical review of the literature. Int J Clin Pract 2009;63: 1061–7.

Wang X, Wang RH, et al., Genetic interactions between Brca1 and Gadd45a in centrosome duplication, genetic stability, and neural tube closure. J Biol Chem 2004;279: 29606–14.

Watanabe M, Osada J, et al., Mice deficient in cystathionine beta-synthase: animal models for mild and severe homocyst(e)inemia. Proc Natl Acad Sci USA 1995;92: 1585–9.

Wlodarczyk BJ, Tang LS, et al., Spontaneous neural tube defects in splotch mice supplemented with selected micronutrients. Toxicol Appl Pharmacol 2006;213: 55–63.

Yang Q, Cogswell ME, et al., Folic acid source, usual intake, and folate and vitamin B-12 status in US adults: National Health and Nutrition Examination Survey (NHANES) 2003–2006. Am J Clin Nutr 2010;91: 64–72.

Zeisel SH, Choline: critical role during fetal development and dietary requirements in adults. Annu Rev Nutr 2006;26: 229–50.

Zhao R, Matherly LH, et al., Membrane transporters and folate homeostasis: intestinal absorption and transport into systemic compartments and tissues. Expert Rev Mol Med 2009;11: e4.

6.2 Folate in human reproductive performance

John M. Twigt; Joop S.E Laven; Regine P.M. Steegers-Theunissen

6.2.1 Introduction

The natural B-vitamin folate is of significant importance for cellular metabolism, fulfilling a multitude of roles in various processes ranging from cell cycle regulation, amino acid biosynthesis, DNA nucleotide synthesis and protein processing (Bliek, 2008). Therefore, it is not surprising that folate deficiency potentially results in many derangements in growth and development with important implications also for reproduction (Molloy and Scott, 2001). Folic acid is a synthetic derivative of folate which is more resilient against oxidation than naturally occurring folates. Folic acid enters the folate cycle by reduction into dihydrofolate by dihydrofolatereductase (DHFR) (Fig 6.4). By means of the intertwined folate- and methionine-cycle (►Fig. 6.4), folates are predominantly utilized in one-carbon metabolism for the synthesis of three out of four DNA-nucleotides (adenine, guanine and thymine) and metabolism of the amino acids, methionine, serine, glycine and cysteine. Many enzymes involved in folate metabolism require cofactors for normal functioning. Methionine synthase is a zinc protein and requires vitamin B12 (cobalamin) as a cofactor and vitamin B6 (pyridoxine) is an important cofactor for the trans-sulfuration pathway. Furthermore, vitamin B2 is needed for adequate synthesis of 5,10-methylene-tetrahydrofolate-reductase (MTHFR) and zinc is also necessary for adequate uptake of folates from the jejunum (Rawlings and Barrett, 1997; Ulrey, 2005).

Humans do not have the ability to endogenously synthesize folates. The demand for folates therefore has to be met entirely by dietary intake. Green leafy vegetables, beans or liver are important natural sources of folates. Alternatively, in several countries grain, cereal and bread products are increasingly often fortified with folic acid, making these products a rich source of folic acid. Natural folate is present in food as 5-methyl-tetrahydrofolate (5-mTHF) with a polyglutamate tail. In the jejunum, 5-methyl-THF-polyglutamate is hydrolyzed to 5-methyl-THF-monoglutamate by glutamate carboxypeptidase II. Because of its low pH optimum, the proton-coupled folate transporter favors folate transport into the enterocytes of the jejunum. Within the enterocytes, 5-methyl-THF-monoglutamate is converted into 5-mTHF and thereafter released into the circulation (Zhao, 2009). In peripheral tissue, several mechanisms for 5-mTHF uptake exist. Folate receptors (FR) exist in three isoforms, α, β and γ, that bind circulating 5-mTHF. The FR-folate complex is internalized by endocytosis and subsequent acidification of the compartment leads to dissociation of 5-mTHF from

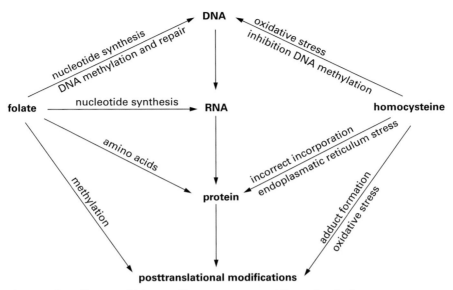

Fig. 6.3: The influence of folate and homocysteine on different levels, from gene to gene product.

the receptor. The mechanism of export from the endosome is likely to be facilitated by the proton-coupled folate transporter. FRα is important for the placental transport of 5-mTHF. In peripheral tissue, however, the reduced folate carrier is the most predominant mechanism for 5-mTHF uptake (Henderson, 1995; Prasad, 1998; Zhao, 2009) (▶Fig. 6.4).

Intracellular, the methyl moiety of 5-mTHF is used by methionine synthase to re-methylate homocysteine (Hcy) to methionine and form tetrahydrofolate (THF). Methionine is further metabolized into S-adenosyl-methionine (SAM) by methionine adenosyltransferase. SAM is the ultimate methyl-donor for virtually all methylation reactions. After transmethylation of SAM, S-adenosyl-homocysteine (SAH) is formed. By means of a reversible reaction, SAH is hydrolyzed to Hcy and adenosine by S-adenosyl-homocysteine hydrolase. A folate independent remethylation pathway for Hcy is present by means of betaine-homocysteine methyltransferase that utilizes a methyl group from betaine to form dimethylglycine and methionine. Approximately 50% of homocysteine is metabolized via the remethylation pathway. The remainder is metabolized via the trans-sulfuration pathway. In this pathway the non-essential amino acid cysteine is required for the synthesis of the important endogenous anti-oxidant glutathione. This pathway is, however, tissue specific, with all necessary enzymes only being expressed in the liver, small intestine, kidney and pancreas (Brosnan, 2004).

After partition of the methyl group, THF is further metabolized via the folate cycle (▶Fig. 6.4) in several ways. (1) THF reacts with formate to form 10-formyl-THF, which either dehydrates to 5,10-methenyl-THF, which is then metabolized to 5,10-methylene-THF (5,10-mTHF), or is allocated to the formation of purines. (2) THF reacts with serine, catalyzed by serine hydroxymethyltransferase to form glycine and 5,10-mTHF. In a reaction catalyzed by MTHFR, 5,10mTHF is reduced to 5-mTHF which can then be used for the re-methylation of homocysteine into methionine. MTHFR forms the conjunction between the methionine and folate cycle, here it is determined whether

5,10-mTHF is utilized for 5-mTHF production or *de novo* synthesis of thymidylate from deoxyuridylate.

A multitude of genes coding for enzymes are required for adequate folate metabolism. Single nucleotide polymorphisms have been identified which affect the efficiency of one-carbon metabolism. However, only polymorphisms in the MTHFR and methionine synthetase reductase (MTRR) gene have shown to be of clinical significance in folate metabolism and later pathology. In the gene coding for the MTHFR enzyme a C→T substitution at position 677 results in a thermolabile variant of the enzyme (Frosst, 1995), The frequency of this polymorphism is dependent on geographical location and varies between 0.1 and 0.5 (Blom, 2009). Homozygotes for this mutation have a 70% reduced MTHFR activity, resulting in hyperhomocysteinemia and DNA hypomethylation (Friso, 2002; Castro, 2004). A 66A→G polymorphism in the MTRR gene has an estimated allele frequency of 0.39–0.59 (Blom, 2009) and results in reduced activity of the MTRR enzyme (Wilson, 1999). The product of the MTRR gene maintains methionine synthase in its active state. It should be noted, however, that enzymatic deficiencies owing to these polymorphisms are only clinically relevant when nutritional deficiency of cobalamin (MTRR) or folates (MTHFR) are co-existent.

The pathogenicity of folate deficiency can, in theory, be elicited in various ways (▶Fig. 6.3). Owing to its nature, highly proliferating tissues are particularly vulnerable, with a high rate of genomic and epigenomic replication and RNA- and protein synthesis. These processes are all dependent on the availability of one-carbon groups provided by the folate pathway. DNA methylation is an epigenetic mechanism. Methylation of cytosine residues in CG repeats, named CpG-islands, exert regulatory properties on gene transcription by interfering with the binding of factors necessary for gene transcription. A sufficient folate supply is necessary for adequate DNA methylation, with hypomethylation giving rise to altered gene expression (Wainfan and Poirier, 1992). Folates also influence factors important for the maintenance of DNA integrity. Efficacy of nucleotide excision repair mechanisms and *de novo* DNA synthesis is modulated by the availability of thymidine triphosphate. Owing to folate deficiency, increasing amounts of deoxyuridine triphosphate is misincorporated into DNA (James, 1997; Pogribny, 1997). Finally, cytosine hypomethylation promotes the deamination of cytosine to uracil, thereafter further stressing uracil-specific repair mechanisms and reducing DNA stability (Pogribny, 1995).

As shown earlier, folate substrate or cofactor deficiency (vitamin B2, B6 and B12 and zinc) results in the accumulation of Hcy. Therefore, the Hcy level in blood serum is regarded as a sensitive marker for the functioning of folate metabolism. Despite its necessity, excess Hcy can exert harmful effects in several ways. Reactive Hcy metabolites can form adducts with lysine residues in proteins or can be misincorporated into proteins as a substitute for methionine, thereby potentially affecting protein function (Jakubowski, 2004). Secondly, it has long been acknowledged that Hcy could disturb the redox balance of the cell by the generation of reactive oxygen species (ROS) (Zou and Banerjee, 2005). An adequate redox balance is required for normal physiology, and many reproductive processes (Agarwal, 2008). An excess of ROS results in oxidative stress, which indiscriminately can affect the functionality of all cellular constituents. Finally, the equilibrium between Hcy and adenosine and SAH is favored towards SAH, SAH is a potent inhibitor of most SAM-dependent methyltransferases (Finkelstein, 2007). DNA hypomethylation, therefore, not only occurs in the situation of

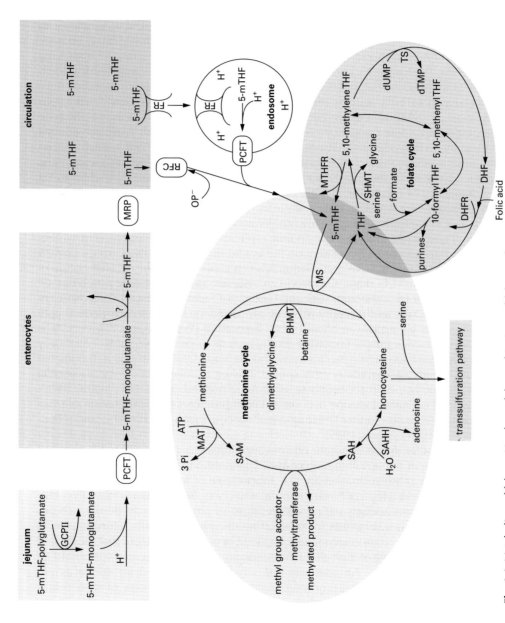

Fig. 6.4: Metabolism of folates; Uptake and the methionine and folate cycle.

reduced availability of SAM owing to reduced Hcy remethylation, but also owing to the inhibitory effect of SAH on methyltransferases (James, 2002).

The interdependency of all factors involved in folate metabolism make it difficult to discern which is an intermediate and which is an actual effector. However, the down-stream effects of these pathological processes have in common that they independently affect genomic, epigenomic and proteomic integrity (►Fig. 6.3) which are essential for normal cellular functioning.

6.2.2 Preconception folate in females

At birth, females have a resting pool of immature oocytes that have arrested in the diplotene stage of the meiotic prophase I. The oocyte is surrounded by a single layer of pregranulosa cells; together this is called the primordial follicle. During the process of follicular growth and maturation an antrum is formed which is filled with fluid. The follicular fluid is the microenvironment in which the developing oocyte resides. It is a plasma exudate that reflects follicular cell metabolism. As a result the magnitude of folate or folic acid ingestion affects 5-mTHF and homocysteine levels in follicular fluid (Steegers-Theunissen, 1993; Boxmeer, 2008). Continuously a cohort of follicles initiate the process of maturation, at the end of the monthly menstrual cycle one follicle and its oocyte have reached the maturity suitable for ovulation and consequent fertiliza-tion. The process of maturation initiation of a follicle and ovulation takes approximately three months (Hohmann, 2005), during which there is an increased need of nutrients. In the primordial follicle stage, the oocyte genome is relatively hypomethylated (Reik, 2001). During oocyte maturation the epigenome is re-established and there is active transcription of DNA and protein synthesis, processes for which an adequate supply of methyl groups from methionine and folate is an absolute prerequisite. The oocyte is the main source of organelles, proteins and other macromolecules found in the early embryo (Picton, 1998).

An adequate folate balance can potentially reduce the risk or overcome female subfertility (Czeizel, 1996; Westphal, 2004; Ebisch, 2007; Chavarro, 2008). Follic-ular sensitivity to gonadotrophins is, in part, modulated by proper functioning of the methionine cycle. Low MTHFR activity has been associated with low follicu-lar activity (Thaler, 2006; Rosen, 2007; Hecht, 2009) and consequently high Hcy levels are associated with an inadequate ovarian response to gonadotrophins in sheep (Kanakkaparambil, 2008). Furthermore, raised levels of Hcy in follicular fluid have a detrimental effect on oocyte and embryo quality (Szymański and Kazdepka-Ziemińska, 2003; Ebisch, 2006; Boxmeer, 2009a). An adequate redox balance influ-ences follicular development and ovulation (Agarwal, 2008), and a disruption of this balance has been shown to induce follicular atresia (Tsai-Turton and Luderer, 2006) and decrease sensitivity of the follicle to gonadotrophins (Margolin, 1990; Tilly and Tilly, 1995; Thaler, 2006).

6.2.3 Preconception folate in men

In men, preconception folate status potentially influences semen quality. During the mitotic phase of spermatogenesis methylation marks that are present have to be main-tained (Trasler, 2009). Also, the genome and cellular machinery is replicated adding to the increased demand for one-carbon groups from the folate- and methionine cycle. During mitosis and meiosis new methylation marks are acquired. The pattern of methylation is specific for the differentiation state of the spermatocyte and the entire epigenome is completely established at the pachytene stage of meiosis (Oakes, 2007).

Observational studies have indicated that males with a low dietary folate intake have a higher frequency of sperm aneuploidy (Young, 2008), increased levels of sperm DNA damage (Boxmeer, 2009b) and a low sperm density and count (Wallock, 2001), which is associated with a higher rate of subfertility. Furthermore, high thiol levels, including Hcy, in the ejaculate have been associated with male subfertility (Ebisch, 2006). By contrast, combined supplementation of folate and zinc sulfate increases the total normal sperm count by 76% (Wong, 2002). Despite the influence on folate metabolism, the MTHFR 677C→T polymorphism is only a risk factor when there is a co-existent folate deficiency (Ebisch, 2003; Lee, 2006).

Similar to follicular maturation, ROS are important second messengers during spermatogenesis (Donnelly, 2000). Spermatocytes have a high content of polyunsaturated fatty acids, lack DNA repair mechanisms and have no antioxidant defense (Kao, 2008). Therefore, the developing spermatocyte is exceptionally prone to disturbances in the redox balance resulting in oxidative stress, which can arise owing to hyperhomocysteinemia. In general, subfertile men have higher levels of ROS in semen, which is associated with lower sperm motility, fertilizing capacity and sperm DNA integrity (Yumura, 2009).

6.2.4 Postconception folate in females

During embryogenesis, folate-dependent processes are of importance for normal development. As has just been covered, at the point of fertilization the entire epigenome has been attained by both gametes. This pattern is specific for the oocyte and spermatocyte and, excluding imprinted genes, needs to be synchronized. Almost the entire DNA methylation pattern is erased after fertilization. With the exception of imprinted genes the genome is de-methylated at the blastocyst stage (Nafee, 2008). During subsequent cleavages from the blastocyst stage onward the DNA is re-methylated in a lineage specific manner (Nafee, 2008). The importance of an adequate supply of methyl groups during the periconception period is demonstrated by a phenotype of hypertension, obesity and diabetes in predominantly male offspring exposed to a low methionine diet during early pregnancy (Sinclair, 2007; Heijmans, 2008). Approximately 8 days post-fertilization placentation begins. Crucial for normal placentation is the invasion of trophoblasts into the endometrial epithelium (Jones and DeCherney, 2007). Excess levels of Hcy induces trophoblast apoptosis and inhibits trophoblast invasion into endometrial epithelium (Di Simone, 2003). As a possible result of excess Hcy, oxidative stress occurs that inhibits normal placentation and alters placental gene expression (Hempstock, 2003; Cindrova-Davies, 2007). Also in experimental settings folate deficiencies inhibit normal placentation and results in a higher fetal morbidity and mortality (Li, 2005; Pickell, 2009). Before circulation is established the embryo resides in a hypoxic environment, during which it is most susceptible to oxidative stress (Burton, 2007). During embryogenesis, ROS are important second messenger in the regulation of transcription factors (Dennery, 2007). Derangement hereof affects successful embryonic development and can result in miscarriages (Agarwal, 2008). This is also reflected by the lower embryo quality after *in vitro* embryo cultures, where embryos endure higher than normal levels of oxidative stress (Martín-Romero, 2008).

6.2.5 Folate and the fetus

A maternal deficiency of folate during the periconception period is associated with several congenital malformations of the fetus. Generally, congenital malformations are considered to be of multifactorial origin, being subject to both genetic and environmental influences. Neural crest cells are progenitors of structures most commonly affected by folate deficiencies. Relative to other embryonic progenitor cells, neuroepithelium cells have a high expression of folate receptors, indicating their dependency on a sufficient folate supply (Rosenquist and Finnell, 2001). *In vitro* studies have indicated that neural crest cells are sensitive to fluctuations in folate and Hcy concentrations (Boot, 2003).

Nutrients necessary for early fetal development are acquired from uterine secretions or, after proper placenta development, from the maternal circulation. Syncytiotrophoblasts form the endothelium of the placental vasculature (Jauniaux, 2006). On the apical membrane of the syncytiotrophoblast FR-α is expressed, which binds circulating 5-mTHF with high affinity. At the basolateral membrane 5-mTHF is transported from the syncytiotrophoblast into the fetal circulation facilitated by the reduced folate carrier. Theoretically this mechanism allows for the build-up of a high concentration gradient, securing fetal 5-mTHF supply, even in a folate deficient environment (Henderson, 1995; Prasad, 1998).

Historically, neural tube defects (NTD) pose the greatest example of congenital malformations owing to folate deficiency. A five-times reduction in NTD occurrence can be achieved by periconception folic acid supplement use by the mother (van der Linden, 2006b). Additionally, food folic acid fortification programs have shown a population-wide reduction in NTD occurrence ranging from 26 to 50% (Mills and Signore, 2004). Hyperhomocysteinemia in the mother has most widely been drawn on as risk indicator for NTD, with elevated levels being elicited by reduced availability of 5-mTHF owing to polymorphisms in genes involved in folate metabolism and uptake or nutritional folate deficiency. Many functional polymorphisms, in genes essential for folate uptake and metabolism have been investigated, nevertheless only the polymorphisms MTRR66A→G and MTHFR677C→T have been shown to increase the rate of NTD (van der Linden, 2006a,b). *In vitro* studies have indicated that direct interference with the efficiency of methylation reactions increases the occurrence of NTD (Afman, 2003, 2005; Dunlevy, 2006). In addition, oxidative stress alters expression of genes necessary for neural tube closure and increase the occurrence of NTD (Chang, 2003; Seonghun, 2007). Interestingly, a 70% reduction in NTD occurrence can be achieved by strong adherence to a Mediterranean diet alone (Vujkovic, 2009).

As the most frequently occurring congenital malformation, congenital heart defects (CHD) have been associated with a maternal deficiency of folate intake and/or metabolism. A 6% drop in the birth prevalence of CHD has been noted after the mandatory fortification of food with folic acid (Ionescu-Ittu, 2009), the underlying mechanism of this association is, however, still lacking. MTHFR deficiency owing to the 677C→T polymorphism and oxidative stress have been associated with CHD in an experimental setting (Li, 2005; Fisher, 2007; Pickell, 2009) and an excess of Hcy inhibits proper septation of the developing heart (Boot, 2004). Nevertheless, in the patient population only hyperhomocysteinemia in the mother posed a 4.4-times higher risk of CHD occurrence where MTHFR deficiency alone seems not to be a risk factor for congenital heart defects in offspring (Verkleij-Hagoort, 2007; van Driel, 2008). The common effect of reduced DNA methylation hereof has not been established as an etiologic factor in CHD occurrence.

Orofacial clefts (OFC) pose a heterogeneous group of malformations ranging from the relatively mild cleft lip to the more severe cleft palate with or without cleft lip. The occurrence of OFC has been related to folate deficiency in a multitude of studies (Johnson and Little, 2008). However, folate supplementation or MTHFR polymorphisms now seem not to be associated with the birth prevalence of OFC (Verkleij-Hagoort, 2007; Johnson and Little, 2008).

DNA hypomethylation can induce meiotic segregation errors which can give rise to trisomy 21 in offspring, causing Down syndrome (DS) (James, 1999). This association has led to the investigation of folate deficiency in DS occurrence. Despite a plausible biological mechanism, many contradicting observations have been made (Eskes, 2006) and no significant connection between maternal MTHFR deficiency or elevated homocysteine levels and DS exists (Zintzaras, 2007; Santos-Rebouças, 2008).

6.2.6 Folate metabolism and pregnancy complications

Between 50% and 60% of all conceptions fail to survive until the end of the first trimester of pregnancy (Norwitz, 2001). The placenta is a highly vascularized organ, therefore Hcy and causes underlying hyperhomocysteinemia have been proposed as a risk factor for placenta-linked pregnancy complications. Predominant among these are fetal growth restriction, pre-eclampsia, placental abruption and habitual abortion. In experimental studies there have been associations between MTHFR polymorphisms, folate deficiency and pregnancy complications (Li, 2005; Pickell, 2009). Nevertheless, experimental findings are not unanimously reflected in clinical findings, where fetal growth restriction (Facco, 2009), pre-eclampsia (Lin and August, 2005) and habitual abortion (Ren and Wang, 2006) are not associated with the MTHFR 677C→T polymorphism. Maternal Hcy status does, however, associate with the occurrence of placenta-related pregnancy complications (Goddijn-Wessel, 1996; Ray and Laskin, 1999; Nelen, 2000; Eskes, 2001; Cotter, 2003) and folic acid use during pregnancy reduced the risk of low-birthweight and small-for-gestational-age fetuses (Timmermans, 2009). In the case of pre-eclampsia, however, it is not clear whether the hyperhomocysteinemic state is the cause or effect of the pathological process (Mignini, 2005). Only hyperhomocysteinemia and not MTHFR polymorphisms as a risk factor can be explained by the fact that the methylation pathway is restored by folic acid use, which is widely recommend to all pregnant women in the western world.

6.2.7 Conclusion

Evidence is accumulating on the significance of an adequate methylation pathway during human reproduction. Because various essential pathways are affected by a shortage of folate, research into the etiology, pathophysiology and prevention of adverse reproductive outcome is complicated. This is further complicated by the fact that intervention studies during human pregnancies are nearly impossible, which necessitates inference from *in vitro* and animal models or observational studies.

Research into single nutrients and gene polymorphisms is a necessity to identify new risk factors and helps to explain underlying biological mechanisms. This type of research, however, is best suited for highly controlled animal- and *in vitro* studies. In epidemiological studies the rational is to focus on associations between adverse reproductive outcome and the compounded biomarkers of the folate- and methionine cycle, i.e., homocysteine, S-adenosyl methionine, S-adenosyl homocysteine, vitamin B12, and DNA and histone methylation patterns (van Driel, 2009). In addition to folate, many cofactors and proper functioning genes are needed for the provision of methyl-groups. Because intrinsically biomarkers and methylation patterns of the genome are adjusted for factors influencing these determinants, both measurements are useful to assess the long- and short-term folate status.

Despite growing knowledge on epigenetic mechanisms and intriguing evidence in animals, at present little is known about the relation between adverse reproductive outcome and epigenetics in human. The epigenome is at the crossroad of environmental exposure and gene expression profiles. Therefore, epigenetics pose an interesting field of future research, which can aid in the identification of both genetic and environmental exposures underlying adverse reproductive outcome associated with methylation cycle deficiencies.

References

Afman LA, Blom HJ, Put NMJVD, Straaten HWMV, Homocysteine interference in neurulation: a chick embryo model. Birth Defects Res A Clin Mol Teratol 2003;67: 421–28.

Afman LA, Blom HJ, Drittij M-J, Brouns MR, van Straaten HWM, Inhibition of transmethylation disturbs neurulation in chick embryos. Brain Res Dev Brain Res 2005;158: 59–65.

Agarwal A, Gupta S, Sekhon L, Shah R, Redox considerations in female reproductive function and assisted reproduction: from molecular mechanisms to health implications. Antioxid Redox Signal 2008;10: 1375–403.

Bliek BJB, Steegers-Theunissen RPM, Blok LJ, Santegoets LAM, Lindemans J, Oostra BA, Steegers EAP, de Klein A, Genome-wide pathway analysis of folate-responsive genes to unravel the pathogenesis of orofacial clefting in man. Birth Defects Res A Clin Mol Teratol 2008;82: 627–35.

Blom HJ, Folic acid, methylation and neural tube closure in humans. Birth Defects Res A Clin Mol Teratol 2009;85: 295–302.

Boot MJ, Steegers-Theunissen RPM, Poelmann RE, van Iperen L, Lindemans J, Gittenberger-De Groot AC, Folic acid and homocysteine affect neural crest and neuroepithelial cell outgrowth and differentiation in vitro. Dev Dyn 2003;227: 301–8.

Boot MJ, Steegers-Theunissen RPM, Poelmann RE, van Iperen L, Gittenberger-de Groot AC, Cardiac outflow tract malformations in chick embryos exposed to homocysteine. Cardiovasc Res 2004;64: 365–73.

Boxmeer JC, Brouns RM, Lindemans J, Steegers EAP, Martini E, Macklon NS, Steegers-Theunissen RPM, Preconception folic acid treatment affects the microenvironment of the maturing oocyte in humans. Fertil Steril 2008;89: 1766–70.

Boxmeer JC, Macklon NS, Lindemans J, Beckers NGM, Eijkemans MJC, Laven JSE, Steegers EAP, Steegers-Theunissen RPM, IVF outcomes are associated with biomarkers of the homocysteine pathway in monofollicular fluid. Hum Reprod 2009a;24: 1059–66.

Boxmeer JC, Smit M, Utomo E, Romijn JC, Eijkemans MJC, Lindemans J, Laven JSE, Macklon NS, Steegers EAP, Steegers-Theunissen RPM, Low folate in seminal plasma is associated with increased sperm DNA damage. Fertil Steril 2009b;92: 548–56.

Brosnan J, Jacobs R, Stead L, Brosnan M, Methylation demand: a key determinant of homocysteine metabolism. Acta Biochim Pol 2004;51: 405–13.

Burton G, Jauniaux E, Charnock-Jones D, Human early placental development: potential roles of the endometrial glands. Placenta 2007;28: 64–9.

Castro R, Rivera I, Ravasco P, Camilo M, Jakobs C, Blom H, de Almeida I, 5,10-methylenetetra-hydrofolate reductase (MTHFR) 677C→T and 1298A→C mutations are associated with DNA hypomethylation. J Med Genet 2004;41: 454–8.

Chang TI, Horal M, Jain SK, Wang F, Patel R, Loeken MR, Oxidant regulation of gene expression and neural tube development: Insights gained from diabetic pregnancy on molecular causes of neural tube defects. Diabetologia 2003;46: 538–45.

Chavarro JE, Rich-Edwards JW, Rosner BA, Willett WC, Use of multivitamins, intake of B vitamins, and risk of ovulatory infertility. Fertil Steril 2008;89: 668–76.

Cindrova-Davies T, Yung H-W, Johns J, Spasic-Boskovic O, Korolchuk S, Jauniaux E, Burton GJ, Charnock-Jones DS, Oxidative stress, gene expression, and protein changes induced in the human placenta during labor. Am J Pathol 2007;171: 1168–79.

Cotter A, Molloy A, Scott J, Daly S, Elevated plasma homocysteine in early pregnancy: a risk factor for the development of nonsevere preeclampsia. Am J Obstet Gynecol 2003;189: 391–4.

Czeizel A, Métneki J, Dudás I, The effect of preconceptional multivitamin supplementation on fertility. Int J Vitam Nutr Res 1996;66: 55–8.

Dennery PA, Effects of oxidative stress on embryonic development. Birth Defects Res C Embryo Today 2007;81: 155–62.

Di Simone N, Maggiano N, Caliandro D, Riccardi P, Evangelista A, Carducci B, Caruso A, Homocysteine induces trophoblast cell death with apoptotic features. Biol Reprod 2003;69: 1129–34.

Donnelly ET, McClure N, Lewis SEM, Glutathione and hypotaurine in vitro: effects on human sperm motility, DNA integrity and production of reactive oxygen species. Mutagenesis 2000; 15: 61–8.

Dunlevy LPE, Burren KA, Chitty LS, Copp AJ, Greene NDE, Excess methionine suppresses the methylation cycle and inhibits neural tube closure in mouse embryos. FEBS Lett 2006;580: 2803–7.

Ebisch IMW, Peters WHM, Thomas CMG, Wetzels AMM, Peer PGM, Steegers-Theunissen RPM, Homocysteine, glutathione and related thiols affect fertility parameters in the (sub)fertile couple. Hum Reprod 2006;21: 1725–33.

Ebisch IMW, van Heerde WL, Thomas CMG, van der Put N, Wong WY, Steegers-Theunissen RPM, C677T methylenetetrahydrofolate reductase polymorphism interferes with the effects of folic acid and zinc sulfate on sperm concentration. Fertil Steril 2003;80: 1190–4.

Ebisch IMW, Thomas CMG, Peters WHM, Braat DDM, Steegers-Theunissen RPM, The importance of folate, zinc and antioxidants in the pathogenesis and prevention of subfertility. Hum Reprod Update 2007;13: 163–74.

Eskes TKAB, Clotting disorders and placental abruption: homocysteine – a new risk factor. Eur J Obstet Gynecol Reprod Biol 2001;95: 206–12.

Eskes TKAB, Abnormal folate metabolism in mothers with Down syndrome offspring: review of the literature. Eur J Obstet Gynecol Reprod Biol 2006;124: 130–3.

Facco FMD, You WMD, Grobman WMDMBA, Genetic thrombophilias and intrauterine growth restriction: a meta-analysis. Obstet Gynecol 2009;113: 1206–16.

Finkelstein JD, Metabolic regulatory properties of S-adenosylmethionine and S-adenosylhomocysteine. Clin Chem Lab Med 2007;45: 1694–9.

Fisher SA, The developing embryonic cardiac outflow tract is highly sensitive to oxidant stress. Dev Dyn 2007;236: 3496–502.

Friso S, Choi S-W, Girelli D, Mason JB, Dolnikowski GG, Bagley PJ, Olivieri O, Jacques PF, Rosenberg IH, Corrocher R, Selhub J, A common mutation in the 5,10-methylenetetrahydrofolate reductase gene affects genomic DNA methylation through an interaction with folate status. Proc Natl Acad Sci USA 2002;99: 5606–11.

Frosst P, Blom H, Milos R, Goyette P, Sheppard C, Matthews R, Boers G, den Heijer M, Kluijtmans L, van den Heuvel L, A candidate genetic risk factor for vascular disease: a common mutation in methylenetetrahydrofolate reductase. Nat Genet 1995;10: 111–3.

Goddijn-Wessel TAW, Wouters MGAJ, van den Molen EF, Spuijbroek MDEH, Steegers-Theunissen RPM, Blom HJ, Boers GHJ, Eskes TKAB, Hyperhomocysteinemia: a risk factor for placental abruption or infarction. Eur J Obstet Gynecol Reprod Biol 1996;66: 23–9.

Hecht S, Pavlik R, Lohse P, Noss U, Friese K, Thaler CJ, Common 677C→T mutation of the 5,10-methylenetetrahydrofolate reductase gene affects follicular estradiol synthesis. Fertil Steril 2009;91: 56–61.

Heijmans BT, Tobi EW, Stein AD, Putter H, Blauw GJ, Susser ES, Slagboom PE, Lumey LH, Persistent epigenetic differences associated with prenatal exposure to famine in humans. Proc Natl Acad Sci USA 2008;105: 17046–9.

Hempstock J, Jauniaux E, Greenwold N, Burton GJ, The contribution of placental oxidative stress to early pregnancy failure. Hum Pathol 2003;34: 1265–75.

Henderson G, Perez T, Schenker S, Mackins J, Antony A, Maternal-to-fetal transfer of 5-methyltetrahydrofolate by the perfused human placental cotyledon: evidence for a concentrative role by placental folate receptors in fetal folate delivery. J Lab Clin Med 1995;126: 184–203.

Ionescu-Ittu R, Marelli AJ, Mackie AS, Pilote L, Prevalence of severe congenital heart disease after folic acid fortification of grain products: time trend analysis in Quebec, Canada. Br Med J 2009;338: b1673.

Jakubowski H, Molecular basis of homocysteine toxicity in humans. Cell Mol Life Sci 2004;61: 470–87.

James SJ, Miller BJ, Basnakian AG, Pogribny IP, Pogribna M, Muskhelishvili L, Apoptosis and proliferation under conditions of deoxynucleotide pool imbalance in liver of folate/methyl deficient rats. Carcinogenesis 1997;18: 287–93.

James SJ, Pogribna M, Pogribny IP, Melnyk S, Hine RJ, Gibson JB, Yi P, Tafoya DL, Swenson DH, Wilson VL, Gaylor DW, Abnormal folate metabolism and mutation in the methylenetetrahydrofolate reductase gene may be maternal risk factors for Down syndrome. Am J Clin Nutr 1999;70: 495–501.

James SJ, Melnyk S, Pogribna M, Pogribny IP, Caudill MA, Elevation in S-Adenosylhomocysteine, DNA hypomethylation: potential epigenetic mechanism for homocysteine-related pathology. J Nutr 2002;132: 2361–6.

Jauniaux E, Poston L, Burton GJ, Placental-related diseases of pregnancy: involvement of oxidative stress and implications in human evolution. Hum Reprod Update 2006;12: 747–55.

Johnson CY, Little J, Folate intake, markers of folate status and oral clefts: is the evidence converging? Int J Epidemiol 2008;37: 1041–58.

Jones E, DeCherney A, In: Boron W, Boulpaep E, editors. Medical physiology: a cellular and molecular approach. Philadelphia: WB Saunders; 2007.

Kanakkaparambil R, Singh R, Li D, Webb R, Sinclair KD, B-Vitamin and homocysteine status determines ovarian response to gonadotropin treatment in sheep. Biol Reprod 2008;80: 743–52.

Kao S-H, Chao H-T, Chen H-W, Hwang TIS, Liao T-L, Wei Y-H, Increase of oxidative stress in human sperm with lower motility. Fertil Steril 2008;89: 1183–90.

Lee H-C, Jeong Y-M, Lee SH, Cha KY, Song S-H, Kim NK, Lee KW, Lee S, Association study of four polymorphisms in three folate-related enzyme genes with non-obstructive male infertility. Hum Reprod 2006;21: 3162–70.

Li D, Pickell L, Liu Y, Wu Q, Cohn JS, Rozen R, Maternal methylenetetrahydrofolate reductase deficiency and low dietary folate lead to adverse reproductive outcomes and congenital heart defects in mice. Am J Clin Nutr 2005;82: 188–95.

Lin J, August P, Genetic thrombophilias and preeclampsia: a meta-analysis. Obstet Gynecol 2005;105: 182–92.

Margolin Y, Aten RF, Behrman HR, Antigonadotropic and antisteroidogenic actions of peroxide in rat granulosa cells. Endocrinology 1990;127: 245–50.

Martín-Romero F, Miguel-Lasobras E, Domínguez-Arroyo J, González-Carrera E, Alvarez I, Contribution of culture media to oxidative stress and its effect on human oocytes. Reprod Biomed Online 2008;17: 652–61.

Mignini L, Latthe P, Villar J, Kilby MD, Carroli G, Khan K, Mapping the theories of preeclampsia: the role of homocysteine. Obstet Gynecol 2005;105: 411–25.

Mills JL, Signore C, Neural tube defect rates before and after food fortification with folic acid. Birth Defects Res A Clin Mol Teratol 2004;70: 844–5.

Molloy A, Scott J, Folates and prevention of disease. Public Health Nutr 2001;4: 601–9.

Nafee TM, Farrell WE, Carroll WD, Fryer AA, Ismail KM, Epigenetic control of fetal gene expression. BJOG 2008;115: 158–68.

Nelen WLDM, Blom HJ, Steegers EAP, den Heijer M, Eskes TKAB, Hyperhomocysteinemia and recurrent early pregnancy loss: a meta-analysis. Fertil Steril 2000;74: 1196–9.

Norwitz ER, Schust DJ, Fisher SJ, Implantation and the survival of early pregnancy. N Eng J Med 2001;345: 1400–8.

Oakes CC, La Salle S, Smiraglia DJ, Robaire B, Trasler JM, Developmental acquisition of genome-wide DNA methylation occurs prior to meiosis in male germ cells. Dev Biol 2007;307: 368–79.

Pickell L, Li D, Brown K, Mikael LG, Wang X-L, Wu Q, Luo L, Jerome-Majewska L, Rozen R, Methylenetetrahydrofolate reductase deficiency and low dietary folate increase embryonic delay and placental abnormalities in mice. Birth Defects Res A Clin Mol Teratol 2009;85: 531–41.

Picton H, Briggs D, Gosden R, The molecular basis of oocyte growth and development. Mol Cell Endocrinol 1998;145: 27–37.

Pogribny IP, Basnakian AG, Miller BJ, Lopatina NG, Poirier LA, James SJ, Breaks in genomic DNA and within the p53 gene are associated with hypomethylation in livers of folate/methyl-deficient rats. Cancer Res 1995;55: 1894–901.

Pogribny IP, Muskhelishvili L, Miller BJ, James SJ, Presence and consequence of uracil in preneoplastic DNA from folate/methyl-deficient rats. Carcinogenesis 1997;18: 2071–6.

Prasad PD, Leibach FH, Ganapathy V, Transplacental transport of water-soluble vitamins: a review. Placenta 1998;19: 243–57.

Rawlings ND, Barrett AJ, Structure of membrane glutamate carboxypeptidase. Biochim Biophys Acta 1997;1339: 247–52.

Ray JG, Laskin CA, Folic acid and homocyst(e)ine metabolic defects and the risk of placental abruption, pre-eclampsia and spontaneous pregnancy loss: a systematic review. Placenta 1999;20: 519–29.

Reik W, Dean W, Walter J, Epigenetic reprogramming in mammalian development. Science 2001;103: 35–47.

Ren A, Wang J, Methylenetetrahydrofolate reductase C677T polymorphism and the risk of unexplained recurrent pregnancy loss: a meta-analysis. Fertil Steril 2006;86: 1716–22.

Rosen MP, Shen S, McCulloch CE, Rinaudo PF, Cedars MI, Dobson AT, Methylenetetrahydrofolate reductase (MTHFR) is associated with ovarian follicular activity. Fertil Steril 2007;88: 632–38.

Rosenquist T, Finnell R, Genes, folate and homocysteine in embryonic development. Proc Nutr Soc 2001;60: 53–61.

Santos-Rebouças CB, Corrêa JC, Bonomo A, Fintelman-Rodrigues N, Moura KCV, Rodrigues CSC, Santos JM, Pimentel MMG, The impact of folate pathway polymorphisms combined to nutritional deficiency as a maternal predisposition factor for Down syndrome. Dis Markers 2008;25: 149–57.

Seonghun R, Roni K, Amram S, Asher O, Nitroxide radicals protect cultured rat embryos and yolk sacs from diabetic-induced damage. Birth Defects Res A Clin Mol Teratol 2007;79: 604–11.

Sinclair KD, Allegrucci C, Singh R, Gardner DS, Sebastian S, Bispham J, Thurston A, Huntley JF, Rees WD, Maloney CA, Lea RG, Craigon J, McEvoy TG, Young LE, DNA methylation, insulin resistance, and blood pressure in offspring determined by maternal periconceptional B vitamin and methionine status. Proc Nutr Soc Sci USA 2007;104: 19351–6.

Steegers-Theunissen R, Steegers E, Thomas C, Hollanders H, Peereboom-Stegeman J, Trijbels F, Eskes T, Study on the presence of homocysteine in ovarian follicular fluid. Fertil Steril 1993;60: 1006–10.

Szymański W, Kazdepka-Ziemińska A, Effect of homocysteine concentration in follicular fluid on a degree of oocyte maturity. Ginekol Pol 2003;74: 1392–6.

Thaler CJ, Budiman H, Ruebsamen H, Nagel D, Lohse P, Effects of the common 677C→T mutation of the 5,10-Methylenetetrahydrofolate Reductase (MTHFR) gene on ovarian responsiveness to recombinant follicle-stimulating hormone. Am J Reprod Immunol 2006;55: 251–8.

Tilly JL, Tilly KI, Inhibitors of oxidative stress mimic the ability of follicle-stimulating hormone to suppress apoptosis in cultured rat ovarian follicles. Endocrinology 1995;136: 242–52.

Timmermans S, Jaddoe VWV, Hofman A, Steegers-Theunissen RgPM, Steegers EAP, Periconception folic acid supplementation, fetal growth and the risks of low birth weight and preterm birth: the Generation R Study. Br J Nutr 2009;102: 777–85.

Trasler JM, Epigenetics in spermatogenesis. Mol Cell Endocrinol 2009;306: 33–6.

Tsai-Turton M, Luderer U, Opposing effects of glutathione depletion and follicle-stimulating hormone on reactive oxygen species and apoptosis in cultured preovulatory rat follicles. Endocrinology 2006;147: 1224–36.

Ulrey CL, Liu L, Andrews LG, Tollefsbol TO, The impact of metabolism on DNA methylation. Hum Mol Genet 2005;14: 139–47.

van der Linden I, den Heijer M, Afman L, Gellekink H, Vermeulen S, Kluijtmans L, Blom H, The methionine synthase reductase 66A>G polymorphism is a maternal risk factor for spina bifida. J Mol Med 2006a;84: 1047–54.

van der Linden IJM, Afman LA, Heil SG, Blom HJ, Genetic variation in genes of folate metabolism and neural-tube defect risk. Birth Defects Res A Clin Mol Teratol 2006b;65: 204–15.

van Driel L, de Jonge R, Helbing W, van Zelst B, Ottenkamp J, Steegers E, Steegers-Theunissen R, Maternal global methylation status and risk of congenital heart diseases. Obstet Gynecol 2008;2: 277–83.

van Driel L, Eijkemans M, de Jonge R, de Vries J, van Meurs J, Steegers E, Steegers-Theunissen R, Body Mass Index is an important determinant of methylation biomarkers in women of reproductive ages. J Nutr 2009;139: 2315–21.

Verkleij-Hagoort A, Bliek J, Sayed-Tabatabaei F, Ursem N, Steegers E, Steegers-Theunissen R, Hyperhomocysteinemia and MTHFR polymorphisms in association with orofacial clefts and congenital heart defects: a meta-analysis. Am J Med Genet A 2007;143A: 952–60.

Vujkovic M, Steegers EA, Looman CW, Ocké MC, van der Spek PJ, Steegers-Theunissen RP, The maternal Mediterranean dietary pattern is associated with a reduced risk of spina bifida in the offspring. BJOG 2009;116: 408–15.

Wainfan E, Poirier LA, Methyl groups in carcinogenesis: effects on DNA methylation and gene expression. Cancer Res 1992;52: 2071–7.

Wallock LM, Tamura T, Mayr CA, Johnston KE, Ames BN, Jacob RA, Low seminal plasma folate concentrations are associated with low sperm density and count in male smokers and nonsmokers. Fertil Steril 2001;75: 252–9.

Westphal L, Polan M, Trant A, Mooney S, A nutritional supplement for improving fertility in women: a pilot study. J Reprod Med 2004;49: 289–93.

Wilson A, Platt R, Wu Q, Leclerc D, Christensen B, Yang H, Gravel RA, Rozen R, A common variant in methionine synthase reductase combined with low cobalamin increases risk for spina bifida. Mol Genet Metab 1999;67: 317–23.

Wong WY, Merkus HMWM, Thomas CMG, Menkveld R, Zielhuis GA, Steegers-Theunissen RPM, Effects of folic acid and zinc sulfate on male factor subfertility: a double-blind, randomized, placebo-controlled trial. Fertil Steril 2002;77: 491–8.

Young SS, Eskenazi B, Marchetti FM, Block G, Wyrobek AJ, The association of folate, zinc and antioxidant intake with sperm aneuploidy in healthy non-smoking men. Hum Reprod 2008;23: 1014–22.

Yumura Y, Iwasaki A, Saito K, Ogawa T, Hirokawa M, Effect of reactive oxygen species in semen on the pregnancy of infertile couples. Int J Urol 2009;16: 202–7.

Zhao R, Matherly L, Goldman I, Membrane transporters and folate homeostasis: intestinal absorption and transport into systemic compartments and tissues. Expert Rev Mol Med 2009;11: e4.

Zintzaras E, Maternal gene polymorphisms involved in folate metabolism and risk of Down syndrome offspring: a meta-analysis. Hum Mol Genet 2007;52: 943–53.

Zou C-G, Banerjee R, Homocysteine and redox signaling. Antioxid Redox Signal 2005;7: 547–59.

6.3 Folate fortification for prevention of neural tube defects

Elizabeth B. Gorman; Richard H. Finnell

6.3.1 Introduction

Birth defects are a global problem that affect approximately 6% of all births causing the deaths of 3.3 million children under the age of five annually (Christianson et al., 2006). Indeed, birth defects are one, if not the leading healthcare concern for the youngest members of our societies. Furthermore, all women are at risk of having a baby with a birth defect, regardless of their age, race, income, or socioeconomic status and, in most cases, the cause of any given birth defect is unknown.

It has been widely appreciated for more than 50 years that folates, essential B-vitamins, are crucial for embryonic development. Animal models subjected to folate deprivation during pregnancy often give birth to malformed offspring (Nelson et al., 1952; Baird et al., 1954). As long ago as 1965 it was suggested that folate deficiency might play a role in the etiology of the common serious congenital malformations of the brain and spinal cord known as neural tube defects (NTDs) (Hibbard et al., 1965). Multiple rigorous studies were conducted in the 1980s and 1990s on folic acid (FA) supplementation, either with or without a multivitamin, and risk of NTD-affected pregnancy (Smithells et al., 1980; Laurence et al., 1981; Mulinare et al., 1988; Bower and Stanley, 1989; Vergel et al., 1990; Wald et al., 1991; Czeizel and Dudas, 1992; Werler et al., 1993; Shaw et al., 1995; Berry et al., 1999). The results of these studies were so striking that several trials had to be stopped prematurely so that all women could be advised to take FA supplements (Wald et al., 1991; Czeizel and Dudas, 1992). With these studies came the realization that the majority of NTD-affected pregnancies could be prevented by folate supplementation and this has been one of the greatest successes of modern birth defects research.

This chapter discusses selected national folate intake recommendations and how these have altered folate consumption and the prevalence of NTD-affected pregnancies. This is followed by a discussion of several folate fortification programs and their impact on NTD-affected pregnancies. Next, other consequences of folate fortification programs are considered. Finally, vitamin B12 fortification will be discussed as well as a possible mechanism of action of folate and vitamin B12 during development.

6.3.2 Neural tube defects (NTDs)

The incidence of NTDs worldwide varies from 0.17 to 6.39 per 1000 live births , making NTDs the second most common structural birth defect (Bowman et al., 2009). NTDs result from incomplete closure of the neural tube around the 28th day of pregnancy leading to severe abnormalities of the brain and/or spinal cord (Greene and Copp, 2009). The most prevalent NTDs are spina bifida, where incomplete closure occurs at the caudal end of the neural tube affecting the spine and anencephaly, where the incomplete closure occurs at the rostral end of the neural tube affecting the brain. Anencephaly is universally fatal, whereas spina bifida can be survivable with adequate medical care but with life-long neurological, orthopedic and urological disabilities (Greene et al., 2009). Other less common forms of NTDs include encephalocele, craniorachischisis and iniencephaly. Amazingly, one single factor, maternal folate status, can have dramatic affects on the incidence of NTDs. Equally dramatic is the fact that we have been able to achieve this remarkable reduction in the prevalence of NTDs with folate supplementation in the absence of having any mechanistic understanding how this might occur.

6.3.3 Vitamin B9

Vitamin B9 is an essential water-soluble vitamin that cannot be synthesized *de novo* in humans, so it must be obtained through the diet or by supplementation. The synthetic form of vitamin B9 found in supplements is folic acid (FA), whereas the natural forms are the folates. Leafy vegetables, legumes, citrus fruits, liver and baker's yeast are rich natural sources of folates. 5-Methyltetrahydrofolate (5-methyl-THF) is the physiologically active form of vitamin B9 whose major metabolic role is to carry one-carbon units (▶Fig. 6.5). One-carbon metabolism involves such important molecules as purines and thymidylate for nucleotide biosynthesis, amino acids for protein biosynthesis and methyl groups for the methylation of lipids, nucleotides and proteins. All these critical building blocks are undoubtedly crucial during the rapid cellular proliferation that occurs during gestation.

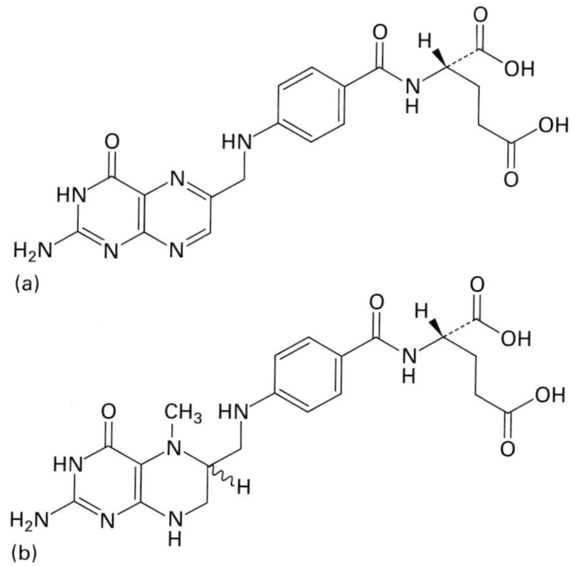

Fig. 6.5: Chemical structures of (a) folic acid and (b) 5-methyltetrahydrofolate.

6.3.4 One-carbon metabolism

During one-carbon metabolism, methylenetetrahydrofolate reductase (MTHFR) catalyzes the irreversible reduction of 5,10-methylenetetrahydrofolate (5,10-methylene-THF) to 5-methyl-THF. 5-Methyl-THF is the methyl donor required for the conversion of homocysteine to the amino acid methionine via the enzyme methionine synthase (MTR) which requires vitamin B12 as a cofactor. 5,10-Methylene-THF can be regenerated from the THF produced in the MTR reaction by the donation of a methyl group from the amino acid serine in a reaction catalyzed by the enzyme serine hydroxymethyl transferase (SHMT). The methionine produced from homocysteine in the MTR reaction can serve as a precursor of S-adenosylmethionine (SAM), which is the principal methyl donor for the methylation of lipids, nucleotides and proteins. THF can be condensed with formate to yield 10-formyl-THF, the precursor of the purines which are required in nucleotide biosynthesis. Additionally, thymidylate synthase (TS) can catalyze the transfer of a methyl group from the 5,10-methylene-THF to methylate deoxyuridylate monophosphate producing thymidylate which is necessary for DNA biosynthesis (Beaudin and Stover, 2009; Stover, 2009) (▶Fig. 6.6). With folates having key roles in multiple biochemical pathways, there are many events during embryogenesis that could be compromised by folate deficiency resulting in aberrant development.

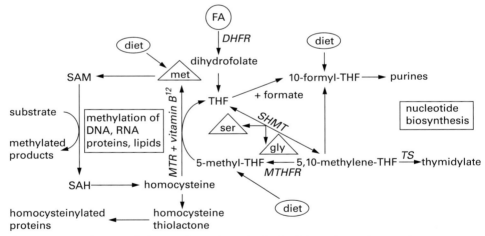

Fig. 6.6: One-carbon metabolism. Folic acid (FA) is obtained through supplementation or the consumption of fortified foods, whereas natural folates are obtained from dietary sources exclusive of fortified products. Whatever the entry point, folates/FA is crucial to the reactions necessary for nucleotide and protein biosynthesis as well as methylation reactions. Abbreviations: 5-methyl-THF, 5-methyltetrahydrofolate; 5,10-methylene-THF, 5,10-methylenetetrahydrofolate; 10-formyl-THF, 10-formyltetrahrdrofolate; FA, folic acid; MTR, methionine synthase; MTHFR, methylenetetrahydrofolate reductase; SAH, S-adenosylhomocysteine; SAM, S-adenosylmethionine; SHMT, serine hydroxymethyl transferase; THF, tetrahydrofolate; and TS, thymidylate synthase. Enzymes are in italics and the amino acids necessary for protein biosynthesis are in outlined by triangles.

6.3.5 Folic acid supplementation recommendations

Tab. 6.1: Seven national recommendations of folate consumption for the prevention of NTDs. All countries recommended daily folic acid supplements except Finland which recommended a healthy diet including many folate rich foods. Supplements of 400 µg of folic acid were recommended for all countries except the Netherlands which recommended 500 µg. The efficacy of the recommendations is presented as the percentage of the follow-up population meeting the recommendation by the follow-up date.

Date	Country	Target population	Follow-up date	Follow-up population	Efficacy	Reference
1992	USA	Childbearing-aged women	1995	Same	25	(MMWR, 1995)
1992	UK	Preconception through 1st trimester	2002–2004	Same	29	(Botto et al., 2005; Brough et al., 2009)
1993	Netherlands	4 weeks before to 8 weeks after conception	1996–2007	Women who want to become pregnant	Increasing from 5 to 36	(Botto et al., 2005; Weggemans et al., 2009)
1993	Ireland	Preconception through 1st trimester	2000	Pregnant women	18	(Oleary et al., 2001; Botto et al., 2005)
1993	China	Preconception through 1st trimester	1993–1995	Pregnant women	81 to 87	(Berry et al., 1999)
1995	Finland	Pregnant women	1998–1999	Same	56	(Botto et al., 2005; Arkkola et al., 2006)
1998	Norway	Childbearing-aged women	2000–2003	Pregnant women	10	(Botto et al., 2005; Nilsen et al., 2006)

For the first time, a birth defect could be efficiently and inexpensively prevented by maternal supplementation with a simple vitamin – FA. In recognition of this, many nations worldwide developed recommendations for folate consumption by women in their reproductive years. The specifics of the recommendations vary, but typically include daily intake of 400 µg of FA periconceptionally.

The recommendations for seven nations (USA, UK, The Netherlands, Ireland, China, Finland and Norway) are presented in ▶Tab. 6.1. These recommendations were made between 1992 and 1998 and target various subsections of the female population. All policies were for daily supplementation with 400 µg of FA except Norway, which recommended 500 µg and Finland, which recommended 400 µg folates through a healthy diet containing folate-rich foods. Follow-up studies were conducted before any changes in folate recommendations (e.g., in the USA before voluntary fortification commenced in 1996). The efficacy of the recommendations is presented as the percentage of the follow-up population meeting the recommendation.

There are some problems inherent to FA supplementation recommendations for the prevention of NTDs. Recommendations targeting pregnant women will miss women who do not yet know they are pregnant. Because neural tube closure occurs before pregnancy is clinically evident, this is a considerable number. Recommendations targeting women who plan to become pregnant will also miss a substantial number of women because a large portion of pregnancies in most countries are unplanned (Busby et al., 2005). Additionally, many women do not know the importance of folates in the reduction of NTD-affected pregnancies and even those who do, might not be willing to take supplements (MMWR, 1999). These issues seriously limit the success of the national folate supplementation recommendations.

In the absence of FA fortification many women do not consume the desired target levels of folates during very early embryogenesis that are recommended by the national policies. The folate consumption follow-up data presented in ▶Tab. 6.1 is from immediately to 10 years after each national recommendation. The percentage of women in the follow-up populations who were consuming the recommended daily dose of folates during the recommended time ranged from 5% to 87% with the majority of the national recommendations falling far short of their goals.

The real test of any national folate consumption recommendation is if they have decreased the number of NTD-affected pregnancies. At the onset of most of the folate supplementation recommendations, the prevalence of NTDs was already declining in the UK and Ireland (Busby et al., 2005), so the continuation of this trend after the recommendations cannot be attributed to the success of either. This evidence and that of other studies suggests that during 1988 to 1998, recommendations alone did not significantly influence trends in NTD-affected pregnancies in Norway, Finland, The Netherlands, UK, or Ireland (Botto et al., 2005). China, by contrast, has had great success in three provinces where they counseled consumption of 400 µg FA daily from premarital exam through the first trimester of pregnancy, resulting in a 16–85% reduction in NTD-affected pregnancies (Berry et al., 1999). Because the majority of countries did not see significant reductions in NTD-affected pregnancies resulting from FA recommendations only, it was evident that the target population was not being reached and recommendations were insufficient to effect the desired reduction in NTD births.

6.3.6 Folic acid fortification

The largely disappointing results of national FA supplementation recommendations paved the way for a multitude of FA fortification programs that were started around the world. These programs are voluntary, mandatory, or voluntary on some food items and mandatory on others. Voluntary fortification allows manufacturers to add vitamins and/or minerals to their food products, whereas mandatory fortification requires it.

Six FA fortification programs in four countries and their affect on the prevalence of NTDs are shown in ▶Tab. 6.2. The partial fortification program listed for Canada starting in 1997 was voluntary from 1997 to 1998 and then mandatory from 1998 to 2000. The enriched cereal grain products fortified in the USA and Canada include flour, rice,

Tab. 6.2: Six folic acid (FA) fortification programs in four countries for the prevention of neural tube defects (NTDs).

Date of fortification and type	Country	Products fortified	Amount of FA fortified with	Follow-up time period	Reduction in NTDs (%)	Reference
1996, voluntary	USA	Enriched cereal grain	140 µg per 100 g	1997–1998	Spina bifida 18, Anencephaly 16	(Williams et al., 2002)
1997, partial	Canada	Enriched cereal grain	60 to 270 µg per 100 g	1997–2000	31	(De Wals et al., 2007)
1998, mandatory	USA	Enriched cereal grain	140 µg per 100 g	1998–1999	Spina bifida 31, Anencephaly 16	(Williams et al., 2002)
1998, mandatory	Canada	Enriched cereal grain	150 to 270 µg per 100 g	2000–2002	46	(De Wals, et al., 2007)
2000, mandatory	Chile	Wheat flour	220 µg per 100 g	2001–2002	43	(Hertrampf and Cortes, 2008)
2004, mandatory	Brazil	Wheat and corn flour	150 µg per 100 g	2005–2006	29	(Pacheco et al., 2009)

pasta and cornmeal (Fletcher et al., 2004). The USA data are from 24 of 27 birth defects surveillance systems participating in the National Birth Defects Prevention Network (Williams et al., 2002). The Canadian data are from seven provinces (De Wals et al., 2007). The Chilean data are from nine hospitals in Santiago (Hertrampf and Cortes, 2008). The Brazilian data are from the city of Recife and this reduction of NTDs was reported as not statistically significant (Pacheco et al., 2009).

The influence on the prevalence of NTD-affected pregnancies in the four countries with the longest running FA fortification programs was mixed, but so too were the adoption strategies that they used to develop their fortification programs. Furthermore, all the genetic and environmental factors involved in the etiology of NTDs could modify the effects of FA such that the fortification outcomes would be similarly modified by factors unique to each country. However, for the USA and Canada, where data exist from two different types of fortification program, mandatory fortification lead to a greater reduction in NTD-affected pregnancies. As of January 2008, 52 countries have now adopted mandatory wheat-flour fortification (MMWR, 2008).

6.3.7 Folic acid fortification concerns

Recently, several articles have been written describing concerns about the effects on the general population of folate fortification and these are reviewed in (Smith et al., 2008). Most of these concerns have arisen after the fact, making mandatory folate fortification one huge uncontrolled experiment in the countries that have gone that route. The most compelling of these concerns include cancer, drug interactions and vitamin B12 (cobalamin)/folate balance.

Initial concerns about colon cancer and folate fortification developed when colon cancer rates started increasing in the USA, Canada and Chile after mandatory folate fortification (Mason et al., 2007; Hirsch et al., 2009). Because folate is crucial for the metabolism of rapidly growing cells, the availability of additional folic acid to pre-existing cancers raises a serious concern. However, studies have also shown that moderate doses of folates are involved in the prevention of colon cancer through nucleotide biosynthesis for DNA repair and methylation for both gene silencing and the suppression of repetitive DNA of viral origin (Sanjoaquin et al., 2005). The most recent evidence suggests a dual role of folates in cancer with moderate intake before the establishment of neoplastic foci having a protective effect, whereas excessive intake afterwards increasing tumor growth (Hubner and Houlston, 2009).

Several pharmaceuticals target folate/one-carbon metabolism and upon widespread mandatory fortification, concerns have arisen about the continued efficacy of these drugs. Studies have suggested the need for increased doses of methotrexate for rheumatoid arthritis treatment (Arabelovic et al., 2007) and a reduction in the effectiveness of pemetrexed in cancer treatment with high levels of FA supplementation (Chattopadhyay et al., 2007). However, at current USA FA fortification levels, adults who consume 400 µg of FA per day or less are unlikely to risk high levels of FA consumption (Yang et al., 2010). Meanwhile, other studies have shown no change in intake of phenytoin, a seizure disorder medication, before and after FA fortification (Ray et al., 2005). Finally, the 2009 U.S. Preventive Services Task Force, who have done a much more exhaustive review than is presented here, found no evidence of drug interactions initiated by FA fortification (U.S. Preventive Services Task Force, 2009).

Concerns have also been raised about unbalancing folate and vitamin B12 levels. Studies have suggested that high folate levels in combination with vitamin B12 deficiency pose particular problems. Masking of vitamin B12 deficiency by FA can occur because FA can 'cure' the anemia resulting from vitamin B12 deficiency, thus delaying diagnosis of vitamin B12 deficiency until after permanent neurological damage has occurred (Rampersaud et al., 2003). Further, when folate concentrations are elevated, the effects of vitamin B12 deficiency are more severe (Miller et al., 2009). However, FA supplementation under sufficient vitamin B12 status has the beneficial effect of improved cognitive function in the elderly (Morris et al., 2007). Rather than cease FA fortification, an alternative solution would be to prevent vitamin B12 deficiency and thus eliminate both its associated anemia and neurological impairment.

6.3.8 Additional folic acid fortification benefits

Folate deficiency has long been known to have adverse effects on the health of the general population, including anemia and neuropathy. In the USA, before FA fortification, 2.3% of school-age children, 24.5% of adults, and 10.8% of the elderly were folate deficient. Since folate fortification, these deficiencies have been dramatically reduced (McLean et al., 2008).

Stroke is a leading cause of death in developed countries resulting in an estimated 666,000 deaths yearly throughout the world (Bonita, 1992). Hyperhomocysteinemeia has been linked to insufficient B vitamin consumption which has been associated with increased risk of stroke (Sanchez-Moreno et al., 2009). Although stroke mortality was already decreasing in the USA and Canada before FA fortification, this decrease accelerated in both nations after FA fortification, whereas no such acceleration has been observed in England and Wales, two countries without mandatory fortification programs (Yang et al., 2006). Even though inconclusive results have been reported (Bonaa et al., 2006; Wang et al., 2007), the great potential for nutrition playing a significant role in cerebral vascular disease bears further study.

Several studies have been performed on the effect of FA supplementation on adverse pregnancy outcomes other than NTDs. The results of these studies have been ambiguous and are reviewed in (Molloy et al., 2008). Some more recent studies suggest that FA could have a preventative role in early spontaneous preterm birth (Bukowski et al., 2009), pre-eclampsia (Wen et al., 2008a), severe congenital heart disease (Ionescu-Ittu et al., 2009), placental abruption, growth restriction and fetal death (Wen et al., 2008b).

Many of the phenomena, both beneficial and of concern, which various studies have tried to connect with folate are complex; probably involving environmental, genetic and epigenetic components. Additionally, these effects are probably modified by different sources of folates (natural folates, FA fortified products, or FA supplements). This could explain some of the heterogeneity in results from different studies.

6.3.9 Vitamin B12 fortification

By co-fortifying bread with FA and B12, concerns about the folate/B12 balance could be alleviated (Winkels et al., 2008). Further, B12 deficiency might play its own role in NTD-affected pregnancies because several studies of maternal B12 levels and NTD-affected pregnancies have revealed an association between low B12 in mothers of affected fetuses compared with controls (Li et al., 2009). B12 is an important cofactor for methionine synthase in the reaction that re-methylates homocysteine to methionine (Stead et al., 2004) as depicted in ▶Fig. 6.6, and, as with folate deficiency, B12 deficiency results in the accumulation of homocysteine (Li et al., 2009).

6.3.10 Potential mechanisms

6.3.10.1 NTDs, homocysteinylation and autoimmunity

The underlying mechanism(s) by which adequate nutrition, specifically folate and B12 status, protects developing embryos remains unknown and is currently the subject of considerable scientific investigation. When MTR activity is inhibited by folate or vitamin B12 deficiency, excess homocysteine is converted to homocysteine thiolactone, which can react with the lysine residues of proteins. These homocysteinylated proteins can be altered in function (Jakubowski et al., 2009) and are likely to be recognized as neo-self antigens which can induce an autoimmune response (Eggleton et al., 2008). It has been known for a long time that antibodies can play a role in a variety of adverse pregnancy outcomes in animal models (Brent, 1964; Barrow and Taylor, 1971) and antibodies to FR (da Costa et al., 2003) and B12 (Seetharam et al., 1997) have been specifically identified for such a role. Considering that during development multiple changes are occurring in response to the dynamic physiologic needs of a rapidly growing embryo, nutritional status might alter crucial proteins during critical points of embryogenesis through homocysteinylation and autoantibodies.

Another possible mechanism for the protective effects of maternal folate status on embryonic development is that of DNA methylation. During early embryogenesis genomic DNA is re-methylated (Reik et al., 2001). Methylation patterns play a crucial role in gene expression and thus the continued development of embryos. Because folate is a key player in the methylation cycle (►Fig. 6.6), maternal folate status could contribute to neural tube closure (Blom, 2009).

6.3.11 Conclusions

A plethora of studies have demonstrated irrevocably that maternal folic acid (FA) supplementation can prevent up to 70% of NTD-affected pregnancies. This led to a variety of national recommendations for folate intake by women in their reproductive years. Unfortunately, recommendations were unable to substantially reduce the occurrence of NTDs. When folate supplementation strategies proved inadequate, several nations instituted FA food fortification programs. These programs were, and are still generally considerably to be more effective in reducing NTD-affected pregnancies than voluntary supplementation. Since their introduction, concerns have arisen as to potential side effects, particularly with respect to cancer, drug interactions, and the balance of folates and vitamin B12. Current data suggest that the moderate FA doses achieved through FA fortification will not cause these adverse affects. Additionally, there could be other benefits to folate fortification. FA fortification has definitely led to a vast reduction in folate deficiency, and other potential health benefits could include reducing the occurrences of other adverse pregnancy outcomes and lowering the incidences of stroke. Vitamin B12 co-fortification might reduce concerns about the folate/B12 balance and have other beneficial effects. The underlying process(es) by which folic acid and B12 facilitate this reduced risk, however, remain unknown. It could be that the elevated levels of homocysteine associated with these deficiencies leads to homocysteinylation of nutrient transport receptors and/or other developmentally relevant proteins. This homocysteinylation might directly interfere with development or could elicit a deleterious autoimmune response. Regardless, the data gap of how nutrient supplementation, such as with the folates, prevents adverse pregnancy outcomes, such as NTDs, needs to be resolved to develop more effective and safe strategies to prevent these devastating birth defects.

References

Knowledge and use of folic acid by women of childbearing age – United States, 1995. MMWR Morb Mortal Wkly Rep 1995;44: 716–8.

Knowledge and use of folic acid by women of childbearing age – United States, 1995 and 1998. MMWR Morb Mortal Wkly Rep 1999;48: 325–7.

Trends in wheat-flour fortification with folic acid and iron – worldwide, 2004 and 2007. MMWR Morb Mortal Wkly Rep 2008;57: 8–10.

Folic acid for the prevention of neural tube defects: U.S. Preventive Services Task Force recommendation statement. Ann Intern Med 2009;150: 626–31.

Arabelovic S, Sam G, et al., Preliminary evidence shows that folic acid fortification of the food supply is associated with higher methotrexate dosing in patients with rheumatoid arthritis. J Am Coll Nutr 2007;26: 453–5.

Arkkola T, Uusitalo U, et al., Dietary intake and use of dietary supplements in relation to demographic variables among pregnant Finnish women. Br J Nutr 2006;96: 913–20.

Baird CD, Nelson MM, et al., Congenital cardiovascular anomalies induced by pteroylglutamic acid deficiency during gestation in the rat. Circ Res 1954;2: 544–54.

Barrow MV, Taylor WJ, The production of congenital defects in rats using antisera. J Exp Zool 1971;176: 41–59.

Beaudin AE, Stover PJ, Insights into metabolic mechanisms underlying folate-responsive neural tube defects: a minireview. Birth Defects Res A Clin Mol Teratol 2009;85: 274–84.

Berry RJ, Li Z, et al., Prevention of neural-tube defects with folic acid in China. China-U.S. Collaborative Project for Neural Tube Defect Prevention. N Engl J Med 1999;341: 1485–90.

Blom HJ, Folic acid, methylation and neural tube closure in humans. Birth Defects Res A Clin Mol Teratol 2009;85: 295–302.

Bonaa KH, Njolstad I, et al., Homocysteine lowering and cardiovascular events after acute myocardial infarction. N Engl J Med 2006;354: 1578–88.

Bonita R, Epidemiology of stroke. Lancet 1992;339: 342–4.

Botto LD, Lisi A, et al., International retrospective cohort study of neural tube defects in relation to folic acid recommendations: are the recommendations working? Br Med J 2005;330: 571.

Bower C, Stanley FJ, Dietary folate as a risk factor for neural-tube defects: evidence from a case-control study in Western Australia. Med J Aust 1989;150: 613–9.

Bowman RM, Boshnjaku V, et al., The changing incidence of myelomeningocele and its impact on pediatric neurosurgery: a review from the Children's Memorial Hospital. Childs Nerv Syst 2009;25: 801–6.

Brent RL, The production of congenital malformations using tissue antisera. II. The spectrum and incidence of malformations following the administration of kidney antiserum to pregnant rats. Am J Anat 1964;115: 525–41.

Brough L, Rees GA, et al., Social and ethnic differences in folic acid use preconception and during early pregnancy in the UK: effect on maternal folate status. J Hum Nutr Diet 2009;22: 100–7.

Bukowski R, Malone FD, et al., Preconceptional folate supplementation and the risk of spontaneous preterm birth: a cohort study. PLoS Med 2009;6: e1000061.

Busby A, Abramsky L, et al., Preventing neural tube defects in Europe: population based study. Br Med J 2005;330: 574–5.

Chattopadhyay S, Tamari R, et al., Commentary: a case for minimizing folate supplementation in clinical regimens with pemetrexed based on the marked sensitivity of the drug to folate availability. Oncologist 2007;12: 808–15.

Christianson A, Howson CP, et al., March of Dimes global report on birth defects. White Plains: March of Dimes Research Foundation; 2006.

Czeizel AE, Dudas I, Prevention of the first occurrence of neural-tube defects by periconceptional vitamin supplementation. N Engl J Med 1992;327: 1832–5.

da Costa M, Sequeira JM, et al., Antibodies to folate receptors impair embryogenesis and fetal development in the rat. Birth Defects Res A Clin Mol Teratol 2003;67: 837–47.

De Wals P, Tairou F, et al., Reduction in neural-tube defects after folic acid fortification in Canada. N Engl J Med 2007;357: 135–42.

Eggleton P, Haigh R, et al., Consequence of neo-antigenicity of the 'altered self'. Rheumatology (Oxford) 2008;47: 567–71.

Fletcher RJ, Bell IP, et al., Public health aspects of food fortification: a question of balance. Proc Nutr Soc 2004;63: 605–14.

Greene ND, Copp AJ, Development of the vertebrate central nervous system: formation of the neural tube. Prenat Diagn 2009;29: 303–11.

Greene ND, Stanier P, et al., Genetics of human neural tube defects. Hum Mol Genet 2009;18: R113–29.

Hertrampf E, Cortes F, National food-fortification program with folic acid in Chile. Food Nutr Bull 2008;29(2 Suppl): S231–7.

Hibbard BM, Hibbard ED, et al., Folic acid and reproduction. Acta Obstet Gynecol Scand 1965;44: 375–400.

Hirsch S, Sanchez H, et al., Colon cancer in Chile before and after the start of the flour fortification program with folic acid. Eur J Gastroenterol Hepatol 2009;21: 436–9.

Hubner RA, Houlston RS, Folate and colorectal cancer prevention. Br J Cancer 2009;100: 233–9.

Ionescu-Ittu R, Marelli AJ, et al., Prevalence of severe congenital heart disease after folic acid fortification of grain products: time trend analysis in Quebec, Canada. Br Med J 2009;338: b1673.

Jakubowski H, Perla-Kajan J, et al., Genetic or nutritional disorders in homocysteine or folate metabolism increase protein N-homocysteinylation in mice. FASEB J 2009;23: 1721–7.

Laurence KM, James N, et al., Double-blind randomised controlled trial of folate treatment before conception to prevent recurrence of neural-tube defects. Br Med J (Clin Res Ed) 1981;282: 1509–11.

Li F, Watkins D, et al., Vitamin B(12) and birth defects. Mol Genet Metab 2009;98: 166–72.

Mason JB, Dickstein A, et al., A temporal association between folic acid fortification and an increase in colorectal cancer rates may be illuminating important biological principles: a hypothesis. Cancer Epidemiol Biomarkers Prev 2007;16: 1325–9.

McLean E, de Benoist B, et al., Review of the magnitude of folate and vitamin B12 deficiencies worldwide. Food Nutr Bull 2008;29(2 Suppl): S38–51.

Miller JW, Garrod MG, et al., Metabolic evidence of vitamin B-12 deficiency, including high homocysteine and methylmalonic acid and low holotranscobalamin, is more pronounced in older adults with elevated plasma folate. Am J Clin Nutr 2009;90: 1586–92.

Molloy AM, Kirke PN, et al., Effects of folate and vitamin B12 deficiencies during pregnancy on fetal, infant, and child development. Food Nutr Bull 2008;29(2 Suppl): S101–11; discussion S112–5.

Morris MS, Jacques PF, et al., Folate and vitamin B-12 status in relation to anemia, macrocytosis, and cognitive impairment in older Americans in the age of folic acid fortification. Am J Clin Nutr 2007;85: 193–200.

Mulinare J, Cordero JF, et al., Periconceptional use of multivitamins and the occurrence of neural tube defects. J Am Med Assoc 1988;260: 3141–5.

Nelson MM, Asling CW, et al., Production of multiple congenital abnormalities in young by maternal pteroylglutamic acid deficiency during gestation. J Nutr 1952;48: 61–79.

Nilsen RM, Vollset SE, et al., Patterns and predictors of folic acid supplement use among pregnant women: the Norwegian Mother and Child Cohort Study. Am J Clin Nutr 2006;84: 1134–41.

Oleary M, Donnell RM, et al., Folic acid and prevention of neural tube defects in 2000 improved awareness – low peri-conceptional uptake. Ir Med J 2001;94: 180–1.

Pacheco SS, Braga C, et al., Effects of folic acid fortification on the prevalence of neural tube defects. Rev Saude Publica 2009;43: 565–71.

Rampersaud GC, Kauwell GP, et al., Folate: a key to optimizing health and reducing disease risk in the elderly. J Am Coll Nutr 2003;22: 1–8.

Ray JG, Langman LJ, et al., Absence of effect of folic acid flour fortification on anticonvulsant drug levels. Am J Med 2005;118: 444–5.

Reik W, Dean W, et al., Epigenetic reprogramming in mammalian development. Science 2001;293: 1089–93.

Sanchez-Moreno C, Jimenez-Escrig A, et al., Stroke: roles of B vitamins, homocysteine and antioxidants. Nutr Res Rev 2009;22: 49–67.

Sanjoaquin MA, Allen N, et al., Folate intake and colorectal cancer risk: a meta-analytical approach. Int J Cancer 2005;113: 825–8.

Seetharam B, Christensen EI, et al., Identification of rat yolk sac target protein of teratogenic antibodies, gp280, as intrinsic factor-cobalamin receptor. J Clin Invest 1997;99: 2317–22.

Shaw GM, Schaffer D, et al., Periconceptional vitamin use, dietary folate, and the occurrence of neural tube defects. Epidemiology 1995;6: 219–26.

Smith AD, Kim YI, et al., Is folic acid good for everyone? Am J Clin Nutr 2008;87: 517–33.

Smithells RW, Sheppard S, et al., Possible prevention of neural-tube defects by periconceptional vitamin supplementation. Lancet 1980;1(8164): 339–40.

Stead LM, Jacobs RL, et al., Methylation demand and homocysteine metabolism. Adv Enzyme Regul 2004;44: 321–33.

Stover PJ, One-carbon metabolism-genome interactions in folate-associated pathologies. J Nutr 2009;139: 2402–5.

Vergel RG, Sanchez LR, et al., Primary prevention of neural tube defects with folic acid supplementation: Cuban experience. Prenat Diagn 1990;10: 149–52.

Wald N, Sneddon J, et al., Prevention of neural tube defects: results of the Medical Research Council Vitamin Study. MRC Vitamin Study Research Group. Lancet 1991;338(8760): 131–7.

Wang X, Qin X, et al., Efficacy of folic acid supplementation in stroke prevention: a meta-analysis. Lancet 2007;369(9576): 1876–82.

Weggemans RM, Schaafsma G, et al., Toward an optimal use of folic acid: an advisory report of the Health Council of the Netherlands. Eur J Clin Nutr 2009;63: 1034–6.

Wen SW, Chen XK, et al., Folic acid supplementation in early second trimester and the risk of preeclampsia. Am J Obstet Gynecol 2008a;198: 45e1–7.

Wen SW, Zhou J, et al., Maternal exposure to folic acid antagonists and placenta-mediated adverse pregnancy outcomes. Can Med Assoc J 2008b;179: 1263–8.

Werler MM, Shapiro S, et al., Periconceptional folic acid exposure and risk of occurrent neural tube defects. J Am Med Assoc 1993;269: 1257–61.

Williams LJ, Mai CT, et al., Prevalence of spina bifida and anencephaly during the transition to mandatory folic acid fortification in the United States. Teratology 2002;66: 33–9.

Winkels RM, Brouwer IA, et al., Bread cofortified with folic acid and vitamin B-12 improves the folate and vitamin B-12 status of healthy older people: a randomized controlled trial. Am J Clin Nutr 2008;88: 348–55.

Yang Q, Botto LD, et al., Improvement in stroke mortality in Canada and the United States, 1990 to 2002. Circulation 2006;113: 1335–43.

Yang Q, Cogswell ME, et al., Folic acid source, usual intake, and folate and vitamin B-12 status in US adults: National Health and Nutrition Examination Survey (NHANES) 2003–2006. Am J Clin Nutr 2010;91(1): 64–72.

6.4 Folate in dementia and cognitive dysfunction

Torbjörn K. Nilsson; Nils-Olof Hagnelius

6.4.1 Introduction

Neuropsychiatric diseases are responsible for approximately one third of the total disease burden in Europe, dementia and cognitive disorders constitute a significant part of these diseases. This chapter will mainly deal with folate in the dementias, but for their interest in illuminating possible mechanisms, will also mention some general cognitive studies. There has been a growing interest in the topic as shown by the number of articles devoted to it in recent years. In this chapter we chose as a matter of principle not to quote reviews, but instead tried to identify methodologically important or interesting themes which we illustrate by selected original papers. We address the issue along the following lines:

- folate transport to the cerebrospinal fluid;
- possible mechanisms for an association of folate with dementia;
- model diseases, genetic or acquired;
- cross-sectional studies;
- prospective studies;
- therapeutic or prophylactic trials.

6.4.2 Definitions in dementia research

Mild cognitive impairment (MCI) is a controversial term to indicate subjects with more memory impairment than in normal aging, but not as much as in a subject with Alzheimer's disease (AD), i.e., they are between normal aging and dementia (Petersen et al., 1999).

Dementia is a term for a non-specific disease syndrome (set of symptoms) which could be caused by many different disease processes or trauma.

Dementia is an acquired, protracted (>6 months according to International Classification of Diseases, 10th revision), significant deterioration in cognitive capacities. Memory disturbance is obligate, deterioration in language, attention, thinking and problem solving, and executive problems are the most prominent areas of symptoms. The degree of difficulties should interfere with daily social activities and represent a significant deterioration compared with the premorbid level.

Dementia diseases have become one of the great causes of death in the USA [see data for 2004 (US National Center for Health Statistics, 2007)]. However, a delay of onset of AD of 5 years would reduce the affected population by 50% (Khachaturian, 1992). One man in 6, and almost 1 woman in 3, will suffer from dementia during their lifetime (Breteler et al., 1998). The basic mechanisms behind AD and other primary degenerative dementias are not known. Malnutrition leading to deficiency of macro- and micronutrients has been recognized as the cause of dementia in some cases (Salvioli et al., 1998), e.g., B-vitamin deficiency. Atrophic gastritis, a usual condition in the elderly, might cause vitamin B12 deficiency owing to malabsorption. Deficiency of B-vitamins could also be owing to side effects of pharmacotherapy, e.g., methotrexate treatment of rheumatoid arthritis or psoriasis.

Definite risk factors (scientifically proven to be causal) are: age, ApoE ε4 allele and family history of dementia. The main dementia risk factor is old age (Fratiglioni et al., 1997). ApoE ε4 is considered a major susceptibility marker for AD. It is associated with an earlier age of AD onset and increased amyloid plaque load (Mann et al., 1997). Whereas the ε4 allele is present in a large proportion of the populations of Europe, all other mutations causing early-onset Alzheimer dementia explain altogether approximately 1–2%. Examples are the *APP* gene, the *Presenilin 1* and the *Presenilin 2* gene mutations.

Furthermore, there are some protective factors against dementia. To live an active life, have a long education, perform daily exercise, drink a glass of red wine/day (Kivipelto et al., 2008) and a good social network with many contacts help to keep your mind better preserved.

Dementia that occurs as a result of another physical disease or injury is classified as secondary dementia. The most common of these disorders is vascular dementia (VaD). It accounts for approximately 20% of all dementias.

VaD usually has its origin in atherosclerotic changes of the vessels inside or outside the brain, but it can also be caused by severe vascular inflammation or result from very low blood pressure. Alois Alzheimer in his first case report described that Auguste Deter had suffered from atherosclerotic changes in the larger vascular tissues (Alzheimer et al., 1995). In recent years it has been argued that AD is perhaps not the most common dementia disease, but rather a combination of both AD and VaD (Aguero-Torres et al., 2006), and vascular mechanisms are by some scientists regarded as risk factors not only for VaD but also for AD (Kalaria, 2000; Skoog, 2000; Aguero-Torres et al., 2006; Knopman, 2006; Cechetto et al., 2008). Risk factors that VaD and AD share include age, atherosclerosis, stroke and TIA, diabetes mellitus, smoking, ApoE ε4 and raised total plasma homocysteine (Hcy) (Braekhus and Engedal, 2004). An association between atrial fibrillation, hypertension and angina with more rapid decline in AD has been described, whereas the use of antihypertensive medication, coronary artery bypass grafting (CABG) and diabetes mellitus were associated with less rapid decline (Mielke et al., 2007). Small vessel dementia is probably caused by changes in the small penetrating end arteries in the depth of the brain, these changes probably relate to, e.g., hypertension (Andin, 2007). Large vessel dementia is caused by infarction (or bleeding) in the large cortical vessels. However, a recent review does not support the influence of traditional vascular risk factors on AD with the exception of exercise and physical function, APOE ε4, diabetes and cholesterol (Purnell et al., 2009). As can be gleaned from the above, the possibility of a link between folate intake and dementia, mediated by vascular mechanisms, would fit in well with some major trends in current dementia research. However, this link has so far not been systematically pursued.

The only major cardiovascular risk factor system that has not been extensively studied as a risk factor for vascular dementia is the hemostatic system. Only a few papers have been published, which do propose it as a possible pathogenetic factor in dementia, particularly vascular dementia (Mari et al., 1996; Bots et al., 1998; Hagnelius et al., 2010).

6.4.3 Folate transport to the cerebrospinal fluid

6.4.3.1 The blood-brain barriers

The central nervous system (CNS) is protected from harmful influences in several ways. A part of this protection is constituted by special types of blood vessels with a high density of tight junctions. Generally we refer to these special vessels as the blood-brain barrier (BBB). The transport of nutrients to the neurons and other cells in the brain has to manage the BBB. Some micronutrient utilizes active transportation, e.g., folate and vitamin C. Folate transport occurs in the choroid plexus, a small tissue in the brain ventricles that also produces the vast majority (~75%) of cerebrospinal fluid (CSF). This way is the only route to support the brain with folate and vitamin C. The function of CSF is also to reduce the brain weight, protect from trauma, to supply the brain with nutrients, and to remove products from brain metabolism.

Tab. 6.3: The four barriers (compartments) in CNS.

Neurovascular unit	Blood-brain barrier (BBB)
Choroid plexus	Blood-CSF barrier (B-CSF-B)
Meninges	Arachnoid barrier (a second blood CSF barrier)
Neuroependyma	In the fetus, the ependymal lining is competent differing CSF from brain tissue
	Adult lining permits free passage of liquor and brain extra cellular fluid

There are three main compartments in the central nervous system, blood, CSF and brain tissue. These compartments are separated by four barriers (▶Tab. 6.3). Failure of the integrity of BBB occurs in cerebral vascular disease such as stroke and might be of importance in the development of dementia disease, particularly VaD.

6.4.3.2 CSF-folate

Early case reports concerning the rare genetic disorder Hereditary Folate Malbsorption, characterised by very low or undetectable CSF levels, stressed that the affected children presented not only with megaloblastic anemia from 2–3 months of age, but also with mental retardation (Poncz et al., 1981).

There is now manifest knowledge that folate is of utmost importance in nervous system development. The first authors to describe CSF-folate concentration in a brief, but widely quoted abstract from 1961 were Herbert and Zalusky (1961). The concentration of folate in the cerebrospinal fluid is approximately two to four times higher than in serum (Herbert and Zalusky, 1961; Wells and Casey, 1967; Alperin and Haggard, 1970). This relation remains constant in the presence of serum folate deficiency (Reynolds et al., 1972) although it has been shown that in subjects with high serum folate levels the CSF-to-serum folate ratio actually drops and could fall under 1.00 (Hagnelius et al., 2008). To achieve this 2- to 4-fold CSF/S-ratio, folate is actively transported from the blood to the CSF via folate receptors in the choroid plexus. Spector and Lorenzo (1975) reported that the folate level in brain was maintained even in severe folate deficiency.

Folate Receptor-α (FR-α) and the recently described Proton-Coupled Folate Transporter (PCFT) seems to work in tandem and thus both are required to maintain the CSF/serum folate gradient (Wollack et al., 2008). The CSF/serum folate ratio could represent a measure of the transport of folate to the CSF compartment. In cognitively healthy patients, CSF-folate has been shown to correlate negatively with age in the interval between 40 years and 99 years (Bottiglieri et al., 2000). Botez and Bachevalier (1981) found that the CSF-folate deficient patients which clinically responded best to folate treatment, were the ones who also had the most pronounced rise in CSF-folate. However, they found no difference in CSF-folate restitution between younger and older people. A predictor of the rise in CSF-folate after treatment was the initial CSF-folate value, where a low value predicted a high rise in CSF-folate level.

In a study by Serot et al. it was found that CSF-folate was significantly lower in AD subjects than in age-matched controls (Serot et al., 2001). By contrast, we found the

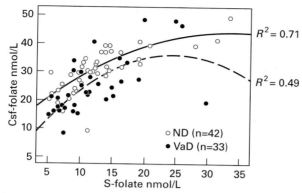

Fig. 6.7: shows the relation between CSF-folate and serum folate. The uptake is saturable (Hagnelius et al., 2008), as also shown by Spector and Lorenzo (1975), Wu and Pardridge (1999) and Obeid et al. (2007). ND, not demented; VaD, patients with vascular dementia.

transport of folate to CSF to be reduced in dementia patients with a vascular component as a cause of their dementia compared with non-dementia (►Fig. 6.7) and also with Alzheimer subjects (Hagnelius et al., 2008). There was a pronounced negative correlation between the CSF/serum folate ratio ($R_{Csf/S}$) and serum folate.

Dysfunction in some of the only partly known mechanisms involved in folate transport could be responsible, e.g., (i) regulation of the choroid plexus pump mechanism or in the (ii) folate receptor expression or the (iii) reduced folate carrier function or (iv) reduced function in the newly discovered proton-coupled folate transporter. Although not very probable, (v) increased demand of cerebral folate could also be an explanation. Finally, it could depend on (vi) leakage of folate out of the CSF compartment across a partly damaged brain-CSF barrier (B-CSF-B). The B-CSF-B damage hypothesis apparently found support in the fact that there was significantly higher albumin ratio in the VaD+Mixed dementia subgroup.

$R_{Csf/S}$ is normally tightly regulated by serum folate, but is also affected by the integrity of the B-CSF-B. By contrast, metabolic and inflammatory markers were unrelated to the $R_{Csf/S}$. The $R_{Csf/S}$ was significantly lower in patients with VaD+Mixed dementia than in ND or AD subjects. We interpret the difference in $R_{Csf/S}$ as sign of a defect, confined to the VaD+Mixed dementia subgroup, in the transport of folate through the choroid plexus.

Folates enter the cells through three carrier-mediated transport systems. Reduced Folate Carrier (RFC) is a classic facilitated transport protein with micromolar (µM) affinity that transports reduced folates across the cell membrane. The RFC is found in virtually all cells and exists in both soluble and membrane-bound forms. Some cells, particularly choroid plexus epithelial cells, also express the FR-α which exhibits pM affinity for folic acid. The glycosylphosphatidylinositol (GPI) anchored FR-α actively transports folates from blood to the CSF by endocytosis (Rothberg et al., 1990). The third kind of folate transporter is the recently discovered Proton Coupled Folate Transporter (PCFT) (Qiu et al., 2006). One function of PCFT is to maintain the CSF-folate gradient in a tandem-like reaction where FR-α is the other part (Wollack et al., 2008).

6.4.4 Possible mechanisms for an association of folate with dementia and cognition in general

Much of the evidence available comes from studies based on plasma total Hcy as a biomarker of folate and/or cobalamin deficiency, because folate intake studies are not as common and suffer from methodological difficulties. The problem here is that total Hcy itself is not specific for folate deficiency although it does reflect intracellular metabolic availability of folate. In the literature there are different opinions as to whether total Hcy itself is neurotoxic or if neurotoxicity is owing to related to reactive oxygen species (Ho et al., 2002), e.g., homocysteic acid which is well known to induce neuronal death when interacting with the NMDA-receptors (Becker et al., 2007). The methyl folate trap theory, originally formulated by Herbert in 1962 (Herbert and Zalusky, 1962), explained the biological protection to methyl group deficiency in kwashiorkor (e.g., methionine deficiency). Vitamin B12 plays no role in the DNA synthesis but nevertheless hematological complications are owing to vitamin B12 deficiency. The folate trap theory explains why vitamin B12 deficiency often results in a functional folate deficiency status, through trapping of 5-THF and thus blocking its further metabolism in e.g., the purine synthesis and thereby giving rise to symptoms such as megaloblastic anemia. The folate trap hypothesis has not been demonstrated in humans with vitamin B12 deficiency except for an occasional case report (Smulders et al., 2006). Vegetarians might, however, illustrate the problem because they often have falsely normal serum folate levels which are metabolically insufficient owing to their subnormal or marginal B12 levels (Herrmann et al., 2003). In a situation with vitamin B12 deficiency, administration of folic acid, which induces cell division and the use of methionine in protein synthesis, impairs methylation of myelin and precipitates or exacerbates subacute combined degeneration of the spinal cord (Reynolds et al., 1993).

Thus, mechanisms can be broadly divided into 'folate-deficiency'-based and 'homocysteine-toxicity' hypotheses. However, such a division could be more theoretical than real. There might even be links between Hcy/folate metabolism and traditional beta-amyloid pathogenetic mechanisms (Chan and Shea, 2007; Sontag et al., 2007).

One major mechanism at play might well be developmental plasticity, the concept that the fetal environment (for instance availability of folate) shapes a fetal growth trajectory (Barker, 2004). Lower fetal growth is associated with problems such as hyperactivity, inattention and conduct problems in the child (Schlotz et al., 2007). Studies seem to support a role of maternal serum folate in protecting against offspring hyperactivity and adjustment problems (Schlotz et al., 2010). Stretching out the time-frame of neurocognitive developmental programming to encompass later childhood, we have studied academic achievement (objectively assessed by sum of school grades in the final year of the compulsory 9-year school) in Swedish 15-year-old adolescents, and found that sum of grades was significantly and positively related to folate intake (▶Fig. 6.8), and significantly negatively to total Hcy levels. These associations held up even when adjusted for several strong predictors of school grades, such as smoking, mother's education level, or parental income (▶Fig. 6.8). Because a higher level of intellectual capacity in mid-life delays or postpones the development of dementia (Fratiglioni and Rocca, 2001), we thus believe that the early-life folate environment could play a role even later in life. Needless to say, such a hypothesis needs much more supportive evidence than is available at present but we look forward to addressing the problem in further prospective studies.

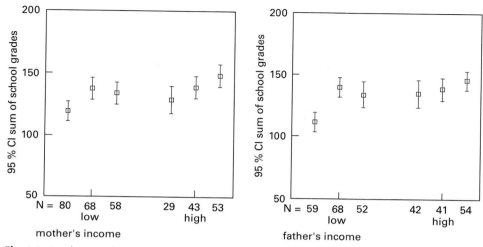

Fig. 6.8: Academic achievement measured as sum of school grades in 15-year-old adolescents according to tertiles of folate intake estimated by a 24 h food intake recall questionnaire. Results are shown separately for pupils with low- and high-income parents, as a measure of socioeconomic level.

Vascular damage caused by Hcy itself or by a lack of folate could promote dementia by the vascular pathway. Therefore, studies that primarily addressed the relation between homocysteine/folate and cerebrovascular disease (ischemic stroke) might be of importance. Lars Brattström et al. in 1984 for the first time described an association between moderate hyperhomocysteinemia and ischemic stroke in a case-control study (Brattström et al., 1984). The vascular pathway found further support in the Canadian study by Ebly et al., where they found an association between stroke and low serum folate as well as an association between low serum folate and dementia (Ebly et al. 1998).

A memorable year in linking vascular stroke with dementia was 2002, with several major studies appearing (Korczyn, 2002; Maxwell et al., 2002; Miller et al., 2002).

In recent years, total Hcy has been proposed as an independent risk factor for dementia and AD (McCaddon et al., 1998; Seshadri et al., 2002; Smith, 2008). Zylberstein et al. found an association between mid-life homocysteine and late-life dementia in women. However, the effect of high Hcy became apparent first after 22 years of duration. They found no interaction between total Hcy and folate for the outcome of dementia (Zylberstein et al., 2009).

6.4.5 Model diseases, genetic or acquired

Hereditary folate malabsorption (HFM) is a rare disorder which manifests itself in childhood with megaloblastic anemia, failure to thrive, diarrhea and severe, progressive neurological symptoms including seizures and peripheral neuropathy (Geller et al., 2002). In 2006, the mechanism was found to consist of point mutations in the gene for proton-coupled folate transporter, *PCFT* (Qiu et al., 2006; Zhao et al., 2007). The longest follow-up time, approximately 26 years, regards a patient with HFM diagnosed already when she was a few months old and treated ever since, first briefly with oral folic acid (which did not correct the hematological and other defects) and then intramuscular injections of folic acid, later changed to i.m. 5-formyltetrahydrofolate. The important message from this patient is that thanks to the treatment with folate supplementation, her cognitive abilities developed normally through childhood, according to the authors, demonstrated by her particular skills in mathematics at school, and further by her obtaining an MBA degree as an adult. The molecular defect in the *PCFT* gene (a rare sequential double mutation, c.197–198GC>AA, for which the parents were heterozygous and the patient homozygous) was also demonstrated in the same paper (Min et al., 2008).

In 2009 (Steinfeld et al., 2009), described a couple of mutations in *FOLR1*, the gene for the other high-affinity folate transporter, folate receptor-alpha, which were also associated with a syndrome of folate deficiency particularly in the CNS, and linked to neurological symptoms including seizures and motor disturbances. All three subjects were children aged 3–5 and all responded to treatment with folinic acid with significant clinical improvements.

Cerebral folate deficiency is an acquired cause of reduced folate transport into the cerebrospinal fluid owing to autoimmunity, which has been proposed by Ramaekers and co-workers (Ramaekers et al., 2005; Bonkowsky et al., 2008). The patients have been children with rather severe neurological symptoms such as developmental delay, motor disturbances, seizures, mental retardation and autistic features, owing to low 5-methyltetrahydrofolate concentrations in CSF, but not in other body compartments. According to these authors this was owing to autoantibodies directed against folate receptor-alpha thereby causing a blocked transport of folate through the B-CSF-B barrier.

A problem with the listed model disorders of folate transport is that they manifest themselves already in early childhood and the neurological symptoms are thus not really those of dementia in the elderly, and none of the described patients has reached old age yet. We have to assume that model disorders that do cause an increased risk for dementia at old age do not manifest themselves at early ages, or do so only insidiously, and are thus probably not accompanied by dramatic laboratory anomalies in the blood or CSF. They will therefore be theoretically difficult to detect. However, the genetic influence on serum folate levels is known to be considerable. A recent paper found the heritability to be >50% (Nilsson et al., 2009). The genetic influence on homocysteine and cobalamin levels was of comparable magnitude. This supports continuous efforts to look for mutations in the folate transporting genes. Thus, we have re-sequenced the 5′-part of the *FOLR1* gene (Nilsson and Börjel, 2004; Börjel et al., 2006; Böttiger et al., 2007) and discovered several novel mutations which we also studied both in non-demented elderly and demented subjects (Böttiger et al., 2007). Two common polymorphisms, *FOLR1* g.1314G>A and g.1928C>T with gene frequencies of 5% and 13%, respectively, did not differ significantly between non-demented and demented; The rare mutations *FOLR1* g.1816delC and g.1841G>A were found to always occur together, thus presumably forming a doubly mutated haplotype of the *FOLR1* gene. This haplotype had a 3-fold higher prevalence among the demented than the non-demented elderly, although this difference did not reach statistical significance. A power analysis indicates that a samples size of $n = 1553$ will be needed to demonstrate a significant association. Because we ourselves already had $n=591$, such a sample size appears within reach through future multicenter collaboration. Further re-sequencing of the *FOLR1* gene could reveal additional low-frequency loci.

6.4.6 Cross-sectional studies

Strachan and Henderson in 1967 presented two cases with dementia and megaloblastic anemia owing to folate deficiency. The two cases resolved (both the hematological problems and the dementia) after folic acid treatment (Strachan and Henderson, 1967). In 1973 Sneath and co-workers presented a paper where they confirmed earlier findings that low red cell folate was associated to dementia (Sneath et al., 1973).

Many more cross-sectional studies have appeared over the years than prospective studies and full detail will be restricted to the latter group of papers (next section). However, several seminal early case-control papers will be mentioned here. In 1983 Goodwin et al. described for the first time epidemiological evidence linking low vitamin B12 and folate status in blood with decline in neurocognitive functions in the elderly (Goodwin et al., 1983). Homocysteine was not analyzed or discussed in their paper. Lindenbaum et al. linked hyperhomocysteinemia, vitamin B12 deficiency and neuro-psychiatric symptoms (Lindenbaum et al., 1988). Karin Nilsson et al. were also early in linking hyperhomocysteinemia to dementia in their case-control studies, (Nilsson et al., 1996). They suggested that patients with a vascular cause of their dementia or a history of occlusive disease had higher total Hcy.

A memorable year in the dementia-homocysteine relationship context was 1998. Several authors linked hyperhomocysteinemia to dementia in their case-control studies. Clarke et al. found that pathologically confirmed AD cases, after adjustment for age, sex, social class, smoking and Apo E ε4 allele, were associated with low levels of the vitamins folate and B12 and elevated serum homocysteine concentrations (Clarke et al., 1998). The OR for Alzheimer type dementia was 3.3 (95% CI, 1.8–6.3) when comparing the top third of serum folate with the low third. They also concluded that the total Hcy level was stable over time, and it had a lack of relationship with disease duration, suggesting that the findings of higher serum total Hcy concentration hardly could be a consequence of the disease. Ebly et al. studied a group of 1171 subjects from the Canadian Study of Health and Aging, and found low levels of serum folate in all types of dementia, low serum folate was also a single explanatory variable for stroke (Ebly et al., 1998). Andrew McCaddon et al. were also early in linking hyperhomocystein-emia to dementia (McCaddon et al., 1998).

The finding by Serot and co-workers finding of low CSF-folate in AD patients has already been mentioned above (Serot et al., 2001). Hultberg et al. found that folate deficiency is common among psychogeriatric patients (Hultberg et al., 2002). They also suggested that serum folate better reflects folate deficiency than blood folate does, whereas Ramos et al. found that red blood cell folate was directly related to cognitive function and inversely associate with dementia (Ramos et al., 2005). Tettamanti et al. found that subclinical folate deficiency could represent a risk factor for cognitive decline in the elderly and that it also could contribute to the development of dementia (Tettamanti et al., 2006). In a study in the USA by Haan and co-workers, they found a significant association between elevated plasma total Hcy and cognitive impairment without dementia or with dementia with a Hazard Ratio of 2.39 (95% CI 1.11–5.16),

(Haan et al., 2007). Serum B12 but not red blood cell folate was also associated with cognitive decline. However, the fortification of flour with folic acid, mandatory in the USA since 1998, has reduced the prevalence of folate deficiency and brought a decline in total Hcy with approximately 15% after 1998. This complicates the interpretation of US studies on the folate/dementia relationship and limits the transferability of their results to other populations.

6.4.7 Prospective studies

Many prospective studies have addressed major cardiovascular endpoints but only a handful has directly concerned dementia as the endpoint. Often, Hcy rather than serum folate or folate intake has been in the focus of the authors (only adjusting for folate as a covariate) making it hard to judge the role of folate itself. Nevertheless, in AD patients, a linear correlation between brain atrophy of the neocortex and low serum folate levels has been described in the important Nun study (Snowdon et al., 2000). A Swedish paper suggested an association between folate and vitamin B12 deficiency and AD (Wang et al., 2001). In the MacArthur study on successful aging, Kado et al. found in a 7-year follow up of signs of cognitive decline that high Hcy was positively and serum folate negatively associated with cognitive decline (i.e., high folate was protective) and that the folate effect seemed independent of Hcy concentrations (Kado et al., 2005), whereas Dufouil et al. found in their 2- and 4-year follow ups that Hcy, independently of folate, was associated with a slight decline in Mini Mental State Examination scores (Dufouil et al., 2003).

In 1092 initially non-demented subjects from the Framingham Cohort, Seshadri et al. found that cognitively intact persons in the highest baseline quartile of total Hcy (>14 μmol/l), 8 years later almost doubled their risk of developing dementia or AD (Seshadri et al., 2002). Adjustments were made for age, sex, ApoE genotype, vascular risk factors other than total Hcy (smoking, alcohol, diabetes mellitus, systolic blood pressure and BMI), and plasma levels of the B-vitamins folate, B12 and B6. They concluded that hyperhomocysteinemia is an independent risk factor for the development of dementia and AD. In a 5-year-long prospective study (from the Canadian Study of Health and Aging) the main result was that people with the lowest folate quartile showed a trend towards both poorer health and cognitive outcome compared with the highest quartile (Maxwell et al., 2002). Ravaglia et al. in 2003 reported similar findings from Italy as Seshadri (Ravaglia et al., 2003). However, neither the study by Seshadri nor the study by Ravaglia found a significant association between serum folate levels and cognitive function. Zylberstein and co-workers in Gothenburg followed 1368 women for 24 years and found total Hcy to be an independent predictor of dementias. In this study the hazard ratio for AD (2.1) was higher than that for any dementia (1.7), and the highest HR was for AD without cerebrovascular disease (2.4). In a subsequent study these authors analyzed the possible impact of MTHFR genotypes on the associations of total Hcy with dementia and found that the 1298A>C polymorphism was protective against dementia (Zylberstein, 2009). They did not find any association with the more well-known MTHFR 677C>T polymorphism, however. None of these three studies therefore support any particular importance of folate.

Middleton et al. reported from Canada that serum folate was significantly related to incident AD and cerebrovascular outcomes in adjusted (but not unadjusted!) analyses, but adding exercise to the models abolished folate as a significant predictor (Middleton et al., 2007). Luchsinger et al. presented recently a prospective paper where they found a reduced risk of AD in subjects with high folate intake independent of other risk factors (Luchsinger et al., 2008).

However, another recent study of over 5000 subjects aged 65 years and older reported no association between folate, vitamin B12 or vitamin B6 and dementia or AD (Nelson et al., 2009).

As stated above in 6.4.4, vascular risk factors could be very important in promoting dementia both of VaD and AD type. Therefore the general prospective cardiovascular risk factor studies should be taken into account here. Thus, in the extensive Norwegian homocysteine study, the Hordaland homocysteine study, total Hcy was found to be a strong predictor of both cardiovascular and non-cardiovascular mortality in an elderly population (Vollset et al., 2001). In the large study of women from Gothenburg, with 24 years follow up, total Hcy was an independent predictor of both AMI and death from AMI (Zylberstein et al., 2004). In the same cohort, total Hcy was associated with lacunar brain infarcts but not with white matter lesions (Zylberstein et al., 2008). In a prospective study from northern Sweden, low serum folate was an independent predictor of a first myocardial infarction in both men and women (Van Guelpen et al., 2009). That study also demonstrated for the first time that this association was independent of both total Hcy and kidney function. There is now convincing epidemiologic evidence that low serum folate and elevated total Hcy both predicts and precedes cardiovascular disease.

6.4.8 Therapeutic or prophylactic trials

Up to 2009 there have been only a few prospective randomized controlled studies that have investigated the effect of B-vitamin supplementation on cognition. We are of the opinion that the strength of the conclusions drawn from such trials should be related to whether the patients treated represented a subpopulation in real need of folate supplementation, or whether patients at all levels of serum folate or plasma Hcy were included in the trial. The latter is often the case, as for instance, in several prophylactic trials in stroke or restenosis.

Durga and co-workers reported results from the FACIT study on healthy people, 50–70 years of age, with raised total Hcy level (>13 µmol/l) where a 3-year-long supplementation with 0.8 mg folic acid/day gave significant better results in the supplemented group versus the placebo group concerning, e.g., memory storage and information-processing speed (Durga et al., 2007).

The Taiwanese study by Sun et al. from 2007, was a 26-week double-blind prospective trial of 89 mild to moderate AD patients (45 men, 44 women) with normal vitamin B12, folate and total Hcy levels. All patients were receiving acetylcholinesterase inhibitor treatment. The subjects were randomized to either supplementation with vitamin B12 (500 µg), vitamin B6 (5 mg), folic acid (1 mg), other vitamins, and iron or to placebo. No statistically significant nor any clinically significant beneficial treatment effects on cognition (measured with the Alzheimer's Disease Assessment Scale – Cognitive part, ADAS-Cog) or Activity of Daily Life (ADL) function were found between the groups after 26 weeks, but total Hcy was significantly reduced by approximately 25% (Sun et al., 2007).

A second study on demented subjects was presented in late 2008 (Aisen et al., 2008). This randomized double-blind, placebo-controlled multicenter study enrolled 409 participants with mild to moderate AD with normal folic acid, vitamin B12 and total Hcy levels; 340 completed the study (202 in the active-treatment group and 138 in the placebo group). During the 18-month-long trial period the total Hcy level was significantly reduced in the active-treatment group (26%) but there were no significant reduction on cognitional decline, as measured with ADAS-Cog. In the placebo group, total Hcy was reduced by 9%. Furthermore, the active-treatment group had a higher quantity of adverse events, including depression and blurred vision.

In a pilot study comprising 41 subjects with probable AD on cholinesterase inhibitors Connoly et al. found an improvement in instrumental ADL functions and in social behavior in the group substituted with 1 mg folic acid/day compared with the placebo group, during the 6-month-long trial (Connelly et al., 2008). There was a raised baseline total Hcy (18.39 μmol/l).

Dietary folate intake has also been suggested to reduce cognitive performance in older persons (Morris et al., 2005), but the balance between intakes of folate and vitamin B12 in a population exposed to mandatory folate fortification could be shifted in such a way as to reduce the transferability of such findings which perhaps do not apply at all in other populations.

The extensive Cochrane review by Malouf et al. saw some evidence for and against folate substitution to prevent cognitive decline or dementia deterioration, with or without vitamin B12 (Malouf and Grimley Evans, 2008). In line with this, A.D. Smith wrote an important review concluding that we need new large-scale randomized total Hcy lowering trials to see if a proportion of dementias could be prevented (Smith, 2008).

6.4.9 Conclusion

We now have several possible mechanisms that could mediate a role of folate in dementia, including vascular and Hcy-related pathways. There are model diseases of both genetic and acquired types. The high hereditability of serum folate promises that more such states might soon be uncovered. Developmental programming, including good folate intake in childhood, could perhaps provide protection against, or at least delay, onset of dementia. We have many case-control studies and some prospective studies making the case for folate, but there are also some prominent negative studies. We do not have enough therapeutic trials with relevant inclusion criteria. We know too little about folate availability within the CNS although we begin to see that this could matter. Above all, we do not have enough nutritional studies addressing the role of early and mid-life folate nutrition, well preceding the overt dementia phase in the elderly. Nevertheless, the case for a role of folate in dementia is building steadily.

References

10 Leading Causes of Death in the U.S. (2004), US National Center for Health Statistics, 2007 (From: http://www.infoplease.com/ipa/A0005110.html/ Accessed June 21, 2009.).

Aguero-Torres H, Kivipelto M, von Strauss, E, Rethinking the dementia diagnoses in a population-based study: what is Alzheimer's disease and what is vascular dementia? A study from the Kungsholmen project. Dement Geriatr Cogn Disord 2006;22: 244–9.

Aisen PS, Schneider LS, Sano M, Diaz-Arrastia R, van Dyck CH, Weiner MF, Bottiglieri T, Jin S, Stokes KT, Thomas RG, Thal LJ, High-dose B vitamin supplementation and cognitive decline in Alzheimer disease: a randomized controlled trial. J Am Med Assoc 2008;300: 1774–83.

Alperin JB, Haggard ME, Cerebrospinal fluid folate (CFA) and the blood brain barrier. Clin Res 1970;18: 40.

Alzheimer A, Stelzmann RA, Schnitzlein HN, Murtagh FR, An English translation of Alzheimer's 1907 paper, 'Über eine eigenartige ErkRankung der Hirnrinde', Clin Anat1995;8: 429–31.

Andin, U, Vascular dementia: classification and clinical correlates. Lund, Sweden: Department of Clinical Sciences, Lund University; 2007.

Barker DJ, The developmental origins of chronic adult disease. Acta Paediatr 2004;93(Suppl): 26–33.

Becker A, Vezmar S, Linnebank M, Pels H, Bode U, Schlegel U, Jaehde U, Marked elevation in homocysteine and homocysteine sulfinic acid in the cerebrospinal fluid of lymphoma patients receiving intensive treatment with methotrexate. Int J Clin Pharmacol Ther 2007;45: 504–15.

Bonkowsky JL, Ramaekers VT, Quadros EV, Lloyd M, Progressive encephalopathy in a child with cerebral folate deficiency syndrome. J Child Neurol 2008;23: 1460–3.

Botez MI, Bachevalier J, The blood-brain barrier and folate deficiency. Am J Clin Nutr 1981;34: 1725–30.

Bots ML, Breteler MM, van Kooten F, Haverkate F, Meijer P, Koudstaal PJ, Grobbee DE, Kluft, C, Coagulation and fibrinolysis markers and risk of dementia. The Dutch Vascular Factors in Dementia Study. Haemostasis 1998;28: 216–22.

Bottiglieri T, Reynolds EH, Laundy M, Folate in CSF and age, J Neurol Neurosurg Psychiatry 2000;69: 562.

Braekhus A, Engedal, K, Vascular dementia – an ill-defined concept, Tidsskr Nor Laegeforen 2004;124: 1097–9.

Brattström LE, Hardebo JE, Hultberg BL, Moderate homocysteinemia – a possible risk factor for arteriosclerotic cerebrovascular disease. Stroke 1984;15: 1012–6.

Breteler MM, Ott A, Hofman A, The new epidemic: frequency of dementia in the Rotterdam Study. Haemostasis 1998;28: 117–23.

Börjel AK, Yngve A, Sjöström M, Nilsson TK, Novel mutations in the 5′-UTR of the FOLR1 gene. Clin Chem Lab Med 2006;44: 161–7.

Böttiger AK, Hagnelius N-O, Nilsson TK, Mutations in exons 2 and 3 of the FOLR1 gene in demented and non-demented elderly subjects. Int J Mol Med 2007;20: 653–62.

Cechetto DF, Hachinski V, Whitehead SN, Vascular risk factors and Alzheimer's disease. Expert Rev Neurother 2008;8: 743–50.

Chan A, Shea TB, Folate deprivation increases presenilin expression, gamma-secretase activity, and Abeta levels in murine brain: potentiation by ApoE deficiency and alleviation by dietary S-adenosyl methionine. J Neurochem 2007;102, 753–60.

Clarke R, Smith AD, Jobst KA, Refsum H, Sutton L, Ueland PM, Folate, vitamin B12, and serum total homocysteine levels in confirmed Alzheimer disease. Arch Neurol 1998;55: 1449–55.

Connelly PJ, Prentice NP, Cousland G, Bonham J, A randomised double-blind placebo-controlled trial of folic acid supplementation of cholinesterase inhibitors in Alzheimer's disease. Int J Geriatr Psychiatry 2008;23: 155–60.

Dufouil C, Alperovitch A, Ducros V, Tzourio C, Homocysteine, white matter hyperintensities, and cognition in healthy elderly people. Ann Neurol 2003;53: 214–21.

Durga J, van Boxtel MP, Schouten EG, Kok FJ, Jolles J, Katan MB, Verhoef P, Effect of 3-year folic acid supplementation on cognitive function in older adults in the FACIT trial: a randomised, double blind, controlled trial. Lancet 2007;369: 208–16.

Ebly EM, Schaefer JP, Campbell NR, Hogan DB, Folate status, vascular disease and cognition in elderly Canadians. Age Ageing 1998;27: 485–91.

Fratiglioni L, Rocca WA, Epidemiology of dementia, Amsterdam: Elsevier; 2001.

Fratiglioni L, Viitanen M, von Strauss E, Tontodonati V, Herlitz A, Winblad B, Very old women at highest risk of dementia and Alzheimer's disease: incidence data from the Kungsholmen Project, Stockholm. Neurology 1997;48: 132–8.

Geller J, Kronn D, Jayabose S, Sandoval C, Hereditary folate malabsorption: family report and review of the literature. Medicine 2002;81: 51–68.

Goodwin JS, Goodwin JM, Garry PJ, Association between nutritional status and cognitive functioning in a healthy elderly population. J Am Med Assoc 1983;249: 2917–21.

Haan MN, Miller JW, Aiello AE, Whitmer RA, Jagust WJ, Mungas DM, Allen LH, Green R, Homocysteine, B vitamins, and the incidence of dementia and cognitive impairment: results from the Sacramento Area Latino Study on Aging. Am J Clin Nutr 2007;85: 511–7.

Hagnelius N-O, Wahlund LO, Nilsson TK, CSF/serum folate gradient: physiology and determinants with special reference to dementia. Dement Geriatr Cogn Disord 2008;25: 516–23.

Hagnelius N-O, Boman K, Nilsson TK, Fibrinolysis and von Willebrand factor in Alzheimer's disease and vascular dementia – a case-referent study. Thromb Res 2010;126:35–38.

Herbert V, Zalusky R, Selective concentration of folic acid activity in cerebro-spinal fluid. Federation Proceedings 1961;20: 453.

Herbert V, Zalusky R, Interrelations of vitamin B12 and folic acid metabolism: folic acid clearance studies. J Clin Invest 1962;41: 1263–76.

Herrmann W, Schorr H, Obeid R, Geisel J, Vitamin B-12 status, particularly holotranscobalamin II and methylmalonic acid concentrations, and hyperhomocysteinemia in vegetarians. Am J Clin Nutr 2003;78: 131–6.

Ho PI, Ortiz D, Rogers E, Shea TB, Multiple aspects of homocysteine neurotoxicity: glutamate excitotoxicity, kinase hyperactivation and DNA damage. J Neurosci Res 2002;70: 694–702.

Hultberg B, Nilsson K, Isaksson A, Gustafson L, Folate deficiency is a common finding in psychogeriatric patients. Aging Clin Exp Res 2002;14: 479–84.

Kado DM, Karlamangla AS, Huang MH, Troen A, Rowe JW, Selhub J, Seeman TE, Homocysteine versus the vitamins folate, B(6), and B(12) as predictors of cognitive function and decline in older high-functioning adults: MacArthur Studies of Successful Aging. Am J Med 2005;118: 161–7.

Kalaria RN, The role of cerebral ischemia in Alzheimer's disease. Neurobiol Aging 2000;21: 321–30.

Khachaturian Z, The five-five, ten-ten plan for Alzheimer's disease, Neurobiol Aging 1992;13: 197–8; discussion 199.

Kivipelto M, Rovio S, Ngandu T, Kareholt I, Eskelinen M, Winblad B, Hachinski V, Cedazo-Minguez A, Soininen H, Tuomilehto J, Nissinen A, Apolipoprotein E epsilon4 magnifies lifestyle risks for dementia: a population based study, J Cell Mol Med 2008;12: 2762–71.

Knopman DS, Dementia and cerebrovascular disease. Mayo Clin Proc 2006;81: 223–30.

Korczyn AD, Homocysteine, stroke, and dementia, Stroke 2002;33: 2343–4.

Lindenbaum J, Healton EB, Savage DG, Brust JC, Garrett TJ, Podell ER, Marcell PD, Stabler SP, Allen RH, Neuropsychiatric disorders caused by cobalamin deficiency in the absence of anemia or macrocytosis. N Engl J Med 1988;318: 1720–8.

Luchsinger JA, Tang MX, Miller J, Green R, Mayeux R, Higher folate intake is related to lower risk of Alzheimer's disease in the elderly. J Nutr Health Aging 2008;12: 648–50.

Malouf M, Grimley Evans J, Folic acid with or without vitamin B12 for the prevention and treatment of healthy elderly and demented people. Cochrane Database Syst Rev 2008;CD004514.

Mann DM, Iwatsubo T, Pickering-Brown SM, Owen F, Saido TC, Perry RH, Preferential deposition of amyloid beta protein (Abeta) in the form Abeta40 in Alzheimer's disease is associated with a gene dosage effect of the apolipoprotein E E4 allele. Neurosci Lett 1997;221: 81–4.

Mari D, Parnetti L, Coppola R, Bottasso B, Reboldi GP, Senin U, Mannucci PM, Hemostasis abnor-malities in patients with vascular dementia and Alzheimer's disease. Thromb Haemost 1996;75: 216–8.

Maxwell CJ, Hogan DB, Ebly EM, Serum folate levels and subsequent adverse cerebrovascular outcomes in elderly persons. Dement Geriatr Cogn Disord 2002;13: 225–34.

McCaddon A, Davies G, Hudson P, Tandy S, Cattell H, Total serum homocysteine in senile demen-tia of Alzheimer type. Int J Geriatr Psychiatry 1998;13: 235–9.

Middleton LE, Kirkland SA, Maxwell CJ, Hogan DB, Rockwood K, Exercise: a potential con-tributing factor to the relationship between folate and dementia. J Am Geriatr Soc 2007;55: 1095–8.

Mielke MM, Rosenberg PB, Tschanz J, Cook L, Corcoran C, Hayden KM, Norton M, Rabins PV, Green RC, Welsh-Bohmer KA, Breitner JC, Munger R, Lyketsos CG, Vascular factors predict rate of progression in Alzheimer disease. Neurology 2007;69:1850–8.

Miller JW, Green R, Mungas DM, Reed BR, Jagust WJ, Homocysteine, vitamin B6, and vascular disease in AD patients. Neurology 2002;58: 1471–5.

Min SH, Oh SY, Karp GI, Poncz M, Zhao R, Goldman ID, The clinical course and genetic defect in the PCFT gene in a 27-year-old woman with hereditary folate malabsorption. J Pediatr 2008;153: 435–7.

Morris MC, Evans DA, Bienias JL, Tangney CC, Hebert LE, Scherr PA, Schneider JA, Dietary folate and vitamin B12 intake and cognitive decline among community-dwelling older persons. Arch Neurol 2005;62: 641–5.

Nelson C, Wengreen HJ, Munger RG, Corcoran CD, Dietary folate, vitamin B-12, vitamin B-6 and incident Alzheimer's disease: the Cache County Memory, Health and Aging Study. J Nutr Health Aging 2009;13: 899–905.

Nilsson TK, Börjel AK, Novel insertion and deletion mutations in the 5'-UTR of the folate receptor-alpha gene: an additional contributor to hyperhomocysteinemia? Clin Biochem 2004;37: 224–9.

Nilsson K, Gustafson L, Fäldt R, Andersson A, Brattström L, Lindgren A, Israelsson B, Hultberg B, Hyperhomocysteinaemia – a common finding in a psychogeriatric population. Eur J Clin Invest 1996;26: 853–9.

Nilsson SE, Read S, Berg S, Johansson B, Heritabilities for fifteen routine biochemical values: findings in 215 Swedish twin pairs 82 years of age or older. Scand J Clin Lab Invest 2009;69: 562–9.

Obeid R, Kostopoulos P, Knapp JP, Kasoha M, Becker G, Fassbender K, Herrmann W, Biomarkers of folate and vitamin B12 are related in blood and cerebrospinal fluid. Clin Chem 2007;53: 326–33.

Petersen RC, Smith GE, Waring SC, Ivnik RJ, Tangalos EG, Kokmen E, Mild cognitive impairment: clinical characterization and outcome. Arch Neurol 1999;56: 303–8.

Poncz M, Colman N, Herbert V, Schwartz E, Cohen AR, Therapy of congenital folate malabsorp-tion. J Pediatr 1981;98: 76–9.

Purnell C, Gao S, Callahan CM, Hendrie HC, Cardiovascular risk factors and incident Alzheimer disease: a systematic review of the literature. Alzheimer Dis Assoc Disord 2009;23: 1–10.

Qiu A, Jansen M, Sakaris A, Min SH, Chattopadhyay S, Tsai E, Sandoval C, Zhao R, Akabas MH, Goldman ID, Identification of an intestinal folate transporter and the molecular basis for heredi-tary folate malabsorption, Cell 2006;127: 917–28.

Ramaekers VT, Rothenberg SP, Sequeira JM, Opladen T, Blau N, Quadros EV, Selhub J, Autoanti-bodies to folate receptors in the cerebral folate deficiency syndrome. N Engl J Med 2005;352: 1985–91.

Ramos MI, Allen LH, Mungas DM, Jagust WJ, Haan MN, Green R, Miller JW, Low folate status is associated with impaired cognitive function and dementia in the Sacramento Area Latino Study on Aging. Am J Clin Nutr 2005;82: 1346–52.

Ravaglia G, Forti P, Maioli F, Muscari A, Sacchetti L, Arnone G, Nativio V, Talerico T, Mariani E, Homocysteine and cognitive function in healthy elderly community dwellers in Italy. Am J Clin Nutr 2003;77: 668–73.

Reynolds EH, Bottiglieri T, Laundy M, Stern J, Payan J, Linnell J, Faludy J, Subacute combined degeneration with high serum vitamin B12 level and abnormal vitamin B12 binding protein. New cause of an old syndrome. Arch Neurol 1993;50: 739–42.

Reynolds EH, Gallagher BB, Mattson RH, Bowers M, Johnson AL, Relationship between serum and cerebrospinal fluid folate. Nature 1972;240: 155–7.

Rothberg KG, Ying YS, Kolhouse JF, Kamen BA, Anderson RG, The glycophospholipid-linked folate receptor internalizes folate without entering the clathrin-coated pit endocytic pathway. J Cell Biol 1990;110: 637–49.

Salvioli G, Ventura P, Pradelli JM, Impact of nutrition on cognition and affectivity in the elderly: a review. Arch Gerontol Geriatr 1998;Suppl 5: 459–68.

Schlotz W, Jones A, Phillips NM, Godfrey KM, Phillips DI, Size at birth and motor activity during stress in children aged 7 to 9 years. Pediatrics 2007;120: e1237–44.

Schlotz W, Jones A, Phillips DI, Gale CR, Robinson SM, Godfrey KM, Lower maternal folate status in early pregnancy is associated with childhood hyperactivity and peer problems in offspring. J Child Psychol Psychiatry 2010;51: 594–602.

Serot JM, Christmann D, Dubost T, Bene MC, Faure GC, CSF-folate levels are decreased in late-onset AD patients. J Neural Transm 2001;108: 93–9.

Seshadri S, Beiser A, Selhub J, Jacques PF, Rosenberg IH, D'Agostino RB, Wilson PW, Wolf PA, Plasma homocysteine as a risk factor for dementia and Alzheimer's disease. N Engl J Med 2002;346: 476–83.

Skoog I, Vascular aspects in Alzheimer's disease. J Neural Transm Suppl 2000;59: 37–43.

Smith AD, The worldwide challenge of the dementias: a role for B vitamins and homocysteine? Food Nutr Bull 2008;29: S143–72.

Smulders YM, Smith DE, Kok RM, Teerlink T, Swinkels DW, Stehouwer CD, Jakobs C, Cellular folate vitamer distribution during and after correction of vitamin B12 deficiency: a case for the methylfolate trap. Br J Haematol 2006;132: 623–9.

Sneath P, Chanarin I, Hodkinson HM, McPherson CK, Reynolds EH, Folate status in a geriatric population and its relation to dementia. Age Ageing 1973;2: 177–82.

Snowdon DA, Tully CL, Smith CD, Riley KP, Markesbery WR, Serum folate and the severity of atrophy of the neocortex in Alzheimer disease: findings from the Nun study. Am J Clin Nutr 2000;71: 993–8.

Sontag E, Nunbhakdi-Craig V, Sontag JM, Diaz-Arrastia R, Ogris E, Dayal S, Lentz SR, Arning E, Bottiglieri T, Protein phosphatase 2A methyltransferase links homocysteine metabolism with tau and amyloid precursor protein regulation. J Neurosci 2007;27: 2751–9.

Spector R, Lorenzo AV, Folate transport in the central nervous system. Am J Physiol 1975;229: 777–82.

Steinfeld R, Grapp M, Kraetzner R, Dreha-Kulaczewski S, Helms G, Dechent P, Wevers R, Grosso S, Gartner J, Folate receptor alpha defect causes cerebral folate transport deficiency: a treatable neurodegenerative disorder associated with disturbed myelin metabolism. Am J Hum Genet 2009;85: 354–63.

Strachan RW, Henderson JG, Dementia and folate deficiency. Q J Med 1967;36: 189–204.

Sun Y, Lu CJ, Chien KL, Chen ST, Chen RC, Efficacy of multivitamin supplementation containing vitamins B6 and B12 and folic acid as adjunctive treatment with a cholinesterase inhibitor in Alzheimer's disease: a 26-week, randomized, double-blind, placebo-controlled study in Taiwanese patients. Clin Ther 2007;29: 2204–14.

Tettamanti M, Garri MT, Nobili A, Riva E, Lucca U, Low folate and the risk of cognitive and functional deficits in the very old: the Monzino 80-plus study. J Am Coll Nutr 2006;25: 502–8.

Van Guelpen B, Hultdin J, Johansson I, Witthoft C, Weinehall L, Eliasson M, Hallmans G, Palmqvist R, Jansson JH, Winkvist A, Plasma folate and total homocysteine levels are associated with the risk of myocardial infarction, independently of each other and of renal function. J Intern Med 2009;266: 182–95.

Wang HX, Wahlin A, Basun H, Fastbom J, Winblad B, Fratiglioni L, Vitamin B(12) and folate in relation to the development of Alzheimer's disease. Neurology 2001;56: 1188–94.

Wells DG, Casey HJ, *Lactobacillus casei* CSF folate activity. Br Med J 1967;3: 834–7.

Wollack JB, Makori B, Ahlawat S, Koneru R, Picinich SC, Smith A, Goldman ID, Qiu A, Cole PD, Glod J, Kamen B, Characterization of folate uptake by choroid plexus epithelial cells in a rat primary culture model. J Neurochem 2008;104: 1494–503.

Vollset SE, Refsum H, Tverdal A, Nygård O, Nordrehaug JE, Tell GS, Ueland PM, Plasma total homocysteine and cardiovascular and noncardiovascular mortality: the Hordaland Homocysteine Study. Am J Clin Nutr 2001;74: 130–6.

Wu D, Pardridge WM, Blood-brain barrier transport of reduced folic acid. Pharm Res 1999;16: 415–9.

Zhao R, Min SH, Qiu A, Sakaris A, Goldberg GL, Sandoval C, Malatack JJ, Rosenblatt DS, Goldman ID, The spectrum of mutations in the PCFT gene, coding for an intestinal folate transporter, that are the basis for hereditary folate malabsorption. Blood 2007;110: 1147–52.

Zylberstein D, Homocysteine and cardiovascular morbidity and dementia in women. Thesis, paper IV. Göteborg: Göteborgs universitet; 2009. pp. 1–13.

Zylberstein DE, Bengtsson C, Bjorkelund C, Landaas S, Sundh V, Thelle D, Lissner L, Serum homocysteine in relation to mortality and morbidity from coronary heart disease: a 24-year follow-up of the population study of women in Gothenburg. Circulation 2004;109: 601–6.

Zylberstein DE, Skoog I, Bjorkelund C, Guo X, Hulten B, Andreasson LA, Palmertz B, Thelle DS, Lissner L, Homocysteine levels and lacunar brain infarcts in elderly women: the prospective population study of women in Gothenburg. J Am Geriatr Soc 2008;56: 1087–91.

Zylberstein DE, Lissner L, Bjorkelund C, Mehlig K, Thelle DS, Gustafson D, Ostling S, Waern M, Guo X, Skoog I, Midlife homocysteine and late-life dementia in women. A prospective population study. Neurobiol Aging 2009; doi:10.1016/j.neurobiolaging.2009.02.024.

6.5 The role of folate in methotrexate-induced neurotoxicity, antiepileptic treatment and depression

Alexander Semmler; Michael Linnebank

6.5.1 Methotrexate metabolic actions

Methotrexate (MTX) is a antifolate drug widely used in the treatment of various forms of cancer including leukemia and solid tumors as well as metastatic and primary brain tumors.

Methotrexate in serum is approximately 50% protein bound. Renal excretion is the primary route of elimination and is dependent on dosage and route of administration. With intravenous administration, 80–90% of the administered dose is excreted unchanged in the urine within 24 h. MTX primarily enters the cell through active transport mediated by the reduced folate carrier 1 (RFC1). At high extracellular concentrations, MTX also enters cells via passive diffusion of the drug. Once in the cell, MTX exerts its antiproliferative effect by interference with the folate/homocysteine cycle mainly through inhibition of dihydrofolate reductase (DHFR). This leads to a lack of 5,10-methylenetetrahydrofolate, which is necessary for nucleic acid synthesis and thus will lead to the death of highly proliferative cells (Goldman and Matherly, 1985) (►Fig. 6.9).

High-dose MTX (HD-MTX) refers to MTX doses that range from 1 to 12 g/m² or even higher. The goals of HD-MTX are to increase MTX concentrations in pharmacological sanctuaries [e.g., central nervous system (CNS), testes], and to increase passive cellular MTX uptake in resistant tumor cells.

The MTX doses used in the treatment of inflammatory diseases such as rheumatoid arthritis are considerably lower and the efficacy and toxicity of low-dose oral MTX is probably mediated by different mechanisms (Wessels et al., 2008).

6.5.2 Clinical presentation of MTX-induced neurotoxicity

Methotrexate dosage and efficacy is mainly limited by complications affecting the CNS. Although many studies attributed these limitations of MTX therapy, the pathological basis of MTX-induced neurotoxicity are not fully understood.

MTX-induced neurotoxicity can present as acute or chronic encephalopathy. Acute MTX-induced encephalopathy develops within 1–14 days after high dose intravenous or intrathecal application of methotrexate and presents with a clinical picture varying from altered mental status to paresis and seizures (Inaba et al., 2008). Acute neurotoxicity has been observed in up to 15% of cancer patients after HD MTX (Jaffe et al., 1985; Rubnitz et al., 1998). Many stay without permanent neurological squela, but fatal outcome was also reported (Brock and Jennings, 2004). Chronic encephalopathy develops within 1 year after treatment and might permanently impair neurological function. Children cured of leukemia, who received high-dose MTX or intrathecal MTX and

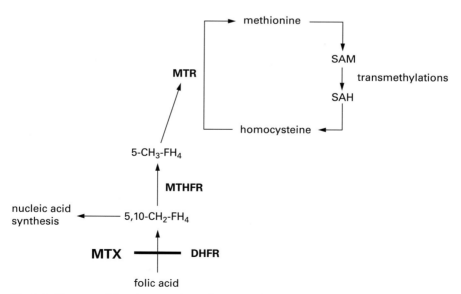

Fig. 6.9: Diagram of the pharmacological MTX mechanism. The folate derivates are synthesized by methylenetetrahydrofolate reductase (MTHFR) and (DHFR). The lack of the folate derivates leads to disturbances of nucleic acid synthesis as well as homocysteine metabolism.

cranial irradiation show a decrease of IQ of more than 15 points after therapy (Ochs et al., 1991; Montour-Proulx et al., 2005). Brain MRI of patients with MTX-induced encephalopathy show transient abnormalities in diffusion-weighted images and continuous abnormalities in T2 and FLAIR imaging located in the cerebral white matter (Rubnitz et al., 1998; Atra et al., 2004; Inaba et al., 2008).

6.5.3 Pathogenesis of MTX-neurotoxicity

MTX is an inhibitor of dihydrofolate reductase (DHFR) preventing the formation of 5,10-methylenetetrahydrofolate and, consecutively, of 5-methyltetrahydrofolate. This results in an inhibition of purine and thymidine biosynthesis causing an S-phase cell cycle arrest, which accounts for the antiproliferative effect of MTX (Tsurusawa et al., 1988). Inhibition of DHFR additionally inhibits remethylation of homocysteine to methionine, which, in turn, causes accumulation of neurotoxic homocysteine and depletion of S-adenosylmethionine (SAM). SAM is an important universal methyl donor in the maintenance of the myelin sheath and membrane stability of CNS cells, as well as a wide variety of other important methylation reactions (Finkelstein, 2000) (▶Fig. 6.9).

The occurrence of acute MTX-toxicity is associated with a significant reduction of SAM concentrations in the cerebrospinal fluid (CSF) of patients treated with high dose MTX and/or intrathecal MTX up to 45 days after MTX application (Surtees et al., 1998; Becker et al., 2007; Vezmar et al., 2009). Anecdotally, acute MTX-neurotoxicity could be reverted by substitution of multiple folate metabolites (Ackermann et al., 2010).

To decrease the toxic effects of MTX, 'leucovorin rescue', which is the substitution of folinic acid (a precursor of 5,10-methylenetetrahydofolate), is initiated 36 h after MTX infusion. In recent years the dosage of folinic acid is adjusted to MTX plasma concentrations, e.g., the dosage of leukovorin is between 30 and 75 mg/m² body surface 36 h after MTX infusion according to the MTX plasma level. Leukovorin rescue is repeated every 6 h until plasma MTX reaches concentrations under 0.1 μmol/l. When MTX is followed by rescue, patients regularly do not show signs of neurotoxicity and have normal CSF SAM concentrations 14 days after MTX application (Vezmar et al., 2009). Reducing the dose of folinic acid below a critical level will result in neurotoxicity, even with low doses of MTX (Cohen, 2004, 2007b). However, it has been suggested that high leucovorin doses will reduce the cure rate in leukemia by decreasing the antiproliferative effects of high-dose MTX treatment, despite the fact that the leukovorin dosage was correlated with high MTX levels, which are expected to give a better prognosis (Cohen, 2004; Skarby et al., 2006). This has led to lowering leucovorin dose in treatment protocols with the risk of an increased rate of acute and chronic neurotoxicity (Skarby et al., 2006; Cohen, 2007a). Accordingly, attempts to facilitate MTX-based chemotherapies and to reduce neurotoxicity in treatment protocols for primary CNS lymphoma by omitting intraventricular treatment is associated with early relapses (Pels et al., 2009). This further underlines the importance of neuroprotective strategies, which do not endanger the efficacy of MTX-based protocols.

6.5.4 Why is MTX-neurotoxicity predominantly a white matter disease?

Myelin basic protein (MBP) is a major myelin protein that accounts for 35% of the total myelin protein. It is a 170-amino acid protein in humans. Post-translational modifications determine the nature of the secondary structure of MBP and its ability to form stable myelin multilayers (Amur et al., 1986). MBP has a methylated arginine at position 107. The methylated arginine is a mixture of mono-, and symmetrically dimethylated methyl-formations (Kim et al., 1997). Methylation of MBP is implemented by a specific methyl-transferase (Miyake, 1975). The activity of this methyltransferase increases during active myelination, suggesting that MBP methylation is a process associated with myelination (Crang and Jacobson, 1982). Methylation of MPB is important for the formation and main-tenance of MBP. Inhibition of the MBP arginine methyltransferase prevents the formation of a compact myelin (Amur et al., 1986). Methylated MBP arginine also increases the interaction between MBP and myelin lipids (Young et al., 1987). In subacute combined degeneration of the spinal cord in humans, demyelination results from a deficiency in vitamin B12, which decreases the amount of the major methyl-donor, SAM, with a subse-quent decrease in methylation of MBP (Surtees, 1993). Therefore, methylation of MBP at a single arginine is important in the formation and maintenance of compact myelin and this could be a link between MTX-induced white matter changes and depletion of brain SAM levels.

6.5.5 Does MTX-neurotoxicity vary with genetic predisposition and dietary vitamin status?

Folate metabolism is not only influenced by drugs such as methotrexate, but also by the availability of dietary vitamins and genetic variants, which increase liability towards MTX-neurotoxicity. We studied a sample of 68 patients receiving MTX-based polyche-motherapy with and without intraventricular treatment for primary CNS lymphoma ana-lyzing ten genetic functional variants of the methionine metabolism. We observed that the TT-genotype of methylenetetrahydrofolate reductase (MTHFR) c.677C>T, the AA-genotype of MTHFR c.1298A>C and the GG-genotype of transcobalamin 2 c.776C>G were associated with the appearance of CNS white matter changes (WMC) after MTX treatment (Linnebank et al., 2005, 2009). Because at least the genetic variants MTHFR c.677C>T and transcobalamin c.776C>G might result in reduced production of SAM and increased levels of neurotoxic homocysteine, these observations further point towards a crucial role of SAM and probably of homocysteine in the development of MTX neuro-toxicity (Linnebank et al., 2005, 2009). Other rare genetic variants of the homocysteine metabolism could also contribute to liability towards MTX neurotoxicity (Linnebank et al., 2007).

Pre-therapeutic folate and vitamin B12 levels speculatively influence occurrence of MTX-induced neurotoxicity. Folic acid supplementation has become routine in low-dose MTX therapy for patients with rheumatoid arthritis, because it was shown that folate supplementation reduces the risk of MTX-side effects (Whittle and Hughes, 2004). However, it is not known, if similar folate supplementation would alter prognosis of HD-MTX therapy also. Interestingly, the toxicity of permetrexed, an antifolate can-cer drug similar to MTX that also inhibits DHFR, correlates with homocysteine plasma levels before therapy (Niyikiza et al., 2002). Homocysteine is considered a 'vitamin deficiency marker', as it will rise in case of folate or vitamin B12 deficiency.

Folate fortification (the addition of folate to grain products to increase the supply of the general population with folate) is associated with increasing MTX dosages in the treatment of patients with rheumatoid arthritis (Arabelovic et al., 2007). There are no data, however, on folate fortification and efficacy or side-effects of HD-MTX in cancer therapy. The occurrence of side-effects of antifolate drugs, particularly of HD-MTX, has been unpredictable up to date. Speculatively, pre-therapeutic homocysteine plasma levels and the individual genetic profile could help to identify patients that are at risk of toxicity before treatment. Vitamin supplementation might lead to a better safety profile of antifolate cancer therapy. If future studies confirm the association of biochemical and genetic factors related with homocysteine metabolism, a biochemical and genetic 'risk profile' might be established yielding individualized MTX-protocols.

The dosage and effectiveness of MTX is limited by its neurotoxic side-effects, which are significantly reduced by the substitution of folinic acid ('leucovorin rescue'). Genetic predisposition and pre-therapeutic folate and vitamin B12 levels might influence MTX neurotoxicity.

6.5.6 Folate and antiepileptic drugs

Antiepileptic drugs (AED) are frequently used in the treatment of epilepsy, psychiatric diseases or pain syndromes. The prevalence of these diseases is high, and the majority of patients are on life-long medication with AED.

Since the original description by Mannheimer in 1952 of two cases with megaloblastic anemia occurring as a probable side effect of anticonvulsant drug therapy with hydantoin derivates (Mannheimer et al., 1952), a series of studies have suggested that treatment with AED, such as valproate, carbamazepine or phenytoin, is associated with reduced mean serum levels of folate and vitamin B12 and that this might mediate AED side effects (Vilaseca et al., 2000; Karabiber et al., 2003; Gidal et al., 2005; Attilakos et al., 2006; Sener et al., 2006). AED side effects often limit the dosage of AEDs. Typical AED side effects such as fatigue, osteoporosis, peripheral neuropathies, atherosclerosis, cerebellar ataxia, increased seizure frequency, neuropsychological impairment, and teratogenesis (Vermeulen and Aldenkamp, 1995; Genton, 2000; Kaaja et al., 2003; Meador et al., 2006, 2009; Kantola-Sorsa et al., 2007; Sirven et al., 2007; Sheth et al., 2008; Tan et al., 2009) are possibly owing to their interference with folate and vitamin B12 metabolism.

Interestingly, folic acid originally had a reputation for powerful excitatory properties and provoking seizures particularly when applied in very high doses and when the blood-brain barrier is circumvented (Hommes et al., 1973; Guidolin et al., 1998). As a result, the idea that some AEDs are antiepileptic because they are folic acid antagonists emerged and the search for new AEDs included medications that demonstrated folic acid antagonism. Lamotrigine, an AED marketed in the 1990s, is one such medication (Sander and Patsalos, 1992).

In a large sample of 2730 patients treated with AEDs, we found that patients treated with carbamazepine, gabapentin, oxcarbazepine, phenytoin or valproate had significantly more often subnormal serum folate levels than untreated patients or controls. The association of carbamazepine and valproate with low folate levels revealed a dose-dependency, whereas the association of gabapentin, oxcarbazepine and phenytoin did not. Although intake of primidone and topiramate was not associated with folate levels *per se*, the daily dose of these AED negatively correlated with folate levels. Additionally, treatment with phenobarbital, pregabalin, primidone or topiramate was associated with reduced mean vitamin B12 levels. Subnormal folate levels and vitamin B12 levels were associated with lower red blood cell count, higher mean corpuscular volume, higher mean corpuscular hemoglobin, higher lymphocyte counts, higher platelet counts, and higher homocysteine plasma levels (Linnebank et al., in press).

The elevation of homocysteine plasma levels might be of particular importance in patients with epilepsy, because homocysteine is a neurotoxic excitatory amino acid functioning at the N-methyl-D-aspartate (NMDA) receptor. Thus, reduced mean folate and elevated homocysteine levels associated with AED treatment could promote seizures and neuronal damage contributing to the brain atrophy observed in 20–50% of patients with epilepsy (Gorgone et al., 2009). In addition, elevated homocysteine levels could underlie the increased risk of atherosclerosis observed in epilepsy patients (Tan et al., 2009). Further, elevated homocysteine and lowered folate concentrations can represent a risk factor for the occurrence of an interictal (occurring between seizures) psychosis (Monji et al., 2005).

In summary, treatment with any of the commonly used AEDs other than levetiracetam and benzodiazepines, but in particular with carbamazepine, gabapentin, phenytoin and primidone, is associated with subnormal or lower mean serum levels of folate or vitamin B12. Because this might mediate AED side effects and decrease AED efficacy, regular controls of folate and vitamin B12 serum levels are recommended in patients on AED treatment. Prophylactic supplementation could be considered as an alternative to regular measurements and selective substitution in patients treated with AED in our view. The prophylactic supplementation of folate is of importance in women of childbearing age who are treated with AED. This is why folic acid supplementation for women of childbearing age, who are on any AED treatment, is particularly indicated and is urgently recommended by the specialist societies (Wilson et al., 2003; Crawford, 2005).

6.5.7 Valproic acid and neural tube defects

There is evidence that valproic acid (VPA) might have a greater teratogenic potential than other AEDs. This was first suggested about 30 years ago by a case series of neural tube defects in children exposed to VPA *in utero* (Bjerkedal et al., 1982). Later it was confirmed, that maternal usage of VPA is associated with a high number of major congenital malformations in the offspring (Samren et al., 1997). Some studies also demonstrated a relation to VPA dosage, with a significantly increased a daily dose of >1000 mg VPA being associated with a significantly higher teratogenic risk (Meador et al., 2006). There is clear evidence for the value of folate supplementation with 0.4 mg folic acid daily in preventing neural tube defects in the general population (Pitkin, 2007). Beyond these general recommendations there is not sufficient evidence that the risk for neural tube defects can be further reduced in women taking AEDs (Kaaja et al., 2003; Yerby, 2003; Harden et al., 2009). Nevertheless, some authors recommend high-dose folic acid (up to 4 mg daily) in women of child-bearing age taking VPA or other enzyme-inducing AEDs such as carbamazepine or phenytoin (Kluger and Meador, 2008). Frequent controls of the serum AED level as well as appropriate screening for neural tube defects in pregnant women by alpha-fetoprotein levels and ultrasonography is recommended.

Antiepileptic drugs can lower folate and vitamin B12 and raise homocysteine concentrations in the blood. Folate and vitamin B12 levels should be routinely monitored in patients treated with antiepileptic drugs. In case of abnormal results, vitamins should be substituted.

In women of childbearing age on AED medication, folate should be substituted with at least 0.4 mg daily. VPA should be avoided if possible. If VPA is necessary for seizure control a daily dosage below 1000 mg could be less problematical than higher doses.

6.5.8 Folate and depression

Unipolar depression is one of the ten leading illnesses of global disease burden and is the most frequent psychiatric disease (Lopez et al., 2006). Depression is underdiagnosed and undertreated, particularly in older patients (VanItallie, 2005). The link between folate and depression has been shown by early reports demonstrating a correlation between the occurrence of neuropsychiatric disorders and folate deficiency in patients with megaloblastic anemia (Shorvon et al., 1980).

Since these initial findings, evidence accumulated that low folate status is associated with depression: reduced folate levels have been demonstrated in up to 56% of patients with a major depressive disorder (Bottiglieri et al., 2000a; Morris et al., 2003; Coppen and Bolander-Gouaille, 2005; Gilbody et al., 2007b; Ng et al., 2009). Low folate is also linked with the severity and length of a depressive episode (Alpert and Fava, 1997; Coppen and Bolander-Gouaille, 2005). Treatment of depression has a delayed or weaker effect in presence of folate deficiency (Alpert and Fava, 1997; Godfrey et al., 1990; Wesson et al., 1994; Rosche et al., 2003). Pre-treatment with folic acid (Godfrey et al., 1990) as well as the simultaneous administration of folic acid and fluoxetine leads to a significantly improved efficacy (Coppen and Bailey, 2000; Papakostas et al., 2005), and low folate levels increase the risk of suffering a depressive relapse during fluoxetine therapy (Papakostas et al., 2004). These associations are stronger when moderately decreased folate levels are combined with additional risk factors such as the TT genotype of MTFR c.677C>T, which promotes the disturbed reduction of 5,10-methylenetetrahydrofolate to 5-methyltetrahydrofolate (Gilbody et al., 2007a).

The connection between low folate levels and depressive disorders might be owing to the SAM- and folate-dependent synthesis of neurotransmitters including the monoamines serotonin (5-HT), norepinephrine (NE) and dopamine (DA) (Stahl, 2007, 2008). A lack of those neurotransmitters can result in depression, and antidepressants act through boosting the action of one or more of these neurotransmitters. Reduced folate levels could lead to a lack of 5-HT, NE and DA via different biochemical pathways. Firstly, the active metabolite of folate, 5-methyltetrahydrofolate (5-MTHF) together with vitamin B12 participates in the remethylation of homocysteine into methionine, which is transferred to its downstream metabolite S-adenosylmethionine (SAM), donor of methyl-groups in the formation of the monoamine neurotransmitters (Losada and Rubio, 1989; Otero-Losada and Rubio, 1989). Oral and intravenous SAM administration showed a mood-enhancing effect (Bottiglieri et al., 1990), and its antidepressant effect might even be comparable with that of the classical tricyclical antidepressants (Bressa, 1994).

The second important connection between reduced folate levels and reduced brain neurotransmitter levels could be tetrahydrobiopterin (BH4). BH4 is a nutrient, rate-limiting co-factor for hydroxylase enzymes involved in the biosynthesis of the neurotransmitters.

Folate is important in the synthesis and regeneration of BH4, which is highly susceptible to oxidation (Antoniades et al., 2006).

The importance of folate levels for the development of depression can vary greatly between patient populations, e.g., they might be of particular importance for the elderly, because the prevalence of folate deficiency increases with age (Selhub et al., 1993; Clarke et al., 2004). The impact of folate fortification on the prevalence of depression and other diseases for which folate might be relevant remains to be elucidated. Whereas serum and CSF concentrations of folate and vitamin B12 fall, those of homocysteine rise with age (Bottiglieri et al., 2000b). The cause of vitamin deficiency in higher age is unclear and has been variously ascribed to chronic illnesses, side effects of medications, malabsorption, increased demand and poor diet (Reynolds, 2002). In elderly Europeans, the average intake of folate is clearly below the recommended daily dose of 400 µg/day (Fabian and Elmadfa, 2008).

Although several categories of antidepressants are available, approximately 30–40% of patients suffer from depression refractory to therapy (Miller and O'Callaghan, 2005). Therapy with folic acid should be taken into account as adjunctive treatment and could be beneficial even in cases with normal blood folate levels (Passeri et al., 1993; Fava and Davidson, 1996; Stahl, 2007).

Folate deficiency favors depression and affects its duration and degree of clinical severity. Folic acid has antidepressant characteristics of its own and improves the therapeutic efficacy of antidepressant drugs. In cases of actual folate deficiency, folic acid administration can be particularly effective. In addition, SAM might have antidepressant effects.

References

Ackermann R, Semmler A, Maurer GD, Hattingen E, Fornoff F, Steinbach JP & Linnebank M, Methotrexate-induced myelopathy responsive to substitution of multiple folate metabolites. J Neurooncol 2010; 97: 425–7.

Alpert JE, Fava M, Nutrition and depression: the role of folate. Nutr Rev 1997;55: 145–9.

Amur SG, Shanker G, Cochran JM, Ved HS, Pieringer RA, Correlation between inhibition of myelin basic protein (arginine) methyltransferase by sinefungin and lack of compact myelin formation in cultures of cerebral cells from embryonic mice. J Neurosci Res 1986;16: 367–76.

Antoniades C, Shirodaria C, Warrick N, Cai S, de Bono J, Lee J, Leeson P, Neubauer S, Ratnatunga C, Pillai R, Refsum H, Channon KM, 5-methyltetrahydrofolate rapidly improves endothelial function and decreases superoxide production in human vessels: effects on vascular tetrahydrobiopterin availability and endothelial nitric oxide synthase coupling. Circulation 2006;114: 1193–201.

Arabelovic S, Sam G, Dallal GE, Jacques PF, Selhub J, Rosenberg IH, Roubenoff R, Preliminary evidence shows that folic acid fortification of the food supply is associated with higher methotrexate dosing in patients with rheumatoid arthritis. J Am Coll Nutr 2007;26: 453–5.

Atra A, Pinkerton CR, Bouffet E, Norton A, Hobson R, Imeson JD, Gerrard M, Acute neurotoxicity in children with advanced stage B-non-Hodgkin's lymphoma and B-acute lymphoblastic leukaemia treated with the United Kingdom children cancer study group 9002/9003 protocols. Eur J Cancer 2004;40: 1346–50.

Attilakos A, Papakonstantinou E, Schulpis K, Voudris K, Katsarou E, Mastroyianni S, Garoufi A, Early effect of sodium valproate and carbamazepine monotherapy on homocysteine metabolism in children with epilepsy. Epilepsy Res 2006;71: 229–32.

Becker A, Vezmar S, Linnebank M, Pels H, Bode U, Schlegel U, Jaehde U, Marked elevation in homocysteine and homocysteine sulfinic acid in the cerebrospinal fluid of lymphoma patients receiving intensive treatment with methotrexate. Int J Clin Pharmacol Ther 2007;45: 504–15.

Bjerkedal T, Czeizel A, Goujard J, Kallen B, Mastroiacova P, Nevin N, Oakley G Jr, Robert E, Valproic acid and spina bifida. Lancet 1982;2: 1096.

Bottiglieri T, Godfrey P, Flynn T, Carney MW, Toone BK, Reynolds EH, Cerebrospinal fluid S-adenosylmethionine in depression and dementia: effects of treatment with parenteral and oral S-adenosylmethionine. J Neurol Neurosurg Psychiatry 1990;53: 1096–8.

Bottiglieri T, Laundy M, Crellin R, Toone BK, Carney MW, Reynolds EH, Homocysteine, folate, methylation, and monoamine metabolism in depression. J Neurol Neurosurg Psychiatry 2000a; 69: 228–32.

Bottiglieri T, Reynolds EH, Laundy M, Folate in CSF and age. J Neurol Neurosurg Psychiatry 2000b;69: 562.

Bressa GM, S-adenosyl-l-methionine (SAMe) as antidepressant: meta-analysis of clinical studies. Acta Neurol Scand Suppl 1994;154: 7–14.

Brock S, Jennings HR, Fatal acute encephalomyelitis after a single dose of intrathecal methotrexate. Pharmacotherapy 2004;24: 673–6.

Clarke R, Grimley Evans J, Schneede J, Nexo E, Bates C, Fletcher A, Prentice A, Johnston C, Ueland PM, Refsum H, Sherliker P, Birks J, Whitlock G, Breeze E, Scott JM, Vitamin B12 and folate deficiency in later life. Age Ageing 2004;33: 34–41.

Cohen IJ, Defining the appropriate dosage of folinic acid after high-dose methotrexate for childhood acute lymphatic leukemia that will prevent neurotoxicity without rescuing malignant cells in the central nervous system. J Pediatr Hematol Oncol 2004;26: 156–63.

Cohen IJ, Comparison of long-term neurocognitive outcomes in young children with acute lymphatic leukemia treated with cranial radiation or high-dose or very high-dose intravenous methotrexate. J Clin Oncol 2007a;25: 734–5; author reply 735.

Cohen IJ, Prevention of high-dose-methotrexate neurotoxicity by adequate folinic acid rescue is possible even after central nervous system irradiation. Med Hypotheses 2007b;68: 1147–53.

Coppen A, Bailey J, Enhancement of the antidepressant action of fluoxetine by folic acid: a randomised, placebo controlled trial. J Affect Disord 2000;60: 121–30.

Coppen A, Bolander-Gouaille C, Treatment of depression: time to consider folic acid and vitamin B12. J Psychopharmacol 2005;19: 59–65.

Crang AJ, Jacobson W, The relationship of myelin basic protein (arginine) methyltransferase to myelination in mouse spinal cord. J Neurochem 1982;39: 244–7.

Crawford P, Best practice guidelines for the management of women with epilepsy. Epilepsia 2005;46 Suppl 9: 117–24.

Fabian E, Elmadfa I, Nutritional situation of the elderly in the European Union: data of the European Nutrition and Health Report (2004). Ann Nutr Metab 2008;52 Suppl 1: 57–61.

Fava M, Davidson KG, Definition and epidemiology of treatment-resistant depression. Psychiatr Clin North Am 1996;19: 179–200.

Finkelstein JD, Pathways and regulation of homocysteine metabolism in mammals. Semin Thromb Hemost 2000;26: 219–25.

Genton P, When antiepileptic drugs aggravate epilepsy. Brain Dev 2000;22: 75–80.

Gidal BE, Tamura T, Hammer A, Vuong A, Blood homocysteine, folate and vitamin B-12 concentrations in patients with epilepsy receiving lamotrigine or sodium valproate for initial monotherapy. Epilepsy Res 2005;64: 161–6.

Gilbody S, Lewis S, Lightfoot T, Methylenetetrahydrofolate reductase (MTHFR) genetic polymorphisms and psychiatric disorders: a HuGE review. Am J Epidemiol 2007a;165: 1–13.

Gilbody S, Lightfoot T, Sheldon T, Is low folate a risk factor for depression? A meta-analysis and exploration of heterogeneity. J Epidemiol Community Health 2007b;61: 631–7.

Godfrey PS, Toone BK, Carney MW, Flynn TG, Bottiglieri T, Laundy M, Chanarin I, Reynolds EH, Enhancement of recovery from psychiatric illness by methylfolate. Lancet 1990;336: 392–5.

Goldman ID, Matherly LH, The cellular pharmacology of methotrexate. Pharmacol Ther 1985;28: 77–102.

Gorgone G, Caccamo D, Pisani LR, Curro M, Parisi G, Oteri G, Ientile R, Rossini PM, Pisani F, Hyperhomocysteinemia in patients with epilepsy: does it play a role in the pathogenesis of brain atrophy? A preliminary report. Epilepsia 2009;50 Suppl 1: 33–6.

Guidolin L, Vignoli A, Canger R, Worsening in seizure frequency and severity in relation to folic acid administration. Eur J Neurol 1998;5: 301–3.

Harden CL, Pennell PB, Koppel BS, Hovinga CA, Gidal B, Meador KJ, Hopp J, TingTY, Hauser WA, Thurman D, Kaplan PW, Robinson JN, French JA, Wiebe S, Wilner AN, Vazquez B, Holmes L, Krumholz A, Finnell R, Shafer PO & Le Guen CL, Management issues for women with epilepsy—focus on pregnancy (an evidence-based review): III. Vitamin K, folic acid, blood levels, and breast-feeding: Report of the Quality Standards Subcommittee and Therapeutics and Technology Assessment Subcommittee of the American Academy of Neurology and the American Epilepsy Society. Epilepsia 2009;50: 1247–55.

Hommes OR, Obbens EA, Wijffels CC, Epileptogenic activity of sodium-folate and the blood-brain barrier in the rat. J Neurol Sci 1973;19: 63–71.

Inaba H, Khan RB, Laningham FH, Crews KR, Pui CH, Daw NC, Clinical and radiological charac-teristics of methotrexate-induced acute encephalopathy in pediatric patients with cancer. Ann Oncol 2008;19: 178–84.

Jaffe N, Takaue Y, Anzai T, Robertson R, Transient neurologic disturbances induced by high-dose methotrexate treatment. Cancer 1985;56: 1356–60.

Kaaja E, Kaaja R, Hiilesmaa V, Major malformations in offspring of women with epilepsy. Neurol-ogy 2003;60: 575–9.

Kantola-Sorsa E, Gaily E, Isoaho M, Korkman M, Neuropsychological outcomes in children of mothers with epilepsy. J Int Neuropsychol Soc 2007;13: 642–52.

Karabiber H, Sonmezgoz E, Ozerol E, Yakinci C, Otlu B, Yologlu S, Effects of valproate and carba-mazepine on serum levels of homocysteine, vitamin B12, and folic acid. Brain Dev 2003;25: 113–5.

Kim S, Lim IK, Park GH, Paik WK, Biological methylation of myelin basic protein: enzymology and biological significance. Int J Biochem Cell Biol 1997;29: 743–51.

Kluger BM, Meador KJ, Teratogenicity of antiepileptic medications. Semin Neurol 2008;28: 328–35.

Linnebank M, Pels H, Kleczar N, Farmand S, Fliessbach K, Urbach H, Orlopp K, Klockgether T, Schmidt-Wolf IG, Schlegel U, MTX-induced white matter changes are associated with polymor-phisms of methionine metabolism. Neurology 2005;64: 912–3.

Linnebank M, Malessa S, Moskau S, Semmler A, Pels H, Klockgether T, Schlegel U, Acute methotrex-ate-induced encephalopathy – causal relation to homozygous allelic state for MTR c.2756A>G (D919G)? J Chemother 2007;19: 455–7.

Linnebank M, Moskau S, Jurgens A, Simon M, Semmler A, Orlopp K, Glasmacher A, Bangard C, Vogt-Schaden M, Urbach H, Schmidt-Wolf IG, Pels H, Schlegel U, Association of genetic variants of methionine metabolism with methotrexate-induced CNS white matter changes in patients with primary CNS lymphoma. Neuro Oncol 2009;11: 2–8.

Linnebank M, Moskau S, Semmler A, Widman G, Stoffel-Wagner B, Weller M, Elger CE, Antiepileptic drugs interact with folate and vitamin B12 serum levels. Ann Neurol (in press).

Lopez AD, Mathers CD, Ezzati M, Jamison DT, Murray CJ, Global and regional burden of disease and risk factors, 2001: systematic analysis of population health data. Lancet 2006;367: 1747–57.

Losada ME, Rubio MC, Acute effects of S-adenosyl-L-methionine on catecholaminergic central function. Eur J Pharmacol 1989;163: 353–6.

Mannheimer E, Pakesch F, Reimer EE, Vetter H, Hemopoietic complications of hydantoin therapy of epilepsy. Med Klin (Munich) 1952;47: 1397–1401.

Meador KJ, Baker GA, Finnell RH, Kalayjian LA, Liporace JD, Loring DW, Mawer G, Pennell PB, Smith JC, Wolff MC, In utero antiepileptic drug exposure: fetal death and malformations. Neurology 2006;67: 407–12.

Meador KJ, Baker GA, Browning N, Clayton-Smith J, Combs-Cantrell DT, Cohen M, Kalayjian LA, Kanner A, Liporace JD, Pennell PB, Privitera M, Loring DW, Cognitive function at 3 years of age after fetal exposure to antiepileptic drugs. N Engl J Med 2009;360: 1597–605.

Miller DB, O'Callaghan JP, Depression, cytokines, and glial function. Metabolism 2005;54: 33–8.

Miyake M, Methylases of myelin basic protein and histone in rat brain. J Neurochem 1975;24: 909–15.

Monji A, Yanagimoto K, Maekawa T, Sumida Y, Yamazaki K, Kojima K, Plasma folate and homocysteine levels may be related to interictal 'schizophrenia-like' psychosis in patients with epilepsy. J Clin Psychopharmacol 2005;25: 3–5.

Montour-Proulx I, Kuehn SM, Keene DL, Barrowman NJ, Hsu E, Matzinger MA, Dunlap H, Halton JM, Cognitive changes in children treated for acute lymphoblastic leukemia with chemotherapy only according to the Pediatric Oncology Group 9605 protocol. J Child Neurol 2005;20: 129–33.

Morris MS, Fava M, Jacques PF, Selhub J, Rosenberg IH, Depression and folate status in the US Population. Psychother Psychosom 2003;72: 80–7.

Ng TP, Feng L, Niti M, Kua EH, Yap KB, Folate, vitamin B12, homocysteine, and depressive symptoms in a population sample of older Chinese adults. J Am Geriatr Soc 2009;57: 871–6.

Niyikiza C, Baker SD, Seitz DE, Walling JM, Nelson K, Rusthoven JJ, Stabler SP, Paoletti P, Calvert AH, Allen RH, Homocysteine and methylmalonic acid: markers to predict and avoid toxicity from pemetrexed therapy. Mol Cancer Ther 2002;1: 545–52.

Ochs J, Mulhern R, Fairclough D, Parvey L, Whitaker J, Ch'ien L, Mauer A, Simone J, Comparison of neuropsychologic functioning and clinical indicators of neurotoxicity in long-term survivors of childhood leukemia given cranial radiation or parenteral methotrexate: a prospective study. J Clin Oncol 1991;9: 145–51.

Otero-Losada ME, Rubio MC, Acute changes in 5-HT metabolism after S-adenosyl-L-methionine administration. Gen Pharmacol 1989;20: 403–6.

Papakostas GI, Petersen T, Mischoulon D, Green CH, Nierenberg AA, Bottiglieri T, Rosenbaum JF, Alpert JE, Fava M, Serum folate, vitamin B12, and homocysteine in major depressive disorder, Part 2: predictors of relapse during the continuation phase of pharmacotherapy. J Clin Psychiatry 2004;65: 1096–8.

Papakostas GI, Petersen T, Lebowitz BD, Mischoulon D, Ryan JL, Nierenberg AA, Bottiglieri T, Alpert JE, Rosenbaum JF, Fava M, The relationship between serum folate, vitamin B12, and homocysteine levels in major depressive disorder and the timing of improvement with fluoxetine. Int J Neuropsychopharmacol 2005;8: 523–8.

Passeri M, Cucinotta D, Abate G, Senin U, Ventura A, Stramba Badiale M, Diana R, La Greca P, Le Grazie C, Oral 5′-methyltetrahydrofolic acid in senile organic mental disorders with depression: results of a double-blind multicenter study. Aging (Milano) 1993;5: 63–71.

Pels H, Juergens A, Glasmacher A, Schulz H, Engert A, Linnebank M, Schackert G, Reichmann H, Kroschinsky F, Vogt-Schaden M, Egerer G, Bode U, Schaller C, Lamprecht M, Hau P, Deckert M, Fimmers R, Bangard C, Schmidt-Wolf IG, Schlegel U, Early relapses in primary CNS lymphoma after response to polychemotherapy without intraventricular treatment: results of a phase II study. J Neurooncol 2009;91: 299–305.

Pitkin RM, Folate and neural tube defects. Am J Clin Nutr 2007;85: 285S–8S.

Reynolds EH, Folic acid, ageing, depression, and dementia. Br Med J 2002;324: 1512–5.

Rosche J, Uhlmann C, Froscher W, Low serum folate levels as a risk factor for depressive mood in patients with chronic epilepsy. J Neuropsychiatry Clin Neurosci 2003;15: 64–6.

Rubnitz JE, Relling MV, Harrison PL, Sandlund JT, Ribeiro RC, Rivera GK, Thompson SJ, Evans WE, Pui CH, Transient encephalopathy following high-dose methotrexate treatment in childhood acute lymphoblastic leukemia. Leukemia 1998;12: 1176–81.

Samren EB, van Duijn CM, Koch S, Hiilesmaa VK, Klepel H, Bardy AH, Mannagetta GB, Deichl AW, Gaily E, Granstrom ML, Meinardi H, Grobbee DE, Hofman A, Janz D, Lindhout D, Maternal use of antiepileptic drugs and the risk of major congenital malformations: a joint European prospective study of human teratogenesis associated with maternal epilepsy. Epilepsia 1997;38: 981–90.

Sander JW, Patsalos PN, An assessment of serum and red blood cell folate concentrations in patients with epilepsy on lamotrigine therapy. Epilepsy Res 1992;13: 89–92.

Selhub J, Jacques PF, Wilson PW, Rush D, Rosenberg IH, Vitamin status and intake as primary determinants of homocysteinemia in an elderly population. JAMA 1993;270: 2693–2698.

Sener U, Zorlu Y, Karaguzel O, Ozdamar O, Coker I, Topbas M, Effects of common anti-epileptic drug monotherapy on serum levels of homocysteine, vitamin B12, folic acid and vitamin B6. Seizure 2006;15: 79–85.

Sheth RD, Binkley N, Hermann BP, Progressive bone deficit in epilepsy. Neurology 2008;70: 170–6.

Shorvon SD, Carney MW, Chanarin I, Reynolds EH, The neuropsychiatry of megaloblastic anaemia. Br Med J 1980;281: 1036–8.

Sirven JI, Fife TD, Wingerchuk DM, Drazkowski JF, Second-generation antiepileptic drugs' impact on balance: a meta-analysis. Mayo Clin Proc 2007;82: 40–7.

Skarby TV, Anderson H, Heldrup J, Kanerva JA, Seidel H, Schmiegelow K, High leucovorin doses during high-dose methotrexate treatment may reduce the cure rate in childhood acute lymphoblastic leukemia. Leukemia 2006;20: 1955–62.

Stahl SM, Novel therapeutics for depression: L-methylfolate as a trimonoamine modulator and antidepressant-augmenting agent. CNS Spectr 2007;12: 739–44.

Stahl SM, L-Methylfolate: a vitamin for your monoamines. J Clin Psychiatry 2008;69: 1352–3.

Surtees R, Biochemical pathogenesis of subacute combined degeneration of the spinal cord and brain. J Inherit Metab Dis 1993;16: 762–70.

Surtees R, Clelland J, Hann I, Demyelination and single-carbon transfer pathway metabolites during the treatment of acute lymphoblastic leukemia: CSF studies. J Clin Oncol 1998;16: 1505–1511.

Tan TY, Lu CH, Chuang HY, Lin TK, Liou CW, Chang WN, Chuang YC, Long-term antiepileptic drug therapy contributes to the acceleration of atherosclerosis. Epilepsia 2009;50: 1579–86.

Tsurusawa M, Niwa M, Katano N, Fujimoto T, Flow cytometric analysis by bromodeoxyuridine/DNA assay of cell cycle perturbation of methotrexate-treated mouse L1210 leukemia cells. Cancer Res 1988;48: 4288–93.

VanItallie TB, Subsyndromal depression in the elderly: underdiagnosed and undertreated. Metabolism 2005;54: 39–44.

Vermeulen J, Aldenkamp AP, Cognitive side-effects of chronic antiepileptic drug treatment: a review of 25 years of research. Epilepsy Res 1995;22: 65–95.

Vezmar S, Schusseler P, Becker A, Bode U, Jaehde U, Methotrexate-associated alterations of the folate and methyl-transfer pathway in the CSF of ALL patients with and without symptoms of neurotoxicity. Pediatr Blood Cancer 2009;52: 26–32.

Vilaseca MA, Monros E, Artuch R, Colome C, Farre C, Valls C, Cardo E, Pineda M, Anti-epileptic drug treatment in children: hyperhomocysteinaemia, B-vitamins and the 677C→T mutation of the methylenetetrahydrofolate reductase gene. Eur J Paediatr Neurol 2000;4: 269–77.

Wessels JA, Huizinga TW, Guchelaar HJ, Recent insights in the pharmacological actions of methotrexate in the treatment of rheumatoid arthritis. Rheumatology (Oxford) 2008;47: 249–55.

Wesson VA, Levitt AJ, Joffe RT, Change in folate status with antidepressant treatment. Psychiatry Res 1994;53: 313–22.

Whittle SL, Hughes RA, Folate supplementation and methotrexate treatment in rheumatoid arthritis: a review. Rheumatology (Oxford) 2004;43: 267–71.

Wilson RD, Davies G, Desilets V, Reid GJ, Summers A, Wyatt P, Young D, The use of folic acid for the prevention of neural tube defects and other congenital anomalies. J Obstet Gynaecol Can 2003;25: 959–73.

Yerby MS, Management issues for women with epilepsy: neural tube defects and folic acid supplementation. Neurology 2003;61: S23–6.

Young PR, Vacante DA, Waickus CM, Mechanism of the interaction between myelin basic protein and the myelin membrane; the role of arginine methylation. Biochem Biophys Res Commun 1987;145: 1112–8.

6.6 Folate in chronic alcoholism and alcoholic liver disease

Charles H. Halsted; Farah Esfandiari; Valentina Medici

6.6.1 Folate deficiency in chronic alcoholism

6.6.1.1 Incidence of chronic alcoholism in the US

Although approximately two-thirds of all people over age 14 consume alcohol to some extent, alcohol abuse in which alcohol consumption increases risk of medical complications is found in approximately 5% of the US population, more in men than women, and greatest in young adults (Grant et al., 2006). In 2004, the estimated lifetime prevalence of alcohol abuse in the adult population of six representative western European countries was 4.1% (7.4% in men and 1% in women) (Alonso et al., 2004). The concentration of alcohol varies among alcoholic beverages, and one 'drink' is defined as containing 12–15 g of alcohol which is found in one 12-ounce (360 ml) bottle of beer, 100 ml of wine, or two ounces (30 ml) of hard liquor. Using these definitions, chronic alcoholism with increased risk of medical complications becomes significant after two to three drinks per day in men and one to two drinks per day in women (Mann et al., 2003).

6.6.1.2 Incidence of folate deficiency among chronic alcoholics

Chronic alcoholics are a target population for folate deficiency, because they typically eat poor diets and can exhibit abnormal intestinal absorption and metabolism of folates. Before dietary fortification of the US diet with folic acid in 1998, the incidence of low serum folate levels in chronic alcoholic patients admitted to municipal hospitals was recorded at approximately 80% (Herbert et al., 1963; Baker et al., 1964), and with low red cell folate levels and megaloblastic anemia in approximately 40% (Savage et al., 1986). Folic acid fortification of the diet has reduced the overall incidence of folate deficiency in the US, which is defined as less than 3 ng/ml for serum folate and less than 140 ng/ml for red blood cell folate, to less than 1% and less than 6% of the population (Pfeiffer et al., 2007). However, we do not know how this policy has affected the incidence of folate deficiency among chronic alcoholics. By contrast, more recent studies from European countries without policies of food folate fortification found low serum folate levels in approximately one-third of chronic alcoholics in Spain (Blasco et al., 2005), whereas low red cell folate levels were found in two-thirds of chronic alcoholics in Portugal (Cravo et al., 2000).

6.6.1.3 Causes of folate deficiency in chronic alcoholism

There are multiple proven and potential causes of folate deficiency in chronic alcoholism (►Tab. 6.4), that relate to pathways of folate homeostasis (Halsted et al., 2010). Folates exist in the diet mainly as a mixture of methylated and oxidized polyglutamyl folates, but also in the monoglutamyl form as folic acid which is often added as a supplement to breakfast cereals and to all grains in the US at a concentration of 140 µg per 100 g. Folates are absorbed in the upper part of the small intestine by a two-stage process in which polyglutamyl folates are first hydrolyzed to their monoglutamyl derivatives by intestinal folate hydrolase which resides on the brush border membrane, followed by active transport across the intestinal brush border membrane, intracellular methylation, and additional transport across the basolateral membrane (Chandler et al., 1991). There are two candidate membrane transporters, the well-characterized reduced folate carrier (RFC) (Nguyen et al., 1997) and the more recently described proton coupled folate transporter (PCFT) (Qiu et al., 2006), each of which might work independently or together. After circulating through the portal vein to the liver, methylated folate (5-methyltetrahydrofolate or 5-MTHF) is transported across the hepatocyte membrane by one or more candidate transporters: RFC, PCFT, or folate binding protein (FBP). Within the hepatocyte, monoglutamyl 5-MTHF is then converted back to the polyglutamyl form for storage and metabolism. Subsequently, approximately 10% of the liver folate pool undergoes biliary secretion as 5-MTHF, then is mostly re-absorbed again in the jejunum with approximately 0.1% fecal excretion (Steinberg et al., 1979). The remaining non-hepatic folate pool circulates in the blood as 5-MTHF for uptake by body tissues. Renal folate excretion is regulated by glomerular filtration and efficient tubular reabsorption RFC; where approximately 1% is excreted daily in the urine (Williams et al., 1982). Therefore, folate deficiency could come about through inadequate diet, intestinal malabsorption, deficient hepatic uptake and/or storage, abnormal biliary secretion, and/or decreased renal tubular conservation.

6.6.1.3.1 Dietary inadequacy of folate

For economic reasons, binge drinking alcoholics typically limit their intake of non-alcoholic calories, and therefore decrease the likelihood to consume foods high in folate, such as fortified grains and green vegetables. Furthermore, except for beer, alcoholic beverages do not contain folate (Darby et al., 1979). Although alcohol is a source of calories at 7 kcal per gram, excessive alcohol use increases body energy expenditure and inhibits the metabolism of dietary fat (Halsted et al., 2004), whereas those who

Tab. 6.4: Causes of folate deficiency in chronic alcoholics.

Inadequate intake of foods containing folate

Intestinal malabsorption of dietary folate

Decreased uptake and storage of absorbed folate by the liver

Increased renal excretion of circulating folate

Possible increased oxidative destruction of folate molecule

develop alcoholic liver disease are typically anorectic with significant self-imposed dietary restriction (Mendenhall et al., 1984).

6.6.1.3.2 Intestinal malabsorption of folate

The upper small intestine is exposed to high concentrations of ethanol after rapid ingestion of the equivalent of three alcoholic beverages (Halsted et al., 1973), and one study showed ultrastructural changes in jejunal absorbing cells following large doses of ethanol in normal volunteers (Rubin et al., 1972). By contrast, in the presence of severe folate deficiency, the intestinal mucosa in chronic alcoholism demonstrates significant changes that include shortening of villi and enlargement of crypt cell nuclei similar to findings of megaloblastic changes in the bone marrow (Hermos et al., 1972). Furthermore, approximately one-third of binge-drinking alcoholics have intermittent or chronic diarrhea which has been shown to relate to reversible disaccharidase deficiency (Perlow et al., 1977), altered small bowel motility (Robles et al., 1974), and decreased absorption of water and electrolytes (Mekhjian et al., 1977). These studies provide background for the hypothesis that chronic alcoholics are at increased risk for folate malabsorption as a cause of folate deficiency.

Our laboratory conducted a series of clinical and animal experiments to determine whether folate absorption is compromised by chronic alcoholism. According to the quantitative appearance of the ^{3}H isotope in blood and urine, the absorption of ^{3}H-labeled folic acid was decreased in recently drinking chronic alcoholics compared with healthy subjects, but not by acute ethanol ingestion in a healthy subject (Halsted et al., 1967). A subsequent study that used the triple lumen tube technique to measure ^{3}H-folic acid uptake from the jejunum found decreased absorption in folate-deficient alcoholics that normalized with abstinence and nutritious diet (Halsted et al., 1971). After intragastric gavage of ^{3}H-folic acid, the fecal excretion of the ^{3}H label was increased and its body retention was decreased in macaque monkeys that had been fed daily ethanol with a nutritious diet for 2 years, consistent with intestinal malabsorption of folic acid (Romero et al., 1981). Studies in a chronic ethanol-fed micropig model found decreased expression of intestinal RFC carrier for monoglutamyl folate (Villanueva et al., 2001). Other studies in ethanol-fed miniature pigs found decreased activity of intestinal folate hydrolase and uptake of polyglutamyl folate from isolated jejunal segments (Naughton et al., 1989; Reisenauer et al., 1989). Together these studies indicate that chronic alcoholism decreases the intestinal absorption of folate by inhibitory effects on intestinal folate hydrolase that regulate the digestion of polyglutamyl folate to monoglutamyl folate and on RFC that regulates the transport of monoglutamyl folate across the intestinal brush border membrane.

6.6.1.3.3 Abnormal liver uptake and storage of folate

The liver is the major storage and metabolic organ for folates in the polyglutamyl form, in which the monoglutamyl 5-MTHF form of folate is taken up by the liver, and then converted to the polyglutamyl form for storage. Subsequently, folate is reconverted to the monoglutamyl 5-MTHF form for export to the bile and systemic circulation. Thus, decreased liver folate content could result from decreased uptake across the liver cell membrane, decreased production of storage and metabolic polyglutamyl folates, or increased biliary secretion or efflux to the circulation. Experiments with chronic ethanol-fed monkeys found decreased hepatic uptake of parenteral ^{3}H-folic acid, whereas the chromatographic patterns of subsequent labeled intrahepatic polyglutamyl folates were unchanged, consistent with decreased hepatocyte membrane transport of folic acid but unchanged intrahepatic metabolism (Tamura et al., 1981). Another study of the fate of injected ^{3}H-folic acid in these alcoholic monkeys showed decreased liver retention together with increased fecal excretion, consistent with increased biliary excretion of folate (Tamura et al., 1983). However, others found reduced biliary folate excretion in ethanol-fed rats (Hillman et al., 1977). The uptake of monoglutamyl folate by the liver cell membrane from the portal vein could be regulated by one or more transport proteins. Our laboratory demonstrated the presence of RFC and FBP in pig liver plasma membranes (Villanueva, 1998, 2001), and others found transcripts of PCFT in mouse liver (Qui et al., 2007). The membrane uptake of labeled 5-MTHF and folic acid are optimal at an acid pH (Horne et al., 1990; Zhao et al., 2005), which is similar to the pH optimum for PCFT (Qui, et al., 2007). RFC kinetics were not affected by ethanol feeding of micropigs (Villanueva et al., 2001), and the effects of ethanol exposure on PCFT expression and kinetics are not known.

6.6.1.3.4 Abnormal renal excretion of folate

5-MTHF is primarily excreted in the urine at approximately 1% of the body pool per day, by a process involving glomerular filtration followed by regulated renal tubular re-absorption (Williams et al., 1982). Studies in both humans and rats have shown up to 40% increase in urine excretion of labeled folic acid following alcohol consumption (Williams et al., 1982; Russell et al., 1983; McMartin et al., 1989), whereas increased urinary folate excretion was considered a major cause of developing folate deficiency in ethanol-fed monkeys (Tamura et al., 1983). Renal tubular brush border membranes demonstrate transcripts and/or protein levels of FBP, RFC and PCFT (Villanueva et al., 1998; Villanueva et al., 2001; Qiu et al., 2007), but definitive effects of chronic ethanol exposure on these transporters have not been established.

6.6.1.3.5 Potential oxidative destruction of folate molecule

Experimental observations suggest that acute exposure to ethanol has an immediate destructive effect on the folate molecule. In a classical clinical experiment on two folate-deficient chronic alcoholics with megaloblastic anemia, Sullivan and Herbert (1964) found that the reticulocyte response to small doses of either oral or parenteral folic acid could be arrested rapidly by the ingestion of intoxicating amounts of ethanol. Later, it was shown that serum folate levels fell precipitously in response to acute ethanol ingestion in normal human volunteers (Eichner et al., 1973). Although it is possible that ethanol might have impaired the release of folate from liver storage sites, others showed *in vitro* that MTHF was cleaved to its component pteridine ring and *p*-aminobenzoylglutamate side chain in the presence of xanthine oxidase and the acetaldehyde product of ethanol metabolism (Shaw et al., 1989), although it is unclear whether this process occurs *in vivo*.

6.6.2 Alcoholic liver disease

6.6.2.1 Incidence, determinants and mortality

Alcoholic liver disease (ALD) occurs in approximately 5% of chronic alcoholics and affects approximately two million people in the US population where it is the 7th leading cause of death in the 45–65 year age group (National Institute of Alcoholism and Alcohol Abuse, 2000). There is no evidence that the incidence of ALD has decreased in the US following institution of mandatory supplementation of the diet with folic acid. ALD represents 4.0% of the global burden of disease, which varies by region in accordance with alcohol consumption. For example, ALD represents 1–3% of the disease burden of the poorest developing countries , 6.8% of disease burden in developed western countries and 12.1% in formerly socialist countries (Room et al., 2005). Worldwide, the incidence of ALD is dependent upon individual alcohol usage, regardless of cultural and national background and of beverage of choice. For example, a German study determined that the risk of ALD with cirrhosis was related to the absolute amount of alcohol consumed over a defined period of time, as defined by the multiple of the estimated daily amount and duration of drinking (Lelbach, 1975).

6.6.2.2 Incidence and potential causes of folate deficiency in ALD

Folate deficiency is more common in ALD patients than in chronic alcoholics without liver disease (Blasco et al., 2005). In addition to the probable effect of ALD on uptake of folic acid by the liver as described above, the storage of folate in the liver is reduced in ALD. This was shown in a study of ALD patients where the provision of a low folate diet resulted in rapid development of folate deficiency with megaloblastic anemia in 4 weeks compared with the 22 weeks to develop folate deficiency by diet in a non-drinking human subject (Herbert et al., 1962; Eichner et al., 1971).

6.6.2.3. Potential role of folate deficiency in causation of ALD

Although clinical folate deficiency is a prominent feature in patients with ALD, circumstantial evidence indicates that it might also promote the onset of this disease. Based on findings that folate-dependent metabolism of methionine in the liver is markedly altered in experimental ALD (Barak et al., 1987; Trimble et al., 1993; Halsted et al., 1996), our laboratory conducted studies in ethanol-fed micropigs that were grouped to receive folate deficient diets or folate replete diets with or without ethanol at 40% of kcal. In contrast to a prior study that showed development of ALD after 52 weeks of ethanol with folate-replete diets (Halsted et al., 1993), micropigs receiving ethanol with folate-deficient diets developed pathological features of ALD after only 14 weeks (Halsted et al., 2002). Whereas ethanol exposure has multiple effects on folate homeostasis as described above, the mechanisms for the potentiating effect of folate deficiency on development of ALD are related to alterations in folate-dependent hepatic methionine metabolism. However, it cannot be inferred from the micropig study that provision of adequate folic acid in the diet has a preventive effect on development of ALD.

6.6.3 Folate and methionine metabolism in the liver

▶Fig. 6.10 depicts reactions of folate that are related to hepatic methionine metabolism and DNA synthesis and could play significant roles in the pathogenesis of ALD. These reactions can be categorized as those primarily involving folate, transmethylation and trans-sulfuration of homocysteine.

6.6.3.1 Folate metabolism in the liver

As shown in ▶Fig. 6.10, dietary folate is metabolized to dihydrofolate (DHF) and tetrahydrofolate (THF) in the liver. Both of these compounds are also produced endogenously by thymidine synthase (TS) and methionine synthase (MS). THF is substrate for generation of 5,10-methylene tetrahydrofolate (5,10-MTHF), which, in turn, is substrate for 5-methyltetrahydrofolate (5-MTHF) by way of methyl tetrahydrofolate reductase (MTHFR). 5,10-MTHF is also a substrate for TS, which regulates DNA nucleotide balance through synthesis of deoxythymidine monophosphate (dTMP) from deoxyuridine monophosphate (dUMP).

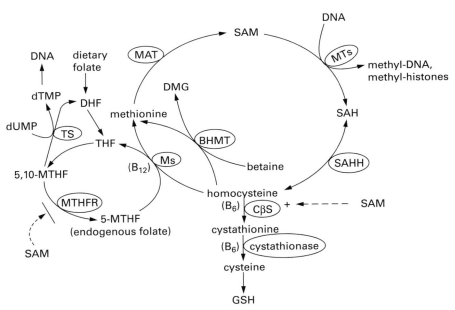

Fig. 6.10: Liver metabolism of folate and methionine. B⁶, vitamin B6; B¹², vitamin B12, BHMT, betaine homocysteine methyltransferase; CβS, cystathionine beta synthase; DHF, dihydrofolate; DMG, dimethylglycine; dUMP, deoxyuridine monophosphate; dTMP, deoxythymidine monophosphate; GSH, glutathione; MAT, methionine adenosyltransferase; MS, methionine synthase; MT, methyltransferase; 5,10-MTHF, 5,10 methylenetetrahydrofolate; 5-MTHF, methyltetrahydrofolate; MTHFR, methylene tetrahydrofolate reductase; SAM, S-adenosylmethionine; SAH, S-adenosylhomocysteine; SAHH, S-adenosylhomocysteine hydrolase; THF, tetrahydrofolate; TS, thymidine synthase.

6.6.3.2 Transmethylation reactions

Turning to methionine metabolism (▶Fig. 6.10), 5-MTHF is the substrate for methionine synthase (MS), which transfers the methyl group of 5-MTHF to homocysteine to produce methionine. Because vitamin B12 is a co-factor for MS, deficiencies of both vitamin B12 and substrate folate as 5-MTHF can elevate levels of homocysteine by impairing its conversion to methionine, and thereby reduce levels of downstream transmethylation products. However, a rescue pathway, betaine homocysteine methyl transferase (BHMT) produces methionine from betaine and homocysteine. Methionine is metabolized in the liver to S-adenosylmethionine (SAM) through methionine adenosyltransferase (MAT) which is encoded in the liver by the gene *MAT1A*. SAM plays a key regulatory role in many reactions that include down-regulation of MTHFR and up-regulation of cystathionine beta synthase (CβS) in the trans-sulfuration pathway. However, its principal role is as a methyl donor for all methyltransferases (MTs), that include substrates DNA and histones, as described below in the epigenetics section. Methylation of DNA by SAM controls the expression of all genes, which are silenced by methylation with adequate SAM, but are activated by hypomethylation such as might occur in SAM deficiency. S-Adenosylhomocysteine (SAH) is the product of all MT reactions. Because SAH inhibits most MT reactions, the SAM/SAH ratio is a useful descriptor of methylation capacity because the K_m for SAM and the K_i for SAH in the DNMT1 [(cytosine-5)-methyltransferase 1] reaction are identical at 1.4 μM/l (Clarke et al., 2001). Hence, SAM has two potential regulatory functions for DNA. SAM regulates DNA synthesis by its negative control on the activity of MTHFR, thereby assuring adequate 5,10-MTHF for the TS reaction and assuring proper DNA nucleotide balance. SAM also regulates gene expression through DNA methylation. Thus, when SAM is deficient, the MTHFR reaction will up-regulate to generate more 5-MTHF, at the same time leading to less 5,10-MTHF substrate for TS with resultant nucleotide imbalance, whereas less SAM for DNA methylation could increase the expression of potentially injurious genes involved in liver injury. SAH is further metabolized by SAH hydrolase (SAHH) to homocysteine in a bi-directional reaction. Hence, when homocysteine is in excess, more SAH will be produced, and *vice versa*.

6.6.3.3 Trans-sulfuration reactions

As shown in ▶Fig. 6.10, the trans-sulfuration pathway eliminates excess homocysteine by a series of reactions that lead to the product glutathione (GSH), which is the principal antioxidant in the liver. SAM facilitates the activity of the initial enzyme CβS, and vitamin B6 is a co-factor for the activities of both CβS and cystathionase. Approximately 70% of the product cysteine is rapidly converted to GSH, the remainder going to alternate pathways.

6.6.3.4 Effects of ethanol on methionine metabolism and relationship to ALD in experimental animal models

Many studies of experimental ALD have shown associations of defects in hepatic methionine metabolism within different pathways of liver injury. Regarding transmethylation, ethanol-fed rats and micropigs were shown to develop increased homocysteine levels together with reduced MS activity and increased compensatory BHMT activity

(Barak et al., 1987; Trimble et al., 1993), together with decrease in liver SAM, increase in liver SAH and reduced production of dTMP (Halsted et al., 1996). Decreased expression of liver MAT and reduced levels of SAM were associated with increased DNA strand breaks in intragastric ethanol-fed mice (Lu et al., 2000). Elevated SAH is a consequence of its enhanced production from elevated homocysteine through bi-directional SAHH, and was associated with increased hepatocellular apoptosis and DNA fragmentation in ethanol-fed rats (Kharbanda et al., 2005) and increased sensitivity to the ethanol-related cytokine tumor necrosis factor (TNFα) in ethanol-fed mice (Song et al., 2004). Betaine, which is an alternate substrate for homocysteine lowering (▶Fig. 6.10), prevented ethanol effects on elevating SAH (Barak et al., 2003) as well as hepatocellular apoptosis (Kharbanda et al., 2005) . In other experiments, betaine prevented ethanol-induced apoptosis and steatosis as well as the increase in their regulatory endoplasmic reticulum (ER) enzymes in intragastric-fed mice (Ji et al., 2003). Ethanol feeding of micropigs activated specific genes in the ER pathways of apoptosis and steatosis in correlation with changes in SAM, SAH and their ratio (Esfandiari et al., 2005).

6.6.3.5 Effects of clinical ALD on liver methionine metabolism

Two studies demonstrated elevated serum homocysteine levels in chronic alcoholic patients, that were highest in binge drinkers compared with those who had abstained from alcohol for at least 72 h (Hultberg et al., 1993; Bleich et al., 2005). Transient elevated serum homocysteine levels in chronic alcoholics can be attributed to an observed inhibitory effect of the alcohol metabolite acetaldehyde on methionine synthase activity (Kenyon et al., 1998). By contrast, the gene expressions of *MS*, *MAT1* and *CβS* were reduced in liver biopsies from ALD patients (Avila et al., 2000; Lee et al., 2004). These findings would account for elevated serum homocysteine in these patients as well as reduced levels of liver SAM and GSH, and were consistent with findings in chronic ethanol-fed micropigs with ALD (Villanueva et al., 2004). A clinical study of 81 ALD patients compared with healthy controls found elevated serum homocysteine and cystathionine that correlated with biochemical tests of liver function, consistent with a block in the trans-sulfuration pathway of homocysteine excretion (Look et al., 2000). Two separate European clinical trials found that the provision of SAM as a diet supplement in ALD patients increased levels of GSH in liver biopsies (Vendemiale et al., 1989) and improved either 2-year mortality or the requirement for liver transplantation (Mato et al., 1999).

6.6.3.6 Evidence for aberrant methionine metabolism in pathogenesis of ALD

There are several reasons why alcohol-induced aberrant methionine metabolism could be integral to the pathogenesis of ALD. First, elevated homocysteine is a potent activator of the ER stress pathway that induces fatty liver through promoting lipogenesis, as well as apoptosis, or death of hepatocytes (Esfandiari et al., 2005). Second, elevated homocysteine is metabolized through the reverse SAHH pathway to SAH, which is a potent inhibitor of DNA and other methyltransferase reactions (Yi et al., 2000). Together with reduced SAM, and hence reduced SAM to SAH ratio, reduced DNA methylation has the potentially potent effect of the activation of potentially injurious genes

(Clarke et al., 2001). This was demonstrated in a recent study of genetically altered ethanol-fed mice that associated up-regulation of ER-induced lipogenesis and apoptosis genes with both a decrease in the liver SAM to SAH ratio and abnormal histone methylation patterns (Esfandiari et al., 2010). Third, because of the regulatory role of SAM in the activity of CβS (►Fig. 6.10), ethanol-induced reduction in SAM secondarily reduces CβS activity and production of antioxidant GSH through the trans-sulfuration pathway. Liver levels of GSH were correlated with those of SAM in ethanol-fed micropigs (Halsted et al., 2002), and were sustained at normal levels by supplementing diets with SAM in both ethanol-fed baboons and micropigs (Lieber et al., 1990; Villanueva et al., 2007). Lastly, two recent studies in the ethanol-fed micropig showed that SAM supplementation maintained normal liver histology while normalizing the SAM to SAH ratio, GSH levels, and expressions of ER stress genes for lipogenesis and apoptosis and of genes that produce reactive oxidant species (ROS) (Esfandiari et al., 2007; Villanueva et al., 2007).

6.6.4 Epigenetic effects of ethanol and folate deficiency in ALD

Epigenetics is the study of post-synthetic modifications of either DNA or chromatin, which is a complex of DNA, histones and non-histone proteins. The fundamental unit of chromatin is the polymer nucleosome, which is composed of 147 base pairs of DNA wrapped around an octamer of histone core proteins. Chromatin remodeling can be initiated by the addition of methyl groups to DNA or by post-translational modifications of the amino acids that make up histones (Kouzarides et al., 2007). The methylation of transcriptional control regions in the specific CpG-rich regions of DNA, called CpG islands, is an epigenetic modification of DNA that can inappropriately silence or down-regulate gene expression. Conversely, hypomethylation could lead to accentuated expression of selected genes, which, e.g., in ALD, could promote pathways of steatosis and other aspects of liver injury. In the context of hepatic methionine metabolism, the level of the methyl donor SAM is crucial for the function of DNA methyltransferases, which transfer a methyl group from SAM to cytosine in CpG dinucleotides (►Fig. 6.10) while generating its product SAH, a potent inhibitor of DNMT reactions.

Post-translational histone modifications cooperate with DNA methylation to repress or activate gene expression (Fuks et al., 2005). These modifications include acetylation and methylation of lysine (K) residues within histones H3 and H4 (Vakoc et al., 2006). Hyperacetylation of histones H3 and H4 in promoter regions is associated with gene activation, whereas histone methylation can be correlated with either transcriptional activation or repression. For example, methylation of H3K4 is associated with transcriptionally active promoter regions, whereas methylation of H3K9 and H3K27 are linked to heterochromatin formation and gene repression (Vakoc et al., 2006). A combination of acetylated histone and trimethylated H3K4 can be detected in transcription sites of active genes (Kim et al., 2009).

The relationship of epigenetics to chronic alcoholism and ALD is summarized in a recent review (Shukla et al., 2008). For example, the exposure of primary rat hepatocytes to ethanol caused reduced H3K9 methylation together with an increase of H3K4 methylation in the regulatory region of many up-regulated genes relevant to alcohol metabolism (Pal-Bhadra et al., 2007). In chronic ethanol-fed rats, reduced histone H3K9 was associated with inhibition of the ubiquitin proteosome pathway

(Oliva et al., 2009), whereas histone H3K4 and H3K27 were increased in association with increased activation of selected genes relevant to liver injury (Bardag-Gorce et al., 2009). In a recent study of genetically altered mice, intragastric ethanol feeding promoted decrease inliver SAM/SAH ratio, together with reduction in H3K9 methylation in promoter regions of activated genes associated with apoptosis and lipid synthesis (Esfandiari et al., 2010).

6.6.5 Summary

The dietary vitamin folate is involved in many aspects of chronic alcoholism and ALD. The risk of folate deficiency is increased by chronic alcohol consumption owing to decreased intestinal absorption, reduced liver uptake, and increased urinary excretion of this vitamin, whereas liver folate storage is reduced in ALD. Liver folate is integral to methionine metabolism, which is closely linked to regulation of DNA metabolism potential pathways of lipogenesis and liver cell death. Folate deficiency accelerates the development of experimental ALD through changes in methionine metabolism, which, in turn, control the epigenetic regulation of DNA and histones involved in the expressions of genes related to liver injury. However, there is no evidence to date that supplementation of the diet with folic acid can prevent the onset of ALD in chronic alcoholic individuals.

References

Alonso JAM, Bernert S, Bruffaerts R, Brugha TS, Bryson H, de Girolamo G, Graaf R, Demyttenaere K, Gasquet I, Haro JM, Katz SJ, Kessler RC, Kovess V, Lépine JP, Ormel J, Polidori G, Russo LJ, Vilagut G, Almansa J, Arbabzadeh-Bouchez S, Autonell J, Bernal M, Buist-Bouwman MA, Codony M, Domingo-Salvany A, Ferrer M, Joo SS, Martínez-Alonso M, Matschinger H, Mazzi F, Morgan Z, Morosini P, Palacín C, Romera B, Taub N, Vollebergh WA, Prevalence of mental disorders in Europe: results from the European Study of the Epidemiology of Mental Disorders (ESEMeD) project. Acta Psychiatr Scand 2004;109: 21–7.

Avila MA, Berasain C, Torres L, Martin-Duce A, Corrales FJ, Yang H, Prieto J, et al., Reduced mRNA abundance of the main enzymes involved in methionine metabolism in human liver cirrhosis and hepatocellular carcinoma. J Hepatol 2000;33: 907–14.

Baker H, Frank O, Ziffer H, Goldfarb S, Leevy CM, Sobotka H, Effect of hepatic disease on liver B-complex vitamin titers. Am J Clin Nutr 1964;14: 1–6.

Barak AJ, Beckenhauer HC, Tuma DJ, Badakhsh S, Effects of prolonged ethanol feeding on methionine metabolism in rat liver. Biochem Cell Biol 1987;65: 230–3.

Barak AJ, Beckenhauer HC, Mailliard ME, Kharbanda KK, Tuma DJ, Betaine lowers elevated s-adenosylhomocysteine levels in hepatocytes from ethanol-fed rats. J Nutr 2003;133: 2845–8.

Bardag-Gorce F, Oliva J, Dedes J, Li J, French BA, French SW, Chronic ethanol feeding alters hepatocyte memory which is not altered by acute feeding. Alcohol Clin Exp Res 2009;33: 684–92.

Blasco C, Caballeria J, Deulofeu R, Lligona A, Pares A, Lluis JM, Gual A, et al., Prevalence and mechanisms of hyperhomocysteinemia in chronic alcoholics. Alcohol Clin Exp Res 2005;29: 1044–8.

Bleich S, Carl M, Bayerlein K, Reulbach U, Biermann T, Hillemacher T, Bonsch D, et al., Evidence of increased homocysteine levels in alcoholism: the Franconian alcoholism research studies (FARS). Alcohol Clin Exp Res 2005;29: 334–6.

Chandler CJ, Harrison DA, Buffington CA, Santiago NA, Halsted CH, Functional specificity of jejunal brush-border pteroylpolyglutamate hydrolase in pig. Am J Physiol 1991;260: G865–72.

Clarke S, Banfield K, S-adenosylmethionine-dependent methyltransferases. In: Carmel R, Jacobsen D, editors. Homocysteine in health and disease. Cambridge: Cambridge University Press; 2001. pp. 63–8.

Cravo ML, Camilo ME, Hyperhomocysteinemia in chronic alcoholism: relations to folic acid and vitamins B(6) and B(12) status. Nutrition 2000;16: 296–302.

Darby W, The nutrient contributions of fermented beverages. In: Gastineau CH DW, Turner TB, editors. Fermented food beverages in nutrition. New York: Academic Press; 1979. pp. 61–79.

Eichner ER, Hillman RS, The evolution of anemia in alcoholic patients. Am J Med 1971;50: 218–32.

Eichner ER, Hillman RS, Effect of alcohol on serum folate level. J Clin Invest 1973;52: 584–91.

Esfandiari F, Villanueva JA, Wong DH, French SW, Halsted CH, Chronic ethanol feeding and folate deficiency activate hepatic endoplasmic reticulum stress pathway in micropigs. Am J Physiol Gastrointest Liver Physiol 2005;289: G54–63.

Esfandiari F, You M, Villanueva JA, Wong DH, French SW, Halsted CH, S-Adenosylmethionine attenuates hepatic lipid synthesis in micropigs fed ethanol with a folate-deficient diet. Alcohol Clin Exp Res 2007;31: 1231–9.

Esfandiari F, Medici V, Wong DH, Jose S, Dolatshahi M, Quinlivan E, Dayal S, Lentz SR, Tsukamoto H, Zhang YH, French SW, Halsted CH, Epigenetic regulation of hepatic endoplasmic reticulum stress pathways in the ethanol-fed cystathionine beta synthase-deficient mouse. Hepatology 2010;51: 932–41.

Fuks F, DNA methylation and histone modifications: teaming up to silence genes. Curr Opin Genet Dev 2005;15: 490–5.

Grant BF, Stinson FS, Chou P, Dufour MC, Pickering MS, The 12-month prevalence and trends in DSM-IV Alcohol Abuse and Dependence: United States, 1991–1992 and 2001–2002. Alcohol Res Health 2006;29: 79–93.

Halsted CH, Nutrition and alcoholic liver disease. Semin Liver Dis 2004;24: 289–304.

Halsted C, Medici V, Esfandiari F, Influence of alcohol on folate status and methionine metabolism in relation to alcoholic liver disease. In: LB Bailey, editor. Folate in health and disease. 2nd ed. Boca Raton, FL: CRC Press; 2010. pp. 429–48.

Halsted CH, Griggs RC, Harris JW, The effect of alcoholism on the absorption of folic acid (H3-PGA) evaluated by plasma levels and urine excretion. J Lab Clin Med 1967;69: 116–31.

Halsted CH, Robles EA, Mezey E, Decreased jejunal uptake of labeled folic acid (3 H-PGA) in alcoholic patients: roles of alcohol and nutrition. N Engl J Med 1971;285: 701–6.

Halsted CH, Robles EA, Mezey E, Distribution of ethanol in the human gastrointestinal tract. Am J Clin Nutr 1973;26: 831–4.

Halsted CH, Villanueva J, Chandler CJ, Ruebner B, Munn RJ, Parkkila S, Niemela O, Centrilobular distribution of acetaldehyde and collagen in the ethanol-fed micropig. Hepatology 1993;18: 954–60.

Halsted CH, Villanueva J, Chandler CJ, Stabler SP, Allen RH, Muskhelishvili L, James SJ, et al., Ethanol feeding of micropigs alters methionine metabolism and increases hepatocellular apoptosis and proliferation. Hepatology 1996;23: 497–505.

Halsted CH, Villanueva JA, Devlin AM, Niemela O, Parkkila S, Garrow TA, Wallock LM, et al., Folate deficiency disturbs hepatic methionine metabolism and promotes liver injury in the ethanol-fed micropig. Proc Natl Acad Sci USA 2002;99: 10072–7.

Herbert V, Experimental nutritional folate deficiency in man. Trans Assoc Am Physicians 1962;75: 307–20.

Herbert V, Zalusky R, Davidson CS, Correlation of folate deficiency with alcoholism and associated macrocytosis, anemia, and liver disease. Ann Intern Med 1963;58: 977–88.

Hermos JA, Adams WH, Liu YK, Sullivan LW, Trier JS, Mucosa of the small intestine in folate-deficient alcoholics. Ann Intern Med 1972;76: 957–65.

Hillman RS, McGuffin R, Campbell C, Alcohol interference with the folate enterohepatic cycle. Trans Assoc Am Physicians 1977;90: 145–56.

Horne DW, Na+ and pH dependence of 5-methyltetrahydrofolic acid and methotrexate transport in freshly isolated hepatocytes. Biochim Biophys Acta 1990;1023: 47–55.

Hultberg B, Berglund M, Andersson A, Frank A, Elevated plasma homocysteine in alcoholics. Alcohol Clin Exp Res 1993;17: 687–9.

Ji C, Kaplowitz N, Betaine decreases hyperhomocysteinemia, endoplasmic reticulum stress, and liver injury in alcohol-fed mice. Gastroenterology 2003;124: 1488–99.

Kenyon SH, Nicolaou A, Gibbons WA, The effect of ethanol and its metabolites upon methionine synthase activity in vitro. Alcohol 1998;15: 305–9.

Kharbanda KK, Rogers DD 2nd, Mailliard ME, Siford GL, Barak AJ, Beckenhauer HC, Sorrell MF, et al., Role of elevated S-adenosylhomocysteine in rat hepatocyte apoptosis: protection by betaine. Biochem Pharmacol 2005;70: 1883–90.

Kim JK, Samaranayake M, Pradhan S, Epigenetic mechanisms in mammals. Cell Mol Life Sci 2009;66: 596–612.

Kouzarides T, Chromatin modifications and their function. Cell 2007;128: 693–705.

Lee TD, Sadda MR, Mendler MH, Bottiglieri T, Kanel G, Mato JM, Lu SC, Abnormal hepatic methionine and glutathione metabolism in patients with alcoholic hepatitis. Alcohol Clin Exp Res 2004;28: 173–81.

Lelbach WK, Cirrhosis in the alcoholic and its relation to the volume of alcohol abuse. Ann N Y Acad Sci 1975;252: 85–105.

Lieber CS, Casini A, DeCarli LM, Kim CI, Lowe N, Sasaki R, Leo MA, S-Adenosyl-L-methionine attenuates alcohol-induced liver injury in the baboon. Hepatology 1990;11: 165–72.

Look MP, Riezler R, Reichel C, Brensing KA, Rockstroh JK, Stabler SP, Spengler U, et al., Is the increase in serum cystathionine levels in patients with liver cirrhosis a consequence of impaired homocysteine transsulfuration at the level of gamma-cystathionase? Scand J Gastroenterol 2000;35: 866–72.

Lu SC, Huang ZZ, Yang H, Mato JM, Avila MA, Tsukamoto H, Changes in methionine adenosyltransferase and S-adenosylmethionine homeostasis in alcoholic rat liver. Am J Physiol Gastrointest Liver Physiol 2000;279: G178–85.

Mann R, Smart RG, Govoni R, The epidemiology of alcoholic liver disease. Alcohol Res Health 2003;27: 209–19.

Mato JM, Camara J, Fernandez de Paz J, Caballeria L, Coll S, Caballero A, Garcia-Buey L, et al., S-Adenosylmethionine in alcoholic liver cirrhosis: a randomized, placebo-controlled, double-blind, multicenter clinical trial. J Hepatol 1999;30: 1081–9.

McMartin KE, Collins TD, Eisenga BH, Fortney T, Bates WR, Bairnsfather L, Effects of chronic ethanol and diet treatment on urinary folate excretion and development of folate deficiency in the rat. J Nutr 1989;119: 1490–7.

Mekhjian H, May ES, Acute and chronic effects of ethanol on fluid transport in the small intestine. Gastroenterology 1977;72: 1280–6.

Mendenhall CL, Anderson S, Weesner RE, Goldberg SJ, Crolic KA, Protein-calorie malnutrition associated with alcoholic hepatitis. Veterans Administration Cooperative Study Group on Alcoholic Hepatitis. Am J Med 1984;76: 211–22.

National Institute of Alcoholism and Alcohol Abuse. Tenth special report to the US Congress on alcohol and health. Rockville, MD; 2000.

Naughton CA, Chandler CJ, Duplantier RB, Halsted CH, Folate absorption in alcoholic pigs: in vitro hydrolysis and transport at the intestinal brush border membrane. Am J Clin Nutr 1989;50: 1436–41.

Nguyen TT, Dyer DL, Dunning DD, Rubin SA, Grant KE, Said HM, Human intestinal folate transport: cloning, expression, and distribution of complementary RNA, Gastroenterology 1997;112: 783–91.

Oliva J, Dedes J, Li J, French SW, Bardag-Gorce F, Epigenetics of proteasome inhibition in the liver of rats fed ethanol chronically. World J Gastroenterol 2009;15: 705–12.

Pal-Bhadra M, Bhadra U, Jackson DE, Mamatha L, Park PH, Shukla SD, Distinct methylation patterns in histone H3 at Lys-4 and Lys-9 correlate with up- & down-regulation of genes by ethanol in hepatocytes. Life Sci 2007;81: 979–87.

Perlow W, Baraona E, Lieber CS, Symptomatic intestinal disaccharidase deficiency in alcoholics. Gastroenterology 1977;1977: 680–4.

Pfeiffer CM, Johnson CL, Jain RB, Yetley EA, Picciano MF, Rader JI, Fisher KD, et al., Trends in blood folate and vitamin B-12 concentrations in the United States, 1988–2004. Am J Clin Nutr 2007;86: 718–27.

Qiu A, Jansen M, Sakaris A, Min SH, Chattopadhyay S, Tsai E, Sandoval C, et al., Identification of an intestinal folate transporter and the molecular basis for hereditary folate malabsorption. Cell 2006;127: 917–28.

Qiu A, Min SH, Jansen M, Malhotra U, Tsai E, Cabelof DC, Matherly LH, et al., Rodent intestinal folate transporters (SLC46A1): secondary structure, functional properties, and response to dietary folate restriction. Am J Physiol Cell Physiol 2007;293: C1669–78.

Reisenauer AM, Buffington CA, Villanueva JA, Halsted CH, Folate absorption in alcoholic pigs: in vivo intestinal perfusion studies. Am J Clin Nutr 1989;50: 1429–35.

Robles EA, Mezey E, Halsted CH, Schuster MM, Effect of ethanol on motility of the small intestine. Johns Hopkins Med J 1974;135: 17–24.

Romero JJ, Tamura T, Halsted CH, Intestinal absorption of [³H]folic acid in the chronic alcoholic monkey. Gastroenterology 1981;80: 99–102.

Room R, Babor T, Rehm J, Alcohol and public health. Lancet 2005;365: 519–30.

Rubin E RB, Lindenbaum J, Gerson CD, Walker G, Lieber CS, Ultrastructural changes in the small intestine induced by ethanol. Gastroenterology 1972;63: 801–14.

Russell RM, Rosenberg IH, Wilson PD, Iber FL, Oaks EB, Giovetti AC, Otradovec CL, et al., Increased urinary excretion and prolonged turnover time of folic acid during ethanol ingestion. Am J Clin Nutr 1983;38: 64–70.

Savage D, Lindenbaum J, Anemia in alcoholics. Medicine (Baltimore) 1986;65: 322–38.

Shaw S, Jayatilleke E, Herbert V, Colman N, Cleavage of folates during ethanol metabolism. Role of acetaldehyde/xanthine oxidase-generated superoxide. Biochem J 1989;257: 277–80.

Shukla SD, Velazquez J, French SW, Lu SC, Ticku MK, Zakhari S, Emerging role of epigenetics in the actions of alcohol. Alcohol Clin Exp Res 2008;32: 1525–34.

Song Z, Zhou Z, Uriarte S, Wang L, Kang YJ, Chen T, Barve S, et al., S-Adenosylhomocysteine sensitizes to TNF-alpha hepatotoxicity in mice and liver cells: a possible etiological factor in alcoholic liver disease. Hepatology 2004;40: 989–97.

Steinberg SE, Campbell CL, Hillman RS, Kinetics of the normal folate enterohepatic cycle. J Clin Invest 1979;64: 83–8.

Sullivan LW, Herbert V, Suppression of hematopoiesis by ethanol. J Clin Invest 1964;43: 2048–62.

Tamura T, Halsted CH, Folate turnover in chronically alcoholic monkeys. J Lab Clin Med 1983;101: 623–8.

Tamura T, Romero JJ, Watson JE, Gong EJ, Halsted CH, Hepatic folate metabolism in the chronic alcoholic monkey. J Lab Clin Med 1981;97: 654–61.

Trimble KC, Molloy AM, Scott JM, Weir DG, The effect of ethanol on one-carbon metabolism: increased methionine catabolism and lipotrope methyl-group wastage. Hepatology 1993;18: 984–9.

Vakoc CR, Sachdeva MM, Wang H, Blobel GA, Profile of histone lysine methylation across transcribed mammalian chromatin. Mol Cell Biol 2006;26: 9185–95.

Vendemiale G, Altomare E, Trizio T, Le Grazie C, Di Padova C, Salerno MT, Carrieri V, et al., Effects of oral S-adenosyl-L-methionine on hepatic glutathione in patients with liver disease. Scand J Gastroenterol 1989;24: 407–15.

Villanueva J, Ling EH, Chandler CJ, Halsted CH, Membrane and tissue distribution of folate binding protein in pig. Am J Physiol 1998;275: R1503–10.

Villanueva JA, Devlin AM, Halsted CH, Reduced folate carrier: tissue distribution and effects of chronic ethanol intake in the micropig. Alcohol Clin Exp Res 2001;25: 415–20.

Villanueva JA, Esfandiari F, White ME, Devaraj S, French SW, Halsted CH, S-Adenosylmethionine attenuates oxidative liver injury in micropigs fed ethanol with a folate-deficient diet. Alcohol Clin Exp Res 2007;31: 1934–43.

Villanueva JA, Halsted CH, Hepatic transmethylation reactions in micropigs with alcoholic liver disease. Hepatology 2004;39: 1303–10.

Williams W, Hueng KC, Renal tubular transport of folic acid and methotrexate in the monkey. Am J Physiol 1982;242: F484–90.

Yi P, Melnyk S, Pogribna M, Pogribny IP, Hine RJ, James SJ, Increase in plasma homocysteine associated with parallel increases in plasma S-adenosylhomocysteine and lymphocyte DNA hypomethylation. J Biol Chem 2000;275: 29318–23.

Zhao R, Hanscom M, Goldman ID, The relationship between folate transport activity at low pH and reduced folate carrier function in human Huh7 hepatoma cells. Biochim Biophys Acta 2005;1715: 57–64.

6.7 Folate and cancer risk

Karen E. Christensen; Joel B. Mason; Rima Rozen

6.7.1 Introduction

Folate, or vitamin B9, is well known for its role in the prevention of anemia and birth defects, and could be a determining factor in other common disorders such as cardiovascular disease and neuropsychiatric disturbances (see other chapters in this book). However, this vitamin also appears to play an important role in the prevention and progression of cancer. Moreover, inhibitors of folate metabolism have been an important cornerstone of cancer treatment for some decades, and genetic variants of folate-dependent enzymes might impact on the efficacy of these agents.

The relation between folate and cancer risk has been most extensively investigated for colorectal cancer (CRC); its effect on the risk of developing other cancers, such as leukemia, lung cancer and breast cancer has also been studied but the findings are not, as yet, conclusive. In general, the impact of folate on cancer risk seems to depend on the timing of the intervention: it appears to prevent the development of new tumors but, paradoxically, could also promote the growth of existing neoplasms. Injudicious intake of large amounts of folic acid, which might occur when individuals are consuming several sources of the vitamin in the form of supplements and fortified foods, could be producing this promotional effect in some societies. Indeed, it has been speculated that mandatory fortification of grain products in the USA, Canada and over 50 other countries, which has been so successful in reducing the incidence of neural tube defects (De Wals et al., 2007), might have resulted in the accelerated progression of subclinical tumors into clinically significant ones in some instances, even though over the long term it might contribute to prevention of the cancer. In this chapter, we will review the mechanisms by which folate modulates tumor formation or growth, and the impact of dietary or genetic variation in folate metabolism on cancer risk in the population.

6.7.2 Mechanisms of carcinogenesis

6.7.2.1 Biochemical role of folate

The term 'folate' encompasses all one-carbon substituted and glutamylated derivatives of folic acid, the synthetic folate found in vitamins and fortified foods. The biologically active form of folic acid, tetrahydrofolate (THF), is an enzyme cofactor that carries one-carbon units for use in several biosynthetic reactions. One-carbon units are transferred to and from THF, interconverted between various oxidation states and used in the synthesis of nucleotides and amino acids. The role of folate in the synthesis of the amino acid methionine is particularly noteworthy because methionine generates the ubiquitous methyl donor S-adenosylmethionine (SAM), which transfers its methyl group in numerous reactions including DNA and protein methylation and phospholipid and neurotransmitter synthesis.

Folate-mediated one-carbon metabolism can be simplistically divided into two segments: the methylation cycle and nucleotide synthesis (▶Fig. 6.11). The two segments are bridged by the enzyme methyleneTHF reductase (MTHFR), which catalyses the irreversible reduction of methyleneTHF to methylTHF, committing one-carbon folates to the methylation cycle. In the methylation cycle, methyl groups are transferred from methylTHF to the toxic amino acid homocysteine (Hcy), regenerating methionine which can then be used to make SAM. When SAM participates in a methylation reaction (e.g., methylation of DNA or phospholipid synthesis), S-adenosylhomocysteine (SAH) is generated, which is, in turn, metabolized to produce Hcy and complete the cycle. Three of the four nucleotides in DNA require folate for *de novo* synthesis. The synthesis of thymidylate (dTMP) from uridylate (dUMP) by thymidylate synthase (TS) requires methyleneTHF whereas the multi-step synthesis of the purine nucleotides adenylate and guanylate requires two molecules of formylTHF per nucleotide.

Folate is required to support DNA synthesis and thus supports the proliferation of cells. Folate deficiency could lead to both genetic and epigenetic changes that either initiate or promote the development of cancer by mechanisms discussed in Sections 6.7.2.2 and 6.7.2.3. Conversely, excess quantities of folate could enhance the proliferation of neoplastic cells, thereby accelerating tumor growth (discussed in Section 6.7.2.4).

6.7.2.2 Uracil misincorporation and DNA strand breaks

Uracil is normally found in DNA owing to the spontaneous hydrolysis of cytosine to uracil, a common event that can result in a C→T transition if not repaired (Barnes and Lindahl, 2004). Abnormally high amounts of uracil might be found in DNA when folate is lacking because decreased availability of methyleneTHF for the thymidylate synthase reaction could increase deoxyuridylate (dUTP) relative to deoxythymidylate (dTTP) in nucleotide pools. This excess of dUTP leads to the mistaken incorporation of uracil in place of thymidine. The nucleotide pools in cells are only large enough to support DNA synthesis for a few minutes (Meuth, 1989); therefore, altered dUTP:dTTP ratios caused by folate deficiency can quickly affect DNA synthesis and repair. Misincorporated uracil from all sources is repaired by several base excision repair systems that excise uracil and replace it with the proper nucleotide (Barnes and Lindahl,

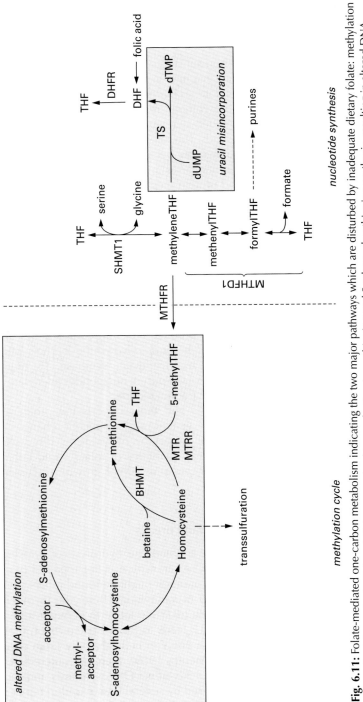

Fig. 6.11: Folate-mediated one-carbon metabolism indicating the two major pathways which are disturbed by inadequate dietary folate: methylation and nucleotide synthesis. Folate deficiency can lead to a reduction in methionine and S-adenosylmethionine synthesis, resulting in altered DNA methylation. An increase in homocysteine can lead to the accumulation of S-adenosylhomocysteine and also impair methylation reactions. Folate deficiency can limit the conversion of uridylate to thymidylate. The accumulation of dUMP can result in excess uracil incorporation into DNA, leading to potentially carcinogenic DNA damage. Abbreviations: DHF, dihydrofolate; DHFR, dihydrofolate reductase; MTHFD1, methyleneTHF dehydrogenase-methenylTHF cyclohydrolase-formylTHF synthetase; MTHFR, methyleneTHF reductase; MTR, methionine synthase; MTRR, methionine synthase reductase; THF, tetrahydrofolate; TS, thymidylate synthase.

2004). However, single-strand breaks are generated during this repair process, and if large amounts of uracil are incorporated into DNA, highly mutagenic double-strand breaks can occur (Dianov et al., 1991; Blount et al., 1997). DNA double-strand breaks can result in chromosomal translocations, inhibition of gene expression, deletion of tumor suppressor genes, and amplification of oncogenes (Ciappio and Mason, 2010). Conversely, strand breaks can lead to the elevated expression of tumor suppressor genes (Crott et al., 2007).

Low folate levels have been found to increase uracil incorporation and DNA strand breaks in cultured cells (Duthie and Hawdon, 1998; Duthie et al., 2000b; Crott et al., 2001). Folate deficiency in culture also resulted in decreased repair of DNA damage (James et al., 1994; Duthie and Hawdon, 1998; Duthie et al., 2000b), which would further increase the accumulation of mutations and other types of instability in the genome. In animal models, folate deficiency has also been observed to cause increased dUTP:dTTP ratios, uracil incorporation, DNA strand breaks and base excision repair (Pogribny et al., 1997b; Choi et al., 1998; Duthie et al., 2000a; Knock et al., 2008). Uracil misincorporation has been linked to tumor development in mice; folate-deficient BALB/c mice have increased dUTP:dTTP ratios and DNA strand breaks in the intestine, and are at an increased risk of developing intestinal tumors (Knock et al., 2008).

Uracil misincorporation might also enhance tumorigenesis in humans; a borderline association between uracil misincorporation and the recurrence of colorectal adenoma (CRA) has been reported (Hazra et al., 2010). Low blood folate levels have been associated with increased dUTP:dTTP and uracil misincorporation in human lymphocytes that could be reversed by folate supplementation (Blount et al., 1997; Jacob et al., 1998; Basten et al., 2006). However, this relation was not observed in either lymphocytes or rectal mucosa in another study (Hazra et al., 2010), and supplementation with very large doses of folic acid were reported in one study to even increase the uracil content of DNA in rectal mucosa (van den Donk et al., 2007a). Similarly, DNA strand breaks in lymphocytes have been observed with folate deficiency in some studies (Blount et al., 1997), but not others (Fenech et al., 1998; Basten et al., 2006). The relation between folate and uracil misincorporation could be influenced by several factors. Age might be an important modifier, because uracil misincorporation owing to folate deficiency has been found to be enhanced in the colon of older rats (Choi et al., 2003). Uracil misincorporation could also be affected by folate-related single nucleotide polymorphisms (SNPs), such as the MTHFR 677 C→T variant (discussed in Section 6.7.4.1), and other genetic factors (Knock et al., 2006, 2008; DeVos et al., 2008). Folate fortification (Hazra et al., 2010) and vitamin B12 levels (Fenech et al., 1998; Kapiszewska et al., 2005) could also be significant confounders.

6.7.2.3 DNA methylation

DNA is methylated by DNA methyltransferases (DNMTs) on the pyrimidine ring of cytosine residues of CpG dinucleotides (a cytosine followed by a guanine). CpGs are not evenly distributed in the genome. They are usually located in CpG-rich regions referred to as CpG islands, which are often found in, and around, gene promoters (Gronbaek et al., 2007; Esteller, 2008). The methylation of DNA is implicated in the regulation of gene expression, as well as maintaining the integrity and organization of the genome.

Global hypomethylation of the genome combined with local hypermethylation of CpG islands in gene promoters is a common feature in neoplastic cells (Gronbaek et al., 2007; Esteller, 2008). Genomic hypomethylation might be one of the earliest changes in carcinogenesis, and has been found to increase with cancer progression (Esteller, 2008). Hypomethylation seems to make DNA more prone to mitotic recombination, leading to potentially carcinogenic chromosome breaks, translocations and loss of alleles (Gronbaek et al., 2007; Esteller, 2008). Hypomethylation could also result in the expression of genes normally silenced by imprinting, promoting de-differentiation and tumorigenesis in tissues (Sakatani et al., 2005; Esteller, 2008). These mechanisms might contribute both to tumor initiation and the progression of cancers. Folate deficiency could result in methylation changes by restricting the availability of 5-methylTHF, which is utilized in the synthesis of methionine and generation of SAM, or by increasing the levels of SAH, an inhibitor of SAM-dependent methyltransferases (Hoffman et al., 1979). Although SAH usually generates homocysteine, hyperhomocysteinemia can reverse the catalytic reaction of the SAH hydrolase and result in generation of SAH; hyperhomocysteinemia is commonly observed in folate deficiency.

Folate deficiency can cause genomic DNA hypomethylation in cells (Duthie et al., 2000b; Wasson et al., 2006), animal models (Balaghi and Wagner, 1993) and human lymphocytes and colonic mucosa (Jacob et al., 1998; Rampersaud et al., 2000; Pufulete et al., 2005). In rat liver, genomic hypomethylation was associated with genome-wide DNA strand break accumulation (Pogribny et al., 1995), a possible mechanism for carcinogenesis. Colorectal cancer patients were reported to have lower blood folate levels and increased DNA hypomethylation in colonic mucosa as compared with controls (Pufulete et al., 2003). In this study, genomic hypomethylation was associated with a significantly increased risk for CRA and a borderline increased risk of CRC, suggesting that hypomethylation could contribute to tumorigenesis (Pufulete et al., 2003). However, the relation between folate deficiency and genomic hypomethylation is not always observed, and might be modified by several factors. Genomic hypomethylation was observed in the liver of rats fed a severely folate-deficient diet (Balaghi and Wagner, 1993) and in the colon of mice fed a diet mildly deficient in folate and other B vitamins (Liu et al., 2007). Mild folate deficiency alone in mouse colon (Liu et al., 2007) and moderate folate deficiency in rat colon and liver (Kim et al., 1995) were not associated with hypomethylation. The timing of the administration of folate-deficient diets (Lawrance et al., 2009), the duration of the deficiency (Pogribny et al., 1997a; Sohn et al., 2003), and the age of the animals (Keyes et al., 2007) could affect the methylation response to folate deficiency.

Age might also increase sensitivity to folate deficiency in humans. DNA hypomethylation in lymphocytes has been linked to low folate levels in older subjects in controlled feeding studies (Jacob et al., 1998; Rampersaud et al., 2000) and in colonic mucosa in a cross-sectional study (Pufulete et al., 2005). However, lymphocyte DNA hypomethylation was not observed in cross-sectional studies of younger adults (Basten et al., 2006; Fenech et al., 1998). Folate-related SNPs, such as the MTHFR 677 C→T variant (see Section 6.7.4.1), might also influence the association of folate levels and DNA hypomethylation (Friso et al., 2002; Stern et al., 2000; Sohn et al., 2009).

Local hypermethylation of gene promoters that silence the expression of tumor suppressor genes has been observed in many cancers (Agrawal et al., 2007). This phenomenon could be linked to the increased expression of DNMT1 in many tumors (Etoh et al.,

2004; Wang et al., 2009). Hypermethylation of the H-cadherin promoter in response to low folate levels has been reported in human nasopharyngeal carcinoma cells in culture (Jhaveri et al., 2001) and hypermethylation of the p16[INK4A] promoter in head and neck squamous cell carcinoma was increased in patients with low dietary folate intake (Kraunz et al., 2006). As with genomic hypomethylation, the extent of local hypermethylation increases with age. Hypermethylation of the ESR1 (estrogen receptor 1) promoter increased in the colorectal mucosa of aged mice (Belshaw et al., 2005); similarly, increased local hypermethylation of the retinoic acid receptor beta 1 and 2 genes in colon and of a panel of epigenetic sites in liver was observed in older patients (Youssef et al., 2004; Nishida et al., 2008). The MTHFR 677 C→T variant also influenced hypermethylation of a panel of promoters in response to lower folate intake in colorectal adenomas (van den Donk et al., 2007b). Increased expression of DNMT1 has been observed in cells cultured in low folate medium (Hayashi et al., 2007). Because DNMT1 could be recruited to sites of DNA damage (Mortusewicz et al., 2005), the increase in DNA damage owing to folate deficiency might serve to attract the methyltransferase and contribute to hypermethylation.

6.7.2.4 Folate as an agent that supports tumor growth

Folate is involved in several processes that support the growth and proliferation of cells, such as nucleotide synthesis, methylation and amino acid synthesis. As such, higher levels of folate could support growth of tumors. Administration of folic acid was observed to adversely affect the clinical course of leukemia patients in the 1940s by accelerating expansion of the cancerous clone of cells (Farber, 1949; Heinle and Welch, 1948). In fact, several chemotherapeutic agents used in the treatment of cancers disrupt folate metabolism, such as methotrexate (MTX) and 5-fluorouracil (5FU). The relation between folic acid and tumor growth is of particular interest owing to the widespread use of supplements containing folic acid as well as the voluntary and mandatory fortification of grain products in some countries (see Section 6.7.3.3).

Work with animal models has helped to elucidate the relation between folate and cancer. As previously mentioned, in mice with no genetic predisposition to cancer or exposure to carcinogens, prolonged folate deficiency can increase risk for intestinal tumors (Knock et al., 2006). However, in rodent models that carry a strong predisposition to forming intestinal neoplasms (owing to genetic alterations or carcinogen exposure), tumor development is often limited by folate deficiency and accelerated by folate supplementation, depending on the timing of the dietary intervention (Baggott et al., 1992; Le Leu et al., 2000; Song et al., 2000; Kotsopoulos et al., 2005; Lawrance et al., 2007; Lawrance et al., 2009; Lindzon et al., 2009). In summary, inadequate folate intake in the early stages of tumorigenesis could serve to initiate or promote tumor development whereas limited folate intake following tumor initiation might limit tumor growth.

Aside from supporting rapidly proliferating cells, there is some concern regarding the presence of unmetabolized folic acid in blood (Kalmbach et al., 2008). Several possible carcinogenic mechanisms associated with unmetabolized folic acid have been suggested, such as inhibition of folate transporters or folate-dependent enzymes, inhibition of nucleotide synthesis, and reduced natural killer (NK) cell cytotoxicity (Smith et al., 2008). However, there are no data at this time indicating that folic acid has idiosyncratic functions as a tumor-promoting agent that are not possessed by the other, more natural co-enzymatic forms of the vitamin.

6.7.3 Folate intake and cancer risk – epidemiological studies

The effect of folate intake on cancer risk has been examined in both prospective cohort and case-control studies. Cancers in certain sites appear to be more sensitive to folate status than others. In addition, cancer risk associated with folate deficiency varies between populations, and is probably modified by genetic factors, intake of other nutrients and age. In many cases, pooled and meta-analyses of the data are available and have increased the power to identify associations between folate intake and cancer risk (Sanjoaquin et al., 2005; Lewis et al., 2006; Larsson et al., 2007; Chen et al., 2010).

6.7.3.1 Folate deficiency and colorectal cancer (CRC)

Many studies have identified an inverse relation between dietary folate and CRC risk. The consensus of these studies is supported by the results of a meta-analysis of five cohort and seven case-control studies published between 1991 and 2004, which found that CRC risk was reduced by ~25% in individuals with high dietary folate intake (Sanjoaquin et al., 2005). However, total folate intake (food plus supplements), when examined in three cohort and three case-control studies, had no significant effect on CRC risk (Sanjoaquin et al., 2005).

The inverse relation of folate and CRC has been reported for two large prospective cohort studies. In a cohort of Swedish women, high dietary folate was observed to protect against colon but not rectal cancer; this effect was more pronounced in smokers than non-smokers (Larsson et al., 2005). In a cohort of American women, there was an inverse association between dietary folate and CRC risk in subjects not taking vitamin supplements; total folate (food plus supplements) and multivitamin use were not significantly associated with CRC risk (Zhang et al., 2006). This finding echoes that of the earlier meta-analysis (Sanjoaquin et al., 2005).

Several case-control studies nested inside large cohorts have permitted investigation of the relation between pre-diagnosis plasma/serum folate and CRC risk. High serum folate has been reported to prevent CRC (Kato et al., 1999; Ma et al., 1997) and CRC specific mortality (Wolpin et al., 2008). This protective effect might be enhanced by homozygosity for the MTHFR 677C→T variant (see Section 6.7.4.1) and negated by alcohol intake (Ma et al., 1997). Similarly, low RBC folate has been shown to significantly increase the risk of advanced adenomas and hyperplastic polyps, particularly in smokers and/or individuals with the MTHFR 677C→T variant (Ulvik et al., 2001). High dietary folate was also found to protect against increased CRA risk owing to alcohol intake (Hermann et al., 2009). The epidemiologic interactions observed between folate and alcohol are consistent with the fact that alcohol is a potent inhibitor of 1-carbon metabolism (Mason and Choi, 2005). By contrast, pre-diagnosis plasma folate and CRC risk formed a bell-shaped curve in a Swedish study; folate levels in the lowest and highest quintiles were protective compared with the middle range (Van Guelpen et al., 2006).

6.7.3.2 Folate deficiency and other cancers

Risk for other gastrointestinal cancers could also be affected by dietary folate intake. A recent meta-analysis showed that higher levels of dietary folate significantly reduced the risk for both esophageal squamous cell carcinoma and esophageal adenocarcinoma

(Larsson et al., 2006). High dietary folate was also found to protect against pancreatic cancers in the same analysis (Larsson et al., 2006) and might also decrease risk for gastric cancer. The relation with gastric cancer varied with geography; high folate intake was protective in the USA, but had no effect on risk in Europe or elsewhere (Larsson et al., 2006).

Studies of breast cancer risk and folate intake have produced mixed results. Two meta-analyses found that folate intake was not associated with breast cancer risk in prospective cohort studies, but that high folate intake significantly reduced breast cancer risk in case-control studies (Larsson et al., 2007; Lewis et al., 2006). Perhaps the inconsistency in the studies is explained by an interaction with alcohol because one of the aforementioned meta-analyses indicated that the reduced risk could be confined to women with increased alcohol consumption (Larsson et al., 2007). Many of the studies included in the meta-analyses suggested that high folate intake might be protective only after menopause (Larsson et al., 2007), as observed in subsequent Swedish and American prospective studies (Cho et al., 2007; Ericson et al., 2007).

Although high dietary folate intake has been reported to reduce lung cancer risk (Voorrips et al., 2000), a pooled analysis of eight cohort studies did not find strong evidence for a protective effect against lung cancer (Cho et al., 2006). Similarly, folate supplements were not reported to affect lung cancer risk in a large prospective cohort study (Slatore et al., 2008).

6.7.3.3 Folate supplementation/fortification and cancer risk

High levels of folic acid intake, owing to supplementation and/or food fortification, could encourage the growth of tumors that would not otherwise develop into clinically significant lesions (see Section 6.7.2.4). In recent years, supplemental folic acid has been investigated in randomized clinical trials as a homocysteine lowering agent for the prevention of cardiovascular disease (CVD) because hyperhomocysteinemia has become recognized as a risk factor for CVD (Humphrey et al., 2008). In one large study of folic acid supplementation in CVD patients, supplementation resulted in a significantly increased occurrence of cancer, particularly lung and CRC (Ebbing et al., 2009). However, in two other similar CVD studies, no significant effect of folic acid supplements on cancer rates was observed (Bonaa et al., 2006; Lonn et al., 2006).

Folic acid supplements have also been investigated as a chemopreventive agent for CRC/CRA in randomized clinical trials, with mixed results. One small trial found that folic acid decreased CRA recurrence (Jaszewski et al., 2008); a non-significant protective effect was reported in a second small trial (Paspatis and Karamanolis, 1994). However, a large trial with a dose of folic acid more similar to that found in the North American diet (0.5 mg/day) found no effect of folic acid on CRA recurrence (Logan et al., 2008). Two longer studies that tested the effects of 1 mg folic acid/day on CRA prevention had conflicting results. One found that, although folic acid did not increase overall CRA recurrence, it did raise the risk of having advanced or multiple lesions, and increased the incidence of prostate cancer (Cole et al., 2007). The other reported that supplemental folic acid reduced CRA recurrence in patients with low folate levels before treatment, had no effect on those whose folate levels were already elevated, and did not increase risk of advanced or multiple lesions (Wu et al., 2009). A meta-analysis of some of these studies concluded that folic acid supplementation for up to 3 years did not increase the risk of CRA, but longer periods of supplementation increased CRA risk, particularly for advanced lesions (Fife et al., 2009). It should be noted, however, that the increased risk over the past 3 years was dictated entirely by the data from the Cole et al. (2007) trial because that is the only one to have extended over such a long period.

The effect of mandatory folic acid fortification of grain products on cancer incidence has also been examined. It has been suggested that fortification in the USA and Canada could have contributed to an increase in CRC rates that occurred in the 1990s (Mason et al., 2007). However, recent studies have also suggested that fortification could have reduced breast cancer incidence in North America (Reddy et al., 2009), and that high levels of folate intake over the long term (including folic acid supplements) might reduce breast cancer risk (Maruti et al., 2009). Clearly, the relation between high folic acid intake and cancer remains controversial, and more data are required before any firm conclusions can be made.

6.7.4 Impact of polymorphisms in folate-related genes on cancer risk

6.7.4.1 MTHFR 677C→T

The MTHFR 677C→T (A222V) variant is the most studied polymorphism in folate metabolism (Frosst et al., 1995). The frequency of the TT genotype is 10–15% in many North American and European populations. The A222V protein is thermolabile with reduced activity (Frosst et al., 1995; Yamada et al., 2001). However, the mutant enzyme can be stabilized by folate (Yamada et al., 2001); consequently the effects of the variant could be overcome by additional folate (Jacques et al., 1996; Hustad et al., 2007). Reduced MTHFR activity is associated with decreased plasma folate, altered distribution of folate derivatives, and increased Hcy (Frosst et al., 1995; Bagley and Selhub, 1998; Friso et al., 2002; Davis et al., 2005; Quinlivan et al., 2005; Fredriksen et al., 2007; Hustad et al., 2007; DeVos et al., 2008; Yang et al., 2008).

As discussed below, studies of the 677C→T variant and CRC generally suggest that the TT genotype is protective. Reduced MTHFR activity spares methyleneTHF which could enhance thymidylate synthesis; the consequent reduction in uracil misincorporation could be the mechanism by which this SNP protects against cancer. Increased thymidylate synthesis (Quinlivan et al., 2005) and reduced uracil misincorporation have been reported in TT individuals (Kapiszewska et al., 2005; DeVos et al., 2008), but have not been observed consistently (Crott et al., 2001; Narayanan et al., 2004).

Abnormal methylation owing to the 677C→T variant could also contribute to modification of cancer risk. Genomic DNA hypomethylation was increased in TT individuals, particularly in combination with low folate status (Stern et al., 2000; Friso et al., 2002), although this was not observed in a study that did not stratify based on folate levels (Narayanan et al., 2004). Altered DNA methylation might explain the loss of protection against cancer observed in TT individuals with low folate status (see below).

Several recent meta-analyses have addressed the relation between the MTHFR 677C→T SNP and cancer risk, particularly risk of CRC. Overall, they conclude that the 677TT genotype reduces CRC risk by approximately 20% (Kono and Chen, 2005; Huang et al., 2007; Hubner and Houlston, 2007). This protective effect was similar for both colon and rectal cancer but might vary between populations (Huang et al., 2007;

Hubner and Houlston, 2007). Folate status could modify the effect of this variant; the protective effect was seen in folate-replete but not folate-deficient individuals (Chen et al., 1996; Ma et al., 1997). However, in other studies, folate levels did not influence the protective effect of the TT genotype (Van Guelpen et al., 2006). The reduced CRC risk associated with this variant might also vary with gender (de Vogel et al., 2009) and is abolished in individuals with higher alcohol consumption (Chen et al., 1996; Ma et al., 1997). The reduction of CRC risk could also be a factor of age; this variant has been found to delay the age of diagnosis of CRC patients (Shannon et al., 2002; Reeves et al., 2009).

In contrast to CRC, most studies suggest that the variant might not modify CRA risk (Kono and Chen, 2005; Huang et al., 2007) or recurrence (Hubner et al., 2006; Levine et al., 2008), although a couple of studies have reported that the TT genotype increases risk for CRA at low folate levels, and decreases risk at high folate levels (Levine et al., 2000; Ulvik et al., 2001). If one assumes the stance of the majority, however, that the variant has no impact on adenoma occurrence, these observations collectively suggest that homozygosity for the variant prevents CRA from developing into CRC. The effect of the variant on CRA risk could be modified by diet.

The 677TT genotype was reported to increase risk for gastric cancer in five meta-analyses (Larsson et al., 2006; Zintzaras, 2006b; Boccia et al., 2008; Dong et al., 2008; Sun et al., 2008). This risk could depend on folate status; it was significantly increased in individuals with low folate levels, but not in those with high levels (Boccia et al., 2008; Sun et al., 2008). The effect of the variant might also vary with ethnicity; the increased risk was significant for Asians, but not Europeans (Boccia et al., 2008; Zintzaras, 2006b). The TT genotype could also increase risk for esophageal and pancreatic cancers (Larsson et al., 2006).

Other meta-analyses suggest that the 677TT genotype could protect against acute lymphoblastic leukemia (ALL) (Robien and Ulrich, 2003; Pereira et al., 2006; Zintzaras et al., 2006), but that it has no effect on lung cancer risk (Mao et al., 2008). No clear relation between this variant and breast cancer risk has emerged (Lewis et al., 2006; Lissowska et al., 2007; Macis et al., 2007; Zintzaras, 2006a). The 677C→T SNP has been investigated as a risk factor for many other cancers, but additional studies are required for clarification.

6.7.4.2 Other polymorphisms in folate-related genes

Associations between other folate-related polymorphisms and cancer are considerably less conclusive than those related to the 677 variant. The MTHFR 1298A→C variant (E429A) (Weisberg et al., 1998) is also common; the frequency of the CC genotype is approximately 10% in North America. This variant is in linkage disequilibrium with the 677C→T SNP; the compound 677TT 1298CC genotype is rarely observed (Ogino and Wilson, 2003). The 1298 variant has a much milder biochemical phenotype than the 677 variant: it only modestly affects enzyme activity and does not appear to affect plasma folate or Hcy levels (Weisberg et al., 1998; Yang et al., 2008).

The results for CRC risk have been contradictory; one recent meta-analysis found that the CC genotype protects against CRC (Huang et al., 2007), whereas another found no significant effect (Kono and Chen, 2005). As with the 677C→T variant, this variant does not appear to influence risk for CRA (Huang et al., 2007). A lack of association between the 1298A→C variant and cancer risk has been reported in meta-analyses investigating gastric cancer (Boccia et al., 2008; Sun et al., 2008), lung cancer (Mao et al., 2008), and breast cancer (Zintzaras, 2006a; Lissowska et al., 2007). Two meta-analyses on ALL risk had contradictory results; one reported no effect of the CC genotype (Pereira et al., 2006), whereas the other reported a protective effect, particularly in children with the 677CC genotype (Zintzaras et al., 2006).

The TS (thymidylate synthase) 2R/3R polymorphism is a variation in the number of 28 base pair repeats in the 5′ untranslated region of the gene and might affect TS expression (Horie et al., 1995). The effect of this variant on plasma folate and Hcy levels is not clear. The 2R/2R genotype is found in ~20% of the North American population (Ulrich et al., 2005) and could reduce CRC risk, particularly in men or individuals with low folate intake (Chen et al., 2003; Ulrich et al., 2005). This variant does not appear to affect risk for CRA, which suggests that it could impede tumor progression (Chen et al., 2004; Ulrich et al., 2002). However, this variant might influence cancer treatment outcomes (see Section 6.7.5).

Many other folate-related SNPs have been investigated as potential risk factors for cancer, including SNPs in MTHFD1, MTR, MTRR, DHFR and SHMT1. Some studies of these SNPs found associations with a variety of cancers [for review see Chen et al. (2010) and Christensen and Rozen (2010)]. It is clear at this time that genetic variation in folate metabolism might have an impact on cancer risk, but the data are still limited.

6.7.5 Influence of folate intake and genetic variation on cancer treatment

Anti-folate chemotherapeutics such as methotrexate (MTX) have been used in the treatment of cancer for decades. MTX primarily inhibits DHFR and is also known to inhibit TS, MTHFR and folate-dependent enzymes in the purine synthesis pathway (Robien, 2005). MTX is used in the treatment of leukemia, lymphoma, breast cancer, head and neck cancer and osteosarcoma, and, at lower doses, in rheumatoid arthritis and psoriasis (Robien, 2005). Other anti-folates such as pemetrexed have similar targets and uses. 5-Fluorouracil (5FU) is often included in discussions of anti-folate chemotherapeutics because it is an inhibitor of TS. These drugs abrogate folate metabolism which disrupts DNA replication in rapidly dividing cells, resulting in inhibition of proliferation or cell death.

The effect of dietary folate intake on anti-folate chemotherapy has not been extensively investigated, and therefore the effects, if any, are largely unknown [for review, see Robien (2005)]. Most pharmacologic studies of folate are focused on the prevention of toxic side effects in rapidly dividing hematopoietic and intestinal mucosal cells. Although dietary folate could influence treatment outcome for applications that use lower doses of anti-folates [reviewed in Smith et al. (2008)], the chemotherapeutic doses in cancer treatment greatly exceed levels that would be expected to be influenced by normal folate intakes, and might therefore be less affected. However, there are concerns that supra-physiological folic acid levels that can result from combined folate fortification and high-dose supplementation could facilitate drug resistance (Smith et al., 2008). In the era of folate fortification and common supplement use, the interaction of folate intake and chemotherapeutic outcome requires further investigation.

Polymorphisms in folate-related genes could affect treatment outcome with anti-folate chemotherapeutics (De Mattia and Toffoli, 2009). The MTHFR 677TT genotype has been associated with increased MTX toxicity (Chiusolo et al., 2002; Toffoli et al.,

2003). However, because this effect is not consistently observed (Kishi et al., 2003), further investigation is required before making clinical recommendations based on genotype. The TT genotype has been reported to reduce the efficacy of MTX; increased likelihood of relapse and worse survival outcomes have been observed (Krajinovic et al., 2004; Aplenc et al., 2005; Chiusolo et al., 2007). These adverse outcomes might be alleviated through folate supplementation, in the form of folic acid or 5-formylTHF (Robien et al., 2004; De Mattia and Toffoli, 2009).

Chemotherapy with 5FU involves the formation of a ternary complex between TS, 5FU and methyleneTHF; this complex inhibits enzyme activity. The MTHFR 677 C→T variant could influence 5FU treatment by increasing the supply of methyleneTHF and consequently the formation of the complex. Improved treatment outcomes have been observed in patients with the TT genotype (Cohen et al., 2003; Etienne et al., 2004; Jakobsen et al., 2005). There appears to be no association between this variant and tumor recurrence or survival (Wisotzkey et al., 1999; Lurje et al., 2008; Afzal et al., 2009). Mixed results have been reported for investigation of this SNP and 5FU toxicity (Cohen et al., 2003; Afzal et al., 2009; Gusella et al., 2009). The TS 2R/2R genotype has been reported to increase the 5FU sensitivity of tumor cells *in vitro* (Yawata et al., 2005), and could improve 5FU treatment outcomes in CRC patients (Iacopetta et al., 2001; Marsh et al., 2001), although these effects are not consistently observed. At present, there are no meta-analyses of the TS variants and cancer risk or treatment outcomes.

6.7.6 Conclusions

The relation between folate intake and cancer risk is complex, and might be difficult to elucidate unless several factors, such as age, genetic variation, and all sources of folate (food and supplements) are taken into account. Nonetheless, a diet rich in folate appears to reduce the risk of colorectal cancer, possibly by limiting tumor initiation; the impact on risk for other types of cancers is not yet conclusive. However, folic acid supplementation after the development of a tumor might not be beneficial and additional studies are clearly warranted to test this hypothesis, particularly in populations with folate fortification and high vitamin supplement use. The association between genetic polymorphisms in folate metabolism and cancer risk or cancer therapy is an important area of continued research that could lead to personalized recommendations for folate intake or cancer treatment.

References

Afzal S, Jensen SA, Vainer B, Vogel U, Matsen JP, Sorensen JB, Andersen PK, Poulsen HE, MTHFR polymorphisms and 5-FU-based adjuvant chemotherapy in colorectal cancer. Ann Oncol 2009;20: 1660–6.

Agrawal A, Murphy RF, Agrawal DK, DNA methylation in breast and colorectal cancers. Mod Pathol 2007;20: 711–21.

Aplenc R, Thompson J, Han P, La M, Zhao H, Lange B, Rebbeck T, Methylenetetrahydrofolate reductase polymorphisms and therapy response in pediatric acute lymphoblastic leukemia. Cancer Res 2005;65: 2482–7.

Baggott JE, Vaughn WH, Juliana MM, Eto I, Krumdieck CL, Grubbs CJ, Effects of folate deficiency and supplementation on methylnitrosourea-induced rat mammary tumors. J Natl Cancer Inst 1992;84: 1740–4.

Bagley PJ, Selhub J, A common mutation in the methylenetetrahydrofolate reductase gene is associated with an accumulation of formylated tetrahydrofolates in red blood cells. Proc Natl Acad Sci USA 1998;95: 13217–20.

Balaghi M, Wagner C, DNA methylation in folate deficiency: use of CpG methylase. Biochem Biophys Res Commun 1993;193: 1184–90.

Barnes DE, Lindahl T, Repair and genetic consequences of endogenous DNA base damage in mammalian cells. Annu Rev Genet 2004;38: 445–76.

Basten GP, Duthie SJ, Pirie L, Vaughan N, Hill MH, Powers HJ, Sensitivity of markers of DNA stability and DNA repair activity to folate supplementation in healthy volunteers. Br J Cancer 2006;94: 1942–7.

Belshaw NJ, Elliott GO, Williams EA, Mathers JC, Buckley L, Bahari B, Johnson IT, Methylation of the ESR1 CpG island in the colorectal mucosa is an 'all or nothing' process in healthy human colon, and is accelerated by dietary folate supplementation in the mouse. Biochem Soc Trans 2005;33: 709–11.

Blount BC, Mack MM, Wehr CM, MacGregor JT, Hiatt RA, Wang G, Wickramasinghe SN, Everson RB, Ames BN, Folate deficiency causes uracil misincorporation into human DNA and chromosome breakage: implications for cancer and neuronal damage. Proc Natl Acad Sci USA 1997;94: 3290–5.

Boccia S, Hung R, Ricciardi G, Gianfagna F, Ebert MP, Fang JY, Gao CM, Gotze T, Graziano F, Lacasana-Navarro M, Lin D, Lopez-Carrillo L, Qiao YL, Shen H, Stolzenberg-Solomon R, Takezaki T, Weng YR, Zhang FF, van Duijn CM, Boffetta P, Taioli E, Meta- and pooled analyses of the methylenetetrahydrofolate reductase C677T and A1298C polymorphisms and gastric cancer risk: a huge-GSEC review. Am J Epidemiol 2008;167: 505–16.

Bonaa KH, Njolstad I, Ueland PM, Schirmer H, Tverdal A, Steigen T, Wang H, Nordrehaug JE, Arnesen E, Rasmussen K, Homocysteine lowering and cardiovascular events after acute myocardial infarction. N Engl J Med 2006;354: 1578–88.

Chen J, Giovannucci E, Kelsey K, Rimm EB, Stampfer MJ, Colditz GA, Spiegelman D, Willett WC, Hunter DJ, A methylenetetrahydrofolate reductase polymorphism and the risk of colorectal cancer. Cancer Res 1996;56: 4862–4.

Chen J, Hunter DJ, Stampfer MJ, Kyte C, Chan W, Wetmur JG, Mosig R, Selhub J, Ma J, Polymorphism in the thymidylate synthase promoter enhancer region modifies the risk and survival of colorectal cancer. Cancer Epidemiol Biomarkers Prev 2003;12: 958–62.

Chen J, Kyte C, Chan W, Wetmur JG, Fuchs CS, Giovannucci E, Polymorphism in the thymidylate synthase promoter enhancer region and risk of colorectal adenomas. Cancer Epidemiol Biomarkers Prev 2004;13: 2247–50.

Chen J, Xu X, Liu A, Ulrich CM, Folate and cancer: epidemiological perspective. In: Bailey LB, editor. Folate in health and disease, 2nd ed. Boca Raton, FL: CRC Press; 2010. pp. 205–34.

Chiusolo P, Reddiconto G, Casorelli I, Laurenti L, Sora F, Mele L, Annino L, Leone G, Sica S, Preponderance of methylenetetrahydrofolate reductase C677T homozygosity among leukemia patients intolerant to methotrexate. Ann Oncol 2002;13: 1915–8.

Chiusolo P, Reddiconto G, Farina G, Mannocci A, Fiorini A, Palladino M, La Torre G, Fianchi L, Sora F, Laurenti L, Leone G, Sica S, MTHFR polymorphisms' influence on outcome and toxicity in acute lymphoblastic leukemia patients. Leuk Res 2007;31: 1669–74.

Cho E, Hunter DJ, Spiegelman D, Albanes D, Beeson WL, van den Brandt PA, Colditz GA, Feskanich D, Folsom AR, Fraser GE, Freudenheim JL, Giovannucci E, Goldbohm RA, Graham S, Miller AB, Rohan TE, Sellers TA, Virtamo J, Willett WC, Smith-Warner SA, Intakes of vitamins A, C and E and folate and multivitamins and lung cancer: a pooled analysis of 8 prospective studies. Int J Cancer 2006;118: 970–8.

Cho E, Holmes M, Hankinson SE, Willett WC, Nutrients involved in one-carbon metabolism and risk of breast cancer among premenopausal women. Cancer Epidemiol Biomarkers Prev 2007;16: 2787–90.

Choi SW, Kim YI, Weitzel JN, Mason JB, Folate depletion impairs DNA excision repair in the colon of the rat. Gut 1998;43: 93–9.

Choi SW, Friso S, Dolnikowski GG, Bagley PJ, Edmondson AN, Smith DE, Mason JB, Biochemical and molecular aberrations in the rat colon due to folate depletion are age-specific. J Nutr 2003;133: 1206–12.

Christensen KE, Rozen R, Genetic variation: effect on folate metabolism and health. In: Bailey LB, editor. Folate in health and disease, 2nd ed. Boca Raton, FL: CRC Press; 2010. pp. 75–110.

Ciappio ED, Mason JB, Folate and carcinogenesis: basic mechanisms. In: Bailey LB, editor. Folate in health and disease, 2nd ed. Boca Raton, FL: CRC Press; 2010. pp. 235–62.

Cohen V, Panet-Raymond V, Sabbaghian N, Morin I, Batist G, Rozen R, Methylenetetrahydrofolate reductase polymorphism in advanced colorectal cancer: a novel genomic predictor of clinical response to fluoropyrimidine-based chemotherapy. Clin Cancer Res 2003;9: 1611–5.

Cole BF, Baron JA, Sandler RS, Haile RW, Ahnen DJ, Bresalier RS, McKeown-Eyssen G, Summers RW, Rothstein RI, Burke CA, Snover DC, Church TR, Allen JI, Robertson DJ, Beck GJ, Bond JH, Byers T, Mandel JS, Mott LA, Pearson LH, Barry EL, Rees JR, Marcon N, Saibil F, Ueland PM, Greenberg ER, Folic acid for the prevention of colorectal adenomas: a randomized clinical trial. J Am Med Assoc 2007;297: 2351–9.

Crott JW, Mashiyama ST, Ames BN, Fenech MF, Methylenetetrahydrofolate reductase C677T polymorphism does not alter folic acid deficiency-induced uracil incorporation into primary human lymphocyte DNA in vitro. Carcinogenesis 2001;22: 1019–25.

Crott JW, Liu Z, Choi S-W, Mason JB, Folate depletion in human lymphocytes up-regulates p53 expression despite marked induction of strand breaks in exons 5–8 of the gene. Mutat Res/Genet Toxicol Environ Mutagen 2007;626: 171–9.

Davis SR, Quinlivan EP, Shelnutt KP, Maneval DR, Ghandour H, Capdevila A, Coats BS, Wagner C, Selhub J, Bailey LB, Shuster JJ, Stacpoole PW, Gregory JF III, The methylenetetrahydrofolate reductase 677C→T polymorphism and dietary folate restriction affect plasma one-carbon metabolites and red blood cell folate concentrations and distribution in women. J Nutr 2005;135: 1040–4.

De Mattia E, Toffoli G, C677T and A1298C MTHFR polymorphisms, a challenge for antifolate and fluoropyrimidine-based therapy personalisation. Eur J Cancer 2009;45: 1333–51.

de Vogel S, Wouters KA, Gottschalk RW, van Schooten FJ, de Goeij AF, de Bruine AP, Goldbohm RA, van den Brandt PA, Weijenberg MP, van Engeland M, Genetic variants of methyl metabolizing enzymes and epigenetic regulators: associations with promoter CpG island hypermethylation in colorectal cancer. Cancer Epidemiol Biomarkers Prev 2009;18: 3086–96.

De Wals P, Tairou F, Van Allen MI, Uh SH, Lowry RB, Sibbald B, Evans JA, Van den Hof MC, Zimmer P, Crowley M, Fernandez B, Lee NS, Niyonsenga T, Reduction in neural-tube defects after folic acid fortification in Canada. N Engl J Med 2007;357: 135–42.

DeVos L, Chanson A, Liu Z, Ciappio ED, Parnell LD, Mason JB, Tucker KL, Crott JW, Associations between single nucleotide polymorphisms in folate uptake and metabolizing genes with blood folate, homocysteine, and DNA uracil concentrations. Am J Clin Nutr 2008;88: 1149–58.

Dianov GL, Timchenko TV, Sinitsina OI, Kuzminov AV, Medvedev OA, Salganik RI, Repair of uracil residues closely spaced on the opposite strands of plasmid DNA results in double-strand break and deletion formation. Mol Gen Genet 1991;225: 448–52.

Dong LM, Potter JD, White E, Ulrich CM, Cardon LR, Peters U, Genetic susceptibility to cancer: the role of polymorphisms in candidate genes. J Am Med Assoc 2008;299: 2423–36.

Duthie SJ, Hawdon A, DNA instability (strand breakage, uracil misincorporation, and defective repair) is increased by folic acid depletion in human lymphocytes in vitro. FASEB J 1998;12: 1491–7.

Duthie SJ, Grant G, Narayanan S, Increased uracil misincorporation in lymphocytes from folate-deficient rats. Br J Cancer 2000a;83: 1532–7.

Duthie SJ, Narayanan S, Blum S, Pirie L, Brand GM, Folate deficiency in vitro induces uracil misincorporation and DNA hypomethylation and inhibits DNA excision repair in immortalized normal human colon epithelial cells. Nutr Cancer 2000b;37: 245–51.

Ebbing M, Bonaa KH, Nygard O, Arnesen E, Ueland PM, Nordrehaug JE, Rasmussen K, Njolstad I, Refsum H, Nilsen DW, Tverdal A, Meyer K, Vollset SE, Cancer incidence and mortality after treatment with folic acid and vitamin B12. J Am Med Assoc 2009;302: 2119–26.

Ericson U, Sonestedt E, Gullberg B, Olsson H, Wirfalt E, High folate intake is associated with lower breast cancer incidence in postmenopausal women in the Malmo Diet and Cancer cohort. Am J Clin Nutr 2007;86: 434–43.

Esteller M, Epigenetics in cancer. N Engl J Med 2008;358: 1148–59.

Etienne MC, Formento JL, Chazal M, Francoual M, Magne N, Formento P, Bourgeon A, Seitz JF, Delpero JR, Letoublon C, Pezet D, Milano G, Methylenetetrahydrofolate reductase gene polymorphisms and response to fluorouracil-based treatment in advanced colorectal cancer patients. Pharmacogenetics 2004;14: 785–92.

Etoh T, Kanai Y, Ushijima S, Nakagawa T, Nakanishi Y, Sasako M, Kitano S, Hirohashi S, Increased DNA methyltransferase 1 (DNMT1) protein expression correlates significantly with poorer tumor differentiation and frequent DNA hypermethylation of multiple CpG islands in gastric cancers. Am J Pathol 2004;164: 689–99.

Farber S, Some observations on the effect of folic acid antagonists on acute leukemia and other forms of incurable cancer. Blood 1949;4: 160–7.

Fenech M, Aitken C, Rinaldi J, Folate, vitamin B12, homocysteine status and DNA damage in young Australian adults. Carcinogenesis 1998;19: 1163–71.

Fife J, Raniga S, Hider PN, Frizelle FA, Folic acid supplementation and colorectal cancer risk; a meta-analysis. Colorectal Dis 2009; Epub ahead of print.

Fredriksen A, Meyer K, Ueland PM, Vollset SE, Grotmol T, Schneede J, Large-scale population-based metabolic phenotyping of thirteen genetic polymorphisms related to one-carbon metabolism. Hum Mutat 2007;28: 856–65.

Friso S, Choi SW, Girelli D, Mason JB, Dolnikowski GG, Bagley PJ, Olivieri O, Jacques PF, Rosenberg IH, Corrocher R, Selhub J, A common mutation in the 5,10-methylenetetrahydrofolate reductase gene affects genomic DNA methylation through an interaction with folate status. Proc Natl Acad Sci USA 2002;99: 5606–11.

Frosst P, Blom HJ, Milos R, Goyette P, Sheppard CA, Matthews RG, Boers GJ, den Heijer M, Kluijtmans LA, van den Heuvel LP, Rozen R, A candidate genetic risk factor for vascular disease: a common mutation in methylenetetrahydrofolate reductase. Nat Genet 1995;10: 111–3.

Gronbaek K, Hother C, Jones PA, Epigenetic changes in cancer. Acta Pathol Microbiol Immunol Scand 2007;115: 1039–59.

Gusella M, Frigo AC, Bolzonella C, Marinelli R, Barile C, Bononi A, Crepaldi G, Menon D, Stievano L, Toso S, Pasini F, Ferrazzi E, Padrini R, Predictors of survival and toxicity in patients on adjuvant therapy with 5-fluorouracil for colorectal cancer. Br J Cancer 2009;100: 1549–57.

Hayashi I, Sohn KJ, Stempak JM, Croxford R, Kim YI, Folate deficiency induces cell-specific changes in the steady-state transcript levels of genes involved in folate metabolism and 1-carbon transfer reactions in human colonic epithelial cells. J Nutr 2007;137: 607–13.

Hazra A, Selhub J, Chao WH, Ueland PM, Hunter DJ, Baron JA, Uracil misincorporation into DNA and folic acid supplementation. Am J Clin Nutr 2010;91: 160–5.

Heinle RW, Welch AD, Experiments with pteroylglutamic acid and pteroylglutamic acid deficiency in human leukemia. J Clin Invest 1948;27: 539.

Hermann S, Rohrmann S, Linseisen J, Lifestyle factors, obesity and the risk of colorectal adenomas in EPIC-Heidelberg. Cancer Causes Control 2009;20: 1397–408.

Hoffman DR, Cornatzer WE, Duerre JA, Relationship between tissue levels of S-adenosylmethionine, S-adenylhomocysteine, and transmethylation reactions. Can J Biochem 1979;57: 56–65.

Horie N, Aiba H, Oguro K, Hojo H, Takeishi K, Functional analysis and DNA polymorphism of the tandemly repeated sequences in the 5′-terminal regulatory region of the human gene for thymidylate synthase. Cell Struct Funct 1995;20: 191–7.

Huang Y, Han S, Li Y, Mao Y, Xie Y, Different roles of MTHFR C677T and A1298C polymorphisms in colorectal adenoma and colorectal cancer: a meta-analysis. J Hum Genet 2007;52: 73–85.

Hubner RA, Muir KR, Liu JF, Sellick GS, Logan RF, Grainge M, Armitage N, Chau I, Houlston RS, Folate metabolism polymorphisms influence risk of colorectal adenoma recurrence. Cancer Epidemiol Biomarkers Prev 2006;15: 1607–13.

Hubner RA, Houlston RS, MTHFR C677T and colorectal cancer risk: A meta-analysis of 25 populations. Int J Cancer 2007;120: 1027–35.

Humphrey LL, Fu R, Rogers K, Freeman M, Helfand M, Homocysteine level and coronary heart disease incidence: a systematic review and meta-analysis. Mayo Clin Proc 2008;83: 1203–12.

Hustad S, Midttun O, Schneede J, Vollset SE, Grotmol T, Ueland PM, The methylenetetrahydrofolate reductase 677C→T polymorphism as a modulator of a B vitamin network with major effects on homocysteine metabolism. Am J Hum Genet 2007;80: 846–55.

Iacopetta B, Grieu F, Joseph D, Elsaleh H, A polymorphism in the enhancer region of the thymidylate synthase promoter influences the survival of colorectal cancer patients treated with 5-fluorouracil. Br J Cancer 2001;85: 827–30.

Jacob RA, Gretz DM, Taylor PC, James SJ, Pogribny IP, Miller BJ, Henning SM, Swendseid ME, Moderate folate depletion increases plasma homocysteine and decreases lymphocyte DNA methylation in postmenopausal women. J Nutr 1998;128: 1204–12.

Jacques PF, Bostom AG, Williams RR, Ellison RC, Eckfeldt JH, Rosenberg IH, Selhub J, Rozen R, Relation between folate status, a common mutation in methylenetetrahydrofolate reductase, and plasma homocysteine concentrations. Circulation 1996;93: 7–9.

Jakobsen A, Nielsen JN, Gyldenkerne N, Lindeberg J, Thymidylate synthase and methylenetetrahydrofolate reductase gene polymorphism in normal tissue as predictors of fluorouracil sensitivity. J Clin Oncol 2005;23: 1365–9.

James SJ, Basnakian AG, Miller BJ, In vitro folate deficiency induces deoxynucleotide pool imbalance, apoptosis, and mutagenesis in Chinese hamster ovary cells. Cancer Res 1994;54: 5075–80.

Jaszewski R, Misra S, Tobi M, Ullah N, Naumoff JA, Kucuk O, Levi E, Axelrod BN, Patel BB, Majumdar AP, Folic acid supplementation inhibits recurrence of colorectal adenomas: a randomized chemoprevention trial. World J Gastroenterol 2008;14: 4492–8.

Jhaveri MS, Wagner C, Trepel JB, Impact of extracellular folate levels on global gene expression. Mol Pharmacol 2001;60: 1288–95.

Kalmbach RD, Choumenkovitch SF, Troen AM, D'Agostino R, Jacques PF, Selhub J, Circulating folic acid in plasma: relation to folic acid fortification. Am J Clin Nutr 2008;88: 763–8.

Kapiszewska M, Kalemba M, Wojciech U, Milewicz T, Uracil misincorporation into DNA of leukocytes of young women with positive folate balance depends on plasma vitamin B12 concentrations and methylenetetrahydrofolate reductase polymorphisms. A pilot study. J Nutr Biochem 2005;16: 467–78.

Kato I, Dnistrian AM, Schwartz M, Toniolo P, Koenig K, Shore RE, Akhmedkhanov A, Zeleniuch-Jacquotte A, Riboli E, Serum folate, homocysteine and colorectal cancer risk in women: a nested case-control study. Br J Cancer 1999;79: 1917–22.

Keyes MK, Jang H, Mason JB, Liu Z, Crott JW, Smith DE, Friso S, Choi SW, Older age and dietary folate are determinants of genomic and p16-specific DNA methylation in mouse colon. J Nutr 2007;137: 1713–7.

Kim YI, Christman JK, Fleet JC, Cravo ML, Salomon RN, Smith D, Ordovas J, Selhub J, Mason JB, Moderate folate deficiency does not cause global hypomethylation of hepatic and colonic DNA or c-myc-specific hypomethylation of colonic DNA in rats. Am J Clin Nutr 1995;61: 1083–90.

Kishi S, Griener J, Cheng C, Das S, Cook EH, Pei D, Hudson M, Rubnitz J, Sandlund JT, Pui CH, Relling MV, Homocysteine, pharmacogenetics, and neurotoxicity in children with leukemia. J Clin Oncol 2003;21: 3084–91.

Knock E, Deng L, Wu Q, Leclerc D, Wang XL, Rozen R, Low dietary folate initiates intestinal tumors in mice, with altered expression of G2-M checkpoint regulators polo-like kinase 1 and cell division cycle 25c. Cancer Res 2006;66: 10349–56.

Knock E, Deng L, Wu Q, Lawrance AK, Wang XL, Rozen R, Strain differences in mice highlight the role of DNA damage in neoplasia induced by low dietary folate. J Nutr 2008;138: 653–8.

Kono S, Chen K, Genetic polymorphisms of methylenetetrahydrofolate reductase and colorectal cancer and adenoma. Cancer Sci 2005;96: 535–42.

Kotsopoulos J, Medline A, Renlund R, Sohn KJ, Martin R, Hwang SW, Lu S, Archer MC, Kim YI, Effects of dietary folate on the development and progression of mammary tumors in rats. Carcinogenesis 2005;26: 1603–12.

Krajinovic M, Lemieux-Blanchard E, Chiasson S, Primeau M, Costea I, Moghrabi A, Role of polymorphisms in MTHFR and MTHFD1 genes in the outcome of childhood acute lymphoblastic leukemia. Pharmacogenomics J 2004;4: 66–72.

Kraunz KS, Hsiung D, McClean MD, Liu M, Osanyingbemi J, Nelson HH, Kelsey KT, Dietary folate is associated with p16(INK4A) methylation in head and neck squamous cell carcinoma. Int J Cancer 2006;119: 1553–7.

Larsson SC, Giovannucci E, Wolk A, A prospective study of dietary folate intake and risk of colorectal cancer: modification by caffeine intake and cigarette smoking. Cancer Epidemiol Biomarkers Prev 2005;14: 740–3.

Larsson SC, Giovannucci E, Wolk A, Folate intake, MTHFR polymorphisms, and risk of esophageal, gastric, and pancreatic cancer: a meta-analysis. Gastroenterology 2006;131: 1271–83.

Larsson SC, Giovannucci E, Wolk A, Folate and risk of breast cancer: a meta-analysis. J Natl Cancer Inst 2007;99: 64–76.

Lawrance AK, Deng L, Brody LC, Finnell RH, Shane B, Rozen R, Genetic and nutritional deficiencies in folate metabolism influence tumorigenicity in Apcmin/+ mice. J Nutr Biochem 2007;18: 305–12.

Lawrance AK, Deng L, Rozen R, Methylenetetrahydrofolate reductase deficiency and low dietary folate reduce tumorigenesis in Apc min/+ mice. Gut 2009;58: 805–11.

Le Leu RK, Young GP, McIntosh GH, Folate deficiency reduces the development of colorectal cancer in rats. Carcinogenesis 2000;21: 2261–5.

Levine AJ, Siegmund KD, Ervin CM, Diep A, Lee ER, Frankl HD, Haile RW, The methylenetetrahydrofolate reductase 677C→T polymorphism and distal colorectal adenoma risk. Cancer Epidemiol Biomarkers Prev 2000;9: 657–63.

Levine AJ, Wallace K, Tsang S, Haile RW, Saibil F, Ahnen D, Cole BF, Barry EL, Munroe DJ, Ali IU, Ueland P, Baron JA, MTHFR genotype and colorectal adenoma recurrence: data from a double-blind placebo-controlled clinical trial. Cancer Epidemiol Biomarkers Prev 2008;17: 2409–15.

Lewis SJ, Harbord RM, Harris R, Smith GD, Meta-analyses of observational and genetic association studies of folate intakes or levels and breast cancer risk. J Natl Cancer Inst 2006;98: 1607–22.

Lindzon GM, Medline A, Sohn KJ, Depeint F, Croxford R, Kim YI, Effect of folic acid supplementation on the progression of colorectal aberrant crypt foci. Carcinogenesis 2009;30: 1536–43.

Lissowska J, Gaudet MM, Brinton LA, Chanock SJ, Peplonska B, Welch R, Zatonski W, Szeszenia-Dabrowska N, Park S, Sherman M, Garcia-Closas M, Genetic polymorphisms in the one-carbon metabolism pathway and breast cancer risk: a population-based case-control study and meta-analyses. Int J Cancer 2007;120: 2696–703.

Liu Z, Choi SW, Crott JW, Keyes MK, Jang H, Smith DE, Kim M, Laird PW, Bronson R, Mason JB, Mild depletion of dietary folate combined with other B vitamins alters multiple components of the Wnt pathway in mouse colon. J Nutr 2007;137: 2701–8.

Logan RF, Grainge MJ, Shepherd VC, Armitage NC, Muir KR, Aspirin and folic acid for the prevention of recurrent colorectal adenomas. Gastroenterology 2008;134: 29–38.

Lonn E, Yusuf S, Arnold MJ, Sheridan P, Pogue J, Micks M, McQueen MJ, Probstfield J, Fodor G, Held C, Genest J, Jr., Homocysteine lowering with folic acid and B vitamins in vascular disease. N Engl J Med 2006;354: 1567–77.

Lurje G, Zhang W, Yang D, Groshen S, Hendifar AE, Husain H, Nagashima F, Chang HM, Fazzone W, Ladner RD, Pohl A, Ning Y, Iqbal S, El-Khoueiry A, Lenz HJ, Thymidylate synthase haplotype is associated with tumor recurrence in stage II and stage III colon cancer. Pharmacogenet Genomics 2008;18: 161–8.

Ma J, Stampfer MJ, Giovannucci E, Artigas C, Hunter DJ, Fuchs C, Willett WC, Selhub J, Hennekens CH, Rozen R, Methylenetetrahydrofolate reductase polymorphism, dietary interactions, and risk of colorectal cancer. Cancer Res 1997;57: 1098–102.

Macis D, Maisonneuve P, Johansson H, Bonanni B, Botteri E, Iodice S, Santillo B, Penco S, Gucciardo G, D'Aiuto G, Rosselli Del Turco M, Amadori M, Costa A, Decensi A, Methylenetetrahydrofolate reductase (MTHFR) and breast cancer risk: a nested-case-control study and a pooled meta-analysis. Breast Cancer Res Treat 2007;106: 263–71.

Mao R, Fan Y, Jin Y, Bai J, Fu S, Methylenetetrahydrofolate reductase gene polymorphisms and lung cancer: a meta-analysis. J Hum Genet 2008;53: 340–8.

Marsh S, McKay JA, Cassidy J, McLeod HL, Polymorphism in the thymidylate synthase promoter enhancer region in colorectal cancer. Int J Oncol 2001;19: 383–6.

Maruti SS, Ulrich CM, White E, Folate and one-carbon metabolism nutrients from supplements and diet in relation to breast cancer risk. Am J Clin Nutr 2009;89: 624–33.

Mason JB, Choi SW, Effects of alcohol on folate metabolism: implications for carcinogenesis. Alcohol 2005;35: 235–41.

Mason JB, Dickstein A, Jacques PF, Haggarty P, Selhub J, Dallal G, Rosenberg IH, A temporal association between folic acid fortification and an increase in colorectal cancer rates may be illuminating important biological principles: a hypothesis. Cancer Epidemiol Biomarkers Prev 2007;16: 1325–9.

Meuth M, The molecular basis of mutations induced by deoxyribonucleoside triphosphate pool imbalances in mammalian cells. Exp Cell Res 1989;181: 305–16.

Mortusewicz O, Schermelleh L, Walter J, Cardoso MC, Leonhardt H, Recruitment of DNA methyltransferase I to DNA repair sites. Proc Natl Acad Sci USA 2005;102: 8905–9.

Narayanan S, McConnell J, Little J, Sharp L, Piyathilake CJ, Powers H, Basten G, Duthie SJ, Associations between two common variants C677T and A1298C in the methylenetetrahydrofolate reductase gene and measures of folate metabolism and DNA stability (strand breaks, misincorporated uracil, and DNA methylation status) in human lymphocytes in vivo. Cancer Epidemiol Biomarkers Prev 2004;13: 1436–43.

Nishida N, Nagasaka T, Nishimura T, Ikai I, Boland CR, Goel A, Aberrant methylation of multiple tumor suppressor genes in aging liver, chronic hepatitis, and hepatocellular carcinoma. Hepatology 2008;47: 908–18.

Ogino S, Wilson RB, Genotype and haplotype distributions of MTHFR677C>T and 1298A>C single nucleotide polymorphisms: a meta-analysis. J Hum Genet 2003;48: 1–7.

Paspatis GA, Karamanolis DG, Folate supplementation and adenomatous colonic polyps. Dis Colon Rectum 1994;37: 1340–1.

Pereira TV, Rudnicki M, Pereira AC, Pombo-de-Oliveira MS, Franco RF, 5,10-Methylenetetrahydrofolate reductase polymorphisms and acute lymphoblastic leukemia risk: a meta-analysis. Cancer Epidemiol Biomarkers Prev 2006;15: 1956–63.

Pogribny IP, Basnakian AG, Miller BJ, Lopatina NG, Poirier LA, James SJ, Breaks in genomic DNA and within the p53 gene are associated with hypomethylation in livers of folate/methyl-deficient rats. Cancer Res 1995;55: 1894–901.

Pogribny IP, Miller BJ, James SJ, Alterations in hepatic p53 gene methylation patterns during tumor progression with folate/methyl deficiency in the rat. Cancer Lett 1997a;115: 31–8.

Pogribny IP, Muskhelishvili L, Miller BJ, James SJ, Presence and consequence of uracil in preneoplastic DNA from folate/methyl-deficient rats. Carcinogenesis 1997b;18: 2071–6.

Pufulete M, Al-Ghnaniem R, Leather AJ, Appleby P, Gout S, Terry C, Emery PW, Sanders TA, Folate status, genomic DNA hypomethylation, and risk of colorectal adenoma and cancer: a case control study. Gastroenterology 2003;124: 1240–8.

Pufulete M, Al-Ghnaniem R, Rennie JA, Appleby P, Harris N, Gout S, Emery PW, Sanders TA, Influence of folate status on genomic DNA methylation in colonic mucosa of subjects without colorectal adenoma or cancer. Br J Cancer 2005;92: 838–42.

Quinlivan EP, Davis SR, Shelnutt KP, Henderson GN, Ghandour H, Shane B, Selhub J, Bailey LB, Stacpoole PW, Gregory JF, III, Methylenetetrahydrofolate Reductase 677C→T Polymorphism and Folate Status Affect One-Carbon Incorporation into Human DNA Deoxynucleosides. J Nutr 2005;135: 389–96.

Rampersaud GC, Kauwell GP, Hutson AD, Cerda JJ, Bailey LB, Genomic DNA methylation decreases in response to moderate folate depletion in elderly women. Am J Clin Nutr 2000;72: 998–1003.

Reddy P, Hogarth M, Li CS, Miller JW, Green R, Breast Cancer Incidence: A Possible Relationship to Folic Acid Fortification? Laboratory Investigation 2009;89: 64A.

Reeves SG, Meldrum C, Groombridge C, Spigelman AD, Suchy J, Kurzawski G, Lubinski J, McElduff P, Scott RJ, MTHFR 677 C>T and 1298 A>C polymorphisms and the age of onset of colorectal cancer in hereditary nonpolyposis colorectal cancer. Eur J Hum Genet 2009;17: 629–35.

Robien K, Folate during antifolate chemotherapy: what we know ... and do not know. Nutr Clin Pract 2005;20: 411–22.

Robien K, Ulrich CM, 5,10-Methylenetetrahydrofolate reductase polymorphisms and leukemia risk: a HuGE minireview. Am J Epidemiol 2003;157: 571–82.

Robien K, Ulrich CM, Bigler J, Yasui Y, Gooley T, Bruemmer B, Potter JD, Radich JP, Methylenetetrahydrofolate reductase genotype affects risk of relapse after hematopoietic cell transplantation for chronic myelogenous leukemia. Clin Cancer Res 2004;10: 7592–8.

Sakatani T, Kaneda A, Iacobuzio-Donahue CA, Carter MG, de Boom Witzel S, Okano H, Ko MS, Ohlsson R, Longo DL, Feinberg AP, Loss of imprinting of Igf2 alters intestinal maturation and tumorigenesis in mice. Science 2005;307: 1976–8.

Sanjoaquin MA, Allen N, Couto E, Roddam AW, Key TJ, Folate intake and colorectal cancer risk: a meta-analytical approach. Int J Cancer 2005;113: 825–8.

Shannon B, Gnanasampanthan S, Beilby J, Iacopetta B, A polymorphism in the methylenetetrahydrofolate reductase gene predisposes to colorectal cancers with microsatellite instability. Gut 2002;50: 520–4.

Slatore CG, Littman AJ, Au DH, Satia JA, White E, Long-term use of supplemental multivitamins, vitamin C, vitamin E, and folate does not reduce the risk of lung cancer. Am J Respir Crit Care Med 2008;177: 524–30.

Smith AD, Kim YI, Refsum H, Is folic acid good for everyone? Am J Clin Nutr 2008;87: 517–33.

Sohn KJ, Stempak JM, Reid S, Shirwadkar S, Mason JB, Kim YI, The effect of dietary folate on genomic and p53-specific DNA methylation in rat colon. Carcinogenesis 2003;24: 81–90.

Sohn KJ, Jang H, Campan M, Weisenberger DJ, Dickhout J, Wang YC, Cho RC, Yates Z, Lucock M, Chiang EP, Austin RC, Choi SW, Laird PW, Kim YI, The methylenetetrahydrofolate reductase C677T mutation induces cell-specific changes in genomic DNA methylation and uracil misincorporation: A possible molecular basis for the site-specific cancer risk modification. Int J Cancer 2009;124: 1999–2005.

Song J, Sohn KJ, Medline A, Ash C, Gallinger S, Kim YI, Chemopreventive effects of dietary folate on intestinal polyps in Apc+/-Msh2-/- mice. Cancer Res 2000;60: 3191–9.

Stern LL, Mason JB, Selhub J, Choi SW, Genomic DNA hypomethylation, a characteristic of most cancers, is present in peripheral leukocytes of individuals who are homozygous for the C677T polymorphism in the methylenetetrahydrofolate reductase gene. Cancer Epidemiol Biomarkers Prev 2000;9: 849–53.

Sun L, Sun YH, Wang B, Cao HY, Yu C, Methylenetetrahydrofolate reductase polymorphisms and susceptibility to gastric cancer in Chinese populations: a meta-analysis. Eur J Cancer Prev 2008;17: 446–52.

Toffoli G, Russo A, Innocenti F, Corona G, Tumolo S, Sartor F, Mini E, Boiocchi M, Effect of methylenetetrahydrofolate reductase 677C→T polymorphism on toxicity and homocysteine plasma level after chronic methotrexate treatment of ovarian cancer patients. Int J Cancer 2003;103: 294–9.

Ulrich CM, Bigler J, Bostick R, Fosdick L, Potter JD, Thymidylate synthase promoter polymorphism, interaction with folate intake, and risk of colorectal adenomas. Cancer Res 2002;62: 3361–4.

Ulrich CM, Curtin K, Potter JD, Bigler J, Caan B, Slattery ML, Polymorphisms in the reduced folate carrier, thymidylate synthase, or methionine synthase and risk of colon cancer. Cancer Epidemiol Biomarkers Prev 2005;14: 2509–16.

Ulvik A, Evensen ET, Lien EA, Hoff G, Vollset SE, Majak BM, Ueland PM, Smoking, folate and methylenetetrahydrofolate reductase status as interactive determinants of adenomatous and hyperplastic polyps of colorectum. Am J Med Genet 2001;101: 246–54.

van den Donk M, Pellis L, Crott JW, van Engeland M, Friederich P, Nagengast FM, van Bergeijk JD, de Boer SY, Mason JB, Kok FJ, Keijer J, Kampman E, Folic acid and vitamin B-12 supplementation does not favorably influence uracil incorporation and promoter methylation in rectal mucosa DNA of subjects with previous colorectal adenomas. J Nutr 2007a;137: 2114–20.

van den Donk M, van Engeland M, Pellis L, Witteman BJ, Kok FJ, Keijer J, Kampman E, Dietary folate intake in combination with MTHFR C677T genotype and promoter methylation of tumor suppressor and DNA repair genes in sporadic colorectal adenomas. Cancer Epidemiol Biomarkers Prev 2007b;16: 327–33.

Van Guelpen B, Hultdin J, Johansson I, Hallmans G, Stenling R, Riboli E, Winkvist A, Palmqvist R, Low folate levels may protect against colorectal cancer. Gut 2006;55: 1461–6.

Voorrips LE, Goldbohm RA, Brants HA, van Poppel GA, Sturmans F, Hermus RJ, van den Brandt PA, A prospective cohort study on antioxidant and folate intake and male lung cancer risk. Cancer Epidemiol Biomarkers Prev 2000;9: 357–65.

Wang W, Gao J, Man XH, Li ZS, Gong YF, Significance of DNA methyltransferase-1 and histone deacetylase-1 in pancreatic cancer. Oncol Rep 2009;21: 1439–47.

Wasson GR, McGlynn AP, McNulty H, O'Reilly SL, McKelvey-Martin VJ, McKerr G, Strain JJ, Scott J, Downes CS, Global DNA and p53 region-specific hypomethylation in human colonic cells is induced by folate depletion and reversed by folate supplementation. J Nutr 2006;136: 2748–53.

Weisberg I, Tran P, Christensen B, Sibani S, Rozen R, A second genetic polymorphism in methylenetetrahydrofolate reductase (MTHFR) associated with decreased enzyme activity. Mol Genet Metab 1998;64: 169–72.

Wisotzkey JD, Toman J, Bell T, Monk JS, Jones D, MTHFR (C677T) polymorphisms and stage III colon cancer: response to therapy. Mol Diagn 1999;4: 95–9.

Wolpin BM, Wei EK, Ng K, Meyerhardt JA, Chan JA, Selhub J, Giovannucci EL, Fuchs CS, Prediagnostic plasma folate and the risk of death in patients with colorectal cancer. J Clin Oncol 2008;26: 3222–8.

Wu K, Platz EA, Willett WC, Fuchs CS, Selhub J, Rosner BA, Hunter DJ, Giovannucci E, A randomized trial on folic acid supplementation and risk of recurrent colorectal adenoma. Am J Clin Nutr 2009;90: 1623–31.

Yamada K, Chen Z, Rozen R, Matthews RG, Effects of common polymorphisms on the properties of recombinant human methylenetetrahydrofolate reductase. Proc Natl Acad Sci USA 2001;98:14853–8.

Yang QH, Botto LD, Gallagher M, Friedman JM, Sanders CL, Koontz D, Nikolova S, Erickson JD, Steinberg K, Prevalence and effects of gene-gene and gene-nutrient interactions on serum folate and serum total homocysteine concentrations in the United States: findings from the third National Health and Nutrition Examination Survey DNA Bank. Am J Clin Nutr 2008;88: 232–46.

Yawata A, Kim SR, Miyajima A, Kubo T, Ishida S, Saito Y, Nakajima Y, Katori N, Matsumoto Y, Fukuoka M, Ohno Y, Ozawa S, Sawada J, Polymorphic tandem repeat sequences of the thymidylate synthase gene correlates with cellular-based sensitivity to fluoropyrimidine antitumor agents. Cancer Chemother Pharmacol 2005;56: 465–72.

Youssef EM, Estecio MR, Issa JP, Methylation and regulation of expression of different retinoic acid receptor beta isoforms in human colon cancer. Cancer Biol Ther 2004;3: 82–6.

Zhang SM, Moore SC, Lin J, Cook NR, Manson JE, Lee IM, Buring JE, Folate, vitamin B6, multivitamin supplements, and colorectal cancer risk in women. Am J Epidemiol 2006;163: 108–15.

Zintzaras E, Methylenetetrahydrofolate reductase gene and susceptibility to breast cancer: a meta-analysis. Clin Genet 2006a;69: 327–36.

Zintzaras E, Association of methylenetetrahydrofolate reductase (MTHFR) polymorphisms with genetic susceptibility to gastric cancer: a meta-analysis. J Hum Genet 2006b;51: 618–24.

Zintzaras E, Koufakis T, Ziakas PD, Rodopoulou P, Giannouli S, Voulgarelis M, A meta-analysis of genotypes and haplotypes of methylenetetrahydrofolate reductase gene polymorphisms in acute lymphoblastic leukemia. Eur J Epidemiol 2006;21: 501–10.

7 Vitamin B12 – Cobalamin

7.1 Vitamin B12

Mustafa Vakur Bor; Ebba Nexo

7.1.1 Vitamin B12 and the active forms of the vitamin

Vitamin B12 (cobalamin) belongs to a group of compounds named corrinoids. The vitamin is composed of a corrin ring surrounding a central cobalt (Co) atom that is bound to both a lower and an upper ligand (►Fig. 7.1). The lower ligand consists of a benzimidazole group that through a ribose-phosphate group is attached to the corrin ring. The upper ligand is unique for each form of the vitamin. In the active forms, the upper ligand is either a methyl or a 5′-deoxyadenosyl group [for a review on vitamin B12 chemistry, see Pratt (1972)].

Both methylcobalamin and 5′-deoxyadenosylcobalamin are synthesized in the cells through removal of the upper ligand initially attached to the Co atom. Whereas 5′-deoxyadenosylcobalamin dominates in most tissues, methylcobalamin is the dominating form in plasma and milk [for review, see Ginsing (1983)]. Both 5′-deoxyadenosylcobalamin and methylcobalamin are light sensitive and upon exposure to light – as, e.g., during preparation of food – the two active forms are converted to aquo (hydroxo) cobalamin. Because the aquo group is a relatively low affinity ligand for Co it is easily exchanged with other ligands such as cyanide. Actually, vitamin B12 is cyanocobalamin, but the term vitamin B12 is often used to denote all active forms of the vitamin, independent of the upper ligand [for review, see Pratt (1972) and Chanarin (1990)].

Aquo- and cyanocobalamin are the most common forms of the vitamin employed in vitamin pills and for treatment of vitamin B12 deficiency. In addition, aquocobalamin is employed in megadoses for the treatment of cyanide poisoning (Zerbe, 1993). The mechanism of the latter is that cyanide displaces the aquo group from the Co atom. The amount of vitamin employed far exceeds the binding capacity of the cobalamin binding proteins in plasma, and because of that the vitamin is filtered freely in the kidney and excreted in the urine together with the cyanide group.

Corrinoids other than cobalamins, such as cobinamide have been identified both in stools and in the circulation, but no physiological functions in humans have been described for these compounds (Allen, 2008; Hardlei, 2009).

7.1.2 Vitamin B12 intake, turnover and requirements

A normal western mixed diet supplied at least 4–6 µg of vitamin B12 per day (Institute of Medicine, 1998). The bioavailability of the vitamin present in food is considered to be high, but the uptake from a single serving is limited to 1.5–2.5 µg owing to a rate limiting capacity for absorption of the vitamin. A second dose given 4–6 h after a first

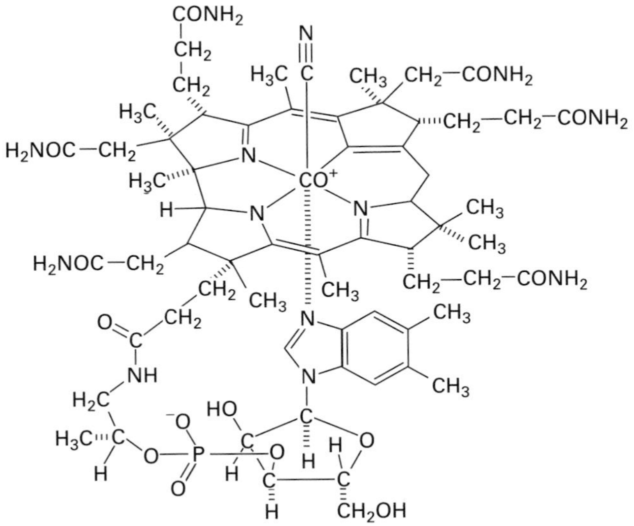

Fig 7.1: Vitamin B12.

can be absorbed with the same efficacy. Thus, the total absorption of vitamin B12 from three meals could be up to 6 µg or more daily (Chanarin, 1990).

Vitamin B12 is lost by excretion, from desquamated cells and from breakdown of the vitamin. Studies employing labelled vitamin B12 and whole body counting suggest a daily loss of vitamin B12 of between 2 and 5 µg in subjects on a mixed diet and with a body pool of 5 mg vitamin B12. An alternative approach for calculation of the daily loss is based on the observation that it takes 2–5 years to develop overt vitamin B12 deficiency with megaloblastic anaemia in patients that has undergone total gastrectomy and thereby lost the ability to absorb vitamin B12. Employing this approach suggests a daily loss of 3–6 µg of vitamin B12 (Chanarin, 1990). It is debatable whether the daily need for vitamin B12 is as high as the amount of the vitamin lost every day would indicate. This is because in healthy individuals part of the vitamin lost through the bile is reabsorbed.

The official daily requirement for vitamin B12 expressed as the Recommended Dietary Allowances (RDAs) is 2.4 µg/day for adults in US according to the last recommendations set by the Food and Nutrition Board in 1998 (Institute of Medicine, 1998). The requirement does not differ according to sex, but it is slightly higher for pregnant and lactating women. Because of the increased risk of food-bound vitamin B12 malabsorption in older adults, it is currently recommended that adults over 50 years of age get most of the RDA from fortified food or vitamin B12 containing supplements. For infants under the age of 1 year, adequate intake (AI) is considerably lower than the intake recommended for adults. The RDA (▶Tab. 7.1) is based on rather old data and more recent studies suggest that 4–7 µg per day would be more appropriate for healthy adults (Bor, 2010).

Vitamin B12 is abundant in seafood and in liver (▶Tab. 7.2), but absent from vegetables and legumes (Institute of Medicine, 1998; US Department of Agriculture, 2004). However, if such nutrients are eaten under circumstances where foods are contaminated with microorganisms the individual might still obtain some vitamin B12.

Tab. 7.1: Recommended dietary allowance (RDA) for vitamin B12.

Life stage	Age	Micrograms/day
Infants	0–6 months	0.4 (AI)[a]
Infants	7–12 months	0.5 (AI)
Children	1–3 years	0.9
Children	4–8 years	1.2
Children	9–13 years	1.8
Adolescents	14–18 years	2.4
Adults	19–50 years	2.4
Adults	51 years and older	2.4[b]
Pregnancy (females)	all ages	2.6
Lactating (females)	all ages	2.8

[a]AI: adequate intake.

[b]Vitamin B12 intake should be from fortified foods and supplements owing to the age-related increase in food-bound malabsorption.

Tab. 7.2: Selected food sources of vitamin B12.

Food	Micrograms per serving	Percent DV[a]
Liver, beef, braised, 1 slice	48	800
Clams, cooked, breaded and fried, 85 g	34	570
Trout, rainbow, wild, cooked, 85 g	5.4	90
Salmon, sockeye, cooked, 85 g	4.9	80
Trout, rainbow, farmed, cooked, 85 g	4.2	50
Beef, top sirloin, broiled, 85 g	2.4	40
Cheeseburger, double patty and bun, 1 sandwich	1.9	30
Yogurt, plain, 1 cup	1.4	25
Haddock, cooked, 85 g	1.2	20
Tuna, white, 85 g	1.0	15
Milk, 1 cup	0.90	15
Cheese, Swiss, 28 g	0.90	15

[a]DV: daily value. DVs were developed by the US Food and Drug Administration (FDA) to help consumers determine the level of various nutrients in a standard serving of food in relation to their approximate requirement for it. The DV for vitamin B12 is 6.0 µg. The table is modified from the US Department of Agriculture's Nutrient Database website (http://www.nal.usda.gov/fnic/foodcomp/search/, where a comprehensive list of foods containing vitamin B12 is provided: (http://www.nal.usda.gov/fnic/foodcomp/Data/SR20/nutrlist/sr20w418.pdf.)

Vitamin B12 is stable and is not destroyed during preparation of the food. As mentioned above the upper ligand of the vitamin might change, but this is of no importance because the active forms are produced in the cell independent of the initial nature of the upper ligand.

No toxic or adverse effects have been associated with intake of large quantities of vitamin B12 from food or supplements in healthy people (Institute of Medicine, 1998; Lonn, 2006). Because of that, no tolerable upper intake level has been set by the Food and Nutrition Board. It should, however, be mentioned that the risk of getting cancer is slightly increased in patients with ischemic heart disease following prolonged intake of high doses of folate (0.8 mg/day) plus vitamin B12 (0.4 mg/day) (Ebbing, 2009). The issue is discussed also in Chapter 6.

The newborn obviously receives vitamin B12 from the milk of the mother. However, there is some uncertainty as to the daily supply of the vitamin because the high content of the vitamin B12 binding protein haptocorrin in milk has proven to give rise to both spuriously high and low concentrations of vitamin B12 when the content of vitamin B12 in milk is measured employing standard laboratory methods for measurement of the vitamin (Lildballe, 2009).

7.1.3 Uptake, transport and utilisation of vitamin B12

Absorption of vitamin B12 from food requires normal function of the stomach, pancreas, and the small intestine. Upon preparation of the food the proteins binding the vitamin are partly destroyed, but stomach acid and gastro-intestinal enzymes are also considered to play an important role in the release of vitamin B12 from food. Once the vitamin is present in its free from it is bound to a binding protein, haptocorrin, present in saliva. Haptocorrin protects the vitamin from the acid surroundings in the stomach, but in the alkaline environment of intestine haptocorrin is degraded by pancreatic enzymes, and the vitamin liberated from food and that recycled through the bile is recognised by intrinsic factor, a glycoprotein synthesized in the parietal cells of the stomach. Intrinsic factor binds only the forms of the vitamin that are active within the body, thereby ensuring that inactive forms (analogues) in the diet or from the bile are excreted rather than absorbed (Chanarin, 1990).

The complex of intrinsic factor and vitamin B12 is recognized in the distal ileum by cubam. Cubam is a receptor complex consisting of cubillin that binds intrinsic factor and amnionless that is requested for internalization [for review, see Moestrup (2006)]. After internalization vitamin B12 is liberated and transported into the blood most probably by an ATP-dependent carrier (Beedholm-Ebsen, 2010). Vitamin B12 can also be absorbed by passive diffusion, but this process is very inefficient – only approximately 1% of a given dose of vitamin B12 is absorbed passively (Chanarin, 1990).

In the blood vitamin B12 meets transcobalamin and haptocorrin. Because unsaturated transcobalamin is the more abundant of the two, most of the newly absorbed vitamin is attached to this protein. However, most of the circulating cobalamin is attached to haptocorrin. This is explained by the fact that the turnover of transcobalamin is very fast as compared with the turnover of haptocorrin [for review, see Nexø (1997)].

Transcobalamin transports vitamin B12 to the cells of the body. At the cellular membrane the transcobalamin bound vitamin is recognized by a recently identified specific receptor and the complex is internalized (Quadros, 2009). After enzymatic cleavage of transcobalamin in the lysosomes the vitamin is finally modified to methyl- and 5'-deoxyadenosylcobalamin (Chanarin, 1990).

Methylcobalamin is formed in the cytoplasm and together with folate it plays a role in the one carbon metabolism, more precisely as a coenzyme for methionine synthase. Methionine synthase catalyses the conversion of homocysteine to methionine and methionine is required for the formation of S-adenosylmethionine, a universal methyl donor for almost 100 different substrates, including DNA, RNA, hormones, proteins, and lipids. 5'-deoxyadenosylcobalamin is formed in the mitochondria and is a coenzyme for methylmalonyl-CoA mutase that converts L-methylmalonyl-CoA to succinyl-CoA in the degradation of propionate, an essential biochemical reaction in fat and protein metabolism [for review, see Banerjee (2003)].

Little is known concerning the further metabolism of cobalamin, but recent studies suggest that eventually vitamin B12 is metabolised to form inactive forms of vitamin B12 (analogues) that are removed from the body by the plasma protein haptocorrin (Hardlei, 2009). Haptocorrin is cleared by the asialoreceptor in the liver, and thereby the analogues are removed from the body through the bile (Chanarin, 1990).

Clarification of the mechanism for uptake and metabolism of vitamin B12 has in part been guided by examination of rare diseases affecting various steps of the metabolic pathways of vitamin B12. The earliest example relates to the discovery of the vitamin. More than 100 years ago a dreadful disease consisting of neurological symptoms and a severe anaemia eventually leading to death of a typically middle-aged person was known as pernicious anaemia (Minot, 1926). Eventually it was realised that it was caused by an autoimmune induced lack of a gastric protein named intrinsic factor. The lack of this protein impaired the absorption of vitamin B12, a vitamin that finally was isolated in the middle of the 20th century (see Section 7.3.1). Later also an inborn lack of intrinsic factor has been described (Tanner, 2005). Both acquired and inherited lack of intrinsic factor can be totally circumvented by injection of vitamin B12 or by oral administration of milligramme doses of the vitamin.

The discovery of receptors needed to absorb the intrinsic factor bound vitamin B12 was hinted also by a distinct but relatively rare condition. A clinical entity was observed in young to teenage children consisting of anaemia and/or failure to thrive. Upon laboratory examinations the children proved to lack the capacity to absorb vitamin B12 despite a normal secretion of intrinsic factor and in addition many of them displayed proteinuria. The children fully recovered upon treatment with vitamin B12 except for a persistent proteinuria. The condition has been named Immerslund-Gräsbeck's syndrome in honour of the two discoverers (see Section 7.3.3.2) [for review, see Gräsbeck (2006)]. Today we know that the disorder is caused by a genetic defect in one of the two receptors responsible for the intestinal uptake of vitamin B12, cubilin and amnionless. The receptors are present also in the proximal tubules of the kidney where they are involved in the uptake of proteins present in the ultrafiltrate and this explains why a defect in the receptors might induce both malabsorption of vitamin B12 and in some of the patients also a proteinuria [for review, see Moestrup (2006)].

Also, the function of transcobalamin has been supported by a clinical condition. Children lacking the protein show signs of vitamin B12 deficiency including anaemia and failure to thrive typically within the first months of life [for review, see Ratschmann (2009)]. Most often the plasma level of cobalamin is within the normal range despite a high level of the metabolic marker of vitamin B12 deficiency, methylmalonic acid. The lack of transcobalamin impairs the capacity to transport vitamin B12 from the intestine and into all the cells of the body. The normal level of plasma cobalamin is explained by a normal absorption of the vitamin combined with a normal concentration of the circulating haptocorrin. It is difficult to understand how children lacking transcobalamin can survive *in utero* and appear normal at birth. Only very few studies examining such children at birth have been reported, but they indicate that already at this stage the child displays metabolic changes suggesting vitamin B12 deficiency (Ratschmann, 2009). If diagnosed and treated with daily injections of vitamin B12 the patients will develop almost normally. If left undiagnosed the children will develop lasting neurological damage.

Several other very rare metabolic diseases have helped in elucidating the intracellular metabolism of vitamin B12, and although a complete account of this is outside the scope of the current chapter a few features are to be mentioned (see Section 7.3.3.3). For many years the general believe was that neurological signs of vitamin B12 deficiency and the demyelization of neural tissues were related to an impaired metabolism of methylmalonic acid caused by an impaired production of 5'-deoxyadenosylcobalamin. However, children with inherited lack of synthesis of only this form of vitamin B12 show severe acidosis, but no sign of neurological disturbances. In contrary children who are unable to synthesize methylcobalamin display both haematological and neurological symptoms. So today it is generally accepted that lack of methylcobalamin is responsible for both the haematological and the neurological impairments related to vitamin B12 deficiency [for review, see Carmel (2003)].

A few patients lacking haptocorrin have been identified by coincidence in patients presenting with a low level of plasma cobalamin but without any signs of vitamin B12 deficiency. No other phenotype has been associated with the lack of haptocorrin and thus so far it is questionable whether this protein has any important role to play in the metabolism of vitamin B12 [for review, see Carmel (2009)].

7.1.4 When should vitamin B12 deficiency be suspected?

Signs and symptoms related to vitamin B12 deficiency are covered in detail in Section 7.3.2.3 and a comprehensive account of acquired vitamin B12 deficiency is given in Section 7.3.4.

In brief, vitamin B12 deficiency should be considered in all patients with unexplained neurological symptoms and in all patients presenting with an unexplained macrocytic anaemia. A special awareness should be given to elderly people above the age of 60 years in whom latent vitamin B12 deficiency is believed to be present in 10–20% of the population. Other important groups are patients with gastrointestinal conditions that limit the absorption of the vitamin. This includes patients with chronic gastrointestinal diseases, and patients treated with drugs that are believed to interfere with the absorption of the vitamin, such as proton inhibitors and possibly oral antidiabetics.

7.1.5 Laboratory diagnosis of vitamin B12 deficiency

The laboratory tests to be performed to clarify whether a patient suffers from vitamin B12 deficiency depend on the initial clinical picture. If the patient is severely anaemic and the initial tests suggest a macrocytic anaemia perhaps even with polynucleated neo-trophils the only additional test needed to ensure the diagnosis is plasma cobalamin. If plasma cobalamin is low the diagnosis is confirmed. If not, folate deficiency or malignant diseases should be suspected.

Most patients with suspected vitamin B12 deficiency do not have anaemia, but rather present themselves with vague non-specific symptoms such as neurological or intestinal complains (see Section 7.3.4 and 7.3.5). In this case several laboratory tests have to be considered. A few comments on each of the tests are summarized in the following paragraphs.

7.1.5.1 Plasma cobalamin

Plasma cobalamin is a useful initial diagnostic test for vitamin B12 deficiency owing to its widespread availability, low costs and the fact that most doctors are familiar with the test. Plasma cobalamin denotes the sum of all cobalamins in plasma, both the part available for the cells that is bound to transcobalamin (20–30%) and the major part that is bound to the plasma protein of unknown function, haptocorrin (70–80%). Before measurement of plasma cobalamins all the binding proteins have to be destroyed and endogenous cobalamin is converted to cyanocobalamin. Most often this is done by exposing the sample to a basic solution and to cyanide. Once present in its free form cobalamin can be measured by various principles. The earliest assays were based on the growth of microorganisms, and at a few laboratories such tests are still in use. Most assays today are run on large automatic equipments and based on the competition between labelled vitamin B12 and cobalamin present in the sample for binding to intrinsic factor. The design of the assay shows some variation among various manufacturers and so do the interval of reference. Because of this, it is important to employ the reference interval supplied by the laboratory that runs the assay [for review, see Vogeser (2007)].

Decreased values that are values well below the lower level of the interval of reference most often indicate vitamin B12 deficiency. Two exceptions should be mentioned. First, pregnant women show a physiological decline in plasma cobalamin so that the values at term are only approximately 50% of the value observed for non-pregnant women (Morkbak, 2007). This is caused both by haemodilution and by a decrease in circulating haptocorrin. Second, as mentioned above, a few patients lack haptocorrin and therefore have a low level of plasma cobalamin despite no signs of deficiency (Carmel, 2009).

Intermediate values that are values around the lower limits of the interval of reference should warrant further examination of the patient employing other markers of vitamin B12 deficiency such as methylmalonic acid (see Section 7.1.5.3 and 7.3.2).

Increased values that are values above the upper limit of the reference interval are a common feature. The cause for such an increase is likely to be related to alterations in one or both of the two binding proteins. An increased level of haptocorrin is seen in several malignant diseases including chronic myeloid leukaemia, polycytemia vera and occasionally solid malignant tumours. Notably, haptocorrin serves as a tumour marker in patients with fibrolaminar hepatoma (Maniaci, 2009). An unexpected level of plasma cobalamin to values above 1000 pmol/l could therefore warrant examination of haptocorrin, and if the concentration is increased a malignant disease should be excluded. An increased level of plasma cobalamin might also be caused by an increase in transcobalamin and most often caused by the presence of auto antibodies against the protein, a condition of unknown origin but apparently not related to an increased risk of developing vitamin B12 deficiency (Chanarin, 1990).

7.1.5.2 Plasma holotranscobalamin

Plasma holotranscobalamin (holoTC, active B12) is a measure of the amount of cobalamin attached to transcobalamin and thereby the part of the circulating cobalamin that is available for the cells of the body. Two types of methods for measurement of holoTC are in use, one that measures the amount of holoTC by a transcobalamin specific ELISA after removal of unsaturated transcobalamin (Nexo, 2002) and one that directly measures transcobalamin saturated with cobalamin (Brady, 2008). Only the latter method is available on an automatic platform.

From a theoretical point of view holoTC (active B12) should be the first marker to show alterations in early vitamin B12 deficiency, and clinical studies performed so far show holoTC to be a slightly better marker of vitamin B12 deficiency than plasma cobalamin (Clarke 2007). So far methods for measurement of holoTC are available only on one automated platform and because of that the clinical experience from the use of holoTC measurements in daily practice is limited.

HoloTC might prove very useful for examination of the capacity to absorb oral vitamin B12 as discussed below. In addition measurement of holoTC could prove useful for diagnosing vitamin B12 deficiency during pregnancy because in contrast to plasma cobalamin it remains stable during an uneventful pregnancy (Morkbak, 2007).

7.1.5.3 Plasma methylmalonic acid

Plasma methylmalonic acid (MMA) accumulates when vitamin B12 is lacking and it is currently the most specific marker of vitamin B12 deficiency. The metabolite is measured employing chromatographic methods such as GC-MS (Schneede, 2005), but so far no methods have been established on automatic platforms. Because of that analysis of MMA is not widely available.

The upper limit for the reference interval has been indicated as values between 0.28 and 0.55 µmol/l. The uncertainty concerning the exact value does not relate to methodological issues but rather to the reference populations included for the establishment of the interval (Vogiatzoglou, 2009). In our laboratory we employ 0.28 µmol/l as the upper limit of the reference interval and values above 0.75 µmol/l are considered to indicate vitamin B12 deficiency in patients with a normal kidney function, see below.

Measurement of MMA in the urine has been employed and it is still used in many laboratories, particularly in relation to screening of newborns for metabolic disorders. The relative diagnostic usefulness of determination of MMA in urine rather than in serum has been assessed in a few studies in the 1990s. The conclusion was that measurement urine samples might be useful if the goal is to detect grossly elevated levels of MMA such as in metabolic diseases (McCann, 1996).

In the interpretation of MMA in serum one has to take into consideration that MMA is correlated to kidney function and thereby to serum creatinine even within the normal range of the analyte (see Section 7.3.6). In addition, age by itself seems to be correlated with an increase in MMA not caused by vitamin deficiency (Vogiatzoglou, 2009).

Increased values to above 0.75 µmol/l strongly support vitamin B12 deficiency, if impaired kidney function can be excluded.

Intermediate values ranging from 0.28 to 0.75 µmol/l are rather frequently observed and are unlikely to be of clinical importance if observed in a patient with no other signs or symptoms suggesting vitamin B12 deficiency.

Decreased values are seen in conditions with an increased filtration rate because MMA is freely filtered in the urine. No clinical condition has been related to a decreased value of MMA.

7.1.5.4 Plasma total homocysteine

Plasma total homocysteine denotes the sum of all compounds in plasma that can be reduced to form homocysteine. Homocysteine is increased in patients with vitamin B12, folate and/or vitamin B6 deficiency [for review, see Refsum (2004)]. In countries without fortification with folic acid an increased level of homocysteine is most often caused by folate deficiency and because of that the analyte is described in Chapter 6.

7.1.5.5 Diagnostic strategy

There is no general consensus as how to use the tests mentioned above when evaluating a patient with suspected vitamin B12 deficiency. In our laboratory the initial step is to measure plasma cobalamin (interval of reference 200–600 pmol/l). A plasma cobalamin level below 125 pmol/l confirms the suspicion of vitamin B12 deficiency. If plasma cobalamin is between 125 and 225 pmol/l MMA is analysed and vitamin B12 deficiency is confirmed, if MMA is above 0.75 µmol/l or judged to be unlikely if MMA is below 0.29 µmol/l. If the level of MMA is between 0.29 and 0.75 µmol/l we recommend repeat measurements of plasma cobalamin and possibly MMA after a year unless obvious clinical signs indicate vitamin B12 deficiency and thereby a need for immediate action (Hvas, 2006).

Several studies have indicated that holoTC (active B12) performs better than cobalamin for identifying individuals judged to have vitamin B12 deficiency (Clarke, 2007). Thus holoTC (active B12) could eventually replace plasma cobalamin, but until it is more widely available this is unlikely to be the case. Homocysteine could be used instead of MMA, but is less helpful because it is increased also in relation to folate and vitamin B6 deficiency.

Recently an algorithm that combines the results of holoTC (active B12), cobalamin MMA and homocysteine has been presented (Fedosov, 2010). The approach is interesting, but so far its clinical usefulness remains to be proven.

It is a special challenge to diagnose vitamin B12 deficiency in patients with an impaired kidney function and in elderly patients. A more than 50% increase in MMA is observed between young (20 years of age) and elderly (80 years of age) individuals and in addition MMA increase by approximately 50% when the creatinine level increase from, e.g., 100 to 200 µmol/l. Cobalamin and holoHC show little change with age whereas holoTC (active B12) also shows a more than 50% increase when creatinine increase from 100 to 200 µmol/l (Hvas, 2005). The implication of these relations are that a decreased cobalamin or holoTC are likely to indicate vitamin B12 deficiency also in the elderly and in patients with kidney disease whereas a moderately increased MMA is of less diagnostic value in these patients.

In patients where the laboratory data and the clinical picture do not fit together some help can be rendered by analysing the level of transcobalamin and haptocorrin, but currently these analyses are available only in our laboratory and in a few other laboratories worldwide.

7.1.6 Clarifying the cause of vitamin B12 deficiency

Once a patient has been diagnosed with vitamin B12 deficiency the cause is to be clarified. It is of importance to elucidate whether the patient is unable to absorb the vitamin and therefore in need of a lifelong substitution either with injections or with milligramme doses of daily oral vitamin B12.

Several laboratory tests could help in elucidating whether vitamin B12 malabsorption is caused by a decreased production of intrinsic factor. The tests are summarized in ▶Tab. 7.3. The availability and the clinical usefulness of most of these tests are, however, debatable.

The Schillings test, the classic test elucidating whether labelled vitamin B12 alone or in combination with intrinsic factor is absorbed from an oral dose, is no longer in routine use owing to difficulties in obtaining radiolabelled vitamin B12 and intrinsic factor. Recently an alternative vitamin B12 absorption test (CobaSorb) has been evaluated in both healthy individuals and in patients (Bor, 2005; Hvas, 2007; Bhat, 2009).

In the CobaSorb test holoTC is measured before (day 0) and 2 days after (day 2) daily intake of 3 times 9 μg of cyanocobalamin (CNCbl). An increase in holoTC between day 0 and day 2 of more than 22% and 10 pmol/l indicates active absorption. The sensitivity of the CobaSorb test has been judged excellent. By contrast, the specificity depends on the baseline concentration of holoTC, and use of this test is not recommended if the baseline holoTC concentration is above 65 pmol/l. An improved version of this test, C-CobaSorb, has resolved this problem and thereby markedly improved the specificity. In C-CobaSorb TC-bound CNCbl is measured at baseline and 24 h after intake of 3 times 9 μg CNCbl. This approach is possible because most of the CNCbl administered as the test dose remains unchanged during intestinal absorption (Hardlei, 2010).

Currently the CobaSorb tests can be performed only employing free vitamin B12 (CNCbl) as the test dose. If in the future a suitable source of intrinsic factor can be obtained, it will also be feasible to use the CobaSorb test to show whether patients who

Tab. 7.3: Laboratory tests used for elucidating the cause of vitamin B12 deficiency.

	Advantage	Disadvantage
Plasma-intrinsic factor-antibodies	Specificity ~100%	Sensitivity ~60%
Plasma-gastrin and pepsinogen	High sensitivity	Low specificity
Plasma-parietal cell antibodies	Sensitivity ~85%	Low specificity
CobaSorb (vitamin B12 uptake)	High sensitivity and specificity	End-point test (holoTC, active B12) is not widely available

are unable to absorb the free vitamin will have a normal absorption if intrinsic factor is supplied. Obviously the tests will also be helpful for studying the capacity to absorb food bound vitamin B12 provided a suitable proxy for the food-bound vitamin can be developed.

Another feasible vitamin B12 absorption test has recently been described. The test employs acceleration mass spectrometry to assess the absorption and kinetics of carbon-14- labelled vitamin B12. So far results for this test have only been reported for a few healthy individuals (Carkeet, 2006).

7.1.7 Concluding remarks

The understanding concerning the uptake and metabolism of vitamin B12 is detailed as compared with current knowledge for many of the other vitamins. Possibly as a consequence the awareness of vitamin B12 deficiency is relatively high among physicians and a relatively large number of laboratory tests are available to guide the diagnostic procedure.

Important issues for the years to come will be to re-evaluate the RDA for vitamin B12 and to clarify the optimal strategy for prevention and treatment of vitamin B12 deficiency.

Another exiting area is the possibility of using the pathway for vitamin B12 as a carrier to ensure cellular delivery of drugs, such as insulin (Petrus, 2007) and of compounds that can allow visualization and possibly treatment of tumours (Waibel, 2008). Time will show whether this new era of vitamin B12 research will prove useful in the clinic.

References

Allen RH, Stabler SP, Identification and quantitation of cobalamin and cobalamin analogues in human feces. Am J Clin Nutr 2008;87: 1324–35.

Banerjee R, Ragsdale SW, The many faces of vitamin B12: catalysis by cobalamin-dependent enzymes. Annu Rev Biochem 2003;72: 209–47.

Beedholm-Ebsen R, van de Wetering K, Hardlei T, Nexø E, Borst P, Moestrup SK, Identification of multidrug resistance protein 1 (MRP1/ABCC1) as a molecular gate for cellular export of cobalamin. Blood 2010;115: 1632–9.

Bhat DS, Thuse NV, Lubree HG, Joglekar CV, Naik SS, Ramdas LV, Johnston C, Refsum H, Fall CH, Yajnik CS, Increases in plasma holotranscobalamin can be used to assess vitamin B-12 absorption in individuals with low plasma vitamin B-12. J Nutr 2009;139: 2119–23.

Bor MV, Cetin M, Aytac S, Altay C, Nexo E, Nonradioactive vitamin B12 absorption test evaluated in controls and in patients with inherited malabsorption of vitamin B12. Clin Chem 2005;51: 2151–5.

Bor MV, von Castel-Roberts KM, Kauwell GP, Stabler SP, Allen RH, Maneval DR, Bailey LB, Nexo E, Daily intake of 4 to 7 microg dietary vitamin B-12 is associated with steady concentrations of vitamin B-12-related biomarkers in a healthy young population. Am J Clin Nutr 2010;91: 571–7.

Brady J, Wilson L, McGregor L, Valente E, Orning L, Active B12: a rapid, automated assay for holotranscobalamin on the Abbott AxSYM analyzer. Clin Chem 2008;54: 567–73.

Carkeet C, Dueker SR, Lango J, Buchholz BA, Miller JW, Green R, et al., Human vitamin B12 absorption measurement by accelerator mass spectrometry using specifically labeled (14)C-cobalamin. Proc Natl Acad Sci USA 2006;103: 5694–9.

Carmel R, Green R, Rosenblatt DS, Watkins D, Update on cobalamin, folate, and homocysteine. Hematology Am Soc Hematol Educ Program 2003;62–81

Carmel R, Parker J, Kelman Z, Genomic mutations associated with mild and severe deficiencies of transcobalamin I (haptocorrin) that cause mildly and severely low serum cobalamin levels. Br J Haematol 2009;147: 386–91.

Chanarin I, The megaloblastic anaemias, 3rd ed. London: Blackwell Scientific Publications; 1990.

Clarke R, Sherliker P, Hin H, Nexo E, Hvas AM, Schneede J, Birks J, Ueland PM, Emmens K, Scott JM, Molloy AM, Evans JG, Detection of vitamin B12 deficiency in older people by measuring vitamin B12 or the active fraction of vitamin B12, holotranscobalamin. Clin Chem 2007;53: 963–70.

Ebbing M, Bønaa KH, Nygård O, Arnesen E, Ueland PM, Nordrehaug JE, Rasmussen K, Njølstad I, Refsum H, Nilsen DW, Tverdal A, Meyer K, Vollset SE, Cancer incidence and mortality after treatment with folic acid and vitamin B12. J Am Med Assoc 2009;302: 2119–26.

Fedosov SN, Metabolic signs of vitamin B(12) deficiency in humans: computational model and its implications for diagnostics. Metabolism 2010 [Epub ahead of print].

Gräsbeck R, Imerslund-Gräsbeck syndrome (selective vitamin B(12) malabsorption with proteinuria). Orphanet J Rare Dis 2006;1: 17.

Gimsing P, Nexo E, The forms of cobalamins in biological materials. In: Hall CA, editor. The cobalamins. New York: Churchill Livingstone; 1983.

Hardlei TF, Nexo E, A new principle for measurement of cobalamin and corrinoids, used for studies of cobalamin analogs on serum haptocorrin. Clin Chem 2009;55: 1002–10.

Hardlei TF, Mørkbak AL, Bor MV, Bailey LB, Hvas AM, Nexo E, Assessment of vitamin B(12) absorption based on the accumulation of orally administered cyanocobalamin on transcobalamin. Clin Chem 2010;56: 432–6.

Hvas AM, Nexo E, Holotranscobalamin – a first choice assay for diagnosing early vitamin B deficiency? J Intern Med. 2005;257: 289–98.

Hvas AM, Nexo E, Diagnosis and treatment of vitamin B12 deficiency – an update. Haematologica 2006;91: 1506–12.

Hvas AM, Morkbak AL, Nexo E, Plasma holotranscobalamin compared with plasma cobalamins for assessment of vitamin B12 absorption; optimisation of a non-radioactive vitamin B12 absorption test (CobaSorb). Clin Chim Acta 2007;376: 150–4.

Institute of Medicine, Dietary reference intakes: thiamin, riboflavin, niacin, vitamin B6, folate, vitamin B12, pantothenic acid, biotin, and choline. Washington, DC: National Acadamy Press; 1998.

Lildballe DL, Hardlei TF, Allen LH, Nexo E, High concentrations of haptocorrin interfere with routine measurement of cobalamins in human serum and milk. A problem and its solution. Clin Chem Lab Med 2009;47: 182–7.

Lonn E, Yusuf S, Arnold MJ, Sheridan P, Pogue J, Micks M, McQueen MJ, Probstfield J, Fodor G, Held C, Genest J Jr, Homocysteine lowering with folic acid and B vitamins in vascular disease. N Engl J Med. 2006;354: 1567–77.

Maniaci V, Davidson BR, Rolles K, Dhillon AP, Hackshaw A, Begent RH, Meyer T, Fibrolamellar hepatocellular carcinoma: prolonged survival with multimodality therapy. Eur J Surg Oncol 2009;35: 617–21.

McCann MT, Thompson MM, Gueron IC, Lemieux B, Giguère R, Tuchman M, Methylmalonic acid quantification by stable isotope dilution gas chromatography-mass spectrometry from filter paper urine samples. Clin Chem 1996;42: 910–4.

Minot GR, Murphy WP, Treatment of pernicious anemia by a special diet. Yale J Biol Med 1926;74: 341–53.

Moestrup SK, New insights into carrier binding and epithelial uptake of the erythropoietic nutrients cobalamin and folate. Curr Opin Hematol 2006;13: 119–23.

Morkbak AL, Hvas AM, Milman N, Nexo E, Holotranscobalamin remains unchanged during pregnancy. Longitudinal changes of cobalamins and their binding proteins during pregnancy and postpartum Haematologica 2007;92: 1711–2.

Nexø E, Cobalamin binding proteins. In: Kräutler B, Arigoni D, Golding BT, editors. Vitamin B12 and B12-proteins. Germany: Wiley-VCH; 1997. pp. 459–75.

Nexo E, Christensen AL, Hvas AM, Petersen TE, Fedosov SN, Quantification of holo-transcobalamin, a marker of vitamin B12 deficiency. Clin Chem 2002;48: 561–2.

Pratt JM, Inorganic chemistry of vitamin B$_{12}$. New York: Academic Press; 1972.

Petrus AK, Vortherms AR, Fairchild TJ, Doyle RP, Vitamin B12 as a carrier for the oral delivery of insulin. Chem Med Chem 2007;2: 1717–21.

Quadros EV, Nakayama Y, Sequeira JM, The protein and the gene encoding the receptor for the cellular uptake of transcobalamin-bound cobalamin. Blood 2009;113:186–92.

Ratschmann R, Minkov M, Kis A, Hung C, Rupar T, Mühl A, Fowler B, Nexo E, Bodamer OA, Transcobalamin II deficiency at birth. Mol Genet Metab 2009;98:285–8.

Refsum H, Smith AD, Ueland PM, Nexo E, Clarke R, McPartlin J, et al., Facts and recommendations about total homocysteine determinations: an expert opinion. Clin Chem 2004;50: 3–32.

Schneede J, Ueland PM, Novel and established markers of cobalamin deficiency: complementary or exclusive diagnostic strategies. Semin Vasc Med 2005;5: 140–55.

Tanner SM, Li Z, Perko JD, Öner C, Çetin M, Altay Ç, et al., Hereditary juvenile cobalamin deficiency caused by mutations in the intrinsic factor gene. Proc Natl Acad Sci USA 2005;102: 4130–3.

US Department of Agriculture, USDA national nutrient database for standard reference, release 17: Nutrient Data Laboratory homepage; 2004. Available from: http://www.nal.usda.gov/fnic/foodcomp.

Vogeser M, Lorenzl S, Comparison of automated assays for the determination of vitamin B12 in serum. Clin Biochem 2007;40: 1342–5.

Vogiatzoglou A, Oulhaj A, Smith AD, Nurk E, Drevon CA, Ueland PM, Vollset SE, Tell GS, Refsum H, Determinants of plasma methylmalonic acid in a large population: implications for assessment of vitamin B12 status. Clin Chem 2009;55: 2198–206.

Waibel R, Treichler H, Schaefer NG, van Staveren DR, Mundwiler S, Kunze S, Küenzi M, Alberto R, Nüesch J, Knuth A, Moch H, Schibli R, Schubiger PA, New derivatives of vitamin B12 show preferential targeting of tumors. Cancer Res 2008;68: 2904–11.

Zerbe NF, Wagner BK, Use of vitamin B12 in the treatment and prevention of nitroprusside-induced cyanide toxicity. Crit Care Med 1993;21: 465–7.

7.2 Worldwide and infantile vitamin B12 deficiency

Sally P. Stabler

7.2.1 Introduction

There are different definitions which can be applied when describing vitamin B12 deficiency worldwide. The spectrum of B12 deficiency covers asymptomatic elevations of methylmalonic acid (MMA) and/or total homocysteine to life-threatening megaloblastic anemia and/or myelopathy. In addition, clinical syndromes of glossitis, megaloblastic gut changes, infertility, psychiatric illness and in infants, failure to thrive with unique neurological abnormalities can result from deficiency (Stabler and Allen, 2004). It is not actually known what the minimum of absorbed vitamin B12 is necessary to sustain life. Diets containing only 0.3–0.65 μg/day, and injections of 0.1 μg have been shown to cure megaloblastic anemia (Baker and Mathan, 1981). Although populations can exist on such marginal diets, serum vitamin B12 and the vitamin B12-dependent metabolites are probably abnormal. It is also probable that some individuals would sustain neurological damage and certainly such limiting amounts could prevent adequate growth and development in children.

The serum vitamin B12 and in some cases, holotranscobalamin II (holo TCII) concentration are often used to define the adequacy of B12 nutrition of a population but both tests are most predictive of status at the extremes of the range of values (Allen, 2009, McLean et al., 2008). There are both false-positive low values (Stabler et al., 1990) and false-negative normal values when simultaneous elevated MMA is used as the criteria for deficiency (Lindenbaum et al., 1990). Concentrations of MMA are extremely sensitive to the withdrawal of vitamin B12 in subjects with pernicious anemia (PA) and thus, are perhaps too sensitive for assigning clinically important deficiency. For instance, careful studies of dietary B12 intake against MMA values show that the RDA for US adults set at 2.4 µg/day actually does not result in the lowest population MMA value. In fact, intakes above 4.0 µg/day seem to decrease MMA further, but clinical deficiency is unlikely if the RDA is absorbed (Bor et al., 2010). MMA elevations occur also in renal insufficiency, which is prevalent in the senior population and possibly in bacterial overgrowth gut conditions, which might complicate interpretation in some populations (Lindenbaum et al., 1990). Clinical deficiency is best proven by an unequivocal response to vitamin B12 treatment with a fall in red cell mean cell volume and increase in hemoglobin. However, subjects with primarily neurological complications of vitamin B12 deficiency might not have much change in blood counts and some B12-deficient myelopathies are irreversible (Lindenbaum et al., 1988). Worldwide data on the causes of megaloblastic pancytopenia are scarce and often different vitamin deficiencies are lumped together in the reports. It must also be remembered that foods containing vitamin B12 are also those rich in iron, zinc and protein, all of which are necessary for adequate hematopoesis. Thus, response to treatment with single nutrients is rarely striking in dietary deficiency (Allen et al., 2009b).

Vitamin B12 deficiency is caused by either selective malabsorption of vitamin B12 or inadequate dietary intake (Stabler and Allen, 2004; Elmadfa and Singer, 2009). The autoimmune disease PA owing to atrophic gastritis with loss of gastric intrinsic factor is prevalent in all populations. Occasionally, said to be most common in northern Europeans, it is now well known that the incidence of PA in persons of African descent is as high as in Europeans (Carmel and Johnson, 1978). There are increasing reports from the Middle East, China and other countries in Asia showing that PA is a frequent cause of megaloblastic anemia (Stabler and Allen, 2004). It is very probable that the role of PA in worldwide vitamin deficiency has been under-recognized in the past. The role of PA versus dietary deficiency will be emphasized in the following discussions of different geographic areas.

The calculation of dietary B12 is another useful tool for estimating intake and therefore predicting population-wide deficiency. Vitamin B12 is mostly present in animal source food. Therefore, the frequencies and quantities of meat, fish, dairy and egg products are studied. General categories such as 'meat' are less useful because there are marked differences in poultry sources as compared with ruminant animals and between muscle and organ meats. Seafoods range widely from shellfish (very high) to invertebrates and fish which are similar to ruminants (Stabler and Allen, 2004). The quantity of meat or eggs consumed per person varies widely, even when people describe themselves as non-vegetarian. In addition, some fermented plant products and condiments could have substantial amounts of vitamin B12, which might explain why serum B12 concentrations can be higher than expected from a dietary listing. There is incomplete knowledge about the type and quantity of corrinoids present in such products because it is also probable that inactive cobalamin analogs (products of bacterial synthesis) could also be present (Stabler and Allen, 2004). Analysis of B12 intake in vegetarian populations in the USA and other parts of the world could also be complicated by intake of fortified supplements, foods and energy drinks.

In summary, B12 deficiency can be defined as biochemical abnormalities, population serum B12 concentrations or by the prevalence of B12-deficient clinical syndromes. Recent reviews describe these approaches in detail (Stabler and Allen, 2004; McLean et al., 2008). Thus, emphasis will be placed on reports from the past 5 years in this review.

7.2.2 Vitamin B12 deficiency by geographic area

7.2.2.1 North America

The high level of food security and widespread use of vitamin supplements in the USA and Canada leads to median intakes of B12 of 3–4 µg and 4–7 µg/day, respectively (NAS, 2000). The risk of vitamin B12 deficiency appears to be mainly in special populations. Dietary deficiency is seen in vegetarians, both vegans and those who describe themselves as lacto-ovo vegetarians. A recent study in Florida shows that MMA was significantly higher in the lowest quintiles of vitamin B12 intake and only leveled off at relatively high intakes of 4–7 µg/day (Bor et al., 2010). The mean serum B12 values from NHANES 1999–2004 were 374 and 417 pmol/l for men and women, respectively (Ganji and Kafai, 2009). However, the 2.5 percentile was significantly lower in those greater than 60 years old at 136 pmol/l (Pfeiffer et al., 2007). Studies in seniors have shown a high prevalence of elevated MMA with lower serum vitamin B12 (Lindenbaum et al., 1994; Johnson et al., 2003). Risk of elevated MMA and low B12 is higher in white Americans than those of African descent (Stabler et al., 1999).

A study in Boston showed a prevalence of 2.9% of positive intrinsic factor antibodies in seniors suggesting PA (Krasinski et al., 1986). PA has been estimated at between 25 and 15 per 100 000 in various cities in the USA. African American and Latin American females presented with younger age (Carmel and Johnson, 1978).

7.2.2.2 Europe

Vitamin B12 deficiency and PA have long been studied in Europe. The prevalence of PA has ranged in different reports from 50 to 200 per 100 000 (Stabler and Allen, 2004). Mean vitamin B12 intake was relatively high, 5–7.3 µg in a large cohort from Norway in both middle-aged and elderly subjects. This was accompanied by relatively high mean vitamin B12 ranging from 335 to 358 pmol/l in the same group (Vogiatzoglou et al., 2009a). MMA increased greater than 750 nmol/l (suggesting deficiency) in 0.9% of the elderly and approximately 5% were greater than 370 nmol/l (Vogiatzoglou et al., 2009b). A survey from the European Nutrition and Health Report estimated vitamin B12 intake from six Western European countries revealing that mean intake was high, 4–7 µg/day (Fabian and Elmadfa, 2008). Serum B12 was compared in immigrant Albanians versus Greeks and was significantly lower in the

Albanians 135 versus 165 pmol/l with 88% of the former considered suboptimal. The differences were attributed to the low animal protein intake by the immigrants (Schulpis et al., 2004). A report from Kazakhstan revealed that 25% of 20 patients with megaloblastic anemia had isolated vitamin B12 deficiency and 20% had combined folate and vitamin B12 deficiency. This population was high meat consuming, thus, PA probably contributed to the deficiency (Akilzhanova et al., 2006).

There have been many studies of European vegetarians (Stabler and Allen, 2004). Total homocysteine has been shown to be higher in vegetarians versus omnivores in studies from Germany, Italy, the UK (Stabler and Allen, 2004) and recently Slovakia (Krajcovicova-Kudlackova et al., 2007) and Austria (Majchrzak et al., 2006).

In summary, the intake of vitamin B12 in omnivorous populations in Europe is fairly high. However, there is much lower intake in those who follow vegetarian diets and possibly in immigrant communities to the western European countries.

7.2.2.3 Mexico, Central and South America

Many studies from rural Mexico have shown high prevalence of dietary vitamin B12 deficiency because of low intake of animal source food (Allen, 2004). A nationwide survey of anemia in children using data from the late 1990s from Mexico found that anemia was very prevalent and related mainly to iron deficiency, and not intake of B12 (Villalpando et al., 2003). A survey of vitamin nutrition of indigenous children in boarding schools in Mexico showed that 22% of the boys and 18.5% of the girls had serum B12 values less than 148 pmol/l and the mean values were less than the 5th percentile of children in NHANES. Although animal source foods were served one to seven times per week, it is possible that the quantities were too low for adequate intake (Monárrez-Espino et al., 2004). A dietary study of 130 healthy, non-pregnant women in Morales, Mexico showed that the median vitamin B12 intake was 3.7 µg/day but 15.4% consumed less than 2 µg/day. Serum B12 was an important determinant of homocysteine values (Torres-Sánchez et al., 2006).

Several studies have shown that there was a high prevalence of vitamin B12 deficiency in Guatemala (Allen, 2004). In a more recent study from a low-income neighborhood in Guatemala of mother-infant pairs it was shown that approximately 37% of the mothers were B12 deficient (less than 148 pmol/l) as compared with 30% of the infants. Large numbers were also marginally deficient. These low B12 levels were correlated with lower hemoglobin, ferritin and plasma folate. However, the mean intake of vitamin B12 in the mothers was 3.15 µg/day and not correlated with the serum B12 (Jones et al., 2007). A lower prevalence of vitamin B12 deficiency (less than 148 pmol/l) was found in 12% of the population of an indigenous community from the Amazon in Venezuela (Garcia-Casal et al., 2008). A larger study from Venezuela showed 11.4% prevalence of deficiency (less than 148 pmol/l) although in the subgroup of pregnant women it was 35% (Garcia-Casal et al., 2005). The mean serum B12 was less than 148 pmol/l in 10% of a cohort of Brazilian women of child-bearing age and 22% had elevated MMA greater than 271 nmol/l with low-normal vitamin B12 concentration. There was coexisting iron deficiency suggesting that low intake of animal protein was the cause of the vitamin B12 deficiency (Barbosa et al., 2008). There are few data about the contribution of vitamin B12 deficiency to megaloblastic anemia from the Americans although the studied cohorts of PA in the USA include many Caribbean and Mexican

Hispanics and persons of African descent (Savage et al., 1994b). Severe megaloblastic anemia was overwhelmingly caused by vitamin B12 deficiency in a series from a public hospital in Brazil. However, it is probable that patients with anemia might have been pretreated with folic acid skewing the results (Guerra-Shinohara et al., 2007).

7.2.2.4 Middle East

Vitamin B12 deficiency both dietary and PA is a common cause of megaloblastic anemia in countries from the Middle East (Ali et al., 1970; Moussa et al., 2000; Harakati, 1996). A study of vegetarians as compared with omnivorous, young, Turkish females found that 27% of the former had lower serum vitamin B12 and higher homocysteine as compared with 16% of the omnivores. The mean intake in the omnivores for B12 was 3.73 µg, but the serum B12 was considerably lower than mean values from the USA (Karabudak et al., 2008). A cross-sectional study of 1698 Turkish patients greater than 65 years old showed mean vitamin B12 values of approximately 236 pmol/l, which is approximately 100 less than in the USA from NHANES, 2003–2006. Total homocysteine values were considerably higher averaging approximately 17 µmol/l (Halil, 2008). Mean serum B12 in a control group of Turkish children was also on the low side, 168 pmol/l (Atabek et al., 2006). A random sample of Turkish adults, mean age 55, had mean vitamin B12 in men of 278 pmol/l, which is less than the 5% cutoff for B12 in NHANES in the USA. In a large cross-sectional population-based study from Iran low serum vitamin B12 (<177 pmol/l) was found in 26% of men and 27% of women although mean intake was 2.9 and 2.2 µg/day for male and females respectively (Fakhrzadeh et al., 2006).

7.2.2.5 Indian sub-continent

Vegetarianism is often followed in India, for both religious and economic reasons and the high prevalence of vitamin B12 deficiency has previously been well documented (Antony, 2003). Megaloblastic anemia is a common cause of pancytopenia and anemia, however, many studies have not provided information on vitamin B12 versus folate deficiency. A prospective study of anemia in a hospital in Delhi, India revealed a prevalence of 2.7% of megaloblastic anemia, caused by pure B12 deficiency in 65% and combined deficiency of B12 and folate in 12%. The etiology was not investigated, although the peak age incidence of 10–30 years would be unlikely for PA (Khanduri and Sharma, 2007). The low intake of vitamin B12 is particularly of concern for women during pregnancy. A study of consecutive cases to a hospital in Lahore, Pakistan showed a median maternal vitamin B12 of 102 pmol/l. The associated vitamin B12 cord levels were 176 pmol/l. Although vitamin B12 status was low, there was no relation with intrauterine growth retardation in infants (Lindblad et al., 2005).

Vitamin B12 was less than 148 pmol/l in 14% and total homocysteine greater than 15 µmol/l in 14% of toddlers from Pune, India and there was a strong negative correlation between homocysteine and vitamin B12 in the entire group (Hanumante et al., 2008). Vitamin B12 500 µg was given orally every other day in a randomized trial of 40 lacto-vegetarian, Indian women and the supplementation increased serum vitamin B12 from 125 to 215 pmol/l in 2 weeks and decreased plasma total homocysteine from 18.4 to 13.4 µmol/l and increased blood hemoglobin concentration from 11.9 to 12.2 g/dl (Yajnik et al., 2007). Detailed neurological testing was reported for a group of 36 vitamin

B12 deficient patients from India, 31 of whom were vegetarians and only four consumed more than 500 ml of milk per day. Antiparietal cell antibodies were found in 50% and one had vitiligo, therefore low vitamin B12 intake was interacting with the onset of PA. Reversible cognitive impairment was found in 47% of these patients confirming clinical significance (Kalita and Misra, 2008). The relative prevalence of B12 versus folate deficiency in Indian children hospitalized with megaloblastic anemia revealed a pure B12 deficiency in 32%, pure folate deficiency in 20% and 30% had low levels of both vitamins. The maternal vitamin B12 levels correlated with those in the children and 73% of the mothers had low B12 (Chandra et al., 2002). A follow-up study showed that the clinical neurological abnormalities and therapeutic responses were not different between those who appeared to have an autoimmune versus nutritional vitamin B12 deficiency (Misra and Kalita, 2007). Male, rural, urban and slum dwellers around Pune, India were compared and were found to have low plasma vitamin B12, 119, 145 and 89 pmol/l, respectively, and elevated total homocysteine, 14.6, 14.2 and 23.7 µmol/l, respectively. Vitamin B12 deficiency impacted the hematological findings and hemoglobin was independently associated with the plasma B12 and ferritin (Yajnik et al., 2006).

A report from Pakistan found that 79% of a retrospective cohort of macrocytic anemia had vitamin B12 deficiency defined by serum less than 148 pmol/l and gastrointestinal abnormalities were present in approximately 40% (Iqbal et al., 2009).

The antenatal serum vitamin B12 in 1165 women in Katmandu, Nepal was between 228 and 246 pmol/l and increased by 49.6 pmol/l in a group given a micronutrient supplement which contained 2.6 µg vitamin B12. However, homocysteine values did not significantly change despite the presence also of folic acid in the preparation (Christian et al., 2006).

7.2.2.6 Africa

Historically, folate deficiency has been thought to be the major cause of megaloblastic anemia in Africa, but more recent studies have shown that PA is a frequent cause of megaloblastic anemia in Africa (Savage et al., 1994a). There are also some areas of dietary vitamin B12 deficiency. Vitamin B12 deficiency was found in 30% of anemic children but also 15.6% of control children as defined by serum vitamin B12 less than 148 pmol/l (200 ng/ml) in a study from Malawi. The B12 deficiency was associated with macrocytosis and an intake of fewer meat-containing meals, 1.9 versus 2.7 per month (Calis et al., 2008). Elevated MMA was found in 18.4% and low vitamin B12, 12.2%, of a group of pregnant women attending an antenatal clinic in Nigeria with a statistically significant inverse relation between serum vitamin B12 and MMA (Vanderjagt et al., 2009). The mean serum B12 concentrations were found to be significantly lower in rural dwellers in northern Nigeria as compared with the urban dwellers but the intake of vitamin B12 ranged from 2.9 µg in urban females to a high of 6.9 µg for rural males, suggesting adequate B12 intake (Glew et al., 2004). No significant difference in B12 values was found between British women and men and Gambian non-pregnant, non-lactating female (Moore et al., 2006). Relatively low mean vitamin B12 levels were found in both HIV-positive and -negative South African breast-feeding women, approximately 200 pmol/l (Papathakis et al., 2007). Mean plasma vitamin B12 trended higher in a population of Ethiopian women who ate the traditional food enset as compared with a maize-based diet, 291 versus 238 pmol/l, although plasma MMA was not different and was higher than expected for the entire group, mean 407 nmol/l. This fermented food contained a significant amount of vitamin B12, presumably the product of bacterial synthesis (Gibson et al., 2008). Serum homocysteine was found to be fairly low, 6.8 µmol and serum B12 relatively high 614.7 pmol/l in fertile women in Burkina Faso in West Africa. Because the diet was said to have poor protein content the question was raised of whether fermented foods containing B12 could have been ingested (Chillemi et al., 2005). The mean vitamin B12 levels were 160 pmol/l and only 1% were less than 111 pmol/l in 279 pregnant women from eastern Sudan. Apparently, the diet included little animal source food, but the authors speculated that consumption of fermented food similar to those eaten in Ethiopia could have contributed to the lack of vitamin B12 deficiency (Abdelrahim et al., 2009).

Unusual arterial or venous thrombosis attributed to severe hyperhomocysteinemia from PA was a presenting complaint in a report of four Moroccan patients (Limal et al., 2006). A large series of 478 patients with megaloblastic anemia from Tunisia showed that 98% had low serum B12 levels less than 131 pmol/l and pure folate deficiency of 1.2%. The median age of 45 years is strikingly lower than populations in Europe and the USA and the crude incidence was 16.6 cases per 1 000 000. PA was proven by a schilling test in approximately 90% of those undergoing further testing (Maktouf et al., 2006). Hyperhomocysteinemia was associated with venous thrombosis and low serum vitamin B12 (less than 148 pmol/l) in 35.8% versus 13.1% in a case-controlled study of Tunisian patients who also had low animal protein intake (Omar et al., 2007). The mean vitamin B12 intake of Egyptian lactating mothers was relatively high, 4.17 µg/day because of a subgroup who ate organ meat and liver. This skewed the data so that only 25.8% of the total study group had an intake of greater than 2.5 µg with 59% consuming between 0–1.5 µg/day (Aziz et al., 2005).

Many feeding studies have been performed in Africa and effects on growth, development, anemia and other parameters studied (Allen et al., 2009b) and it has been concluded that multiple micronutrient supplementation provides the most benefit. The intake of animal source food significantly decreased the odds for low plasma vitamin B12 level (less than 148 pmol/l) in a cohort of Kenyan schoolchildren. A feeding intervention of 1 µg of B12/day significantly improved plasma vitamin B12 concentration. The average intake previous to the intervention had been 0.51 µg/day, of which 70% was from milk (McLean et al., 2007). A freshly made yogurt preparation raised plasma vitamin B12 and folate and lowered plasma homocysteine and urinary MMA as compared with a control commercial yogurt preparation in school-aged Egyptian children (Mohammad et al., 2006).

7.2.2.7 Asia

Dietary intake of vitamin B12 in Japan, Korea, China (Gao et al., 2003) and Southeast Asia (Vu et al., 2009) has been previously reported to be generally adequate with the exception of vegetarians (Stabler and Allen, 2004). A recent study of pregnant women in Japan showed an intake between 5.5 and 7.9 µg/day with corresponding low plasma homocysteine values ranging from 5 to 5.9 µmol/l and vitamin B12 values ranging from 405 (first trimester) to 265 pmol/l (third trimester) (Takimoto et al., 2007). The large Japan Public Health Center Prospective Study showed an intake of 6.5–11.1 µg/day and that dietary B12 and folate and vitamin B6 were protective factors for coronary heart disease (Ishihara et al., 2008).

Reports describing PA and B12 deficient megaloblastic anemia have been rare from China, although a report from Hong Kong suggested an incidence of PA 5.5 per 1000/year, which would be probably the low estimate (Chui et al., 2001). A more recent report from a neurology department found that 19.7% of elderly inpatients had vitamin B12 deficiency defined as a vitamin B12 less than 139 pmol/l and total homocysteine greater than 15 μmol/l. Extensive testing showed that the patients had neurological abnormalities but only 9.8% had megaloblastic anemia (Wang et al., 2009). Proven or probable pernicious anemia was the cause of megaloblastic anemia in 224 Chinese patients out of 296 seen from 1994 to 2005 at a hospital in Hong Kong. The median age, sex ratio and clinical features were very similar to those seen in PA patients from Europe (Wun Chan, 2006). The same group brought attention to 20 Chinese patients with megaloblastic anemia who presented with MCV less than 99 fl because of thalassemia trait and iron deficiency. Their observations are important because thalassemia is highly prevalent in Asia and patients with PA could be missed using criteria that were developed in northern Europeans (Chan et al., 2007). Neural-tube defects were associated with low meat, egg and milk intake, lower vitamin B12 and higher homocysteine in a study from Shanxi Provence, which has a very high incidence of neural-tube defects. Very few case women ate meat more than three times per week or eggs or milk more than five times per week (Zhang et al., 2009).

Low vitamin B12 levels (less than 160 pmol/l) were found in only 1% of a population of patients presenting for upper gastrointestinal endoscopy at a hospital in Vietnam and the *Helicobacter pylori*-positive patients were four times more likely to have been B12 deficient. Thus, the authors concluded that B12 deficiency might be uncommon in Vietnam (v Nguyen et al., 2006). The mean plasma vitamin B12 was high (494 pmol/l) in 489 urban and rural Vietnamese women and only 3% had low plasma B12. Consumption of meat, fish and fish sauce was common in the population (Hien, 2008).

In summary, pernicious anemia is being recognized as a major cause of megaloblastic anemia in Asia where it could have been under-reported in the past. Dietary vitamin B12 appears to be adequate except in vegetarian populations and in a few areas with little animal food availability.

7.2.2.8 Oceania

The prevalence of very low serum vitamin B12 was 6.3% in a cohort of 2901 older Australians and was accompanied by elevated total homocysteine in 51.6% of that group (Flood et al., 2006). The median serum B12 in children from Australia in micronutrient studies at baseline was relatively high at approximately 370 pmol/l and increased 50 pmol/l with the feeding of 1.5 μg B12/day for a year (NEMO Study Group, 2007). Data are not available from the Pacific Islands for prevalence of dietary B12 deficiency or pernicious anemia.

7.2.3 Infantile B12 deficiency

The vitamin B12 status of infants is determined both by the vitamin B12 that was accessible to the fetus during gestation and in the exclusively breast-fed infant the supply in the mother's milk. The Food and Nutrition Board set a requirement of 0.4 μg/day for infants and the average breast milk B12 concentration was reported as 0.42 μg/l (Allen, 2002).

Megaloblastic anemia and developmental abnormalities have been described in breast-fed infants from vitamin B12 deficient Asian Indian mothers more than 50 years ago (Dikshit, 1957). The increase in exclusive breast-feeding worldwide including developed countries has led to the recognition of the vitamin B12-deficient infant whose mother has undiagnosed PA, post-gastric bypass (Celiker and Chawla, 2009), or other gastrointestinal malabsorption or vegetarian diet. Vitamin B12 status in infants can be assessed by serum vitamin B12 levels and urinary or serum MMA and homocysteine. The plasma MMA rises in the days after birth and remains generally much higher than in older children or adults for up to 6 months, which makes application of adult-derived normal ranges problematic for infants (Monsen et al., 2003). Sensitive infant screening methods utilizing blood spot gas chromatography/mass spectrometry or tandem mass spectrometry are revealing infants with methylmalonic aciduria owing to maternal vitamin B12 deficiency. A study from Brazil showed that four of 234 infants with organic acidemia had maternal vitamin B12 deficiency as a cause (Wajner et al., 2009). Many of these infants could have had metabolic abnormalities before presenting at the usual 4–12-month period with failure to thrive, neurological and developmental abnormalities and in some cases megaloblastic anemia (Campbell et al., 2005; Marble et al., 2008).

The clinical syndrome in the vitamin B12-deficient infant varies from that in adults (Dror et al., 2008). Because of rapid brain growth in the first year of life the neurological consequences are devastating with disorders of consciousness, movement and failure of or delayed myelination shown on brain imaging studies (Black, 2008). Megaloblastic anemia might or might not be present similar to adults with B12 deficiency. The mothers are often strikingly normal with subclinical B12 deficiency, although metabolic abnormalities such as elevated MMA or homocysteine are found. The poor outcome in these infants was described many years ago (Graham et al., 1992). A recent review (Dror et al., 2008) discusses the clinical findings in 48 infants. The cases showed high prevalence of developmental delay, hypotonia, lethargy, convulsions and abnormal EEGs. The vast majority were less than 10th percentile for weight, approximately half less than the 10th percentile for head circumference and a significant percent had frank cerebral atrophy. Long-term developmental impairment was frequently reported (Dror et al., 2008). There were 40 B12-deficient breast-fed infants and toddlers studied in a cohort recognized over 4 years from 5000 children referred for suspected metabolic disease to a University Hospital (Honzik et al., 2010). The most common symptom was failure to thrive (40%) with feeding difficulties and vomiting, hypotonia, hydrocephaly, developmental delay and regression. A subgroup of patients with a mean B12 of 123 pmol/l had few clinical symptoms but were diagnosed based on elevated urinary MMA or plasma total homocysteine. The subgroup of severely affected infants had a mean B12 of 69 pmol/l and extreme elevations of urinary MMA (1704 mg/g creatinine) and plasma homocysteine (99 μmol/l). Anemia was present in 63% and was megaloblastic in 28%. Mothers were on vegetarian diets, ($N = 5$) had gastrocopy-proven chronic gastritis ($N = 9$) and Schilling test was abnormal in eight of the 17. Breast milk B12 was low, 47 versus 82 pmol/l comparing six of the mothers versus seven healthy controls. Only two of the 17 mothers had mild anemia, one macrocytic. Plasma total homocysteine was elevated in the 16 measured, but plasma MMA was not measured. Although the first clinical symptoms appeared at a mean age of 5.4 months, there was a previous gradual growth failure which is probably one of the earliest signs of B12 deficiency in infants. The infants responded quickly to B12, however, several developed seizures and mild-to-moderate mental retardation and delayed speech development were observed later in some of the patients. Low socioeconomic status with extremely low animal source food intake appeared to be the cause of vitamin B12 deficiency in a series of 27 infants with severe megaloblastic anemia owing to B12 deficiency diagnosed between 2000 and 2008 in Turkey (Zengin et al., 2009). Only one of the mothers was thought to have pernicious anemia although the diagnostic criteria were not given.

Every year more case reports of the B12-deficient infant appear. In summary, the breast-fed infant is vulnerable to vitamin B12 deficiency. A high degree of suspicion is needed to prevent tragic delay of diagnosis because the mothers are frequently asymptomatic, without megaloblastic anemia or other symptoms. Educational efforts directed towards identifying those individuals at risk such as history of other autoimmunity, gastrointestinal abnormalities and/or dietary limitations of animal source food should be implemented in obstetrics clinics. High dose oral vitamin B12 or infantile vitamin B12 supplementation would also be of benefit in populations thought to be at risk if diagnostic capabilities were not available.

References

Abdelrahim II, Adam GK, Mohmmed AA, Salih MM, Ali NI, Elbashier MI, Adam I, Anaemia, folate and vitamin B12 deficiency among pregnant women in an area of unstable malaria transmission in eastern Sudan. Trans R Soc Trop Med Hyg 2009;103: 493–6.

Akilzhanova A, Takamura N, Aoyagi K, Karazhanova L, Yamashita S, Folic acid deficiency: main etiological factor of megaloblastic anemia in Kazakhstan? Am J Hematol 2006;81: 471.

Ali SA, al-Yusuf AR, Salem SN, el-Ghamrawy E, Zagulaul S, Pernicious anaemia among Arabs in Kuwait. J Clin Pathol 1970;23: 577–9.

Allen LH, Impact of vitamin B-12 deficiency during lactation on maternal and infant health. Adv Exp Med Biol 2002;503: 57–67.

Allen LH, Folate and vitamin B12 status in the Americas. Nutr Rev 2004;62: S29–33; discussion S34.

Allen LH, How common is vitamin B-12 deficiency? Am J Clin Nutr 2009;89: 693S–6S.

Allen LH, Peerson JM, Olney DK, Provision of multiple rather than two or fewer micronutrients more effectively improves growth and other outcomes in micronutrient-deficient children and adults. J Nutr 2009;139: 1022–30.

Antony AC, Vegetarianism and vitamin B-12 (cobalamin) deficiency. Am J Clin Nutr 2003;78: 3–6.

Atabek ME, Pirgon O, Karagozoglu E, Plasma homocysteine levels in children and adolescents with type 1 diabetes. Indian Pediatr 2006;43: 401–7.

Aziz SA, Hussein L, Evaluation of vitamin B12 status in Egypt IV: food consumption patterns among lactating mothers and their impact on the intake of the vitamin. Int J Food Sci Nutr 2005;56: 455–62.

Barbosa PR, Stabler SP, Trentin R, Carvalho FR, Luchessi AD, Hirata RD, Hirata MH, Allen RH, Guerra-Shinohara EM, Evaluation of nutritional and genetic determinants of total homocysteine, methylmalonic acid and S-adenosylmethionine/S-adenosylhomocysteine values in Brazilian childbearing-age women. Clin Chim Acta 2008;388: 139–47.

Baker SJ, Mathan VI, Evidence regarding the minimal daily requirement of dietary vitamin B12. Am J Clin Nutr 1981;34: 2423–33.

Black MM, Effects of vitamin B12 and folate deficiency on brain development in children. Food Nutr Bull 2008;29: S126–31.

Bor MV, von Castel-Roberts KM, Kauwell GP, Stabler SP, Allen RH, Maneval DR, Bailey LB, Nexo E, Daily intake of 4 to 7 µg dietary vitamin B-12 is associated with steady concentrations of vitamin B-12-related biomarkers in a healthy young population. Am J Clin Nutr 2010;91: 571–7.

Calis JC, Phiri KS, Faragher EB, Brabin BJ, Bates I, Cuevas LE, de Haan RJ, Phiri AI, Malange P, Khoka M, Hulshof PJ, van Lieshout L, Beld MG, Teo YY, Rockett KA, Richardson A, Kwiatkowski DP, Molyneux ME, van Hensbroek MB, Severe anemia in Malawian children. N Engl J Med 2008;358: 888–99.

Campbell CD, Ganesh J, Ficicioglu C, Two newborns with nutritional vitamin B12 deficiency: challenges in newborn screening for vitamin B12 deficiency. Haematologica 2005;90: ECR45.

Carmel R, Johnson CS, Racial patterns in pernicious anemia. Early age at onset and increased frequency of intrinsic-factor antibody in black women. N Engl J Med 1978;298: 647–50.

Celiker MY, Chawla A, Congenital B12 deficiency following maternal gastric bypass. J Perinatol 2009;29: 640–2.

Chan CW, Liu SY, Kho CS, Lau KH, Liang YS, Chu WR, Ma SK, Diagnostic clues to megaloblastic anaemia without macrocytosis. Int J Lab Hematol 2007;29: 163–171.

Chandra J, Jain V, Narayan S, Sharma S, Singh V, Kapoor AK, Batra S, Folate and cobalamin deficiency in megaloblastic anemia in children. Indian Pediatr 2002;39: 453–7.

Chui CH, Lau FY, Wong R, Soo OY, Lam CK, Lee PW, Leung HK, So CK, Tsoi WC, Tang N, Lam WK, Cheng G, Vitamin B12 deficiency--need for a new guideline. Nutrition 2001;17: 917–20.

Christian P, Jiang T, Khatry SK, LeClerq SC, Shrestha SR, West KP Jr, Antenatal supplementation with micronutrients and biochemical indicators of status and subclinical infection in rural Nepal. Am J Clin Nutr 2006;83: 788–94.

Chillemi R, Simpore J, Persichilli S, Minucci A, D'Agata A, Musumeci S, Elevated levels of plasma homocysteine in postmenopausal women in Burkina Faso. Clin Chem Lab Med 2005;43: 765–71.

Dikshit AK, Nutritional dystrophy and anemia. Ind J Child Health 1957;6: 132–6.

Dror DK, Allen LH, Effect of vitamin B12 deficiency on neurodevelopment in infants: current knowledge and possible mechanisms. Nutr Rev 2008;66: 250–5.

Elmadfa I, Singer I, Vitamin B-12 and homocysteine status among vegetarians: a global perspective. Am J Clin Nutr 2009;89: 1693S–8S.

Fabian E, Elmadfa I, Nutritional situation of the elderly in the European Union: data of the European Nutrition and Health Report (2004). Ann Nutr Metab 2008;52: 57–61.

Fakhrzadeh H, Ghotbi S, Pourebrahim R, Nouri M, Heshmat R, Bandarian F, Shafaee A, Larijani B, Total plasma homocysteine, folate, and vitamin B12 status in healthy Iranian adults: the Tehran homocysteine survey (2003–2004)/a cross-sectional population based study. BMC Public Health 2006;6: 29.

Flood VM, Smith WT, Webb KL, Rochtchina E, Anderson VE, Mitchell P, Prevalence of low serum folate and vitamin B12 in an older Australian population. Aust N Z J Public Health 2006;30: 38–41.

Ganji V, Kafai MR, Demographic, lifestyle, and health characteristics and serum B vitamin status are determinants of plasma total homocysteine concentration in the post-folic acid fortification period, 1999–2004. J Nutr 2009;139: 345–52.

Gao X, Yao M, McCrory MA, Ma G, Li Y, Roberts SB, Tucker KL, Dietary pattern is associated with homocysteine and B vitamin status in an urban Chinese population. J Nutr 2003;133: 3636–42.

Garcia-Casal MN, Osorio C, Landaeta M, Leets I, Matus P, Fazzino F, Marcos E, High prevalence of folic acid and vitamin B12 deficiencies in infants, children, adolescents and pregnant women in Venezuela. Eur J Clin Nutr 2005;59: 1064–70.

Garcia-Casal MN, Leets I, Bracho C, Hidalgo M, Bastidas G, Gomez A, Pena A, Perez H, Prevalence of anemia and deficiencies of iron, folic acid and vitamin B12 in an indigenous community from the Venezuelan Amazon with a high incidence of malaria. Arch Latinoam Nutr 2008;58: 12–8.

Gibson RS, Abebe Y, Stabler S, Allen RH, Westcott JE, Stoecker BJ, Krebs NF, Hambidge KM, Zinc, gravida, infection, and iron, but not vitamin B-12 or folate status, predict hemoglobin during pregnancy in Southern Ethiopia. J Nutr 2008;138: 581–6.

Glew RH, Conn CA, Vanderjagt TA, Calvin CD, Obadofin MO, Crossey M, Vanderjagt DJ, Risk factors for cardiovascular disease and diet of urban and rural dwellers in northern Nigeria. J Health Popul Nutr 2004;22: 357–69.

Graham SM, Arvela OM, Wise GA, Long-term neurologic consequences of nutritional vitamin B12 deficiency in infants. J Pediatr 1992;121: 710–4.

Guerra-Shinohara EM, Morita OE, Pagliusi RA, Blaia-d'Avila VL, Allen RH, Stabler SP, Elevated serum S-adenosylhomocysteine in cobalamin-deficient megaloblastic anemia. Metabolism 2007;56: 339–47.

Hanumante NM, Wadia RS, Deshpande SS, Sanwalka NJ, Vaidya MV, Khadilkar AV, Vitamin B12 and homocysteine status in asymptomatic Indian toddlers. Indian J Pediatr 2008;75: 751–3.

Harakati MS, Pernicious anemia in Arabs. Blood Cells Mol Dis 1996;22: 98–103.

Honzik T, Adamovicova M, Smolka V, Magner M, Hruba E, Zeman J, Clinical presentation and metabolic consequences in 40 breastfed infants with nutritional vitamin B(12) deficiency – What have we learned? Eur J Paediatr Neurol 2010 [E-pub ahead of print].

Iqbal SP, Kakepoto GN, Iqbal SP, Gastrointestinal abnormalities in vitamin B12 deficient patients with megaloblastic anemia. J Coll Physicians Surg Pak 2009;19: 672–3.

Ishihara J, Iso H, Inoue M, Iwasaki M, Okada K, Kita Y, Kokubo Y, Okayama A, Tsugane S; JPHC Study Group. Intake of folate, vitamin B6 and vitamin B12 and the risk of CHD: the Japan Public Health Center-Based Prospective Study Cohort I, J Am Coll Nutr 2008;27:127–36.

Johnson MA, Hawthorne NA, Brackett WR, Fischer JG, Gunter EW, Allen RH, Stabler SP, Hyperhomocysteinemia and vitamin B-12 deficiency in elderly using Title IIIc nutrition services. Am J Clin Nutr 2003;77: 211–20.

Jones KM, Ramirez-Zea M, Zuleta C, Allen LH, Prevalent vitamin B-12 deficiency in twelve-month-old Guatemalan infants is predicted by maternal B-12 deficiency and infant diet. J Nutr 2007;137: 1307–13.

Kalita J, Misra UK, Vitamin B12 deficiency neurological syndromes: correlation of clinical, MRI and cognitive evoked potential. J Neurol 2008;255: 353–59.

Karabudak E, Kiziltan G, Cigerim N, A comparison of some of the cardiovascular risk factors in vegetarian and omnivorous Turkish females. J Hum Nutr Diet 2008;21: 13–22.

Khanduri U, Sharma A, Megaloblastic anaemia: prevalence and causative factors. Natl Med J India 2007;20: 172–5.

Krajcovicova-Kudlackova M, Blazicek P, Mislanova C, Valachovicova M, Paukova V, Spustova V, Nutritional determinants of plasma homocysteine. Bratisl Lek Listy 2007;108: 510–5.

Krasinski SD, Russell RM, Samloff IM, Jacob RA, Dallal GE, McGandy RB, Hartz SC, Fundic atrophic gastritis in an elderly population. Effect on hemoglobin and several serum nutritional indicators. J Am Geriatr Soc 1986;34: 800–6.

Limal N, Scheuermaier K, Tazi Z, Sene D, Piette JC, Cacoub P, Hyperhomocysteinaemia, thrombosis and pernicious anaemia. Thromb Haemost 2006;96: 233–5.

Lindblad B, Zaman S, Malik A, Martin H, Ekström AM, Amu S, Holmgren A, Norman M, Folate, vitamin B12, and homocysteine levels in South Asian women with growth-retarded fetuses. Acta Obstet Gynecol Scand 2005;84:1055–61.

Lindenbaum J, Healton EB, Savage DG, Brust JC, Garrett TJ, Podell ER, Marcell PD, Stabler SP, Allen RH, Neuropsychiatric disorders caused by cobalamin deficiency in the absence of anemia or macrocytosis. N Engl J Med 1988;318: 1720–8.

Lindenbaum J, Savage DG, Stabler SP, Allen RH, Diagnosis of cobalamin deficiency: II, Relative sensitivities of serum cobalamin, methylmalonic acid, and total homocysteine concentrations. Am J Hematol 1990;34: 99–107.

Lindenbaum J, Rosenberg IH, Wilson PW, Stabler SP, Allen RH, Prevalence of cobalamin deficiency in the Framingham elderly population. Am J Clin Nutr 1994;60: 2–11.

Majchrzak D, Singer I, Männer M, Rust P, Genser D, Wagner KH, Elmadfa I, B-vitamin status and concentrations of homocysteine in Austrian omnivores, vegetarians and vegans. Ann Nutr Metab 2006;50: 485–91.

Maktouf C, Bchir A, Louzir H, Mdhaffer M, Elloumi M, Ben Abid H, Meddeb B, Makni F, Laatiri A, Soussi T, Hafsia A, Dellagi K, Megaloblastic anemia in North Africa. Haematologica 2006;91: 990–1.

Marble M, Copeland S, Khanfar N, Rosenblatt DS, Neonatal vitamin B12 deficiency secondary to maternal subclinical pernicious anemia: identification by expanded newborn screening. J Pediatr 2008;152: 731–3.

McLean ED, Allen LH, Neumann CG, Peerson JM, Siekmann JH, Murphy SP, Bwibo NO, Demment MW, Low plasma vitamin B-12 in Kenyan school children is highly prevalent and improved by supplemental animal source foods. J Nutr 2007;137: 676–82.

McLean E, de Benoist B, Allen LH, Review of the magnitude of folate and vitamin B12 deficiencies worldwide. Food Nutr Bull 2008;29: S38–51.

Misra UK, Kalita J, Comparison of clinical and electrodiagnostic features in B12 deficiency neurological syndromes with and without antiparietal cell antibodies. Postgrad Med J 2007;83: 124–7.

Mohammad MA, Molloy A, Scott J, Hussein L, Plasma cobalamin and folate and their metabolic markers methylmalonic acid and total homocysteine among Egyptian children before and after nutritional supplementation with the probiotic bacteria Lactobacillus acidophilus in yoghurt matrix. Int J Food Sci Nutr 2006;57: 470–80.

Monárrez-Espino J, Martínez H, Martínez V, Greiner T, Nutritional status of indigenous children at boarding schools in northern Mexico. Eur J Clin Nutr 2004;58: 532–40.

Monsen AL, Refsum H, Markestad T, Ueland PM, Cobalamin status and its biochemical markers methylmalonic acid and homocysteine in different age groups from 4 days to 19 years. Clin Chem 2003;49: 2067–75.

Moore SE, Mansoor MA, Bates CJ, Prentice AM, Plasma homocysteine, folate and vitamin B(12) compared between rural Gambian and UK adults. Br J Nutr 2006;96: 508–15.

Moussa NA, Awad MO, Yahya TM, Pernicious anaemia and neurophysiological studies in Arabs. Int J Clin Pract 2000;54: 152–4.

National Academy of Sciences, Institute of Medicine. Dietary reference intakes for thiamin, riboflavin, niacin, vitamin B6, folate, vitamin B12, pantothenic acid, biotin and choline, Ch. 9. Washington, DC: National Acadamic Press; 2000. pp. 305–56. http://nap.edu/openbook/0309065542/html/306.html

NEMO Study Group. Osendarp SJ, Baghurst KI, Bryan J, Calvaresi E, Hughes D, Hussaini M, Karyadi SJ, van Klinken BJ, van der Knaap HC, Lukito W, Mikarsa W, Transler C, Wilson C, Effect of a 12-mo micronutrient intervention on learning and memory in well-nourished and marginally nourished school-aged children: 2 parallel, randomized, placebo-controlled studies in Australia and Indonesia. Am J Clin Nutr 2007;86: 1082–93.

Omar S, Ghorbel IB, Feki H, Souissi M, Feki M, Houman H, Kaabachi N, Hyperhomocysteinemia is associated with deep venous thrombosis of the lower extremities in Tunisian patients. Clin Biochem 2007;40: 41–5.

Papathakis PC, Rollins NC, Chantry CJ, Bennish ML, Brown KH, Micronutrient status during lactation in HIV-infected and HIV-uninfected South African women during the first 6 mo after delivery. Am J Clin Nutr 2007;85: 182–92.

Pfeiffer CM, Johnson CL, Jain RB, Yetley EA, Picciano MF, Rader JI, Fisher KD, Mulinare J, Osterloh JD, Trends in blood folate and vitamin B-12 concentrations in the United States, 1988–2004. Am J Clin Nutr 2007;86: 718–27.

Savage D, Gangaidzo I, Lindenbaum J, Kiire C, Mukiibi JM, Moyo A, Gwanzura C, Mudenge B, Bennie A, Sitima J, Stabler SP, Allen RH, Vitamin B12 deficiency is the primary cause of megaloblastic anaemia in Zimbabwe. Br J Haematol 1994a;86: 844–50.

Savage DG, Lindenbaum J, Stabler SP, Allen RH, Sensitivity of serum methylmalonic acid and total homocysteine determinations for diagnosing cobalamin and folate deficiencies. Am J Med 1994b;96: 239–46.

Schulpis KH, Michalakakou K, Gavrili S, Karikas GA, Lazaropoulou C, Vlachos G, Bakoula C, Papassotiriou I, Maternal-neonatal retinol and alpha-tocopherol serum concentrations in Greeks and Albanians. Acta Paediatr 2004;93: 1075–80.

Stabler SP, Allen RH, Vitamin B12 deficiency as a worldwide problem. Annu Rev Nutr 2004;24: 299–26.

Stabler SP, Allen RH, Savage DG, Lindenbaum J, Clinical spectrum and diagnosis of cobalamin deficiency. Blood 1990;76: 871–81.

Stabler SP, Allen RH, Fried LP, Pahor M, Kittner SJ, Penninx BW, Guralnik JM, Racial differences in prevalence of cobalamin and folate deficiencies in disabled elderly women. Am J Clin Nutr 1999;70: 911–9.

Takimoto H, Mito N, Umegaki K, Ishiwaki A, Kusama K, Abe S, Yamawaki M, Fukuoka H, Ohta C, Yoshiike N, Relationship between dietary folate intakes, maternal plasma total homocysteine and B-vitamins during pregnancy and fetal growth in Japan. Eur J Nutr 2007;46: 300–6.

Torres-Sánchez L, Chen J, Díaz-Sánchez Y, Palomeque C, Bottiglieri T, López-Cervantes M, López-Carrillo L, Dietary and genetic determinants of homocysteine levels among Mexican women of reproductive age. Eur J Clin Nutr 2006;60: 691–7.

v Nguyen T, van Oijen MG, Janssen MJ, Laheij RJ, Jansen JB, van Asten H, Vitamin B12 deficiency in patients with upper gastrointestinal symptoms in the Mekong Delta, Vietnam. Dig Liver Dis 2006;38: 438–9.

Vanderjagt DJ, Ujah IA, Patel A, Kellywood J, Crossey MJ, Allen RH, Stabler SP, Obande OS, Glew RH, Subclinical vitamin B12 deficiency in pregnant women attending an antenatal clinic in Nigeria. J Obstet Gynaecol 2009;29: 288–95.

Villalpando S, Shamah-Levy T, Ramírez-Silva CI, Mejía-Rodríguez F, Rivera JA, Prevalence of anemia in children 1 to 12 years of age. Results from a nationwide probabilistic survey in Mexico. Salud Publica Mex 2003;45: S490–8.

Vogiatzoglou A, Smith AD, Nurk E, Berstad P, Drevon CA, Ueland PM, Vollset SE, Tell GS, Refsum H, Dietary sources of vitamin B-12 and their association with plasma vitamin B-12 concentrations in the general population: the Hordaland Homocysteine Study. Am J Clin Nutr 2009a;89: 1078–87.

Vogiatzoglou A, Oulhaj A, Smith AD, Nurk E, Drevon CA, Ueland PM, Vollset SE, Tell GS, Refsum H, Determinants of plasma methylmalonic acid in a large population: implications for assessment of vitamin B12 status. Clin Chem 2009b;55: 2198–206.

Vu TT, Nguyen TL, Nguyen CK, Nguyen TD, Skeaff CM, Venn BJ, Walmsley T, George PM, McLean J, Brown MR, Green TJ, Folate and vitamin B12 status of women of reproductive age living in Hanoi City and Hai Duong Province of Vietnam. Public Health Nutr 2009;12: 941–6.

Wajner M, Coelho Dde M, Ingrassia R, de Oliveira AB, Busanello EN, Raymond K, Flores Pires R, de Souza CF, Giugliani R, Vargas CR, Selective screening for organic acidemias by urine organic acid GC-MS analysis in Brazil: fifteen-year experience. Clin Chim Acta 2009;400: 77–81.

Wang YH, Yan F, Zhang WB, Ye G, Zheng YY, Zhang XH, Shao FY, An investigation of vitamin B12 deficiency in elderly inpatients in neurology department. Neurosci Bull 2009;25: 209–15.

Wun Chan JC, YU Liu HS, Sang Kho BC, Yin Sim JP, Hang Lau TK, Luk YW, Chu RW, Fung Cheung FM, Tat Choi FP, Kwan Ma Es, Pernicious anemia in Chinese: a study of 181 patients in a Hong Kong hospital. Medicine (Baltimore) 2006;85: 129–38.

Yajnik CS, Deshpande SS, Lubree HG, Naik SS, Bhat DS, Uradey BS, Deshpande JA, Rege SS, Refsum H, Yudkin JS, Vitamin B12 deficiency and hyperhomocysteinemia in rural and urban Indians. J Assoc Physicians India 2006;54: 775–82.

Yajnik CS, Lubree HG, Thuse NV, Ramdas LV, Deshpande SS, Deshpande VU, Deshpande JA, Uradey BS, Ganpule AA, Naik SS, Joshi NP, Farrant H, Refsum H, Oral vitamin B12 supplementation reduces plasma total homocysteine concentration in women in India. Asia Pac J Clin Nutr 2007;16: 103–9.

Zengin E, Sarper N, Caki Kiliç S, Clinical manifestations of infants with nutritional vitamin B deficiency due to maternal dietary deficiency. Acta Paediatr 2009;98: 98–102.

Zhang T, Xin R, Gu X, Wang F, Pei L, Lin L, Chen G, Wu J, Zheng X, Maternal serum vitamin B12, folate and homocysteine and the risk of neural tube defects in the offspring in a high-risk area of China. Public Health Nutr 2009;12: 680–6.

7.3 Cobalamin deficiency

Wolfgang Herrmann; Rima Obeid

7.3.1 Introduction

The discovery of cobalamin (Cbl; vitamin B12) was, after several years of intensive studies on pernicious anemia (PA), a previously fatal disease. In the early 1920s Minot and Murphy demonstrated that they were able to cure PA by whole liver extract. Later, it was shown that liver is an important source of Cbl. Animals can obtain Cbl by consuming foods contaminated with synthesizing bacteria and then incorporate the vitamin into their body organs. Foods of animal source are the only natural source of Cbl in the human diet. Cbl is synthesized exclusively in microorganisms, and in humans it is an essential component in methyl group transfer and cell division. Cbl belongs to a group of compounds of similar chemical structure but completely different biological functions. The vitamin is crucially involved in the proliferation, maturation and regeneration of cells. Cbl maintains low homocysteine (Hcy) levels by transferring a methyl group from 5-methyltetrahydrofolate (5-MTHF) to Hcy converting it into methionine.

Cbl consists of a corrinoid molecule with cobalt in the centre of this molecule. The synthetic forms of Cbl are cyanocobalamin and hydroxycobalamin. There are only two forms of Cbl that have biological activity as cofactors in enzyme reactions (▶Fig. 7.2). These are adenosylcobalamin (AdoCbl) and methylcobalamin (MeCbl) (Herzlich and Herbert, 1988). In mammalian metabolism, Cbl is required for only two key enzymatic reactions. The first reaction occurs in the cytosol and involves synthesis of methionine from Hcy. Methionine synthase and its cofactor MeCbl catalyze this reaction. The second pathway takes place in the mitochondria and involves isomerization of methylmalonyl-CoA to succinyl-CoA. This reaction is catalyzed by methylmalonyl-CoA mutase with AdoCbl as a cofactor (Stroinsky and Schneider, 1987). The excess of methymalonyl-CoA is converted into methylmalonic acid (MMA). Cbl deficiency leads

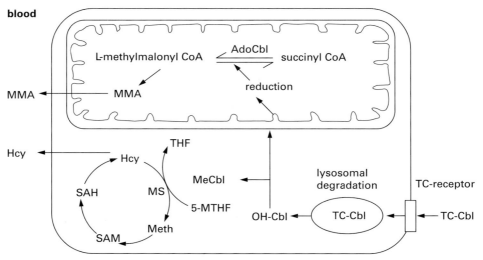

Fig. 7.2: The metabolic pathways enhanced by cobalamin (see text for details). Hcy, homocysteine; Met, methionine; SAH, S-adenosylhomocysteine; SAM, S-adenosylmethionine; MeCbl, methylcobalamin; AdoCbl, adenosylcobalamine; Meth, methionine; MS, methionine synthase; MMA, methylmalonic acid; THF, Tetralhydrofolate; MTHF, methyltetrahydrofolate; TC, transcobalamin.

to enhanced conversion of methylmalonyl-CoA into MMA and elevation of the latter compound in the blood. Therefore, concentrations of MMA and total (t) Hcy in plasma can reflect Cbl status.

7.3.2. Cobalamin hemostasis and deficiency

Dietary Cbl is bound to food proteins and must be released before that the vitamin can be absorbed. The release of Cbl from its food-binding proteins is achieved by the action of gastric acid and proteolytic enzymes in the stomach. In the stomach Cbl is captured by haptocorrin (transcobalamin I), an R-binder protein made in the saliva and stomach. In the upper small intestine, pancreatic enzymes and an alkaline pH degrade the haptocorrin-Cbl complex. The free vitamin is then captured by intrinsic factor (IF), another Cbl binding protein. The IF-Cbl complex is transported to the terminal ileum where the complex is recognized and internalized by specific membrane receptors of the enterocytes (intrinsic factor receptor). The receptor-mediated absorption of Cbl is a saturable process and a maximal amount of 3 µg of the vitamin per meal is thought to be internalized via this pathway. After absorption of Cbl-IF complex into the enterocytes, the complex is degraded and Cbl is transferred to a third binding protein, transcobalamin (transcobalamin II, TC). TC is synthesized within the enterocytes and is the only binder that can deliver Cbl into cells via TC-receptor. The TC-Cbl complex is released into the portal circulation and is subsequently recognized by TC-receptors that are expressed by all cell types. The part of Cbl which is bound to TC is named holotranscobalamin (holoTC) (Carmel, 1985). Only 6–20% of total plasma Cbl is present as holoTC (Hall, 1977). The remaining part of Cbl is bound to haptocorrin and is called holohaptocorrin (holoHC) (England et al., 1976). Despite that haptocorrin binds almost 80% of total plasma Cbl, the functions of this protein are not well investigated.

A considerable amount of Cbl is secreted into the bile. Two-thirds of the secreted Cbl in the bile is reabsorbed in the ileum. The liver contains most of the Cbl (2–3 mg) in the body (Markle, 1996). The kidney and the brain are also two important organs that accumulate Cbl. The kidney can release Cbl in case of short-term depletion of the vitamin. Cbl is excreted into urine and this can be reabsorbed in the proximal tubules via a specific receptor (megalin/cubilin) (Moestrup et al., 1996). The major route by which Cbl is lost from the body is through the feces.

7.3.2.1 Staging and diagnosis of cobalamin deficiency

The observations by Herbert et al. (Herbert, 1994) suggest that cobalamin deficiency is a proceeding process which develops through different stages. In the early stages, plasma and cells become depleted of the vitamin causing a lowered serum concentration of holoTC whereas functional metabolic markers for Cbl deficiency, such as tHcy and MMA, are still within the normal range and clinical signs of the deficiency are missing (Herbert et al., 1990; Lindgren et al., 1999). If the negative balance continues, the metabolic markers tHcy and MMA become elevated in plasma. This is explained by impairment of the Cbl-dependent enzymes (methionine synthase and methylmalonyl-CoA mutase). Clinical signs of Cbl deficiency become obvious in late stages (macrocytic anemia, neurological symptoms).

Owing to the latent nature of Cbl deficiency and the possible irreversible neurological damage, an early diagnosis is crucial (Weir and Scott, 1999). On the one hand, because a single reliable diagnostic approach for ruling out Cbl deficiency is not available (Herrmann et al., 2001b, 2003c), the assessment of the different markers (reflecting the metabolic status and Cbl stores) is favored and provides in that way a valuable diagnostic tool for Cbl status. On the other hand, megaloblastic anemia and neurological symptoms are neither sensitive nor they are specific for Cbl deficiency. Additionally, elevated MMA and tHcy as metabolic signs of deficiency can be observed in the absence of hematological or clinical manifestations. Concentration of total Cbl in serum is also too insensitive for diagnosing Cbl deficiency (Herrmann et al., 2000, 2001b). Measurements of holoTC, MMA and tHcy in plasma provide sensitive and specific laboratory tools. However, these markers have also limitations in some clinical conditions such as renal insufficiency or folate deficiency (see Chapters 7.3.5 and 7.3.6).

7.3.2.2 Cobalamin deficiency causes folate trap

Because of the role of Cbl in folate metabolism, Cbl deficiency can cause a secondary folate deficiency. Cbl deficiency inhibits the activity of methionine synthase, and causes the retention of 5-MTHF. 5-MTHF becomes trapped because the transfer of the methyl group is inhibited (▶Fig. 7.3). The level of folate in serum or plasma of Cbl deficient subjects could be normal to high normal, however, this is mostly as 5-MTHF. This phenomenon is called 'folate trap'. Folate and Cbl deficiency have similar clinical (megaloblastic red cells) and metabolic (elevation of tHcy) signs. This

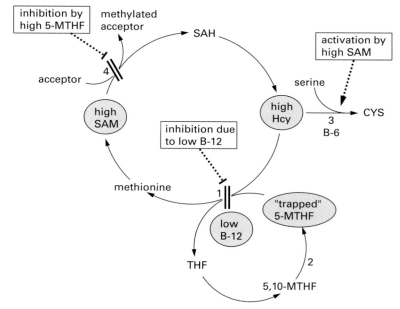

Fig. 7.3: Homocysteine metabolism in Cbl deficiency. Low Cbl causes an inhibition of Hcy remethylation and thus induces trapping of 5-MTHF. The increased folate concentration inhibits the transmethylation reaction leading to elevated SAM levels. High SAM concentrations activate the trans-sulfuration pathway. Cbl, cobalamin; Hcy, homocysteine; SAH, S-adenosylhomocysteine; SAM, S-adenosylmethionine; CYS, cystathionine; THF, tetrahydrofolate; 5-MTHF, 5-methyl-tetrahydrofolate; 5,10-MTHF, 5,10-methylenetetrahydrofolate). 1, methionine synthase; 2, N5,N10-methylene-tetrahydrofolatereductase; 3, cystathionine-β-synthase; 4, glycine-N-methyltransferase).

explains why Cbl deficient subjects were frequently treated with folate. This treatment might relieve the hematological symptoms thus allowing the neurological signs of Cbl deficiency to progress. Folate treatment itself is not the cause of worsening neurological symptoms in cobalamin-deficient people. ►Fig. 7.4 shows how cobalamin-deficient people (vegetarians in this case) show high concentrations of plasma tHcy and folate.

7.3.2.3 Cobalamin deficient state

Cbl deficiency can be either clinically manifested or subtle. Clinical symptoms of Cbl deficiency include neurological and hematological signs (see Chapter 7.3.4.4.1 and 7.3.5.5.1). Neurological symptoms are considered a late manifestation of the disease; they are often presented without significant hematological signs. The typical hematological symptoms of Cbl deficiency occur also late in the course of the disease and might or might not occur along with the neurological signs. The exact prevalence of clinically significant Cbl deficiency is not known; the range of symptoms is wide and the new markers enable the detection of vitamin deficiency

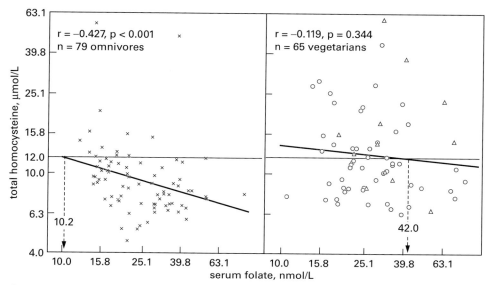

Fig. 7.4: Scatterplot showing concentrations of tHcy in relation to serum folate in omnivorous (left plot) and vegetarians (right plot). Numbers on the axis are anti-Log.

notably more often. Subtle Cbl deficiency cannot be described as a disease condition, because during this phase, metabolic markers of Cbl status are increased without clinical manifestations. However, this condition is common and can evolve to clear deficiency.

Cbl deficiency (either clear or subtle) is common worldwide and is more widespread in the population than it has been assumed so far (Sipponen et al., 2003; Clarke et al., 2004). In developed countries, Cbl deficiency was thought to be restricted to patients with malabsorption, intestinal resection, or those who do not ingest a sufficient amount of the vitamin (Carmel, 1997; Herrmann et al., 2003c). However, recent studies have shown that these conditions are not rare and they can cause Cbl deficiency in a large number of elderly people and vegetarians. In developing countries, Cbl deficiency has been shown to be common in children, middle age and elderly people (Refsum et al., 2001; Rogers et al., 2003; Herrmann et al., 2009a). Cbl deficiency is often unrecognized because the clinical manifestations are subtle or because deficient people cannot be recognized by using of insensitive markers such as total Cbl. Early diagnosis of Cbl deficiency is essential for preventing irreversible neurological damage (Graham et al., 1992; Masalha et al., 2001). This has been made possible by available laboratory biomarkers such as holoTC and MMA.

Functional Cbl deficiency can be defined in terms of serum or plasma concentrations of tHcy, Cbl, holoTC and MMA. However, the diagnostic utility and performance of these parameters are not equally good. Hyperhomocysteinemia (HHcy) (tHcy > 12 μmol/l) can also be caused by folate or vitamin B6 deficiency which should be excluded before making a decision about Cbl deficiency. Concentrations of total Cbl in plasma have been long used as a first line parameter; because of low cost and wide availability of this test. Limitations of this test include low sensitivity (increased false negative results) and limited specificity, particularly when plasma Cbl concentrations <400 pmol/l (Herrmann et al., 2003c; Loikas et al., 2003). In line with this, people with Cbl concentrations within the reference range (>156 pmol/l) can show clinical signs of Cbl deficiency (Lesho and Hyder, 1999) or raised concentrations of MMA (>300 nmol/l) and lowered concentrations of holoTC (<35 pmol/l) (Herrmann et al., 2003c). A lowered serum holoTC concentration is the earliest marker of Cbl deficiency and signals that the body does not have sufficient Cbl and that the Cbl stores are emptying as a result of the negative balance of Cbl (Herrmann et al., 2003c). Lowered holoTC combined with raised MMA and tHcy levels are indicative of metabolically manifested Cbl deficiency. Clinical signs might already be present but can still be missing (Kuzminski et al., 1998).

7.3.2.4 Prevalence and risk groups for cobalamin deficiency

Insufficient intake or disrupted absorption of Cbl will result in Cbl deficiency. The National Research Council of the US National Academy of Sciences has recommended that adults should ingest 2.4 µg daily (Institute of Medicine, 2000). The recommended dietary intake (RDI) is based on the calculation of the amount of Cbl that is necessary to sustain a normal hematological status (normal hemoglobin and MCV) and to maintain remission in PA. At the time when the recommended dietary intake was set, no studies had investigated the direct link between Cbl intake and MMA concentrations. New results have shown that the plasma concentration of MMA and tHcy falls when Cbl is ingested, whereas the holoTC concentration rises (Bor et al., 2006). A minimum daily intake of 6 µg Cbl results in an optimal plasma concentration of the investigated biomarkers (Bor et al., 2006). More recent studies have shown that the recommended daily intake of Cbl should be newly determined and seems too low, particularly for older people.

   The prevalence of subtle Cbl deficiency is high when sensitive and relatively specific laboratory markers are used such as MMA, holoTC and tHcy (Obeid et al., 2004; Herrmann et al., 2005a). Risk groups for Cbl deficiency (▶Tab. 7.4) include: patients with unexplained anemia; patients with unexplained neuropsychiatric symptoms; patients with gastrointestinal manifestations, including stomatitis, anorexia and diarrhea; elderly people (Obeid et al., 2004); vegetarians (Herrmann et al., 2003c); patients with gastrointestinal disorders, such as Crohn's disease or infection with *Heliobacter pylori*; and patients with stomach resection (Baik and Russell, 1999). Further risk groups for Cbl deficiency are persons with an increased vitamin requirement – such as pregnant and breastfeeding women, patients with autoimmune disorders or persons with HIV infection. Furthermore, persons who regularly take proton pump inhibitors can also develop Cbl deficiency. Cbl deficiency is also widespread in patients with renal disorders (more details below) (Obeid et al., 2005b). There are currently no follow-up studies showing how many people who are classified as having subtle deficiency will develop clinically manifested deficiency. In the general population, the prevalence of Cbl deficiency (defined by clinical or metabolic markers) in younger people is 5–7% (Herrmann et al., 2003b).

Tab. 7.4: Risk populations and conditions associated with cobalamin deficiency.

Group	Causes and remarks
Vegetarian, vegan	Low Cbl intake
Neonates and breast-fed infants of vegetarian mothers	Low Cbl absorption with breast milk
Elderly people	Pernicious anemia, achlorhydria, malabsorption caused by other gastrointestinal disorders (gastric or intestinal surgery, gastritis, *Helicobacter pylori*, atrophy, bacterial overgrowth), alcohol
Neurodegenerative and neuropsychiatric disorders	Neuropathies, dementia, Alzheimer's disease, cognitive disorders, schizophrenia
Chronic atrophic corpus gastritis	Malabsorption of Cbl; Crohn's disease
Disorders of the terminal ileum	Ileal lymphoma, ileal resection, bacterial overgrowth of the ileum
Macrocytic anemia	Low absorption of Cbl or pernicious anemia
Chronic alcoholism	Low or disrupted absorption of Cbl
Medication	Proton pump inhibitors, H_2 receptor agonists, inhalation of nitrous oxide
AIDS associated myelopathy	Abnormal Cbl dependent transmethylation

7.3.3 Inherited causes of cobalamin deficiency

The most important inherited disorders of Cbl absorption, transport, metabolism, or utilization are presented in ▶Tab. 7.5.

7.3.3.1 Congenital transcobalamin deficiency

These are disorders of Cbl transport or absorption. A congenital recessive defect causes a lack of the binding protein, TC. Although babies are born asymptomatic, severe hematological and neurological manifestations are expressed few days to weeks after birth. This case is characterized by irritation, failure to thrive, and severe elevation of MMA in blood and urine of affected children. In most cases, high doses of Cbl can improve clinical symptoms (Hakami et al., 1971; Cooper and Rosenblatt, 1987; Bibi et al., 1999; Teplitsky et al., 2003). Haptocorrin deficiency (deficiency of R-binder) has also been recently reported and is associated with a very low total serum Cbl. Nevertheless, subjects who express this phenotype remain asymptomatic and concentrations of holoTC remain within the normal range (Lin et al., 2001).

7.3.3.2 Imerslund-Gräsbeck syndrome

Imerslund-Gräsbeck syndrome (IGS) or selective Cbl malabsorption is a rare autosomal recessive disorder characterized by Cbl deficiency and megaloblastic anemia

Tab. 7.5: Hereditary disorders of cobalamin absorption, transport, metabolism or utilization.

Defect	Affected enzyme or step	Metabolic abnormalities	Therapeutic strategies
Congenital pernicious anemia (intrinsic factor deficiency)	Cobalamin absorption	↑tHcy, ↑MMA	Cobalamin + intrinsic factor
Imerslund-Gräsbeck syndrome	Selective cobalamin malabsorption	proteinurea, ↑tHcy, ↑MMA	Cobalamin injection
Transcobalamin II deficiency	Defective transport of cobalamin into the blood stream and into the cells	↑tHcy, ↑MMA	High doses of systemic cobalamin
Methylmalonic aciduria	Methylmalonyl CoA mutase deficiency (mut^0, mut$^-$)	↑MMA, acidosis	Protein restriction (limiting the amino acids that use the propionate pathway)
Cbl A and Cbl B diseases	Failure to synthesize adenosylcobalamin	↑MMA	Cobalamin injections
Cbl E and Cbl G diseases	Failure to synthesize methylcobalamin	↑tHcy, ↓methionine	Cobalamin injections + betaine
Cbl C and Cbl D diseases	Failure to synthesize adenosylcobalamin and methylcobalamin	↑MMA, ↑tHcy	Cobalamin injections + betaine
Cbl F disease	Failure to release cobalamin from the lysosome	↑MMA, ↑tHcy	Cobalamin injections

(Gräsbeck, 2006). This disease is characterized by proteinuria and lose of Cbl in urine (Ben-Ami et al., 1990). Cbl malabsorption in this case is related to a defective cubulin, the receptor for IF-Cbl complex that is expressed in the enterocytes and the renal tubulus. Cbl absorption tests show low absorption, not corrected by administration of IF. The symptoms appear from 4 months up to several years after birth. The syndrome was first described in Finland and Norway where the prevalence is approximately 1:200 000 births. In most cases, the molecular basis of the selective malabsorption and proteinuria involves a mutation in one of two genes, cubilin (*CUBN*) on chromosome 10 or amnionless (*AMN*) on chromosome 14. Both proteins are components of the intestinal receptor for the Cbl-IF complex and the receptor mediating the tubular reabsorption of protein from the primary urine. Management includes life-long Cbl injections, and with this regimen, the patients stay healthy for decades.

7.3.3.3 Disorders of cobalamin utilization

Methylmalonic aciduria is related to a functional defect or a deficiency of the mitochondrial enzyme, methylmalonyl CoA mutase. Methylmalonic aciduria or methylmalonic acidemia is an autosomal recessive metabolic disorder (Radmanesh et al., 2008). It stems from several genotypes (Matsui et al., 1983); all forms of the disorder are usually diagnosed in the early neonatal period, presenting progressive encephalopathy, and secondary hyperammonemia. The disorder can result in death if undiagnosed or left untreated. Culturing fibroblasts from those patients have shown that some patients do not response to Cbl treatment, and others have a residual enzyme activity and response to Cbl treatment. Cbl mutant A and B are related to adenosylcobalamin deficiency and cause methylmalonic aciduria. Cbl A defect is related to a failure in a reduction step and the second disorder is caused by a failure to transfer adenosyl to Cbl. Cbl mutant C, D and F diseases are associated with combined adenosylcobalamin and methylcobalamin deficiencies. Therefore, patients have usually homocystinuria, hypomethioninemia and methylmalonic aciduria. The C and D defects involve a defective reductase step, whereas the F mutant involves inability of releasing Cbl from the lysosome. The last two disorders in Cbl utilization are Cbl mutant E and G that are related to methylcobalamin deficiency. Methylmalonic acidemia has varying diagnoses, treatment requirements and prognoses, which are determined by the specific genetic mutation causing the inherited form of the disorder (Matsui et al., 1983). A severe nutritional deficiency of Cbl can also result in methylmalonic acidemia (Higginbottom et al., 1978). When the amount of Cbl is insufficient for the conversion of cofactor methylmalonyl-CoA into succinyl-CoA, the build-up of unused methylmalonyl-CoA eventually leads to methylmalonic acidemia. This diagnosis is often used as an indicator of Cbl deficiency in serum.

7.3.4. Acquired causes of cobalamin deficiency

7.3.4.1 Food cobalamin malabsorption

Food cobalamin malabsorption is the most common cause of Cbl deficiency in elderly people (Carmel, 1995). There are several diseases that could cause Cbl malabsorption which is characterized by failure to release Cbl from food or from intestinal transport proteins, particularly in the presence of hypochlorhydria where absorption of 'unbound' Cbl is still normal. Food Cbl malabsorption is distinguished by Cbl deficiency in the presence of sufficient food Cbl and a negative Schilling test which excludes malabsorption or PA (Carmel, 1995; Andres et al., 2003b) (▶Tab. 7.6). It has been reported that 60–70% of elderly subjects with Cbl deficiency suffer from food Cbl malabsorption (Andres et al., 2004, 2005) which is primarily seen in gastric atrophy. More than 40% of people over 80 years of age are affected by gastric atrophy that could be related to H. pylori infection (Andres et al., 2003b; Carmel, 1995). Factors which contribute to food Cbl malabsorption in elderly subjects comprise chronic carriage of H. pylori and intestinal microbial proliferation which is demonstrated by antibiotic treatment (Suter et al., 1991; Kaptan et al., 2000); long-term ingestion of biguanides (metformin) (Bauman et al., 2000; Andres et al., 2002), H2-receptor antagonists and proton pump inhibitors (Howden, 2000; Andres et al., 2003a; Hirschowitz et al., 2008); histamine(2) receptor antagonists (Ruscin et al., 2002); chronic alcoholism (Kaltenbach et al., 1995); gastric surgery; partial pancreatic exocrine failure and Sjögren's syndrome (Andres et al., 2003b; Marinella, 2008).

Tab. 7.6: When cobalamin malabsorption should be suspected.

Atrophic gastritis, chronic *Helicobacter pylori* infection

HIV infection

Chronic alcoholism

Medications that alter gastrointestinal pH such as H2-receptor antagonists, proton pump inhibitors, or biguanides

Gastrectomy, gastric bypass surgery

Pancreatic failure

Unexplained cobalamin deficiency

HoloTC not increased in blood after low oral dose of free cobalamin (up to 30 µg/day)

Sufficient dietary intake, no organic disease but consistent evidence for a metabolic deficiency

Type B chronic atrophic gastritis is related to *H. pylori* infection and is known to cause Cbl malabsorption. This disorder results in a low acid-pepsin production and food Cbl malabsorption. The release of Cbl from food protein is decreased in the case of lowered gastric acidity (Doscherholmen et al., 1977). Importantly, because the production of IF is not affected in Type B atrophic gastritis, affected subjects could benefit from crystalline Cbl. Oral Cbl therapy (3–5 mg/week) was effective in treatment of food-Cbl malabsorption (Andres et al., 2001b).

Celiac disease and tropical spree are also associated with Cbl deficiency. In both cases, recurrent diarrhea causes severe damage to the gastrointestinal tract and interferes with Cbl absorption by the enterocytes. Finally several drugs are known to alter gastrointestinal pH thus causing Cbl malabsorption. ▶Tab. 7.7 summarizes the most important acquired causes of Cbl deficiency.

7.3.4.2 Cobalamin deficiency related to pernicious anemia

PA distinguished by antibodies against IF is the most famous disorder of Cbl absorption and one of the most frequent among elderly patients (up to 50% of the cases) (Andres et al., 2000). In PA as an autoimmune disease, the gastric mucosa, particularly fundal mucosa, will be destroyed by a cell-mediated autoimmune process (Toh et al., 1997). Atrophic gastritis is an autoimmune condition that eventually manifests itself as PA. Antibodies against parietal cells or those against IF are considered characteristics of the disease. Parietal cell antibodies can cause lack of IF and thus Cbl deficiency. In this case, Cbl cannot be absorbed because of the lack of IF. Furthermore, IF antibodies are only detected in about 50% of patients with PA whereas parietal cell antibodies which target the H+/K+ adenosine triphosphatase alpha and beta subunits, are more frequent and found in >90% of PA patients; but their specificity is much lower (50%) (Toh et al., 1997). In a recent study on patients with atrophic gastritis, Cbl deficiency and macrocytic anemia were found in about 50% of the cases and IF antibodies were detected

Tab. 7.7: Acquired causes of cobalamin deficiency.

Disease or condition	Mechanism
Restricted intake	Vegetarians, children of vegetarian mothers, poverty, malnutrition, anorexia nervosa
Increased demands	Bleeding, pregnancy, lactation
Medications	Changing gastrointestinal pH, interaction with vitamin absorption or metabolism
Anti H2 receptor	
Proton pump inhibitors	
Oral contraceptives	
Pernicious anemia (type A atrophic gastritis)	anti-IF antibodies
Antiparital cell antibodies	Lack of IF
Type B atrophic gastritis (*H. pylori*)	Changing gastrointestinal pH
Other gastrointestinal morbidities	Interact with the vitamin absorption
Terminal ileal diseases	
Pancreatic insufficiency	
Ileal or gastric resection	
Celiac disease, tropical spree	
Colitis ulcerosa, Morbus Crohn	

in 27% but parietal cell antibodies were positive in 81% of the atrophic body gastritis patients (Lahner et al., 2009).

Hypergastrinemia has also been associated with PA. It is indicative of PA (sensitivity >80%, specificity <50%) and a positive Schilling test together with IF antibodies confirm the diagnosis (specificity >99%) (Pruthi and Tefferi, 1994). Furthermore, PA is associated with many autoimmune disorders, including vitiligo, dysthyroidia, Addison's disease and Sjögren's syndrome (Chan et al., 2009). It is also associated with an increased frequency of gastric neoplasms: adenocarcinomas, lymphomas and carcinoid tumors (Pruthi and Tefferi, 1994). PA is regarded as the most distinct feature and sequela of autoimmune atrophic gastritis (presence of parietal cell antibodies in 60–90% of cases) which is seen as an independent risk factor for the development of gastric cancer (Neesse et al., 2009). A prospective longitudinal study of Chinese PA patients found that IF antibodies positive patients contracted cancer approximately three times more often than IF antibodies negative patients during follow-up (Chan et al., 2008). Twenty percent of all cancers were gastric carcinoma. It is concluded that IF antibodies positive PA patients have a higher risk of developing all types of cancers and cancer related deaths than IF antibodies negative patients. Furthermore, a recent population based study of autoimmune condition revealed that multiple myeloma was also associated with an increased risk for PA (Anderson et al., 2009).

7.3.4.3 Cobalamin deficiency and immune dysfunction

An increased incidence of tuberclosis in vegetarians, impaired antibody responses to pneumococcal vaccine in elderly patients having a low Cbl status, and abnormal lymphocyte subpopulations in Cbl deficient subjects with megaloblastic anemia supports a role for Cbl in immune function (Solomon, 2007). As mentioned above, autoimmune gastritis and PA are common autoimmune disorders, being present in up to 2% of the general population. In addition, patients with Type 1 diabetes mellitus also have an increased prevalence of associated organ-specific autoimmune diseases such as PA (Alonso et al., 2009).

There is also an association of Cbl deficiency and HIV. In a retrospective review of a HIV-infected outpatient cohort, within 2 years of their initial HIV presentation, about 10% developed a low serum Cbl (Hepburn et al., 2004). In another study on HIV-infected patients low vitamin Cbl and red blood cell folate concentrations were observed in 20% and 10% of the patients (Remacha et al., 2003). Therefore, low serum Cbl levels occur commonly among HIV-infected patients, even at early disease stages without overt symptoms of Cbl deficiency. Antiretroviral therapy might cause a secondary increase of serum Cbl concentrations that might not be used as a marker for cobalamin status in this case. Additionally, low serum concentrations of Cbl have been associated with increased neurological abnormalities and more rapid HIV disease progression (Tang and Smit, 1998).

To clarify the role of Cbl in the immunological function, serum complement C3, IgM, IgG, IgE contents, splenocytes expression of CD4, CD8 and CD4 positive intracellular IFN-gamma and IL-4 were examined in Cbl-deficient mice, and the effect of the administration of MeCbl was studied. These results suggest that Cbl deficiency causes CD4+CD8- T cells shift from the T helper type 1 to the T helper type 2, which participate in the IgE production and elevate CD4+CD8-/CD4-CD8+ ratio. Therefore, vitamin B12 plays a role in maintaining the immune function (Funada et al., 2000, 2001).

Sjögren's syndrome is an autoimmune disorder in which immune cells attack and destroy the exocrine glands that produce tears and saliva (Delaleu et al., 2008). In a study by Andres et al. (Andres et al., 2001a), Sjögren's syndrome was the cause of 3.75% of cases with familial Cbl malabsorption and 2.4% of all cases of Cbl deficiency. The pathogenesis of this association is not known, but several mechanisms could be involved, such as a low haptocorrin level related to cellular immune infiltration of salivary glands, achlorhydria related to gastric infiltration and/or mild pancreatic insufficiency (Sheikh and Shaw-Stiffel, 1995).

7.3.4.4 Cobalamin deficiency related to a low intake or increased requirement of the vitamin

7.3.4.4.1 Cobalamin deficiency and vegetarian life style

Chronic low intake of Cbl can cause severe deficiency. Cbl deficiency takes years to develop, even when one stops to ingest the vitamin. This is related to the relatively large body stores of Cbl, in addition to the effective enterohepatic circulation that ensures reabsorption of the vitamin. Natural Cbl sources in the human diet are restricted to foods of animal origin (Herbert, 1988). Subjects who adhere to a life long strict vegetarian diet develop Cbl deficiency (Herbert, 1994; Herrmann et al., 2003c). Because milk and eggs contain a low amount of Cbl, the intake of Cbl in a lacto- and lacto-ovo-vegetarian diet might be sufficient. Nevertheless, studies have shown that Cbl status (indicated by MMA, holoTC, and tHcy) was lower in lacto- and lacto-ovo-vegetarians compared with omnivorous subjects (Herrmann et al., 2003c). In addition, metabolic signs of Cbl deficiency were more common in vegans compared with lacto- and lacto-ovo-vegetarians (Herrmann et al., 2003c). Chronic low intake of Cbl and its deficiency could be endemic in developing countries and is related to poverty and malnutrition in this case (Refsum et al., 2001; Herrmann et al., 2003a, 2009b; Rogers et al., 2003).

Cbl status is directly correlated with dietary intake and length of time following a vegetarian diet (Chanarin et al., 1985; Miller et al., 1991). Serum concentrations of MMA, holoTC, tHcy and total Cbl are related to the type of the diet (►Tab. 7.8). According to the strictness of the diet, approximately 30–60% of vegetarian subjects might have metabolic evidence indicating Cbl deficiency (Rauma et al., 1995; Donaldson, 2000). Vegan subjects had the lowest Cbl status. This is expected, because a vegan diet includes no types of animal foods. Although lacto- and lacto-ovo-vegetarians consume some animal foods (egg, milk and milk products), metabolic signs of Cbl deficiency were also common in this group (Herrmann et al., 2003c) (►Tab. 7.8). This group of vegetarians show intermediate Cbl status compared with vegans and omnivorous (Herrmann et al., 2003c). In this study 45% of subjects with low holoTC and elevated MMA had normal serum Cbl levels (►Fig. 7.5). Additionally, low doses of Cbl such as the one usually found in the multivitamin preparations are not likely to prevent the depletion of the vitamin in individuals who ingest little or no animal products.

The most common cause of vitamin deficiency at early childhood is being born or lactated by a vitamin-deficient mother. A serious neurological syndrome and developmental disorders have been described in few exclusively breast-fed infants of strict vegetarian

Tab. 7.8: Cobalamin status in vegetarian and non-vegetarian subjects.

	Omnivorous (n = 79)	LOV/LV (n = 66)	Vegan (n = 29)
Cobalamin, pmol/l	287 (190/471)	192 (127/450)[a]	148 (99/314)[a,b]
HoloTC, pmol/l	54 (16/122)	23 (3/155)[a]	10 (2/78)[a,b]
MMA, nmol/l	161 (95/357)	355 (138/1948)[a]	708 (193/3470)[1,2]
tHcy, μmol/l	8.8 (5.5/16.1)	10.6 (6.4/27.7)[a]	12.8 (5.9/57.1)[a]
Folate, nmol/l	21.8 (14.5/51.5)	28.8 (16.1/77)[a]	31.8 (19.7/78.1)[1]

Data are median (5th/95th). $p < 0.05$: [a]compared with omnivorous controls; [b]comparing LOV/LV with vegans. LOV/LV, lacto-ovo/lacto-vegetarians.

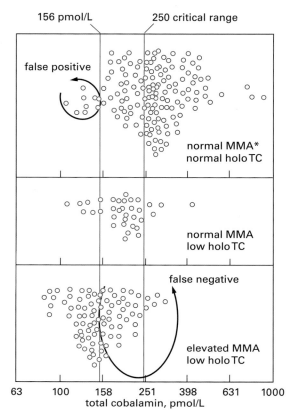

Fig. 7.5: Serum concentrations of cobalamin in subjects with normal holoTC and MMA and in those with at least one pathological test. Only subjects with normal concentration of serum creatinine are included in this figure. *Normal cobalamin status defined as MMA ≤ 271 nmol/L/ holo TC > 35 pmol/L.

mothers who were Cbl deficient (Higginbottom et al., 1978; Kuhne et al., 1991). Cbl deficiency in infants is associated with a marked developmental regression, poor brain growth or a poor intellectual outcome. Other signs include impaired communicative reactions and fine and gross motor functions. Low Cbl status had also negative influence on school achievement in schoolchildren. Prolonged insufficient intake of the vitamin is also a common case of Cbl deficiency in children. Adolescents previously consumed a macrobiotic diet had lower scores in some measures of cognitive performance as compared with adolescents who consumed an omnivorous diet from birth onwards (Louwman et al., 2000). Cbl deficiency should be suspected in children with unexplained neurological symptoms, failure to thrive, or poor intellectual performance. Attention should be paid to familial factors (maternal vitamin status), and predisposing environmental factors (poverty, vegetarian diet).

Cbl induced macrocytosis can be masked when iron status is in a state of negative balance (Van der Weyden et al., 1972; Spivak, 1982). In vegetarians, hematological parameters in relation to Cbl and iron status have been studied by our group (Obeid et al., 2002). Lower lymphocytes and platelets counts and higher MCV were found in some Cbl deficient subjects. Significantly higher MCV was seen in Cbl deficient subjects who had higher iron status than that in Cbl-deficient subjects with lower iron status. Macrocytosis (MCV >97 fl) was presented in only 5% of the vegetarian subjects. Megaloblastic anemia was not invariably presented in long-term Cbl deficient subjects (Carmel et al., 1987; Refsum et al., 2001). Folic acid in excess can ameliorate the megaloblastic shape of red blood cells in Cbl-deficient subjects (Hoffbrand and Jackson, 1993).

7.3.4.4.2 Cobalamin deficiency during pregnancy and early life

The requirements for B vitamins (folate, Cbl, and vitamin B6) are exceptionally high during pregnancy as a result of increased maternal metabolic rate and fetal demands (Heller et al., 1973). Maternal nutritional status before and during pregnancy is the main determinant of the nutritional status of the offspring (Bjorke Monsen et al., 2001; Murphy et al., 2004). Folate, Cbl and vitamin B6 function as cofactors in one-carbon metabolism, DNA synthesis and numerous methylation reactions. These metabolic pathways are particularly active in developing embryos. Cbl deficiency can occur in women who do not ingest a sufficient amount of the vitamin. Metabolic and clinical signs of Cbl deficiency have been reported in newborn babies from strict vegetarian mothers or in breast-fed infants from deficient mothers (Dagnelie et al., 1989; Graham et al., 1992; Schneede et al., 1994; Bjorke Monsen et al., 2001). These conditions were partly reversible after Cbl supplementation. The content of Cbl in mother milk was related to markers of Cbl deficiency in the infants (Bjorke Monsen et al., 2001). This explains the finding that exclusively breast-fed babies from deficient mothers are at increased risk for developing metabolic and clinical signs of deficiency.

Several studies investigated B vitamin status in pregnant women and their newborns (Guerra-Shinohara et al., 2002; Molloy et al., 2002; Obeid et al., 2005d). Studies of neonates (aged 3 days to 6 months) have shown markedly higher serum concentrations of plasma tHcy and MMA in these infants than in older children (Monsen et al., 2003). Moreover, concentrations of plasma tHcy and MMA were higher in newborns 6 weeks after birth than at birth (Bjorke Monsen et al., 2001). However, most neonates remain virtually asymptomatic. Elevated concentrations of plasma tHcy in neonates are related to higher concentrations of MMA, cystathionine, or methionine (Monsen et al., 2003; Refsum et al., 2004). By contrast, in the case of older children, metabolic changes were associated with lower concentrations of Cbl rather than folate (Monsen et al., 2003). Therefore, a transient inadequate Cbl status and a disturbed transmethylation at this age have been suspected (Monsen et al., 2003; Refsum et al., 2004).

Concentrations of MMA were found to be higher in cord blood than in maternal blood and the concentrations of cord blood MMA were predicted by cord Cbl and maternal MMA and Cbl concentrations (Obeid et al., 2005d). Moreover, lower cord MMA was associated with larger differences between cord blood and maternal concentrations of Cbl, but not with higher maternal concentrations of Cbl (▶Fig. 7.6). These results suggest a rate-limiting step in the transplacental transport of Cbl. Because most pregnant

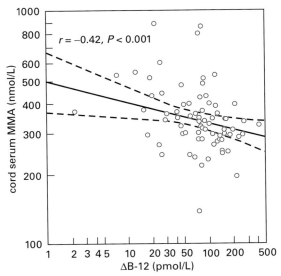

Fig. 7.6: Scatterplot representing the correlation between concentrations of MMA in cord serum and the difference in Cbl concentrations between cord and maternal sera (ΔB12). The correlation coefficient and *p* value are according to Spearman's test. Data on both the *x* and the *y* axes are anti-log.

women receive folic acid containing supplements containing 0–3 µg Cbl/day, special emphasis should be placed on ensuring adequate intake of Cbl during pregnancy.

MMA elevation in newborns from non-deficient mothers might also be a part of a general adaptation of the newborn to extrauterine life, in which the activities of many enzymes are under stress and must independently satisfy the high metabolic rate during postnatal life. Some authors argue that elevated concentrations of MMA that are reversible by Cbl supplementation in many newborns might indicate a low Cbl status (Ueland and Monsen, 2003). However, Cbl supplement could enhance the expression or function of Cbl dependent enzymes thus lowering MMA.

7.3.5 Cobalamin deficiency in elderly people

Cbl deficiency in geriatric population has gained a particular importance in recent years (Baik and Russell, 1999; Obeid et al., 2004). Serum concentration of Cbl decreases with age and that of MMA and tHcy increase. The incidence rate of Cbl deficiency in the elderly ranges between 10 and 40%, depending on the marker used to rule out the deficiency (Lindenbaum et al., 1994; Herrmann et al., 2000; Morris et al., 2002; Sipponen et al., 2003). Several age-related physiological factors could negatively influence the absorption of the vitamin from the intestine.

On the one hand, the decline in Cbl status with age could not be explained by a low dietary intake of the vitamin. In most studies on elderly people, the daily ingested amount of Cbl was above the RDI for Cbl. This deficiency is not presumed to be associated with dietary causes but rather with malabsorption (Howard et al., 1998). Fifty-three percent of elderly patients from the Strasbourg study who had Cbl deficiency had malabsorption problems and 33% had PA; in only 2% was Cbl deficiency related to insufficient dietary intake, and in 11% the etiology of the Cbl deficiency remained unexplained (Henoun et al., 2005). However, because the current RDI for Cbl in elderly people is low, dietary deficiencies are underestimated.

On the other hand, it is well recognized that low Cbl status in the elderly is associated with an increased incidence of PA (type A atrophic gastritis), and type B atrophic gastritis. In western countries, approximately 2–3% of free living elderly people (>60 years) had undiagnosed PA (Krasinski et al., 1986; Carmel, 1996). Ethnic differences in the incidence of PA and the age of onset have been reported (Carmel and Johnson, 1978). In one study on elderly subjects [n = 228, mean age 81 (69–90) years] we found that 16% had a low serum concentration of holoTC and an elevated MMA, which indicate a relatively late stage of Cbl deficiency (Herrmann et al., 2005a). Seven percent of the elderly subjects had only low holoTC that might suggest a depletion state where the functional metabolic markers (MMA and tHcy) are normal. Furthermore, 20% of the elderly subjects had an elevated concentration of MMA but a normal holoTC, in addition to a higher concentration of serum creatinine. The relation between holoTC and MMA has been examined in relation to age and renal function (Obeid et al., 2004) (▶Fig. 7.7). In general, elderly people display higher MMA concentrations in ranges of holoTC comparable with that in younger subjects. This phenomenon was more pronounced in elderly with renal insufficiency. The latter findings suggest that cellular Cbl-delivery could be challenged in elderly with renal insufficiency, leading to MMA increment and holoTC retention.

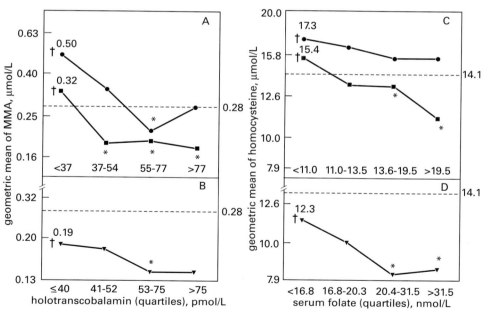

Fig. 7.7: (A and B) geometric means of MMA in quartiles of holoTC: (C and D), geometric means of tHcy in quartiles of folate.▼, younger adults (n = 74); ■, older adults with creatinine within the reference interval (n = 130); ●, older adults with increased creatinine (n = 98). *, p < 0.05 compared with the reference group († indicates the reference group, ANOVA and Tamhane tests).

Using synthetic Cbl preparations can protect elderly persons from symptoms of deficiency (Rajan et al., 2002a). Dietary intake of Cbl does not provide any information on Cbl status because malabsorption is a common and important factor (Herrmann and Obeid, 2009). The incidence of *H. pylori* is high in elderly people and can lead to atrophic gastritis, and in turn to Cbl malabsorption, owing to disrupted production of hydrochloric acid (Sipponen et al., 2003). *H. pylori* was found in 56% of patients with Cbl deficiency (Kaptan et al., 2000). In 40% of the patients, serum concentrations of Cbl rose after treatment for *H. pylori* infection. According to recent reports, long-term treatment of *H. pylori* (1 year) resulted in a significant rise in mean Cbl (from 146 to 271 pmol/l) and a fall in mean tHcy concentrations (from 41 to 13 μmol/l) (Marino et al., 2007).

Elderly people seem to be resistant to low oral doses of Cbl (Rajan et al., 2002b). Serum concentrations of MMA were not normalized in most Cbl-deficient elderly people who received crystalline Cbl in doses between 25 and 100 μg (Rajan et al., 2002b). The RDI of Cbl for older adults (2.4 μg/day) is far below the dose likely to normalize serum concentrations of the metabolites in elderly people.

Disturbed renal function in elderly population should be considered when judging Cbl status. A low Cbl status in elderly people with renal insufficiency might be overlooked by using holoTC or Cbl as a sole marker determining Cbl status, because these markers are mostly within the reference range. Contrary, the occurrence of low Cbl status might be overestimated using the MMA test, because an unknown portion of this increment is related to renal insufficiency. The presence of a low serum concentration of holoTC and an elevated MMA in elderly people strongly suggest Cbl deficiency, but the absence of the combined results might not exclude a deficiency. A significant reduction of MMA after Cbl treatment might indicate a pre-treatment low status of the vitamin.

7.3.5.1 Diseases associated with cobalamin deficiency

7.3.5.1.1 Cobalamin deficiency and neurological complications

Low concentrations of folate, Cbl and/or B6 are common in dementia patients (Obeid and Herrmann, 2006; Herrmann et al., 2007e). Cobalamin and folate are very important for the synthesis of DNA and different methylation reactions that take place in the brain (methylation of DNA, RNA, myelin, phospholipids, receptors and neurotransmitters). According to this, patients with neuropsychiatric disorders had reduced levels of SAM as the active methyl group donor in cerebrospinal fluid (Weir and Scott, 1999). Additionally, in Alzheimer's disease (AD) patients, the SAM levels post-mortem were very low in the brain and cerebrospinal fluid (Morrison et al., 1996; Weir and Scott, 1999). Disorders of methylation capacity might enhance formation of β-amyloid and tau proteins in brains of AD patients (Scarpa et al., 2003). In subjects older than 70 years, the incidence of AD doubled with low Cbl (<150 pmol/l) in comparison with subjects with higher vitamin concentrations (Wang et al., 2001). Dementia has also been linked to low serum concentrations of holoTC, the metabolically active form of Cbl (McCaddon et al., 2001). Low concentrations of Cbl in serum and/or cerebrospinal fluid were found in patients with dementia (Clarke et al., 1998). Additionally, serum concentrations of B-vitamins were negatively related to deficits in neurocognitive tests (Graham et al., 1997). The association between Cbl deficiency and depression has also been documented in elderly women (Penninx et al., 2000). Moreover, peripheral neuropathy occurred in 40% of Cbl-deficient subjects (Shorvon et al., 1980). Cbl deficiency can cause lesions in spinal cord, peripheral nerves and cerebrum, and improvements have been reported after initiation of vitamin treatment (Masalha et al., 2001; Lorenzl et al., 2003). The neurological symptoms in older people, whose high tHcy and/or low Cbl concentrations were normalized through substitution with B vitamins, tended to improve after long-term follow-up treatment (Bjorkegren and Svardsudd, 2004; McCaddon, 2006). The most common symptoms are sensory disturbances in the extremities, memory loss, dementia and psychosis.

7.3.5.1.2 Cobalamin deficiency and osteoporosis

Osteoporosis is a frequent disease of elderly persons with often devastating consequences for the affected individuals (Cummings and Melton, 2002; Melton III, 2003). Recent epidemiologic studies have linked low circulating Cbl and high tHcy concentrations to low bone mineral density (BMD) and fragility fractures, typical symptoms of osteoporosis (Dhonukshe-Rutten et al., 2003, 2005a; McLean et al., 2004, 2008; van Meurs et al., 2004). Experimental *in vivo* and *in vitro* studies suggest direct effects of Hcy and Cbl on bone and bone metabolism (Herrmann et al., 2007a,c,d, 2008; Ozdem et al., 2007). Kim et al., demonstrated that Cbl stimulates proliferation and functional maturation of human bone marrow stromal osteoprogenitor cells and UMR106 osteoblastic cells as assessed by [^{3}H]thymidine incorporation and bone alkaline phosphatase activity (Kim et al., 1996). It was concluded that a suppressed activity of osteoblasts might contribute to osteoporosis and fractures in patients with Cbl deficiency. Studies on human osteoclasts revealed a distinct activation of osteoclasts with decreasing concentrations of folate, Cbl and B6 (Herrmann et al., 2007a). Therefore, Cbl seems to have a regulatory role in bone resorption. Accordingly, Carmel et al., reported lower concentrations of the bone formation markers bone alkaline phosphatase and osteocalcin in Cbl-deficient patients compared with subjects with adequate vitamin status (Carmel et al., 1988).

Despite convincing evidence from experimental studies, clinical studies investigating Cbl status, fracture risk and BMD are not consistent. Some studies found an association between Cbl and fracture risk or BMD whereas others did not observe such an association (Herrmann et al., 2007b). However, the importance of Cbl for bone health has been supported by clinical data where patients with low Cbl status or PA exhibited low BMD, increased fracture rate and accelerated bone turnover that could be improved by Cbl supplementation (Carmel et al., 1988; Goerss et al., 1992; Melton and Kochman, 1994).

Considering the potential association between Cbl and bone health it can be assumed that vegetarians might be particularly prone to disturbances of bone metabolism, accelerated bone loss and fragility fractures (Chiu et al., 1997). Data regarding bone health in vegetarians, however, are conflicting. Whereas some studies have reported decreased BMD in vegetarians (Chiu et al., 1997; Dhonukshe-Rutten et al., 2005b;

Fontana et al., 2005) others did not (Ellis et al., 1972; Wang et al., 2008). An association between Cbl status and BMD in vegetarians was first observed in a group of formerly macrobiotic-fed adolescents (Dhonukshe-Rutten et al., 2005b). Decreased levels of total Cbl and high concentrations of MMA were associated with low BMD. The EPIC-Oxford study including 9420 vegetarians and 1126 vegans revealed an increased fracture risk in vegans only (Appleby et al., 2007). In a recent study on vegetarians (Herrmann et al., 2009b), we demonstrated that vegetarians with low Cbl status (holoTC <35 pmol/l and MMA >271 nmol/l) had significantly higher plasma concentrations of the bone turnover markers bone alkaline phosphatase, osteocalcin, pro-collagen type I N-terminal peptide and C-terminal telopeptides of collagen 1. The inconsistent findings from different studies might be related to the duration and the strictness of the vegetarian diet on the one hand, and to the status of vitamin D, another important vitamin for bone metabolism, on the other hand. Additionally, chronic cobalamin deficiency occurring in childhood age, where bone formation is highly active, might have devastating effects on bone health. Furthermore, long-standing cobalamin deficiency might have significant effects on bone health in elderly people, where bone formation is less active.

7.3.6 Cobalamin deficiency and renal insufficiency

Cbl deficiency is common in renal patients. Nevertheless, diagnosing Cbl deficiency in renal patients remains a challenge. Renal insufficiency causes elevation of MMA and total Hcy (Savage et al., 1994; Stabler et al., 1996; Herrmann et al., 2001a). Unexpectedly low serum concentrations of Cbl or holoTC are uncommon in patients with renal insufficiency (Herrmann et al., 2005a). However, renal patients show significant metabolic improvements (reduction of MMA) after treatment with Cbl (Obeid et al., 2005c). The reasons for elevated serum Cbl (total Cbl and holoTC) in renal patients are not known. An abnormal distribution of holoTC (Carmel et al., 2001), a disturbed receptor activity for renal transcobalamin uptake and the possibility that transcobalamin is functionally altered by renal failure are possible explanations for accumulation of Cbl in serum of renal patients.

   Cbl deficiency is a major health problem in elderly population who also have a high prevalence of renal insufficiency which markedly affects Cbl-dependent metabolism (Lindenbaum et al., 1994; Morris et al., 2002; Sipponen et al., 2003). In one study on older subjects, 20% had an elevated concentration of MMA and a normal holoTC, in addition to an elevated concentration of serum creatinine (Herrmann et al., 2005b). This typical metabolic profile associated with impaired renal function might complicate and delay the laboratory diagnosis of Cbl deficiency. This could suggest that the retention of holoTC might be a general phenomenon in subjects with renal insufficiency. We studied the relation between holoTC and MMA in young subjects and in elderly people according to their renal function (Obeid et al., 2004) (►Fig. 7.7). According to the results, elderly people had, compared with younger subjects, a comparable holoTC range whereas their MMA concentrations were significantly higher. This was even more distinct in elderly subjects who suffered from renal insufficiency. The latter findings support the hypothesis that cellular Cbl-delivery might be restricted in elderly patients with renal insufficiency, leading to an increment of MMA and holoTC retention. In line with this suggestion, elderly people seemed to be resistant to low oral doses of Cbl (Rajan et al., 2002b).

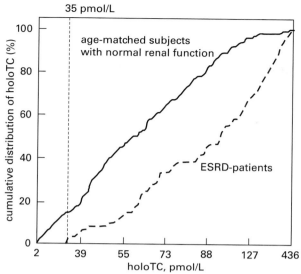

Fig. 7.8: The cumulative distribution of serum concentrations of holoTC in dialysis patients compared with age-matched controls with normal renal function (normal creatinine).

Chronic hemodialysis patients are a group of high risk for Cbl deficiency (Henning et al., 2001; Herrmann et al., 2003b). In one study, we observed higher concentrations of holoTC in patients on hemodialysis than in normal subjects (median holoTC 100 vs 61 pmol/l) which at first seemed inconsistent with the supposed Cbl deficiency (Herrmann et al., 2005a). Furthermore, the distribution of serum concentrations of holoTC was shifted towards a higher range compared with a group of age-matched subjects with normal renal function (▶Fig. 7.8). By contrast, serum concentrations of MMA were severely elevated in dialysis patients (median MMA 987 nmol/l; normal <271 nmol/l). However, it is not known how much of the MMA elevation comes from Cbl deficiency and how much comes from renal insufficiency (Lindgren, 2002).

As mentioned above, reasons behind holoTC increment in renal patients are not fully understood. Dialysis patients have a negligible residual renal function. Therefore, holoTC is neither filtered nor reabsorbed in the proximal tubule. This could participate in the retention of holoTC in plasma compartments. Additionally, the short half-life of holoTC in serum and the accumulation of this portion in renal failure might suggest an increment in the rate of its synthesis. We found that severely increased concentrations of MMA in renal patients were associated with high serum concentrations of holoTC. In addition, intervention studies on renal patients demonstrated that supra-physiological doses of Cbl significantly reduce serum MMA (▶Fig. 7.9) and normalize tHcy, despite normal pre-treatment serum concentration of the vitamin (Henning et al., 2001; Hoffer and Elian, 2004; Obeid et al., 2005c). Thus, serum Cbl levels within the reference range in renal patients are not likely to ensure Cbl delivery into the cells. These findings suggest that cellular uptake of holoTC faces a resistance in the peripheral tissues which participate in its retention and have been proven in cell culture experiments (Obeid et al., 2005a). It is concluded that Cbl uptake might be impaired in renal patients.

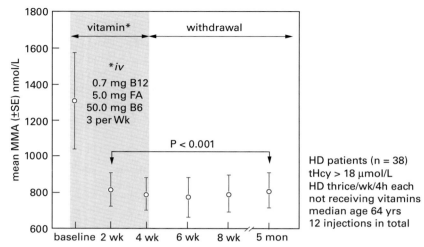

Fig. 7.9: Response of MMA to vitamin treatment in dialysis patients. SE; standard error. HD; hemodialysis.

7.3.7 Conclusions

Cbl deficiency is widespread among elderly people, patients with unexplained anemia, patients with unexplained neuropsychiatric symptoms, vegetarians, patients with intestinal diseases (such as Crohn's disease, infection with *H. pylori*, or stomach resection), and patients with gastrointestinal manifestations (stomatitis, anorexia and diarrhea). Food Cbl malabsorption is the most common cause of Cbl deficiency in elderly people and is characterized by the inability to release Cbl from food or from transporting proteins in the presence of sufficient food Cbl. Cbl malabsorption related to an autoimmune disease (PA) is also common in elderly people.

Further risk groups for Cbl deficiency are persons with an increased vitamin requirement – such as pregnant and breast-feeding women, patients with autoimmune disorders or persons with HIV infection. Metabolic and clinical signs of Cbl deficiency have been reported in newborn babies from strict vegetarian mothers or in breast-fed infants from deficient mothers. The most common cause of vitamin deficiency at early childhood is being born or lactated by a vitamin-deficient mother (vegetarian life style). Cbl deficiency in infants is associated with a marked developmental regression, poor brain growth or poor intellectual outcome. Furthermore, persons who regularly take proton pump inhibitors can also develop Cbl deficiency. Cbl deficiency is also widespread in patients with renal dysfunction, despite normal plasma concentrations of Cbl or holoTC. These markers do not indicate Cbl deficiency in renal patients because of raised serum concentrations of MMA and total Hcy which can be lowered by Cbl supplementation.

Total serum Cbl is a late, relatively insensitive and unspecific biomarker of deficiency that does not reflect recent variations in Cbl status. HoloTC, the metabolically active portion of Cbl, is an early laboratory parameter that becomes decreased in case of a negative Cbl balance. Serum concentration of MMA is a functional Cbl marker that increases when the Cbl stores are depleted. Because the clinical manifestations of Cbl deficiency are unspecific, people at risk should be identified be treated, and should regularly test their Cbl status.

The neurological symptoms of Cbl deficiency can be irreversible. Early detection is therefore important and depends on using the available laboratory metabolic markers. Recent epidemiologic studies have linked low circulating Cbl to low bone BMD and fragility fractures, typical symptoms of osteoporosis. Experimental *in vivo* and *in vitro* studies suggest direct effects of Cbl on bone and bone metabolism.

References

Alonso N, Soldevila B, Sanmarti A, Pujol-Borrell R, Martinez-Caceres E, Regulatory T cells in diabetes and gastritis. Autoimmun Rev 2009;8: 659–62.

Anderson LA, Gadalla S, Morton LM, Landgren O, Pfeiffer R, Warren JL, Berndt SI, Ricker W, Parsons R, Engels EA, Population-based study of autoimmune conditions and the risk of specific lymphoid malignancies. Int J Cancer 2009;125: 398–405.

Andres E, Goichot B, Schlienger JL, Food cobalamin malabsorption: a usual cause of vitamin B12 deficiency. Arch Intern Med 2000;160: 2061–2.

Andres E, Goichot B, Perrin AE, Vinzio S, Demangeat C, Schlienger JL, Sjogren's syndrome: a potential new aetiology of mild cobalamin deficiency. Rheumatology (Oxford) 2001a;40: 1196–7.

Andres E, Kurtz JE, Perrin AE, Maloisel F, Demangeat C, Goichot B, Schlienger JL, Oral cobalamin therapy for the treatment of patients with food- cobalamin malabsorption. Am J Med 2001b;111: 126–9.

Andres E, Noel E, Goichot B, Metformin-associated vitamin B12 deficiency. Arch Intern Med 2002;162: 2251–2.

Andres E, Noel E, Abdelghani MB, Vitamin B(12) deficiency associated with chronic acid suppression therapy. Ann Pharmacother 2003a;37: 1730.

Andres E, Perrin AE, Demangeat C, Kurtz JE, Vinzio S, Grunenberger F, Goichot B, Schlienger JL, The syndrome of food-cobalamin malabsorption revisited in a department of internal medicine. A monocentric cohort study of 80 patients. Eur J Intern Med 2003b;14: 221–6.

Andres E, Loukili NH, Noel E, Kaltenbach G, Abdelgheni MB, Perrin AE, Noblet-Dick M, Maloisel F, Schlienger JL, Blickle JF, Vitamin B12 (cobalamin) deficiency in elderly patients. Can Med Assoc J 2004;171: 251–9.

Andres E, Affenberger S, Vinzio S, Kurtz JE, Noel E, Kaltenbach G, Maloisel F, Schlienger JL, Blickle JF, Food-cobalamin malabsorption in elderly patients: clinical manifestations and treatment. Am J Med 2005;118: 1154–9.

Appleby P, Roddam A, Allen N, Key T, Comparative fracture risk in vegetarians and nonvegetarians in EPIC-Oxford. Eur J Clin Nutr 2007;61: 1400–6.

Baik HW, Russell RM, Vitamin B12 deficiency in the elderly. Annu Rev Nutr 1999;19: 357–77.

Bauman WA, Shaw S, Jayatilleke E, Spungen AM, Herbert V, Increased intake of calcium reverses vitamin B12 malabsorption induced by metformin. Diabetes Care 2000;23: 1227–31.

Ben-Ami M, Katzuni E, Koren A, Imerslund syndrome with dolichocephaly. Pediatr Hematol Oncol 1990;7: 177–81.

Bibi H, Gelman-Kohan Z, Baumgartner ER, Rosenblatt DS, Transcobalamin II deficiency with methylmalonic aciduria in three sisters. J Inherit Metab Dis 1999;22: 765–72.

Bjorke Monsen AL, Ueland PM, Vollset SE, Guttormsen AB, Markestad T, Solheim E, Refsum H, Determinants of cobalamin status in newborns. Pediatrics 2001;108: 624–30.

Bjorkegren K, Svardsudd K, A population-based intervention study on elevated serum levels of methylmalonic acid and total homocysteine in elderly people: results after 36 months of follow-up. J Intern Med 2004;256: 446–52.

Bor MV, Lydeking-Olsen E, Moller J, Nexo E, A daily intake of approximately 6 microg vitamin B-12 appears to saturate all the vitamin B-12-related variables in Danish postmenopausal women. Am J Clin Nutr 2006;83: 52–8.

Carmel R, The distribution of endogenous cobalamin among cobalamin-binding proteins in the blood in normal and abnormal states. Am J Clin Nutr 1985;41: 713–9.

Carmel R, Malabsorption of food-cobalamin. In: Wickramasinghe SN, editor. *Baillière's clinical haematology. Megaloblastic anaemia, vol. 8.* London: Baillière Tindall; 1995. pp. 639–55.

Carmel R, Prevalence of undiagnosed pernicious anemia in the elderly. Arch Intern Med 1996;156: 1097–100.

Carmel R, Cobalamin, the stomach, and aging. Am J Clin Nutr 1997;66: 750–9.

Carmel R, Johnson CS, Racial patterns in pernicious anemia. Early age at onset and increased frequency of intrinsic-factor antibody in black women. N Engl J Med 1978;298: 647–50.

Carmel R, Sinow RM, Karnaze DS, Atypical cobalamin deficiency. Subtle biochemical evidence of deficiency is commonly demonstrable in patients without megaloblastic anemia and is often associated with protein-bound cobalamin malabsorption. J Lab Clin Med 1987;109: 454–63.

Carmel R, Lau KH, Baylink DJ, Saxena S, Singer FR, Cobalamin and osteoblast-specific proteins. N Engl J Med 1988;319: 70–5.

Carmel R, Vasireddy H, Aurangzeb I, George K, High serum cobalamin levels in the clinical setting–clinical associations and holo-transcobalamin changes. Clin Lab Haematol 2001;23: 365–71.

Chan JC, Liu HS, Kho BC, Lau TK, Li VL, Chan FH, Leong IS, Pang HK, Lee CK, Liang YS, Longitudinal study of Chinese patients with pernicious anaemia. Postgrad Med J 2008;84: 644–50.

Chan JC, Liu HS, Kho BC, Lau TK, Li VL, Chan FH, Leong IS, Pang HK, Lee CK, Liang YS, Pattern of thyroid autoimmunity in Chinese patients with pernicious anemia. Am J Med Sci 2009;337: 432–7.

Chanarin I, Malkowska V, O'Hea AM, Rinsler MG, Price AB, Megaloblastic anaemia in a vegetarian Hindu community. Lancet 1985;2: 1168–72.

Chiu JF, Lan SJ, Yang CY, Wang PW, Yao WJ, Su LH, Hsieh CC, Long-term vegetarian diet and bone mineral density in postmenopausal Taiwanese women. Calcif Tissue Int 1997;60: 245–9.

Clarke R, Smith AD, Jobst KA, Refsum H, Sutton L, Ueland PM, Folate, vitamin B12, and serum total homocysteine levels in confirmed Alzheimer disease. Arch Neurol 1998;55: 1449–55.

Clarke R, Grimley EJ, Schneede J, Nexo E, Bates C, Fletcher A, Prentice A, Johnston C, Ueland PM, Refsum H, Sherliker P, Birks J, Whitlock G, Breeze E, Scott JM, Vitamin B12 and folate deficiency in later life. Age Ageing 2004;33: 34–41.

Cooper BA, Rosenblatt DS, Inherited defects of vitamin B12 metabolism. Annu Rev Nutr 1987;7: 291–320.

Cummings SR, Melton LJ, Epidemiology and outcomes of osteoporotic fractures. Lancet 2002;359: 1761–7.

Dagnelie PC, van Staveren WA, Vergote FJ, Dingjan PG, van den BH, Hautvast JG, Increased risk of vitamin B-12 and iron deficiency in infants on macrobiotic diets. Am J Clin Nutr 1989;50: 818–24.

Delaleu N, Immervoll H, Cornelius J, Jonsson R, Biomarker profiles in serum and saliva of experimental Sjogren's syndrome: associations with specific autoimmune manifestations. Arthritis Res Ther 2008;10: R22.

Dhonukshe-Rutten RA, Lips M, de JN, Chin APM, Hiddink GJ, Van DM, de Groot LC, van Staveren WA, Vitamin B-12 status is associated with bone mineral content and bone mineral density in frail elderly women but not in men. J Nutr 2003;133: 801–7.

Dhonukshe-Rutten RA, Pluijm SM, de Groot LC, Lips P, Smit JH, van Staveren WA, Homocysteine and vitamin B12 status relate to bone turnover markers, broadband ultrasound attenuation, and fractures in healthy elderly people. J Bone Miner Res 2005a;20: 921–9.

Dhonukshe-Rutten RA, Van DM, Schneede J, de Groot LC, van Staveren WA, Low bone mineral density and bone mineral content are associated with low cobalamin status in adolescents. Eur J Nutr 2005b;44: 341–7.

Donaldson MS, Metabolic vitamin B12 status on a mostly raw vegan diet with follow-up using tablets, nutritional yeast, or probiotic supplements. Ann Nutr Metab 2000;44: 229–34.

Doscherholmen A, Ripley D, Chang S, Silvis SE, Influence of age and stomach function on serum vitamin B12 concentration. Scand J Gastroenterol 1977;12: 313–9.

Ellis FR, Holesh S, Ellis JW, Incidence of osteoporosis in vegetarians and omnivores. Am J Clin Nutr 1972;25: 555–8.

England JM, Down MC, Wise IJ, Linnell JC, The transport of endogenous vitamin B12 in normal human serum. Clin Sci Mol Med 1976;51: 47–52.

Fontana L, Shew JL, Holloszy JO, Villareal DT, Low bone mass in subjects on a long-term raw vegetarian diet. Arch Intern Med 2005;165: 684–9.

Funada U, Wada M, Kawata T, Mori K, Tamai H, Isshiki T, Onoda J, Tanaka N, Tadokoro T, Maekawa A, Vitamin B-12-deficiency affects immunoglobulin production and cytokine levels in mice. Int J Vitam Nutr Res 2001;71: 60–5.

Funada U, Wada M, Kawata T, Mori K, Tamai H, Kawanishi T, Kunou A, Tanaka N, Tadokoro T, Maekawa A, Changes in CD4+CD8-/CD4-CD8+ ratio and humoral immune functions in vitamin B12-deficient rats. Int J Vitam Nutr Res 2000;70: 167–71.

Goerss JB, Kim CH, Atkinson EJ, Eastell R, O'Fallon WM, Melton LJ III, Risk of fractures in patients with pernicious anemia. J Bone Miner Res 1992;7: 573–9.

Graham IM, Daly LE, Refsum HM, Robinson K, Brattstrom LE, Ueland PM, Palma-Reis RJ, Boers GH, Sheahan RG, Israelsson B, Uiterwaal CS, Meleady R, McMaster D, Verhoef P, Witteman J, Rubba P, Bellet H, Wautrecht JC, de Valk HW, Sales Luis AC, Parrot-Rouland FM, Tan KS, Higgins I, Garcon D, Andria G, Plasma homocysteine as a risk factor for vascular disease. The European Concerted Action Project. J Am Med Assoc 1997;277: 1775–81.

Graham SM, Arvela OM, Wise GA, Long-term neurologic consequences of nutritional vitamin B12 deficiency in infants. J Pediatr 1992;121: 710–4.

Gräsbeck R, Imerslund-Grasbeck syndrome (selective vitamin B(12) malabsorption with proteinuria). Orphanet J Rare Dis 2006;1: 17.

Guerra-Shinohara EM, Paiva AA, Rondo PH, Yamasaki K, Terzi CA, D'Almeida V, Relationship between total homocysteine and folate levels in pregnant women and their newborn babies according to maternal serum levels of vitamin B12. Br J Obstst Gynaecol 2002;109: 784–91.

Hakami N, Neiman PE, Canellos GP, Lazerson J, Neonatal megaloblastic anemia due to inherited transcobalamin II deficiency in two siblings. N Engl J Med 1971;285: 1163–70.

Hall CA, The carriers of native vitamin B12 in normal human serum. Clin Sci Mol Med 1977;53: 453–7.

Heller S, Salkeld RM, Korner WF, Vitamin B6 status in pregnancy. Am J Clin Nutr 1973;26: 1339–48.

Henning BF, Zidek W, Riezler R, Graefe U, Tepel M, Homocyst(e)ine metabolism in hemodialysis patients treated with vitamins B6, B12 and folate. Res Exp Med (Berl) 2001;200: 155–68.

Henoun LN, Noel E, Ben AM, Locatelli F, Blickle JF, Andres E, Cobalamin deficiency due to non-immune atrophic gastritis in elderly patients. A report of 25 cases. J Nutr Health Aging 2005;9: 462.

Hepburn MJ, Dyal K, Runser LA, Barfield RL, Hepburn LM, Fraser SL, Low serum vitamin B12 levels in an outpatient HIV-infected population. Int J STD AIDS 2004;15: 127–33.

Herbert V, Vitamin B-12: plant sources, requirements, and assay. Am J Clin Nutr 1988;48: 852–8.

Herbert V, Staging vitamin B-12 (cobalamin) status in vegetarians. Am J Clin Nutr 1994;59: 1213S–22S.

Herbert V, Fong W, Gulle V, Stopler T, Low holotranscobalamin II is the earliest serum marker for sub-normal vitamin B12 (cobalamin) absorption in patients with AIDS. Am J Hematol 1990;34: 132–9.

Herrmann W, Schorr H, Bodis M, Knapp JP, Muller A, Stein G, Geisel J, Role of homocysteine, cystathionine and methylmalonic acid measurement for diagnosis of vitamin deficiency in high-aged subjects. Eur J Clin Invest 2000;30: 1083–9.

Herrmann W, Schorr H, Geisel J, Riegel W, Homocysteine, cystathionine, methylmalonic acid and B-vitamins in patients with renal disease. Clin Chem Lab Med 2001a;39: 739–46.

Herrmann W, Schorr H, Purschwitz K, Rassoul F, Richter V, Total homocysteine, vitamin B-12, and total antioxidant status in vegetarians. Clin Chem 2001b;47: 1094–101.

Herrmann W, Obeid R, Jouma M, Hyperhomocysteinemia and vitamin B-12 deficiency are more striking in Syrians than in Germans – causes and implications. Atherosclerosis 2003a;166: 143–50.

Herrmann W, Obeid R, Schorr H, Geisel J, Functional vitamin B12 deficiency and determination of holotranscobalamin in populations at risk. Clin Chem Lab Med 2003b;41: 1478–1488.

Herrmann W, Schorr H, Obeid R, Geisel J, Vitamin B-12 status, particularly holotranscobalamin II and methylmalonic acid concentrations, and hyperhomocysteinemia in vegetarians. Am J Clin Nutr 2003c;78: 131–6.

Herrmann W, Schorr H, Obeid R, Makowski J, Fowler B, Kuhlmann MK, Disturbed homocysteine and methionine cycle intermediates s-adenosylhomocysteine and s-adenosylmethionine are related to degree of renal insufficiency in type 2 diabetes. Clin Chem 2005b;51: 891–7.

Herrmann M, Schmidt J, Umanskaya N, Colaianni G, Al-Marrawi F, Widmann T, Zallone A, Wildemann B, Herrmann W, Stimulation of osteoclast activity by low B-vitamin concentrations. Bone 2007a;41: 584–91.

Herrmann M, Peter SJ, Umanskaya N, Wagner A, Taban-Shomal O, Widmann T, Colaianni G, Wildemann B, Herrmann W, The role of hyperhomocysteinemia as well as folate, vitamin B(6) and B(12) deficiencies in osteoporosis: a systematic review. Clin Chem Lab Med 2007b;45: 1621–32.

Herrmann M, Umanskaya N, Wildemann B, Colaianni G, Schmidt J, Widmann T, Zallone A, Herrmann W, Accumulation of homocysteine by decreasing concentrations of folate, vitamin B12 and B6 does not influence the activity of human osteoblasts in vitro. Clin Chim Acta 2007c;384: 129–34.

Herrmann M, Wildemann B, Claes L, Klohs S, Ohnmacht M, Taban-Shomal O, Hubner U, Pexa A, Umanskaya N, Herrmann W, Experimental hyperhomocysteinemia reduces bone quality in rats. Clin Chem 2007d;53: 1455–61.

Herrmann W, Herrmann M, Obeid R, Hyperhomocysteinaemia: a critical review of old and new aspects. Curr Drug Metab 2007e;8: 17–31.

Herrmann M, Umanskaya N, Wildemann B, Colaianni G, Widmann T, Zallone A, Herrmann M, Stimulation of osteoblast activity by homocysteine. J Cell Mol Med 2008;12: 1205–10.

Herrmann W, Obeid R, Holotranscobalamin – an early marker for laboratory diagnosis of vitamin B12 deficiency. Eur Haematol 2009a;2: 2–6.

Herrmann W, Obeid R, Schorr H, Geisel J, The usefulness of holotranscobalamin in predicting vitamin B12 status in different clinical settings. Curr Drug Metab 2005a;6: 47–53.

Herrmann W, Obeid R, Schorr H, Hübner U, Geisel J, Sand-Hill M, Nayyar A, Herrmann M, Enhanced bone metabolism in vegetarians – the role of vitamin B12 deficiency. Clin Chem Lab Med 2009b;47: 1381–7.

Herzlich B, Herbert V, Depletion of serum holotranscobalamin II. An early sign of negative vitamin B12 balance. Lab Invest 1988;58: 332–7.

Higginbottom MC, Sweetman L, Nyhan WL, A syndrome of methylmalonic aciduria, homocystinuria, megaloblastic anemia and neurologic abnormalities in a vitamin B12-deficient breast-fed infant of a strict vegetarian. N Engl J Med 1978;299: 317–23.

Hirschowitz BI, Worthington J, Mohnen J, Vitamin B12 deficiency in hypersecretors during long-term acid suppression with proton pump inhibitors. Aliment Pharmacol Ther 2008;27: 1110–21.

Hoffbrand AV, Jackson BF, Correction of the DNA synthesis defect in vitamin B12 deficiency by tetrahydrofolate: evidence in favour of the methyl-folate trap hypothesis as the cause of megaloblastic anaemia in vitamin B12 deficiency. Br J Haematol 1993;83: 643–7.

Hoffer LJ, Elian KM, Parenteral vitamin B12 therapy of hyperhomocysteinemia in end-stage renal disease. Clin Invest Med 2004;27: 10–3.

Howard JM, Azen C, Jacobsen DW, Green R, Carmel R, Dietary intake of cobalamin in elderly people who have abnormal serum cobalamin, methylmalonic acid and homocysteine levels. Eur J Clin Nutr 1998;52: 582–7.

Howden CW, Vitamin B12 levels during prolonged treatment with proton pump inhibitors. J Clin Gastroenterol 2000;30: 29–33.

Institute of Medicine, Dietary reference intakes for thiamin, riboflavin, niacin, vitamin B6, folate, vitamin B12, pantothenic acid, biotin, and choline. 2000; pp. 150–95.

Kaltenbach G, Andres E, Imler M, Ileal malabsorption of vitamin B12 in the chronic alcoholics. Gastroenterol Clin Biol 1995;19: 544–5.

Kaptan K, Beyan C, Ural AU, Cetin T, Avcu F, Gulsen M, Finci R, Yalcin A, *Helicobacter pylori* – is it a novel causative agent in vitamin B12 deficiency? Arch Intern Med 2000;160: 1349–53.

Kim GS, Kim CH, Park JY, Lee KU, Park CS, Effects of vitamin B12 on cell proliferation and cellular alkaline phosphatase activity in human bone marrow stromal osteoprogenitor cells and UMR106 osteoblastic cells. Metabolism 1996;45: 1443–6.

Krasinski SD, Russell RM, Samloff IM, Jacob RA, Dallal GE, McGandy RB, Hartz SC, Fundic atrophic gastritis in an elderly population. Effect on hemoglobin and several serum nutritional indicators. J Am Geriatr Soc 1986;34: 800–6.

Kuhne T, Bubl R, Baumgartner R, Maternal vegan diet causing a serious infantile neurological disorder due to vitamin B12 deficiency. Eur J Pediatr 1991;150: 205–8.

Kuzminski AM, Del Giacco EJ, Allen RH, Stabler SP, Lindenbaum J, Effective treatment of cobalamin deficiency with oral cobalamin. Blood 1998;92: 1191–8.

Lahner E, Norman GL, Severi C, Encabo S, Shums Z, Vannella L, Fave GD, Annibale B, Reassessment of intrinsic factor and parietal cell autoantibodies in atrophic gastritis with respect to cobalamin deficiency. Am J Gastroenterol 2009;104: 2071–9.

Lesho EP, Hyder A, Prevalence of subtle cobalamin deficiency. Arch Intern Med 1999; 159: 407.

Lin JC, Borregaard N, Liebman HA, Carmel R, Deficiency of the specific granule proteins, R-binder/transcobalamin I and lactoferrin, in plasma and saliva: a new disorder. Am J Med Genet 2001;100:145–51.

Lindenbaum J, Rosenberg IH, Wilson PW, Stabler SP, Allen RH, Prevalence of cobalamin deficiency in the Framingham elderly population. Am J Clin Nutr 1994;60: 2–11.

Lindgren A, Elevated serum methylmalonic acid. How much comes from cobalamin deficiency and how much comes from the kidneys? Scand J Clin Lab Invest 2002;62: 15–9.

Lindgren A, Kilander A, Bagge E, Nexo E, Holotranscobalamin – a sensitive marker of cobalamin malabsorption. Eur J Clin Invest 1999;29: 321–9.

Loikas S, Lopponen M, Suominen P, Moller J, Irjala K, Isoaho R, Kivela SL, Koskinen P, Pelliniemi TT, RIA for serum holo-transcobalamin: method evaluation in the clinical laboratory and reference interval. Clin Chem 2003;49: 455–62.

Lorenzl S, Vogeser M, Muller-Schunk S, Pfister HW, Clinically and MRI documented funicular myelosis in a patient with metabolical vitamin B12 deficiency but normal vitamin B12 serum level. J Neurol 2003;250: 1010–11.

Louwman MW, Van Dusseldorp M, van der Vijver FJ, Thomas CM, Schneede J, Ueland PM, Refsum H, van Staveren WA, Signs of impaired cognitive function in adolescents with marginal cobalamin status. Am J Clin Nutr 2000;72: 762–9.

Marinella MA, Anemia following Roux-en-Y surgery for morbid obesity: a review. South Med J 2008;101: 1024–31.

Marino MC, de Oliveira CA, Rocha AM, Rocha GA, Clementino NC, Antunes LF, Oliveira RA, Martins AS, Del Puerto HL, D'Almeida V, Galdieri L, Pedroso ER, Cabral MM, Nogueira AM, Queiroz DM, Long-term effect of *Helicobacter pylori* eradication on plasma homocysteine in elderly patients with cobalamin deficiency. Gut 2007;56: 469–74.

Markle HV, Cobalamin. Crit Rev Clin Lab Sci 1996;33: 247–56.

Masalha R, Chudakov B, Muhamad M, Rudoy I, Volkov I, Wirguin I, Cobalamin-responsive psychosis as the sole manifestation of vitamin B12 deficiency. Isr Med Assoc J 2001;3: 701–3.

Matsui SM, Mahoney MJ, Rosenberg LE, The natural history of the inherited methylmalonic acidemias. N Engl J Med 1983;308: 857–61.

McCaddon A, Homocysteine and cognitive impairment; a case series in a General Practice setting. Nutr J 2006;5: 6.

McCaddon A, Hudson P, Davies G, Hughes A, Williams JH, Wilkinson C, Homocysteine and cognitive decline in healthy elderly. Dement Geriatr Cogn Disord 2001;12: 309–13.

McLean RR, Jacques PF, Selhub J, Tucker KL, Samelson EJ, Broe KE, Hannan MT, Cupples LA, Kiel DP, Homocysteine as a predictive factor for hip fracture in older persons. N Engl J Med 2004;350: 2042–9.

McLean RR, Jacques PF, Selhub J, Fredman L, Tucker KL, Samelson EJ, Kiel DP, Cupples LA, Hannan MT, Plasma B vitamins, homocysteine, and their relation with bone loss and hip fracture in elderly men and women. J Clin Endocrinol Metab 2008;93: 2206–12.

Melton LJ III, Adverse outcomes of osteoporotic fractures in the general population. J Bone Miner Res 2003;18: 1139–41.

Melton ME, Kochman ML, Reversal of severe osteoporosis with vitamin B12 and etidronate therapy in a patient with pernicious anemia. Metabolism 1994;43: 468–9.

Miller DR, Specker BL, Ho ML, Norman EJ, Vitamin B-12 status in a macrobiotic community. Am J Clin Nutr 1991;53: 524–9.

Moestrup SK, Birn H, Fischer PB, Petersen CM, Verroust PJ, Sim RB, Christensen EI, Nexo E, Megalin-mediated endocytosis of transcobalamin-vitamin-B12 complexes suggests a role of the receptor in vitamin-B12 homeostasis. Proc Natl Acad Sci USA 1996;93: 8612–7.

Molloy AM, Mills JL, McPartlin J, Kirke PN, Scott JM, Daly S, Maternal and fetal plasma homocysteine concentrations at birth: the influence of folate, vitamin B12, and the 5,10-methylenetetrahydrofolate reductase 677C→T variant. Am J Obstet Gynecol 2002;186: 499–503.

Monsen AL, Refsum H, Markestad T, Ueland PM, Cobalamin status and its biochemical markers methylmalonic acid and homocysteine in different age groups from 4 days to 19 years. Clin Chem 2003;49: 2067–75.

Morris MS, Jacques PF, Rosenberg IH, Selhub J, Elevated serum methylmalonic acid concentrations are common among elderly Americans. J Nutr 2002;132: 2799–803.

Morrison LD, Smith DD, Kish SJ, Brain S-adenosylmethionine levels are severely decreased in Alzheimer's disease. J Neurochem 1996;67: 1328–31.

Murphy MM, Scott JM, Arija V, Molloy AM, Fernandez-Ballart JD, Maternal homocysteine before conception and throughout pregnancy predicts fetal homocysteine and birth weight. Clin Chem 2004;50: 1406–12.

Neesse A, Michl P, Barth P, Vieth M, Langer P, Ellenrieder V, Gress TM, Multifocal early gastric cancer in a patient with autoimmune atrophic gastritis and iron deficiency anaemia. Z Gastroenterol 2009;47: 223–7.

Obeid R, Geisel J, Schorr H, Hubner U, Herrmann W, The impact of vegetarianism on some haematological parameters. Eur J Haematol 2002;69: 275–9.

Obeid R, Herrmann W, Mechanisms of homocysteine neurotoxicity in neurodegenerative diseases with special reference to dementia. FEBS Lett 2006;580: 2994–3005.

Obeid R, Kuhlmann M, Kirsch CM, Herrmann W, Cellular uptake of vitamin B12 in patients with chronic renal failure. Nephron Clin Pract 2005a;99: c42–8.

Obeid R, Kuhlmann MK, Kohler H, Herrmann W, Response of homocysteine, cystathionine, and methylmalonic acid to vitamin treatment in dialysis patients. Clin Chem 2005b;51: 196–201.

Obeid R, Kuhlmann MK, Kohler H, Herrmann W, Response of homocysteine, cystathionine, and methylmalonic acid to vitamin treatment in dialysis patients. Clin Chem 2005c;51: 196–201.

Obeid R, Munz W, Jager M, Schmidt W, Herrmann W, Biochemical indexes of the B vitamins in cord serum are predicted by maternal B vitamin status. Am J Clin Nutr 2005d;82: 133–9.

Obeid R, Schorr H, Eckert R, Herrmann W, Vitamin B12 status in the elderly as judged by available biochemical markers. Clin Chem 2004;50: 238–41.

Ozdem S, Samanci N, Tasatargil A, Yildiz A, Sadan G, Donmez L, Herrmann M, Experimental hyperhomocysteinemia disturbs bone metabolism in rats. Scand J Clin Lab Invest 2007;67: 748–56.

Penninx BW, Guralnik JM, Ferrucci L, Fried LP, Allen RH, Stabler SP, Vitamin B(12) deficiency and depression in physically disabled older women: epidemiologic evidence from the Women's Health and Aging Study. Am J Psychiatry 2000;157: 715–21.

Pruthi RK, Tefferi A, Pernicious anemia revisited. Mayo Clin Proc 1994;69: 144–50.

Radmanesh A, Zaman T, Ghanaati H, Molaei S, Robertson RL, Zamani AA, Methylmalonic acidemia: brain imaging findings in 52 children and a review of the literature. Pediatr Radiol 2008;38: 1054–61.

Rajan S, Wallace JI, Beresford SA, Brodkin KI, Allen RA, Stabler SP, Screening for cobalamin deficiency in geriatric outpatients: prevalence and influence of synthetic cobalamin intake. J Am Geriatr Soc 2002a;50: 624–30.

Rajan S, Wallace JI, Brodkin KI, Beresford SA, Allen RH, Stabler SP, Response of elevated methylmalonic acid to three dose levels of oral cobalamin in older adults. J Am Geriatr Soc 2002b;50: 1789–95.

Rauma AL, Torronen R, Hanninen O, Mykkanen H, Vitamin B-12 status of long-term adherents of a strict uncooked vegan diet ('living food diet') is compromised. J Nutr 1995;125: 2511–5.

Refsum H, Yajnik CS, Gadkari M, Schneede J, Vollset SE, Orning L, Guttormsen AB, Joglekar A, Sayyad MG, Ulvik A, Ueland PM, Hyperhomocysteinemia and elevated methylmalonic acid indicate a high prevalence of cobalamin deficiency in Asian Indians. Am J Clin Nutr 2001;74: 233–41.

Refsum H, Grindflek AW, Ueland PM, Fredriksen A, Meyer K, Ulvik A, Guttormsen AB, Iversen OE, Schneede J, Kase BF, Screening for serum total homocysteine in newborn children. Clin Chem 2004;50: 1769–84.

Remacha AF, Cadafalch J, Sarda P, Barcelo M, Fuster M, Vitamin B-12 metabolism in HIV-infected patients in the age of highly active antiretroviral therapy: role of homocysteine in assessing vitamin B-12 status. Am J Clin Nutr 2003;77: 420–4.

Rogers LM, Boy E, Miller JW, Green R, Sabel JC, Allen LH, High prevalence of cobalamin deficiency in Guatemalan schoolchildren: associations with low plasma holotranscobalamin II and elevated serum methylmalonic acid and plasma homocysteine concentrations. Am J Clin Nutr 2003;77: 433–40.

Ruscin JM, Page RL, Valuck RJ, Vitamin B(12) deficiency associated with histamine(2)-receptor antagonists and a proton-pump inhibitor. Ann Pharmacother 2002;36: 812–6.

Savage DG, Lindenbaum J, Stabler SP, Allen RH, Sensitivity of serum methylmalonic acid and total homocysteine determinations for diagnosing cobalamin and folate deficiencies [see comments]. Am J Med 1994;96: 239–46.

Scarpa S, Fuso A, D'Anselmi F, Cavallaro RA, Presenilin 1 gene silencing by S-adenosylmethionine: a treatment for Alzheimer disease? FEBS Lett 2003;541: 145–8.

Schneede J, Dagnelie PC, van Staveren WA, Vollset SE, Refsum H, Ueland PM, Methylmalonic acid and homocysteine in plasma as indicators of functional cobalamin deficiency in infants on macrobiotic diets. Pediatr Res 1994;36: 194–201.

Sheikh SH, Shaw-Stiffel TA, The gastrointestinal manifestations of Sjogren's syndrome. Am J Gastroenterol 1995;90: 9–14.

Shorvon SD, Carney MW, Chanarin I, Reynolds EH, The neuropsychiatry of megaloblastic anaemia. Br Med J 1980;281: 1036–8.

Sipponen P, Laxen F, Huotari K, Harkonen M, Prevalence of low vitamin B12 and high homocysteine in serum in an elderly male population: association with atrophic gastritis and *Helicobacter pylori* infection. Scand J Gastroenterol 2003;38: 1209–16.

Solomon LR, Disorders of cobalamin (vitamin B12) metabolism: emerging concepts in pathophysiology, diagnosis and treatment. Blood Rev 2007;21: 113–30.

Spivak JL, Masked megaloblastic anemia. Arch Intern Med 1982;142: 2111–4.

Stabler SP, Lindenbaum J, Allen RH, The use of homocysteine and other metabolites in the specific diagnosis of vitamin B-12 deficiency. J Nutr 1996;126: 1266S–72S.

Stroinsky A, Schneider Z, Cobamide dependant enzymes. In: Schneider Z, Stroinsky A, editors. Comprehensive B-12. Berlin: de Gruyter; 1987. pp. 225–66.

Suter PM, Golner BB, Goldin BR, Morrow FD, Russell RM, Reversal of protein-bound vitamin B12 malabsorption with antibiotics in atrophic gastritis. Gastroenterology 1991;101: 1039–45.

Tang AM, Smit E, Selected vitamins in HIV infection: a review. AIDS Patient Care STDS 1998;12: 263–73.

Teplitsky V, Huminer D, Zoldan J, Pitlik S, Shohat M, Mittelman M, Hereditary partial transcobalamin II deficiency with neurologic, mental and hematologic abnormalities in children and adults. Isr Med Assoc J 2003;5: 868–72.

Toh BH, van D, I, Gleeson PA, Pernicious anemia. N Engl J Med 1997;337: 1441–8.

Ueland PM, Monsen AL, Hyperhomocysteinemia and B-vitamin deficiencies in infants and children. Clin Chem Lab Med 2003;41: 1418–26.

Van der Weyden M, Rother M, Firkin B, Megaloblastic maturation masked by iron deficiency: a biochemical basis. Br J Haematol 1972;22: 299–307.

van Meurs JB, Dhonukshe-Rutten RA, Pluijm SM, van der Klift M, de Jonge R, Lindemans J, de Groot LC, Hofman A, Witteman JC, van Leeuwen JP, Breteler MM, Lips P, Pols HA, Uitterlinden AG, Homocysteine levels and the risk of osteoporotic fracture. N Engl J Med 2004;350: 2033–41.

Vitali C, Bombardieri S, Jonsson R, Moutsopoulos HM, Alexander EL, Carsons SE, Daniels TE, Fox PC, Fox RI, Kassan SS, Pillemer SR, Talal N, Weisman MH, Classification criteria for Sjogren's syndrome: a revised version of the European criteria proposed by the American-European Consensus Group. Ann Rheum Dis 2002;61: 554–8.

Wang HX, Wahlin A, Basun H, Fastbom J, Winblad B, Fratiglioni L, Vitamin B(12) and folate in relation to the development of Alzheimer's disease. Neurology 2001;56: 1188–94.

Wang YF, Chiu JS, Chuang MH, Chiu JE, Lin CL, Bone mineral density of vegetarian and non-vegetarian adults in Taiwan. Asia Pac J Clin Nutr 2008;17: 101–6.

Weir DG, Scott JM, Brain function in the elderly: role of vitamin B12 and folate. Br Med Bull 1999;55: 669–82.

7.4 Signs and symptoms of vitamin B12 (cobalamin) deficiency: a critical review of the literature

Emmanuel Andrès

7.4.1 Introduction

Vitamin B12 (cobalamin) deficiency is a common and potentially life-threatening disorder. However, owing to its insidious onset as well as its atypical and at times non-specific clinical presentations, the deficiency often remains undiagnosed

(Lindenbaum et al., 1994; Andrès et al., 2004, 2007). Owing to the seriousness of potential complications (particularly haematological and neurological disorders), it is essential that the clinician has a sound understanding of the presenting signs and symptoms. The aim of this article is to provide an exhaustive and critical review of the various clinical presentations suggestive of cobalamin deficiency, as reported in the literature.

7.4.2 Pathophysiology

The recommended daily intake of vitamin B12 varies from 2 to 5 µg, depending on the guidelines used in different countries. Vitamin B12 is exclusively found in foods of animal origin. A balanced diet generally provides enough vitamin B12 to largely exceed the body's daily requirement (Andrès et al., 2005, 2007; Snow, 1999). The existence of an enterohepatic cycle allows cobalamin to be spared. In times of deficit, Megalin, a receptor expressed in the renal proximal tubules, is responsible for the reabsorption of vitamin B12 excreted in the urine. The body's vitamin B12 reserves are thus very abundant, which accounts for the often late and insidious onset of clinical signs of deficiency (which appear after 7 years on average), as well as the frequent discrepancy between the extent of the biochemical abnormalities, notably anaemia, and the paucity of clinical signs (Nicolas and Guéant, 1994; Andrès et al., 2005). The major steps of vitamin B12 metabolism are summarised in ►Fig. 7.10.

Vitamin B12 is a ubiquitous coenzyme involved in important intracellular enzyme reactions (Federici et al., 2007), in particular those leading to DNA and methionine synthesis from homocysteine (►Fig. 7.10) (Koury and Ponka, 2004; Scalabrino et al., 2007; Solomon, 2007). Hence, if there is a deficit in vitamin B12, these vital processes cannot be maintained – resulting in the development of symptoms of deficiency. Impairment of DNA synthesis results in a 'maturation blockade' which essentially affects rapidly dividing cells, such as red blood cells and those of the skin and mucous membranes. From a haematological perspective, the block in DNA synthesis combined with a relative preservation of RNA synthesis results in 'nucleocytoplasmic asynchrony'. Intramedullary 'cell abortion' occurs owing to ineffective haematopoiesis and megaloblastosis. Both are associated with clinical and biochemical features which could initially be mistaken for other conditions, such as haemolytic anaemia, thrombotic microangiopathy, or acute leukosis (Koury and Ponka, 2004; Federici et al., 2007; Scalabrino et al., 2007; Solomon, 2007).

The underlying mechanism by which cobalamin deficiency affects the nervous system is complex and poorly understood. The most widely accepted theory is that an alteration in methionine synthesis leads to defective production of myelin, which is associated with nerve conduction abnormalities (Scott and Weir, 1981; Andrès et al., 2001; Scalabrino and Peracchi, 2006; Federici et al., 2007). The role of vitamin B12 in regulating the synthesis and activity of several neurotrophic cytokines has also been proposed. This role is thought to be independent of the coenzyme activity of vitamin B12 (Scalabrino and Peracchi, 2006; Solomon, 2007; Scalabrino et al., 2008). Recent studies involving patients with neurological symptoms associated with vitamin B12 deficiency have revealed an increase in serum and cerebrospinal fluid levels of neurotoxic cytokines, namely: neurotoxic tumour necrosis factor (TNF)-alpha, nerve growth factor (NGF), and soluble CD40 ligand. In addition, there was a concomitant decrease in

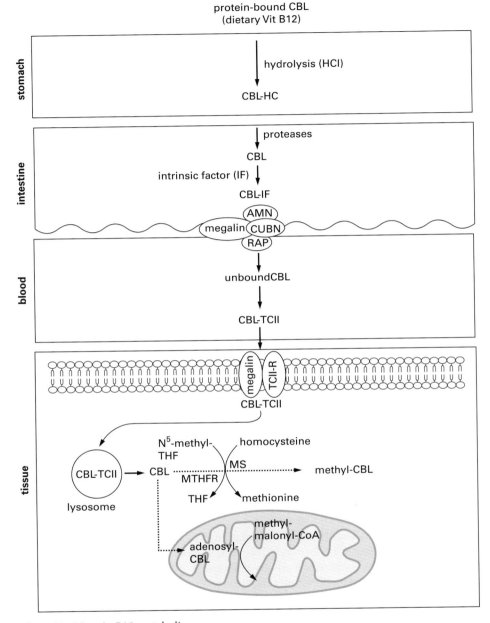

Fig. 7.10: Vitamin B12 metabolism.

CBL: Cobalamin
HC: hoptocorin
CUBN: cubilin
AMN: amnionless
RAP: receptor-associated protein

TCII: transcobalomin II
TCII-R: transcobalomin II receptor
THF: tetrahydrofolate
MTHF: Methyltetrahydrofolate reductase
MS: methionine synthatse

certain neurotrophic cytokines, such as neurotrophic epidermal growth factor (EGF) and interleukin (IL)-6. After correcting the vitamin B12 deficiency, levels of these cytokines returned to normal (Scalabrino et al., 2007).

7.4.3 Clinical presentations of vitamin B12 deficiency

The use of strict criteria to define vitamin B12 deficiency (▶Tab. 7.9) has resulted in more stringent control of the medical literature and increased recognition of previously unknown clinical presentations of cobalamin deficiency (Andrès et al., 2005). The main signs, symptoms and syndromes related to cobalamin deficiency that are reported in the literature are presented in ▶Tab. 7.10. The presentation of vitamin B12 deficiency is often multisystemic in nature and can vary greatly in severity. Haematological and neurological features usually predominate the clinical picture, in addition to symptoms related to epithelial cell involvement (Stabler et al., 1990; Andrès et al., 2005, 2007; Carmel and Serrai, 2006; Maktouf et al., 2007).

7.4.3.1 Haematopoietic disorders

Presentations involving the haematopoietic system range from asymptomatic patients with incidental abnormalities found on performing a full blood count, to severe complications reflecting profound pancytopaenia, or even atypical presentations which could initially present in the same way as acute haemolysis or haematological malignancies (Stabler et al., 1990; Andrès et al., 2005; Carmel and Serrai, 2006; Federici et al., 2007; Maktouf et al., 2007). ▶Tab. 7.11 shows the frequency of the main abnormalities observed in our Strasbourg cohort involving more than 200 patients (Federici et al., 2007). Megaloblastic macrocytic anaemia was the most frequent abnormality found. Typically, macrocytosis is very pronounced during cobalamin deficiency, and generally higher than 110–120 fl in the case of Biermer's disease (pernicious anaemia). As it is often associated with leukopaenia or thrombocytopenia of varying severity, the blood count frequently reveals a pancytopaenia. Hypersegmentation of neutrophils (right shift in the Arneth count) is also very common, and must be looked for on the blood film. This parameter is often missed owing to the use of automatic devices. Clinically, the anaemia related to vitamin B12 deficiency develops progressively (vitamin B12 reserves of approx. 5–10 years). Often the tint of the skin is sallow and can appear slightly jaundiced owing to the associated haemolytic component. The hair looks grey and the face is puffy (Dreyfus et al., 1992; Lee and Herbert, 1999; Federici et al., 2007).

Tab. 7.9: Definition of vitamin B12 deficiency.

Serum vitamin B12 levels <150 pmol/l (<200 pg/ml) *and* clinical features and/or hematological anomalies related to cobalamin deficiency
Serum vitamin B12 levels <150 pmol/l on two separate occasions
Serum vitamin B1 levels <150 pmol/l *and* total serum homocysteine levels >13 µmol/l *or* methylmalonic acid levels >0.4 µmol/l (in the absence of renal failure and folate and vitamin B6 deficiencies)
Low serum holotranscobalamin levels <35 pmol/l

Tab. 7.10: Main signs and symptoms of vitamin B12 deficiency.

Hematological manifestations	Neuro-psychiatric manifestations	Digestive manifestations	Other manifestations
Frequent: macrocytosis, hypersegmentation of the neutrophils, aregenerative macrocytary anemia, LDH and bilirubin elevation, medullary megaloblastosis ('blue spinal cord')	*Frequent*: polyneurites (particularly sensitive ones), ataxia, Babinski's phenomenon	*Classic*: Hunter's glossitis, jaundice, LDH and bilirubin elevation ('intramedullary destruction')	*Under study*: atrophy of the vaginal mucosa and chronic vaginal and urinary infections (particularly mycosis), hypofertility and repeated miscarriages, venous thromboembolic disease, angina (hyperhomocysteinaemia), osteoporosis
Rare: isolated thrombocytopenia and neutropaenia, pancytopaenia	*Classic*: combined sclerosis of the spinal cord		
Very rare: haemolytic anemia, thrombotic microangiopathy (presence of schistocytes)	*Rare*: cerebellar syndromes affecting the cranial nerves including optic neuritis, optic atrophy, urinary and/or faecal incontinence	*Debatable*: abdominal pain, dyspepsia, nausea, vomiting, diarrhoea, disturbances in intestinal functioning	
	Under study: changes in the higher functions, even dementia, stroke and atherosclerosis (hyperhomocystein-aemia), parkinsonian syndromes, depression, multiple sclerosis	*Rare*: resistant and recurring mucocutaneous ulcers	

On examination of the bone marrow, megaloblastosis gives it a bluish appearance owing to hyperbasophilia. In the red cell line, anisocytosis and ovalocytosis are noted and are associated with nuclear hypersegmentation of polynuclear neutrophils (Dreyfus et al., 1992; Lee and Herbert, 1999). At times, intramedullary 'abortion' could lead to a haemolytic picture, with clinical and biochemical results suggestive of haemolytic anaemia, such as increased bilirubin levels, decreased haptoglobin and markedly elevated serum lactate dehydrogenase. Following supplementation, the LDH has been reported to normalise rapidly (Andrès and Kaltenbach, 2003; Andrès et al., 2003a,b, 2005). In addition to the conditions mentioned above, vitamin B12 deficiency might also present in a similar manner to thrombotic microangiopathy, where haemolytic anaemia, thrombocytopenia, and schizocytosis coexist. This scenario is observed in approximately 10% of patients (Federici et al., 2007).

Tab. 7.11: Main hematological abnormalities and manifestations in 201 patients with documented vitamin B12 deficiency.

	Number of patients (%)
Anemia	74 (37%)
Anemia and macrocytosis	68 (33.8%)
Isolated macrocytosis	34 (17%)
Leukopaenia	28 (14%)
Neutropaenia	6 (3%)
Thrombocytopaenia	20 (10%)
Pancytopaenia	10 (5%)
Pseudothrombotic microangiopathy	5 (2.5%)
Haemolytic anaemia	3 (1.5%)
No abnormality	56 (28%)

From a practical perspective, it is worth noting that following cobalamin supplementation these abnormalities fully and rapidly disappear, usually within a few days or weeks and without leaving any lasting sequelae. There is also a full recovery seen in the full blood count (and in the absence of this, the diagnosis of vitamin B12 deficiency should be questioned) (Federici et al., 2007). Within approximately 1 week reticulocytosis occurs, whereas mean globular volume normalises within 1 month and haemoglobin concentration in 2–3 months.

7.4.3.2 Disorders of the nervous system

The neurological features found in vitamin B12 deficiency are extremely variable. Neurological symptoms could predominate over haematological findings or be isolated without any abnormality of the full blood count. In the case series published by Lindenbaum et al., which included 141 patients with neuropsychiatric conditions related to cobalamin-deficiency, anaemia and macrocytosis were absent in 28% of cases. (Lindenbaum et al., 1988). From our own experience, which involves over 300 patients with a median age of 71 years, neuropsychiatric presentations were isolated and indicative of vitamin B12 deficiency in one-quarter of the cases studied (Federici et al., 2007).

The most common neurological disorders include: polyneuritis (which is frequently purely sensory in nature), ataxia and a positive Babinski sign. Nowadays, combined sclerosis of the spinal cord, previously considered the most classical presentation, is rarely observed. In this condition, a posterior cord syndrome is associated with abnormalities of the pyramidal tract (Scott and Weir, 1981; Lindenbaum et al., 1988; Andrès et al., 2001, 2005; Gochard et al., 2009). The main clinical findings (in particular neuropsychiatric symptoms), which were observed in our series of more than 92 patients aged over 65 years, are presented in ▶Tab. 7.12 (Andrès et al., 2007). Painful spinothalamic tract involvement, cerebellar ataxia, sphincter disorders, and retrobulbar optic neuritis are other possible presentations.

Tab. 7.12: Neuro-psychiatric manifestations in 92 patients with vitamin B12 deficiency related to food-cobalamin malabsorption.

Mean age (years)	76 ± 8
Sex ratio (female/male)	2
Neuropsychiatric signs and symptoms	70%
Sensitive polyneuritis	45%
Cognitive impairment	23%
Asthenia and lethargy	21%

With regard to imaging studies, MRI scanning could reveal a T2 hypersignal at the higher levels of the spinal cord, most often in the cervico-thoracic area. This could be associated with oedematous enlargement of the cord at the level of T1. However, patients with several marked clinical features have had normal MRI scan reports, suggesting that radiological abnormalities occur later in the disease process (Berger and Quencer, 1991; Larner et al., 1997). The predominance of non-specific white matter changes often renders the diagnosis difficult, particularly when differentiating between degenerative demyelinating diseases (Andrès et al., 2001).

Other presentations including parkinsonian syndrome, depression, manic states, psychoses, obsessive-compulsive disorder and sleep disorders have also been described, but the causal relation has not yet been demonstrated. A statistical relation between cobalamin deficiency and cognitive disorders has been reported. However, study findings regarding improvement of higher brain functional disturbances following supplementation were conflicting. Our research team was not able to demonstrate any appreciable, clinically significant improvement, other than a mean improvement of 2 points on the Folstein Mini Mental State examination, which was mainly seen in cases of established or progressive dementia (Saracaceanu et al., 1997; Abyad, 2002; Andrès and Kaltenbach, 2003; Andrès et al., 2003a,b; Starr et al., 2005; Gochard et al., 2009).

Generally, improvement in neuropsychiatric disorders is less marked if the symptoms have been present for a long time, hence the necessity for early diagnosis and prompt cobalamin supplementation (Savage and Lindenbaum, 1995; Gochard et al., 2009). However, the absence of any improvement following supplementation should provoke the clinician to question the relation between the reported symptoms and vitamin B12 deficiency. In our experience, 30% of patients with neuropsychiatric symptoms did not respond to cyanocobalamin supplementation (despite good treatment compliance). Such symptoms could well have been owing to causes other than cobalamin deficiency, particularly in elderly subjects with multiple co-morbidities (Andrès et al., 2005, 2007).

7.4.3.3 Epithelial cell involvement

Disorders involving the epithelial layer commonly occur in the GI tract. The main difficulty exists when differentiating between symptoms related to cobalamin deficiency itself and those which are owing to the gastro-intestinal disorder responsible for the deficiency. Hunter's glossitis is the most typical feature. The tongue appears bald, dry, and smooth and the patient experiences pain when eating. Other symptoms such as vomiting, dyspepsia, diarrhoea, or functional digestive disorders have also been observed, although the relation with vitamin B12 deficiency has not yet been proven (Andrèset al., 2005).

Other presentations of vitamin B12 deficiency involving epithelial cells include recurrent mucocutaneous ulcers, vaginal atrophy and repeated genitourinary infections owing to the weakened urinary mucosal barrier (Andrès et al., 2005).

7.4.3.4 Vascular system involvement

Vitamin B12 deficiency is one of the causes of hyperhomocysteinaemia, which is recognised as an independent risk factor for venous thromboembolic disease, with a relative risk ranging from 1.5 to 2, depending on the study. However, only a few cases of venous thrombosis associated with cobalamin deficiency have been reported in the literature (Den Heijer et al., 1998; Wald et al., 2002). This might be accounted for by the relatively low levels of hyperhomocysteinaemia found secondary to vitamin B12 deficiency (in our experience, approximately 20–30 μmol/l on average), but also, to some extent, by the poor understanding of this complication. In the literature, most diagnoses of vitamin B12 deficiency that were confirmed in patients with deep venous thrombosis were observed in cases of Biermer's disease or those presenting with an insufficient exogenous vitamin B12 intake. From a practical perspective, vitamin B12 deficiency must be considered when thrombosis is associated with aregenerative anaemia, macrocytosis or haemolysis, or neuropsychiatric conditions. However, in the presence of marked homocysteinaemia (exceeding 80 or 100 μmol/l), other potential causes should be sought, such as: renal insufficiency, advanced age, folate deficiency, hypo/hyperthyroidism, homozygous mutations of C677T methylene tetrahydrofolate reductase in addition to hereditary causes such as deficiencies of other enzymes involved in the conversion of homocysteine to methionine, e.g., cystathionine and beta-synthase (▶Fig. 7.10) (Kharchafi et al., 2002). The treatment of thrombosis related to vitamin B12 deficiency is based on standard anticoagulation therapy and cobalamin supplementation, there are no other specific guidelines at present. It is worth noting that cobalamin supplementation could play a protective role against future recurrent thrombotic events (Ammouri et al., 2009).

It has been suggested that atherosclerosis and cerebral vascular accidents have also occurred as a result of hyperhomocysteinaemia related to vitamin B12 deficiency. However, the relation is not well documented and remains a matter of debate, even if it is an interesting point of discussion in terms of the aetiology involved (Andrès et al., 2005; Kumar et al., 2009). Results from studies involving vitamin B12 supplementation do not correspond well with epidemiological data. Theoretically, even a moderate hyperhomocysteinaemia exerts procoagulant effects on vascular endothelial cells whilst also acting on vascular smooth muscle and promoting the initiation and progression of atherothrombotic processes. However, in eight clinical trials involving 24 000 subjects, vitamin B supplementation was compared with placebo and standard management; the results showed that supplementation had no positive impact on myocardial infarction, stroke, or cardiovascular mortality (http://www.cochrane.org/reviews/index.htm). It is also noteworthy that a recent meta-analysis by Wang et al., provides evidence for significant stroke reduction by B-vitamin supplementation (B12, B6, B9) (Wang et al., 2007). ▶Tab. 7.10 summarizes the major clinical presentations according to their frequency and causal relation with cobalamin deficiency.

7.4.4 Factors influencing the presenting features of vitamin B12 deficiency

7.4.4.1 Age

The aetiology and clinical presentation of vitamin B12 deficiency are dependent on the patients' age.

In the neonate, congenital anomalies of vitamin B12 metabolism such as intrinsic factor deficiency, Imerslund disease, transcobalamin abnormalities and intracellular abnormalities are the predominant causes of vitamin B12 deficiency (►Fig. 7.10). Moreover, apart from the typical haematological features, examination of the bone marrow in the neonate could reveal elective medullary hypoplasia of the erythroblastic cell line or global medullary hypoplasia. The granular cell line might exhibit hyperplasia, often accompanied by suggestive giant metamyelocytes. Pseudo-thrombotic microangiopathy, which is frequently encountered in the neonate, might initially be mistaken for haemolytic uraemic syndrome (Zittoun, 1998).

In the elderly, food-cobalamin malabsorption syndrome (60%) and Biermer's disease (15–20%) are the most frequent causes of vitamin B12 deficiency (Andrès et al., 2007). Clinical symptoms are similar to those observed in younger subjects, but the onset is often insidious. As a result, the diagnosis is often not made until the advanced stages of disease, when major haematological and neurological complications are already present (Dali-Youcef and Andrès, 2009). In a study by Vogel et al., which included 79 patients with food-cobalamin malabsorption syndrome, dementia was the most common presenting condition leading to diagnosis in subjects over 75 years (Vogel et al., 2008). Reflex abnormalities were also more frequent with advanced age. In addition, vitamin B12 and haemoglobin plasma levels were lower in elderly subjects.

7.4.4.2 Aetiology of disease

Macrocytosis and anaemia appear to be more pronounced in patients with Biermer's disease in comparison with those with food-cobalamin malabsorption syndrome. The lower mean serum vitamin B12 levels found in Biermer's disease have been proposed as a potential explanation for this, although severity of the haematological abnormalities has not been shown to correlate well with the serum vitamin B12 levels (Andrès and Kaltenbach, 2003; Andrès et al., 2003a,b Loukili et al., 2004). Certain causes of vitamin B12 deficiency, such as a vegetarian diet and atrophic gastritis, are also frequently associated with iron deficiency. As a consequence, mean globular volume is lower in patients with these additional factors than in isolated vitamin B12 deficiency alone, and at times it could be associated with a trend towards a microcytosis (Obeid et al., 2002). In patients with Biermer's disease, Hershko et al., identified younger age group and female gender as significant factors that were associated with iron deficiency (Hershko et al., 2006).

7.4.4.3 Pregnancy and lactation

Physiological needs are increased during pregnancy and lactation (Andrès et al., 2005). Vitamin B12 deficiency in pregnant women has been suggested as a highly probable cause of recurrent miscarriages owing to hyperhomocysteinaemia, which leads to prematurity and foetal abnormalities (affecting the nervous system in particular) (Frenkel and Yardley, 2000; Refsum, 2001; Andrès et al., 2005; Molloy et al., 2008). Rare cases, which present with similar symptoms to HELLP syndrome, have also been reported (Hartong et al., 2007). Pronounced vitamin B12 deficiency has been found in neonates born to mothers presenting with vitamin B12 deficiency during pregnancy or lactation (Andrès et al., 2009).

7.4.5 Clinical presentations and treatment

The treatment of established vitamin B12 deficiency is based upon the administration of intramuscular cyanocobalamin. Its efficacy on the resolution of clinical signs and symptoms has been proven. Likewise, oral cyanocobalamin given at treatment doses has been shown to exhibit a similar efficacy to intramuscular cyanocobalamin, resulting in significantly increased levels of serum vitamin B12 and improvements in haematological parameters. However, the efficacy of oral cobalamin in the treatment of severe neurological disease has not yet been sufficiently documented. Therefore, in these patients cobalamin must still be administered via the parenteral route (Andrès et al., 2009).

References

Abyad A, Prevalence of vitamin B12 deficiency among demented patients and cognitive recovery with cobalamin replacement. J Nutr Health Aging 2002;6: 254–60.

Ammouri W, Tazi Mezalek Z, Harmouche H, Aouni M, Adnaoui M, Analyse de quatre observations de thromboses veineuses révélant une maladie de Biermer. Rev Med Interne 2009;30(2 Suppl): S64.

Andrès E, Kaltenbach G, Prevalence of vitamin B12 deficiency among demented patients and cognitive recovery with cobalamin replacement. J Nutr Health Aging 2003;7: 309–10.

Andrès E, Renaux V, Campos F, Opréa C, Sonntag-Fohrer C, Warter JM, Dufour P, Maloisel F, Troubles neurologiques isolés révélant une maladie de Biermer chez le sujet jeune Rev Med Interne 2001;22: 389–93.

Andrès E, Noel E, Maloisel F, Hematological findings in the syndrome of food-cobalamin malabsorption. Am J Med 2003a;115: 592.

Andrès E, Perrin AE, Demengeat C, Kurtz JE, Vinzio S, Grunenberger F et al., The syndrome of food-cobalamin malabsorption revisited in a department of internal medicine. A monocentric cohort study of 80 patients. Eur J Intern Med 2003b;14: 221–6.

Andrès E, Loukili NH, Noel E, Kaltenbach G, Abdelgheni MB, Perrin AE et al., Vitamin B12 (cobalamin) deficiency in elderly patients. Can Med Assoc J 2004;171: 251–9.

Andrès E, Affenberger S, Vinzio S, Noel E, Kaltenbach G, Schlienger JL, Carences en vitamine B12 chez l'adulte: étiologies, manifestations cliniques et traitement. Rev Med Interne 2005;26: 938–46.

Andrès E, Vidal-Alaball J, Federici L, Loukili NH, Zimmer J, Kaltenbach G, Clinical aspects of cobalamin deficiency in elderly patients. Epidemiology, causes, clinical manifestations, and treatment with special focus on oral cobalamin therapy. Eur J Intern Med 2007;18: 456–62.

Andrès E, Serraj K, Mecili M, Ciobanu E, Vogel T, Weitten T, Mise au point sur la vitamine B12 administrée par voie orale. Ann Endocrinol 2009;70: 455–61.

Berger JR, Quencer R, Reversible myelopathy with pernicious anemia: clinical/MRN correlation. Neurology 1991;41: 947–8.

Carmel R, Sarrai M, Diagnosis and management of clinical and subclinical cobalamin deficiency: advances and controversies. Curr Hematol Rep 2006;5: 23–33.

Dali-Youcef N, Andrès E, An update on cobalamin deficiency in adults. Quart J Med 2009;102: 17–28.

Den Heijer M, Rosendaal FR, Blom HJ, Gerrits WB, Bos GM, Hyperhomocysteinemia and venous thrombosis: a meta-analysis. Thromb Haemost 1998;80: 874–7.

Dreyfus B, Breton-Gorius J, Reyes F, Rochant H, Rosa J, Vernant JP, In: L'Hématologie de Bernard Dreyfus. Paris: Flammarion Médecine-Sciences; 1992. pp. 524–5.

Federici L, Henoun Loukili N, Zimmer J, Affenberger S, Maloisel F, Andrès E, Manifestations hématologiques de la carence en vitamine B12: données personnelles et revue de la littérature. Rev Med Interne 2007;28: 225–31.

Frenkel EP, Yardley DA, Clinical and laboratory features and sequelae of deficiency of folic acid (folate) and vitamin B12 (cobalamin) in pregnancy and gynecology. Hematol Oncol Clin North Am 2000;14: 1079–100.

Gochard A, Mondon K, De Toffol B, Autret A, Carence en vitamine B12, ataxie cérébelleuse et troubles cognitifs. Rev Neurol 2009;165: 1095–8

Hartong SC, Steegers EA, Visser W, Hemolysis, elevated liver enzymes and low platelets during pregnancy due to Vitamin B12 and folate deficiencies. Eur J Obstet Gynecol Reprod Biol 2007;131: 241–2.

Hershko C, Ronson A, Souroujon M, Maschler Z, Heyd J, Patz J, Variable hematological presentation of autoimmune gastritis: age-related progression from iron deficiency to cobalamin depletion. Blood 2006;107: 1673–9.

Kharchafi A, Oualim Z, Amezyane T, Mahassin F, Ghafir D, Ohayon V, Archane MI, Maladie de Biermer et thrombose veineuse. À propos de deux observations. Rev Med Interne 2002;23: 563–6.

Koury MJ, Ponka P, New insights into erythropoiesis: the roles of folate, vitamin B12, and iron. Annu Rev Nutr 2004;24: 105–31.

Kumar J, Garg G, Sundaramoorthy E, Prasad PV, Karthikeyan G, Ramakrishnan L, Ghosh S, Sengupta S, Vitamin B12 deficiency is associated with coronary artery disease in an Indian population. Clin Chem Lab Med 2009;47: 334–8.

Larner AJ, Zeman AZ, Allen CM, Antoun NM, MRI appearances in subacute combined degeneration of the spinal cord due to vitamin B12 deficiency. J Neurol Neurosurg Psychiatry 1997;62: 99–100.

Lee GR, Herbert V, Pernicious anemia. In: Lee GR, Foerster J, Lukens J, Paraskevas F, Greer JP, Rodgers GM, editors. Wintrobe's clinical hematology, 10th ed. Philadelphia, PA: Williams & Wilkins; 1999. pp. 941–7.

Lindenbaum J, Healton EB, Savage DG, Brust, JCM., Garrett TJ, Podell ER et al., Neuropsychiatric disorders caused by cobalamin deficiency in the absence of anemia or macrocytosis. N Engl J Med 1988;318: 1720–8.

Lindenbaum J, Rosenberg IH, Wilson PWF, Stabler SP, Allen RH, Prevalence of cobalamin deficiency in the Framingham elderly population. Am J Clin Nutr 1994;60: 2–11.

Loukili NH, Noel E, Blaison G, Goichot B, Kaltenbach G, Rondeau M et al., Données actuelles sur la maladie de Biermer. À propos d'une étude rétrospective de 49 observations. Rev Med Interne 2004;25: 556–61.

Maktouf C, Bchir F, Louzir H, Elloumi M, Ben Abid H, Mdhaffer M et al., Clinical spectrum of cobalamin deficiency in Tunisia. Ann Biol Clin 2007;65: 135–42.

Molloy AM, Kirke PN, Brody LC, Scott JM, Mills JL, Effects of folate and vitamin B12 deficiencies during pregnancy on fetal, infant, and child development. Food Nutr Bull 2008;29(Suppl 2): S101–11.

Nicolas JP, Guéant JL, Absorption, distribution et excrétion de la vitamine B12. Ann Gastroenterol Hepatol (Paris) 1994;30: 270–82.

Obeid R, Geisel J, Schorr H, Hubner U, Herrmann W, The impact of vegetarianism on some haematological parameters. Eur J Haematol 2002;69: 275–9.

Refsum H, Folate, vitamin B12 and homocysteine in relation to birth defects and pregnancy outcome. Br J Nutr 2001;85(Suppl 2): S109–13.

Saracaceanu E, Tramoni AV, Henry JM, An association between subcortical dementia and pernicious anemia: a psychiatric mask. Compr Psychiatry 1997;38: 349–51.

Savage DG, Lindenbaum J, Neurological complications of acquired cobalamin deficiency: clinical aspects. Bailliere's Clin Haematol 1995;8: 657–78.

Scalabrino G, Peracchi M, New insights into the pathophysiology of cobalamin deficiency. Trends Mol Med 2006;12: 247–54.

Scalabrino G, Veber D, Mutti E, New pathogenesis of the cobalamin-deficient neuropathy. Med Secoli 2007;19: 9–18.

Scalabrino G, Veber D, Mutti E, Experimental and clinical evidence of the role of cytokines and growth factors in the pathogenesis of acquired cobalamin-deficient leukoneuropathy. Brain Res Rev 2008;59: 42–54.

Scott JM, Weir DG, The methyl folate trap. Lancet 1981;2: 337–40.

Snow C, Laboratory diagnosis of vitamin B12 and folate deficiency. A guide for the primary care physician. Arch Intern Med 1999;159: 1289–98.

Solomon LR, Disorders of cobalamin (vitamin B12) metabolism: emerging concepts in pathophysiology, diagnosis and treatment. Blood Rev 2007;21: 113–30.

Stabler SP, Allen RH, Savage DG, Lindenbaum J, Clinical spectrum and diagnosis of cobalamin deficiency. Blood 1990;76: 871–81.

Starr JM, Pattie A, Whiteman MC, Deary IJ, Whalley LJ, Vitamin B12, serum folate, and cognitive change between 11 and 79 years. J Neurol Neurosurg Psychiatry 2005;76: 291–2.

Vogel T, Federici L, Kaltenbach G, Berthel M, Andrès E, Carence en vitamine B12 par mal digestion ou non dissociation de la vitamine B12 de ses protéines porteuses: évaluation comparative des caractéristiques cliniques et paracliniques en fonction de l'âge. Rev Med Interne 2008;29(Suppl 1): S70–1.

Wald SW, Law M, Morris JK, Homocysteine and cardiovascular disease: evidence on causality from a meta-analysis. Br Med J 2002;325: 1202–6.

Wang X, Qin X, Demirtas H, Li J, Mao G, Huo Y et al., Efficacy of folic acid supplementation in stroke prevention: a meta-analysis. Lancet 2007;369: 1876–82.

Zittoun J, Manifestations hématologiques des anomalies congénitales des folates et des cobalamines. Revue Française Lab 1998;303: 45–8.

7.5 Vitamin B12 supplementation, how much, how often, how long?

Rima Obeid; Wolfgang Herrmann

7.5.1. Introduction

Management of cobalamin (Cbl) deficiency depends on the physiological or pathophysiological reasons that caused it. Therefore, it is crucial to define these reasons before starting the treatment. An additional important issue to be considered is management of subclinical Cbl deficiency or the one characterized by metabolic abnormalities in the absence of clinical or hematological signs. The most important task before treating Cbl deficiency is, therefore, to document the clinical and metabolic abnormalities and judge their connection to the deficiency and their response to treatment.

7.5.1.1 Conditions that cause cobalamin deficiency

A typical western diet provides between 3 and 30 µg of Cbl per day, which might be sufficient for maintaining normal Cbl status in people who can absorb the vitamin. In a study on 173 elderly people, low dietary intake of Cbl (<2 µg) was recorded in only three people (1.7%) (Howard et al., 1998). The bioavailability of Cbl is affected by storage and cooking of the foods, other co-administered compounds such as alcohol and medications, and also by several common pathophysiological conditions such as malabsorptive disorders. Therefore, Cbl deficiency can occur in people thought to be ingesting a sufficient amount of the vitamin.

The recommended dietary allowance of 2.4 µg/day has been set based on the lowest amount of Cbl necessary for remission of the hematological signs (megaloblastic anemia) in a group of patients with severe Cbl deficiency (Institute of Medicine, 2000). More recent studies accessing blood concentrations of modern markers of Cbl, suggested that the daily requirements for Cbl should be set at >6 µg (Bor et al., 2006).

The intrinsic factor system operating in the terminal ileum can efficiently absorb tiny amounts of Cbl in the diet. Diseases affecting any step in this absorptive device are expected to limit the absorption of vitamin B12 via intrinsic factor. The state of Cbl depletion starts when the daily loss of Cbl exceeds the daily intake or the daily absorbed amount (▶Tab. 7.13). The depletion takes a few years to progress to deficiency. A pre-clinical deficiency that is characterized by metabolic abnormalities, is a widespread condition that deserves more attention from clinicians. Long-term follow-up studies on the progression of the metabolic abnormalities into clinically evident deficiency are not available. However, many experts support treating such cases to prevent the progression of the deficiency into clinically manifested and probably irreversible condition. See also Chapter 7.3 (Herrmann and Obeid) for more details.

7.5.2 Metabolic signs of cobalamin deficiency, advantages and limitations

Concentrations of holotranscobalamin (holoTC), methylmalonic acid (MMA) and total Hcy help detecting asymptomatic cases of Cbl deficiency (Savage et al., 1994; Stabler, 1995). These markers show more sensitivity and specificity for detecting Cbl deficiency compared with hematologic or neurologic signs. Laboratory markers of

Tab. 7.13: Common causes of low cobalamin status or higher requirements.

Acquired cobalamin deficiency	Causes
Low intake	Poverty
	Avoiding foodstuff of animal origin, adherence to a strict vegetarian diet
	Newborns from deficient mothers
Impaired absorption	Pernicious anemia
	Food cobalamin malabsorption
	Atrophic gastritis, *Helicobacter pylori*, partial or total gastrectomy, Zollinger-Ellison syndrome, pancreatic insufficiency, intestinal overgrowth, sprue, alcohol abuse, medications
Aging	Cobalamin-resistance
Renal disease	Blood toxins
	Decreased renal cobalamin metabolism
	Cobalamin resistance
Diabetes mellitus	Cobalamin resistance
	Related to advanced glycation end products
HIV	Increased requirements
Pregnancy	Increased requirements

Cbl (MMA, total Hcy) have become indispensable tools for setting and confirming a diagnosis or monitoring the treatment. Nevertheless, the limitation of the available laboratory markers in some clinical conditions should be kept in mind (Chapter 7.1, Nexo et al.).

There is currently no firm evidence showing that individuals expressing metabolic signs of Cbl deficiency will transfer to a deficient state within a few years. However, studies on people following a vegetarian diet have shown that the strictness and the duration of the diet were related to the degree of the metabolic abnormalities (Herrmann et al., 2005). Therefore, it is believed that people who show metabolic abnormalities related to Cbl deficiency should be either supplemented with Cbl or recommended to modify their diet to obtain a sufficient amount of the vitamin. Diet modifications are, however, less effective and reinforce the importance of metabolic maintenance on regular basis.

7.5.3 Cobalamin treatment

There is no consensus on the frequency, route of administration, duration of treatment, and the dose used for treating Cbl deficiency. This review will therefore present several points of view before developing final recommendations concerning treating Cbl deficiency.

7.5.3.1 Pharmacologic preparations

Different pharmacologic preparations of Cbl have been used, including cyano-, hydroxo-, adenosyl- and methyl-cobalamin. Cyanocobalamin is a widely used form. This form requires conversion into metabolically active compounds *in vivo*. Hydroxocobalamin is the form preferred in Europe. This compound is thought to be less stable than cyanocobalamin, but has a slower metabolism which allows less frequent injections (Tudhope et al., 1967). One study has shown that i.m. injection of 200 µg of hydroxocobalamin was better retained in the circulation than 200 µg of cyanocobalamin suggesting that hydroxocobalamin might have longer half-life in the body than cyanocobalamin (Hall et al., 1984). However, these observations were done on plasma Cbl in healthy people. In addition, most injections today contain ≥0.5 mg Cbl, hence, any differences that might be related to Cbl form will be compensated for by the high dose.

Earlier observations suggest that cyanocobalamin is rather unstable in multi-vitamin mineral pills and is converted into Cbl analogs (Kondo et al., 1982) that could interfere with Cbl transport (Fedosov et al., 2007). Additionally, cyanocobalamin might be contraindicated in patients with tobacco abuse. Hydroxo- or methyl-cobalamin is favored over cyanocobalamin in people with certain genetic defects who are not able to convert cyanocobalamin. The recently identified protein, MMACHC, is responsible for releasing Cbl from its cyanocobalamin form. This step is a prerequisite for the assimilation of Cbl with the corresponding enzymes (methionine synthase and methylmalonyl CoA-mutase) (Kim et al., 2008). Patients with inborn errors of Cbl metabolism belonging to the Cbl C group lack this protein and show no improvement on cyanocobalamin treatment in contrast to hydroxocobalamin (Andersson et al., 1998; Bartholomew et al., 1988). However, this condition is considered rare and cyanocobalamin remains a widely used Cbl derivative.

Few studies are available that utilized the direct co-enzyme forms, methyl- or adenosyl-cobalamin (Sato et al., 2005; James et al., 2009). Methylcobalamin is a direct coenzyme form and the form required by methionine synthase for methylation of homocysteine into methionine. Old studies suggested that methylcobalamin might be retained by the body better than cyanocobalamin (Okuda et al., 1973). Studies comparing pharmaceutical Cbl forms regarding absorption, bioavailability and effectiveness in lowering MMA or tHcy are not available. Methylcobalamin (75 µg/kg per day) has been injected subcutaneously for children with autistic disorders (James et al., 2009). This product has been found to improve disturbances in methionine metabolism related to oxidative stress and to improve speech and cognition in treated patients (James et al., 2009). Nevertheless, available studies are open-non-controlled making difficult to speculate that the direct co-enzyme form is more effective than the precursor forms. Methylcobalamin is the form preferred in Japan, but again there is no firm evidence showing its superiority compared with other available products.

7.5.3.2 Route and schedule of administration

7.5.3.2.1 Route of administration

There is no consensus on the route and schedule of Cbl treatment. Regardless of these two issues, long time monitoring is one key point that should be considered to optimize the treatment in each newly diagnosed Cbl deficiency case. The between-individual response to treatment varies widely (Tudhope et al., 1967) and is not predictable even in the same disease group. However, the intra-individual response is relatively constant thus stressing the importance of individual decision regarding the treatment model.

Many experts prefer to start with high parenteral doses (1–5 mg) for quick replenishment of the body stores and then the intervals between the injections can be widened (Bastrup-Madsen et al., 1983). A shift to oral treatment or even use of oral treatment to bridge the intervals between the injections over the first few months can be tested (Carmel, 2008). Starting with relatively higher doses of Cbl administered parenterally helps to delay relapse in many patients who discontinue the treatment. A higher amount of Cbl can be retained by the body after injection than after oral supplementation. This explains the fact that relapse is faster after oral than after parenteral Cbl treatment.

Oral supplementation has gained more attention over injections in treating Cbl deficiency, because of its lower cost and better patient compliance. The costs and potential savings of switching a group of elderly people from parenteral Cbl to high-dose oral therapy have been evaluated (van Walraven et al., 2001). The estimated costs including drugs, injections, pharmacists' fees, and injection-associated physician visits were much lower using oral Cbl compared with injections (van Walraven et al., 2001). Oral treatment has been popular in Sweden in the past 40 years (Berlin et al., 1968; Berlin, 1985) and accounted for more than 70% of the Cbl prescribed in Sweden in 2000 (Nilsson et al., 2005). Unexpectedly, in a survey done in 1991 in Minnesota, USA, more than 90% of the 245 medical health practitioners participating in this survey believed that patients with pernicious anemia cannot absorb oral Cbl.

Moreover, approximately 95% were unaware that oral preparations were available for treating pernicious anemia (Lederle, 1991).

The effectiveness of Cbl in correcting the deficiency should be the main criteria when choosing the route of administration. Numerous studies have tested oral Cbl treatment in Cbl-deficient people (Berlin et al., 1968; Kuzminski et al., 1998). It has been estimated that approximately 1.2% (mean) of any oral dose of Cbl arrives the blood by simple diffusion, a pathway that is IF-independent. The IF-system is responsible for binding approximately 1–2 μg Cbl. Studies have shown that oral doses of Cbl (less than 1 mg) in patients with PA were not successful in maintaining serum Cbl and delaying relapse. Because of the strong variations of the absorbed amount of free-Cbl, a high oral dose (1–2 mg) daily is recommended to ensure sufficient Cbl absorption (Butler et al., 2006). Many components of the meal can disturb absorption of the vitamin and thus it is recommended that oral supplement of Cbl should not be administered with meals.

In several non-controlled studies, remission or improvement of hematological symptoms or neurological complications were documented after oral Cbl supplementation with daily doses between 0.3 and 2.0 mg. In one study, no hematological or neurological relapses occurred during long-term treatment with 1 mg oral Cbl given to patients with pernicious anemia (Magnus, 1986). In a randomized controlled trial, the effect of oral (1 mg twice/day) versus i.m. cyanocobalamin (1 mg on days 1, 3, 7, 10, 14, 21, 30, 60, and 90) was compared for treating patients with Cbl deficiency (defined as serum Cbl <160 pg/ml or 118 pmol/l) (Kuzminski et al., 1998). Both treatment arms showed equally effective reduction in plasma concentration of the metabolic markers MMA and tHcy, and improvement of hematological and neurological signs in approximately equal proportion. Some patients with pernicious anemia (*Abs* against IF) showed an increase in serum Cbl and lowering of MMA and tHcy comparable with other deficient patients without pernicious anemia suggesting that many patients with malabsorptive disorders could benefit from oral treatment (Kuzminski et al., 1998). In a further study, 30 patients with food-Cbl malabsorption were treated with oral cyanocobalamin 250, 500 or 1000 μg/day (Andres et al., 2003). All patients showed normalization of serum Cbl, improvement in macrocytosis, and 54% showed remission of anemia symptoms.

In an open controlled randomized study on patients with megaloblastic anemia related to Cbl deficiency, 1 mg Cbl (either orally or i.m.) were used each day for 10 days, then once per week for 4 weeks then once per month for life (Bolaman et al., 2003). Hematologic and neurologic improvements were recorded in both treatment arms, without finding a difference between the two routes at the end of the study (after 90 days) (Bolaman et al., 2003). However, neither metabolic markers nor holoTC were measured in this study to see if the treatment was effective in normalizing the biochemical markers and overcome the depletion. Longer duration of follow-up is also necessary before such a therapy regimen can be recommended.

The effectiveness of long-term biweekly 1 mg oral cyanocobalamin was tested in a non-controlled study on patients with inherited defects in cubilin or amnionless receptors (*n* = 12) and those lacking intrinsic factor (*n* = 4) (Bor et al., 2008). With the exception of four patients who stopped the treatment for at least 1 year before the study, every patient had been following this schedule of treatment for at least 6 years when they were tested for their blood MMA, tHcy, Cbl and holoTC. Subjects treated as described showed one or more abnormal markers in blood (MMA >510 nmol/l, tHcy >22 µmol/l, Cbl <126 pmol/l, and holoTC <21 pmol/l) (Bor et al., 2008). Therefore, long-term oral cyanocobalamin (1 mg) biweekly was not sufficient for normalizing the metabolic markers although it was effective in correcting the hematologic signs (Bor et al., 2008). The study by Bor et al., is one of the few that tested blood concentrations of MMA and Cbl. This stresses the importance of monitoring the treatment using the metabolic markers to judge the effectiveness of the treatment.

A shift from intramuscular to oral Cbl treatment has been retrospectively studied on 60 patients with Cbl deficiency (Roth et al., 2004). Patients were treated with parenteral Cbl for a mean of 4 years, and then shifted to oral Cbl and followed for a mean of 3 years. The mean concentrations of serum Cbl and hematologic markers were similar after parenteral and oral Cbl. Two patients on oral Cbl were found to have low concentrations of serum Cbl (Roth et al., 2004). Metabolic markers (MMA, tHcy) were not evaluated to judge the treatment on a long-term basis.

Cbl substitution to people with low intake seems to restore the metabolic dysfunction associated with the deficiency of the vitamin. Accordingly, concentrations of serum Cbl and urinary MMA were tested in vegans consuming a Cbl-deprived diet for at least 2 years (Donaldson, 2000). Vegans supplemented with sublingual cyanocobalamin showed metabolic improvements after 3 months of follow up. Vegans who received nutritional yeast (estimated to contain 5 µg Cbl/day) showed a significant reduction of urinary excretion of MMA, but mean urinary concentration of MMA was much higher after 3 months than that in vegans treated with sublingual cyanocobalamin. Finally, vegans who took a probiotic formula or flora food showed almost no improvement in urinary MMA excretion suggesting that this supplement form cannot recover Cbl depletion related to low dietary intake (Donaldson, 2000).

Our investigations on vegetarians from Germany and the Netherland have shown that lacto- and lacto-ovo vegetarians and vegans who used over-the-counter multivitamins containing between 1.0 and 3.5 µg Cbl had better Cbl status compared with those not using supplements (Herrmann et al., 2003). Nevertheless, multivitamins containing such a low amount of Cbl were not effective in normalizing Cbl status in vegetarians (Herrmann et al., 2003), suggesting that depleted people might require higher amounts of Cbl to normalize blood Cbl markers (mainly MMA).

Taken together, Cbl injection is often used in the first few days or weeks and then an oral therapy (between 1 and 2 mg/day) can be tested for long-time therapeutic goals. However, because not all patients show a sufficient response to oral Cbl treatment, determination of serum concentrations of the metabolic markers (tHcy and MMA) should be performed to ensure the effectiveness of the therapy.

7.5.3.2.2 Schedule of treatment (start, how often, how long)

In the USA the usual treatment depends on injection of 1 mg cyanocobalamin daily for the first week followed by weekly injections for the next month then monthly injections (Pruthi et al., 1994). In Denmark, the treatment starts usually with a depot preparation of cyanocobalamin weekly for 4 weeks (Bastrup-Madsen et al., 1983), then every third month.

It is widely accepted that the treatment of Cbl deficiency should always begin with large doses of the vitamin (usually i.m.) with the aim of filling the depleted stores.

▶Tab. 7.14 shows a summary of a suggested schedule for treating Cbl deficiency. Using 1 mg as a single injection is followed by a retention of approximately 15% (150 µg) of the Cbl in the body. This dose might be sufficient to correct anemia. There is no consensus regarding the use of injections or oral treatment. For example, Bolaman et al., used 1 mg Cbl (either orally or i.m.) each day for 10 days, then once per week for 4 weeks then once per month for life (Bolaman et al., 2003). This schedule seemed effective in correcting hematological and neurological signs of Cbl deficiency at follow-up points (30–90 days) in 100% and approximately 77% of the study population, respectively.

Tab. 7.14: Suggested schema for treating patients with overt cobalamin deficiency.

Schedule	Comments
Starting	
Start with injections (1 mg cyano-, hydroxo-cobalamin or other forms)	Starting with oral cobalamin might delay improvement.
Continuing	
Continue injecting cobalamin at least until clinical symptoms recover	Recovery of neurological symptoms if present occurs within 1–6 months. Symptoms which persist 6–12 months after adequate treatment are probably not reversible.
Other treatment choices	
Bridge the injections with oral cobalamin (at least 1–2 mg/day)	Might later try to completely shift to oral therapy or to bridge the time between injections.
	Oral cobalamin should be given before the meal, because many components can affect the absorption.
	Diet modifications or 5–20 µg cobalamin daily are probably ineffective.
	Doses of 80–150 µg daily improves cobalamin status but are insufficient to maintain it or correct the biochemical imbalance, particularly in older people or in inherited disorders.
	Doses of 100–500 µg might be sufficient in some patients, but are not successful in the long term, because of the wide individual variations in the amount absorbed, particularly when taken with meals.

(Continued)

Tab. 7.14 (*Continued*)

Schedule	Comments
	Doses of 1–2 mg/day are required for successful long-term results.
Monitoring	
Monitor treatment by measuring the metabolic markers (MMA, tHcy)	Monitoring the treatment is the best way to avoid relapse.
	Hematological signs (MCV, anemia, and hypersegmentation) are not the gold standard for remission, because they are not uniquely expressed and are affected by iron and folate deficiencies.
Monitoring holoTC after oral supplement can help identifying people who are less likely to benefit from oral supplements	HoloTC increases in blood only 6–8 hours after oral supplements.
Monitoring holoTC can help identifying people in the depletion phase, before the biochemical markers increased	HoloTC is thought to be the first parameter to indicate cobalamin depletion.
Total cobalamin is usually not recommended for monitoring the treatment if holoTC test possible	Total cobalamin (80% of it holohaptocorrin) is less sensitive to short term changes in blood cobalamin related to substitution or depletion.
Relapse	
Lower the possibility of relapse	Maintain compliance.
	Relapse might occur after stopping the treatment.
	Relapse in patients using oral supplements is more likely to occur faster than those on injections.
	Relapse with cyanocobalamin is faster than with hydroxocobalamin.

7.5.4 Monitoring the response to treatment

Monitoring the treatment of Cbl deficiency is as important as the treatment, because it helps to confirm the diagnosis and set individual treatment regimens including the route of administration and the dose. Unfortunately, this important part of treating Cbl deficiency is underestimated or misinterrupted. ▶Tab. 7.15 summarizes the most important ways of monitoring Cbl treatment.

7.5.4.1 Monitoring the hematological signs

Several hematological manifestations can accompany Cbl deficiency. In addition to megaloblastic red blood cells, low white blood cell and platelet counts, reticulocytes,

Tab. 7.15: Monitoring cobalamin treatment.

Symptoms	Monitoring	Response	Relapse	Comments
Hematological signs				
Low hemoglobin	Within 1 week of adequate treatment	Increase in reticulocyte count		The response is relatively slow
Increased MCV	Not expensive	Decrease in MCV		Not all patients have hematologic signs
Reticulocytes hypersegmentation		Correction of anemia		Iron or and folate deficiency can interfere with the response to treatment
Low platelets count				
Metabolic markers				
High serum concentration of MMA	Lowered within a few days	MMA is normalized in patients with normal renal function, or considerably reduced (by >200 nmol/l) in patients with renal insufficiency	Occurs after stopping the treatment and depleting the stores of cobalamin	Some authors prefer using urinary MMA, this should be combined with creatinine assay
	The assay is relatively expensive and not widely available, but belongs to the laboratory parameters that are strongly recommended for monitoring		MMA relapse occurs mostly after the concentrations of holoTC decrease, but before the hematological and clinical signs appear	Because plasma or serum MMA are often measured, the reference range for MMA in plasma or serum is widely accepted and known from other studies
High plasma concentration of total Hcy	Lowering total Hcy within a few days	Total Hcy can be normalized	Occurs after stopping the treatment and depleting the stores of cobalamin	

(Continued)

Tab. 7.15 (Continued)

Symptoms	Monitoring	Response	Relapse	Comments
	Parameters that are strongly recommended for monitoring and confirming the diagnosis	Elevated total Hcy that cannot be corrected by cobalamin treatment might be related either to folate deficiency or to in renal insufficiency		
Low concentrations of holoTC or cobalamin	increasing holoTC can be used to verify cobalamin absorption after oral supplementation to ensure that the patients can absorb cobalamin	HoloTC and cobalamin increased in blood very fast after injection	HoloTC is the earliest parameter to decline in the case of depletion	
	holoTC test is not widely available but is becoming more popular	HoloTC increases 6–8 h after oral supplementation for people who absorb cobalamin	Holohaptocorrin holoHC (the major part of total cobalamin) is less sensitive for recent cobalamin deficiency	
Neurological symptoms				
Include a wide spectrum of signs	Symptoms not corrected within 6–12 months of adequate treatment are probably not reversible	Most reversible symptoms improve within 1 month	Possible	Some neurological signs cannot be taken as an index for improvement
		In long-term deficiency, symptoms can be irreversible, but treatment should be maintained to prevent progress of the neurological signs		

hypersegmentation and low hemoglobin have been reported. Hematological remission has been recorded to occur approximately 1 week after starting the treatment (Carmel, 2008). This includes an increase in reticulocyte count, decreased mean corpuscular volume (MCV) and correction of anemia (Bolaman et al., 2003). The response to treatment depends also on the severity of anemia. For example, in a study on 30 patients with Cbl malabsorption, treatment with Cbl caused correction of macrocytosis in all patients and remission of anemia in only 54% of the patients (Andres et al., 2003). In another study on 60 patients with megaloblastic anemia, all hematological parameters were improved after 30 and 90 days of receiving oral or i.m. Cbl (Bolaman et al., 2003).

One very important limitation in depending on the hematological signs to monitor Cbl treatment is the co-existing iron deficiency that could mask the macrocytosis and cause normocytic but hypochromic cells. Moreover, folate deficiency causes similar hematological symptoms and is not corrected by supplying Cbl. Another issue to be considered here is that the hematological symptoms are not uniquely expressed and are indeed inversely related to the neurological symptoms.

7.5.4.2 Monitoring the metabolic response

This part of monitoring the treatment is probably the most important and reliable one. Lowering blood concentrations of MMA and tHcy within 1 week of starting the treatment indicates improvement in Cbl-dependent biological reactions. The metabolic improvements confirm also the diagnosis. Nevertheless, several confounding factors should be considered when starting treatment with Cbl (▶Tab. 7.16).

If the plasma concentration of holoTC does not increase after Cbl injection, this might be related to rare disorders or a deficiency of the carrier protein, transcobalamin. HoloTC increasing in plasma after oral Cbl supplements confirms that this therapeutic

Tab. 7.16: Confounding factors to be considered when treating cobalamin deficiency.

Renal function	Renal function is a major factor determining persistent elevation of MMA after cobalamin treatment. Lowering MMA by >200 nmol/l in renal patients confirms a pre-treatment deficiency.
Iron deficiency	Iron deficiency can mask hematological signs of cobalamin deficiency. After starting cobalamin treatment, the enhanced production of red cells requires controlling iron status. Iron deficiency should be corrected.
Bacterial overgrowth	MMA elevation that cannot be corrected by cobalamin treatment might be related to intestinal bacterial overgrowth. This can be corrected by using a suitable antibiotic.
Folate deficiency	Cobalamin treatment can unmask folate deficiency and combined cobalamin and folate supplementation might be required in severe cobalamin-deficient people.

route can be recommended for long-term substitution of the vitamin. Healthy people show a peak holoTC plasma concentration within few hours (6–8 h) after only one dose (9–200 µg) of the vitamin. This returns to normal at 24 h.

Plasma concentration of total Cbl (80% of it is holohaptocorrin) shows a slower response to oral Cbl supplementation compared with holoTC (Bor et al., 2004). People not showing increased Cbl in plasma after Cbl treatment might have haptocorrin deficiency, a case that is believed to be not rare, but probably without clinical sequela (Carmel, 2003).

When no response of MMA and tHcy can be recorded after supplementing Cbl to people who proposed to be deficient, this might suggest an incorrect diagnosis (Lindenbaum et al., 1990). Elevated concentrations of MMA might be related to intestinal bacterial overgrowth in this case. Moreover, recording the response of MMA and total Hcy is particularly important in patients with end-stage renal disease or elderly people with renal insufficiency. People with renal insufficiency have elevated MMA (typically > 500 nmol/l in end stage renal disease). MMA can be lowered by Cbl injection (Obeid et al., 2005) or oral supplementation (Moelby et al., 2000), but the concentrations of the metabolites cannot be normalized in the majority of the patients. We have suggested that lowering of MMA by >200 nmol/l supports a pretreatment deficiency even when MMA cannot be normalized. The residual increase in concentration of MMA after Cbl treatment might be related to renal dysfunction, or intestinal bacterial overgrowth. Some reports documented an increase in plasma concentration of MMA that is responsive to treatment with antibiotics (Lindenbaum et al., 1990). This can be explained by bacterial production of propionic acid, a substrate for producing MMA. A residual increase in concentration of total Hcy after Cbl treatment might be related either to renal dysfunction or to folate deficiency or both of these conditions.

Concentrations of Cbl and/or holoTC increase in serum after starting Cbl injection, with only few exceptions (e.g. holoTC does not increase in TC-deficient people). Therefore, measurements of these two parameters do not deliver important information on the effectiveness of the treatment in general. Nevertheless, because the rise in serum concentration of the vitamin proceeds the correction of the metabolic abnormalities, both parameters might be very helpful after starting oral Cbl treatment, particularly when uncertainty exists as to whether the patient absorbs the vitamin or not. Serum concentration of holoTC is the earliest marker reflecting changes in Cbl status (Bor et al., 2004). HoloTC assays have been introduced in the year 2002 (Nexo et al., 2002) and meanwhile have been automated. This parameter has great potential to replace the assessment of total Cbl in serum.

Studies conducted by Nexo et al., suggested that the assessment of serum holoTC concentration after administering a low dose of Cbl (27 µg/day) might reflect the ability to absorb Cbl (Bor et al., 2005; Hvas et al., 2006). The test has been also used in combination with recombinant IF. A rise in serum holoTC after cyanocobalamin and IF, but not after cyanocobalamin without IF suggests malabsorption of food Cbl.

Taken together, plasma concentrations of MMA and tHcy are the most reliable markers showing the response to Cbl treatment. Plasma concentration of total Cbl increases but shows more heterogeneity between the studies. HoloTC is an emerging parameter that might be the earliest one to monitor Cbl repletion.

7.5.4.3 Monitoring the neurological symptoms

Neurological symptoms related to Cbl deficiency have been reported to vary and to be only partly reversible. Symptoms include sensitive peripheral neuropathy, cognitive decline, memory disorders, impaired concentration, and loss of sense of vibration (Bolaman et al., 2003). The reversibility of many neurological symptoms depends on the duration of the disease. Many symptoms are not reversible. Residual disability has been reported in 6% of neurological patients (Healton et al., 1991). Symptoms showing no improvement after 6–12 months of treatment are thought to persist (Carmel, 2008). In a study on 60 patients with megaloblastic anemia related to Cbl deficiency, 31 patients had neurological symptoms. Regardless of the route of Cbl treatment, only 16 of 31 patients with manifested neurological symptoms showed improvements after 30 days of treatment (Bolaman et al., 2003).

7.5.5 Relapse of cobalamin deficiency

Relapse in patients treated initially with Cbl might be related to the lack of knowledge about the nature of the disease. Many patients must be motivated to keep taking Cbl supplements and many physicians must carry the responsibility of long-term monitoring to avoid relapse. Relapse occurs within 1–2 years in patients with pernicious anemia who cannot keep their Cbl stores because of the malabsorption and the depletion of Cbl secreted with the pancreatic juice.

7.5.6 Toxicity and side effects

Cbl is a water-soluble vitamin, and any excess can be excreted via the kidney. The toxicity of Cbl is limited. Anaphylactic allergic reactions to Cbl or a preservative compound in the preparation might occur, some of which cannot be prevented by changing the pharmaceutical product. In this case supervision by an allergist is recommended. Another possible side-effect is formation of an autoantibody complex with TC leading to very high plasma concentration of the vitamin. Finally, 16% and 2% of intracellular Cbl was found to be cyanocobalamin in vitamin users and non-users, respectively (Gimsing et al., 1982). The relation of this phenomenon to health aspects has not been established yet.

7.5.7 Cobalamin-responsive disorders without laboratory signs

A major challenge is to decide to treat or not treat people whose clinical symptoms and laboratory test results are conflicting (Solomon, 2005). We believe that Cbl treatment should be started in patients presenting with neurological signs of Cbl deficiency, even if the metabolic markers were normal. Even though such cases are rare, they do exist in the medical literature.

7.5.8 Subtle cobalamin deficiency

Subtle Cbl deficiency is characterized by a low concentration of holoTC and/or metabolic signs related to Cbl deficiency such as elevated concentrations of MMA and total Hcy in the absence of clinical signs. However, low plasma concentration of Cbl in many people is not associated with elevated serum concentrations of MMA or total Hcy. Therefore, recommendation of Cbl supplements would be better based on metabolic dysfunction. Subtle Cbl deficiency is common in elderly people, and can be explained by food-Cbl malabsorption (Campbell et al., 2003). The reported prevalence of low plasma Cbl among elderly people ranges between 5% and 40% and differs according to ethnic origin (Carmel et al., 1999; Joosten et al., 1993; Obeid et al., 2004). However, the intake of crystalline Cbl has been found to be the strongest predictor of Cbl status in elderly people (Campbell et al., 2003), suggesting that the major part of daily Cbl intake should be achieved via crystalline Cbl.

In many studies, the dietary intake of Cbl among elderly people exceeds the Recommended Dietary Intake (RDA) of 2.4 µg/day (van Asselt et al., 1998; Institute of Medicine, 2000). In a study on 105 healthy elderly Dutch people (van Asselt et al., 1998), mild Cbl deficiency (<260 pmol/l and MMA> 320 nmol/l) was detected in 24% and atrophic gastritis in 32%. Only approximately 6% ingested insufficient Cbl. Cbl intake (food and supplements) was higher in people without Cbl deficiency compared with those with Cbl deficiency (median 6.3 vs 4.9 µg/day) (van Asselt et al., 1998). Also, several other studies documented metabolic signs of Cbl deficiency in elderly people (Lindenbaum et al., 1994) that respond to Cbl (Rajan et al., 2002).

Interestingly, serum gastrin was one factor predicting low serum Cbl in elderly people not consuming crystalline Cbl. In people taking crystalline Cbl (as supplements or fortified food), Cbl intake from non-food sources predicted plasma Cbl indicating that even people with atrophic gastritis benefit from crystalline Cbl, but not from food-bound Cbl (Campbell et al., 2003).

The view presented above regarding treatment of subtle Cbl deficiency is not welcomed by all investigators. For example, follow up of 432 people with elevated concentrations of MMA for 1–4 years has shown that MMA improved in 44% of them and worsened in 16% without any treatment (Hvas et al., 2001). Because causes other than Cbl might be responsible for MMA elevation, Cbl deficiency should be usually confirmed by using two parameters (decreased holoTC and increased MMA). Moreover, there are no controlled trials showing how many people with abnormal serum markers can develop true Cbl deficiency; therefore, many experts do not support treating such people.

Assuming that subtle Cbl deficiency should be treated, this means that 190 people of the 432 with elevated MMA will be unnecessarily treated with Cbl to rescue, 242 who might transverse into a true deficiency in the above-mentioned study (Hvas et al., 2001). In our opinion, because of the low toxicity of Cbl and the high costs related to irreversible neurological complications caused by Cbl deficiency, subtle Cbl deficiency should be treated.

7.5.9 A need to revise the recommended dietary allowance

Recent findings stress considering higher recommended daily intake of Cbl in elderly people. Several lines of evidence suggested that the currently recommended dietary intake of Cbl of 2.4 µg/day is too low. First, most elderly people ingest sufficient food-Cbl, but the higher the ingested amount, the lower the possibility is to have elevated plasma MMA and lowered total Cbl (van Asselt et al., 1998). Second, studies have shown that between 4 and 6 µg /day are required for maintaining normal concentrations of

Roth M, Orija I, Oral vitamin B12 therapy in vitamin B12 deficiency. Am J Med 2004;116: 358.

Sato Y, Honda Y, Iwamoto J, Kanoko T, Satoh K, Effect of folate and mecobalamin on hip fractures in patients with stroke: a randomized controlled trial. J Am Med Assoc 2005;293: 1082–8.

Savage DG, Lindenbaum J, Stabler SP, Allen RH, Sensitivity of serum methylmalonic acid and total homocysteine determinations for diagnosing cobalamin and folate deficiencies [see comments]. Am J Med 1994;96: 239–46.

Seal EC, Metz J, Flicker L, Melny J, A randomized, double-blind, placebo-controlled study of oral vitamin B12 supplementation in older patients with subnormal or borderline serum vitamin B12 concentrations. J Am Geriatr Soc 2002;50: 146–51.

Solomon LR, Cobalamin-responsive disorders in the ambulatory care setting: unreliability of cobalamin, methylmalonic acid, and homocysteine testing. Blood 2005;105: 978–85.

Stabler SP, Screening the older population for cobalamin (vitamin B12) deficiency. J Am Geriatr Soc 1995;43: 1290–7.

Tudhope GR, Swan HT, Spray GH, Patient variation in pernicious anaemia, as shown in a clinical trial of cyanocobalamin, hydroxocobalamin and cyanocobalamin-zinc tannate. Br J Haematol 1967;13: 216–28.

van Asselt DZ, de Groot LC, van Staveren WA, Blom HJ, Wevers RA, Biemond I, Hoefnagels WH, Role of cobalamin intake and atrophic gastritis in mild cobalamin deficiency in older Dutch subjects. Am J Clin Nutr 1998;68: 328–34.

van Walraven C, Austin P, Naylor CD, Vitamin B12 injections versus oral supplements. How much money could be saved by switching from injections to pills? Can Fam Physician 2001;47: 79–86.

8 Treatment with B-vitamins and disease outcome

8.1 Folic acid fortification

Joshua W. Miller

8.1.1 Introduction

The ongoing saga of folic acid fortification is an example of both a highly successful public health intervention (for its intended purpose) and a cautionary tale on the complexities and ethics of such interventions. Fully initiated in the United States (U.S.) and Canada as of 1998 for the prevention of neural tube birth defects (NTDs), at least 52 countries and territories have now adopted folic acid fortification programs as of the writing of this chapter (▶Tab. 8.1) (Flour Fortification Initiative, 2010). Notable absentees from this list, however, are all the countries of the European Union. Although there is little disagreement that folic acid fortification is very effective in reducing the incidence of NTDs, questions have been raised about the safety of folic acid based on both theoretical concerns and empirical evidence. There are also concerns about civil liberties and the appropriateness of governments imposing such interventions on their populations.

8.1.2 History

8.1.2.1 The discovery and isolation of folic acid

The story of folic acid begins with the recognition by Wills in the early 1930s (Wills, 1931) of a natural component of yeast (the 'Wills factor') that could prevent megaloblastic anemia of pregnancy, a potentially fatal condition. Later that decade, Stokstad identified a chicken growth factor in yeast that he termed 'factor U' (Stokstad and Manning, 1938). In 1941, Snell working with Mitchell isolated a factor from spinach that could support the growth of the lactic acid bacteria, *Streptococcus faecalis* and *Lactobacillus casei* (Mitchell et al., 1941). They named this factor 'folic acid' based on *folium*, the Latin word for leaf. Isolation of the pure crystalline form of the vitamin was achieved by Stokstad in 1943 (Stokstad, 1943), and it was recognized that the Wills factor, factor U and folic acid were the same substance. Subsequent work during the 1950s and 1960s by many investigators (Bailey, 2007), notably Stokstad and colleagues (Shane et al., 1997), elucidated the components and details of folate metabolism, the inter-relationships between folate, vitamin B12 and methionine/homocysteine metabolism, and the roles of folates in pyrimidine and purine synthesis (▶Fig. 8.1).

8.1.2.2 Fortification of foods with folic acid

In the early 1970s, folic acid-responsive megaloblastic anemia of pregnancy was recognized as a major world health problem (Herbert, 1968). Because of a relative lack of antenatal care and limited use of folic acid supplement pills, even among the

Tab. 8.1: Countries and territories with folic acid fortification as of 2010 (Flour Fortification Initiative, 2010).

Africa	Latin America	South America
Cote d'Ivoire	Belize	Argentina
Egypt	Costa Rica	Bolivia
Ghana	El Salvador	Brazil
Guinea	Guatemala	Chile
Morocco	Honduras	Columbia
Senegal	Mexico	Ecuador
South Africa	Nicaragua	Paraguay
	Panama	Peru
Caribbean	Uruguay	
Barbados		*North America*
Cuba	*Middle East*	Canada
Dominican Republic	Bahrain	United States
Grenada	Iran	
Guadeloupe	Iraq	*Oceania*
Guyana	Jordan	Australia
Haiti	Kuwait	Fiji
Puerto Rico	Oman	
Saint Vincent	Palestine	
	Qatar	
Central/Eastern Europe	Saudi Arabia	
Kazakhstan	Yemen	
Kyrgyzstan		
Turkmenistan	*East/Southeast Asia*	
	Indonesia	
European Union		
None		

economically advantaged, it was proposed that fortification of foods with folic acid could be an effective alternative method of delivering the vitamin to women of child-bearing age (Colman et al., 1974a,b,c). However, no data were available at the time to indicate whether folic acid fortification would be effective.

In a series of elegant publications, Colman and colleagues (Colman et al., 1974a,b,c, 1975a,b,c; Margo et al., 1975) demonstrated the feasibility of fortifying maize meal, rice and bread flour with folic acid to improve folate status in pregnant women.

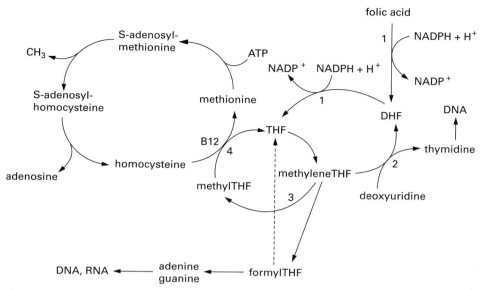

Fig. 8.1: Folate metabolism. Various metabolic forms of folate are required for pyrimidine (thymidine) and purine (adenine, guanine) synthesis, and the remethylation of homocysteine to reform methionine. Folic acid from supplements or fortified foods enters the cell and must go through two rounds of reduction to become metabolically active. Key enzymes: 1, dihydrofolate reductase; 2, thymidylate synthase; 3, methylenetetrahydrofolate reductase; 4, methionine synthase. Abbreviations: DHF, dihydrofolate; THF, tetrahydrofolate; B12, vitamin B12.

South African women in the late stages of pregnancy were fed fortified staple foods containing daily doses of folic acid from 300 to 1000 µg for 25–30 days. Significant increases in red blood cell and serum folate were observed (Colman et al., 1974a,b,c, 1975a,b,c), and megaloblastic anemia was prevented (Colman et al., 1974a,b,c, 1975a,b,c). By contrast, pregnant women who did not receive the fortified foods exhibited slight declines in blood folate levels over the same time frame. Additional studies demonstrated that folic acid was reasonably stable during boiling or baking (Colman et al., 1975a,b,c), and bioavailability of the vitamin was approximately 30–60% of an equivalent amount of folic acid administered in aqueous solution separate from food (Colman et al., 1975a,b,c). These were important findings in the wake of a report by the Joint FAO/WHO Expert Committee on Nutrition espousing the necessity of food fortification programs to correct nutrient deficiencies within populations (FAO/WHO, 1971).

8.1.2.3 Folic acid and the prevention of NTDs

The neural tube is a structure that forms during early vertebral development by invagination of the neural crest cells, which then differentiate into the brain and spinal column. In humans, closure occurs at discontinuous sites along the neural tube with complete closure occurring within 28 days of conception. NTDs are a group of conditions in which there is incomplete closure of the neural tube, often resulting in prenatal or neonatal death or severe disability. The most common NTDs are spina bifida (myelomeningocele), in which the spinal cord is exposed owing to incomplete closure of the spinal column, and anencephaly, in which the brain fails to develop owing to incomplete closure of the cranial region and consequent exposure to amniotic fluid. NTDs are the most common birth defects with a prevalence ranging from ~0.8/1000 births in the U.S. (Honein et al., 2001) to ~14/1000 births in China (Li et al., 2006).

The first indications that folic acid might be important for fetal development came from studies of folate deficiency in rats (Hibbard and Smithells, 1965) and from clinical cases in which pregnant women were given aminopterin, a folate antagonist (Goetsch, 1962; Hibbard and Smithells, 1965). Based on these findings, Hibbard and Smithells hypothesized that fetal malformations resulted from impaired maternal folate metabolism (Hibbard and Smithells, 1965). In 1965, they demonstrated that women who had given birth to a child with a severe birth defect, compared with women who had an unaffected birth, were more likely to exhibit abnormal formiminoglutamic acid excretion after a histidine load (a test of the efficiency of folate metabolism) (Hibbard and Smithells, 1965). The study was limited, however, in that it was not possible to determine if the impaired folate metabolism was owing to inadequate intake, malabsorption, or defective metabolism of the vitamin.

Later in 1976, Smithells et al. (1976) published that a small cohort of women ($n = 6$) who had an NTD-affected birth also had low blood levels of folate, riboflavin and vitamin C during the first trimester of their pregnancies. This led to the hypothesis that NTDs were caused by nutritional deficiencies (Smithells et al., 1976). Smithells and colleagues then conducted a non-randomized trial of a multivitamin supplement consumed daily from approximately 1 month before conception through 2 months post-conception in women who had had a previous NTD-affected pregnancy, the results of which were presented in a series of publications in the late 1970s and early 1980s (Smithells et al., 1980, 1981, 1983; Schorah et al., 1983). Those who received the supplement had an NTD recurrence rate of 0.7% compared with those who had not received the supplement in whom the recurrence rate was 4.7% (Schorah et al., 1983). This landmark study was compelling, but not definitive owing to its non-randomized design, and it did not distinguish which component of the multivitamin was responsible for the reduction in NTD recurrence.

Two subsequent randomized control trials firmly established the specific impact of folic acid on NTD incidence. Laurence et al. (1981) assessed the effect of high-dose folic acid (4 mg/day) on NTD recurrence in a small cohort of women in Wales. Sixty women were randomized to receive the folic acid, of which 44 actually took the supplements. An additional 51 were assigned to receive a placebo. No NTD births occurred in those women that took the folic acid supplements, whereas two NTD births occurred in the group of 16 non-compliant women and four occurred in the placebo group. More compelling were the findings of the MRC Vitamin Study published in 1991 (MRC Vitamin Study Research Group, 1991), which featured a 2×2 factorial design of folic acid supplements (4 mg/day) taken alone or in combination with a multivitamin, compared with the same multivitamin without folic acid, or placebo. In a total study sample of 1817 women who had had a previous NTD-affected pregnancy, there were 1195 recorded births of which 27 were affected by an NTD. A total of nine NTD births were observed in the groups that received folic acid with or without the multivitamin, whereas 22 NTD births occurred in the groups receiving the multivitamin alone or placebo. This amounted to a 72% reduction in recurrence and solidified the role of folic acid in preventing NTDs.

A subsequent randomized control trial in 1992 by Czeizel and Dudas provided additional important information (Czeizel and Dudas, 1992). Hungarian women who had not had a previous NTD-affected pregnancy were given either a supplement containing 0.8 mg folic acid along with 18 other vitamins, minerals and trace elements, or a supplement containing 3 minerals and a low dose of vitamin C. Out of a total of 4753 pregnancies, no NTDs were observed in those who received the multivitamin supplement, whereas six occurred in those who received the mineral/vitamin C supplement. Although this study did not definitively establish that folic acid prevented NTDs, it did suggest that a lower dose of folic acid (0.8 mg/day) might be as effective as the higher doses used in the previous randomized control trials (4 mg/day) (Laurence et al., 1981; MRC Vitamin Study Research Group, 1991), and that folic acid prevented the initial occurrence of NTDs, as well as their recurrence (►Tab. 8.2).

These and other studies (Lumley et al., 2001; Hobbs et al., 2010) provided the impetus for the implementation of folic acid fortification in the U.S. and Canada, fully implemented as of 1998.

8.1.2.4 Implementation of folic acid fortification

A detailed history of the political and bureaucratic machinations that ultimately led to the institution of folic acid fortification in the U.S. and Canada is beyond the scope of this chapter. Readers are referred to historical accounts by Oakley (2009) and Junod (2010). In brief, it is noteworthy to mention that in the early 1990s, despite the mounting evidence indicating that folic acid reduced the incidence of NTDs, two U.S. health

Tab. 8.2: Selected folic acid intervention studies for the prevention of neural tube defects.

Authors	Year	Study design	Findings
Smithells et al. (Smithells et al., 1980, 1981, 1983; Schorah et al., 1983)	1980–1983	Non-randomized, multivitamin with folic acid (0.36 mg)	Reduced rate of NTD recurrence
Laurence et al.	1981	Randomized, double-blind, placebo-controlled folic acid (4 mg)	Reduced rate of NTD recurrence in compliant women
MRC Vitamin Study Research Group	1991	Randomized, double-blind, placebo-controlled, 2×2 design, folic acid (4 mg) ± multivitamin	Reduced rate of NTD recurrence in those taking folic acid with or without the multivitamin
Czeizel and Dudas	1992	Randomized, double-blind, placebo-controlled, multivitamin with folic acid (0.8 mg)	Reduced rate of NTD occurrence

agencies initially came to opposite conclusions. In 1991 and 1992, scientists at the Centers for Disease Control and Prevention (CDC) deliberated and concluded that folic acid fortification was effective, whereas the Food and Drug Administration (FDA) was not convinced (Junod, 2010). Later in 1992, the FDA changed its conclusion after considering additional evidence, and CDC scientists published the following recommendation from the U.S. Public Health Service:

"All women of childbearing age in the United States who are capable of becoming pregnant should consume 0.4 mg of folic acid per day for the purpose of reducing their risk of having a pregnancy affected with spina bifida or other NTDs." (Centers for Disease Control and Prevention, 1992).

Subsequently in 1993, the FDA approved, as allowed by the 1990 Nutrition Labeling and Education Act, the health claim that folic acid reduces the risk of NTDs (Junod, 2010). This ultimately paved the way for the final FDA decision, published in March 1996, to mandate the fortification of all enriched cereal grain products at the level of 140 µg folic acid per 100 g of grain by January, 1998 (Food and Drug Administration, 1996). Notably, the subsequent Canadian decision to follow the U.S. lead on folic acid fortification was apparently made based primarily on economic and business considerations. Because Canadian millers sold much of their flour in the U.S. under the North American Free Trade Agreement, political pressure was brought to initiate fortification in Canada so that the millers would not have to produce separate products for the Canadian and U.S. markets (Oakley, 2009).

8.1.3 Efficacy of folic acid fortification

One of the unfortunate aspects of the folic acid fortification program in the U.S. was that a formal program to monitor its efficacy was not instituted at the time of its initiation in 1998. Such monitoring was mostly left to *ad hoc* analyses performed by interested investigators. Nonetheless, substantial and compelling data have been generated indicating that folic acid fortification has been highly effective for its intended purpose (▶Tab. 8.3).

8.1.3.1 Effect on blood folate concentrations

The earliest reports of the effect of folic acid fortification on blood folate concentrations in the U.S. came from analyses of an HMO cohort in California (Lawrence et al., 1999) and the Framingham Offspring Study cohort in Massachusetts (Jacques et al., 1999). Both studies showed that shortly after the initiation of fortification in 1998, serum folate concentrations had approximately doubled compared with pre-fortification values from earlier in the decade. Moreover, the increase was observed in both non-supplement and supplement users (Jacques et al., 1999). In addition, the prevalence of folate deficiency (defined as serum folate <3 ng/ml) declined from over 20% to ~1% (Jacques et al., 1999). Subsequent analyses of more nationally representative study samples from the National Health and Nutrition Examination Survey (NHANES) confirmed these findings in the general population (Centers for Disease Control and Prevention, 2002; Dietrich et al., 2005; Pfeiffer et al., 2007), and in the target population, women of child-bearing age (Centers for Disease Control and Prevention, 2002; Dietrich et al., 2005). These latter studies showed that the increase was also reflected in red blood

Tab. 8.3: Reported effects of folic acid fortification.

Positive effects

1. Reduced prevalence of folate deficiency[a] (Jacques et al., 1999; Lawrence et al., 1999; Centers for Disease Control and Prevention, 2002; Hertrampf et al., 2003; Chen and Rivera, 2004; Liu et al., 2004; Dietrich et al., 2005; Pfeiffer et al., 2007)

2. Reduced prevalence of hyperhomocysteinemia[a] (Jacques et al., 1999)

3. Reduced incidence and severity of neural tube defects[a] (Honein, 2001; Persad et al., 2002; Williams et al., 2002; Chen and Rivera, 2004; Hertrampf and Cortes, 2004; Liu et al., 2004; López-Camelo et al., 2005; Bol et al., 2006; De Wals et al., 2007; Sayed et al., 2008; Centers for Disease Control and Prevention, 2010)

4. Reduced incidence of neuroblastoma (French et al., 2003)

5. Reduced incidence of stroke mortality (Yang et al., 2006)

Negative effects

1. Increased incidence of colorectal cancer (Mason et al., 2007; Hirsch et al., 2009)

2. Exacerbation of vitamin B12 deficiency (clinically and metabolically) (Morris et al., 2007; Selhub et al., 2007; Miller et al., 2009)

3. Increased incidence of high adiposity and insulin resistance in children exposed *in utero* (Yajnik et al., 2008)

4. Interference with natural killer cell activity (Troen et al., 2006)

5. Inhibition of anti-folate drug efficacy (Arabelovic et al., 2007)

[a]There is general scientific agreement that the effect is causal.

cell folate concentrations. Additional studies in other countries that have initiated folic acid fortification, including Canada, Chile and Costa Rica, show similar improvements in folate status (Hertrampf et al., 2003; Chen and Rivera, 2004; Liu et al., 2004). Importantly, these studies reflect how quickly the folate status of a population can be improved through fortification. Also, the Framingham Offspring study demonstrated that the prevalence of hyperhomocysteinemia (defined as plasma homocysteine >13 μmol/l) decreased by half after fortification, indicating that the observed increases in blood folate levels were accompanied by a change in a folate-dependent metabolite (Jacques et al., 1999).

8.1.3.2 Effect on NTD incidence

The first report on the efficacy of folic acid fortification on NTD incidence in the U.S. was by Honein et al. (2001) who examined birth certificate records from 45 states and Washington, DC. From the pre-fortification period of 1995–1996 to the post-fortification period of 1998–1999, a 19% reduction in total NTD births (3.78/10 000 births to 3.05/10 000 births) was detected, with a 23% reduction in spina bifida and an 11% reduction in anencephaly. Similar reductions in total NTDs, spina bifida and anencephaly were reported by the CDC (Centers for Disease Control and Prevention, 2010) between the pre- and post-fortification periods of 1991–1995 and 1999–2005, also using birth certificate data. Using population-based state surveillance systems, which include in some cases reporting of prenatal NTD diagnoses, Williams et al. (2002) found somewhat higher percent reductions (total NTDs: 26%; spina bifida: 31%; anencephaly: 16%). Using only surveillance data that included prenatal diagnosis, the percent reductions were still higher (total NTDs: 32%; spina bifida: 40%; anencephaly: 19%) (Williams et al., 2002).

In Canada, the percent reductions in NTD incidence have been more dramatic. Total NTDs from seven Canadian provinces declined by 46% (15.8/10 000 births to 8.6/10 000 births) between the periods of 1993–1997 and 2000–2002 (De Wals et al., 2007). The declines were particularly impressive within Nova Scotia (54%) (Persad et al., 2002) and Newfoundland (78%) (Liu et al., 2004). It is important to note, however, that percent reductions are highly dependent on pre-fortification NTD rates, which were higher in Canada than in the U.S. In Nova Scotia and Newfoundland, the rates were very high (25.5/10 000 births and 43.6/10 000 births, respectively) (Liu et al., 2004; Persad et al., 2002). Thus, the higher percent reductions probably represent greater initial need for fortification in Canada than a need for higher levels of fortification in the U.S.

Declines in total NTD rates have been observed in other countries after the initiation of fortification, including Chile (40–55%) (Hertrampf and Cortes, 2004; López-Camelo et al., 2005), Costa Rica (35%) (Chen and Rivera, 2004), and South Africa (30%) (Sayed et al., 2008). In addition, survival of those born with spina bifida has increased in the U.S., suggesting that folic acid fortification reduces the severity of NTDs, as well as the incidence (Bol et al., 2006). Thus, by all accounts, folic acid fortification has significantly reduced the incidence of NTDs and as with the observed improvements in folate status discussed above, the benefit of reduced NTD incidence was achieved in a remarkably short period of time.

8.1.4 Effects of folic acid fortification beyond NTDs

Because of the fundamental roles played by folate and one-carbon metabolism in cellular functions and replication, it is not unexpected that folic acid fortification would have consequences beyond the reduction of NTD incidence. Positive influences on the prevalence of folate deficiency and hyperhomocysteinemia, as cited above, were unsurprising. Other potential positive effects that were anticipated included reduced risk of cancer and reduced risk of vascular disease related to hyperhomocysteinemia. However, concern was also expressed for potential negative effects (Smith et al., 2008). Particular concerns were that excess folic acid could actually promote tumor growth, and would mask vitamin B12 deficiency. Another consideration was that the form of folate used in supplements and for fortification is folic acid, which is a synthetic, unnatural form of the vitamin. Folic acid is fully oxidized and unsubstituted, and must be reduced and biochemically modified intracellularly to become bioactive (►Fig. 8.1). It is not unreasonable to consider the possibility that high intake of such an unnatural substance might have negative consequences.

8.1.4.1 Cancer

The role of folate in cancer is complex. In the form of methylenetetrahydrofolate, folate serves as a substrate for the conversion of deoxyuridine to thymidine, which in turn is incorporated into DNA (►Fig. 8.1). Folate deficiency limits the synthesis of thymidine and leads to misincorporation of uracil into DNA. Mammalian cells have efficient DNA repair mechanisms that remove misincorporated uracil, which is then replaced by thymidine. However, when folate is deficient, thymidine supply is low, which can leave holes or breaks in the DNA base sequence. Such breaks putatively predispose DNA to mutation and initiation of cancer. After cancer initiation, however, the influence of folate changes. Cancer cells, as with every mammalian cell, require folate for DNA synthesis and replication. Consequently, folate deficiency will actually retard tumor proliferation. This is the basis for the use of anti-folate drugs, such as methotrexate (an inhibitor of the enzyme dihydrofolate reductase) and 5-fluorouracil (an inhibitor of the enzyme thymidylate synthase), as cancer chemotherapeutics. Thus, folate deficiency exhibits a 'two-faced' quality such that it can predispose to the initiation of cancer, but retard its progression. With respect to folic acid fortification, we must also consider the converse, i.e., that excess folic acid will both prevent the initiation of cancer, but promote its progression (Kim, 2004; Smith et al., 2008).

Evidence that folic acid fortification might have promoted an increased incidence of colorectal cancer was provided by Mason et al. (2007). Using an ecological study design, rates of colorectal cancer in the U.S. and Canada were examined between 1986 and 2002. Before the initiation of folic acid fortification in both countries, colorectal cancer rates were declining. However, coincident with the institution of fortification between 1996–1998, colorectal cancer rates began to rise for a period of ~3 years before resuming a pattern of reducing incidence in both countries. The increased incidence was estimated to have increased the rate of colorectal cancers by 4–6 per 100 000 people, or as many as 15 000 extra colorectal cancers per year. Although controversial, a biologically plausible interpretation of these findings is that the increased folic acid intake accelerated the progression and subsequent clinical detection of pre-existing colorectal cancers. Other potential explanations for the findings, such as changes in diagnostic criteria and changes in colonoscopy rates, were ruled out as explanations for the data. Thus, this study provides intriguing, although not definitive evidence (owing to the nature of the study design) that folic acid fortification promotes cancer progression. It is important to consider, however, that mortality owing to colorectal cancers was not assessed by Mason et al. (2007), and therefore it is not clear if the increased incidence of colorectal cancer was accompanied by increased mortality.

More recent data from Chile provide additional support that folic acid fortification promotes cancer in populations. Hirsch et al. (2009) examined cancer rates in Chile from 1992 to 2004. After initiation of folic acid fortification in 2000, rates of both colon cancer and breast cancer increased, whereas rates of gastric cancer were unchanged. The increased rate of breast cancer might have been owing to the initiation of a program for early detection of breast cancer and universal access to breast cancer treatment by the Chilean government that occurred at the same time as the initiation of fortification. No such explanation for the increased rate of colon cancer was identified and the authors concluded, consistent with the U.S. and Canada data, that folic acid fortification could have, indeed, promoted colon cancer progression. However, it is important to note that although the colon cancer rate increased, there was no concomitant increase in colon cancer mortality (Hirsch et al., 2009).

Not all reports of the putative effect of folic acid fortification on cancer rates have been negative. In 2003, French et al. reported on the rates of three pediatric cancers in Ontario, Canada before and after the initiation of folic acid fortification (French et al., 2003).

No effect of fortification was observed on infant acute lymphoblastic leukemia or hepatoblastoma. By contrast, the rate of neuroblastoma declined from 1.57 cases per 10 000 births before fortification to 0.62 case per 10 000 births after fortification.

8.1.4.2 Vascular disease

Elevated plasma homocysteine (hyperhomocysteinemia) is now generally accepted as an independent risk factor for cardiovascular, cerebrovascular and peripheral vascular disease (Refsum et al., 1998). Folate, in the form of methyltetrahydrofolate, serves as a substrate in the vitamin B12-dependent conversion of homocysteine to methionine (►Fig. 8.1). Folate deficiency impairs this conversion leading to accumulation of homocysteine within cells and its subsequent export into the blood. As cited above, folic acid fortification resulted in a significant decrease in blood homocysteine levels and the prevalence of hyperhomocysteinemia in the U.S. (Jacques et al., 1999). Only limited evidence is available on whether this decrease in homocysteine levels has affected vascular disease rates. The most compelling data concern stroke mortality.

In 2006, Yang et al. (2006) compared rates of stroke mortality in the U.S. and Canada with those in England and Wales, where folic acid fortification has not been initiated. Between the years 1990 and 2002, stroke mortality rates steadily declined in all four countries. In both the U.S. and Canada, folic acid fortification appeared to influence the rate; in the U.S., the yearly rate of decline in stroke mortality increased from 0.3% pre-fortification to 2.9% post-fortification, whereas in Canada the rate of decline increased from 1.0% to 5.4%. By contrast, the rates of decline in England and Wales did not change over the same time period. The effects of fortification in the U.S. and Canada on stroke mortality were observed in both men and women, and in the U.S. in both whites and blacks.

In contrast to stroke, no evidence has yet been produced that coronary artery disease (CAD) mortality has been affected by folic acid fortification. Anderson et al. in 2004 compared 2-year mortality rates in patients with advanced CAD who underwent coronary angiography before (1994–1997) and after (1998–1999) fortification (Anderson et al., 2004). The post-fortification group had lower median homocysteine and a lower prevalence of hyperhomocysteinemia (defined as >15 µmol/l). In addition, hyperhomocysteinemia remained a significant risk factor for CAD mortality. Nonetheless, no significant difference in overall CAD mortality was observed between the pre- and post-fortification groups. Limitations of this study, however, preclude concluding definitively that folic acid fortification does not affect CAD mortality. In addition to its ecological design and lack of control of confounding factors, the length of follow-up could have been too short to see significant effects. Clearly, more studies are needed to assess the effect of folic acid fortification on vascular disease outcomes.

8.1.4.3 Vitamin B12 deficiency

Deficiencies of both folate and vitamin B12 share the same clinical manifestation, megaloblastic anemia. Megaloblastic anemia results when insufficient folate is available for DNA synthesis and replication of red blood cell precursors in the bone marrow. This can result from dietary folate deficiency, but is also caused by vitamin B12 deficiency. Vitamin B12 is the required cofactor for the conversion of homocysteine to methionine that utilizes methyltetrahydrofolate as the methyl donor (►Fig. 8.1). In the process, tetrahydrofolate is formed. When vitamin B12 is deficient, the homocysteine to methionine conversion is impaired, and folate becomes trapped as methyltetrahydrofolate (the so-called 'methyl-folate trap') (Herbert and Zalusky, 1962). Consequently, methyltetrahydrofolate is not converted into tetrahydrofolate and then methylenetetrahydrofolate, the substrate required for thymidine synthesis. Thus, a functional folate deficiency is created and megaloblastic anemia results when vitamin B12 is deficient.

Over a half-century ago, it was discovered that folic acid supplements could cure megaloblastic anemia caused by vitamin B12 deficiency (Reynolds, 2002). This is because folic acid is converted within the cell first to dihydrofolate, then to tetrahydrofolate and methylenetetrahydrofolate, bypassing the methyl-folate trap (►Fig. 8.1). DNA synthesis and red blood cell precursor replication can then proceed and the megaloblastic anemia is reversed. However, the patient remains vitamin B12 deficient and might go on to develop neurological damage over time unless the B12 deficiency is detected and corrected. In this manner, folic acid supplements can mask vitamin B12 deficiency. With the institution of folic acid fortification, one of the expressed concerns was that vitamin B12 deficiency would be masked, particularly in older adults in which the prevalence of vitamin B12 deficiency is high primarily owing to malabsorption of the vitamin.

In 2007, two publications suggested that folic acid fortification might not mask vitamin B12 deficiency, but in fact could exacerbate it. Using NHANES data from 1999–2002, Morris et al. (2007) evaluated associations between vitamin B12 status and cognitive impairment and anemia in older adults (age ≥60 years). Subjects with low serum vitamin B12 (<148 pmol/l) had elevated odds ratios for anemia (OR: 2.7; 95% CI: 1.7, 4.2) and cognitive impairment (OR: 2.5; 95% CI: 1.6, 3.8), as would be expected. More surprising was that subjects who had a combination of low serum B12 and high serum folate (>59 nmol/l) had elevated odds ratios for both anemia (OR: 3.1; 95% CI: 1.5, 6.6) and cognitive impairment (OR: 2.6; 95% CI: 1.1, 6.1) compared with those who had low serum B12 and normal serum folate (<59 nmol/l). These data suggest that the risk of both anemia and cognitive impairment owing to vitamin B12 deficiency is exacerbated by excess folate intake.

In the second study, Selhub et al. (2007) expanded these clinical findings to include two metabolic indicators of vitamin B12 status, homocysteine and methylmalonic acid. Again using NHANES data from 1999–2002, low serum B12 (<148 pmol/l) was associated with elevated levels of both metabolites, as expected. Moreover, the highest homocysteine and methylmalonic acid levels were observed in those subjects who had low serum B12 and high serum folate. Thus, the same combination of low vitamin B12 and high folate status associated with the highest risk of anemia and cognitive impairment was also associated with the highest levels of metabolic impairment. The associations with homocysteine and methylmalonic acid were confirmed by Miller et al. (2009) in a separate analysis of Hispanic elderly: higher levels of homocysteine and methylmalonic acid were observed in subjects with low plasma B12 (<148 pmol/l) and elevated plasma folate (>45 nmol/l) than in subjects with low B12 and non-elevated folate (≤45 nmol/l). Moreover, subjects with the low B12/high folate combination also had a lower amount of total plasma B12 bound to transcobalamin (holotranscobalamin), the plasma transport protein responsible for delivering vitamin B12 from the site of absorption in the small intestine to all the tissues of the body. However, in contrast to Morris et al. (2007),

Miller et al. (2009) did not observe differences between the low B12/high folate and low B12/non-elevated folate groups in indices of cognitive impairment (Measures of anemia were not available for this study).

The effects of an imbalance between vitamin B12 and folate status might not be confined to anemia and cognitive function in older adults. Because of the high rate of vegetarianism in India, many women have low vitamin B12 status and high folate status during pregnancy. Yajnik et al. (2008), examining data from the Pune Maternal Nutrition Study in India, found that children at age 6 who were exposed *in utero* to an imbalance of low B12 and high folate had greater total fat mass and an increased rate of insulin resistance compared with children exposed to less folate. The authors speculate that the imbalance in vitamin B12 and folate status of the mother leads to epigenetic alterations that pre-dispose the child to fat accumulation and associated risk of insulin resistance (Yajnik et al., 2008).

What might be the mechanism by which high folate status exacerbates vitamin B12 deficiency? One hypothesis is that excess folic acid intake causes the oxidation and consequent inactivation of intracellular vitamin B12 (Selhub et al., 2007). A precedent for this is the irreversible oxidation and inactivation of vitamin B12 that is induced by the anesthetic, nitrous oxide, and which causes severe vitamin B12 deficiency (Drummond and Matthews, 1994). However, a similar effect of folic acid on vitamin B12 has yet to be demonstrated. Another hypothesis is that metabolism of folic acid might lead to excess accumulation of dihydrofolate (Smith et al., 2008). Dihydrofolate is itself an inhibitor of thymidylate synthase (Dolnick and Cheng, 1978) and methylenetetrahydrofolate reductase (Matthews and Baugh, 1980). Inhibition of the former enzyme is what leads to megaloblastic anemia and inhibition of the latter enzyme is thought to affect reactions important for brain function, as well as methylation reactions including DNA methylation.

It must also be considered that because the studies cited above are epidemiological in design, it is not possible to conclude definitively that excess folic acid actually exacerbates vitamin B12 deficiency. A plausible alternative explanation for the data has been put forth by Berry et al. (2007). Individuals who have very high folate status probably consume supplements containing both folic acid and vitamin B12. Despite this, there is still a subset of individuals with high folate status who have low vitamin B12 status. Berry argues that these people are probably those who have severe vitamin B12 malabsorption, such as that caused by pernicious anemia or severe atrophic gastritis. Therefore, grouping together of individuals with the combination of low vitamin B12 and high folate status artificially places those with the most severe vitamin B12 deficiency into the same group. Consequently, this group has the highest apparent risk for metabolic and clinical vitamin B12 deficiency, not owing to excess folic acid, but simply as an artifact of how the population sub-groups are defined. Thus, it remains an open question as to whether or not excess folic acid exacerbates vitamins B12 deficiency.

8.1.4.4 Immune function

The primary form of circulating folate in the blood is methyltetrahydrofolate. Oral folic acid is converted into methyltetrahydrofolate primarily in the jejunum, and then enters the blood. However, it is known that some folic acid can diffuse unmetabolized into the circulation. With the implementation of folic acid fortification, we are now seeing a high percentage of the general population with detectable concentrations of unmetabolized folic acid in serum (Troen et al., 2006; Sweeney et al., 2009). One of the potential consequences of this could be impaired immune function. Troen et al. (2006) assessed natural killer (NK) cell activity in the blood of post-menopausal women with varying intakes of dietary folate and folic acid from supplements. Those women with low overall dietary intake of folate who took a folic acid supplement had better NK activity than those who did not take a supplement. However, in those women who had high dietary folate intake and who also took folic acid supplements, NK activity was impaired relative to those who did not take supplements. Moreover, NK activity in these women was not correlated with total circulating folate, but was inversely correlated with circulating concentrations of unmetabolized folic acid. Thus, excess folic acid from supplements and fortified foods could have negative consequences on immune function. These data also raise the question of whether unmetabolized folic acid affects the function of other cell types.

8.1.4.5 Anti-folate medications

Anti-folate drugs are effective treatments for a variety of conditions, including cancer, epilepsy, malaria, psoriasis and rheumatoid arthritis. These drugs are typically specific inhibitors of one or more folate metabolizing enzymes. Theoretical concerns have been raised that high intake of folic acid from fortified foods could limit the efficacy of anti-folate drugs in the treatment of these disorders. Little data are available, however, that address this issue. One study by Arabelovic et al. (2007) provides preliminary evidence that folic acid fortification has indeed affected anti-folate drug efficacy. Through a retrospective chart review of medical records for patients diagnosed with rheumatoid arthritis, methotrexate dosing levels were compared among rheumatoid arthritis patients from 1988 to 1999. Before the initiation of folic acid fortification, mean weekly methotrexate doses was 12.4 ± 4.0 mg. After folic acid fortification, there was a significant rise in mean weekly methotrexate dose to 16.6 ± 5.1 mg. Although not definitive, this study suggests that folic acid intake is an important consideration for patients on anti-folate medications.

8.1.5 Commentary

For its intended purpose – reduction of the incidence of NTDs – there is little doubt that folic acid fortification is highly effective and one of the most successful public health interventions ever devised. Certainly, tens of thousands of NTDs, with their attendant morbidity, mortality and emotional and financial costs, have been prevented since the mid- to late-1990s. Moreover, it is estimated that ~300 000 births per year are affected by NTDs worldwide, with 50–70% preventable if universal folic acid fortification or periconceptual supplementation could be made available to all. The prevention of NTDs with folic acid is a noble and moral priority.

However, the accumulating evidence suggesting negative consequences of excessive folic acid intake generates a confounding ethical challenge. The basic tenet of medicine – to do no harm – creates a quandary when both action and inaction lead to harm. More challenging is weighing a certainty against possibilities, i.e., the certainty of folic acid fortification preventing NTDs versus the possibilities of excess folic acid intake promoting cancer progression, exacerbating vitamin B12 deficiency, inhibiting immune function, increasing susceptibility to insulin resistance in children exposed in utero, and affecting the efficacy of anti-folate medications. Despite the extent of the evidence of negative effects, we must remember that it is almost exclusively epidemiological evidence, and that all the observed associations are, at this time, just associations. Some of the associations are stronger and more compelling than others, but in no case has causality been definitively established. How do we proceed under these circumstances? The answer depends on who you are.

8.1.5.1 Researchers

Clinicians and scientists on both sides of the folic acid fortification debate have been passionate and persuasive in their positions (Smith et al., 2008; Oakley, 2009). There is a danger, however, that passion might occlude objectivity. It is time that research scientists do what we do best. The epidemiological observations, although not definitive, do generate testable hypotheses, and it is our responsibility to devise and conduct experiments that will objectively examine these hypotheses. In this regard, it is important to remember the five basic epidemiological principles in determining causality:

- *Consistency.* Many of the observed associations between folic acid and pathophysiological and clinical outcomes have not been replicated in more than one or two studies. Will additional epidemiological studies demonstrate the universality of the associations?
- *Strength of the associations.* How much more prevalent is the outcome in those exposed to folic acid compared with those not exposed?
- *Biological gradient.* Does the association between the outcome and folic acid increase with increasing exposure to the vitamin?
- *Temporality.* Does the exposure to folic acid precede the outcome?
- *Biological plausibility.* Based on our understanding of folic acid metabolism, is there a mechanism or mechanisms that explain the observed associations?

Perhaps the most important research yet to be conducted is in the area of biological plausibility. Our understanding of biochemistry and cellular function strongly supports a role for folic acid in promoting cancer cell proliferation and tumor progression. One is reminded that anti-folate chemotherapeutics, such as methotrexate and 5-fluorouracil, were among the first anti-cancer agents and continue to be used today. Mechanisms to explain other putative effects of excess folic acid, e.g., exacerbation of vitamin B12 deficiency or interference with natural killer cell activity, are more speculative. Nonetheless, there are proposed mechanisms, including accumulation of unmetabolized folic acid, inhibition of intracellular folate metabolism and associated functions, and irreversible oxidation of vitamin B12 (Dolnick and Cheng, 1978; Matthews and Baugh, 1980; Drummond and Matthews, 1994; Smith et al., 2008). Testing of these and other hypotheses are a basic and necessary research priority.

It is also important not to 'cherry pick' research findings based on whether or not they support preconceived viewpoints. No epidemiological study is perfect, and random chance or other alternative explanations for observed associations often are conjured to explain away epidemiological findings. This is certainly true for those studies in which negative effects of folic acid are suggested. However, it is also true for studies in which positive effects of folic acid are purported, such as apparent reductions in stroke incidence after the initiation of folic acid fortification in the U.S. and Canada. It is disingenuous to cite these findings as supportive of benefits of folic acid fortification beyond preventing NTDs, whereas at the same time dismissing associations between folic acid and negative outcomes based on flaws in study design. The objective scientist recognizes that among the possible explanations for observed associations between folic acid and all observed outcomes (positive and negative) is that excess folic acid exposure might or might not actually cause the outcome in question.

8.1.5.2 Governments

A notable development in the short history of folic acid fortification is the large number of countries (>50) who have adopted it, following the lead of the U.S. and Canada. Many countries apparently have made this decision without generating data within and relevant to their own populations. It is assumed that what works in the U.S. and Canada will work for them. In light of the potential risks associated with folic acid fortification, this might not be prudent.

In a recent review, Lawrence et al. (2009) examined the rationales for folic acid fortification policies in selected countries. Their analysis reveals important questions that should be asked by governments before instituting such a policy and provides compelling support for adoption of folic acid fortification to be decided on a country-to-country basis. Among the important questions are the following:

- *What is the rate of NTDs within the population?* If the baseline incidence of NTDs is already low, folic acid fortification might have only a small effect on the overall rate, and potentially put a large proportion of the population at risk. New Zealand has been put forth as an example: it is estimated that folic acid fortification will prevent ~8 NTD births per year, while exposing ~525 000 people to excess folic acid per NTD prevented (Smith and Refsum, 2009). Does the benefit outweigh the risk in New Zealand? By contrast, in China, where NTD rates are among the highest in the world, a large proportion of the population is low or deficient in folate, and supplement use is very low. Coupled with the fact that a large scale intervention trial with folic acid has demonstrated a clear and substantial reduction in NTD rates in China (Berry et al., 1999), the benefits could largely outweigh the risks in this country.
- *What is the population's intake of dietary folate and folic acid supplements before fortification?* Negative effects of folic acid might only be manifested when intake exceeds an upper tolerable limit, currently set at 1 mg/day by the Institute of Medicine of the U.S. (Institute of Medicine, 1998). The proportion of supplement users in the U.S. who exceed the upper limit of intake is estimated to be as high as 11% (Choumenkovitch et al., 2001). Berry et al. (2007) have argued that it is individuals who consume both folic acid supplements and folic acid from fortified foods who are responsible for this high rate of excessive intake, and it is these individuals who are driving the risk associated with such high intake. Thus, it can be argued, folic acid fortification should be coupled with policies that limit supplement use.
- *Is fortification feasible within a country?* A key issue is the identification of a staple food that is amenable to fortification and which can be delivered to and is consumed by the target population (i.e., women of child-bearing age). In countries such as the U.S. and Canada, bread and related wheat-based products are almost universally consumed, the technology for large-scale, nation-wide fortification of wheat flour is available, and the infra-structure for distribution is in place. Thus, fortification has

been feasible and successful in these countries. By contrast, in countries in which rice is the staple food and there is not universal consumption of breads and related items, such as China, fortification is a greater challenge. Rice is more difficult to fortify than wheat flour. Moreover, China lacks a national regulatory framework to institute a fortification program (Lawrence et al., 2009) and there could be infra-structural barriers to nation-wide distribution of fortified food products.

- *Other country-to-country considerations.* Other factors might impact the decision to fortify. Recently, there has been increasing appreciation that many populations, partic-ularly in developing countries, have low vitamin B12 status (as indicated by low serum vitamin B12) (Allen et al., 1995; Gielchinsky et al., 2001; Refsum et al., 2001; Rogers et al., 2003). Moreover, low vitamin B12 status is not primarily confined to older adults, as generally observed in the U.S. and Europe, but is seen at all stages of life, including in infants, children and young adults (Allen et al., 1995; Gielchinsky et al., 2001; Refsum et al., 2001; Rogers et al., 2003). The causes of low vitamin B12 status could be owing to low life-long dietary intake, as well as conditions affecting intestinal absorption. Governments might therefore want to consider the potential exacerbation of vitamin B12 deficiency that could be caused by excess folic acid intake. The Pune study in India in which *in utero* exposure to an imbalance of low vitamin B12 and high folic acid was associated with increased insulin resistance later in childhood (Yajnik et al., 2008) suggests that this is a real concern. Other countries might have popula-tions who have libertarian views that are not receptive to governmental interventions that bypass individual choice. This could be a factor in why none of the countries of the European Union have adopted folic acid fortification as of the writing of this chapter.

Factors favoring folic acid fortification that might be characteristic of a country include genetics and religious mores. Hispanic populations have a relatively high prevalence of the MTHFR C677T polymorphism (Guéant-Rodriguez et al., 2006), which increases the requirement for folate and is a contributing factor to the risk of NTDs (van der Put et al., 1995; Botto and Yang, 2000). The high prevalence of this polymorphism in Hispanics might therefore favor the need for folic acid fortification. In Ireland, where the NTD rate is relatively high, abortion is illegal, probably in deference to the religious beliefs of the population. It has been suggested that this places an added burden on the government to prevent NTDs because abortion of affected pregnancies is not an option (Lawrence et al., 2009). This, too, might favor folic acid fortification.

8.1.5.3 Individuals

For physicians and their patients, prescription of folic acid supplements, and even over-all dietary intake of folic acid in the context of fortification, should be considered more carefully. For women of child-bearing age, prenatal care is very important for the health of both the mother and child. One of the staples of such care is the prenatal multivitamin supplement, which contains folic acid. Often a separate folic acid supplement is also prescribed. This practice remained in place even after the implementation of folic acid fortification. Rarely, if ever, is the folate status of a woman measured. Some argue that this is bad medicine. With folic acid fortification, many if not most women of child-bearing age have adequate folate status to provide sufficient protection against NTDs and other birth defects. They therefore do not need extra folic acid supplements, and in light of the potential negative effects of excess folic acid delineated above, such supplements might actually be ill-advised. Good medical practice should include measurement of serum or red blood cell folate, as well as serum vitamin B12, as a component of early prenatal care so that informed decisions can be made on the necessity of folic acid supplements in women residing in countries with folic acid fortification. Other individuals for whom similar considerations should be made are cancer patients and patients with conditions treated with anti-folate medications, such as rheumatoid arthritis and epilepsy.

8.1.6 Conclusion

The issue of folic acid fortification is clearly complex, and is an issue over which reasonable people will disagree. The plea by Oakley that "*...the day soon come when no new children bear the consequences of their governments' failures to implement fully effective prevention programs based on scientific evidence*" (Oakley, 2009) is impassioned and noble. However, the statement by Smith, Kim, and Refsum that "*...it is not justified to assume that the finding of a protective effect of high folate in a whole population necessarily applies to all people within a population*" (Smith et al., 2008) also has substantial merit. The ethical challenge is great: do we limit or discontinue folic acid fortification, and in so doing give enhanced meaning to the idiom, 'throw the baby out with the bath water'? It seems the most prudent course of action is for scientists to continue to carry out the studies and accumulate the data that will allow governments and individuals to make informed, evidence-based decisions. Also, when folic acid fortification is initiated, targeted monitoring programs should be carefully planned and instituted to assess efficacy in improving folate status and reducing NTD incidence, as well as the incidence of both positive and negative collateral effects.

References

Allen LH, Rosado JL, Casterline JE, Martinez H, Lopez P, Muñoz E, Black AK, Vitamin B-12 deficiency and malabsorption are highly prevalent in rural Mexican communities. Am J Clin Nutr 1995;62: 1013–9.

Anderson JL, Jensen KR, Carlquist JF, Bair TL, Horne BD, Muhlestein JB, Effect of folic acid fortification of food on homocysteine-related mortality. Am J Med 2004;116: 158–64.

Arabelovic S, Sam G, Dallal GE, Jacques PF, Selhub J, Rosenberg IH, Roubenoff R, Preliminary evidence shows that folic acid fortification of the food supply is associated with higher methotrexate dosing in patients with rheumatoid arthritis. J Am Coll Nutr 2007;26: 453–5.

Bailey LB, Folic acid. In: Zempleni J, Rucker RB, McCormick DB, Suttie JW, editors. Handbook of vitamins. Boca Raton, FL: CRC Press; 2007. pp. 385–412.

Berry RJ, Li Z, Erickson JD, Li S, Moore CA, Wang H, Mulinare J, Zhao P, Wong LY, Gindler J, Hong SX, Correa A, Prevention of neural-tube defects with folic acid in China: China-U.S. collaborative project for neural tube defect prevention. New Engl J Med 1999;341: 1485–90.

Berry RJ, Carter HK, Yang Q, Cognitive impairment in older Americans in the age of folic acid fortification. Am J Clin Nutr 2007;86: 265–7.

Bol KA, Collins JS, Kirby RS, National Birth Defects Prevention Network, Survival of infants with neural tube defects in the presence of folic acid fortification. Pediatrics 2006;117: 803–13.

Botto LD, Yang Q, 5,10-Methylenetetrahydrofolate reductase gene variants and congenital anomalies: a HuGE review. Am J Epidemiol 2000;151: 862–77.

Centers for Disease Control and Prevention, Recommendations for the use of folic acid to reduce the number of cases of spina bifida and other neural tube defects. Morb Mortal Wkly Rep 1992;41: 1–7.

Centers for Disease Control and Prevention, Folate status in women of childbearing age, by race and ethnicity-United States, 1999–2000. Morb Mortal Wkly Rep 2002;51: 808–10.

Centers for Disease Control and Prevention. http://www.cdc.gov/Features/dsSpinaBifida/ (accessed March 28, 2010).

Chen LT, Rivera MA, The Costa Rican experience: reduction of neural tube defects following food fortification programs. Nutr Rev 2004;62: S40–3.

Choumenkovitch SF, Jacques PF, Nadeau MR, Wilson PW, Rosenberg IH, Selhub J, Folic acid fortification increases red blood cell folate concentrations in the Framingham study. J Nutr 2001;131: 3277–80.

Colman N, Barker M, Green R, Metz J, Prevention of folate deficiency in pregnancy by food fortification. Am J Clin Nutr 1974;27: 339–44.

Colman N, Green R, Stevens K, Metz J, Prevention of folate deficiency by food fortification. VI. The antimegaloblastic effect of folic acid-fortified maize meal. S Afr Med J 1974;48: 1795–8.

Colman N, Larsen JV, Barker M, Barker EA, Green R, Metz J, Prevention of folate deficiency by food fortification. V. A pilot field trial of folic acid-fortified maize meal. S Afr Med J 1974;48: 1763–6.

Colman N, Barker EA, Barker M, Green R, Metz J, Prevention of folate deficiency by food fortification. IV. Identification of target groups in addition to pregnant women in an adult rural population. Am J Clin Nutr 1975;28: 471–6.

Colman N, Green R, Metz J, Prevention of folate deficiency by food fortification. II. Absorption of folic acid from fortified staple foods. Am J Clin Nutr 1975;28: 459–64.

Colman N, Larsen JV, Barker M, Barker EA, Green R, Metz J, Prevention of folate deficiency by food fortification. III. Effect in pregnant subjects of varying amounts of added folic acid. Am J Clin Nutr 1975;28: 465–70.

Czeizel AE, Dudas I, Prevention of the first occurrence of neural-tube defects by periconceptional vitamin supplementation. N Engl J Med 1992;327: 1832–5.

De Wals P, Tairou F, Van Allen MI, Uh SH, Lowry RB, Sibbald B, Evans JA, Van den Hof MC, Zimmer P, Crowley M, Fernandez B, Lee NS, Niyonsenga T, Reduction in neural-tube defects after folic acid fortification in Canada. N Engl J Med 2007;357: 135–42.

Dietrich M, Brown CJ, Block G, The effect of folate fortification of cereal-grain products on blood folate status, dietary folate intake, and dietary folate sources among adult non-supplement users in the United States. J Am Coll Nutr 2005;24: 266–74.

Dolnick BJ, Cheng YC, Human thymidylate synthetase. II. Derivatives of pteroylmono- and -polyglutamates as substrates and inhibitors. J Biol Chem 1978;253: 3563–7.

Drummond JT, Matthews RG, Nitrous oxide inactivation of cobalamin-dependent methionine synthase from *Escherichia coli*: characterization of the damage to the enzyme and prosthetic group. Biochemistry 1994;33: 3742–50.

FAO/WHO Expert Committee on Nutrition. Food fortification. World Health Organization Technical Report Serial No. 477. Geneva, 1971.

Flour Fortification Initiative. http://www.sph.emory.edu/wheatflour/index.php (accessed March 28, 2010).

Food and Drug Administration. Food labeling: health claims and label statements; folate and neural tube defects. Federal Register 1996;61: 8752–81.

French AE, Grant R, Weitzman S, Ray JG, Vermeulen MJ, Sung L, Greenberg M, Koren G, Folic acid food fortification is associated with a decline in neuroblastoma. Clin Pharmacol Therapeut 2003;74: 288–94.

Gielchinsky Y, Elstein D, Green R, Miller JW, Elstein Y, Algur N, Lahad A, Shinar E, Abrahamov A, Zimran A, High prevalence of low serum vitamin B12 in a multi-ethnic Israeli population. Br J Haematol 2001;115: 707–9.

Goetsch C, An evaluation of aminopterin as an abortifacient. Am J Obstet Gynecol 1962;83: 1474–7.

Guéant-Rodriguez RM, Guéant JL, Debard R, Thirion S, Hong LX, Bronowicki JP, Namour F, Chabi NW, Sanni A, Anello G, Bosco P, Romano C, Amouzou E, Arrieta HR, Sánchez BE, Romano A, Herbeth B, Guilland JC, Mutchinick OM, Prevalence of methylenetetrahydrofolate reductase 677T and 1298C alleles and folate status: a comparative study in Mexican, West African, and European populations. Am J Clin Nutr 2006;83: 701–7.

Herbert V, Zalusky R, Interrelations of vitamin B12 and folic acid metabolism: folic acid clearance studies. J Clin Invest 1962;41: 1263–76.

Herbert V, Megaloblastic anemia as a problem in world health. Am J Clin Nutr 1968;21: 1115–20.

Hertrampf E, Cortés F, Erickson JD, Cayazzo M, Freire W, Bailey LB, Howson C, Kauwell GP, Pfeiffer C, Consumption of folic acid-fortified bread improves folate status in women of reproductive age in Chile. J Nutr 2003;133: 3166–9.

Hertrampf E, Cortes F, Folic acid fortification of wheat flour: Chile. Nutr Rev 2004;62: S44–8.

Hibbard ED, Smithells RW, Folic acid metabolism and human embryopathy. Lancet 1965;285: 1254.

Hirsch S, Sanchez H, Albala C, de la Maza MP, Barrera G, Leiva L, Bunout D, Colon cancer in Chile before and after the start of the flour fortification program with folic acid. Eur J Gastroenterol Hepatol 2009;21: 436–9.

Hobbs CA, Shaw GM, Werler MM, Mosley B, Folate status and birth defect risk: epidemiological perspective. In: Bailey LB, editor. Folate in health and disease, 2nd ed. Boca Raton, FL: CRC Press; 2010. pp. 133–53.

Honein MA, Paulozzi LJ, Mathews TJ, Erickson, JD, Wong LYC, Impact of folic acid fortification of the US food supply on the occurrence of neural tube defects. J Am Med Assoc 2001;285: 2981–6.

Institute of Medicine. Folate. In: Dietary reference intakes for thiamin, riboflavin, niacin, vitamin B6, folate, vitamin B12, pantothenic acid, biotin, and choline. Washington, DC: National Academy Press; 1998. pp. 196–305.

Jacques PF, Selhub J, Bostom AG, Wilson PW, Rosenberg IH, The effect of folic acid fortification on plasma folate and total homocysteine concentrations. N Engl J Med 1999;340: 1449–54.

Junod SW, Folic acid fortification: fact and folly. http://www.fda.gov/AboutFDA/WhatWeDo/History/ProductRegulation/SelectionsFromFDLIUpdateSeriesonFDAHistory/ucm091883.htm (accessed March 28, 2010).

Kim YI, Will mandatory folic acid fortification prevent or promote cancer? Am J Clin Nutr 2004;80: 1123–8.

Laurence KM, James N, Miller MH, Tennant GB, Campbell H, Double-blind randomised controlled trial of folate treatment before conception to prevent recurrence of neural-tube defects. Br Med J (Clin Res Ed) 1981;282: 1509–11.

Lawrence JM, Petitti DB, Watkins M, Umekubo MA, Trends in serum folate after food fortification. Lancet 1999;354: 915–6.

Lawrence MA, Chai W, Kara R, Rosenberg IH, Scott J, Tedstone A, Examination of selected national policies towards mandatory folic acid fortification. Nutr Rev 2009;67(Suppl 1): S73–8.

Li Z, Ren A, Zhang L, Ye R, Li S, Zheng J, Hong S, Wang T, Li Z, Extremely high prevalence of neural tube defects in a 4-county area in Shanxi Province, China. Birth Defects Res: A. Clin Mol Teratol 2006;76: 237–4.

Liu S, West R, Randell E, Longerich L, O'Connor KS, Scott H, Crowley M, Lam A, Prabhakaran V, McCourt C, A comprehensive evaluation of food fortification with folic acid for the primary prevention of neural tube defects. BMC Pregnancy Childbirth 2004;4: 20.

Lumley J, Watson L, Watson M, Bower C, Periconceptual supplementation with folate and/or multivitamins for preventing neural tube defects. Cochrane Database Syst Rev 2001; CD001065.

López-Camelo JS, Orioli IM, da Graça Dutra M, Nazer-Herrera J, Rivera N, Ojeda ME, Canessa A, Wettig E, Fontannaz AM, Mellado C, Castilla EE, Reduction of birth prevalence rates of neural tube defects after folic acid fortification in Chile. Am J Med Genet A 2005;135: 120–5.

MRC Vitamin Study Research Group, Prevention of neural tube defects: results of the medical research council vitamin study. Lancet 1991;338: 131–7.

Margo G, Barker M, Fernandes-Costa F, Colman N, Green R, Metz J, Prevention of folate deficiency by food fortification. VII. The use of bread as a vehicle for folate supplementation. Am J Clin Nutr 1975;28:761–3.

Mason JB, Dickstein A, Jacques PF, Haggarty P, Selhub J, Dallal G, Rosenberg IH, A temporal association between folic acid fortification and an increase in colorectal cancer rates may be illuminating important biological principles: a hypothesis. Cancer Epidemiol Biomark Prev 2007;16:1325–9.

Matthews RG, Baugh CM, Interactions of pig liver methylenetetrahydrofolate reductase with methylenetetrahydropteroylpolyglutamate substrates and with dihydropteroylpolyglutamate inhibitors. Biochemistry 1980;19: 2040–5.

Miller JW, Garrod MG, Allen LH, Haan MN, Green R, Metabolic evidence of vitamin B-12 deficiency, including high homocysteine and methylmalonic acid and low holotranscobalamin, is more pronounced in older adults with elevated plasma folate. Am J Clin Nutr 2009;90: 1586–92.

Mitchell HK, Snell EE, Williams RJ, The concentration of 'folic acid'. J Am Chem Soc 1941; 63:2284.

Morris MS, Jacques PF, Rosenberg IH, Selhub J, Folate and vitamin B-12 status in relation to anemia, macrocytosis, and cognitive impairment in older Americans in the age of folic acid fortification. Am J Clin Nutr 2007;85: 193–200.

Oakley GP, The scientific basis for eliminating folic acid-preventable spina bifida: a modern miracle from epidemiology. Ann Epidemiol 2009;19: 226–30.

Persad VL, Van den Hof MC, Dubé JM, Zimmer P, Incidence of open neural tube defects in Nova Scotia after folic acid fortification. Can Med Assoc J 2002;167: 241–5.

Pfeiffer CM, Johnson CL, Jain RB, Yetley EA, Picciano MF, Rader JI, Fisher KD, Mulinare J, Osterloh JD, Trends in blood folate and vitamin B-12 concentrations in the United States, 1988–2004. Am J Clin Nutr 2007;86: 718–27.

Refsum H, Ueland PM, Nygard O, Vollset SE, Homocysteine and cardiovascular disease. Annu Rev Med 1998;49: 31–62.

Refsum H, Yajnik CS, Gadkari M, Schneede J, Vollset SE, Orning L, Guttormsen AB, Joglekar A, Sayyad MG, Ulvik A, Ueland PM, Hyperhomocysteinemia and elevated methylmalonic acid indicate a high prevalence of cobalamin deficiency in Asian Indians. Am J Clin Nutr 2001;74: 233–41.

Reynolds EH, Benefits and risks of folic acid to the nervous system. J Neurol Neurosurg Psychiatry 2002;72: 567–71.

Rogers LM, Boy E, Miller JW, Green R, Sabel JC, Allen LH, High prevalence of cobalamin deficiency in Guatemalan school children: association with elevated serum methylmalonic acid and plasma homocysteine, and low plasma holotranscobalamin II concentrations, Am J Clin Nutr 2003;77: 433–40.

Sayed AR, Bourne D, Pattinson R, Nixon J, Henderson B, Decline in the prevalence of neural tube defects following folic acid fortification and its cost-benefit in South Africa. Birth Defects Res: A Clin Mol Teratol 2008;82: 211–6.

Schorah CJ, Wild J, Hartley R, Sheppard S, Smithells RW, The effect of periconceptional supplementation on blood vitamin concentrations in women at recurrence risk for neural tube defect. Br J Nutr 1983;49: 203–11.

Selhub J, Morris MS, Jacques PF, In vitamin B12 deficiency, higher serum folate is associated with increased total homocysteine and methylmalonic acid concentrations. Proc Natl Acad Sci USA 2007;104: 19995–20000.

Shane B, Carpenter KJ, E.L. Robert Stokstad (1913–1995). J Nutr 1997;127: 199–201.

Smith AD, Kim YI, Refsum H, Is folic acid good for everyone? Am J Clin Nutr 2008;87: 517–33.

Smith AD, Refsum H, Submission to the New Zealand food safety authority regarding the proposal to amend the New Zealand (mandatory fortification of bread with folic acid) food standard 2007. 2009. pp. 1–6.

Smithells RW, Sheppard S, Schorah CJ, Vitamin deficiencies and neural tube defects. Arch Dis Childhood 1976;51: 944–50.

Smithells RW, Sheppard S, Schorah CJ, Seller MJ, Nevin NC, Harris R, Read AP, Fielding DW, Possible prevention of neural-tube defects by periconceptional vitamin supplementation. Lancet 1980;315: 339–40.

Smithells RW, Sheppard S, Schorah CJ, Seller MJ, Nevin NC, Harris R, Read AP, Fielding DW, Apparent prevention of neural tube defects by periconceptual vitamin supplementation. Arch Dis Childhood 1981;56: 911–8.

Smithells RW, Nevin NC, Seller MJ, Sheppard S, Harris R, Read AP, Fielding DW, Walker S, Schorah CJ, Wild J, Further experience of vitamin supplementation for prevention of neural tube defect recurrences. Lancet 1983;321: 1027–31.

Stokstad ELR, Manning PDV, Evidence of a new growth factor required by chicks. J Biol Chem 1938;125: 687–96.

Stokstad ELR, Some properties of a growth factor for Lactobacillus casei. J Biol Chem 1943;149: 573–4.

Sweeney MR, Staines A, Daly L, Traynor A, Daly S, Bailey SW, Alverson PB, Ayling JE, Scott JM, Persistent circulating unmetabolised folic acid in a setting of liberal voluntary folic acid fortification: implications for further mandatory fortification? BMC Public Health 2009;9: 295.

Troen AM, Mitchell B, Sorensen B, Wener MH, Johnston A, Wood B, Selhub J, McTiernan A, Yasui Y, Oral E, Potter JD, Ulrich CM, Unmetabolized folic acid in plasma is associated with reduced natural killer cell cytotoxicity among postmenopausal women. J Nutr 2006;136: 189–94.

Williams LJ, Mai CT, Edmonds LD, Shaw GM, Kirby RS, Hobbs CA, Sever LE, Miller LA, Meaney FJ, Levitt M, Prevalence of spina bifida and anencephaly during the transition to mandatory folic acid fortification in the United States. Teratology 2002;66: 33–9.

Wills L, Treatment of 'pernicious anaemia of pregnancy' and 'tropical anaemia' with special reference to yeast extract as a curative agent. Br Med J 1931;1: 1059–64.

Yajnik CS, Deshpande SS, Jackson AA, Refsum H, Rao S, Fisher DJ, Bhat DS, Naik SS, Coyaji KJ, Joglekar CV, Joshi N, Lubree HG, Deshpande VU, Rege SS, Fall CH, Vitamin B12 and folate concentrations during pregnancy and insulin resistance in the offspring: the Pune Maternal Nutrition Study. Diabetologia 2008;51: 29–38.

Yang Q, Botto LD, Erickson JD, Berry RJ, Sambell C, Johansen H, Friedman JM, Improvement in stroke mortality in Canada and the United States, 1990 to 2002. Circulation 2006;113: 1335–43.

van der Put NM, Steegers-Theunissen RP, Frosst P, Trijbels FJ, Eskes TK, van den Heuvel LP, Mariman EC, den Heyer M, Rozen R, Blom HJ, Mutated methylenetetrahydrofolate reductase as a risk factor for spina bifida. Lancet 1995;346: 1070–1.

8.2 Effects of lowering homocysteine with B-vitamins on vascular and non-vascular disease

Robert Clarke

8.2.1 Introduction

Homocysteine is a sulphur-containing amino acid involved in folate and methionine metabolism (Mudd et al., 1964) and is a potentially modifiable risk factor for cardiovascular disease, venous thromboembolism and all-cause mortality (Mudd, 1985; Clarke, 1991; Boushey, 1995; Danesh and Lewington, 1998; Homocysteine Studies Collaboration, 2002). Observations on vascular disease and thromboembolism in untreated children with homocystinuria, a rare autosomal recessive condition with plasma homocysteine levels greater than 100 µmol/l, prompted the 'homocysteine hypothesis' that moderate elevations of homocysteine could be relevant to vascular disease in the general population (McCully, 1969).

8.2.2 Observational studies of homocysteine and cardiovascular disease

In 1976, Wilcken and Wilcken reported that cases with coronary heart disease (CHD) had higher homocysteine levels than age-matched controls (Wilcken and Wilcken, 1976). In 1991, Clarke et al. demonstrated that the associations of homocysteine with risk of CHD and stroke were independent of established risk factors, such as smoking, elevated cholesterol and blood pressure (Clarke, 1991). Subsequently, these results were replicated by many other retrospective case-control studies and a meta-analysis of all such case-control studies implemented by Boushey et al. (1995) reported that a 5 µmol/l higher measured homocysteine (e.g., 15 vs 10 µmol/l) was associated with an odds ratio (95% confidence interval [95% CI]) for CHD of 1.6 (95% CI: 1.3–1.9). Indeed, it was suggested that the increased risk of CHD associated with a 5 µmol/l higher homocysteine was comparable to that associated with an 0.5 mmol/l higher total cholesterol (Boushey et al., 1995). Moreover, the latter report concluded that elevated homocysteine levels was a causal factor and not an epiphenomenon of atherosclerosis and advocated clinical trials to test the 'homocysteine hypothesis' that folic acid-based vitamin supplements to lower homocysteine levels could prevent vascular disease (Boushey et al., 1995) (▶Tab. 8.4).

Tab. 8.4: Summary of the observational studies of homocysteine and risk of coronary heart disease (CHD), by year of publication.

Year of publication	Author	No. of CHD cases	Main findings for CHD risk
1976	Wilcken	25	First identified association of homocysteine with CHD
1991	Clarke	60	Homocysteine association with CHD identified as being independent of other risk factors
1995	Boushey	2458	5 µmol/l lower homocysteine → 60% lower CHD risk in retrospective studies
1999	Danesh and Lewington	3740	5 µmol/l lower homocysteine → 30% lower lower CHD risk in prospective studies
2002	Homocysteine Studies Collaboration	5073	25% lower usual homocysteine → 10% lower CHD risk in prospective studies

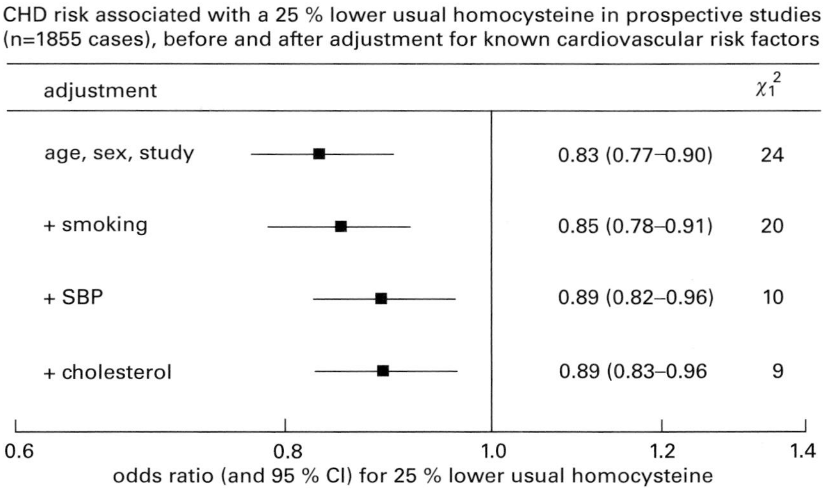

CHD risk associated with a 25 % lower usual homocysteine in prospective studies (n=1855 cases), before and after adjustment for known cardiovascular risk factors

Fig. 8.2: CHD risk associated with a 25% lower usual homocysteine in prospective studies, before and after adjustment for known cardiovascular risk factors.

In the late 1990s, the results of prospective or cohort studies of homocysteine and vascular disease (where blood for homocysteine determinations was collected before the onset of disease in cases) reported results for associations that were much less extreme than those observed in the retrospective studies (where blood for homocysteine determinations was collected after the onset of vascular disease) (Danesh and Lewington, 1998). In 1998 Danesh and Lewington reported that a 5 µmol/l higher measured homocysteine was associated with an odds ratio for CHD of only 1.3 (95% CI: 1.1–1.5) in prospective studies compared with 1.6 (1.4–1.7) in retrospective studies (Danesh and Lewington, 1998). The discrepancy between the results of prospective and retrospective studies was interpreted to indicate 'reverse causality' (i.e., the effect of vascular disease on homocysteine concentrations) (Danesh and Lewington, 1999).

The Homocysteine Studies Collaboration meta-analysis was set up to collect individual participant data from all observational studies of homocysteine and risk of CHD and stroke and provides reliable estimates for the strength of the associations of homocysteine with CHD and stroke after adjustment for known risk factors (Homocysteine Studies Collaboration, 2002). With individual participant data, the Homocysteine Studies Collaboration meta-analysis was able to examine the shape and strength of association of homocysteine with vascular disease after excluding individuals with prevalent vascular disease and adjustment for confounding by other known cardiovascular risk factors (Homocysteine Studies Collaboration, 2002). After excluding individuals with prior disease at enrolment and adjustment for smoking, blood pressure and cholesterol, a 25% lower than usual (i.e., long-term) homocysteine concentration (approx. 3 µmol/l, a difference typically achieved by folic acid supplementation in populations without mandatory fortification of grain products with folic acid) was associated with an 11% (95% CI: 4–17%) lower risk of CHD and a 19% (5–31%) lower risk of stroke (Homocysteine Studies Collaboration, 2002) (▶Fig. 8.2).

The Homocysteine Studies Collaboration meta-analysis did not adjust for the effects of creatinine (as these data were not available in all studies) and was unable to assess the extent to which the association of homocysteine with vascular disease could have been confounded by renal function.

8.2.3 Effects of B-vitamins on homocysteine levels

In populations without folic acid fortification, dietary supplementation with 0.5–5 mg of folic acid typically lowers homocysteine levels by 23%, and in combination with vitamin B12 (mean 0.5 mg) by 30% (Homocysteine Lowering Trialists' Collaboration, 1998). The effects of folic acid are attenuated in populations with mandatory folic acid fortification, where combination therapy typically lowers homocysteine by 20% (Homocysteine Lowering Trialists' Collaboration). Individuals with renal disease typically have homocysteine levels that are approximately twice as great as that in the general population and remain responsive to folic acid with reductions of approximately 25% expected.

8.2.4 Effects of B-vitamins on cardiovascular disease, cancer and mortality

Eight large-scale homocysteine-lowering trials for prevention of cardiovascular disease involving a total of 37 485 participants have reported their results before the end of 2009 (Baker et al., 2002; Lonn et al., 2002; Toole et al., 2004; Bonaa et al., 2006; Jamison et al., 2007; Albert et al., 2008; Ebbing et al., 2008; SEARCH Collaborative Group, 2010). A meta-analysis of the published results of these trials has been conducted and the results have been published previously elsewhere (Clarke et al., 2010). Randomised trials were eligible for inclusion in this meta-analysis if: (i) they involved a randomised comparison of folic acid based B-vitamin supplements for prevention of cardiovascular disease versus placebo; (ii) the relevant treatment arms differed only with respect to the homocysteine-lowering intervention (i.e., they were unconfounded); and (iii) the trial involved 1000 or more participants for a scheduled treatment duration of at least 1 year. Summary data were extracted from all trials completed before the end of 2009 for the present meta-analysis. The comparisons were intention-to-treat analyses of first events during the scheduled treatment period in all participants allocated to folic acid-based B-vitamins or control (irrespective of any other treatment allocated factorially). The main outcomes were coronary events, stroke, cancer and all-cause mortality. Coronary events were defined as the first occurrence of non-fatal myocardial infarction or coronary death; although for several trials the definition of coronary events was restricted to fatal or non-fatal myocardial infarction. Stroke was defined as the first occurrence of either ischemic or hemorrhagic or unclassified strokes. Cancer was defined as any new cancer occurring after randomization, excluding non-melanoma skin cancers.

For each trial, data were abstracted on the number allocated to each treatment and the number of coronary events, stroke events, cancer events, and deaths from any cause by treatment allocation. The expected number of events assuming treatment had no

Tab. 8.5: Selected characteristics of the large homocysteine-lowering trials for prevention of cardiovascular disease.

Year of publication	Trial	No. of participants	Daily dose of B-vitamins		
			Folic acid (mg/day)	B12 (mg/day)	B6 (mg/day)
2002	CHAOS-2	1882	5.0	–	–
2004	VISP	3680	2.5	0.4	25
2006	NORVIT	3749	0.8	0.4	40
2006	HOPE-2	5522	2.5	1.0	5
2007	HOST	2056	40	2.0	100
2007	WENBIT	3090	0.8	0.4	40
2008	WAFACS	5442	2.5	1.0	50
2010	SEARCH	12 064	2.0	1.0	–
2009	ALL	37 485			

effect, and the observed minus expected (o-e) statistics and their variances (v) were calculated for each trial and summed to produce, respectively, a grand total observed minus expected (G) and its variance (V) (Early Breast Cancer Trialists' Collaborative Group, 1990). The one-step estimate of the event rate ratio is G/V. The χ^2-test statistic (χ^2_{n-1}) for heterogeneity between n trials is $S-(G^2/V)$, where S is the sum over all the trials of $(o$-$e)^2/v$ (Cochran, 1954).

Selected characteristics of the large-scale trials for prevention of cardiovascular disease are shown in ▶Tab. 8.5. Six trials recruited individuals with prior CHD or people at high risk of CHD (Baker et al., 2002; Lonn et al., 2002; Bonaa et al., 2006; Albert et al., 2008; Ebbing et al., 2008; SEARCH Collaborative Group, 2010), one trial recruited individuals with prior stroke (Toole et al., 2004) and one trial recruited individuals with chronic renal disease (Jamison et al., 2007). All trials compared the effects of folic acid based B-vitamins with placebo, except the VISP trial that compared the effects of 2.5 mg with 0.02 mg of folic acid (Toole et al., 2004). The daily doses of folic acid used in the trials ranged from 0.8 to 40 mg. All trials included vitamin B12 (dose range 0.4–1 mg) with folic acid, except the CHAOS-2 trial (Baker et al., 2002) that used a daily dose of 5 mg of folic acid alone. Four trials (Lonn et al., 2002; Toole et al., 2004; Jamison et al., 2007; Albert et al., 2008) assessed the effects of combinations of folic acid (dose range: 2.5–40 mg), vitamin B12 (dose range: 0.4–1 mg), and vitamin B6 (dose range: 5–100 mg). Two trials (Bonaa et al., 2006; Ebbing et al., 2008) assessed the effects of vitamin B6 (40 mg) versus placebo independently of folic acid (0.8 mg) plus vitamin B12 (0.4 mg) versus placebo using a factorial design. The meta-analysis assessed the effects of B-vitamins on the risk of vascular and non-vascular events associated with an approximate 25% reduction in homocysteine levels for approximately 5 years.

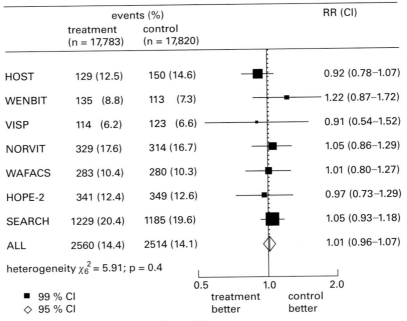

Fig. 8.3: Effects of B-vitamins on coronary heart disease.

8.2.5 Effects on CHD and stroke

Among the 35 603 participants in seven trials with CHD events, there were 5074 CHD events during the scheduled treatment period (one trial did not report results for CHD events (Baker et al., 2002). Allocation to folic acid had no significant effect on risk of CHD events with 2560 among 17 783 (14.4%) allocated to folic acid and 2514 (14.1%) among 17 820 allocated to control, with a hazard ratio (HR) (95%CI) of 1.01 (0.96–1.07) (▶Fig. 8.3). There was no heterogeneity in the effects on CHD between the results of individual trials (test for heterogeneity, $\chi_6^2 = 5.91$; $p = 0.4$).

Despite consistent evidence in observational studies for stronger associations of blood homocysteine levels with risk of stroke than for CHD (Homocysteine Studies Collaboration, 2002), ▶Fig. 8.4 shows that allocation to folic acid had no significant effects on the overall risk of stroke (725 vs 758 stroke events, HR 0.96; 95% CI: 0.87–1.07) either. There was no heterogeneity in the effects on stroke risk between the results of individual trials (test for heterogeneity, $\chi_6^2 = 7.52$; $p = 0.3$).

8.2.6 Effects on cancer incidence and overall mortality

Data were available on 2692 incident cancers among the 29 907 individuals included in seven of the vascular disease trials [one trial did not collect any data on cancer (Baker et al., 2002)]. Cancer events occurred in 1387 (9.3%) of 14 924 allocated to folic acid and 1305 (8.7%) of those allocated control with a HR (95% CI) of 1.08 (95% CI: 0.99–1.17) (▶Fig. 8.5). There was no heterogeneity in the effects on cancer between the results of individual trials (test for heterogeneity, $\chi_4^2 = 2.31$; $p = 0.7$).

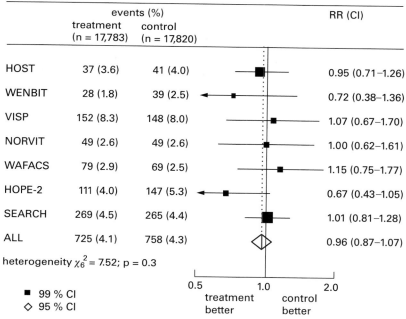

Fig. 8.4: Effects of B-vitamins on stroke.

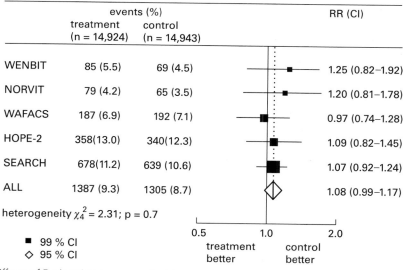

Fig. 8.5: Effects of B-vitamins on cancer incidence.

Data were available on 5128 deaths among the 37 485 participants in eight trials (►Fig. 8.6). Allocation to folic acid was not associated with any significant effects on overall mortality: 2581 deaths (13.8%) among 18 723 allocated folic acid and 2547 deaths (13.6%) among 18 762 allocated as controls, with a hazard ratio (95% CI) of 1.02

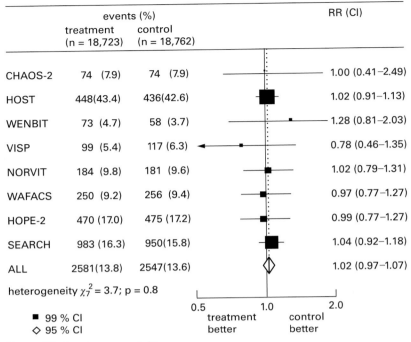

	events (%)		RR (CI)
	treatment (n = 18,723)	control (n = 18,762)	
CHAOS-2	74 (7.9)	74 (7.9)	1.00 (0.41–2.49)
HOST	448(43.4)	436(42.6)	1.02 (0.91–1.13)
WENBIT	73 (4.7)	58 (3.7)	1.28 (0.81–2.03)
VISP	99 (5.4)	117 (6.3)	0.78 (0.46–1.35)
NORVIT	184 (9.8)	181 (9.6)	1.02 (0.79–1.31)
WAFACS	250 (9.2)	256 (9.4)	0.97 (0.77–1.27)
HOPE-2	470 (17.0)	475 (17.2)	0.99 (0.77–1.27)
SEARCH	983 (16.3)	950(15.8)	1.04 (0.92–1.18)
ALL	2581(13.8)	2547(13.6)	1.02 (0.97–1.07)

heterogeneity $\chi_7^2 = 3.7$; p = 0.8

0.5   1.0   2.0
treatment better   control better

■ 99 % CI
◇ 95 % CI

Fig. 8.6: Effects of B-vitamins on mortality.

(95% CI: 0.97–1.07). There was no heterogeneity in the effects on mortality between the results of individual trials (test for heterogeneity, $\chi_7^2 = 3.7$; $p = 0.8$).

8.2.7 Discussion

Although observational studies conducted over two to three decades had demonstrated associations of homocysteine with vascular disease, the results of these studies did not prove causality. Randomised trials were required to assess the efficacy and safety of folic acid for prevention of cardiovascular disease and to assess causality. The initial trials were designed before the results of the Homocysteine Studies Collaboration meta-analysis were available in 2002 (Homocysteine Studies Collaboration, 2002) and hence few of the individual trials had sufficient statistical power to confirm or refute the 10% difference in risk of CHD that was predicted by the Homocysteine Studies Collaboration meta-analysis. The present meta-analysis involving 5074 CHD and 1483 stroke events among 35 603 participants (and 5128 deaths among 37 485 participants) showed that lowering homocysteine levels for approximately 5 years had no beneficial effects on either CHD or stroke. These results refute the findings of a previous meta-analysis of B-vitamin trials that purported to demonstrate that folic acid was effective for the prevention of stroke (Wang et al., 2007). Moreover, these results also differ from a report based on an analysis of secular trends in stroke mortality in the USA and the UK, which attributed the greater reduction in stroke mortality between 1990 and 2002 in the USA compared with that in the UK to the introduction of fortification (Yang et al., 2006). By contrast, the present meta-analysis demonstrated that folic acid supplementation had no significant effect on the risk of stroke.

Concerns have been expressed about the safety of long-term use of folic acid sup-plements, with possible increased risks of cancer (Kim, 2004). Although observational studies had reported inverse associations of dietary intake of folate (or blood levels of folate) with overall cancer, colorectal cancer and breast cancer (Giovannucci, 2002; Zhang et al., 2003; Larsson et al., 2007; Lin et al., 2008), one small trial involving 1021 individuals with a prior history of colorectal adenoma suggested a possible adverse ef-fect of folic acid on both the risk of recurrent colorectal adenoma (Cole et al., 2007) and on prostate cancer (Figueiredo et al., 2009). In addition, an analysis of secular trends of colorectal cancer incidence in the USA and Canada indicating a transient reversal in the downward trends in colorectal cancer incidence after 1995 that were attributed to the introduction of mandatory folic acid fortification in February 1996. (Mason et al., 2007). The results of this meta-analysis for cancer differ from those of a previous trial involving 1021 adenoma participants that suggested a significant hazard for cancer (Cole et al., 2007), particularly prostate cancer (Figueiredo et al., 2009).The present meta-analysis, involving 29 867 individuals with 2692 incident cancer events, demonstrated no statistically significant adverse effects on cancer incidence, overall or in any individual trial. Nevertheless, prolonged follow-up of participants in these trials is required to exclude any longer-term effects of folic acid on risk of cancer.

Large-scale trials and meta-analysis of such trials are required to assess moderate treatment benefits. However, within trials or between trials within meta-analysis, sub-group analysis could result in spurious results owing to the play of chance. Hence, it is important to avoid sub-group analyses to reduce the risk of spurious results except those sub-groups that have been pre-specified on the basis of some prior hypothesis. Replica-tion of the results of trials is also important before making recommendations for clinical practice or public health. The B-Vitamin Treatment Trialists' Collaboration was set up as a prospective meta-analysis involving individual participant data from all large-scale homocysteine-lowering trials (B-Vitamin Treatment Trialists' Collaboration, 2006) to as-sess the effects of B-vitamin supplementation on vascular disease, cancer and mortal-ity, overall and in pre-specified sub-groups and use time-to-event analysis rather than comparison of summary results by treatment allocation. The B-Vitamin Treatment Tri-alists' Collaboration meta-analysis will provide more definitive results, particularly in important pre-specified sub-groups such as those with low folate or high homocysteine levels, and those receiving B-vitamins for a longer duration of treatment. Moreover, the B-Vitamin Treatment Trialists' Collaboration should also provide more reliable evidence for the effects of B-vitamins on cancer (including cancer types) and cause-specific mortality.

If homocysteine levels are not causally related to vascular disease, presumably homo-cysteine levels are related to disease by being a correlate of underlying disease or risk factors that are related to CHD. Apart from the strong correlation of homocysteine levels with folate and vitamin B12, homocysteine levels are strongly correlated with renal function. In retrospect, most of the observational epidemiological studies did not adjust for the effects of renal function when assessing the associations of homocysteine with CHD and stroke. Thus, the discrepant findings of the observational studies of homocys-teine and CHD and stroke and the homocysteine-lowering trials suggest that a correlate of renal impairment might be a therapeutic target for prevention of vascular disease.

The available evidence from published studies suggests that B-vitamins have no ben-eficial effects on risk of CHD, stroke or all-cause mortality or cancer.

Although these results cannot exclude the possibility that more prolonged duration of treatment could be associated with some beneficial effects, albeit this is unlikely as two of the trials were continued for approximately 7 years (Albert et al., 2008; SEARCH Collaborative Group, 2010). Importantly, the available evidence also suggests no evidence of hazard from cancer or cause-specific mortality associated with B-vitamin supplementation, but prolonged follow-up is required to completely refute such concerns. Thus, with the exception of the use of B-vitamins in patients with homocystinuria, the available evidence would suggest that routine use of B-vitamins cannot be recommended for prevention of vascular disease in the general population.

8.2.8 Conclusions

Homocysteine is a sulphur-containing amino acid involved in folate and methionine metabolism that is also a potentially modifiable risk factor for cardiovascular disease. Moderately elevated homocysteine levels have been associated with higher risks of cardiovascular disease, venous thromboembolism and all-cause mortality, but it is unclear if these associations are causal. The 'homocysteine hypothesis' of vascular disease has attracted considerable interest, because homocysteine levels are readily lowered by daily dietary supplementation with folic acid; raising the prospect that dietary supplementation with folic acid-based B-vitamins could prevent cardiovascular disease. Several large-scale trials have been set up to assess the efficacy and safety of B-vitamin supplements for prevention of vascular disease. A meta-analysis of the published results of eight trials involving a total of 37 485 individuals examined the effects of lowering homocysteine with B-vitamins on 5074 coronary heart disease (CHD) events, 1483 stroke events, 2692 incident cancer events and 5128 deaths. Taken together, allocation to B-vitamins lowered homocysteine levels by approximately 25% for an average duration of 5 years. Allocation to B-vitamins had no significant effects on any cardiovascular events, with hazard ratios (95% confidence intervals) of 1.01 (0.96–1.07) for CHD and 0.96 (0.87–1.07) for stroke. Importantly, however, allocation to B-vitamins had no significant adverse effects on cancer [1.08 (0.99–1.17), or for death from any cause [1.02 (0.97–1.07)]. Thus, supplementation with B-vitamins had no significant beneficial effects on the risks of cardiovascular events, and no adverse effects on cancer or overall mortality. A planned meta-analysis based on individual participant data from all the available trials will assess the effects of lowering homocysteine levels in a wide range of subgroups and on additional outcomes. However, the available evidence does not support the routine use of B-vitamins for the prevention of cardiovascular disease or all-cause mortality.

References

Albert CM, Cook NR, Gaziano JM, Zaharris E, MacFadyen J, Danielson E et al., Effect of folic acid and B vitamins on risk of cardiovascular events and total mortality among women at high risk for cardiovascular disease: a randomized trial. J Am Med Assoc 2008;299: 2027–36.

Baker F, Picton D, Blackwood S, Hunt J, Erskine M, Dyas M et al., Blinded comparison of folic acid and placebo in patients with ischaemic heart disease: an outcome trial. Circulation 2002;106:3642.

Bonaa KH, Njolstad I, Ueland PM, Schirmer H, Tverdal A, Steigen T, Wang H, Nordrehaug, JE, Arnesen E, Rasmussen K, and the NORVIT Trial Investigators, Homocysteine lowering and cardiovascular events after acute myocardial infarction. N Engl J Med 2006;354: 1578–88.

Boushey CJ, Beresford SA, Omenn GS, Motulsky AG, A quantitative assessment of plasma homo-cysteine as a risk factor for vascular disease. Probable benefits of increasing folic acid intakes. J Am Med Assoc 1995;274: 1049–57.

B-Vitamin Treatment Trialists' Collaboration, Homocysteine-lowering trials for prevention of car-diovascular events: a review of the design and power of the large randomized trials. Am Heart J 2006;151: 282–7.

Carson NA, Cusworth DC, Dent CE, Field CM, Neill DW, Westall RG, Homocystinuria: a new inborn error of metabolism associated with mental deficiency. Arch Dis Child 1963;38: 425–36.

Clarke R, Daly L, Robinson K, Naughten E, Cahalane S, Fowler B et al., Hyperhomocysteinemia: an independent risk factor for vascular disease. N Engl J Med 1991;324: 1149–55.

Clarke R, Halsey J, Bennett, D, Lewington S, Homocysteine and vascular disease: review of pub-lished results of the homocysteine-lowering trials. J Inherit Metab Dis 2010; in press.

Cochran WG, Some methods for strengthening the common Chi-squared tests. Biometrics 1954; 10: 417–51.

Cole BF, Baron JA, Sandler RS, Haile RW, Ahnen DJ, Bresalier RS et al., Folic acid for the prevention of colorectal adenomas: a randomized clinical trial. J Am Med Assoc 2007;297: 2351–9.

Danesh J, Lewington S, Plasma homocysteine and coronary heart disease: systematic review of published epidemiological studies. J Cardiovasc Risk 1998;5: 229–32.

Early Breast Cancer Trialists' (CTT) Collaborative Group, Treatment of early breast cancer. Vol. 1 Worldwide evidence 1985–1990. Oxford: Oxford University Press; 1990.

Ebbing M, Bleie O, Ueland PM, Nordrehaug JE, Nilsen DW, Vollset SE et al., Mortality and car-diovascular events in patients treated with homocysteine-lowering B vitamins after coronary angiography: a randomized controlled trial. J Am Med Assoc 2008;300: 795–804.

Figueiredo JC, Grau MV, Haile RW, Sandler RS, Summers RW, Bresalier RS et al., Folic acid and risk of prostate cancer: results from a randomized clinical trial. J Natl Cancer Inst 2009;101: 432–5.

Galan P, Briancon S, Blacher J, Czernichow S, Hercberg S, The SU.FOL.OM3 Study: a secondary prevention trial testing the impact of supplementation with folate and B-vitamins and/or Omega-3 PUFA on fatal and non fatal cardiovascular events, design, methods and participants characteris-tics. Trials 2008;9:35.

Giovannucci E, Epidemiologic studies of folate and colorectal neoplasia: a review. J Nutr 2002;132(8 Suppl): 2350S–5S.

Homocysteine Lowering Trialists' Collaboration, Dose-dependent effects of folic acid on blood concentrations of homocysteine: a meta-analysis of the randomized trials. Am J Clin Nutr 2005;82: 806–12.

Homocysteine Studies Collaboration, Homocysteine and risk of ischemic heart disease and stroke a meta-analysis. J Am Med Assoc 2002;288: 2015–22.

Jamison RL, Hartigan P, Kaufman JS, Goldfarb DS, Warren SR, Guarino PD et al., Effect of homocysteine lowering on mortality and vascular disease in advanced chronic kidney dis-ease and end-stage renal disease: a randomized controlled trial. J Am Med Assoc 2007;298: 1163–70.

Kim YI, Will mandatory folic acid fortification prevent or promote cancer? Am J Clin Nutr 2004;80: 1123–8.

Larsson SC, Giovannucci E, Wolk A, Folate and risk of breast cancer: a meta-analysis. J Natl Cancer Inst 2007;99: 64–76.

Lin J, Lee IM, Cook NR, Selhub J, Manson JE, Buring JE et al., Plasma folate, vitamin B-6, vitamin B-12, and risk of breast cancer in women. Am J Clin Nutr 2008;87: 734–43.

Lonn E, Yusuf S, Arnold MJ, Sheridan P, Pogue J, Micks M Sheridan P, Pogue J et al., Homocysteine lowering with folic acid and B-vitamins in vascular disease. N Engl J Med 2006;354: 1567–77.

Mason JB, Dickstein A, Jacques PF, Haggarty P, Selhub J, Dallal G et al., A temporal association between folic acid fortification and an increase in colorectal cancer rates may be illuminating important biological principles: a hypothesis. Cancer Epidemiol Biomarkers Prev 2007;16: 1325–9.

McCully KS, Vascular pathology of homocysteinemia: implications for the pathogenesis of arteriosclerosis. Am J Pathol 1969;56: 111–28.

Mudd SH, Finkelstein JD, Irreverre F, Laster L, Homocystinuria: an enzymatic defect. Science 1964:143:1443–5.

Mudd SH, Skovby F, Levy HL, Pettigrew KD, Wilcken B, Pyeritz RE, Andria G, Boers GH, Bromberg IL, Cerone et al., The natural history of homocystinuria due to cystathionine β-synthase deficiency. Am J Hum Genet 1985;37: 1–31.

Study of the Effectiveness of Additional Reductions in Cholesterol and Homocysteine (SEARCH) Collaborative Group, Randomized comparison of homocysteine-lowering with folic acid plus vitamin B12 versus placebo in 12,064 myocardial infarction survivors. JAMA 2010;303: 2486–94.

Toole JF, Malinow MR, Chambless LE, Spence JD, Pettigrew LC, Howard VJ et al., Lowering homocysteine in patients with ischemic stroke to prevent recurrent stroke, myocardial infarction, and death: the Vitamin Intervention for Stroke Prevention (VISP) randomized controlled trial. J Am Med Assoc 2004;291: 565–75.

Wang X, Qin X, Demirtas H, Li J, Mao G, Huo Y et al., Efficacy of folic acid supplementation in stroke prevention: a meta-analysis. Lancet 2007;369: 1876–82.

Wilcken DEL, Wilcken B, The pathogenesis of coronary artery disease: a possible role for methionine metabolism. J Clin Invest 1976;57: 1079–82.

Yang Q, Botto LD, Erickson JD, Berry RJ, Sambell C, Johansen H et al., Improvement in stroke mortality in Canada and the United States, 1990 to 2002. Circulation 2006;113: 1335–43.

Yap S, Boers GH, Wilcken B, Wilcken DE, Brenton DP, Lee PJ et al., Vascular outcome in patients with homocystinuria due to cystathionine beta-synthase deficiency treated chronically: a multicenter observational study. Arterioscler Thromb Vasc Biol 2001;21: 2080–5.

Zhang SM, Willett WC, Selhub J, Hunter DJ, Giovannucci EL, Holmes MD et al., Plasma folate, vitamin B6, vitamin B12, homocysteine, and risk of breast cancer. J Natl Cancer Inst 2003;95: 373–80.

8.3 B-vitamins in patients with renal disease

Jutta Dierkes; Judith Heinz

8.3.1 Vitamin status in patients with renal disease: the magnitude of the problem

8.3.1.1 The evidence for vitamin deficiencies in renal patients

For some 20 years or even longer, there is a debate whether patients with end-stage renal disease require supplementation with water-soluble vitamins. Despite the common clinical practice of giving water-soluble vitamins, there is surprisingly little medical evidence based on clinical trials or experimental studies concerning this issue. This is also recognized by the EBPG guideline on nutrition (Fouque et al., 2007), that states: *"Due to insufficient evidence from clinical trials for recommending administration of vitamins, the following information only reflects the expert's opinion and cannot be considered as a clinical guideline but a recommendation"*.

Thus, this chapter will summarize the available evidence on B-vitamin status and their health effects in patients with renal diseases.

8.3.1.2 Diagnosis of vitamin deficiencies

Criteria for the diagnosis of vitamin deficiency are specific for every single vitamin. However, some common rules can be applied to most of the B-vitamins. First of all, it has to be stated that in clinical practice, some vitamins (biotin, pantothenic acid, niacin) are hardly measured and therefore data on vitamin status are hardly available. Other vitamins such as folate and cobalamin, are regularly measured using commercial assays.

The measurement of vitamin concentration itself has been questioned in renal patients and instead, the measurement of functional markers such as homocysteine and methylmalonic acid (MMA) has been suggested (Mason, 2003).

It has to be noted that both metabolites are themselves influenced by renal function (Moelby et al., 1992; Lewerin et al., 2007) which limits their use as markers of vitamin status in end-stage renal disease. By contrast, both elevated homocysteine and MMA levels are related to folate and cobalamin concentrations (Robinson et al., 1996; Dierkes et al., 1999a, Herrmann et al., 2001; Obeid et al., 2005; Zoungas et al., 2006). Furthermore, it has been shown that homocysteine and MMA are reduced upon folic acid and cobalamin administration, particularly if the vitamins are applied intravenously (Dierkes et al., 1999a,b; Suliman et al., 1999; Sunder-Plassmann et al., 2000; Henning et al., 2001; Obeid et al., 2005).

However, there are no established cut-offs for these metabolites in renal patients and up to now, most studies report vitamin status determined by the concentration of vitamins in blood or serum/plasma.

The question whether patients suffering from end-stage renal disease do have vitamin deficiencies is difficult to answer. Many studies that have measured folate, e.g., report baseline folate levels in patients who are already receiving vitamin supplements. In addition, most studies did not measure folate levels in all patients of the respective dialysis center, but selected patients for inclusion in clinical studies. Thus, it can be assumed that these patients are not representative for the entire dialysis population and do not reflect the true extent of deficiencies (▶Tab. 8.6).

In the early 1990s, Descombes et al. (1993) investigated the status of folate, cobalamin, thiamine, riboflavin, pyridoxine and biotin in 43 hemodialysis patients (representing 100% of the patients treated in the dialysis center). Whereas thiamine, biotin, riboflavin, folate and cobalamin deficiencies were only occasionally observed, erythrocyte transaminase activation coefficients (indicating pyridoxine status) were in the insufficient range in two-thirds of the dialysis patients.

Folate and cobalamin in unsupplemented patients with ESRD were measured by our group also in the 1990s. In a single dialysis center, 17 of 102 hemodialysis patients received regular vitamin supplementation. We observed low cobalamin levels in 14 out of 102 patients (14%) (Dierkes et al., 1999b), but none of the patients had low serum folate concentrations (Dierkes et al., 1999b). In a subsequent study, we measured also pyridoxal-5-phosphate and observed low levels (<15 nmol/l) in 19 out of 61 hemodialysis patients (31%) (Dierkes et al., 2001). In this later study, the frequencies of cobalamin

Tab. 8.6: Overview of studies that investigated vitamin deficiency in dialysis patients.

Study	No. of patients	Folate	Cobalamin	Vitamin B6	Other vitamins	Regular vitamin supplementation
Descombes et al., 1993	43 (100% of single center)	1.5%	2.5%	65%	Thiamine 5% Riboflavin 0% Biotin 1.7%	Folic acid 2–3 mg/week; vitamin C 400–600 mg/week
Dierkes et al., 1999a,b	102 (100% of single center)	0%	15%	n.d.	n.d.	No vitamin supplementation
Bamonti-Catena et al., 1999	112	63% when serum folate was used; 1.8% when RBC folate was used	Measured, but not specified	n.d.	n.d.	Not specified
Suliman et al., 2000	117 (100% of single center)	0%	0%	n.d.	n.d.	Water soluble vitamins, but no folic acid, no B12
Dierkes et al., 2001	61 (approx. 50% of single center)	7%	18%	31%	Not reported	No supplementation in the month before the study
van Guldener et al., 2000	41 (participants in RCT)	0%	0%	Occasionally		No folic acid supplementation, other vitamins unclear
Billion et al., 2002	55	10%	6%	n.d.	n.d.	No vitamin supplementation
Zoungas et al., 2004	315 multicenter study	6.4%	Not reported	n.d.	n.d.	46% of hemodialysis patients, 22% of peritoneal dialysis patients
Obeid and Herrmann, 2005	38 (out of 75 patients, only those with Hcy >18 μmol/l)	11%	11%	19%	n.d.	Stopped at least 4 weeks before study
Heinz et al., 2009a,b	650 multicenter study	4.3%	3%	37%	Thiamine 0%	30%

n.d., not determined.

deficiency (<200 pmol/l) in unsupplemented patients were similar to the earlier study (18%), and the frequency of low folate levels (<6.4 nmol/l) was 7%.

Suliman et al. (2000) investigated homocysteinemia and nutritional status in a cross-sectional study including all patients treated in a single Swedish dialysis center. Measurements were made in 117 hemodialysis patients, who were all supplemented with water-soluble vitamins including vitamin B6 (10 mg/day), but without folic acid and vitamin B12. The authors observed in all patients plasma levels of folate and vitamin B12 within the normal range. In a Dutch study including hemodialysis patients who were not vitamin supplemented and who participated in a homocysteine lowering trial, baseline data of 41 patients revealed that all patients had folate and cobalamin levels within the reference range (> 3.4 nmol/l and > 120 pmol/l, respectively), and only a few patients (the exact number was not given) had low pyridoxal-5-phosphate levels (van Guldener et al., 2000).

Another study that focused on folate was published by Bamonti-Catena et al. (1999). In 112 hemodialysis patients, both serum folate and erythrocyte folate levels were measured. Interestingly, 63% of patients had low serum folate (<7 nmol/l) but only 1.8% had low RBC folate (<540 nmol/l). This might question either the use of serum folate in hemodialysis patients or the cut-offs for serum folate or RBC folate applied. In a French study, Billion et al. (2002) observed folate deficiency (defined as serum levels <10 nmol/l) in 10% and cobalamin deficiency (<180 pmol/l) in 6% of 55 unsupplemented hemodialysis patients.

It is obvious that many studies on vitamin deficiencies in hemodialysis patients are small, single-center studies which could be subject to selection bias. Larger studies became only recently available and include baseline data of randomized controlled trials with folic acid or multivitamins (Zoungas et al., 2006; Jamison et al., 2007; Vianna et al., 2007; Heinz et al., 2009a,b).

Patients with chronic kidney disease and patients with end-stage renal disease were recruited for a randomized controlled folic acid supplementation trial (ASFAST) by Zoungas et al. (2004). In these patients, 21% of predialysis patients, 46% of hemodialysis patients and 22% of peritoneal dialysis patients received folic acid at baseline, and folate deficiency defined as red blood cell folate <510 nmol/l was observed in 6.4% of patients. At baseline, no data were provided for cobalamin deficiency. During the course of the ASFAST trial with a median follow-up time of 3.6 years, eight out of 159 randomized patients in the placebo group developed folate deficiency (RBC folate <510 nmol/l) and received folic acid, and in 12 patients out of 315 patients in both treatment groups a vitamin B12 deficiency (<160 pmol/l) was detected (Zoungas et al., 2006).

In a large multicenter randomized clinical trial implemented from 2002 to 2008 in Germany, we included 650 hemodialysis patients (Heinz et al., 2009a,b). Approximately 30% of patients received regular vitamin supplementation with water-soluble vitamins, and low blood vitamin concentrations, indicating deficiencies, were as follows: low thiamine levels were not observed, low serum folate levels (<6.4 nmol/l) 4.3%, low plasma pyridoxal-5-phosphate levels (<20 nmol/l) 37%, and low serum cobalamin levels (<150 pmol/l) were observed in 3% (►Fig. 8.7).

In conclusion, the currently available literature does not allow estimation of the exact extent of B-vitamin deficiencies in hemodialysis patients. This is owing to the bias in selection of patients, the lack of appropriate markers to define vitamin deficiency

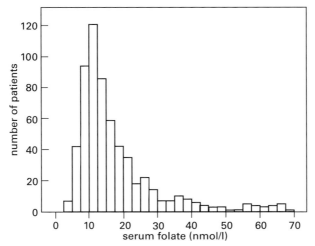

Fig. 8.7: Baseline serum folate levels in 650 patients randomized in a controlled trial with B-vitamins (Heinz et al., 2009a,b). Patients were recruited from 33 dialysis centers in Germany, and approximately 30% of them received vitamin supplements before the study. Values exceeding 30 ng/ml (*n* = 77) are not shown. The cut-off for deficiency was 2.8 ng/ml (6.4 nmol/l).

and the lack of data obtained in patients who were previously not supplemented with B-vitamins.

In addition, there is a considerable lack of data on other vitamins than folate, cobalamin and vitamin B6. Low pyridoxal-5-phosphate can frequently occur, however, there is a current debate whether plasma pyridoxal-5-phosphate truly reflects vitamin B6 status in patients with chronic inflammation (Bates et al., 1999; Friso et al., 2001). Therefore, a high frequency of low plasma pyridoxal-5-phosphate levels in hemodialysis patients might not reflect vitamin B6 deficiency, and vitamin B6 status should be measured in these patients either by the use of whole blood pyridoxal-5-phosphate or by the erythrocyte transaminase activation coefficient (Talwar et al., 2003).

8.3.1.3 Reasons for diminished vitamin status in hemodialysis patients

In the literature, frequently cited reasons for increased vitamin requirements in hemodialysis patients include dietary restrictions, altered metabolism, interactions with drugs and losses during the dialysis process. It is, however, surprising that these issues have not been systematically investigated. Indeed, data supporting an altered metabolism of vitamins are only available for folate (Jennette and Goldman, 1975; Livant et al., 1994). Losses during the dialysis process are reported for vitamin C (Wang et al., 1999), folate (Leblanc et al., 2000; Lasseur et al., 2001; Heinz et al., 2008) and vitamin B6 (Kasama et al., 1996; Leblanc et al., 2000; Heinz et al., 2008). Other vitamins have only been occasionally been addressed (Heinz et al., 2008). Although these studies have all included only low number of patients, it can be concluded that losses occur during dialysis, and that molecular weight and binding to proteins and probably also dialysis membranes affect the magnitude of this effect. More studies are needed that address also long-term effects of high-flux/high-efficiency dialysis on vitamin status.

To our knowledge, the effect of dietary restrictions on reduced intake of vitamins has never been analyzed systematically. In addition, although patients on hemodialysis require several different drugs owing to the dialysis process, but also owing to frequent co-morbidities such as hypertension, dyslipidemia, diabetes, cardiovascular disease, heart failure and other chronic conditions, interactions of drugs with vitamins have not been addressed in hemodialysis patients, as, e.g., in diabetic patients. From these studies, it is known that metformin and omeprazole can interfere with vitamin B12 metabolism (Schenk et al., 1999; Bauman et al., 2000; Ting et al., 2006) but there is a lack of studies in hemodialysis patients.

8.3.2 Health effects of B-vitamin supplements in renal patients

Despite the many unresolved questions whether supplementation with B-vitamins is warranted in dialysis patients or not, some studies addressed specific health effects of B-vitamins. These effects include anemia, neuropathy and cardiovascular disease and mortality.

8.3.2.1 Anemia

Chronic kidney disease is associated with anemia owing to the insufficient production of erythropoietin by the diseased kidneys. Several studies have demonstrated that anemia is associated with increased risk of heart failure and death in renal patients (Foley et al., 1998). Correction of anemia in these patients reduces hospitalization rates and might improve the quality of life (Revicki et al., 1995; Collins et al., 2001). An effective treatment of anemia in patients with renal failure is the administration of recombinant human erythropoietin. However, the hematopoietic response to recombinant human erythropoietin is affected by other conditions, e.g., iron deficiency or inflammatory processes (Hörl et al., 2000; Stenvinkel, 2001). Also, folate and vitamin B12 deficiency could account for hypo-responsiveness to erythropoietin treatment (Breen and Mcdougall, 1999; Drüeke, 2001; Agarwal, 2006). Folic acid is required for one-carbon-transfer reactions and is therefore involved in the DNA synthesis during erythropoiesis. A reduced DNA synthesis results in the manifestation of megaloblastic erythropoiesis and macrocytic anemia (Teschner et al., 2002). Although correction of iron deficiency is an essential part in treatment of anemia, administration of folic acid is not a standard care in patients with end-stage renal disease (KDOQI, 2007). Several small-scale studies have demonstrated that administration of high-dose folic acid can normalize erythrocyte cell volume and allows dose reduction of recombinant human erythropoietin (Pronai et al., 1995; Bamgbola and Kaskel, 2005; Schiffl and Lang, 2006). However, normalization of erythrocyte cell volume and improvement in recombinant human erythropoietin response was only observed in patients with macrocytic anemia, but not for normocytic patients (Schiffl and Lang, 2006; Sepe et al., 2006). Furthermore, the administration of folic acid seems to be not effective in patients with normal red blood cell folate concentrations (Westhuyzen et al., 1993; Blumberg et al., 1998).

In conclusion, folic acid supplementation might be beneficial in treatment of anemia in patients with macrocytic anemia and low level of red blood cell folate. However, it has to be noted that high dose folic acid intake can mask a sub-clinical vitamin B12 deficiency. Hematological symptoms owing to the vitamin B12 deficiency are compensated by folic acid, but the neurological component of the vitamin B12 deficiency persists (Scott et al., 1981; Hoffbrand and Jackson, 1993). Therefore, folic acid supplementation should be done under consideration of vitamin B12 status or in combination with cobalamin supplementation.

8.3.2.2 Neuropathy

Uremic polyneuropathy is a well-known complication in patients with end-stage renal disease and occurs in approximately 60% of hemodialysis patients. Symptoms include: restless legs, spontaneous cramps, distal paresthesias (Bolton and Young, 1990). Early signs of polyneuropathy are an elevation of the vibratory threshold and impaired temperature sensibility most pronounced in the lower extremities (Lindblom and Tegnér, 1985; Tegnér and Lindholm, 1985).

One of the presumed factors for the development of uremic polyneuropathy is the insufficient removal of uremic toxins during the dialysis procedure (Malberti et al., 1991). However, the underlying mechanisms for the nerve damage are not completely clarified. Thus, there are only few therapeutic options to treat polyneuropathy in patients with end-stage renal disease.

Because of the potential influence of B-vitamins on the nerve regeneration and remyelination (Beck, 1988; Kuwabara et al., 1999) it has been examined in several small-scale studies whether there is a relation between uremic polyneuropathy and depletion of B-vitamins (Kuwabara et al., 1999; Moriwaki et al., 2000; Okada et al., 2000). The results of the studies indicate an improvement in symptoms of polyneuropathy owing to supplementation with vitamin B6 in patients treated with high-flux hemodialysis or peritoneal dialysis (Moriwaki et al., 2000; Okada et al., 2000). The results on vitamin B12 in patients with uremic polyneuropathy are contradictory. An oral supplementation with vitamin B12 (500 µg/day) for 4 weeks did not improve polyneuropathy symptoms (Okada et al., 2000). By contrast, long-term intravenous administration of vitamin B12 (1500 µg/week) for 6 months yielded beneficial effects in neuropathy patients (Kuwabara et al., 1999). However, these are results of small studies with heterogeneous study design, particularly with regard to the route of administration of treatment, and the cause of polyneuropathy is complex. Thus far, it is unclear whether the long-term process of polyneuropathy is reversible at all, independent of renal function.

For diagnosis of polyneuropathy the German Society of Neurology recommended laboratory testing for vitamin B12 and serum holo-transcobalamin, as the earliest marker of vitamin B deficiency (Herrmann et al., 2005; Obeid and Herrmann, 2007; Heuß et al., 2009).

In conclusion, there is a potential benefit owing to B-vitamins, which has to be proven in randomized studies.

8.3.2.3 Cardiovascular disease (CVD) and mortality

Renal failure is associated with poor prognosis for survival and cardiovascular complications. Dialysis patients have a higher prevalence of atherosclerosis and a 5–20-fold higher risk for cardiovascular mortality compared with the general population (Foley et al., 1998; Sarnak et al., 2003). In renal transplant recipients cardiovascular mortality is at least twice as high as in the general population. CVD is the most common cause of death, accounting for 35–50% of all-cause mortality in these patients (Sarnak et al., 2003).

The increased cardiovascular risk in patients with impaired renal function can only partially be explained by established risk factors, e.g., hypertension, hypercholesterolemia or overweight (Nishizawa et al., 2001; Klassen et al., 2002; Salahudeen, 2002; Kalantar-Zadeh et al., 2005). In hemodialysis patients, research in CVD has paid attention to non-traditional risk factors, which are associated with impaired glomerular filtration rate, e.g., homocysteine (Kielstein et al., 2008), and interest in B-vitamin status and supplementation has increased owing to the association of low concentrations of folate, cobalamin and/or pyridoxine with elevated concentrations of homocysteine.

8.3.3 Homocysteine as a risk factor for CVD and reduction of homocysteine by B-vitamins

Whereas in the general population homocysteine has been identified as a risk factor for CVD (Homocysteine Studies Collaboration, 2002; Wald et al., 2002), studies in patients with end-stage renal disease are controversial (Bachmann et al., 1995; Robinson et al., 1996; Moustapha et al., 1998; Kunz et al., 1999; Manns et al., 1999; Dierkes et al., 2000; Haraki et al., 2001; Ducloux et al., 2002; Mallamaci et al., 2002; Kalantar-Zadeh et al., 2004; Ducloux et al., 2006). However, a meta-analysis of prospective observational studies in these patients demonstrated that homocysteine is an independent risk factor for CVD and all-cause mortality in dialysis patients not receiving B-vitamins from supplements or fortified foods (Heinz et al., 2009a,b). A positive association between elevated homocysteine level and CVD was also found in renal transplant patients (Ducloux et al., 2000; Marcucci et al., 2000).

Elevated concentrations of homocysteine with typical mean values of 35 μmol/l are commonly found in patients with renal failure (Heinz et al., 2009a,b). The prevalence of hyperhomocysteinemia in patients with end-stage renal disease is nearly 100% with homocysteine concentrations up to 100 μmol/l (Dierkes et al., 2000). It is assumed that the reduced kidney function leads to increased homocysteine level in the plasma, however, the underlying mechanisms are still unclear. Because an impaired intrarenal homocysteine metabolism and a decreased urinary excretion cannot explain hyperhomocysteinemia in patients with renal failure (Refsum et al., 1985; van Guldener et al., 1998a,b), alterations in the sulfur amino acid metabolism owing to uremic conditions are discussed (van Guldener et al., 1999, 2006). Homocysteine concentration in patients with end-stage renal disease treated with dialysis falls after renal transplantation (Arnadottir et al., 1998). The prevalence of hyperhomocysteinemia in transplant patients is 50–60%, whereas in the general population the prevalence is approximately 5% (Malinow et al., 1999; Krmar et al., 2001; Díaz et al., 2005). In patients with end-stage renal disease as well as in transplant recipients the administration of folic acid alone reduces homocysteine level by approximately 30% (Yango et al., 2001; Koyama et al., 2002). It can be assumed that there is an upper limit in folate status above which no further reduction in plasma homocysteine can be achieved. The optimal dose of folic acid in patients with impaired renal function could be between 1 and 5 mg daily (de Vriese et al., 2002). Vitamin B12, when administered alone 1 mg parenterally in a 4-week interval is efficient to decrease plasma homocysteine by 10% (Kaplan et al., 2001). The combined supplementation with folic acid, vitamin B12 and vitamin B6 reduces homocysteine concentration by 30–50% (Suliman et al., 1999; Dierkes et al., 2001; Henning et al., 2001). Close correlations between pre-treatment homocysteine level and therapy effect were observed, in patients with the highest homocysteine level, the largest benefit from treatment was observed (Perna et al., 1997; Kunz et al., 1999; Arnadottir et al., 2000; Sunder-Plassmann et al., 2000). Despite the observed reduction in homocysteine concentration, normalization of plasma homocysteine by vitamin treatment alone in patients with renal failure seems to be rare. However, Obeid et al. showed that the combination of folic acid (5 mg), vitamin B12 (0.7 mg), and vitamin B6 (50 mg) administered intravenously in this study normalized serum concentrations of homocysteine in almost all of the hyperhomocysteinemic dialysis patients (Obeid et al., 2005). Therapy with folic acid is more effective in patients with pre-terminal renal failure and renal transplant recipients compared with patients with end-stage renal disease (Thambyrajah et al., 2000; Bostom et al., 2001). A homocysteine concentration lower than 12 µmol/l after B-vitamin supplementation was observed in 20–65% of pre-dialysis patients (Bostom et al., 1997; Thambyrajah et al., 2000), and only in less than 10% of the dialysis patients (Bostom et al., 2000; Yango et al., 2001).

8.3.4 Observational and intervention studies with B-vitamins with surrogate endpoints

Surrogate endpoints of CVD that have been investigated in B-vitamin studies include endothelial function, arterial stiffness or blood pressure in short-term and medium-term clinical studies (Thambyrajah et al., 2000; van Guldener et al., 2000; Baragetti et al., 2007; Tochihara et al., 2008). The overall result was that folic acid did not improve endothelial function in hemodialysis patients. By contrast, an improvement of flow mediated dilation has been observed in both hemodialyis and in peritoneal dialysis patients after the use of 5-methyltetrahydrofolate, the active metabolite of folic acid (Buccianti et al., 2002; Baragetti et al., 2007) or folinic acid (Anderson et al., 2006).

There was an interesting 'side observation' by van Guldener et al. (2000): the authors observed a decrease in mean arterial pressure upon homocysteine lowering treatment with folic acid for approximately 1 year. An association between folate intake and hypertension has also been suggested in the Nurses' Health Study (Forman et al., 2009). Whether this association reflects a true effect or chance deserves further studies.

8.3.5 Observational studies on vitamin supplementation and mortality

The association between water-soluble vitamins and all-cause mortality has been investigated in two prospective observational studies. A first indication for this association was observed in the Dialysis Outcomes and Practice Patterns Study (DOPPS) I, which was an observational study evaluating the use of water-soluble vitamins among dialysis patients in France, Germany, Italy, Japan, Spain, UK and USA (Fissell et al., 2004). The risk for all-cause mortality was reduced by 16% in patients taking water-soluble vitamins on a routine basis (adjusted RR 0.84; 95% CI, 0.76–0.94; $p = 0.001$). The risk for hospitalization was also lower among patients administered water-soluble vitamins, however, this association was not significant (adjusted RR 0.94; 95% CI, 0.85–1.04; p = 0.24) (Fissell et al., 2004). On facility-level it was demonstrated that a 10% increment of patient use of water-soluble vitamins the facility-level mortality was reduced by 2% (adjusted RR 0.98; 95% CI, 0.95–1.00; p = 0.05) (Fissell et al., 2004). The association between vitamins and all-cause mortality was also confirmed in a further prospective observational study in a cohort of 102 hemodialysis patients with a follow-up period of 4 years. A strong association between the intake of water-soluble vitamins and re-duced total mortality was observed (adjusted HR 0.39; 95% CI, 0.19–0.79); p < 0.01) (Domröse et al., 2007).

However, owing to the non-randomized study design, observational studies have certain limitations. It cannot be excluded that administration of vitamin supplements is a marker for better overall care or a better health and nutritional status. Also, socio-economic factors could have influenced the results. These facts emphasize the need for randomized controlled trials to investigate the effects of a therapy on mortality and morbidity of chronic diseases. Some intervention studies and randomized controlled tri-als on B-vitamins in hemodialysis patients have been conducted and will be described in detail below.

8.3.6 Randomized clinical trials with B-vitamins

There are several intervention studies available examining the effect of a vitamin B sup-plementation on cardiovascular events or total mortality in patients with renal failure whereas four of them fulfilled the criteria for randomized controlled trials (Zoungas et al., 2006; Jamison et al., 2007; Vianna et al., 2007; Heinz et al., 2010). The other studies included different dosages of folic acid or used patients not receiving vitamin supplements on a routine basis as a control group (Righetti et al., 2003, 2006; Wrone et al., 2004) (▶Tab. 8.8).

study	treatment n events/n total	control n events/n total	risk ratio (95 % CI)		
Zoungas 2006	77 / 156	86 / 159		0.91	(0.74, 1.13)
Jamison 2007	129 / 1032	150 / 1024		0.85	(0.69, 1.06)
Vianna 2007	26 / 93	30 / 93		0.87	(0.56, 1.35)
Heinz 2010	83 / 327	89 / 23		0.84	(0.65, 1.07)
total	1608	1599		0.86	(0.76, 0.98)

test for overall effect: Z = 2.24 (p = 0.03); I² = 0 %

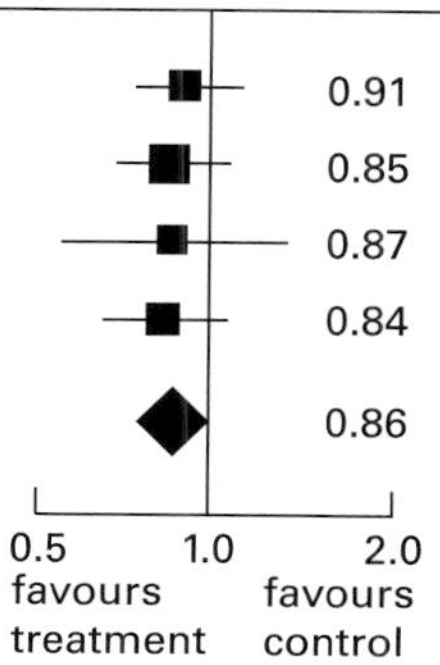

0.5　1.0　2.0
favours treatment　favours control

Fig. 8.8: Effect of B-vitamins on cardiovascular events: randomized controlled trials in patients with chronic kidney disease with the respective risk ratio for of each study and a pooled risk ratio of all studies.

Tab. 8.7: Intervention studies with B-vitamins in patients with renal failure.

Study	Outcome	Follow-up (mean or median)	Intervention	Results
Heinz et al., 2010	Total mortality and non-fatal/fatal CVD	2.1 years	Treatment[a] (2.5 mg FA+10 mg B6+25μg B12) versus control[a] (0.1 mg FA+0.5 mg B6+2μg B12)	Total mortality HR 1.13 (95% CI, 0.85–1.50, p = 0.51) CVD HR 0.80 (95% CI, 0.60–1.07, p = 0.13)
Jamison et al., 2007	Total mortality and non-fatal/fatal CVD	38 months	Treatment (40 mg FA+100 mg B6+2 mg B12) versus placebo	Total mortality HR 1.04 (95% CI, 0.91–1.18, p = 0.60) Myocardial infarction HR 0.86 (95% CI, 0.67–1.08, p = 0.18) Stroke HR 0.90 (95% CI, 0.58–1.40, p = 0.64)
Righetti et al., 2003	Non-fatal CVD	12 months	Treatment (5 mg or 15 mg FA) versus untreated	CVD in treatment group n = 13 of 51 versus CVD in untreated group n = 11 of 30 (p = 0.08) HR n/a
Righetti et al., 2006	Non-fatal/fatal CVD	29 months	Treatment (5 mg FA[b]) versus untreated	CVD in treated group n = 26 of 63 versus CVD in untreated group n = 32 of 51 (p = 0.05) HR n/a
Vianna et al., 2007	Non-fatal/fatal CVD	24 months	Treatment (10 mg FA) versus placebo	CVD in treated group n = 26 of 93 versus CVD in untreated group n = 30 of 93 HR n/a

(*Continued*)

Tab. 8.7 (*Continued*)

Study	Outcome	Follow-up (mean or median)	Intervention	Results
Wrone et al., 2004	Total mortality and non-fatal/fatal CVD (combined endpoint)	24 months	Treatment (5 mg or 15 mg FA)[c] versus 'usual care' (1 mg FA)[c]	CVD/mortality in treated group 39% (5 mg FA) and 47% (15 mg FA) versus CVD in 'usual care' group 44% (1 mg FA) ($p = 0.47$) HR n/a
Zoungas et al., 2006	Non-fatal/fatal CVD	3.6 years	Treatment (15mg FA) vs. placebo	CVD HR 0.95 (95% CI, 0.69–1.30, $p = 0.75$)

[a]All capsules contained further water-soluble vitamins.

[b]In patients with plasma B12 levels <200 ng/l additionally B1 250 mg; B6 250 mg and B12 500 mg.

[c]All capsules contained B1 1.5 mg; B6 12.5 mg; B12 6 μg and further water-soluble vitamins.

CVD, cardiovascular events; FA, folic acid; HR, hazard ratio; CI, confidence interval.

Although in observational studies administration of water-soluble vitamins was associated with a reduction in mortality (Fissell et al., 2004; Domröse et al., 2007) this effect was not observed in intervention trials. In the HOST trial (Homocysteinemia in Kidney and End Stage Renal Disease) supplementation with 40 mg folic acid, 2 mg vitamin B12 and 100 mg vitamin B6 for a median study period of 3.2 years did not improve survival in patients with advanced chronic kidney disease or end-stage renal disease (HR 1.04; 95% CI, 0.91–1.18; $p = 0.6$) (Jamison et al., 2007). Additionally, the results of a *post-hoc* analysis of the large-scale randomized controlled trial HOPE-2 (Heart Outcomes Prevention Evaluation), by which only patients with a glomerular filtration rate <60 ml/min were included in the analysis indicated no reduction in all-cause mortality owing to B-vitamin administration (Mann et al., 2008).

Most of the intervention studies examining the effect of B-vitamins on cardiovascular events resulted in a non-significant reduction of CVD risk (Righetti et al., 2003; Zoungas et al., 2006; Jamison et al., 2007; Vianna et al., 2007; Heinz et al., 2010). However, Rhigetti et al. showed that homocysteine-lowering folate therapy decreases cardiovascular events in dialysis patients (Righetti et al., 2006). Additionally, a significant risk reduction for cardiovascular events of 14% can be found by pooling the results of the available randomized controlled trials in patients with chronic kidney disease and end-stage renal disease (▶Fig. 8.8) (Zoungas et al., 2006; Jamison et al., 2007; Vianna et al., 2007; Heinz et al., 2010).

It has to be mentioned that the lack of a significant effect on CVD risk could be owing to a lack of statistical power. The statistical power of the randomized controlled trials was calculated to show a risk reduction in CVD events of 17–50% (Zoungas et al., 2006; Jamison et al., 2007; Heinz et al., submitted). The results of these studies, however, found a non-significant event reduction by 10–20%. Therefore, the sample sizes were too small to detect significant differences (Bostom et al., 2009). For a statistical power of 0.80, which is taken as the minimum power of a randomized controlled trial, more than 5000 patients had to be included in the study to prove an effect in the magnitude of 10–20%. A trial on the effect of B-vitamins on CVD in kidney transplant recipients is running (Bostom et al., 2009). Thus far, there is no information available about the clinical benefit of B-vitamins in kidney transplant recipients.

References

Agarwal AK, Practical approach to the diagnosis and treatment of anemia associated with CKD in elderly. J Am Med Dir Assoc 2006;7(Suppl 9): S7–12.

Anderson TJ, Sun YH, Hubacek J, Hyndman ME, Verma S, Shewchuk L, Scott-Douglas N, Effects of folinic acid on forearm blood flow in patients with end-stage renal disease. Nephrol Dial Transplant 2006;21: 1927–33.

Arnadottir M, Hultberg B, Wahlberg J, Fellström B, Dimény E, Serum total homocysteine concentration before and after renal transplantation. Kidney Int 1998;54: 1380–4.

Arnadottir M, Gudnason V, Hultberg B, Treatment with different doses of folic acid in haemodialysis patients: effects on folate distribution and aminothiol concentrations. Nephrol Dial Transplant 2000;15: 524–8.

Bachmann J, Tepel M, Raidt H, Riezler R, Graefe U, Langer K, Zidek W, Hyperhomocysteinemia and the risk for vascular disease in hemodialysis patients. J Am Soc Nephrol 1995;6: 121–5.

Bamgbola OF, Kaskel F, Role of folate deficiency on erythropoietin resistance in pediatric and adolescent patients on chronic dialysis. Pediatr Nephrol 2005;20: 1622–9.

Bamonti-Catena F, Buccianti G, Porcella A, Valenti G, Como G, Finazzi S, Maiolo AT, Folate measurements in patients on regular hemodialysis treatment. Am J Kidney Dis 1999;33: 492–7.

Baragetti I, Raselli S, Stucchi A, Terraneo V, Furiani S, Buzzi L, Garlaschelli K, Alberghini E, Catapano AL, Buccianti G, Improvement of endothelial function in uraemic patients on peritoneal dialysis: a possible role for 5-MTHF administration. Nephrol Dial Transplant 2007;22: 3292–7.

Bates CJ, Pentieva KD, Prentice A, Mansoor MA, Finch S, Plasma pyridoxal phosphate and pyridoxic acid and their relationship to plasma homocysteine in a representative sample of British men and women aged 65 years and over. Br J Nutr 1999;81: 191–201.

Bauman WA, Shaw S, Jayatilleke E, Spungen AM, Herbert V, Increased intake of calcium reverses vitamin B12 malabsorption induced by metformin. Diabetes Care 2000;23: 1227–31.

Beck WS, Cobalamin and the nervous system. N Engl J Med 1988;318: 1752–4.

Billion S, Tribout B, Cadet E, Queinnec C, Rochette J, Wheatley P, Bataille P, Hyperhomocysteinaemia, folate and vitamin B12 in unsupplemented haemodialysis patients: effect of oral therapy with folic acid and vitamin B12. Nephrol Dial Transplant 2002;17: 455–61.

Blumberg A, Zehnder C, Huber A, Folic acid supplementation rarely improves erythropoietin response. Nephron 1998;78: 115.

Bolton CF, Young BG, Neurological complications of renal disease. Boston: Butterworth; 1990.

Bostom AG, Gohh RY, Beaulieu AJ, Nadeau MR, Hume AL, Jacques PF, Selhub J, Rosenberg IH, Treatment of hyperhomocysteinemia in renal transplant recipients. A randomized, placebo-controlled trial. Ann Intern Med 1997;127: 1089–92.

Bostom AG, Shemin D, Gohh RY, Beaulieu AJ, Jacques PF, Dworkin L, Selhub J, Treatment of mild hyperhomocysteinemia in renal transplant recipients versus hemodialysis patients. Transplantation 2000;69: 2128–31.

Bostom AG, Shemin D, Gohh RY, Beaulieu AJ, Bagley P, Massy ZA, Jacques PF, Dworkin L, Selhub J, Treatment of hyperhomocysteinemia in hemodialysis patients and renal transplant recipients. Kidney Int Suppl 2001;78:S246–52.

Bostom AG, Carpenter MA, Hunsicker L, Jacques PF, Kusek JW, Levey AS, McKenney JL, Mercier RY, Pfeffer MA, Selhub J; FAVORIT Study Investigators. Baseline characteristics of participants in the Folic Acid for Vascular Outcome Reduction in Transplantation (FAVORIT) Trial. Am J Kidney Dis 2009;53: 121–8.

Breen CP, Macdougall IC, Correction of epoetin-resistant megaloblastic anaemia following vitamin B12 and folate administration. Nephron 1999;83: 374–5.

Buccianti G, Raselli S, Baragetti I, Bamonti F, Corghi E, Novembrino C, Patrosso C, Maggi FM, Catapano AL, 5-methyltetrahydrofolate restores endothelial function in uraemic patients on convective haemodialysis. Nephrol Dial Transplant 2002;17: 857–64.

Collins AJ, Li S, St Peter W, Ebben J, Roberts T, Ma JZ, Manning W, Death, hospitalization, and economic associations among incident hemodialysis patients with hematocrit values of 36 to 39%. J Am Soc Nephrol 2001;12: 2465–73.

De Vriese AS, Verbeke F, Schrijvers BF, Lameire NH, Is folate a promising agent in the prevention and treatment of cardiovascular disease in patients with renal failure? Kidney Int 2002;61: 1199–209.

Descombes E, Hanck AB, Fellay G, Water soluble vitamins in chronic hemodialysis patients and need for supplementation. Kidney Int 1993;43: 1319–28.

Díaz JM, Sainz Z, Gich I, Guirado LL, Puig T, Oliver A, Montañés R, Chuy E, Solà R, Factors involved in baseline hyperhomocysteinemia in renal transplantation. Transplant Proc 2005;37: 3799–801.

Dierkes J, Domröse U, Ambrosch A, Bosselmann HP, Neumann KH, Luley C, Response of hyperhomocysteinemia to folic acid supplementation in patients with end-stage renal disease. Clin Nephrol 1999a;51: 108–15.

Dierkes J, Domröse U, Ambrosch A, Schneede J, Guttormsen AB, Neumann KH, Luley C, Supplementation with vitamin B12 decreases homocysteine and methylmalonic acid but also serum folate in patients with end-stage renal disease. Metabolism 1999b;48: 631–5.

Dierkes J, Domröse U, Bosselmann KP, Neumann KH, Luley C, Homocysteine lowering effect of different multivitamin preparations in patients with end-stage renal disease. J Ren Nutr 2001;11: 67–72.

Domröse U, Heinz J, Westphal S, Luley C, Neumann KH, Dierkes J, Vitamins are associated with survival in patients with end-stage renal disease: a 4-year prospective study. Clin Nephrol 2007;67: 221–29.

Drüeke T, Hyporesponsiveness to recombinant human erythropoietin. Nephrol Dial Transplant 2001;16: S25–8.

Ducloux D, Motte G, Challier B, Gibey R, Chalopin JM, Serum total homocysteine and cardiovascular disease occurrence in chronic, stable renal transplant recipients: a prospective study. J Am Soc Nephrol 2000;11: 134–7.

Ducloux D, Bresson-Vautrin C, Kribs M, Abdelfatah A, Chalopin JM, C-Reactive protein and cardiovascular disease in peritoneal dialysis patients. Kidney Int 2002;62: 1417–22.

Ducloux D, Klein A, Kazory A, Devillard N, Chalopin JM, Impact of malnutrition-inflammation on the association between homocysteine and mortality. Kidney Int 2006;69: 331–5.

Fissell RB, Bragg-Gresham JL, Gillespie BW, Goodkin DA, Bommer J, Saito A, Akiba T, Port FK, Young EW, International variation in vitamin prescription and association with mortality in the Dialysis Outcomes and Practice Patterns Study (DOPPS). Am J Kidney Dis 2004;44: 293–9.

Foley RN, Parfrey PS, Sarnak MJ, Epidemiology of cardiovascular disease in chronic renal disease. J Am Soc Nephrol 1998;9: S16–23.

Forman JP, Stampfer MJ, Curhan GC, Diet and lifestyle risk factors associated with incident hypertension in women. J Am Med Assoc 2009;302: 401–11.

Fouque D, Vennegoor M, ter Wee P, Wanner C, Basci A, Canaud B, Haage P, Konner K, Kooman J, Martin-Malo A, Pedrini L, Pizzarelli F, Tattersall J, Tordoir J, Vanholder R, EBPG guideline on nutrition. Nephrol Dial Transplant 2007;22(Suppl 2): ii45–87.

Friso S, Jacques PF, Wilson PW, Rosenberg IH, Selhub J, Low circulating vitamin B(6) is associated with elevation of the inflammation marker C-reactive protein independently of plasma homocysteine levels. Circulation 2001;103: 2788–91.

Haraki T, Takegoshi T, Kitoh C, Kajinami K, Wakasugi T, Hirai J, Shimada T, Kawashiri M, Inazu A, Koizumi J, Mabuchi H, Hyperhomocysteinemia, diabetes mellitus, and carotid atherosclerosis independently increase atherosclerotic vascular disease outcome in Japanese patients with end-stage renal disease. Clin Nephrol 2001;56: 132–9.

Heinz J, Domröse U, Westphal S, Luley C, Neumann KH, Dierkes J, Washout of water-soluble vitamins and of homocysteine during haemodialysis: effect of high-flux and low-flux dialyser membranes. Nephrology 2008;13: 384–9.

Heinz J, Domröse U, Luley C, Westphal S, Kropf S, Neumann KH, Dierkes J, Influence of a supplementation with vitamins on cardiovascular morbidity and mortality in patients with end-stage renal disease: design and baseline data of a randomized clinical trial. Clin Nephrol 2009a;71: 363–5.

Heinz J, Kropf S, Luley C, Dierkes J, Homocysteine as a risk factor for cardiovascular disease in patients treated by dialysis: a meta-analysis. Am J Kidney Dis 2009b;54: 478–89.

Heinz J, Kropf S, Domröse U, Westphal S, Borucki K, Luley C, Neumann KH, Dierkes J, B-vitamins and the risk for total mortality and cardiovascular disease in end-stage renal disease. Results of a randomized controlled trial. (Submitted). Circulation 2010;A21: 1432–1438.

Henning BF, Zidek W, Riezler R, Graefe U, Tepel M, Homocyst(e)ine metabolism in hemodialysis patients treated with vitamins B6, B12 and folate. Res Exp Med 2001;200: 155–68.

Herrmann W, Schorr H, Geisel J, Riegel W, Homocysteine, cystathionine, methylmalonic acid and B- vitamins in patients with renal disease. Clin Chem Lab Med 2001;39: 739–46.

Herrmann W, Obeid R, Schorr H, Geisel J, The usefulness of holotranscobalamin in predicting vitamin B12 status in different clinical settings. Curr Drug Metab 2005;6: 47–53.

Heuß D, Auer-Grumbach M, Haupt WF, Löscher W, Neundörfer B, Rautenstrauß B, Renaud S, Sommer C, Diagnosis of polyneuropathies Guidelines of the German Society of Neurology. Akt Neurol 2009;36: e3–13.

Hoffbrand AV, Jackson BF, Correction of the DNA synthesis defect in vitamin B12 deficiency by tetrahydrofolate: evidence in favour of the methyl-folate trap hypothesis as the cause of megaloblastic anaemia in vitamin B12 deficiency. Br J Haematol 1993;83: 643–7.

Homocysteine Studies Collaboration, Homocysteine and risk of ischemic heart disease and stroke: a meta-analysis. J Am Med Assoc 2002;288: 2015–22.

Hörl WH, Jacobs C, Macdougall IC, Valderrábano F, Parrondo I, Thompson K, Carveth BG, European best practice guidelines 14–16: inadequate response to epoetin. Nephrol Dial Transplant 2000;15(Suppl 4): S43–50.

Jamison RL, Hartigan P, Kaufman JS, Goldfarb DS, Warren SR, Guarino PD, Gaziano JM; Veterans Affairs Site Investigators, Effect of homocysteine lowering on mortality and vascular disease in advanced chronic kidney disease and end-stage renal disease: a randomized controlled trial. J Am Med Assoc 2007;298: 1163–70.

Jennette JC, Goldman ID, Inhibition of the membrane transport of folates by anions retained in uremia. J Lab Clin Med 1975;86: 834–43.

Kalantar-Zadeh K, Block G, Humphreys MH, McAllister CJ, Kopple JD, A low, rather than a high, total plasma homocysteine is an indicator of poor outcome in hemodialysis patients. J Am Soc Nephrol 2004;15: 442–53.

Kalantar-Zadeh K, Kilpatrick RD, McAllister CJ, Greenland S, Kopple JD, Reverse epidemiology of hypertension and cardiovascular death in the hemodialysis population: the 58th annual fall conference and scientific sessions. Hypertension 2005;45: 811–7.

Kaplan LN, Mamer OA, Hoffer LJ, Parenteral vitamin B12 reduces hyperhomocysteinemia in end-stage renal disease. Clin Invest Med 2001; 24: 5–11.

Kasama R, Koch T, Canals-Navas C, Pitone JM, Vitamin B6 and hemodialysis: the impact of high-flux/high-efficiency dialysis and review of the literature. Am J Kidney Dis 1996;27: 680–6.

KDOQI, Clinical practice guideline and clinical practice recommendations for anemia in chronic kidney disease: 2007 update of hemoglobin target. Am J Kidney Dis 2007;50: 471–530.

Kielstein JT, Salpeter SR, Buckley NS, Cooke JP, Fliser D, Two cardiovascular risk factors in one? Homocysteine and its relation to glomerular filtration rate. A meta-analysis of 41 studies with 27,000 participants. Kidney Blood Press Res 2008;31: 259–67.

Klassen PS, Lowrie EG, Reddan DN, DeLong ER, Coladonato JA, Szczech LA, Lazarus JM, Owen WF Jr., Association between pulse pressure and mortality in patients undergoing maintenance hemodialysis. JAMA 2002;287: 1548–55.

Koyama K, Usami T, Takeuchi O, Morozumi K, Kimura G, Efficacy of methylcobalamin on lowering total homocysteine plasma concentrations in haemodialysis patients receiving high-dose folic acid supplementation. Nephrol Dial Transplant 2002;17: 916–22.

Krmar RT, Ferraris JR, Ramirez JA, Galarza CR, Waisman G, Janson JJ, Llapur CJ, Sorroche P, Legal S, Cámera MI, Hyperhomocysteinemia in stable pediatric, adolescents, and young adult renal transplant recipients. Transplantation 2001;71: 1748–51.

Kunz K, Petitjean P, Lisri M, Chantrel F, Koehl C, Wiesel ML, Cazenave JP, Moulin B, Hannedouche TP, Cardiovascular morbidity and endothelial dysfunction in chronic haemodialysis patients: is homocyst(e)ine the missing link? Nephrol Dial Transplant 1999;14: 1934–42.

Kuwabara S, Nakazawa R, Azuma N, Suzuki M, Miyajima K, Fukutake T, Hattori T, Intravenous methylcobalamin treatment for uremic and diabetic neuropathy in chronic hemodialysis patients. Intern Med 1999;38: 472–5.

Lasseur C, Parrot F, Delmas Y, Level C, Ged C, Redonnet-Vernhet I, Montaudon D, Combe C, Chauveau P, Impact of high-flux/high-efficiency dialysis on folate and homocysteine metabolism. J Nephrol 2001;14: 32–5.

Leblanc M, Pichette V, Geadah D, Ouimet D, Folic acid and pyridoxal-5'-phosphate losses during high-efficiency hemodialysis in patients without hydrosoluble vitamin supplementation. J Ren Nutr 2000;10: 196–201.

Lewerin C, Ljungman S, Nilsson-Ehle H, Glomerular filtration rate as measured by serum cystatin C is an important determinant of plasma homocysteine and serum methylmalonic acid in the elderly. J Intern Med 2007;261: 65–73.

Lindblom U, Tegnér R, Thermal sensitivity in uremic neuropathy. Acta Neurol Scand 1985;71: 290–4.

Livant EJ, Tamura T, Johnston KE Vaughn WH, Bergmann SM, Forehand J, Walthaw J, Plasma folate conjugase activities and folate concentrations in patients receiving hemodialysis. J Nutr Biochem 1994;5: 504–08.

Malberti F, Surian M, Farina M, Vitelli E, Mandolfo S, Guri L, De Petri GC, Castellani A, Effect of hemodialysis and hemodiafiltration on uremic neuropathy. Blood Purif 1991;9: 285–95.

Malinow MR, Bostom AG, Krauss RM, Homocyst(e)ine, diet, and cardiovascular diseases: a statement for healthcare professionals from the Nutrition Committee, American Heart Association. Circulation 1999;99: 178–82.

Mallamaci F, Zoccali C, Tripepi G, Fermo I, Benedetto FA, Cataliotti A, Bellanuova I, Malatino LS, Soldarini A; CREED Investigators. Hyperhomocysteinemia predicts cardiovascular outcomes in hemodialysis patients. Kidney Int 2002;61: 609–14.

Mann JF, Sheridan P, McQueen MJ, Held C, Arnold JM, Fodor G, Yusuf S, Lonn EM; HOPE-2 investigators. Homocysteine lowering with folic acid and B vitamins in people with chronic kidney disease – results of the renal Hope-2 study. Nephrol Dial Transplant 2008;23: 645–53.

Manns BJ, Burgess ED, Hyndman ME, Parsons HG, Schaefer JP, Scott-Douglas NW, Hyperhomocyst(e)inemia and the prevalence of atherosclerotic vascular disease in patients with endstage renal disease. Am J Kidney Dis 1999;34: 669–77.

Marcucci R, Zanazzi M, Bertoni E, Brunelli T, Fedi S, Evangelisti L, Pepe G, Rogolino A, Prisco D, Abbate R, Gensini GF, Salvadori M, Risk factors for cardiovascular disease in renal transplant recipients: new insights. Transpl Int 2000;13(Suppl 1): S419–24.

Mason JB, Biomarkers of nutrient exposure and status in one-carbon (methyl) metabolism. J Nutr. 2003;133(Suppl 3): 941S–7S.

Moelby L, Rasmussen K, Hoegaard-Rasmussen H, Serum methylmalonic acid in uraemia. Scand J Clin Lab Invest 1992;52: 351–4.

Moriwaki K, Kanno Y, Nakamoto H, Okada H, Suzuki H, Vitamin B6 deficiency in elderly patients on chronic peritoneal dialysis. Adv Perit Dial 2000;16: 308–12.

Moustapha A, Naso A, Nahlawi M, Gupta A, Arheart KL, Jacobsen DW, Robinson K, Dennis VW, Prospective study of hyperhomocysteinemia as an adverse cardiovascular risk factor in end-stage renal disease. Circulation 1998;97: 138–41.

Nishizawa Y, Shoji T, Ishimura E, Inaba M, Morii H, Paradox of risk factors for cardiovascular mortality in uremia: is a higher cholesterol level better for atherosclerosis in uremia? Am J Kidney Dis 2001;38(Suppl 1): S4–7.

Obeid R, Herrmann W, Holotranscobalamin in laboratory diagnosis of cobalamin deficiency compared to total cobalamin and methylmalonic acid. Clin Chem Lab Med 2007;45: 1746–50.

Obeid R, Kuhlmann MK, Köhler H, Herrmann W, Response of homocysteine, cystathionine, and methylmalonic acid to vitamin treatment in dialysis patients. Clin Chem 2005;51: 196–201.

Okada H, Moriwaki K, Kanno Y, Sugahara S, Nakamoto H, Yoshizawa M, Suzuki H, Vitamin B6 supplementation can improve peripheral polyneuropathy in patients with chronic renal failure on high-flux haemodialysis and human recombinant erythropoietin. Nephrol Dial Transplant 2000;15: 1410–3.

Perna AF, Ingrosso D, De Santo NG, Galletti P, Brunone M, Zappia V, Metabolic consequences of folate-induced reduction of hyperhomocysteinemia in uremia. J Am Soc Nephrol 1997;8: 1899–905.

Pronai W, Riegler-Keil M, Silberbauer K, Stockenhuber F, Folic acid supplementation improves erythropoietin response. Nephron 1995;71: 395–400.

Refsum H, Helland S, Ueland PM, Radioenzymic determination of homocysteine in plasma and urine. Clin Chem 1985;31: 624–8.

Revicki DA, Brown RE, Feeny DH, Henry D, Teehan BP, Rudnick MR, Benz RL, Health-related quality of life associated with recombinant human erythropoietin therapy for predialysis chronic renal disease patients. Am J Kidney Dis 1995;25: 548–54.

Righetti M, Ferrario GM, Milani S, Serbelloni P, La Rosa L, Uccellini M, Sessa A, Effects of folic acid treatment on homocysteine levels and vascular disease in hemodialysis patients. Med Sci Monit 2003;9: PI19–24.

Righetti M, Serbelloni P, Milani S, Ferrario G, Homocysteine-lowering vitamin B treatment decreases cardiovascular events in hemodialysis patients. Blood Purif 2006;24: 379–86.

Robinson K, Gupta A, Dennis V, Arheart K, Chaudhary D, Green R, Vigo P, Mayer EL, Selhub J, Kutner M, Jacobsen DW, Hyperhomocysteinemia confers an independent increased risk of atherosclerosis in end-stage renal disease and is closely linked to plasma folate and pyridoxine concentrations. Circulation 1996;94: 2743–8.

Salahudeen AK, So, overweight is associated with better survival in dialysis patients! Nephrol Dial Transplant 2002;17: 1151–2.

Sarnak MJ, Levey AS, Schoolwerth AC, Coresh J, Culleton B, Hamm LL, McCullough PA, Kasiske BL, Kelepouris E, Klag MJ, Parfrey P, Pfeffer M, Raij L, Spinosa DJ, Wilson PW; American Heart Association Councils on Kidney in Cardiovascular Disease, High Blood Pressure Research, Clinical Cardiology, and Epidemiology and Prevention, Kidney disease as a risk factor for development of cardiovascular disease: a statement from the American Heart Association Councils on Kidney in Cardiovascular Disease, High Blood Pressure Research, Clinical Cardiology, and Epidemiology and Prevention. Circulation 2003;108: 2154–69.

Schenk BE, Kuipers EJ, Klinkenberg-Knol EC, Bloemena EC, Sandell M, Nelis GF, Snel P, Festen HP, Meuwissen SG, Atrophic gastritis during long-term omeprazole therapy affects serum vitamin B12 levels. Aliment Pharmacol Ther 1999;13: 1343–6.

Schiffl H, Lang SM, Folic acid deficiency modifies the haematopoietic response to recombinant human erythropoietin in maintenance dialysis patients. Nephrol Dial Transplant 2006;21: 133–7.

Scott JM, Dinn JJ, Wilson P, Weir DG, Pathogenesis of subacute combined degeneration: a result of methyl group deficiency. Lancet 1981;2: 334–7.

Sepe V, Adamo G, Giuliano MG, Soccio G, Libetta C, Dal Canton A, High-dose folic acid supplements and responsiveness to rHu-EPO in HD patients. Nephrol Dial Transplant 2006;21: 2036.

Stenvinkel P, The role of inflammation in the anaemia of end-stage renal disease. Nephrol Dial Transplant 2001;16(Suppl 7): S36–40.

Suliman ME, Divino Filho JC, Bàràny P, Anderstam B, Lindholm B, Bergström J, Effects of high-dose folic acid and pyridoxine on plasma and erythrocyte sulfur amino acids in hemodialysis patients. J Am Soc Nephrol 1999;10: 1287–96.

Suliman ME, Qureshi AR, Bárány P, Stenvinkel P, Filho JC, Anderstam B, Heimbürger O, Lindholm B, Bergström J, Hyperhomocysteinemia, nutritional status, and cardiovascular disease in hemodialysis patients. Kidney Int 2000;57: 1727–35.

Sunder-Plassmann G, Födinger M, Buchmayer H, Papagiannopoulos M, Wojcik J, Kletzmayr J, Enzenberger B, Janata O, Winkelmayer WC, Paul G, Auinger M, Barnas U, Hörl WH, Effect of high dose folic acid therapy on hyperhomocysteinemia in hemodialysis patients: results of the Vienna multicenter study. J Am Soc Nephrol 2000;11: 1106–16.

Talwar D, Quasim T, McMillan DC, Kinsella J, Williamson C, O'Reilly DS, Pyridoxal phosphate decreases in plasma but not erythrocytes during systemic inflammatory response. Clin Chem 2003;49: 515–8.

Tegnér R, Lindholm B, Vibratory perception threshold compared with nerve conduction velocity in the evaluation of uremic neuropathy. Acta Neurol Scand 1985;71: 284–9.

Teschner M, Kosch M, Schaefer RM, Folate metabolism in renal failure. Nephrol Dial Transplant 2002;17(Suppl 5): S24–7.

Thambyrajah J, Landray MJ, McGlynn FJ, Jones HJ, Wheeler DC, Townend JN, Does folic acid decrease plasma homocysteine and improve endothelial function in patients with predialysis renal failure? Circulation 2000;102: 871–5.

Ting RZ, Szeto CC, Chan MH, Ma KK, Chow KM, Risk factors of vitamin B(12) deficiency in patients receiving metformin. Arch Intern Med 2006;166: 1975–9.

Tochihara Y, Whiting MJ, Barbara JA, Mangoni AA, Effects of pre-vs. intra-dialysis folic acid on arterial wave reflections and endothelial function in patients with end-stage renal disease. Br J Clin Pharmacol 2008;66: 717–22.

van Guldener C, Donker AJ, Jakobs C, Teerlink T, de Meer K, Stehouwer CD, No net renal extraction of homocysteine in fasting humans. Kidney Int 1998a;54: 166–9.

van Guldener C, Janssen MJ, Lambert J, ter Wee PM, Donker AJ, Stehouwer CD, Folic acid treatment of hyperhomocysteinemia in peritoneal dialysis patients: no change in endothelial function after long-term therapy. Perit Dial Int 1998b;18: 282–9.

van Guldener C, Kulik W, Berger R, Dijkstra DA, Jakobs C, Reijngoud DJ, Donker AJ, Stehouwer CD, De Meer K, Homocysteine and methionine metabolism in ESRD: A stable isotope study. Kidney Int 1999;56: 1064–71.

van Guldener C, Lambert J, ter Wee PM, Donker AJ, Stehouwer CD, Carotid artery stiffness in patients with end-stage renal disease: no effect of long-term homocysteine-lowering therapy. Clin Nephrol 2000;53: 33–41.

van Guldener C, Why is homocysteine elevated in renal failure and what can be expected from homocysteine-lowering? Nephrol Dial Transplant 2006;21: 1161–6.

Vianna AC, Mocelin AJ, Matsuo T, Morais-Filho D, Largura A, Delfino VA, Soares AE, Matni AM, Uremic hyperhomocysteinemia: a randomized trial of folate treatment for the prevention of cardiovascular events. Hemodial Int 2007;11: 210–6.

Wald DS, Law M, Morris JK, Homocysteine and cardiovascular disease: evidence on causality from a meta-analysis. Br Med J 2002;325:1202–06.

Wang S, Eide TC, Sogn EM, Berg KJ, Sund RB, Plasma ascorbic acid in patients undergoing chronic haemodialysis. Eur J Clin Pharmacol 1999;55: 527–32.

Westhuyzen J, Matherson K, Tracey R, Fleming SJ, Effect of withdrawal of folic acid supplementation in maintenance hemodialysis patients. Clin Nephrol 1993;40: 96–9.

Wrone EM, Hornberger JM, Zehnder JL, McCann LM, Coplon NS, Fortmann SP, Randomized trial of folic acid for prevention of cardiovascular events in end-stage renal disease. J Am Soc Nephrol 2004;15: 420–26.

Yango A, Shemin D, Hsu N, Jacques PF, Dworkin L, Selhub J, Bostom AG, Rapid communication: L-folinic acid versus folic acid for the treatment of hyperhomocysteinemia in hemodialysis patients. Kidney Int 2001;59: 324–7.

Zoungas S, Branley P, Kerr PG, Ristevski S, Muske C, Demos L, Atkins RC, Becker G, Fraenkel M, Hutchison BG, Walker R, McNeil JJ, McGrath BP, Atherosclerosis and folic acid supplementation trial in chronic renal failure: baseline results. Nephrology 2004;9: 130–41.

Zoungas S, McGrath BP, Branley P, Kerr PG, Muske C, Wolfe R, Atkins RC, Nicholls K, Fraenkel M, Hutchison BG, Walker R, McNeil JJ, Cardiovascular morbidity and mortality in the Atherosclerosis and Folic Acid Supplementation Trial (ASFAST) in chronic renal failure: a multicenter, randomized, controlled trial. J Am Coll Cardiol 2006;47: 1108–16.

9 Vitamin C – Ascorbic acid

9.1 Vitamin C in human nutrition

Henriette Frikke-Schmidt; Pernille Tveden-Nyborg; Jens Lykkesfeldt

9.1.1 Introduction

Given the insight provided by Nobel laureates Albert Szent-Györgyi and Norman Haworth who discovered and characterized vitamin C (Szent-Györgyi, 1928; Ault et al., 1933; Haworth and Hirst, 1933), or ascorbic acid as they named it owing to its antiscorbutic properties no one today doubts the importance of vitamin C as a ubiquitous and unequivocal part of all life. One aspect that contributes to its particular status is that in contrast to mammals in general, primates, fruit bats, red-vented bulbuls, and guinea pigs are unable to synthesize this simple low molecular weight structure owing to a mutation in the gene coding for L-gulonolactone oxidase, the last enzyme in the biosynthesis of vitamin C. Consequently, we rely on its presence in our diet.

Vitamin C plays a role in numerous biological reactions, many of which are still largely unexplained. It has been suggested that vitamin C be used as a remedy against many diseases as different as common colds and cancer. Even today, there is considerable controversy about the exact role of the vitamin in human nutrition and no agreement has been reached on the amount needed to be consumed for optimum well-being where various authorities have recommended amounts ranging from 30 mg to several grams per day.

The present chapter outlines the basic chemistry of vitamin C, pharmacological aspects, established biological functions of vitamin C and clinical consequences of vitamin C deficiency. Examples of new roles of vitamin C supported by emerging experimental evidence are given and proper laboratory analysis of these labile compounds is discussed.

9.1.2 Biochemistry of vitamin C

9.1.2.1 Forms of vitamin C

L-Ascorbic acid, or reduced vitamin C, is the primary biologically active form of vitamin C. At physiological pH, ascorbic acid is approximately 99.8% ionized and essentially all biological reactions involving vitamin C more specifically involves the monoanion ascorbate (Buettner and Schafer, 2004). The two-electron oxidation product dehydroascorbic acid (DHAA) also has antiscorbutic properties because it is readily converted back to ascorbate *in vivo* by both chemical and enzymatic means (Poulsen et al., 2003). Further oxidation renders the vitamin inactive by leading to the irreversible formation of 2,3-diketogulonate as well as oxalate, threonate and other products (Poulsen et al., 2003). DHAA has a half-life of only a few minutes at physiological pH (Bode et al., 1990). Consequently, highly efficient ways of regenerating ascorbate *in vivo* has evolved. It is obvious that these processes must be of major importance; in particular in species that lack the ability to synthesize ascorbic acid.

9.1.2.2 Vitamin C as an antioxidant

Whereas ascorbate is merely a simple carbohydrate, its ene-diol structure provides it with a complex chemistry (▶Fig. 9.1). Probably its most important chemical property is that ascorbate fulfills the criteria of an effective antioxidant (Carr and Frei, 1999). Thus, it has a very complicated redox chemistry which involves the comparatively stable radical intermediate, ascorbyl free radical (AFR), and is heavily influenced by the acidic properties of the molecule. It has been known for many years that ascorbate is easily oxidized by molecular oxygen, in particular in the presence of transition metals.

In all known biological reactions in which ascorbate acts as a cofactor or as a radical quencher, the molecular mechanism is that of an antioxidant, i.e., it donates reducing equivalents to the biological reaction and is itself oxidized in the process to AFR, two molecules of which disproportionates to one molecule of ascorbic acid (AA) and one of DHAA. To prevent the loss of ascorbate in vivo, DHAA is efficiently reduced back to ascorbate intracellularly, e.g., by erythrocytes, hepatocytes and other tissues. This process is commonly referred to as ascorbate recycling (Washko et al., 1993; May et al., 1995). Consequently, the recycling of ascorbate plays the key role in preserving its antioxidant function. In humans, where relatively small amounts of vitamin C are required through the diet to prevent pathologies such as scurvy, this process is very efficient and of great importance (Lykkesfeldt et al., 2003). May and coworkers have studied ascorbate recycling in erythrocytes in detail and demonstrated that recycling of ascorbate in erythrocytes occurs predominantly via glutathione-dependent dehydroascorbic acid reductases apparently with a small contribution from NADPH-dependent dehydroascorbic acid reductases such as thioredoxin reductase (May et al., 1995, 1996, 1997, 1998, 2000a,b, 2001a,b; Mendiratta et al., 1998a,b).

Vitamin C plays a pivotal role in the antioxidant defense. The molecule has been called the most important water-soluble antioxidant in biological fluids (Frei et al., 1989, 1990) and has earned this honor for several reasons. Chemically speaking, both ascorbate and its one-electron oxidation product AFR have remarkably low one-electron reduction potentials of +282 and −174 mV, respectively (Buettner, 1993), placing ascorbate at the bottom of the antioxidant hierarchy. This means that on top of the ability to reduce virtually all physiologically relevant oxidants, ascorbate is capable of regenerating other antioxidants such as vitamin E from the α-tocopheroxyl radical and glutathione from the glutathiyl radical back into their active states (Buettner and Schafer, 2004). Equally importantly, the relative stability of the AFR renders it a harmless intermediate incapable of inducing free radical damage itself. Instead, at physiological pH, AFR primarily disproportionates via dimer-formation into one molecule of ascorbate and one of DHAA (Buettner and Schafer, 2004).

The electrochemical properties outlined above do indeed suggest that ascorbate is a unique antioxidant. In agreement, both in vitro and in vivo experiments have confirmed that ascorbate plays a key role in the antioxidant defense as a whole. For example, Frei and coworkers have shown under a variety of oxidizing conditions that ascorbate is the only antioxidant capable of completely preventing lipid oxidation in plasma and once ascorbate is depleted; lipid hydroperoxides are formed despite the presence of

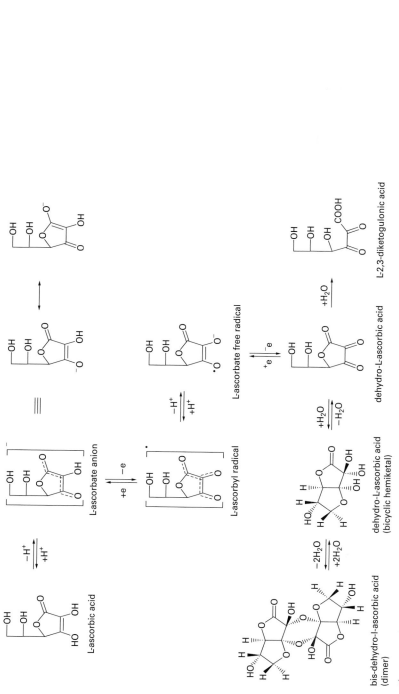

Fig. 9.1: Schematic outline of ascorbic acid oxidation and nomenclature. Abstraction of a hydrogen atom leads to the formation of the ascorbate monoanion. A one-electron oxidation results in ascorbyl radical. The highly resonance-stabilized structure renders it a comparatively long-lived intermediate. Abstraction of a hydrogen atom forms the ascorbate free radical and further oxidation results in the formation of dehydroascorbic acid. In aqueous solution, its preferred structure is a bicyclic hemiketal. Dehydration of an aqueous solution forms a dimer. Hydrolysis and further oxidation irreversibly converts dehydroascorbic acid to 2,3-diketogulonic acid and other compounds all of which have no vitamin C activity.

other plasma antioxidants such as α-tocopherol and beta-carotene (Frei et al., 1988, 1991; Lynch et al., 1994; Gokce and Frei, 1996; McCall and Frei, 1999). We have recently shown *in vivo*, that ascorbate is selectively retained in the brain during vitamin C deficiency in guinea pigs and that it keeps other antioxidants including vitamin E and glutathione reduced during increased oxidative stress in the brain (Lykkesfeldt et al., 2007). Thus, it appears that both *in vivo* and *in vitro* data support the pivotal role of ascorbate as an antioxidant.

9.1.3 Measurement of vitamin C in biological samples

Analytical methodology providing reproducible quantification of ascorbate and DHAA is a necessary prerequisite for the understanding of the biological role of vitamin C as well as using ascorbate and DHAA as biomarkers of oxidative stress. However, precise and accurate measurement of ascorbate and in particular DHAA in biological samples poses a significant challenge in analytical chemistry. One problem is the labile nature of the compounds, but perhaps even more significant is the fact, that they are in chemical and biological equilibrium with each other. Unawareness of these built-in difficulties has led to inconsistent data in the literature and even misleading conclusions. Consequently, for studies of vitamin C, the *ex vivo* stability of the analytes and efficient blocking of their *in vivo* equilibrium should be recognized as equally important on a par with traditional analytical virtues such as specificity, sensitivity, and absence of interfering compounds.

9.1.3.1 Special issues and assay principles

Several assay principles have been employed in the analysis of ascorbate and DHAA over the years and the number of published methods of quantification is almost overwhelming. The methodologies largely fall into three main categories: (i) assays in which ascorbate and DHAA are measured directly in the sample; (ii) measurement following derivatization; and (iii) so-called subtraction methods.

From the chemist's point of view, direct measurement is most often preferable owing to its simplicity. Ascorbate is easily quantified directly, e.g., by means of ultraviolet or electrochemical detection. However for DHAA, an ideal detection method does not exist. Direct detection of DHAA is unspecific and lacks the required sensitivity whereas derivatization procedures amplify the risk of shifting the *in vivo* equilibrium between ascorbate and DHAA. The third alternative, subtraction methods, is commonly based on the direct determination of ascorbate followed by reduction of the sample after which total vitamin C, i.e., ascorbate+DHAA, is measured. Subsequently, the concentration of DHAA is calculated by subtraction, i.e., DHAA = Vitamin C$_{total}$ – Ascorbate. Examples of the opposite strategy, i.e., measurement of DHAA followed by oxidation and measurement of total DHAA, are also known but have not gained much popularity owing to the problems in accurate determination of DHAA. Clearly, each of the three assay principles involves trade-offs.

Means of detection range from simple colorimetric assays to advanced LC-MS. The advantages and drawbacks of various assay principles have been reviewed (Rumsey et al., 2000). The authors concluded that for analysis of biological samples, their preference was high-performance liquid chromatography (HPLC) with coulometric detection (i.e., a subtraction method), owing to its high sensitivity and specificity. However, no method can undo the damage if the samples are not collected, handled or stored properly. Thus, regardless of the equipment and methods employed, meticulous practice is necessary to completely prevent or reproducibly limit *ex vivo* oxidation as much as possible.

9.1.3.1.1 Oxidation of ascorbate

In most biological samples, the concentration of ascorbate is many-fold that of DHAA. Thus in particular in DHAA analysis, control of post-sampling conversion of ascorbate to DHAA is of major importance. Knowledge of reactions and/or conditions leading to DHAA formation and degradation is crucial to the effort of limiting these undesirable events.

Ascorbate is oxidized by molecular oxygen in aqueous solution. In the absence of catalysts, the reaction between ascorbate and O_2 is slow, although pH dependent, ascorbate being more stable at low pH. Ascorbate oxidation is enhanced by the presence of many transition metal ions. Thus, addition of 5 µM copper(II) ions to an aqueous 0.1 mM ascorbate solution or a plasma sample was found to quantitatively oxidize the ascorbate in a few seconds (Lykkesfeldt et al., 1995). As summarized in ►Tab. 9.1, ascorbate oxidation is influenced by several factors (Cooke and Moxon, 1981; Lykkesfeldt and Ames, 1999; Rumsey et al., 2000) some of which can be eliminated or reduced by using the recommended precautions. A further complication is that ascorbate oxidation is concentration dependent, i.e., a sample with low concentration of ascorbate is more prone to oxidation than a sample with high concentration. When sample collection

Tab. 9.1: Some important factors influencing ascorbic acid oxidation and dehydroascorbic acid degradation in biological samples.

Factor	Recommended precaution
Time	Carry out all procedures of sample collection, stabilization, preparation and analysis as quickly as possible without compromising reproducibility or safety
Divalent cation concentration	Use 18.2 MΩ purified water for all applications Use highest quality reagents for all applications Use chelators (e.g., EDTA) in buffers
Temperature	Keep samples and relevant solutions cold Use temperature controlled autosampler (4°C)
pH	Acidify samples – lower pH enhance the stability of both ascorbate and dehydroascorbic acid and maintain the *in vivo* equilibrium
Oxygen concentration	Use nitrogen or helium sparged buffers
Light	Protect experiments from light Use amber vials for analysis
Oxidizing enzymes	Precipitate and remove proteins before sample storage

procedures are properly optimized, time becomes increasingly important. In plasma, oxidation of ascorbate starts almost immediately and exceeds 20% in 1 h in unstabilized plasma or blood samples on ice (Lykkesfeldt et al., 1995).

9.1.3.1.2 Degradation of dehydroascorbic acid

Whereas post-sampling oxidation of ascorbate gives rise to artifactually elevated DHAA concentrations, hydrolysis can reduce the recovery of DHAA and total vitamin C. DHAA is unstable at physiological conditions and is irreversibly hydrolyzed to 2,3-diketogulonic acid and other products with a reported half-life of only 6 min (pH 7.0; 37°C) (Bode et al., 1990). It has been suggested that DHAA underestimation could result from this (Bode et al., 1990), but our results have shown that this effect is probably of minor importance in, e.g., blood and plasma, where no significant loss of total vitamin C was observed for at least 2 h, compared with that of ascorbate oxidation, which amounts to approximately 30–50% of total vitamin C during the same period (Lykkesfeldt et al., 1995). By contrast, in ascorbate recycling experiments, where 6–150 mM DHAA preparations are added to cell suspensions, DHAA hydrolysis could lead to erroneous results owing to decreasing substrate availability. Dissolving DHAA in ice-cold acetate buffer (pH 4.0) immediately before use can, however, alleviate the problem by increasing the stability of DHAA (Lykkesfeldt and Ames, 1999; Lykkesfeldt et al., 2003).

9.1.3.2 Analysis of ascorbic acid and total vitamin C

Assessment of ascorbate concentrations in, e.g., plasma is routinely performed in many laboratories. A wide variety of methods have been presented over the past decades employing spectrophotometry, fluorometry, gas chromatography, enzymatic assays, capillary electrophoresis or HPLC with UV, fluorescence or electrochemical detection [see Rumsey et al. (2000) for review]. In some cases ascorbate is still being measured as DHAA following oxidation and derivatization (Fujita et al., 2001). Most methods of ascorbate measurement, in particular HPLC-based methods, are capable of producing valid results if the proper precautions are taken to ensure sample stability.

Our original method based on reversed-phase HPLC with coulometric detection (Lykkesfeldt et al., 1995) was among the first to emphasize the widely occurring post-sampling ascorbate oxidation as a problem in ascorbate and DHAA analysis and provide practical and validated solutions. The method has later modified to include co-analysis of erythorbic acid and uric acid, the use of uric acid as an endogenous standard for ascorbate oxidation, rapid analysis of 2 min per run as well as more reliable reducing and storage conditions allowing up to 4 days in a cooled autosampler for prepared samples or up to 5 years at −80°C (Lykkesfeldt, 2000, 2002, 2007).

9.1.3.3 Quantification of dehydroascorbic acids

Unfortunately, the difficulties in measuring DHAA and the major risk of artifactual oxidation of ascorbate have been ignored until recently and are only starting to be more widely recognized. Consequently, a considerable proportion of the existing literature on DHAA and even recently published papers continue to report values that clearly show artifactually elevated concentrations of DHAA of up to 25% of the total ascorbate in healthy individuals. By contrast, most experienced researchers in the field agree that in a normal biological sample, e.g., a plasma sample from a healthy non-smoking individual, the concentration of DHAA *in vivo* is very close to nil (Lykkesfeldt et al., 1997). However, artifactual oxidation occurs *ex vivo* during sample collection, preparation and analysis. Even if one is successful in limiting these undesirable events, DHAA concentrations of up to a few percent will commonly be found, regardless of whether a subtraction method or a direct assay is used. Consequently, practice and inclusion of proper controls is the only way of making sure that the assay is performed correctly.

Each assay principle employed for DHAA involves tradeoffs. Pre- or post-column or online derivatization of DHAA in combination with HPLC with fluorescence detection is used, e.g., in analysis of foodstuffs where the concentration of DHAA is considerable (Ali and Phillippo, 1996; Kall and Andersen, 1999). However, the methods are not sensitive enough to quantify the minute amounts found in living biological systems. Mass-spectrometry methods have also been employed in DHAA analysis (Deutsch and Kolhouse, 1993). Although these methods have the ability to quantify small amounts, the sample preparation is tedious and operation requires more expensive equipment and most often specialized staff. Moreover, derivatization techniques in general have the drawback of unintentionally shifting the equilibrium between ascorbate and DHAA instead of preserving it.

As mentioned above, subtraction methodology is commonly used in DHAA analysis. The major drawback of this assay principle is that ascorbate and total ascorbate concentrations are similar and usually many-fold the level of DHAA. Consequently, the resulting DHAA concentration is encumbered with a relatively larger error compared with directly measured concentrations. Another inconvenience of subtraction methods is that often the reducing agent used for the total ascorbate measurement has to be removed before HPLC analysis because of chromatographic interference (Levine et al., 1999). Dithiothreitol (DTT) is a convenient and powerful reducing agent commonly used in total ascorbate analysis (Lykkesfeldt et al., 1995). However, although removal of DTT is usually not necessary before HPLC separation, we found the pH at which samples are usually stored in the autosampler is too low (typically <3) for DTT to have any ability to keep ascorbate reduced (Lykkesfeldt, 2000). Both in the case of removal and inactivity of the reducing agent, the stability of ascorbate in the reduced samples is compromised and rapid analysis is necessary to obtain valid results. By contrast, the reducing agent TCEP appears ideal for total ascorbate measurement (Lykkesfeldt, 2000). It does not interfere with the chromatography and remains active at the pH of 4.5 at which the samples can be stored for several days in a cooled autosampler.

9.1.4 Sources of vitamin C

9.1.4.1 Dietary sources

In general, fruits and vegetables are generous sources of vitamin C and it is estimated that almost 90% of vitamin C intake from an ordinary diet comes from these sources. The content varies from relatively low in fruits such as pears and bananas (less than 10 mg/kg wet weight) to very high in citrus fruits, kiwis and mango (more than 400 mg/kg wet weight). Certain vegetables, e.g., broccoli, tomatoes and peppers are rich in vitamin C whereas others, e.g., carrots, beans and celery contain relatively low amounts (Sinha et al., 1993; Szeto et al., 2002; Gil et al., 2006). Because ascorbate tends to degrade when heated and during storage, the type of processing and preparation procedures typically applied to fruits and vegetables should be considered when judging their suitability as dietary sources of vitamin C. In particular oil-frying at high temperatures might cause the vitamin content to decrease to a small fraction of the original concentration whereas boiling or steaming are less damaging ways of food preparation from a vitamin C point of view (Miglio et al., 2008). Also, the vitamin C content can vary according to growth conditions, season of the year and storage time (Gil et al., 2006; Erdman and Klein, 1982). Yet, five to nine servings of most fruits and vegetables per day is estimated to equal at least 200 mg of vitamin C (Dietary reference intakes, 2000).

One of the most widely acknowledged dietary sources of vitamin C are juices made from citrus fruits. Since the 18th century, where it was used to prevent scurvy during prolonged sea voyages, orange juice has had its place in the human diet and even today, orange juice is the main source of dietary vitamin C in the USA (Subar et al., 1998). As noted above, vitamin C content of juice varies with the applied preparation. Hence, freshly squeezed orange juice contains more vitamin C than juices intended for a long shelf-life, and the ascorbate content will also depend on storage time and temperature (Kabasakalis et al., 2000).

The presence of vitamin C in other dietary products than fruits and vegetables are typically owing to its addition as a preservative to processed foods to protect against oxidation. In a few cases, vitamin C can be obtained from animal sources. This is of importance in areas of the world where vegetation tends to be sparse such as in the arctic regions where fruits and vegetables therefore might not be available in adequate amounts. In these areas, the native people have relied on obtaining their vitamin C from animal sources, e.g., raw liver and whale skin (Fediuk et al., 2002).

9.1.4.2 Vitamin C deficiency

Guidelines developed by the National Survey of Canada have defined severe vitamin C deficiency as a plasma concentration below 11 μmol/l, marginal vitamin C deficiency as a plasma concentration between 11 and 23 μmol/l and hypovitaminosis C covering both by being categorized as plasma concentrations below 23 μmol/l (Smith and Hodges, 1987). In severe deficiency, there is an increased risk of developing scurvy, which is the ultimate and lethal syndrome that develops upon severe and prolonged lack of vitamin C. The earliest signs are fatigue and inflammation of the gums, that become swollen and bleeding, soon to be followed by petechia, joint effusions, impaired wound healing, depression, coiled hair, ecchymoses and eventually death (Jacob and Sotoudeh, 2002). In the western world, scurvy is now considered a rare disease, in the USA affecting mostly those suffering from drug/alcohol abuse or malnutrition (Dietary reference intakes, 2000). This is in contrast to the so-called subclinical vitamin C deficiency covering individuals with hypovitaminosis C who do not experience clinical symptoms known to be directly attributable to poor vitamin C status. In fact, it has been estimated that several hundred million people can be diagnosed as having hypovitaminosis C according to the above guidelines (Schectman et al., 1989; Wrieden et al., 2000; Hampl et al., 2004; Tveden-Nyborg and Lykkesfeldt, 2009).

Development of hypovitaminosis C results from an imbalance between ascorbate intake, turnover and excretion. Because ascorbate functions as a chain-breaking antioxidant or antioxidant cofactor in biological reactions, increased turnover could particularly result from a redox imbalance or so-called oxidative stress. This has been associated with a variety of chronic conditions including cancer, cardiovascular-related disorders, some neurodegenerative diseases or exposure to oxidants in the environment, e.g., pollution, radiation and passive smoking. In all of the above cases, it has been reported that those affected by the specific malignancies/environmental exposure have lower plasma ascorbate status compared with healthy individuals (Block, 1991; Riviere et al., 1998; Block et al., 2002; Aycicek et al., 2005; Lykkesfeldt, 2006; Frikke-Schmidt and Lykkesfeldt, 2009; Harrison and May, 2009; Padhy and Padhi, 2009).

9.1.4.3 Identification of high-risk individuals

The safest way of identifying individuals lacking vitamin C involves analysis of vitamin C content in the blood. However, as more insight and knowledge is acquired concerning the conditions causing depletion of the ascorbate pool, it becomes progressively easier to identify groups of individuals who are at risk of suffering from hypovitaminosis C.

As previously noted, increased oxidant stress has been associated with numerous conditions including obesity, asthma, cancer, hypercholesterolemia, pre-eclampsia, Alzheimer's, diabetes, cardiovascular disease, etc. (Jacob and Sotoudeh, 2002; Myatt and Cui, 2004; Willcox et al., 2004; Vincent et al., 2007; Martino et al., 2008). Hence, individuals suffering from these conditions might be considered at risk of vitamin C deficiency. Furthermore, certain subpopulations tend to have a very low intake of vitamin C. These are typically people of low socioeconomic status, where fruits and vegetables are too expensive for their limited budget, alcoholics, who get most of their calories from alcohol, drug abusers, and in some cases, those voluntarily following very restricted dietary regimes (Dietary reference intakes, 2000). Another well-defined group with a highly increased risk of hypovitaminosis C is smokers and people exposed to passive smoking (Lykkesfeldt, 2006). This is supported by the report that the turnover of ascorbate in heavy smokers is doubled compared with healthy non-smoking controls (Kallner et al., 1981) and that ascorbate oxidation is increased (Lykkesfeldt et al., 1997, 2000, 2003). The same picture is seen in large epidemiological studies of vitamin C, where smoking is a dominant determinant of poor vitamin C status. Some of this difference correlates with smokers eating less fruits and vegetables, yet in studies taking dietary intake into account and comparing smokers to non-smokers with a similar intake of fruits and vegetables, the smokers maintain significantly lower levels of vitamin C (Lykkesfeldt et al., 2000). As a direct consequence of these findings, the latest revision of the dietary reference intake of vitamin C by the Food and Nutrition board under the US National Academy of Sciences recommends that smokers add 35 mg/day to the RDA (Dietary reference intakes, 2000).

9.1.5 Bioavailability issues

9.1.5.1 Oral bioavailability of vitamin C

Upon ingestion, ascorbate is absorbed through the action of the sodium-ascorbate co-transporter 1 (SVCT1) in the entire length of the small intestine (Malo and Wilson, 2000). The pharmacokinetics of vitamin C has been studied in detail by Levine and coworkers (Levine et al., 1996). Oral bioavailability of vitamin C is highly dose dependent and varies between nil and approximately 100% depending on the current vitamin C status of the individual. Daily vitamin C doses of up to approximately 200 mg are completely absorbed whereas the part of doses exceeding approximately 500 mg per day are almost quantitatively excreted (Levine et al., 1996). Once absorbed, the plasma concentration of ascorbate is very tightly regulated. Hence, the body very efficiently takes up ascorbate when needed whereas surplus amounts are just as efficiently excreted maintaining a saturation level of approximately 70 µmol/l if adequate amounts of vitamin C are available (Schectman et al., 1991; Schectman, 1993; Lykkesfeldt et al., 1997; Lykkesfeldt, 2006). This is also reflected in measurements of urinary excretion after vitamin C administration: at daily doses higher than 500 mg, additional ascorbate is practically excreted 100% whereas vitamin C is selectively retained by SVCT1 in the kidney during deficiency (Levine et al., 1996).

In the 2000 revision of the RDA for vitamin C from the Food and Nutrition Board, recommendations to men and women were increased to 90 and 75 mg/day, respectively, whereas smokers were advised to ingest additionally 35 mg/day (Dietary reference intakes, 2000). For the first time, the guideline took into account the biochemical evidence supporting an important role of AA in the defense against oxidative stress. By contrast, previous recommendations have been based primarily on clinical evidence, i.e., the ability to prevent scurvy. The acceptance of biochemical evidence in support of the higher RDA for vitamin C could well result in this becoming further increased because several studies have suggested that approximately 200 mg vitamin C per day is required to reach saturation, i.e., a plasma concentration of 70 µmol/l (Schectman et al., 1991; Schectman, 1993; Lykkesfeldt et al., 1997; Lykkesfeldt, 2006).

9.1.5.2 Dietary sources vs. supplements

There does not seem to be any difference in bioavailability between vitamin C from dietary/'natural' sources or from vitamin supplements. In foods, vitamin C is present as L-ascorbic acid or ascorbate which is the same chemical entity added to supplements. Thus far, no dietary factors regulating the activity of the ascorbate transporter SVCT1 has emerged and this transporter does not rely on the presence of any non-endogenous factors to accumulate ascorbate (Savini et al., 2008). Comparison of six servings of fruits and vegetables per day with a supplement estimated to contain the same amounts of vitamins and minerals also showed no significant effect of the vitamin C source during the intervention period of 25 days (Dragsted et al., 2004). Thus, strictly from a vitamin C point of view, the use of supplements seems to be a satisfactory alternative if the vitamin C content of the diet is inadequate.

9.1.5.3 Intravenous administration of vitamin C

Intravenous bolus administration and infusion of vitamin C has regained interest in recent years. The main reason for using this route of administration is that pharmacological concentrations of vitamin C in the blood can be achieved as the otherwise tightly controlled absorption of vitamin C from the intestine is bypassed. The phenomenon has been illustrated in a study by Padayatta and co-workers where intravenous administration of 1.25 g of vitamin C resulted in a plasma concentration >1 mmol/l (Padayatty et al., 2004). These extreme supraphysiological levels of plasma ascorbate are evaluated for the treatment of cancer because several *in vitro* data suggest that millimolar concentrations of vitamin C are cytotoxic to cancer cells (Leung et al., 1993; Lin et al., 2006; Ha et al., 2009). Emerging data suggest that vitamin C infusion might promote apoptosis in cancer cells *in vivo*. However, controlled clinical trials are required to elaborate on a consistent effect in cancer patients. This topic is covered in more detail in the chapter by Frei and coworkers in this volume.

9.1.5.4 Toxicity of vitamin C

A major concern when working with any compound in pharmacological doses is toxicity. In general, oral administration of up to several grams of vitamin C is considered safe owing to the tightly controlled absorption and excretion mechanisms. The upper tolerable limit has been set to 2 g/day by the Food and Nutrition Board (Dietary reference intakes, 2000) although currently, strong scientific evidence to define and defend a UL for vitamin C is not available (Johnston, 1999). Intravenous loading of patients with ascorbate is also considered relatively safe as compared with side effects that can occur with the use of chemotherapeutics. In some patients, side effects were apparently related to the infusion fluid having a high osmolarity causing osmotic diuresis (Hoffer et al., 2008). The remaining reported side effects primarily relates to patients suffering from renal disease, glucose 6-phosphate deficiency, or hemochromatosis. Concerning renal disease, ascorbate is metabolized to oxalate that could crystallize in the urine causing kidney stone formation, hence the use of high-dose ascorbate is not recommended in cases of renal dysfunction (Padayatty et al., 2006). In patients with glucose 6-phosphate deficiency, ascorbate might cause hemolysis and the excess iron present in plasma in patients suffering from hemochromatosis has been speculated to induce Fenton chemistry causing ascorbate to act as a powerful pro-oxidant (Dietary reference intakes, 2000). This effect, however, has not been documented to take place *in vivo*.

9.1.6 Biological functions of vitamin C

Ascorbate acts as a modulator of several cellular reactions and is a required cofactor of several hydroxylation reactions and in the biosynthesis of catecholamines providing necessary reducing equivalents (Katsuki, 1996; Mandl et al., 2009). One of the most well-investigated mechanisms is the role of vitamin C in collagen synthesis, in which it acts as a cofactor for the Fe(II)-dependent 2-oxoglutarate dependent dioxygenases (2-ODDs), e.g., prolyl and lysyl hydroxylases (Hewitson et al., 2003; Schofield and Zhang, 1999; Mandl et al., 2009). The enzymes catalyze the hydroxylation of unfolded procollagen chains, leading to the creation of a triple helical structure and the formation of mature collagen trimers (Murad et al., 1981a,b). When levels of 2-ODDs are decreased, the procollagen chains are insufficiently hydroxylated preventing the assembly of stable collagen. The inability to synthesize sufficient functional collagen is one of the hallmarks of scurvy and is responsible for several clinical symptoms. In the biosynthesis of carnitine, important for intracellular transport of triglycerides, vitamin C plays an analogous role, serving as a specific antioxidant by maintaining iron in its reduced stage, thereby promoting adequate proline hydroxylation. Several cellular proteins rely on 2-ODD proline hydroxylation to interact, and are therefore dependent on sufficient availability of ascorbate (Myllyharju and Kivirikko, 2004). Inside the nucleus, ascorbate-dependent hydroxylation of transcriptions factors are reported [hypoxia-inducible transcription factors (HIFs)] as able to regulate the transcriptional response of various target genes coding for proteins implicated in, i.e., angiogenesis, iron homeostasis and cell proliferation (Schofield and Ratcliffe, 2004; Metzen, 2007) and have been linked to DNA repair and the demethylation of histones (H3 lysines) (Tsukada et al., 2006).

The role of vitamin C in the brain and central nervous system has become the subject of increased attention. The brain shows the highest concentration of ascorbate compared with other organs reaching concentrations in neurons 10-fold that of reference tissue such as the liver (Rice and Russo-Menna, 1998). Acting as a cofactor, ascorbate provides reducing equivalents for the conversion of dopamine to norepinephrin, catalyzed by the dopamine-β-hydroxylase enzyme (Levine and Morita, 1985). A high level of dopamine in the brain is associated with the generation of reactive oxygen species and has been shown to be cytotoxic in neurons, a toxicity that could be prevented by injections with antioxidants (Berman et al., 1996). In chromaffin cells, ascorbate is secreted in association with catecholamine granules *in vitro* (Levine et al., 1983) and in the human adrenal gland *in vivo* (Padayatty et al., 2007). Data have also associated low levels of ascorbate with increased apoptosis in cells actively synthesizing catecholamines, suggesting that vitamin C plays a key role in sustaining the viability of catecholaminergic cells (Bornstein et al., 2003).

Involvement in the glutamate-ascorbate hetero-exchange system in the brain is also a recognized key function of vitamin C. The neurotransmitter glutamate is released to the extracellular space and can result in neuronal damage through excitatory overload/excitotoxicity, and the concomitant generation of ROS (Rice, 2000). The glutamate-ascorbate hetero-exchange results in glutamate reuptake by neurons combined with a subsequent release of ascorbate to the extracellular space, allowing for a sustained intra- and extracellular ascorbate homeostasis and for ascorbate to reduce extracellular ROS (O'Neill et al., 1983; Miele et al., 1994).

As mentioned earlier, ascorbate has been called the most important water-soluble antioxidant in plasma (Frei et al., 1990) and is linked to the oxidation of low density lipoprotein (LDL) in the subendothelial space of blood vessels playing a putative role in the pathogenesis of atherosclerosis (Steinberg, 1997; Steinberg and Chait, 1998). However, ascorbate appears to play a more specific role in the vasculature. In endothelial cells, eNOS (endothelial nitric oxide synthase) generates nitric oxide (NO) which diffuses to the vessel smooth muscle cells. It modulates the vascular muscle tone and also employs an anti-atherogenic effect on the endothelial cells and platelets (Ignarro et al., 2002). The cofactor tetrahydrobiopterin (BH4) is directly associated with the regulation of eNOS activity and data suggest that vitamin C is specifically responsible for keeping BH4 in its active reduced state (Heitzer et al., 2000; Katusic, 2001).

9.1.6.1 Established and proposed manifestations of vitamin C deficiency

The most well known and established clinical manifestation of vitamin C deficiency is the development of scurvy. The disease has been known for centuries, but was not discovered to be associated with a specific treatment until James Lind conducted his now renowned clinical trial on a group of scorbutic sailors in 1752/53, establishing that the juice from citrus fruits could reverse the illness within a very short time frame (Lind, 1753). Today scurvy is rarely reported and exists primarily in cases of predisposing diseases such as chronic kidney failure, alcoholism and in severe cases of malnutrition. Although some genetic factors might predispose to the development of scurvy (Delanghe et al., 2007), it is agreed that plasma levels below 11 µmol/l increase the risk of developing clinical scurvy and the onset of clinical symptoms typically appears at serum concentrations below 2.5 µmol/l (Hodges et al., 1971; Johnston and Thompson, 1998; Bennett and Coninx, 2005).

As reviewed by us elsewhere, studies in human populations investigating putative effects of vitamin C on vasodilatation, generally concludes that there is a beneficial acute effect of vitamin C in improving vasodilatation, however, evidence of long-term benefits are scarce (Frikke-Schmidt and Lykkesfeldt, 2009) (▶Fig. 9.2). The observed favorable effects support the hypothesis that vitamin C might act to prevent superoxide-mediated oxidation of NO to peroxynitrite, either through the antioxidant capacity of ascorbate or through an as yet undisclosed alternative pathway increasing NO levels in the vascular regime (May and Qu, 2009). However, although intracellular concentrations of ascorbate could potentially be high enough for ascorbate to be able to compete with NO for the reaction with superoxide, the reaction kinetics are unfavorable for ascorbate (Jackson et al., 1998). Thus more recently, it has been shown that vitamin C in physiological amounts can increase the production of NO substantially in cultured human endothelial cells (Heller et al., 1999). As mentioned above, the mechanism is believed to involve a vitamin C-mediated increase in reduced BH4 which increases NO activity via eNOS in a dose-dependent manner (Heller et al., 1999; Heitzer et al., 2000; Huang et al., 2000). High plasma concentrations achieved by infusion have been reported to improve endothelial-dependent vasodilation in, e.g., smokers and patients with type 1 and 2 diabetes and coronary artery disease (Heitzer et al., 1996; Levine et al., 1996; Ting et al., 1996, 1997; Motoyama et al., 1997; Solzbach et al., 1997; Hornig et al., 1998; Ito et al., 1998; Kugiyama et al., 1998; Taddei et al., 1998; Timimi et al., 1998; Chambers et al., 1999; Gokce et al., 1999).

In recent years, increased attention has been placed on the role of vitamin C in the development of the brain. In rats, concentrations of ascorbate increases in the fetal brain during gestation, particularly during the last trimester (Kratzing et al., 1985). In line with this, *in vitro* studies report an essential role of ascorbate in promoting neural differentiation, neurite formation and maturation of neuronal precursor cells (Lee et al., 2003). Because the developing brain is particularly sensitive to changes in redox homeostasis, we have previously hypothesized that vitamin C deficiency is associated with neurological abnormalities owing to neurotoxicity and ROS induced apoptosis (▶Fig. 9.3) (Tveden-Nyborg and Lykkesfeldt, 2009). Children exposed to malnutrition and prenatal hypoxemia show reduced brain size and neuronal numbers as well as lesser arborization of dendrites, connected to learning disabilities in later life (Low et al., 1992; Cordero et al., 1993; Litt et al., 2005; Hack, 2007). Animal models of under nutrition report of reductions in hippocampal neuronal numbers linked to poor performance in spatial memory and cognition (Morgane et al., 1993; Ranade et al., 2008). In juvenile guinea pigs, chronic marginal vitamin C deficiency resulted in significant reductions of hippocampal neurons and impaired spatial memory compared with normal controls, creating a link between vitamin C deficiency and aberrant hippocampal function (Tveden-Nyborg et al., 2009). Epidemiological screenings of human populations have reported as much as 30% of toddlers and mothers to be,

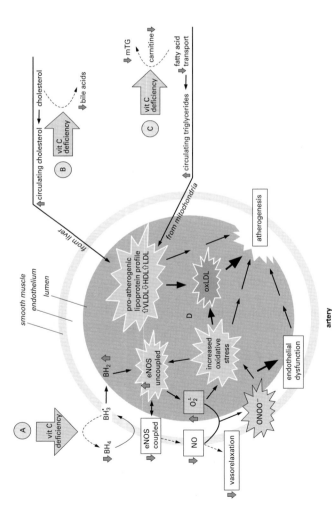

Fig. 9.2: Summary of the potential involvement of vitamin C deficiency in atherogenesis. (A) Ascorbate plays an important role in keeping tetrahydrobiopterin (BH_4) reduced. Lack of vitamin C impairs the reduction of the BH_3-radical (BH_3) to BH_4, and renders its oxidation to dihydrobiopterin (BH_2) the preferred reaction. BH_2 cannot bind to eNOS and the result is eNOS uncoupling. This causes eNOS to produce superoxide rather than NO. Superoxide has a high affinity for NO and their reaction forms the deleterious compound peroxynitrite ($ONOO^-$). The combined effect of these events is endothelial dysfunction. (B) Vitamin C is involved in the conversion of cholesterol to bile acids via the 7α-hydroxylase in the liver. In vitamin C deficiency, less cholesterol will be excreted by this mechanism causing the levels of circulating cholesterol to rise. (C) Vitamin C is a cofactor in the biosynthesis of carnitine. Lack of this cofactor decreases the carnitine mediated transport of triglycerides into the mitochondria (mTG = mitochondrial triglyceride) resulting in an increasingly pro-atherogenic lipoprotein profile. (D) Ascorbate is a powerful antioxidant placed low in the antioxidant hierarchy and could be important for the maintenance of redox balance in the blood stream. Thus, oxidative stress in the vasculature might increase directly by lack of vitamin C. This increase in oxidative stress can both induce endothelial dysfunction and also increase the formation of oxLDL. The combined effect of the resulting redox imbalance is believed to promote atherogenesis. Reproduced from (Frikke-Schmidt and Lykkesfeldt, 2009).

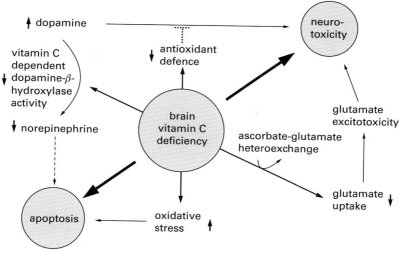

Fig. 9.3: Possible molecular mechanisms of neurotoxicity mediated by vitamin C deficiency. Vitamin C maintains CNS function through various molecular pathways. In vitamin C deficiency, the conversion of dopamine to norepinephrine catalyzed by vitamin C dependent dopamine-β-hydroxylase is impaired resulting in increased concentrations of dopamine. Excess dopamine results in generation of reactive oxygen species which can normally be removed by antioxidant action, but in case of vitamin C deficiency, the defense is unlikely to function optimally and prevent neurotoxicity. Decreased norepinephrine could render the neurons unable to signal triggering apoptotic pathways. Vitamin C deficiency can also induce apoptosis through increased oxidative stress in general. Moreover, the ascorbate-glutamate hetero-exchange system is likely to be affected. This leads to decreased glutamate uptake allowing for extracellular accumulation and excitotoxic neural injury, conducted by an increase of intracellular Ca^{2+}. This, in turn, might elicit apoptotic pathways. Reproduced from (Tveden-Nyborg and Lykkesfeldt, 2009).

to have vitamin C levels below 23 μmol/l, emphasizing the considerable prevalence of marginal vitamin C deficiency (Villalpando et al., 2003; Madruga de Oliveira et al., 2004). However, more detailed studies are necessary to evaluate vitamin C deficiency as a risk factor in brain development, and possibly supporting future supplementation to high-risk individuals.

9.1.6.2 Vitamin C status and disease risk

The possible association between vitamin C status and risk of disease development has been the topic of numerous epidemiological studies.

For cardiovascular disease, independent surveys of more than 8000 US and 22 000 British citizens both found an inverse correlation between serum vitamin C and coronary heart disease (Simon et al., 2001; McFadden et al., 2008). Several large scale population studies have confirmed this tendency of vitamin C as being involved in the prevention of cardiovascular disease (CDV) (Gey et al.,1987a,b, 1993a,b; Steinberg,

1991; Kritchevsky et al., 1995; Nyyssonen et al., 1997; Simon et al., 1998). In a re-examination of the NHANES II data combined with a follow up on vital status 12–16 years later, Loria et al. found that men in the lowest (<28.4 μmol/l) compared with the highest (>73.8 μmol/l) serum ascorbate quartile had a 57% higher risk of death from any cause and a 62% higher risk of dying from cancer (Loria et al., 2000). A similar conclusion was reached by Simon et al. who also found that severe or marginal vitamin C deficiency was significantly associated with all-cause mortality (Simon et al., 2001). In a 20-year follow-up study in the UK, significantly higher risk of mortality from stroke was observed in elderly men and women with severe and marginal vitamin C deficiency separately compared with counterparts with plasma concentrations of vitamin C >28 μmol/l (Gale et al., 1995). The authors concluded that vitamin C status was as strong a predictor of death from stroke as diastolic blood pressure (Gale et al., 1995). An inverse correlation between vitamin C status and stroke was also reported from a study in a rural Japanese population aged 40 years or more (Yokoyama et al., 2000). In a 12-year follow up on the Basel Prospective Study, significantly increased risk of ischemic heart disease and stroke was found in individuals with plasma ascorbate <22.7 μmol/l corresponding to severe or marginal vitamin C deficiency (Gey et al., 1987a,b, 1993a,b).

Whereas epidemiological studies have shown positive correlations between vitamin C status and health, randomized controlled intervention studies have been less convincing. Thus, none of the major clinical studies using mortality or morbidity as end points has found significant positive effects of supplementation with vitamin C (Blot et al., 1993; Heart Protection Study Collaborative Group, 2002; Hercberg et al., 2004; Cook et al., 2007). In agreement, a recent meta-analysis found no positive (or negative) effect of vitamin C supplementation on any major clinical outcome (Bjelakovic et al., 2007). However, a few studies have found effect in selected subpopulations. In the ASAP study, the effect of vitamin C, vitamin E or a combination on carotid intima thickness a marker of an atherosclerotic progression was studied (Salonen et al., 2000). The authors found that 3 years of supplementation with vitamin C and E in combination (but not vitamin C alone) significantly decreased the intima progression rate in men, but not women. Similar results were found at the 6-year follow up, and the authors concluded that supplementation with vitamin C and E in combination slows down atherosclerotic progression in hypercholesterolemic men (Salonen et al., 2003).

The apparent discrepancy between epidemiological studies and randomized controlled trials of vitamin C is puzzling and has been a topic of a recent review (Lykkesfeldt and Poulsen, 2010). Detailed scrutiny of the performed controlled trials has led to the identification of several pitfalls with regard to the examination of the possible benefit of vitamin C supplementation. Thus, the majority of randomized controlled trials does not directly assess the effects of vitamin C, but have used different formulations of multiple antioxidants only permitting a gross estimation of effect originating from isolated components. Moreover, not a single trial has actually used vitamin C deficiency as inclusion criteria. Given the dose-dependent pharmacokinetics of vitamin C described above, it is obvious that effect of vitamin C supplementation can only be expected in individuals that actually absorb the compound. The authors found that only in one of 35 clinical trials with vitamin C, the subjects had vitamin C deficiency at the study start (Lykkesfeldt and Poulsen, 2010). Thus, in spite of the available literature, it remains unclear if supplementation with vitamin C to high-risk individuals is beneficial.

9.1.7 Conclusion

Vitamin C is involved in numerous biological reactions and new functions are still discovered. The so-called antioxidant miracle of the 1980s made vitamin C a popular dietary supplement but whereas considerable literature has identified an inverse correlation between vitamin C status and mortality, the current evidence is primarily of epidemiological nature and thus lacks the ability to establish causality. Increased molecular insight has recently shifted the more or less unspecific antioxidant role of vitamin C as a radical quencher towards a role as a specific irreplaceable mediator in well-defined reactions. Although vitamin C indisputably works as an antioxidant, providing reducing equivalents to the reactions in which it participates, focus should be devoted these specific actions rather than that of various antioxidant cocktails.

Large prospective intervention studies with vitamin C have not been able to establish if vitamin C supplementation promotes health in individuals who are potentially in need of supplementation. However, the studies have convincingly documented that healthy people ingesting a balanced diet with adequate fruit and vegetable content are unlikely to benefit from further supplementation with vitamin C. The lack of knowledge concerning the effects of vitamin C intervention in other subpopulations are mainly owing to inadequate study designs not taking its complex pharmacokinetics into account. At present, studies designed to evaluate the effects of vitamin C supplementation in subgroups expected to benefit from supplementation, e.g., poorly nourished people with a western lifestyle, are required. The fact that a substantial part of the population in developed countries are suffering from subclinical vitamin C deficiency and the potential health problems and expenses for society associated with this condition underline the need for further investigations. Considering the easy and inexpensive cure by which vitamin C deficiency can be resolved makes a good chance of a value-for-money health benefit for a considerable part of the world's population.

References

Ali MS, Phillippo ET, Simultaneous determination of ascorbic, dehydroascorbic, isoascorbic, and dehydroisoascorbic acids in meat-based food products by liquid chromatography with postcolumn fluorescence detection: a method extension. J AOAC Int 1996;79: 803–8.

Ault RG, Baird DK, Carrington HC, Haworth WN, Herbert RW, Hirst EL, Percival EGV, Smith F, Stacey M, Synthesis of D- and L-ascorbic acid and of analogous substances. J Chem Soc 1933; 1419–23.

Aycicek A, Erel O, Kocyigit A, Increased oxidative stress in infants exposed to passive smoking. Eur J Pediatr 2005;164: 775–8.

Bennett M, Coninx R, The mystery of the wooden leg: vitamin C deficiency in East African prisons. Trop Doct 2005;35: 81–4.

Berman SB, Zigmond MJ, Hastings TG, Modification of dopamine transporter function: effect of reactive oxygen species and dopamine. J Neurochem 1996;67: 593–600.

Bjelakovic G, Nikolova D, Gluud LL, Simonetti RG, Gluud C, Mortality in randomized trials of antioxidant supplements for primary and secondary prevention: systematic review and meta-analysis. J Am Med Assoc 2007;297: 842–57.

Block G, Epidemiologic evidence regarding vitamin C and cancer. Am J Clin Nutr 1991;54: 1310S–4S.

Block G, Dietrich M, Norkus EP, Morrow JD, Hudes M, Caan B, Packer L, Factors associated with oxidative stress in human populations. Am J Epidemiol 2002;156: 274–85.

Blot WJ, Li JY, Taylor PR, Guo W, Dawsey S, Wang GQ, Yang CS, Zheng SF, Gail M, Li GY, Nutrition intervention trials in Linxian, China: supplementation with specific vitamin/mineral combinations, cancer incidence, and disease-specific mortality in the general population. J Natl Cancer Inst 1993;85: 1483–92.

Bode AM, Cunningham L, Rose RC, Spontaneous decay of oxidized ascorbic acid (dehydro-L-ascorbic acid) evaluated by high-pressure liquid chromatography. Clin Chem 1990;36: 1807–9.

Bornstein SR, Yoshida-Hiroi M, Sotiriou S, Levine M, Hartwig HG, Nussbaum RL, Eisenhofer G, Impaired adrenal catecholamine system function in mice with deficiency of the ascorbic acid transporter (SVCT2). FASEB J 2003;17: 1928–30.

Buettner GR, The pecking order of free radicals and antioxidants: lipid peroxidation, alpha-tocopherol, and ascorbate. Arch Biochem Biophys 1993;300: 535–43.

Buettner GR, Schafer FQ, Ascorbate as an antioxidant. In: Asard H, May JM, Smirnoff N, editors. Vitamin C: its functions and biochemistry in animals and plants. Oxford: BIOS Scientific Publishers Limited; 2004. pp. 173–88.

Carr A, Frei B, Does vitamin C act as a pro-oxidant under physiological conditions? FASEB J 1999;13: 1007–24.

Chambers JC, McGregor A, Jean-Marie J, Obeid OA, Kooner JS, Demonstration of rapid onset vascular endothelial dysfunction after hyperhomocysteinemia: an effect reversible with vitamin C therapy. Circulation 1999;99: 1156–60.

Cook NR, Albert CM, Gaziano JM, Zaharris E, MacFadyen J, Danielson E, Buring JE, Manson JE, A randomized factorial trial of vitamins C and E and beta carotene in the secondary prevention of cardiovascular events in women: results from the Women's Antioxidant Cardiovascular Study. Arch Intern Med 2007;167: 1610–8.

Cooke JR, Moxon RED, The detection and measurement of vitamin C. In: Counsell JN, Hornig DH, editors. Vitamin C. London: Applied Science Publishers; 1981. pp. 167–89.

Cordero ME, D'Acuna E, Benveniste S, Prado R, Nunez JA, Colombo M, Dendritic development in neocortex of infants with early postnatal life undernutrition. Pediatr Neurol 1993;9: 457–64.

Delanghe JR, Langlois MR, De Buyzere ML, Torck MA, Vitamin C deficiency and scurvy are not only a dietary problem but are codetermined by the haptoglobin polymorphism. Clin Chem 2007;53: 1397–400.

Deutsch JC, Kolhouse JF, Ascorbate and dehydroascorbate measurements in aqueous solutions and plasma determined by gas chromatography-mass spectrometry. Anal Chem 1993;65: 321–6.

Dietary reference intakes for vitamin C, vitamin E, selenium and carotenoids: a report of the Panel on Dietary Antioxidants and Related Compounds, Subcommitties on Upper Reference Levels of Nutrients and of the Interpretation and Use of Dietary Reference Intakes, and the Standing Committee on the Scientific Evaluation of Dietary Reference Intakes, Food and Nutrition Board, Institute of Medicine, National Academy of Sciences. Washington DC: National Academy Press; 2000.

Dragsted LO, Pedersen A, Hermetter A, Basu S, Hansen M, Haren GR, Kall M, Breinholt V, Castenmiller JJ, Stagsted J, Jakobsen J, Skibsted L, Rasmussen SE, Loft S, Sandstrom B, The 6-a-day study: effects of fruit and vegetables on markers of oxidative stress and antioxidative defense in healthy nonsmokers. Am J Clin Nutr 2004;79: 1060–72.

Erdman JW, Klein BP, Harvesting, processing, and cooking influences on vitamin-C in foods. Adv Chem Series 1982; 499–532.

Fediuk K, Hidiroglou N, Madere R, Kuhnlein HV, Vitamin C in Inuit traditional food and women's diets. J Food Compos Anal 2002;15: 221–35.

Frei B, Stocker R, Ames BN, Antioxidant defenses and lipid peroxidation in human blood plasma. Proc Natl Acad Sci U S A 1988;85: 9748–52.

Frei B, England L, Ames BN, Ascorbate is an outstanding antioxidant in human blood plasma. Proc Natl Acad Sci U S A 1989;86: 6377–81.

Frei B, Stocker R, England L, Ames BN, Ascorbate: the most effective antioxidant in human blood plasma. Adv Exp Med Biol 1990;264: 155–63.

Frei B, Forte TM, Ames BN, Cross CE, Gas phase oxidants of cigarette smoke induce lipid peroxidation and changes in lipoprotein properties in human blood plasma. Protective effects of ascorbic acid. Biochem J 1991;277: 133–8.

Frikke-Schmidt H, Lykkesfeldt J, Role of marginal vitamin C deficiency in atherogenesis: in vivo models and clinical studies. Basic Clin Pharmacol Toxicol 2009;104: 419–33.

Fujita Y, Mori I, Yamaguchi T, Hoshino M, Shigemura Y, Shimano M, Spectrophotometric determination of ascorbic acid with iron(III) and p-carboxyphenylfluorone in a cationic surfactant micellar medium. Anal Sci 2001;17: 853–7.

Gale CR, Martyn CN, Winter PD, Cooper C, Vitamin C and risk of death from stroke and coronary heart disease in cohort of elderly people. B Med J 1995;310: 1563–6.

Gey KF, Brubacher GB, Stahelin HB, Plasma levels of antioxidant vitamins in relation to ischemic heart disease and cancer. Am J Clin Nutr 1987a;45: 1368–77.

Gey KF, Stahelin HB, Puska P, Evans A, Relationship of plasma level of vitamin C to mortality from ischemic heart disease. Ann N Y Acad Sci 1987b;498: 110–23.

Gey KF, Moser UK, Jordan P, Stahelin HB, Eichholzer M, Ludin E, Increased risk of cardiovascular disease at suboptimal plasma concentrations of essential antioxidants: an epidemiological update with special attention to carotene and vitamin C. Am J Clin Nutr 1993a;57: 787S–97S.

Gey KF, Stahelin HB, Eichholzer M, Poor plasma status of carotene and vitamin C is associated with higher mortality from ischemic heart disease and stroke: Basel Prospective Study. Clin Invest 1993b;71: 3–6.

Gil MI, Aguayo E, Kader AA, Quality changes and nutrient retention in fresh-cut versus whole fruits during storage. J Agric Food Chem 2006;54: 4284–96.

Gokce N, Frei B, Basic research in antioxidant inhibition of steps in atherogenesis. J Cardiovasc Risk 1996;3: 352–7.

Gokce N, Keaney JF Jr, Frei B, Holbrook M, Olesiak M, Zachariah BJ, Leeuwenburgh C, Heinecke JW, Vita JA, Long-term ascorbic acid administration reverses endothelial vasomotor dysfunction in patients with coronary artery disease. Circulation 1999;99: 3234–40.

Ha YM, Park MK, Kim HJ, Seo HG, Lee JH, Chang KC, High concentrations of ascorbic acid induces apoptosis of human gastric cancer cell by p38-MAP kinase-dependent up-regulation of transferrin receptor. Cancer Lett 2009;277: 48–54.

Hack M, Survival and neurodevelopmental outcomes of preterm infants. J Pediatr Gastroenterol Nutr 2007;45(Suppl 3): S141–2.

Hampl JS, Taylor CA, Johnston CS, Vitamin C deficiency and depletion in the United States: the Third National Health and Nutrition Examination Survey, 1988 to 1994. Am J Public Health 2004;94: 870–5.

Harrison FE, May JM, Vitamin C function in the brain: vital role of the ascorbate transporter SVCT2. Free Radic Biol Med 2009;46: 719–30.

Haworth WN, Hirst EL, Synthesis of ascorbic acid. J Soc Chem Indust (Lond) 1933;52: 645–7.

Heart Protection Study Collaborative Group MRC/BHF Heart Protection Study of antioxidant vitamin supplementation in 20,536 high-risk individuals: a randomised placebo-controlled trial. Lancet 2002;360: 23–33.

Heitzer T, Just H, Munzel T, Antioxidant vitamin C improves endothelial dysfunction in chronic smokers. Circulation 1996;94: 6–9.

Heitzer T, Brockhoff C, Mayer B, Warnholtz A, Mollnau H, Henne S, Meinertz T, Munzel T, Tetrahydrobiopterin improves endothelium-dependent vasodilation in chronic smokers: evidence for a dysfunctional nitric oxide synthase. Circ Res 2000;86: E36–41.

Heller R, Munscher-Paulig F, Grabner R, Till U, L-Ascorbic acid potentiates nitric oxide synthesis in endothelial cells. J Biol Chem 1999;274: 8254–60.

Hercberg S, Galan P, Preziosi P, Bertrais S, Mennen L, Malvy D, Roussel AM, Favier A, Briancon S, The SUVIMAX Study: a randomized, placebo-controlled trial of the health effects of antioxidant vitamins and minerals. Arch Intern Med 2004;164: 2335–42.

Hewitson KS, McNeill LA, Elkins JM, Schofield CJ, The role of iron and 2-oxoglutarate oxygenases in signalling. Biochem Soc Trans 2003;31: 510–5.

Hodges RE, Hood J, Canham JE, Sauberlich HE, Baker EM, Clinical manifestations of ascorbic acid deficiency in man. Am J Clin Nutr 1971;24: 432–43.

Hoffer LJ, Levine M, Assouline S, Melnychuk D, Padayatty SJ, Rosadiuk K, Rousseau C, Robitaille L, Miller WH Jr, Phase I clinical trial of i.v. ascorbic acid in advanced malignancy. Ann Oncol 2008;19: 1969–74.

Hornig B, Arakawa N, Kohler C, Drexler H, Vitamin C improves endothelial function of conduit arteries in patients with chronic heart failure. Circulation 1998;97: 363–8.

Huang A, Vita JA, Venema RC, Keaney JF Jr, Ascorbic acid enhances endothelial nitric-oxide synthase activity by increasing intracellular tetrahydrobiopterin. J Biol Chem 2000;275: 17399–406.

Ignarro LJ, Napoli C, Loscalzo J, Nitric oxide donors and cardiovascular agents modulating the bioactivity of nitric oxide: an overview. Circ Res 2002;90: 21–8.

Ito K, Akita H, Kanazawa K, Yamada S, Terashima M, Matsuda Y, Yokoyama M, Comparison of effects of ascorbic acid on endothelium-dependent vasodilation in patients with chronic congestive heart failure secondary to idiopathic dilated cardiomyopathy versus patients with effort angina pectoris secondary to coronary artery disease. Am J Cardiol 1998;82: 762–7.

Jackson TS, Xu A, Vita JA, Keaney JF Jr, Ascorbate prevents the interaction of superoxide and nitric oxide only at very high physiological concentrations. Circ Res 1998;83: 916–22.

Jacob RA, Sotoudeh G, Vitamin C function and status in chronic disease. Nutr Clin Care 2002;5: 66–74.

Johnston CS, Biomarkers for establishing a tolerable upper intake level for vitamin C. Nutr Rev 1999;57: 71–7.

Johnston CS, Thompson LL, Vitamin C status of an outpatient population. J Am Coll Nutr 1998;17: 366–70.

Kabasakalis V, Siopidou D, Moshatou E, Ascorbic acid content of commercial fruit juices and its rate of loss upon storage. Food Chem 2000;70: 325–8.

Kall MA, Andersen C, Improved method for simultaneous determination of ascorbic acid and dehydroascorbic acid, isoascorbic acid and dehydroisoascorbic acid in food and biological samples. J Chromatogr B Biomed Sci Appl 1999;730: 101–11.

Kallner AB, Hartmann D, Hornig DH, On the requirements of ascorbic acid in man: steady-state turnover and body pool in smokers. Am J Clin Nutr 1981;34: 1347–55.

Katsuki H, Vitamin C and nervous tissue. In vivo and in vitro aspects. Sub-Cellular Biochem 1996;25: 293–311.

Katusic ZS, Vascular endothelial dysfunction: does tetrahydrobiopterin play a role? Am J Physiol Heart Circ Physiol 2001;281: H981–6.

Kratzing CC, Kelly JD, Kratzing JE, Ascorbic acid in fetal rat brain. J Neurochem 1985;44: 1623–4.

Kritchevsky SB, Shimakawa T, Tell GS, Dennis B, Carpenter M, Eckfeldt JH, Peacher-Ryan H, Heiss G, Dietary antioxidants and carotid artery wall thickness. The ARIC Study. Atherosclerosis Risk in Communities Study. Circulation 1995;92: 2142–50.

Kugiyama K, Motoyama T, Hirashima O, Ohgushi M, Soejima H, Misumi K, Kawano H, Miyao Y, Yoshimura M, Ogawa H, Matsumura T, Sugiyama S, Yasue H, Vitamin C attenuates abnormal vasomotor reactivity in spasm coronary arteries in patients with coronary spastic angina. J Am Coll Cardiol 1998;32: 103–9.

Lee JY, Chang MY, Park CH, Kim HY, Kim JH, Son H, Lee YS, Lee SH, Ascorbate-induced differentiation of embryonic cortical precursors into neurons and astrocytes. J Neurosci Res 2003;73: 156–65.

Leung PY, Miyashita K, Young M, Tsao CS, Cytotoxic effect of ascorbate and its derivatives on cultured malignant and nonmalignant cell lines. Anticancer Res 1993;13: 475–80.

Levine GN, Frei B, Koulouris SN, Gerhard MD, Keaney JF Jr, Vita JA, Ascorbic acid reverses endothelial vasomotor dysfunction in patients with coronary artery disease. Circulation 1996;93: 1107–13.

Levine M, Morita K, Ascorbic acid in endocrine systems. Vitamin Horm 1985;42: 1–64.

Levine M, Asher A, Pollard H, Zinder O, Ascorbic acid and catecholamine secretion from cultured chromaffin cells. J Biol Chem 1983;258: 13111–5.

Levine M, Conry-Cantilena C, Wang Y, Welch RW, Washko PW, Dhariwal KR, Park JB, Lazarev A, Graumlich JF, King J, Cantilena LR, Vitamin C pharmacokinetics in healthy volunteers: evidence for a recommended dietary allowance. Proc Natl Acad Sci USA 1996;93: 3704–9.

Levine M, Wang Y, Rumsey SC, Analysis of ascorbic acid and dehydroascorbic acid in biological samples. Methods Enzymol 1999;299: 65–76.

Lin SY, Lai WW, Chou CC, Kuo HM, Li TM, Chung JG, Yang JH, Sodium ascorbate inhibits growth via the induction of cell cycle arrest and apoptosis in human malignant melanoma A375.S2 cells. Melanoma Res 2006;16: 509–19.

Lind J, A treatise on the scurvy in three parts containing an enquiry into the nature, causes and cure of that disease, together with a critical and chronological view of what has been published on the subject. Edinburgh: Sands, Murray and Cochran; 1753.

Litt J, Taylor HG, Klein N, Hack M, Learning disabilities in children with very low birthweight: prevalence, neuropsychological correlates, and educational interventions. J Learn Disabil 2005;38: 130–41.

Loria CM, Klag MJ, Caulfield LE, Whelton PK, Vitamin C status and mortality in US adults. Am J Clin Nutr 2000;72: 139–45.

Low JA, Handley-Derry MH, Burke SO, Peters RD, Pater EA, Killen HL, Derrick EJ, Association of intrauterine fetal growth retardation and learning deficits at age 9 to 11 years. Am J Obstet Gynecol 1992;167: 1499–505.

Lykkesfeldt J, Determination of ascorbic acid and dehydroascorbic acid in biological samples by high-performance liquid chromatography using subtraction methods: reliable reduction with tris[2-carboxyethyl]phosphine hydrochloride. Anal Biochem 2000;282: 89–93.

Lykkesfeldt J, Measurement of ascorbic acid and dehydroascorbic acid in biological samples. In: Maines M, Costa LG, Hodson E, Reed JC, editors. Current protocols in toxicology. New York: John Wiley & Sons; 2002. pp. 7.6.1–15.

Lykkesfeldt J, Smoking depletes vitamin C: Should smokers be recommended to take supplements? In: Halliwell B, Poulsen HE, editors. Cigarette smoke and oxidative stress. Berlin: Springer Verlag; 2006. pp. 237–60.

Lykkesfeldt J, Ascorbate and dehydroascorbic acid as reliable biomarkers of oxidative stress: analytical reproducibility and long-term stability of plasma samples subjected to acidic deproteinization. Cancer Epidemiol Biomarkers Prev 2007;16: 2513–6.

Lykkesfeldt J, Ames BN, Ascorbic acid recycling in rat hepatocytes as measurement of antioxidant capacity: decline with age. Methods Enzymol 1999;299: 83–8.

Lykkesfeldt J, Poulsen HE, Is vitamin C supplementation beneficial? Lessons learned from randomized controlled trials. Br J Nutr 2010;103:1251–9.

Lykkesfeldt J, Loft S, Poulsen HE, Determination of ascorbic acid and dehydroascorbic acid in plasma by high-performance liquid chromatography with coulometric detection – are they reliable biomarkers of oxidative stress? Anal Biochem 1995;229: 329–35.

Lykkesfeldt J, Loft S, Nielsen JB, Poulsen HE, Ascorbic acid and dehydroascorbic acid as biomarkers of oxidative stress caused by smoking. Am J Clin Nutr 1997;65: 959–63.

Lykkesfeldt J, Christen S, Wallock LM, Chang HH, Jacob RA, Ames BN, Ascorbate is depleted by smoking and repleted by moderate supplementation: a study in male smokers and nonsmokers with matched dietary antioxidant intakes. Am J Clin Nutr 2000;71: 530–6.

Lykkesfeldt J, Viscovich M, Poulsen HE, Ascorbic acid recycling in human erythrocytes is induced by smoking in vivo. Free Radic Biol Med 2003;35: 1439–47.

Lykkesfeldt J, Trueba GP, Poulsen HE, Christen S, Vitamin C deficiency in weanling guinea pigs: differential expression of oxidative stress and DNA repair in liver and brain. Br J Nutr 2007;98: 1116–9.

Lynch SM, Morrow JD, Roberts LJ, Frei B, Formation of non-cyclooxygenase-derived prostanoids (F2-isoprostanes) in plasma and low density lipoprotein exposed to oxidative stress in vitro. J Clin Invest 1994;93: 998–1004.

Madruga de Oliveira A, de Carvalho Rondo PH, Barros SB, Concentrations of ascorbic acid in the plasma of pregnant smokers and nonsmokers and their newborns. Int J Vitam Nutr Res 2004;74: 193–8.

Malo C, Wilson JX, Glucose modulates vitamin C transport in adult human small intestinal brush border membrane vesicles. J Nutr 2000;130: 63–9.

Mandl J, Szarka A, Banhegyi G, Vitamin C: update on physiology and pharmacology. Br J Pharmacol 2009;157: 1097–110.

Martino F, Loffredo L, Carnevale R, Sanguigni V, Martino E, Catasca E, Zanoni C, Pignatelli P, Violi F, Oxidative stress is associated with arterial dysfunction and enhanced intima-media thickness in children with hypercholesterolemia: the potential role of nicotinamide-adenine dinucleotide phosphate oxidase. Pediatrics 2008;122: e648–55.

May JM, Qu ZC, Ascorbic acid efflux and re-uptake in endothelial cells: maintenance of intracellular ascorbate. Mol Cell Biochem 2009;325: 79–88.

May JM, Qu ZC, Whitesell RR, Ascorbic acid recycling enhances the antioxidant reserve of human erythrocytes. Biochemistry 1995;34: 12721–8.

May JM, Qu ZC, Whitesell RR, Cobb CE, Ascorbate recycling in human erythrocytes: role of GSH in reducing dehydroascorbate. Free Radic Biol Med 1996;20: 543–51.

May JM, Mendiratta S, Hill KE, Burk RF, Reduction of dehydroascorbate to ascorbate by the selenoenzyme thioredoxin reductase. J Biol Chem 1997;272: 22607–10.

May JM, Qu ZC, Mendiratta S, Protection and recycling of alpha-tocopherol in human erythrocytes by intracellular ascorbic acid. Arch Biochem Biophys 1998;349: 281–9.

May JM, Qu Z, Cobb CE, Extracellular reduction of the ascorbate free radical by human erythrocytes. Biochem Biophys Res Commun 2000a;267: 118–23.

May JM, Qu Z, Morrow JD, Cobb CE, Ascorbate-dependent protection of human erythrocytes against oxidant stress generated by extracellular diazobenzene sulfonate. Biochem Pharmacol 2000b;60: 47–53.

May JM, Qu Z, Cobb CE, Recycling of the ascorbate free radical by human erythrocyte membranes. Free Radic Biol Med 2001a;31: 117–24.

May JM, Qu Z, Morrow JD, Mechanisms of ascorbic acid recycling in human erythrocytes. Biochim Biophys Acta 2001b;1528: 159–66.

McCall MR, Frei B, Can antioxidant vitamins materially reduce oxidative damage in humans? Free Radic Biol Med 1999;26: 1034–53.

McFadden E, Luben R, Wareham N, Bingham S, Khaw KT, Occupational social class, risk factors and cardiovascular disease incidence in men and women: a prospective study in the European Prospective Investigation of Cancer and Nutrition in Norfolk (EPIC-Norfolk) cohort. Eur J Epidemiol 2008;23: 449–58.

Mendiratta S, Qu ZC, May JM, Enzyme-dependent ascorbate recycling in human erythrocytes: role of thioredoxin reductase. Free Radic Biol Med 1998a;25: 221–8.

Mendiratta S, Qu ZC, May JM, Erythrocyte ascorbate recycling: antioxidant effects in blood. Free Radic Biol Med 1998b;24: 789–97.

Metzen E, Enzyme substrate recognition in oxygen sensing: how the HIF trap snaps. Biochem J 2007;408: e5–6.

Miele M, Boutelle MG, Fillenz M, The physiologically induced release of ascorbate in rat brain is dependent on impulse traffic, calcium influx and glutamate uptake. Neuroscience 1994;62: 87–91.

Miglio C, Chiavaro E, Visconti A, Fogliano V, Pellegrini N, Effects of different cooking methods on nutritional and physicochemical characteristics of selected vegetables. J Agric Food Chem 2008;56: 139–47.

Morgane PJ, ustin-LaFrance R, Bronzino J, Tonkiss J, az-Cintra S, Cintra L, Kemper T, Galler JR, Prenatal malnutrition and development of the brain. Neurosci Biobehav Rev 1993;17: 91–128.

Motoyama T, Kawano H, Kugiyama K, Hirashima O, Ohgushi M, Yoshimura M, Ogawa H, Yasue H, Endothelium-dependent vasodilation in the brachial artery is impaired in smokers: effect of vitamin C. Am J Physiol 1997;273: H1644–50.

Murad S, Grove D, Lindberg KA, Reynolds G, Sivarajah A, Pinnell SR, Regulation of collagen synthesis by ascorbic acid. Proc Natl Acad Sci U S A 1981a;78: 2879–82.

Murad S, Sivarajah A, Pinnell SR, Regulation of prolyl and lysyl hydroxylase activities in cultured human skin fibroblasts by ascorbic acid. Biochem Biophys Res Commun 1981b;101: 868–75.

Myatt L, Cui X, Oxidative stress in the placenta. Histochem Cell Biol 2004;122: 369–82.

Myllyharju J, Kivirikko KI, Collagens, modifying enzymes and their mutations in humans, flies and worms. Trends Genet 2004;20: 33–43.

Nyyssonen K, Porkkala-Sarataho E, Kaikkonen J, Salonen JT, Ascorbate and urate are the strongest determinants of plasma antioxidative capacity and serum lipid resistance to oxidation in Finnish men. Atherosclerosis 1997;130: 223–33.

O'Neill RD, Fillenz M, Albery WJ, Goddard NJ, The monitoring of ascorbate and monoamine transmitter metabolites in the striatum of unanaesthetised rats using microprocessor-based voltammetry. Neuroscience 1983;9: 87–93.

Padayatty SJ, Sun H, Wang Y, Riordan HD, Hewitt SM, Katz A, Wesley RA, Levine M, Vitamin C pharmacokinetics: implications for oral and intravenous use. Ann Intern Med 2004;140: 533–7.

Padayatty SJ, Riordan HD, Hewitt SM, Katz A, Hoffer LJ, Levine M, Intravenously administered vitamin C as cancer therapy: three cases. Can Med Assoc J 2006;174: 937–42.

Padayatty SJ, Doppman JL, Chang R, Wang Y, Gill J, Papanicolaou DA, Levine M, Human adrenal glands secrete vitamin C in response to adrenocorticotrophic hormone. Am J Clin Nutr 2007;86: 145–9.

Padhy PK, Padhi BK, Effects of biomass combustion smoke on hematological and antioxidant profile among children (8–13 years) in India. Inhal Toxicol 2009;21: 705–11.

Poulsen HE, Møller P, Lykkesfeldt J, Weimann A, Loft S, Ascorbic acid and DNA damage. In: Asard H, May JM, Smirnoff N, editors. Vitamin C: its functions and biochemistry in animals and plants. Oxford: BIOS Scientific Publishers Limited; 2003. pp. 189–202.

Ranade SC, Rose A, Rao M, Gallego J, Gressens P, Mani S, Different types of nutritional deficiencies affect different domains of spatial memory function checked in a radial arm maze. Neuroscience 2008;152: 859–66.

Rice ME, Ascorbate regulation and its neuroprotective role in the brain. Trends Neurosci 2000;23: 209–16.

Rice ME, Russo-Menna I, Differential compartmentalization of brain ascorbate and glutathione between neurons and glia. Neuroscience 1998;82: 1213–23.

Riviere S, Birlouez-Aragon I, Nourhashemi F, Vellas B, Low plasma vitamin C in Alzheimer patients despite an adequate diet. Int J Geriatr Psychiatry 1998;13: 749–54.

Rumsey SC, Levine M, Vitamin C. In: Song WO, Beecher GR, Eitenmiller RR, editors. Modern analytical methodologies in fat- and water-soluble vitamins. New York: John Wiley & Sons; 2000. pp. 411–45.

Salonen JT, Nyyssonen K, Salonen R, Lakka HM, Kaikkonen J, Porkkala-Sarataho E, Voutilainen S, Lakka TA, Rissanen T, Leskinen L, Tuomainen TP, Valkonen VP, Ristonmaa U, Poulsen HE, Antioxidant Supplementation in Atherosclerosis Prevention (ASAP) study: a randomized trial of the effect of vitamins E and C on 3-year progression of carotid atherosclerosis. J Intern Med 2000;248: 377–86.

Salonen RM, Nyyssonen K, Kaikkonen J, Porkkala-Sarataho E, Voutilainen S, Rissanen TH, Tuomainen TP, Valkonen VP, Ristonmaa U, Lakka HM, Vanharanta M, Salonen JT, Poulsen HE, Six-year effect of combined vitamin C and E supplementation on atherosclerotic progression: the Antioxidant Supplementation in Atherosclerosis Prevention (ASAP) Study. Circulation 2003;107: 947–53.

Savini I, Rossi A, Pierro C, Avigliano L, Catani MV, SVCT1 and SVCT2: key proteins for vitamin C uptake. Amino Acids 2008;34: 347–55.

Schectman G, Estimating ascorbic acid requirements for cigarette smokers. Ann N Y Acad Sci 1993;686: 335–45.

Schectman G, Byrd JC, Gruchow HW, The influence of smoking on vitamin C status in adults. Am J Public Health 1989;79: 158–62.

Schectman G, Byrd JC, Hoffmann R, Ascorbic acid requirements for smokers: analysis of a population survey. Am J Clin Nutr 1991;53: 1466–70.

Schofield CJ, Ratcliffe PJ, Oxygen sensing by HIF hydroxylases. Nat Rev Mol Cell Biol 2004;5: 343–54.

Schofield CJ, Zhang Z, Structural and mechanistic studies on 2-oxoglutarate-dependent oxygenases and related enzymes. Curr Opin Struct Biol 1999;9: 722–31.

Simon JA, Hudes ES, Browner WS, Serum ascorbic acid and cardiovascular disease prevalence in U.S. adults. Epidemiology 1998;9: 316–21.

Simon JA, Hudes ES, Tice JA, Relation of serum ascorbic acid to mortality among US adults. J Am Coll Nutr 2001;20: 255–63.

Sinha R, Block G, Taylor PR, Problems with estimating vitamin C intakes. Am J Clin Nutr 1993;57: 547–50.

Smith JL, Hodges RE, Serum levels of vitamin C in relation to dietary and supplemental intake of vitamin C in smokers and nonsmokers. Ann N Y Acad Sci 1987;498: 144–52.

Solzbach U, Hornig B, Jeserich M, Just H, Vitamin C improves endothelial dysfunction of epicardial coronary arteries in hypertensive patients. Circulation 1997;96: 1513–9.

Steinberg D, Antioxidants and atherosclerosis. A current assessment. Circulation 1991;84: 1420–5.

Steinberg D, Low density lipoprotein oxidation and its pathobiological significance. J Biol Chem 1997;272: 20963–6.

Steinberg FM, Chait A, Antioxidant vitamin supplementation and lipid peroxidation in smokers. Am J Clin Nutr 1998;68: 319–27.

Subar AF, Krebs-Smith SM, Cook A, Kahle LL, Dietary sources of nutrients among US adults, 1989 to 1991. J Am Diet Assoc 1998;98: 537–47.

Szent-Györgyi A, Observations on the function of the peroxidase systems. Biochem J 1928;22: 1387–09.

Szeto YT, Tomlinson B, Benzie IF, Total antioxidant and ascorbic acid content of fresh fruits and vegetables: implications for dietary planning and food preservation. Br J Nutr 2002;87: 55–9.

Taddei S, Virdis A, Ghiadoni L, Magagna A, Salvetti A, Vitamin C improves endothelium-dependent vasodilation by restoring nitric oxide activity in essential hypertension. Circulation 1998;97: 2222–9.

Timimi FK, Ting HH, Haley EA, Roddy MA, Ganz P, Creager MA, Vitamin C improves endothelium-dependent vasodilation in patients with insulin-dependent diabetes mellitus. J Am Coll Cardiol 1998;31: 552–7.

Ting HH, Timimi FK, Boles KS, Creager SJ, Ganz P, Creager MA, Vitamin C improves endothelium-dependent vasodilation in patients with non-insulin-dependent diabetes mellitus. J Clin Invest 1996;97: 22–8.

Ting HH, Timimi FK, Haley EA, Roddy MA, Ganz P, Creager MA, Vitamin C improves endothelium-dependent vasodilation in forearm resistance vessels of humans with hypercholesterolemia. Circulation 1997;95: 2617–22.

Tsukada Y, Fang J, Erdjument-Bromage H, Warren ME, Borchers CH, Tempst P, Zhang Y, Histone demethylation by a family of JmjC domain-containing proteins Nature 2006;439: 811–6.

Tveden-Nyborg P, Lykkesfeldt J, Does vitamin C deficiency result in impaired brain development in infants? Redox Rep 2009;14: 2–6.

Tveden-Nyborg P, Johansen LK, Raida Z, Villumsen CK, Larsen JO, Lykkesfeldt J, Vitamin C deficiency in early postnatal life impairs spatial memory and reduces the number of hippocampal neurons in guinea pigs. Am J Clin Nutr 2009;90: 540–6.

Villalpando S, Montalvo-Velarde I, Zambrano N, Garcia-Guerra A, Ramirez-Silva CI, Shamah-Levy T, Rivera JA, Vitamins A, and C and folate status in Mexican children under 12 years and women 12–49 years: a probabilistic national survey. Salud Publica Mex 2003;45(Suppl 4): S508–19.

Vincent HK, Innes KE, Vincent KR, Oxidative stress and potential interventions to reduce oxidative stress in overweight and obesity. Diabetes Obes Metab 2007;9: 813–39.

Washko PW, Wang Y, Levine M, Ascorbic acid recycling in human neutrophils. J Biol Chem 1993;268: 15531–5.

Willcox JK, Ash SL, Catignani GL, Antioxidants and prevention of chronic disease. Crit Rev Food Sci Nutr 2004;44: 275–95.

Wrieden WL, Hannah MK, Bolton-Smith C, Tavendale R, Morrison C, Tunstall-Pedoe H, Plasma vitamin C and food choice in the third Glasgow MONICA population survey. J Epidemiol Community Health 2000;54: 355–60.

Yokoyama T, Date C, Kokubo Y, Yoshiike N, Matsumura Y, Tanaka H, Serum vitamin C concentration was inversely associated with subsequent 20-year incidence of stroke in a Japanese rural community: The Shibata Study. Stroke 2000;31: 2287–94.

9.2 Vitamin C in human disease prevention

Victoria J. Drake; Balz Frei

9.2.1 Introduction

Vitamin C is an essential nutrient for humans because the body cannot synthesize it; therefore, it must be obtained from dietary sources. It is required for several metabolic reactions, including the biosynthesis of collagen, carnitine, and the neurotransmitter norepinephrine, as well as for the conversion of cholesterol to bile acids. Additionally, vitamin C is a highly effective antioxidant and could function to regenerate vitamin E, another important antioxidant; both vitamins protect biological macromolecules from oxidative damage (Higdon, 2003). Recommendations for dietary intake of vitamin C have been largely based on prevention of marginal and severe deficiency, known as scurvy, rather than on the amount that might be needed to optimize health and prevent chronic disease. This chapter discusses the scientific evidence for the role of vitamin C in the prevention of various human diseases.

9.2.2 Cardiovascular diseases

9.2.2.1 Coronary heart disease

Coronary heart disease (CHD), also known as coronary artery disease and coronary disease, is a major cause of morbidity and mortality worldwide (American Heart Association, 2007). CHD is a narrowing of the coronary arteries that supply blood to the heart; arterial narrowing can result from atherosclerosis within the coronary arteries (Schroeder and Falk, 1995). In addition to increased plasma levels of low-density lipoproteins and decreased levels of high-density lipoproteins, oxidative stress and dysregulation of redox-sensitive gene expression in vascular cells, vascular inflammation, and endothelial dysfunction are important causal factors in the pathogenesis of atherosclerosis (Thomas et al., 2008; Libby et al., 2009). Vitamin C could be an important defense in the pathogenesis of CHD because it is a highly effective antioxidant in human plasma

(Frei et al., 1989); inhibits oxidative modifications of lipoproteins (Retsky et al., 1993); and is important in maintaining normal endothelial function and vasorelaxation (Carr and Frei, 2000). Thus, several epidemiological studies have investigated the relation of vitamin C intake to CHD incidence.

Overall, results of prospective cohort studies examining the association between vitamin C intake from foods or supplements and risk of CHD have been inconsistent. Some (Knekt et al., 1994; Pandey et al., 1995; Sahyoun et al., 1996; Osganian et al., 2003), but not all (Fehily et al., 1993; Rimm et al., 1993; Gale et al., 1995; Kushi et al., 1996; Losonczy et al., 1996; Genkinger et al., 2004), studies have found a protective role of vitamin C. A 2008 meta-analysis analyzed the findings of 14 prospective cohort studies and concluded that higher dietary intakes of vitamin C were associated with a significantly reduced risk of CHD (Ye and Song, 2008). Specifically, those in the top third of dietary vitamin C intake had a 14% lower risk compared with those in the bottom third. However, use of vitamin C supplements was not associated with CHD risk in this pooled analysis, and the authors also did not find a dose-response relation when data from nine studies were analyzed (Ye and Song, 2008). A previous analysis suggested that a threshold for a protective effect could occur at intakes of approximately 100 mg of vitamin C daily (Carr and Frei, 1999). Data from pharmacokinetic studies in healthy, young adults indicate that this dose results in near-saturation with vitamin C of circulating immune cells and, hence, probably tissue cells as well (Levine et al., 1996, 2001). Thus, it has been suggested that vitamin C intake beyond 100 mg/day might not result in much additional benefit with respect to prevention of CHD (Carr and Frei, 1999). This is one possible explanation for the lack of association between vitamin C supplement use and CHD in the above-mentioned meta-analysis (Ye and Song, 2008) and for null findings in randomized controlled trials (RCTs) of vitamin C supplementation in the prevention or treatment of cardiovascular diseases (MRC/BHF, 2002; Waters et al., 2002; Vivekananthan et al., 2003; Zureik et al., 2004; Cook et al., 2007; Sesso et al., 2008).

It is important to note that RCTs conducted thus far with 'antioxidant vitamins', including vitamin C, have had several limitations (Frei, 2004). For example, most trials, whether investigating CAD, cancer, or other chronic diseases, have not determined blood levels of vitamin C before and after supplementation or assessed levels of oxidative stress in the study subjects; therefore, it is impossible to know whether supplementation actually increased vitamin C status or decreased oxidative stress status of the trial participants (Frei, 2004). Future clinical trials should be conducted in subgroups of individuals with low baseline levels of vitamin C. The daily supplemental dose and duration of supplement use are also important considerations in trial design. Intervention trials using only vitamin C supplements are needed because many RCTs have employed a combination of antioxidant vitamins, making it impossible to isolate the effects of supplemental vitamin C alone (Lykkesfeldt and Poulsen, 2010).

Although RCTs are the 'gold standard' used to evaluate the effect of pharmaceutical drugs, such trials are not well-suited to study the effects of nutrients (Heaney, 2008). For example, trials of vitamin supplementation compare low intakes (from diet) with higher intakes (from supplements) in subjects who have a lifelong intake of these vitamins; by contrast, drug trials compare the absence of the drug with its presence in subjects who have not been exposed to this drug before. Therefore, the 'placebo' group in RCTs of vitamin supplements is not a true placebo or 'non-exposed' group, in contrast to the placebo group in RCTs of drugs. This has important implications for the statistical power and data interpretation of these trials, which are commonly overlooked by study investigators. In addition, drug trials are conducted in diseased individuals, whereas primary disease prevention trials using supplemental micronutrients are evaluated in healthy individuals (Heaney, 2008). Finally, 'pharmacokinetic' behavior and metabolism differ greatly between micronutrients (including vitamin C) and xenobiotics (including pharmaceutical drugs) and often have been incompletely characterized to date.

9.2.2.2 Stroke

Stroke is a significant cause of morbidity and mortality in both developed and developing nations. In the USA, almost 90% of all strokes are ischemic, with the remainder being either intracerebral or subarachnoid hemorrhage. The cognitive impairment and dementia that frequently result from stroke are major public health problems (Feigin et al., 2009). Because oxidative stress has been strongly implicated in the pathogenesis of both ischemic and hemorrhagic stroke (Heistad et al., 2009), stroke incidence and severity could be modulated by antioxidant status. Vitamin C is found at high, millimolar concentrations in the brain and thus might have a neuroprotective role (Rice, 2000). Accordingly, several epidemiological studies have examined whether dietary or blood levels of vitamin C are associated with stroke.

Overall, most prospective cohort studies examining dietary intake of vitamin C and risk of stroke have associated higher intake levels with a lower risk. A study that followed 730 elderly adults for 20 years found that dietary intakes >45 mg/day of vitamin C were associated with a significant, 50% reduction in risk of death from stroke when compared with those with intakes <28 mg/day of vitamin C (Gale et al., 1995). Another prospective study in nearly 5200 older adults observed that higher dietary intakes of vitamin C were associated with a significantly lower risk of ischemic stroke (Voko et al., 2003); this inverse association was primarily owing to an observed 73% reduction in risk in cigarette smokers. Smoking is known to increase vitamin C requirements because smokers are under increased oxidative stress and generally have lower vitamin C status than non-smokers (Food and Nutrition Board, 2000). Higher dietary intakes of vitamin C were also related to a lower risk of stroke in a cohort of 1843 middle-aged men, but the association was not statistically significant (Daviglus et al., 1997).

Additionally, a prospective study in a cohort of 26 593 male smokers found a significant, inverse association between dietary vitamin C intake and intracerebral hemorrhage, but no association was observed between dietary vitamin C intake and cerebral infarction or subarachnoid hemorrhage (Hirvonen et al., 2000). Specifically, a median vitamin C intake of 141 mg/day was associated with a 61% lower risk of intracerebral hemorrhage compared with a median intake of 52 mg of vitamin C daily. Although many prospective cohort studies have observed an inverse relation between vitamin C intake and stroke, not all have found a protective effect (Keli et al., 1996; Ross et al., 1997; Ascherio et al., 1999). For instance, total daily intake of vitamin C, from diet and supplements, was not associated with risk for ischemic stroke or hemorrhagic stroke in a cohort of 43 738 men participating in the Health Professionals Follow-up Study (Ascherio et al., 1999).

Food frequency questionnaires and dietary recalls are two methods used to assess dietary intake of vitamin C in epidemiological studies. However, these methods have only a moderate relation with plasma levels of vitamin C (Dehghan et al., 2007).

Compared with dietary intake assessments, fasting blood levels of vitamin C are a more reliable measure of the body's vitamin C status (Levine et al., 1996, 2001). Several studies have investigated whether plasma or serum levels of vitamin C are related to risk of stroke, with many observing an inverse correlation. A prospective study in 730 elderly people found that those with plasma vitamin C concentrations >27.8 µmol/l had a 30% lower risk of death from non-hemorrhagic stroke compared with those with plasma vitamin C concentrations <11.9 µmol/l (Gale et al., 1995). The Second National Health and Nutrition Examination Survey (NHANES II), a national survey of the USA population, analyzed data from 6595 men and women to determine whether serum levels of vitamin C were associated with incidence of self-reported stroke. This survey found that those with serum vitamin C levels between 62.5 µmol/l and 153.3 µmol/l had a 26% lower risk of total stroke compared with those with serum levels between 5.7 µmol/l and 22.7 µmol/l (Simon et al., 1998). Higher serum levels of vitamin C were also associated with a significantly lower risk of total stroke in a cohort of 2121 Japanese adults (Yokoyama et al., 2000). A prospective study in a cohort of 2419 men in Finland found that plasma levels of vitamin C <28.4 µmol/l were associated with a greater than 2-fold increased risk of stroke compared with those with plasma vitamin C levels >65.0 µmol/l (Kurl et al., 2002). Most recently, a prospective cohort study in 20 649 men and women participating in the European Prospective Investigation into Cancer and Nutrition (EPIC)-Norfolk study found that those with plasma vitamin C concentrations ≥66 µmol/l had a 42% lower risk of stroke compared with those with plasma vitamin C concentrations <41 µmol/l (Myint et al., 2008). Collectively, these studies suggest that higher dietary intake levels of vitamin C are protective against stroke.

However, the available population-based studies mainly indicate that taking oral vitamin C supplements is not protective against stroke (Ascherio et al., 1999; Yochum et al., 2000). Additionally, RCTs of vitamin C supplements, often provided in combination with other antioxidant supplements, have generally not found a protective effect on stroke (Mark et al., 1998; Hercberg et al., 2004; Cook et al., 2007; Sesso et al., 2008). As discussed above, data interpretation of these RCTs is hampered by several, inherent limitations. Overall, current research suggests that a vitamin C-rich diet might reduce the risk of stroke, in contrast to vitamin C supplements. Therefore, it is possible that plasma vitamin C concentration is a good indicator of fruit and vegetable consumption, but that vitamin C itself is not protective against stroke, or at least not the only or main component in fruits and vegetables accounting for their beneficial effect on stroke risk.

9.2.2.3 Hypertension

Hypertension is a major public health concern worldwide, afflicting an estimated 26% of the world's population (Kearney et al., 2005). The condition, basically defined as a systolic blood pressure of 140 mmHg or greater or a diastolic blood pressure of 90 mmHg or greater (Lloyd-Jones et al., 2010), is known to increase the risk for cardiovascular and kidney diseases (Whelton, 1994). Dietary modification is important in the prevention of hypertension. Because oxidative stress might contribute to endothelial dysfunction and impaired vasorelaxation, antioxidant vitamins could be beneficial for hypertension. Several observational studies have found inverse associations between blood pressure and dietary intake or blood levels of vitamin C (Yoshioka et al., 1984;

Salonen et al., 1988; Choi et al., 1991; Jacques, 1992a,b,c; Moor de Burgos et al., 1992; Moran et al., 1993; Ness et al., 1996; Toohey et al., 1996; Bates et al., 1998; Block et al., 2008). However, several other dietary factors could contribute to the association. For instance, as mentioned above, vitamin C is a marker of fruit and vegetable intake, and several micronutrients and phytochemicals in fruits and vegetables might influence blood pressure. Thus, it is not known with certainty whether vitamin C is causally related to blood pressure. Intervention trials have mainly focused on disease treatment in individuals with elevated blood pressure rather than on preventing the condition, with positive results in at least one well-designed study (Duffy et al., 1999). Large-scale, long-term studies would be needed to determine whether supplemental vitamin C is effective in the prevention of hypertension.

9.2.3 Cancer

Some observational studies, mainly case-control studies, have associated consumption of fruits and non-starchy vegetables with a reduced risk for several types of cancer, primarily cancers of the digestive tract (i.e., mouth, pharynx, larynx, esophagus and stomach) (World Cancer Research Fund, 2007). Vitamin C is one of many compounds in fruits and vegetables that could possibly be protective against the development of cancer through several different mechanisms, including acting as an antioxidant, recycling vitamin E, stimulating the immune system, and inhibiting carcinogen formation. Several studies have investigated the association of dietary vitamin C intake and cancer. Most case-control studies have observed that dietary vitamin C intake is associated with a decreased risk of cancers of the digestive tract and the lungs (Carr and Frei, 1999); however, case-control studies might be subject to bias owing to their dependence on dietary recall and selection of appropriate control groups. Therefore, prospective cohort studies, which are less prone to bias by such limitations, are given considerably more weight when evaluating the association between diet and disease. Overall, prospective cohort studies in which daily vitamin C intake in the lowest quantile was greater than approximately 85 mg have not found significant effects of vitamin C on cancer risk; protective effects have generally only been observed in those consuming at least 80–110 mg/day of vitamin C (Carr and Frei, 1999). With respect to specific types of cancer, a preventative effect of dietary vitamin C is strongest for cancers of the digestive tract, such as those of the oral cavity, esophagus and stomach (Carr and Frei, 1999).

Cancers of the upper digestive tract are major public health problems worldwide (Chainani-Wu, 2002; World Cancer Research Fund, 2007). In combination with other micronutrients, dietary vitamin C appears to protect against the development of oral, pharyngeal, and esophageal cancer (Chainani-Wu, 2002). Regarding esophageal cancer, case-control studies have consistently shown that consumption of foods containing vitamin C is linked with a lower risk (World Cancer Research Fund, 2007). Moreover, dietary vitamin C intake has been inversely associated with risk of gastric cancer in several studies (Tsugane and Sasazuki, 2007), and a few studies have associated higher blood levels of vitamin C with lower risk of gastric cancer (Stahelin et al., 1991; You et al., 2000; Yuan et al., 2004; Jenab et al., 2006). A protective effect against gastric cancer is biologically plausible because vitamin C can scavenge free radicals produced in the stomach (Drake et al., 1996), inhibit the formation of carcinogenic *N*-nitroso compounds (Mirvish, 1986; Tannenbaum et al., 1991), stimulate immune responses (Kelley and Bendich 1996), and possibly inhibit *Helicobacter pylori* infection – a bacterial infection strongly linked to gastric cancer (Suzuki et al., 2009). Infection with *H. pylori* has been shown to lower vitamin C levels in gastric secretions (Banerjee et al., 1994), and gastric vitamin C levels can be increased with vitamin C supplementation (Waring et al., 1996) or through eradication of the infection (Rokkas et al., 1995). Thus, vitamin C supplementation could be an important adjunct to standard *H. pylori* therapy in reducing the risk of gastric cancer.

Although vitamin C could help protect against cancers of the upper digestive tract, current evidence suggests that dietary vitamin C is not associated with the development of cancers at other sites. An analysis of eight prospective studies found that dietary vitamin C was not related to a decreased risk of lung cancer after the analysis was adjusted for other dietary factors and cigarette smoking (Cho et al., 2006). In addition, the available studies indicate that vitamin C intake from foods is not related to hormone-dependent cancers, including breast, ovarian and prostate cancer. (Carr and Frei, 1999; Willis and Wians, 2003; Zhang, 2004). Some studies have investigated whether the use of vitamin C supplements is associated with cancer development. Prospective studies have generally not observed significant associations between vitamin C supplement use and overall risk of cancer (Shibata et al., 1992), cancer-related mortality (Losonczy et al., 1996), or individual cancers (Hunter et al., 1993; Kushi et al., 1996; Verhoeven et al., 1997; Slatore et al., 2008). However, one study in a cohort of 77 719 older adults found that vitamin C supplement use over a 10-year period was associated with a slight reduction in risk of cancer-related mortality (Pocobelli et al., 2009).

In addition to dietary and supplemental intake, several epidemiological studies have examined the association between plasma levels of vitamin C and risk of various cancers. Plasma concentrations of vitamin C reflect total vitamin C intake from diet and supplements. Although several case-control studies have observed significantly lower plasma levels of vitamin C in cancer subjects compared with control subjects (Stahelin et al., 1984; Romney et al., 1985; Ramaswamy and Krishnamoorthy, 1996; Erhola et al., 1997; Adhikari et al., 2005; Sharma et al., 2009), few prospective studies to date have found significant associations between plasma concentrations of vitamin C and cancer risk (Eichholzer et al., 1996; Sahyoun et al., 1996; Berndt et al., 2005). One prospective study in a cohort of 19 496 adults participating in the EPIC-Norfolk study found that higher plasma vitamin C levels were associated with a significantly lower risk of cancer incidence and cancer-related mortality in men but not in women (Luben et al., 2002).

Although results of observational studies, including case-control and prospective cohort studies, provide information on the relation between diet and disease, it is often difficult to determine if the observed associations can be specifically attributed to vitamin C intake or whether vitamin C is simply a marker of a healthful diet rich in fruits and vegetables. Moreover, causality cannot be established by observational studies. Hence, importance has been placed on obtaining evidence from RCTs. Results of RCTs of vitamin C supplementation have generally not found positive effects with respect to cancer-related endpoints (Blot et al., 1993; Kirsh et al., 2006; Bjelakovic et al., 2008; Gaziano et al., 2009; Lin et al., 2009). However, as mentioned above, such intervention trials have several limitations, making their results difficult to interpret.

9.2.4 Age-related eye diseases

9.2.4.1 Cataracts

Cataracts, the leading cause of age-related visual impairment worldwide, are a clouding and discoloration of the normally clear lens of the eye (Wong and Hyman, 2008; World Health Organization, 2009). Although the condition can manifest as secondary to a chronic disease, such as hypertension or diabetes, long-term exposure to ultraviolet light is a strong risk factor for cataracts (West, 1999; McCarty and Taylor, 2002). Ultraviolet light and cellular free radicals can damage proteins in the eye's lens, causing them to cluster and form the opacities known as cataracts. The opacities that cloud the lens obstruct the passage of light. Cataracts develop slowly and can eventually result in significant impairment of vision. Thus, cataracts become more severe with increasing age.

Because cataracts are thought to result from oxidative damage to the eye, nutritional antioxidants such as vitamin C could help prevent the disease or delay its progression. Moreover, vitamin C accumulates in the lens of the eye (Varma, 1987), and decreased levels of vitamin C within the lens have been linked to an increased severity of the disease (Tessier et al., 1998). A few observational studies have found higher dietary intakes of vitamin C to be associated with a lower risk of cataracts. A prospective study that followed more than 35 000 Japanese adults for 5 years reported that men in the highest quintile of dietary vitamin C intake had a 35% lower risk of cataract diagnosis compared with men in the lowest quintile (Yoshida et al., 2007). In this study, women in the highest quintile of dietary vitamin C intake had a 41% lower risk of cataract diagnosis and a 36% lower risk of cataract extraction (Yoshida et al., 2007). However, other observational studies have found no association between dietary intake of vitamin C and cataracts (Hankinson et al., 1992; Lyle et al., 1999; Cumming et al., 2000), although one of the studies reporting an overall null association found an inverse association in heavy smokers and hypertensives; cigarette smoking and high blood pressure are two established risk factors for cataracts (Lyle et al., 1999).

Studies examining the effect of vitamin C supplement use on cataract development have also reported mixed results. A cross-sectional study in 247 older women participating in the Nurses' Health Study found that vitamin C supplement use for 10 or more years was linked to a 77% lower risk of early lens opacities and an 83% lower risk of moderate lens opacities (Jacques et al., 1997). Use of vitamin C supplements for a shorter duration was not associated with a decreased risk of cataracts in this study (Jacques et al., 1997). Similarly, a prospective study of 50 826 women in the USA observed that those who used vitamin C supplements for 10 or more years had a 45% lower incidence of cataract extraction compared with non-supplement users (Hankinson et al., 1992). However, a more recent prospective study in 24 593 Swedish women who were followed for 8.2 years found that users of vitamin C supplements had a 25% higher incidence of cataract extraction (Rautiainen et al., 2010). In this study, vitamin C supplement use for 10 or more years was associated with a 46% increased incidence of cataract extraction, but the association was not statistically significant (Rautiainen et al., 2010). A much smaller prospective cohort study did not observe vitamin C supplement use to be associated with cataracts (Seddon et al., 1994). In addition, a 7-year randomized, placebo-controlled trial in 4629 adults participating in the Age-Related Eye Disease Study (AREDS) found that a daily antioxidant supplement, which contained 500 mg of vitamin C, 400 IU of vitamin E, and 15 mg of beta-carotene, had no effect on the development and progression of cataracts (AREDS, 2001b).

To date, two studies have reported an inverse association between cataracts and blood levels of vitamin C – an objective measure of dietary vitamin C intake. In NHANES II, each 1 mg/dl (57 µmol/l) incremental increase in serum levels of vitamin C was associated with a 26% lower risk of cataract (Simon and Hudes, 1999). This NHANES II analysis included data from 4001 adults aged 60–74 years. A more recent study of 1112 older adults in North India found those with the highest (≥15 µmol/l) levels of plasma vitamin C had a 36% lower risk of cataract compared with those with the lowest plasma vitamin C levels (≤6.3 µmol/l) (Dherani et al., 2008). The relation between vitamin C intake and cataract development warrants further study to clarify the issues of dose and duration of vitamin C supplementation, as well as duration of follow-up.

9.2.4.2 Age-related macular degeneration

Age-related macular degeneration (AMD) is a major cause of blindness in older adults in industrialized nations. AMD is a progressive disease that involves the degeneration of the macula, the center of the eye's retina, leading to loss of central vision (Congdon et al., 2003). Unlike cataracts, there is no cure for AMD; therefore, studies have investigated possible ways to prevent the disease or delay its progression. Because the retina is a metabolically active tissue and particularly susceptible to oxidative stress, dietary and supplemental antioxidants have been specifically investigated in the prevention and progression of AMD. Epidemiological studies on the association between intake of dietary antioxidants and risk of AMD have reported mixed results. A systematic review and meta-analysis of nine prospective cohort studies found that dietary intake of several antioxidants, including vitamin C, had no significant effect on the primary prevention of AMD (Chong et al., 2007). Additionally, there is little evidence that antioxidants in supplement form help prevent AMD, although they might be beneficial in the treatment of the disease (Evans, 2008). A large intervention trial in patients with AMD, the AREDS found that a combination of antioxidants, containing a daily supplement of 500 mg of vitamin C, 400 IU of vitamin E, and 15 mg of beta-carotene, as well as 80 mg of zinc, slowed both the progression to advanced AMD and the loss of visual acuity over a period of 6.3 years (AREDS, 2001a).

However, this antioxidant combination without zinc has not been associated with significant effects in patients with AMD (AREDS, 2001a,b). To date, no RCTs of AMD incidence or progression have been conducted that used vitamin C supplements only.

9.2.5 Gout

Gout is the most prevalent type of inflammatory arthritis in men, affecting at least 1% of men in western nations (Terkeltaub, 2003). A hallmark of gout is elevated blood concentrations of uric acid (urate). The condition results when urate crystals are deposited in joints, causing inflammation and pain; urate crystal deposition in the kidneys and urinary tract can result in kidney stones (Edwards, 2008). Although there is a hereditary component to gout, dietary and lifestyle modification could potentially help prevent and manage the disease (Choi and Curhan, 2005; Saag and Choi, 2006). Vitamin C has been reported to increase urinary excretion of uric acid, thereby lowering levels of uric acid in blood (del Arbol, 1976; Stein et al., 1976). A few observational studies have examined the relation of dietary intake of vitamin C and gout. One study in 1387 men participating in the Health Professionals Follow-up Study found that total daily intake of vitamin C, from diet and supplements, was inversely associated with serum levels of uric acid (Gao et al., 2008). The inverse association was primarily owing to intake of vitamin C in supplement form (Gao et al., 2008). A prospective cohort study in 46 994 men, who were followed for 20 years, found a dose-dependent protective effect of total vitamin C intake against gout (Choi et al., 2009). In comparison with men who consumed less than 250 mg/day of vitamin C, the risk of gout was 17% lower in men consuming 500–999 mg/day of vitamin C, 32% lower in those consuming 1000–1499 mg/day, and 45% lower in men consuming greater than 1500 mg/day of vitamin C (Choi et al., 2009). In addition to the mentioned observational studies, a RCT in 184 adults reported that vitamin C supplementation of 500 mg daily for 2 months decreased serum levels of uric acid compared with a placebo (Huang et al., 2005).

Thus, the available data indicate that supplemental vitamin C might be beneficial in the prevention of gout, rather than detrimental, although more research is needed on the association.

9.2.6 Common cold

In 1970, Linus Pauling published a book entitled, 'Vitamin C and the Common Cold', which popularized the idea that large doses, sometimes called 'mega-doses', of vitamin C could have use in preventing and treating the common cold (Pauling, 1970). Pauling subsequently published two meta-analyses of early studies on this topic, concluding that supplemental vitamin C use decreases the incidence and severity of the common cold (Pauling, 1971, 2000). Since these publications, there have been many prophylactic trials of vitamin C supplementation on the common cold; most trials have employed daily dosages of 2 g of vitamin C or less. To date, Douglas and colleagues have published three Cochrane reviews on the effect of vitamin C supplementation on the prevention and treatment of the common cold (Douglas et al., 2000, 2004, 2007). The most recent meta-analysis examined the results of 30 placebo-controlled trials of vitamin C supplementation, involving 11 350 individuals, as a prophylaxis for the common cold (Douglas et al., 2007). Individual trials used between 200 mg/day and 3 g/day of supplemental vitamin C for 2 weeks to 5 years, and the placebos in a few studies contained low-dose (≤70 mg/day) vitamin C. This meta-analysis found no significant effect of supplemental vitamin C on incidence of the common cold; however, significant effects were observed in a subgroup of individuals under physical or cold stress. In a subgroup analysis of marathon runners, skiers, and soldiers training in subarctic conditions, vitamin C supplementation was associated with a 50% decrease in cold incidence (Douglas et al., 2007). Additionally, the meta-analysis by Douglas et al. (2007) found that prophylactic use of supplemental vitamin C was associated with an 8.0% reduction of cold duration in adults and a 13.6% reduction of cold duration in children. Thus, currently available evidence indicates that supplemental vitamin C has little impact as a prophylaxis against the common cold in the general population, but it could help prevent colds in individuals under stress.

9.2.7 Conclusions

Data from observational studies indicate that a vitamin C-rich diet could protect against the development of several chronic diseases, including heart disease, stroke, and certain cancers. By contrast, results from RCTs of vitamin C supplementation have been overall disappointing (Lykkesfeldt and Poulsen, 2010), which suggests that the beneficial effect of fruits and vegetables on chronic disease prevention might not be attributable to their vitamin C content. However, these RCTs, although considered the 'gold standard' for establishing safety and efficacy of pharmaceutical drugs, suffer from numerous limitations when applied to micronutrients, including vitamin C (Frei, 2004; Heaney, 2008; Lykkesfeldt and Poulsen, 2010). For example, dose and duration of supplementation, baseline vitamin C and oxidative stress status of study participants, lack of a true placebo group, and incomplete understanding of 'pharmacokinetics' and metabolism of vitamin C render the design of RCTs and the interpretation of their results very problematic.

Current dietary intake recommendations for vitamin C in most nations are set at levels that prevent covert or overt deficiency disease, but appear to be too low for prevention of age-related, chronic diseases. Studies in young, healthy non-smokers have shown that daily intakes of approximately 400 mg of vitamin C fully saturate vitamin C levels in plasma and circulating cells (Levine et al., 2001). Pharmacokinetic studies have not yet been conducted in older adults or in subjects with infections or inflammatory or other diseases; these subpopulations probably require higher intakes of vitamin C to maintain normal body levels. Given the fact that a large percentage of individuals in western societies does not meet dietary intake recommendations for vitamin C, let alone consume vitamin C in amounts that would saturate their body pools, it seems reasonable to recommend a 500-mg daily supplement for all individuals. This level of supplementation does not cause any adverse health effects, maximizes antioxidant protection from vitamin C in the body, and, in combination with a healthful diet abundant in fruits and vegetables, could help protect against the development of various chronic diseases. Large, well-designed, long-term RCTs in subjects with low to marginal dietary vitamin C intakes would be necessary to definitively determine the value of vitamin C supplementation in chronic disease prevention.

References

A randomized, placebo-controlled, clinical trial of high-dose supplementation with vitamins C and E, beta carotene, and zinc for age-related macular degeneration and vision loss: AREDS report no. 8. Arch Ophthalmol 2001a;119: 1417–36.

A randomized, placebo-controlled, clinical trial of high-dose supplementation with vitamins C and E and beta carotene for age-related cataract and vision loss: AREDS report no. 9. Arch Ophthalmol 2001b;119: 1439–52.

Adhikari D, Baxi J, Risal S, Singh PP, Oxidative stress and antioxidant status in cancer patients and healthy subjects, a case-control study. Nepal Med Coll J 2005;7: 112–5.

American Heart Association. Statistical fact sheet – populations. 2007 Update. International cardiovascular disease statistics <http://www.americanheart.org/downloadable/heart/1177593979236FS06INTL07.pdf>. Accessed 1/13/10.

Ascherio A, Rimm EB, Hernan MA, et al., Relation of consumption of vitamin E, vitamin C, and carotenoids to risk for stroke among men in the United States. Ann Intern Med 1999;130: 963–70.

Banerjee S, Hawksby C, Miller S, Dahill S, Beattie AD, McColl KE, Effect of Helicobacter pylori and its eradication on gastric juice ascorbic acid. Gut 1994;35: 317–22.

Bates CJ, Walmsley CM, Prentice A, Finch S, Does vitamin C reduce blood pressure? Results of a large study of people aged 65 or older. J Hypertens 1998;16: 925–32.

Berndt SI, Carter HB, Landis PK, et al., Prediagnostic plasma vitamin C levels and the subsequent risk of prostate cancer. Nutrition 2005;21: 686–90.

Bjelakovic G, Nikolova D, Simonetti RG, Gluud C, Systematic review: primary and secondary prevention of gastrointestinal cancers with antioxidant supplements. Aliment Pharmacol Ther 2008;28: 689–703.

Block G, Jensen CD, Norkus EP, Hudes M, Crawford PB, Vitamin C in plasma is inversely related to blood pressure and change in blood pressure during the previous year in young Black and White women. Nutr J 2008;7: 35.

Blot WJ, Li JY, Taylor PR, et al., Nutrition intervention trials in Linxian, China: supplementation with specific vitamin/mineral combinations, cancer incidence, and disease-specific mortality in the general population. J Natl Cancer Inst 1993;85: 1483–92.

Carr A, Frei B, The role of natural antioxidants in preserving the biological activity of endothelium-derived nitric oxide. Free Radic Biol Med 2000;28: 1806–14.

Carr AC, Frei B, Toward a new recommended dietary allowance for vitamin C based on antioxidant and health effects in humans. Am J Clin Nutr 1999;69: 1086–107.

Chainani-Wu N, Diet and oral, pharyngeal, and esophageal cancer. Nutr Cancer 2002;44: 104–26.

Cho E, Hunter DJ, Spiegelman D, et al., Intakes of vitamins A, C and E and folate and multivitamins and lung cancer: a pooled analysis of 8 prospective studies. Int J Cancer 2006;118: 970–8.

Choi ESK, Jacques PF, Dallal GE, Jacob RA, Correlation of blood pressure with plasma ascorbic acid. Nutr Res 1991;11: 1377–82.

Choi HK, Curhan G, Gout: epidemiology and lifestyle choices. Curr Opin Rheumatol 2005;17: 341–5.

Choi HK, Gao X, Curhan G, Vitamin C intake and the risk of gout in men: a prospective study. Arch Intern Med 2009;169: 502–7.

Chong EW, Wong TY, Kreis AJ, Simpson JA, Guymer RH, Dietary antioxidants and primary prevention of age related macular degeneration: systematic review and meta-analysis. Br Med J 2007;335: 755.

Congdon NG, Friedman DS, Lietman T, Important causes of visual impairment in the world today. J Am Med Assoc 2003;290: 2057–60.

Cook NR, Albert CM, Gaziano JM, et al., A randomized factorial trial of vitamins C and E and beta carotene in the secondary prevention of cardiovascular events in women: results from the Women's Antioxidant Cardiovascular Study. Arch Intern Med 2007;167: 1610–8.

Cumming RG, Mitchell P, Smith W, Diet and cataract: the Blue Mountains Eye Study. Ophthalmology 2000;107: 450–6.

Daviglus ML, Orencia AJ, Dyer AR, et al., Dietary vitamin C, beta-carotene and 30-year risk of stroke: results from the Western Electric Study. Neuroepidemiology 1997;16: 69–77.

Dehghan M, Akhtar-Danesh N, McMillan CR, Thabane L, Is plasma vitamin C an appropriate biomarker of vitamin C intake? A systematic review and meta-analysis. Nutr J 2007;6: 41.

del Arbol JL, Ascorbic acid and uricosuria. Ann Intern Med 1976;85: 829.

Dherani M, Murthy GV, Gupta SK, et al. Blood levels of vitamin C, carotenoids and retinol are inversely associated with cataract in a North Indian population. Invest Ophthalmol Vis Sci 2008;49: 3328–35.

Douglas RM, Chalker EB, Treacy B, Vitamin C for preventing and treating the common cold. Cochrane Database Syst Rev 2000;2: CD000980.

Douglas RM, Hemila H, D'Souza R, Chalker EB, Treacy B, Vitamin C for preventing and treating the common cold. Cochrane Database Syst Rev 2004;4: CD000980.

Douglas RM, Hemila H, Chalker E, Treacy B, Vitamin C for preventing and treating the common cold. Cochrane Database Syst Rev 2007;3: CD000980.

Drake IM, Davies MJ, Mapstone NP, et al., Ascorbic acid may protect against human gastric cancer by scavenging mucosal oxygen radicals. Carcinogenesis 1996;17: 559–62.

Duffy SJ, Gokce N, Holbrook M, et al., Treatment of hypertension with ascorbic acid. Lancet 1999;354: 2048–9.

Edwards NL, The role of hyperuricemia and gout in kidney and cardiovascular disease. Cleve Clin J Med 2008;75(Suppl 5): S13–6.

Eichholzer M, Stahelin HB, Gey KF, Ludin E, Bernasconi F, Prediction of male cancer mortality by plasma levels of interacting vitamins: 17-year follow-up of the prospective Basel study. Int J Cancer 1996;66: 145–50.

Erhola M, Nieminen MM, Kellokumpu-Lehtinen P, Metsa-Ketela T, Poussa T, Alho H, Plasma peroxyl radical trapping capacity in lung cancer patients: a case-control study. Free Radic Res 1997;26: 439–47.

Evans J, Antioxidant supplements to prevent or slow down the progression of AMD: a systematic review and meta-analysis. Eye (Lond) 2008;22: 751–60.

Fehily AM, Yarnell JW, Sweetnam PM, Elwood PC, Diet and incident ischaemic heart disease: the Caerphilly Study. Br J Nutr 1993;69: 303–14.

Feigin VL, Lawes CM, Bennett DA, Barker-Collo SL, Parag V, Worldwide stroke incidence and early case fatality reported in 56 population-based studies: a systematic review. Lancet Neurol 2009;8: 355–69.

Food and Nutrition Board, Institute of Medicine. Vitamin C, dietary reference intakes for vitamin C, vitamin E, selenium, and carotenoids. Washington DC: National Academy Press; 2000. pp. 95–185.

Frei B, Efficacy of dietary antioxidants to prevent oxidative damage and inhibit chronic disease. J Nutr 2004;134: 3196S–8S.

Frei B, England L, Ames BN, Ascorbate is an outstanding antioxidant in human blood plasma. Proc Natl Acad Sci USA 1989;86: 6377–81.

Gale CR, Martyn CN, Winter PD, Cooper C, Vitamin C and risk of death from stroke and coronary heart disease in cohort of elderly people. Br Med J 1995;310: 1563–6.

Gao X, Curhan G, Forman JP, Ascherio A, Choi HK, Vitamin C intake and serum uric acid concentration in men. J Rheumatol 2008;35: 1853–8.

Gaziano JM, Glynn RJ, Christen WG, et al., Vitamins E and C in the prevention of prostate and total cancer in men: the Physicians' Health Study II randomized controlled trial. J Am Med Assoc 2009;301: 52–62.

Genkinger JM, Platz EA, Hoffman SC, Comstock GW, Helzlsouer KJ, Fruit, vegetable, and antioxidant intake and all-cause, cancer, and cardiovascular disease mortality in a community-dwelling population in Washington County, Maryland. Am J Epidemiol 2004;160: 1223–33.

Hankinson SE, Stampfer MJ, Seddon JM, et al., Nutrient intake and cataract extraction in women: a prospective study. Br Med J 1992;305: 335–9.

Heaney RP, Nutrients, endpoints, and the problem of proof. J Nutr 2008;138: 1591–5.

Heistad DD, Wakisaka Y, Miller J, Chu Y, Pena-Silva R, Novel aspects of oxidative stress in cardiovascular diseases. Circ J 2009;73: 201–7.

Hercberg S, Galan P, Preziosi P, et al., The SUVIMAX Study: a randomized, placebo-controlled trial of the health effects of antioxidant vitamins and minerals. Arch Intern Med 2004;164: 2335–42.

Higdon J, Vitamin C, An evidence-based approach to vitamins and minerals: health benefits and intake recommendations. New York: Thieme; 2003. pp. 65–72.

Hirvonen T, Virtamo J, Korhonen P, Albanes D, Pietinen P, Intake of flavonoids, carotenoids, vitamins C and E, and risk of stroke in male smokers. Stroke 2000;31: 2301–6.

Huang HY, Appel LJ, Choi MJ, et al., The effects of vitamin C supplementation on serum concentrations of uric acid: results of a randomized controlled trial. Arthritis Rheum 2005;52: 1843–7.

Hunter DJ, Manson JE, Colditz GA, et al., A prospective study of the intake of vitamins C, E, and A and the risk of breast cancer. N Engl J Med 1993;329: 234–40.

Jacques PF, A cross-sectional study of vitamin C intake and blood pressure in the elderly. Int J Vitam Nutr Res 1992a;62: 252–5.

Jacques PF, Effects of vitamin C on high-density lipoprotein cholesterol and blood pressure. J Am Coll Nutr 1992b;11: 139–44.

Jacques PF, Relationship of vitamin C status to cholesterol and blood pressure. Ann N Y Acad Sci 1992c;669: 205–13; discussion 213–4.

Jacques PF, Taylor A, Hankinson SE, et al., Long-term vitamin C supplement use and prevalence of early age-related lens opacities. Am J Clin Nutr 1997;66: 911–6.

Jenab M, Riboli E, Ferrari P, et al., Plasma and dietary vitamin C levels and risk of gastric cancer in the European Prospective Investigation into Cancer and Nutrition (EPIC-EURGAST). Carcinogenesis 2006;27: 2250–7.

Kearney PM, Whelton M, Reynolds K, Muntner P, Whelton PK, He J, Global burden of hypertension: analysis of worldwide data. Lancet 2005;365: 217–23.

Keli SO, Hertog MG, Feskens EJ, Kromhout D, Dietary flavonoids, antioxidant vitamins, and incidence of stroke: the Zutphen study. Arch Intern Med 1996;156: 637–42.

Kelley DS, Bendich A, Essential nutrients and immunologic functions. Am J Clin Nutr 1996;63: 994S–6S.

Kirsh VA, Hayes RB, Mayne ST, et al., Supplemental and dietary vitamin E, beta-carotene, and vitamin C intakes and prostate cancer risk. J Natl Cancer Inst 2006;98: 245–54.

Knekt P, Reunanen A, Jarvinen R, Seppanen R, Heliovaara M, Aromaa A, Antioxidant vitamin intake and coronary mortality in a longitudinal population study. Am J Epidemiol 1994;139: 1180–9.

Kurl S, Tuomainen TP, Laukkanen JA, et al., Plasma vitamin C modifies the association between hypertension and risk of stroke. Stroke 2002;33: 1568–73.

Kushi LH, Fee RM, Sellers TA, Zheng W, Folsom AR, Intake of vitamins A, C, and E and postmenopausal breast cancer. The Iowa Women's Health Study. Am J Epidemiol 1996;144: 165–74.

Levine M, Conry-Cantilena C, Wang Y, et al., Vitamin C pharmacokinetics in healthy volunteers: evidence for a recommended dietary allowance. Proc Natl Acad Sci USA 1996;93: 3704–9.

Levine M, Wang Y, Padayatty SJ, Morrow J, A new recommended dietary allowance of vitamin C for healthy young women. Proc Natl Acad Sci USA 2001;98: 9842–6.

Libby P, Ridker PM, Hansson GK, Inflammation in atherosclerosis: from pathophysiology to practice. J Am Coll Cardiol 2009;54: 2129–38.

Lin J, Cook NR, Albert C, et al., Vitamins C and E and beta carotene supplementation and cancer risk: a randomized controlled trial. J Natl Cancer Inst 2009;101: 14–23.

Lloyd-Jones D, Adams RJ, Brown TM, et al., Heart disease and stroke statistics – 2010 update. A report from the American Heart Association. Circulation 2010;121: e46–215.

Losonczy KG, Harris TB, Havlik RJ, Vitamin E and vitamin C supplement use and risk of all-cause and coronary heart disease mortality in older persons: the Established Populations for Epidemiologic Studies of the Elderly. Am J Clin Nutr 1996;64: 190–6.

Luben R, Khaw KT, Welch A, et al., Plasma vitamin C, cancer mortality and incidence in men and women: a prospective study. IARC Sci Publ 2002;156: 117–8.

Lykkesfeldt J, Poulsen HE, Is vitamin C supplementation beneficial? Lessons learned from randomised controlled trials. Br J Nutr 2010;103:1251–9.

Lyle BJ, Mares-Perlman JA, Klein BE, Klein R, Greger JL, Antioxidant intake and risk of incident age-related nuclear cataracts in the Beaver Dam Eye Study. Am J Epidemiol 1999;149: 801–9.

Mark SD, Wang W, Fraumeni JF Jr, et al., Do nutritional supplements lower the risk of stroke or hypertension? Epidemiology 1998;9: 9–15.

McCarty CA, Taylor HR, A review of the epidemiologic evidence linking ultraviolet radiation and cataracts. Dev Ophthalmol 2002;35: 21–31.

Mirvish SS, Effects of vitamins C and E on N-nitroso compound formation, carcinogenesis, and cancer. Cancer 1986;58(8 Suppl): 1842–50.

Moor de Burgos A, Wartanowicz M, Ziemlanski S, Blood vitamin and lipid levels in overweight and obese women. Eur J Clin Nutr 1992;46: 803–8.

Moran JP, Cohen L, Greene JM, et al., Plasma ascorbic acid concentrations relate inversely to blood pressure in human subjects. Am J Clin Nutr 1993;57: 213–7.

MRC/BHF Heart Protection Study of antioxidant vitamin supplementation in 20536 high-risk individuals: a randomised placebo-controlled trial. Lancet 2002;360: 23–33.

Myint PK, Luben RN, Welch AA, Bingham SA, Wareham NJ, Khaw KT, Plasma vitamin C concentrations predict risk of incident stroke over 10 y in 20 649 participants of the European Prospective Investigation into Cancer Norfolk prospective population study. Am J Clin Nutr 2008;87: 64–9.

Ness AR, Khaw KT, Bingham S, Day NE, Vitamin C status and blood pressure. J Hypertens 1996;14: 503–8.

Osganian SK, Stampfer MJ, Rimm E, et al., Vitamin C and risk of coronary heart disease in women. J Am Coll Cardiol 2003;42: 246–52.

Pandey DK, Shekelle R, Selwyn BJ, Tangney C, Stamler J, Dietary vitamin C and beta-carotene and risk of death in middle-aged men. The Western Electric Study. Am J Epidemiol 1995;142: 1269–78.

Pauling LC, Vitamin C and the common cold. San Francisco: W.H. Freeman; 1970.

Pauling L, Ascorbic acid and the common cold. Am J Clin Nutr 1971;24: 1294–99.

Pauling L, The significance of the evidence about ascorbic acid and the common cold. Proc Natl Acad Sci USA 1971;68: 2678–81.

Pocobelli G, Peters U, Kristal AR, White E, Use of supplements of multivitamins, vitamin C, and vitamin E in relation to mortality. Am J Epidemiol 2009;170: 472–83.

Ramaswamy G, Krishnamoorthy L, Serum carotene, vitamin A, and vitamin C levels in breast cancer and cancer of the uterine cervix. Nutr Cancer 1996;25: 173–7.

Rautiainen S, Lindblad BE, Morgenstern R, Wolk A, Vitamin C supplements and the risk of age-related cataract: a population-based prospective cohort study in women. Am J Clin Nutr 2010;91: 487–93.

Retsky KL, Freeman MW, Frei B, Ascorbic acid oxidation product(s) protect human low density lipoprotein against atherogenic modification. Anti-rather than prooxidant activity of vitamin C in the presence of transition metal ions. J Biol Chem 1993;268: 1304–9.

Rice ME, Ascorbate regulation and its neuroprotective role in the brain. Trends Neurosci 2000;23: 209–16.

Rimm EB, Stampfer MJ, Ascherio A, Giovannucci E, Colditz GA, Willett WC, Vitamin E consumption and the risk of coronary heart disease in men. N Engl J Med 1993;328: 1450–6.

Rokkas T, Papatheodorou G, Karameris A, Mavrogeorgis A, Kalogeropoulos N, Giannikos N, Helicobacter pylori infection and gastric juice vitamin C levels. Impact of eradication. Dig Dis Sci 1995;40: 615–21.

Romney SL, Duttagupta C, Basu J, et al., Plasma vitamin C and uterine cervical dysplasia. Am J Obstet Gynecol 1985;151: 976–80.

Ross RK, Yuan JM, Henderson BE, Park J, Gao YT, Yu MC, Prospective evaluation of dietary and other predictors of fatal stroke in Shanghai, China. Circulation.1997;96: 50–5.

Saag KG, Choi H, Epidemiology, risk factors, and lifestyle modifications for gout. Arthritis Res Ther 2006;8(Suppl 1): S2.

Sahyoun NR, Jacques PF, Russell RM, Carotenoids, vitamins C and E, and mortality in an elderly population. Am J Epidemiol 1996;144: 501–11.

Salonen JT, Salonen R, Ihanainen M, et al., Blood pressure, dietary fats, and antioxidants. Am J Clin Nutr 1988;48: 1226–32.

Schroeder AP, Falk E, Vulnerable and dangerous coronary plaques. Atherosclerosis 1995;118(Suppl): S141–9.

Seddon JM, Christen WG, Manson JE, et al., The use of vitamin supplements and the risk of cataract among US male physicians. Am J Public Health 1994;84: 788–92.

Sesso HD, Buring JE, Christen WG, et al., Vitamins E and C in the prevention of cardiovascular disease in men: the Physicians' Health Study II randomized controlled trial. J Am Med Assoc 2008;300: 2123–33.

Sharma A, Tripathi M, Satyam A, Kumar L, Study of antioxidant levels in patients with multiple myeloma. Leuk Lymphoma 2009;50: 809–15.

Shibata A, Paganini-Hill A, Ross RK, Henderson BE, Intake of vegetables, fruits, beta-carotene, vitamin C and vitamin supplements and cancer incidence among the elderly: a prospective study. Br J Cancer 1992;66: 673–9.

Simon JA, Hudes ES, Browner WS, Serum ascorbic acid and cardiovascular disease prevalence in U.S. adults. Epidemiology 1998;9: 316–21.

Simon JA, Hudes ES, Serum ascorbic acid and other correlates of self-reported cataract among older Americans. J Clin Epidemiol 1999;52: 1207–11.

Slatore CG, Littman AJ, Au DH, Satia JA, White E, Long-term use of supplemental multivitamins, vitamin C, vitamin E, and folate does not reduce the risk of lung cancer. Am J Respir Crit Care Med 2008;177: 524–30.

Stahelin HB, Gey KF, Eichholzer M, et al., Plasma antioxidant vitamins and subsequent cancer mortality in the 12-year follow-up of the prospective Basel Study. Am J Epidemiol 1991;133: 766–75.

Stahelin HB, Rosel F, Buess E, Brubacher G, Cancer, vitamins, and plasma lipids: prospective Basel study. J Natl Cancer Inst 1984;73: 1463–8.

Stein HB, Hasan A, Fox IH, Ascorbic acid-induced uricosuria. A consequency of megavitamin therapy. Ann Intern Med 1976;84: 385–8.

Suzuki H, Iwasaki E, Hibi T, *Helicobacter pylori* and gastric cancer. Gastric Cancer 2009;12: 79–87.

Tannenbaum SR, Wishnok JS, Leaf CD, Inhibition of nitrosamine formation by ascorbic acid. Am J Clin Nutr 1991;53(1 Suppl): 247S–50S.

Terkeltaub RA, Clinical practice. Gout. N Engl J Med 2003;349: 1647–55.

Tessier F, Moreaux V, Birlouez-Aragon I, Junes P, Mondon H, Decrease in vitamin C concentration in human lenses during cataract progression. Int J Vitam Nutr Res 1998;68: 309–15.

Thomas SR, Witting PK, Drummond GR, Redox control of endothelial function and dysfunction: molecular mechanisms and therapeutic opportunities. Antioxid Redox Signal 2008;10: 1713–65.

Toohey L, Harris MA, Allen KG, Melby CL, Plasma ascorbic acid concentrations are related to cardiovascular risk factors in African-Americans. J Nutr 1996;126: 121–8.

Tsugane S, Sasazuki S, Diet and the risk of gastric cancer: review of epidemiological evidence. Gastric Cancer 2007;10: 75–83.

Varma SD, Ascorbic acid and the eye with special reference to the lens. Ann N Y Acad Sci 1987;498: 280–306.

Verhoeven DT, Assen N, Goldbohm RA, et al., Vitamins C and E, retinol, beta-carotene and dietary fibre in relation to breast cancer risk: a prospective cohort study. Br J Cancer 1997;75: 149–55.

Vivekananthan DP, Penn MS, Sapp SK, Hsu A, Topol EJ, Use of antioxidant vitamins for the prevention of cardiovascular disease: meta-analysis of randomised trials. Lancet 2003;361: 2017–23.

Voko Z, Hollander M, Hofman A, Koudstaal PJ, Breteler MM, Dietary antioxidants and the risk of ischemic stroke: the Rotterdam Study. Neurology 2003;61: 1273–5.

Waring AJ, Drake IM, Schorah CJ, et al., Ascorbic acid and total vitamin C concentrations in plasma, gastric juice, and gastrointestinal mucosa: effects of gastritis and oral supplementation. Gut 1996;38: 171–6.

Waters DD, Alderman EL, Hsia J, et al., Effects of hormone replacement therapy and antioxidant vitamin supplements on coronary atherosclerosis in postmenopausal women: a randomized controlled trial. J Am Med Assoc 2002;288: 2432–40.

West S, Ocular ultraviolet B exposure and lens opacities: a review. J Epidemiol 1999;9(6 Suppl): S97–101.

Whelton PK, Epidemiology of hypertension. Lancet 1994;344: 101–6.

Willis MS, Wians FH, The role of nutrition in preventing prostate cancer: a review of the proposed mechanism of action of various dietary substances. Clin Chim Acta 2003;330: 57–83.

Wong TY, Hyman L, Population-based studies in ophthalmology. Am J Ophthalmol 2008;146: 656–63.

World Cancer Research Fund/American Institute for Cancer Research. Food, nutrition, physical activity, and the prevention of cancer: a global perspective. Washington, DC: AICR; 2007.

World Health Organization, Visual impairment and blindness <http://www.who.int/mediacentre/factsheets/fs282/en/>. Accessed 1/8/10, May 2009.

Ye Z, Song H, Antioxidant vitamins intake and the risk of coronary heart disease: meta-analysis of cohort studies. Eur J Cardiovasc Prev Rehabil 2008;15: 26–34.

Yochum LA, Folsom AR, Kushi LH, Intake of antioxidant vitamins and risk of death from stroke in postmenopausal women. Am J Clin Nutr 2000;72: 476–83.

Yokoyama T, Date C, Kokubo Y, Yoshiike N, Matsumura Y, Tanaka H, Serum vitamin C concentration was inversely associated with subsequent 20-year incidence of stroke in a Japanese rural community. The Shibata study. Stroke 2000;31: 2287–94.

Yoshida M, Takashima Y, Inoue M, et al., Prospective study showing that dietary vitamin C reduced the risk of age-related cataracts in a middle-aged Japanese population. Eur J Nutr 2007;46: 118–24.

Yoshioka M, Matsushita T, Chuman Y, Inverse association of serum ascorbic acid level and blood pressure or rate of hypertension in male adults aged 30–39 years. Int J Vitam Nutr Res 1984;54: 343–7.

You WC, Zhang L, Gail MH, et al., Gastric dysplasia and gastric cancer: *Helicobacter pylori*, serum vitamin C, and other risk factors. J Natl Cancer Inst 2000;92: 1607–12.

Yuan JM, Ross RK, Gao YT, Qu YH, Chu XD, Yu MC, Prediagnostic levels of serum micronutrients in relation to risk of gastric cancer in Shanghai, China. Cancer Epidemiol Biomarkers Prev 2004;13: 1772–80.

Zhang SM, Role of vitamins in the risk, prevention, and treatment of breast cancer. Curr Opin Obstet Gynecol 2004;16: 19–25.

Zureik M, Galan P, Bertrais S, et al., Effects of long-term daily low-dose supplementation with antioxidant vitamins and minerals on structure and function of large arteries. Arterioscler Thromb Vasc Biol 2004;24: 1485–91.

10 Vitamin D – Cholecalciferol

10.1 Vitamin D – biological significance and nutritional aspects

A. Zittermann

10.1.1 Introduction

Vitamin D_3 (cholecaliferol) is unique among vitamins in that humans can produce it themselves in their skin provided they have sufficient exposure to ultraviolet radiation. Vitamin D_3 and vitamin D_2 (ergocalciferol) is also found naturally in some foods (►Fig. 10.1). Because of its skin synthesis, vitamin D_3 is not really a vitamin for humans. The skin of humans and many animals has a high concentration of the sterol cholesterol which is converted by enzymes in the skin to the sterol 7-dehydrocholesterol. Exposure of skin to sunlight for regular intervals results in the photochemical conversion of 7-dehydrocholesterol into previtamin D_3, which is rapidly converted to vitamin D_3. This sunlight-generated vitamin D_3 is a precursor of the active hormonal form of vitamin D_3. Under these circumstances vitamin D is not a vitamin because it has been produced by the body (with the assistance of sunlight). However, if the person or animal lives in the absence of sunlight (e.g., North America and Europe in the winter) or exclusively indoors (institutionalized people), then there is indeed an absolute regular requirement for the fat-soluble vitamin D, that must be met through proper dietary intake (History of vitamin D, 2010).

10.1.2 History

The first scientific description of a vitamin D deficiency, namely rickets, was provided in the 17th century by Daniel Whistler (1645) and Francis Glisson (1650). During the 19th and early 20th century, industrialization and urbanization in Europe and North America were associated with high prevalence of rickets. Up to 40–60% of children living in certain locations during the Industrial Revolution had the problem (Huh and Gordon, 2008). In times when rickets was highly prevalent in Europe, e.g., in 1900, mortality under the age of 5 years was approximately 250/1000 life-born children, than dropped to 50 around 1950, and is now approximately five (Wjst, 2004). In 1909, among infants 18 months or less who had died, histopathological evidence of rickets was found in 96% at autopsy (Rajakumar, 2003), highlighting the strong association of rickets with infant mortality.

It was in 1919/20 that Sir Edward Mellanby, working with dogs raised exclusively indoors recognized that rickets was caused by a deficiency of a trace component present in the diet. He called this fat-soluble substance vitamin A. McCollum and colleagues, however, later discovered that the factor responsible for healing rickets was distinct from vitamin A. McCollum named this new substance vitamin D. In 1923 Goldblatt and Soames identified that when a precursor of vitamin D in the skin (7-dehydrocholesterol) was irradiated with sunlight or ultraviolet light, a substance equivalent to the fat-soluble vitamin was produced. Hess and Weinstock confirmed the dictum that 'light equals

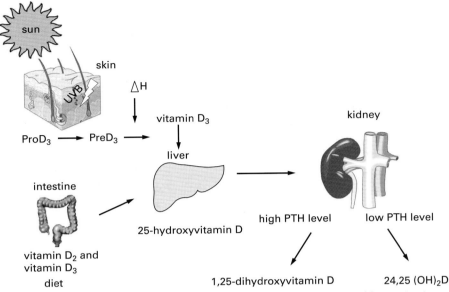

Fig. 10.1: Vitamin D metabolism. (ΔH is the energy that is needed for the conversion of the pre vitamin D3 molecule into vitamin D3 molecule).

vitamin D'. The chemical structures of the vitamins D were determined by Adolf Windaus at the University of Göttingen in Germany. Windaus was awarded the Nobel Prize in Chemistry in 1928 for his work on sterols and their relation to vitamins. However, the chemical structures of the vitamins D were determined in his laboratory not before the 1930s (Wolf, 2004). Vitamin D_2 which could be produced by ultraviolet irradiation of ergosterol was chemically characterized in 1932. Vitamin D_3 was chemically characterized in 1936 when it was shown to result from the ultraviolet irradiation of 7-dehydrocholesterol. Virtually simultaneously, the elusive antirachitic component of cod liver oil was shown to be identical to the newly characterized vitamin D_3. The first Nobel Prize for vitamin D-related research was, however, already awarded to Niels Finsen in 1903. He won the Nobel Prize for Medicine and Physiology for his theory to cure Lupus vulgaris (skin-tuberculosis) using phototherapy. Nowadays it is clear that vitamin D is the key component produced by phototherapy. Vitamin D has not only important anti-rachitic properties but is also a very potent immunomodulator (see below).

10.1.3 Vitamin D metabolism

Skin synthesis of vitamin D_3 usually contributes 80–90% to vitamin D supply in free-living persons. Vitamin D_3 can be produced very effectively by humans when ultraviolet radiation (UVB) from sunlight or artificial sources reaches skin cells. In an investigation by Holick's working group, vitamin D_3 synthesis occurred throughout the year at latitudes of 34°N and below, whereas no production of vitamin D_3 was found in the winter months of November to February at 42°N (Boston) or October to March at 52°N (Edmonton), even if the exposure time was extended to 3 h. In the mid-summer months of June and July, the amount of vitamin D_3 increased to a maximum of approximately

12% at lower latitudes, to 9% in 1 h in Boston and 11% in 3 h in Edmonton. Analyses after exposure of the 7-dehydrocholesterol solution at several places in the southern hemisphere showed concordant results. However, using the MacLaughlin action spectrum of the UV-induced production of previtamin D_3 in human skin, the vitamin D weighted UV in the winter months is roughly 5% of the summer value at mid-latitudes, around 40°N. Thus sufficient vitamin D should be produced in an individual in winter, if whole body UV exposure is performed (Norval et al., 2010). A whole-body exposure to the summer UV spectrum of 15–20 min daily is able to produce up to 250 µg vitamin D (Stamp et al., 1977; Krause et al., 1998). It has been assumed that exposure of arms and legs for 5–30 min between the hours of 10:00 h and 15:00 h twice a week is often adequate. Exposure to sunlight or artificial UVB radiation that is equivalent to 0.5 erythemal dose results in synthesis of 75 µg vitamin D_3 (Holick, 2007). The exact amount of vitamin D_3 production in human skin depends on the geographic latitude, season, time of day, as well as on the weather conditions (cloudiness), amount of air pollution and surface reflection. In addition, clothing habits, lifestyle, and workplace (e.g., indoor vs outdoor), sunscreen use, and sun avoidance practices have a strong impact on vitamin D_3 synthesis. It is also noteworthy that skin type determines a person's effectiveness in producing vitamin D_3. The darker the skin is pigmented, the more ultraviolet radiation is absorbed by melanin and the less vitamin D_3 is produced. Migrant populations and their descendants often have skin types that do not fit to the ambient ultraviolet environment. To achieve a similar effect on vitamin D_3 production compared with a fair-skinned person, the exposure time to ultraviolet radiation in a dark-skinned person living in Europe or North America must be up to six times longer (Clemens et al., 1982). Skin pigmentation is considered an important reason why Afro-Americans have considerably poorer vitamin D status compared with white Americans (Nesby-O'Dell et al., 2002).

Cutaneously synthesized or orally ingested vitamin D is transported in the circulation bound to vitamin D binding protein (DBP). In the blood, only a small fraction is present as free, unbound vitamin D metabolites. The 25-hydroxylation of both vitamin D_2 or vitamin D_3, is the initial step in vitamin D activation. This takes place primarily in the liver. Nevertheless, extra-hepatic sources of 25-hydroxylation have been described in humans as well. They include macrophages, fibroblasts, keratinocytes and arterial endothelial cells (Gascon-Barre, 2005). In the liver, the existence of both a mitochondrial and microsomal 25-hydroxylase has been described. The microsomal enzyme is the physiologically relevant enzyme. It is an enzyme of low capacity and high affinity. By contrast, the mitochondrial enzyme is of high-capacity and low-affinity and is thought to be relevant only under conditions of high vitamin D concentration such as vitamin D intoxication. Liver production of 25-hydroxyvitamin D (25(OH)D) is not significantly regulated. Synthesis of 25(OH)D is primarily dependent on substrate concentration. An important consequence of this lack of physiological regulation of 25(OH)D is that measurement of circulating 25(OH)D is an excellent measure of vitamin D supply. In the kidney, 25(OH)D is further hydroxylated into the active hormonal form 1,25-dihydroxyvitamin D (calcitriol). This step is under control of parathyroid hormone (PTH, see below). Usually, circulating 1,25-dihydroxyvitamin D concentrations are tightly controlled.

The active form of vitamin D, 1,25-dihydroxyvitamin D, is known as a regulator of systemic calcium homeostasis. However, 1,25-dihydroxyvitamin D also plays a pivotal role in the intracellular calcium homeostasis and has pleiotropic effects in various tissues. The biological actions of 1,25-dihydroxyvitamin D are mediated through the vitamin D receptor (VDR). In this context, 1,25-dihydroxyvitamin D functions as a steroid hormone that binds to a cytosolic VDR resulting in a selective demasking of the genome of the nucleolus. VDR is a ligand-dependent transcription factor that belongs to the super family of the nuclear hormone receptors. Binding of 1,25-dihydroxyvitamin D induces conformational changes in VDR which promotes its hetero-dimerization with retinoid X receptor (RXR), followed by translocation of this complex into the nucleus. The RXR-VDR heterodimer binds to the vitamin D responsive elements (VDRE) in promoter regions of 1,25-dihydroxyvitamin D responsive genes, which, in turn, results in the regulatory function of 1,25-dihydroxyvitamin D. The vitamin D receptor (VDR) is nearly ubiquitously expressed, and almost all cells respond to 1,25-dihydroxyvitamin D exposure; approximately 3% of the human genome is regulated, directly and/or indirectly, by the vitamin D endocrine system. Polymorphisms of the VDR have been described for the endonuclease BmsI, Apa I, Taq I and Fok I restriction sites (Zittermann, 2003b).

25(OH)D can also be converted by a renal 24-hydroxylase into 24,25-dihydroxyvitamin D. Circulating 24,25-dihydroxyvitamin D levels are very strongly correlated with circulating 25(OH)D levels. Circulating 25(OH)D levels are, however, approximately ten times higher than serum 24,25-dihydroxyvitamin D levels and are approximately 500–1000 times higher than serum 1,25-dihydroxyvitamin D levels. Several tissues also possess 24-hydroxylase activity resulting in a local production of 24,25-dihydroxyvitamin D from 25(OH)D. It has been hypothesized that 24,25-dihydroxyvitamin D is indispensable for normal calcium and phosphorus homeostasis. Consequently, a cellular receptor for 24,25-dihydroxyvitamin D has been postulated by some investigators (Norman, 1998).

The *de novo* mRNA and protein synthesis induced by the cytosolic calcitriol-VDR complex require periods lasting hours to days. However, rapid 1,25-dihydoxyvitamin D actions have also been observed in several tissues at both the cellular and subcellular level (Norman, 1998). These 1,25-dihydroxyvitamin D actions cannot be explained by receptor-hormone interactions with the genome. Meanwhile, a membrane-bound VDR has been recognized in different cell lines leading to an activation of specific intracellular metabolic pathways within a few minutes. Given the pivotal role of ionized calcium in muscle contraction, nerve-impulse conduction, and other physiological phenomena, such a rapid response could be life-saving for the organism (Nemere and Farach-Carson, 1998).

Cellular uptake of circulating 25(OH)D takes place through megalin-mediated endocytosis of the DBP 25(OH)D complex (Tuohimaa, 2009). Apart from the kidney, 1,25-dihydroxyvitamin D can be locally produced in several tissues that possess VDR and are responsive to this hormone. These tissues include monocytes, dendritic cells, B lymphocytes, colonocytes, vascular smooth muscle cells and endothelial cells. Consequently, for 1,25-dihydroxyvitamin D a paracrine role apart from its calcium-regulating function has been proposed (Bouillon et al., 1998). It has been assumed that local 1,25-dihydroxyvitamin D synthesis depends on substrate availability, e.g., on the concentration of circulating 25(OH)D. Cellular uptake of 25(OH)D in extrarenal tissues is significantly reduced in case of low circulating 1,25-dihyroxyvitamin D, e.g., in patients with renal insufficiency. There is also evidence that at least in some tissues local 1,25-dihydroxyvitamin D production is largely independent from 25(OH)D availability and is mediated by other stimuli (e.g., wound-induced synthesis in keratinocytes and Toll-like receptor 2 mediated production in monocytes) (Liu et al., 2006; Schauber et al., 2007).

Most former research dealing with utilization of vitamins D_2 and D_3 assumed that these two forms are equally potent in mammals including humans. This assumption is based on the fact that the steps of activation into the active hormonal form are identical for vitamins D_2 and D_3. However, during recent years concern arose whether vitamin D_2 is as effective as vitamin D_3 in maintaining circulating concentrations of 25(OH)D (Trang et al., 1998; Armas et al., 2004). These concerns could, however, not be confirmed by all researchers (Holick et al., 2008; Pietras et al., 2009). Nevertheless, an addition concern against the efficacy of vitamin D_2 is the fact that the position 24 of vitamin D_2, in contrast to the similar position in vitamin D_3, can be considered to be highly reactive. The formation of 1,24,25-trihydroxyvitamin D_2 represents an unequivocal deactivation of the vitamin D_2 molecule. Conversely, the comparable vitamin D_3 metabolite, 1,24,25-trihydroxyvitamin D_3, maintains significant activity and must undergo further side-chain oxidation to be rendered totally inactive (Horst et al., 2005).

10.1.4 Relation of vitamin D to calcium and parathyroid hormone

Serum calcium homeostasis is essential for blood coagulation, for activation of various intracellular processes, and for bone health. Therefore, a serum calcium level of 2.5 mmol/l is maintained in all life-forms of vertebrates, aquatic and terrestrial. Together with parathyroid hormone (PTH) and calcitonin, vitamin D carries out the policing job of regulating serum calcium levels in highly evolved mammals. This regulating mechanism is done with astounding efficiency, indicating the importance of serum calcium homeostasis. The regulatory system of calciotropic hormones appears to have developed after transition of life from water (calcium-phosphorus rich environment) to land (environment poor in calcium and phosphorus). This assumption is supported by the fact that in fish PTH is missing and calcitonin is inactive (Rao and Raghuramulu, 1999).

Together with PTH, vitamin D is responsible for maintaining serum calcium levels by increasing intestinal calcium absorption, renal calcium reabsorption, and calcium resorption from bone. Without vitamin D, only 10–15% of dietary calcium and about 60% of phosphorus is absorbed. Vitamin D increases the efficiency of intestinal calcium absorption to 30–40% and phosphorus absorption to approximately 80% (Holick, 2007).

In the case of vitamin D deficiency (25(OH)D below 25 nmol/l), severe secondary hyperparathyroidism (SHPT) (serum PTH >65 pg/ml), and calcium malabsorption are seen. Significant substrate-dependent reduction in serum 1,25-dihydroxyvitamin D levels occur already if the circulating serum 25(OH)D level falls below 30–40 nmol/l (Zittermann, 2006). If vitamin D deficiency is less severe, mild hyperparathyroidism can occur. The increase in serum PTH will stimulate renal synthesis of 1,25-dihydroxyvitamin D to keep calcium absorption and serum calcium within normal limits. Consequently, serum 1,25-dihydroxyvitamin D is maintained within normal limits at the expense of an increase of serum PTH. In line with this, Thomas et al. (1998) have reported an inverse relation between serum 25(OH)D and serum PTH in in-hospital patients who had 25(OH)D levels in the range of 0–75 nmol/l (0–30 ng/ml) (►Fig. 10.2). Serum PTH showed a progressive increase when serum 25(OH)D was below 27.5–37.5 nmol/l (11–15 ng/ml). Results fit well together with the fact that centenarians with undetectable serum 25(OH)D levels have severe SHPT. By contrast, no case of SHPT is seen in elderly subjects with 25(OH)D levels above 100 nmol/l (Zittermann, 2006). No threshold exists between serum 25(OH)D and serum PTH up to a 25(OH)D level of 150 nmol/l. Supplementation

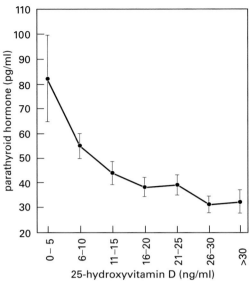

Fig. 10.2: Relation between serum 25-hydroxyvitamin D concentrations and mean (±SE) serum concentrations of parathyroid hormone in medical inpatients. To convert values for 25-hydroxyvitamin D to nmol/l, multiply by 2.5. To convert values for parathyroid hormone to pmol/l, multiply by 0.11 (Thomas et al., 1998).

studies demonstrate that even in subjects with initial serum 25(OH)D levels of already 70 nmol/l an increase in 25(OH)D to approximately 210 nmol/l still resulted in a decrease in serum PTH levels of 24% within 4 months of vitamin D supplementation (Heaney et al., 2003). Generally, elderly subjects have higher PTH levels than younger subjects on a given 25(OH)D level. Consequently, higher 25(OH)D levels are necessary in elderly subjects than in younger adults to suppress serum PTH levels into the low physiologic range. Although the effect of additional vitamin D seems to be highest if serum 25(OH)D is low (►Fig. 10.2), available data also indicate that serum PTH and circulating 1,25-dihydroxyvitamin D does obviously not reach a plateau during a wide range of serum 25(OH)D levels (Zittermann, 2006; Konradsen et al., 2008). It should also be mentioned that even healthy adolescents have already elevated serum PTH levels if their serum 25(OH)D levels are low (Zittermann, 2006). Elevated PTH concentrations have not only been recognized as a risk factor for enhanced bone resorption (Passeri et al., 2003) but also for cardiovascular disease (Hagström et al., 2009).

Serum 25(OH)D is, however, not the only regulator of PTH. If abundant dietary calcium is available, PTH decreases, calcitonin increases, and excess calcium is deposed in bone or excreted via bile and urine. Thus, dietary calcium intake is an important factor influencing serum PTH levels. Calcium supplementation of 1000 mg is able to decrease postprandial serum PTH by 50% within 2 h. With respect to serum calcium homeostasis, high dietary calcium intake and adequate vitamin D status seem to be able to replace each other: this assumption is supported by the fact that in healthy adults with 25(OH)D concentrations below 25 nmol/l, calcium intake of less than 800 mg/day versus more than 1200 mg/day is significantly associated with higher serum PTH

(Steingrimsdottir et al., 2005). By contrast, an improvement in vitamin D status does not suppress PTH levels in individuals with 25(OH)D concentrations between 25 and 50 nmol/l if daily calcium intakes are above 1200 mg (Schleithoff et al., 2007).

Whereas 25(OH)D is an important regulator of PTH, PTH, in turn, stimulates renal 1,25-dihydroxyvitamin D synthesis and thus controls homeostasis of circulating levels of 1,25-dihydroxyvitamin D. However, this control mechanism obviously does not work in all patients. In frail chronically bedridden patients with vitamin D deficiency, e.g., the absence of SHPT was common and persistent (Björkman et al., 2009), whereas the high prevalence of vitamin D deficiency would have suggested a high prevalence of SHPT. In addition, in a group of patients with end-stage heart failure and frequent vitamin D deficiency, both PTH and calcitriol levels were surprisingly low in some severely ill patients (Zittermann et al., 2008). Finally, a dramatic fall in circulating 1,25-dihydroxyvitamin D concentrations (and also intestinal calcium absorption) occurred in a cosmonaut during the German-Russian MIR 97 spaceflight, although these alterations were not paralleled by subsequent changes in serum 25(OH)D or PTH concentrations (Zittermann et al., 2000, ▶Fig. 10.3). Some of these surprising results might be explained by a suppression of 1,25-dihydroxyvitamin D through proinflammatory cytokines such as interleukin-6 and tumor necrosis factor-α (Zittermann et al., 2009b). Another explanation is the liberation of calcium from bone by reduced mechanical forces, resulting in a slight increase in serum calcium and a subsequent suppression in serum PTH. Circulating 1,25-dihydroxyvitamin D concentrations are also low in patients with renal insufficiency, e.g., in patients with glomerular filtration rates below 60 ml/min. Although PTH levels increase in this situation, the accompanying phosphate retention lowers synthesis of 1,25-dihydroxyvitamin D (Zittermann, 2006). This is owing to a hyperphosphatemia-induced increase in concentrations of fibroblast growth factor-23 (FGF-23) (Holick, 2007). FGF-23 is a newly recognized regulator of 1,25-dihydroxyvitamin D. Whereas excess 1,25-dihydroxyvitamin D concentrations are reported in FGF-23 knockout mice (Stubbs et al., 2007), high FGF-23 concentrations are associated with low 1,25-dihydroxyvitamin D concentrations (Antoniucci et al., 2006).

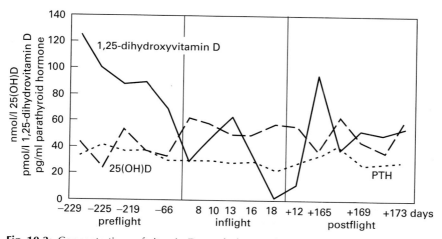

Fig. 10.3: Concentrations of vitamin D metabolites and parathyroid hormone in a German cosmonaut before, during and after the MIR 97 space mission (Zittermann et al., 2000).

In total, available data indicate that 1,25-dihydroxyvitamin D homeostasis in the blood is usually tightly regulated by PTH. However, this regulation obviously does not work in the case of substrate deficiency, e.g., deficient 25(OH)D concentrations, and in the case of elevated concentrations of FGF-23 and/or proinflammatory cytokines.

10.1.5 Stages of vitamin D status and prevalence of vitamin D inadequacy

The measurement of 25(OH)D is the adequate tool for the assessment of vitamin D status in the general population. Nevertheless, there is currently no consensus on adequate/optimal circulating 25(OH)D concentrations. Cut-off values range between 50 nmol/l (Hintzpeter et al., 2008), 90–100 nmol/l (Bischoff-Ferrari et al., 2006), and more than 100 nmol (Gorham et al., 2009). This inconsistency is, in part, owing to different criteria of defining inadequacy. Many researchers do not differentiate between different stages of vitamin D status. However, similar to other vitamins, it is possible to categorize the stages of vitamin D status into deficiency, insufficiency, hypovitaminosis, adequacy and intoxication (▶Tab. 10.1). Generally, in the deficiency range severe vitamin-specific clinical symptoms occur. In the insufficiency range, only vitamin-specific biochemical signs of disturbed metabolic pathways are present. In the stage of hyovitaminosis, body stores of the vitamin are already low and slight metabolic disturbances such as altered biochemical parameters could be present, although these biochemical parameters are usually still in the reference range. In the stage of adequacy no disturbances in body functions that depend on this vitamin do occur. In the toxicity range, excess actions of the vitamin can lead to severe and specific clinical symptoms. Both severe deficiency and severe intoxication can ultimately be lethal. It is noteworthy that the consequences of an insufficient vitamin D status on an individual basis might be mild, but the consequences on a population scale could be more important because of the large number of people who

Tab. 10.1: Categorization of vitamin D status classified according to circulating 25-hydroxyvitamin D concentrations.

Stage	25-hydroxyvitamin D (nmol/l)	Clinical/biochemical alterations
Deficiency	<25	Rickets, osteomalacia, myopathy, calcium malabsorption, severe hyperparathyroidism, low 1,25-dihydroxyvitamin D concentrations, impaired immune and cardiac function, death
Insufficiency	25 to 49.9	Reduced bone mineral density, impaired muscle function, low intestinal calcium absorption rates, elevated PTH levels, slightly reduced 1,25-dihydroxyvitamin D concentration
Hypovitaminosis D	50 to 75–100	Low bodily stores of vitamin D, slightly elevated PTH levels
Adequacy	100 to 375	No disturbances of vitamin D-dependent functions
Intoxication	>375	Intestinal calcium hyperabsorption, hypercalcemia, soft tissue calcification, death

PTH, parathyroid hormone.

are affected. People with long lasting vitamin D insufficiency could have the highest risk to develop vitamin D-related chronic diseases. Although sometimes otherwise stated, there is no difference between an adequate and optimal vitamin D level.

The aforementioned categorization might be helpful for scientific research on vitamin D: patients with vitamin D deficiency who participate in a clinical trial should benefit from vitamin D supplementation by an improvement in vitamin D-dependent clinical symptoms. However, if patients with vitamin D insufficiency are included, only improvements in biochemical parameters can be expected, particularly if the duration of the trial is short and the number of patients included is relatively small. No improvements can be expected if patients who are in the stage of hypovitaminosis D or vitamin D adequacy are included in a vitamin D supplementation trial. These statements seem to be trivial. However, there is currently intensive scientific research in the potential health benefits of vitamin D. Therefore, the different stages of vitamin D status and their relevance for the outcome of scientific investigations should be kept in mind. The problem is that no clear consensus with respect to vitamin D adequacy currently exists. However, despite disagreement concerning adequate/optimal circulating 25(OH)D concentrations, there is general agreement that concentrations below 50 nmol/l must be considered insufficient.

Insufficient vitamin D status is prevalent around the world. In the six regions Asia, Europe, Middle East and Africa, Latin America, North America and Oceania between 50% and more than 90% of people have 25(OH)D concentrations below 50 nmol/l (Mithal et al., 2009). Low vitamin D status is most common in South Asia and the Middle East. Insufficient vitamin D status and even vitamin D deficiency is widespread and is re-emerging as a major health problem globally. Urbanization in combination with modern and also traditional lifestyles such as indoor working, indoor leisure time activities, and traditional Islamic clothing, and in combination with the aging process (institutionalization) is an important risk factor for vitamin D insufficiency/deficiency in large parts of the adult population. In highly urbanized areas, individual daily sun exposure is usually too low to achieve a 25(OH)D level of 75 nmol/l. Diet is not able to close the gap in vitamin D supply (see below). An additional reason for inadequate vitamin D status could involve indoor exposures to UV-A passing through windows, which can break down vitamin D in the blood, whereas windows effectively block UV-B passage (Godar et al., 2009). It has also been hypothesized that vitamin D could be removed from the skin by washing (Helmer et al., 1937).

Urbanization and industrialization has long been known as a major cause of childhood rickets in western countries. Rickets is now on the increase in many developing countries, and is also re-emerging as an important health problem in countries with strong sun avoidance policies and cultures requiring modest dress.

10.1.6 Recommended daily intake, food content and actual intake

10.1.6.1 Recommended intake

▶Tab. 10.2 illustrates the recommended dietary vitamin D intake in different countries according to different age groups. It is important to realize that for infants these recommendations have the goal that dietary vitamin D intake should completely meet their vitamin D requirement. For adults, however, it is assumed that skin synthesis contributes significantly to vitamin D status. This explains, at least in part, the relatively high daily

Tab. 10.2: Recommended dietary vitamin D intakes in the USA, European Union, the Nordic countries (Denmark, Finland, Iceland, Norway, Sweden), and Germany, Austria, and Switzerland (The Scientific Committee for Food, 1993; Standing Committee on the Scientific Evaluation of Dietary Reference Intakes, 1997; Deutsche Gesellschaft für Ernährung, 2000; Holmes et al., 2009).

	Institute of Medicine, USA, 1997; adequate intake (AI)	European community's population reference intake (PRI), 1993	Nordic nutrition recommendation, 2004	D–A–CH– reference values, 2000
6–11 months	5	10–25	10	10
1–3 years	5	0–10	10 (7.5 for 2–3 year olds)	5
4–10 years	5	0–10	7.5	5
11–17 years	5	0–15	7.5	5
18–50 years	5	0–10	7.5	5
51–60 years	10	0–10	7.5	5
61–64 years	10	0–10	10	5
65–70 years	10	10	10	10
>70 years	15	10	10	10
Pregnancy, lactation	5	10	10	5

D-A-CH = Germany, Austria, Switzerland.

vitamin D recommendation for infants compared with adults (if calculated per kg body weight). In addition, the recommendations are based simply on whether the amount is enough to prevent rickets or osteomalacia. Now, we know that vitamin D relates to many other aspects of health (see below). Therefore, the recommended daily intake is not a guideline for optimizing all vitamin D dependent body functions in adults. Thus, there is an urgent need to change current recommendations for adults who live in the absence of sunlight (e.g., institutionalized people, indoor workers, veiled women). Recommendations do not differ between pregnant and non-pregnant women. However, there is evidence for an increased risk of vitamin D deficiency at late pregnancy, most probably because of altered calcium and vitamin D metabolism (Wulf Becker et al., 2004). A substantial oral vitamin D intake (50 or 100 µg daily) in pregnant women with insufficient vitamin D status is not only able to increase circulating 25-hydroxyvitamin D but also significantly increases circulating 1,25-dihydroxyvitamin D concentrations compared with an intake of only 10 µg daily (Hollis and Wagner, 2009), indicating insufficient 1,25-dihydroxyvitamin D concentrations with low dose vitamin D supplementation.

10.1.6.2 Food sources

Animal products constitute the bulk source of vitamin D that occurs naturally in unfortified foods. Fatty salt water fish such as herring, salmon, and sardines are good sources of vitamin D (►Tab. 10.3). In fish, vitamin D is mainly of dietary origin, i.e., phytoplankton

Tab. 10.3: Natural vitamin D content in selected foods (Kluthe and Kassel, 2009).

Food	Vitamin D content (µg/100 g)
Fish, salmon, fresh	16.3
Fish, tuna, canned in oil	3.0
Fish, herring, fresh	26.0
Fish, sardines, in oil	4.0
Fish, eel, smoked	22.0
Butter	1.24
Egg	2.93
Whole milk	0.17
Cheese, Gouda	1.25
Cheese, Parmesan	0.70
Liver, beef	1.0
Cod liver oil	330.0
Mushrooms, shiitake, fresh	2.0
Mushrooms, champignon, fresh	1.94
Mushrooms, morel, fresh	3.0
Fruits (apple)	0.0
Vegetables (kale, broccoli, spinach, tomato, carrots, lettuce)	0.0

and zooplankton, which inhabits the photic zone and thus is capable of photosynthesizing vitamin D_2 and/or vitamin D_3. In low-fat fish such as codfish, the majority of the vitamin D is stored in the liver. This explains the traditionally high vitamin D content of cod liver oil (▶Tab. 10.3). However, most cod liver oil capsules are nowadays standardized in vitamin D content and do not exceed an amount of 10 µg per capsule. Small quantities of vitamin D_3 are also derived from eggs, veal, beef, butter and vegetable oils whereas plants, fruits and nuts are extremely poor sources of vitamin D. Some mushrooms can contain vitamin D_2 if they are exposed to natural or artificial UVB radiation.

10.1.6.3 Food fortification

In the USA, artificial fortification of foods such as milk (both fresh and evaporated), margarine and butter, yoghurt, orange juice, breakfast cereals and chocolate mixes help in meeting the recommended dietary allowance of vitamin D. In consumer's milk, 10 µg of chemically synthesized vitamin D_3 is added per quarter gallon. The same amount is added to orange juice and infant formulas. In the USA, the milk supplementation process started in the 1940s and reduced the incidence of juvenile rickets by 85%. In most European countries food fortification policy with vitamin D is more restrictive than in the USA. For example, most European countries do not fortify consumer's milk with vitamin D. Because the problem of vitamin D deficiency is, however, well recognized, models for optimal food fortification with vitamin D have been developed (Hirvonen et al., 2007).

Tab. 10.4: Daily vitamin D intake (µg) from food only in the USA and Germany in different age groups (Calvo et al., 2004; Deutsche Gesellschaft für Ernährung e.V., 2008).

Age	United States[1]		Germany	
(years)	Males	Females	Males	Females
1–4	–	–	1.20	1.13
4–5	–	–	1.32	1.33
6–7	6.2	5.1	1.40	1.30
7–10	6.2	5.1	1.30	1.20
10–12	6.2	5.1	1.50	1.40
12–13	5.9	4.3	1.9	1.7
13–15	5.9	4.3	2.0	1.6
15–18	5.9	4.3	2.4	1.6
20–49	4.6	3.7	–	–
≥50	4.9	4.0	–	–
65–74	–	–	1.9	1.8
75–84	–	–	2.0	1.6
85–94	–	–	1.7	1.4
95	–	–	1.1	1.6

[1] Whites; – no data available from the reference.

10.1.6.4 Daily vitamin D intake

Daily vitamin D intake is illustrated in ▶Tab. 10.4 for the USA and Germany. It is obvious that vitamin D intake is higher in the USA than in Germany in all age groups. This is most probably owing to differences in fortification policy in the two countries. In Germany, median vitamin D intake is clearly below the recommend intake in all age groups (see also ▶Tab. 10.2). In the USA, particularly people above the age of 50 years have a median vitamin D intake below the recommended USA intake. Daily vitamin D intake is as low as in Germany in various parts of the world. For example, mean daily vitamin D intake is 2.5 µg in women in Lebanon, 30–50 years of age (Gannagé-Yared et al., 2000), below 1.9 µg in geriatric patients in Israel (Goldray et al., 1989), 1.9 µg in adult Tunisian women (Meddeb et al., 2005), 1 µg in Chinese girls, 12–14 years of age (Du et al., 2001) and 0.4 µg in pregnant women in Northern India (Sachan et al., 2005).

10.1.6.5 Vitamin D supplements

As an alternative to food fortification, vitamin D tablets can be used to improve vitamin D status. In the USA, over-the-counter multivitamin tablets contain 10 µg vitamin D (as vitamin D_2 or D_3). Vitamin D supplements contain 10 µg, 20 µg, 25 µg and 50 µg vitamin D_3. In Germany, only vitamin D supplements up to 25 µg vitamin D_3 are available. Higher amounts have to be prescribed. Vitamin D_2 is the only form available by prescription in the USA. In France and the UK both vitamin D forms are available, and in Germany only vitamin D_3 is available by prescription.

The commercial production of vitamin D_3 depends on the availability of either 7-dehydrocholesterol or cholesterol. 7-Dehydrocholesterol can be obtained via organic solvent extraction of animal skins (cow, pig or sheep) followed by an extensive purification. The crystalline 7-dehydrocholesterol is dissolved in an organic solvent and irradiated with ultraviolet light to carry out the transformation (similar to that which occurs in human and animal skin) to produce vitamin D_3. This vitamin D_3 is then purified and crystallized further before it is formulated for use as dietary supplement. Vitamin D_2 is produced from the yeast sterol ergosterol by ultraviolet radiation.

10.1.7 Oral vitamin D intake to attain a desired 25-hydroxyvitamin D concentration

It has been calculated that 1 µg vitamin D increases circulating 25(OH)D levels in adults by approximately 1 nmol/l (Vieth, 2009). This means that an oral intake of 5–10 µg vitamin D, as currently recommended, will increase circulating 25(OH)D by 5–10 nmol/l only. This estimation is in line with the fact that veiled ethnic Danish Moslem women with a calculated daily vitamin D intake of 13.5 µg had mean circulating 25(OH)D concentrations of 17.5 nmol/l only (Glerup et al., 2000). Unsurprisingly, a daily supplement of 10 µg vitamin D is not able to increase circulating 25(OH)D in Finnish adolescent girls during the winter. Daily supplementation with 20 µg vitamin D resulted in a 25(OH)D level which was only 14 nmol/l higher in comparison with unsupplemented girls (Lehtonen-Veromaa et al., 2002). Data are in line with dose-response studies on vitamin D performed in healthy adults (Heaney et al., 2003). Consequently, 50 µg vitamin D daily are necessary to increase circulating 25(OH)D concentrations from 25 to 75 nmol/l on average. However, to maintain a serum level above 75 nmol/l in almost all subjects of a group that has mean initial 25(OH)D levels of 30 nmol, a daily intake of approximately 100–125 µg vitamin D is necessary. If the mean initial circulating 25(OH)D concentration is higher (e.g., 50 nmol/l), a daily vitamin D intake of 75 µg is still necessary to maintain a serum level above 75 nmol/l in almost all subjects (Aloia et al., 2008). Some variation in the increment in circulating 25(OH)D on a given dose can be explained by individual differences in body weight. After whole-body UVB irradiation the incremental increase in vitamin D_3 is 57% lower in obese than in nonobese subjects (Wortsman et al., 2000). Obesity-associated vitamin D insufficiency is probably owing to the decreased bioavailability of vitamin D_3 from cutaneous and dietary sources because of its deposition in body fat compartments. The content of the vitamin D_3 precursor 7-dehydrocholesterol in the skin of obese and nonobese subjects is not significantly different between groups nor is its conversion to previtamin D_3 after irradiation in vitro. The deposition of vitamin D in body fat compartments is one explanation why obese individuals often have lower circulating 25(OH)D concentrations than nonobese individuals (Wortsman et al., 2000; Arunabh et al., 2003). Taking differences in body weight into account, the increment in circulating 25(OH)D after administration of oral vitamin D is very similar in infants, children and adults. Per kg body weight, the respective vitamin D dose for increasing circulating 25(OH)D by 50 nmol/l is 0.5–1.0 µg in adults (Heaney et al., 2003; Schleithoff et al., 2006; Zittermann et al., 2009a), 0.67 µg in children (Zittermann, 2003a) and 1 µg in infants (Wagner et al., 2010).

Compared with oral vitamin D, the potency of oral 25(OH)D in enhancing circulating 25(OH)D is much higher. Per µg dose, oral 25(OH)D increases circulating 25(OH)D by 4 nmol/l on average (Vieth, 2005). Thus the increase in circulating 25(OH)D per µg dose is four time higher for 25(OH)D administration than for vitamin D_3 administration (1 nmol/l). Consequently, only 25% of vitamin D molecules ever become 25(OH)D. At least three-quarters of the molecule of vitamin D that enter the body are removed by some fate. However, in case of low doses of orally administered vitamin D, e.g., 10 µg per day, the increase per µg dose in circulating 25(OH)D can obviously vary between 1 and 4 nmol/l (Aloia et al., 2008), indicating that some people can convert almost all vitamin D into 25(OH)D if necessary.

10.1.8 Vitamin D intoxication

Vitamin D intoxication is associated with hyperabsorption of calcium and phosphorus (Zittermann and Koerfer, 2008). Manifestations of vitamin D toxicity include hypercalcemia, hypercalciuria, ectopic soft tissue calcification, including vascular calcification and nephrocalcinosis and renal failure. The vitamin D and nicotine model is used as a model of arterial calcification. Supra-physiological vitamin D doses (7.5 mg/kg) plus nicotine can rapidly produce calcium and phosphate overload in the young rat. Such treatment produces a lasting 10–40-fold increase in the aortic calcium content, the major site of calcium deposition being on the medial elastic fibers near the lumen. Moreover, aortic phosphate content increases 80–175-fold.

In otherwise healthy humans, however, the risk of vitamin D intoxication is extremely rare (Zittermann, 2003b). Vitamin D intoxications such as hypercalcemia do not occur until oral vitamin D intake and serum 25(OH)D concentrations exceed 250 µg/day (approx. 3–5 µg/kg body weight) and 500 nmol/l, respectively (Zittermann and Koerfer, 2008). Cases of vitamin D intoxication have been observed after the administration of very high therapeutic vitamin D_3 doses, in association with an over-the-counter supplement that contained 26–430 times the vitamin D_3 amount listed by the manufacturer, and in association with an accidentally excessive overfortification of consumers' milk with vitamin D_3. During earlier decades, intermittent high-dose vitamin D (6–15 mg vitamin D_2 several times within the first 18 months of life) has been administered to prevent rickets in central European countries such as the former German Democratic Republic. This amount was equivalent to approximately 25–50 µg vitamin D_2/kg body weight per day. The safety of this regimen has been questioned. Indeed, this strategy resulted in serum 25(OH)D concentrations >500 nmol/l, hypercalcemia and hyperphosphatemia in several cases. It has been suggested that this strategy was responsible for vascular calcification in children (Zittermann and Koerfer, 2008). In British infants, vitamin D intoxication has been described during the late 1940s and early 1950s after heavy enrichment of dried milk powder together with vitamin D-enriched cereals and in addition to the recommendation of a daily vitamin D supplement of 17.5–20.0 µg (Zittermann, 2003b).

There are no reports of vitamin D intoxication in healthy adults after intensive sunlight exposure. Vitamin D in the skin reaches a plateau after only 15–30 min of UVB exposure. Then, vitamin D-inactive substances such as lumisterol and tachysterol are produced, which do not reach the systemic circulation. There are also no reports in the literature about vitamin D intoxication with traditionally consumed foods (Zittermann, 2003b).

References

Aloia JF, Patel M, Dimaano R, Li-Ng M, Talwar SA, Mikhail M, Pollack S, Yeh JK, Vitamin D intake to attain a desired serum 25-hydroxyvitamin D concentration. Am J Clin Nutr 2008;87: 1952–8.

Antoniucci DM, Yamashita T, Portaloe AA, Dietary phosphorus regulates serum fibroblast growth factor-23 concentrations in healthy men. J Clin Endocrinol Metab 2006;91: 3144–9.

Armas LA, Hollis BW, Heaney RP, Vitamin D2 is much less effective than vitamin D3 in humans. J Clin Endocrinol Metab 2004;89: 5387–91.

Arunabh S, Pollack S, Yeh J, Aloia JF, Body fat content and 25-hydroxyvitamin D levels in healthy women. J Clin Endocrinol Metab 2003;88: 157–61.

Bischoff-Ferrari HA, Giovannucci E, Willett WC, Dietrich T, Dawson-Hughes B, Estimation of optimal serum concentrations of 25-hydroxyvitamin D for multiple health outcomes. Am J Clin Nutr 2006;84: 18–28.

Björkman MP, Sorva AJ, Risteli J, Tilvis RS, Low parathyroid hormone levels in bedridden geriatric patients with vitamin D deficiency. J Am Geriatr Soc 2009;57: 1045–50.

Bouillon R, Carmeliet G, Daci E, Segaert S, Verstuyf A, Vitamin D metabolism and action, Osteoporos Int 1998;8: S13–9.

Calvo MS, Whiting SJ, Barton CN, Vitamin D fortification in the United States and Canada: current status and data needs. Am J Clin Nutr 2004;80(6Suppl): 1710S–6S.

Clemens TL, Adams JS, Henderson SL, Holick MF, Increased skin pigment reduces the capacity of skin to synthesise vitamin D3. Lancet 1982;8263: 74–6.

Deutsche Gesellschaft für Ernährung e.V., Ernährungsbericht 2008. Meckenheim: Druck Center Meckenheim GmbH; 2008.

Deutsche Gesellschaft für Ernährung, Österreichische Gesellschaft für Ernährung, Schweizerische Gesellschaft für Ernährungsforschung & Schweizerische Vereinigung für Ernährung (2000) Referenzwerte für die Nährstoffzufuhr. Frankfurt/M, Germany: Umschau Verlag; 2000.

Du X, Greenfield H, Fraser DR, Ge K, Trube A, Wang Y, Vitamin D deficiency and associated factors in adolescent girls in Beijing. Am J Clin Nutr 2001;74: 494–500.

Gannagé-Yared MH, Chemali R, Yaacoub N, Halaby G, Hypovitaminosis D in a sunny country: relation to lifestyle and bone markers. J Bone Miner Res 2000;15: 1856–62.

Gascon-Barre M, The vitamin D 25-hydroxylase. In: Feldman D, Pike JW, Glorieux FH, editors. Vitamin D. 2nd ed. Amsterdam: Elsevier Academic Press, 2005. pp. 47–67.

Glerup H, Mikkelsen K, Poulsen L, Hass E, Overbeck S, Thomsen J, Charles P, Eriksen EF, Commonly recommended daily intake of vitamin D is not sufficient if sunlight exposure is limited. J Intern Med 2000;247: 260–8.

Godar DE, Landry RJ, Lucas AD, Increased UVA exposures and decreased cutaneous Vitamin D(3) levels may be responsible for the increasing incidence of melanoma. Med Hypotheses 2009;72: 434–43.

Goldray D, Mizrahi-Sasson E, Merdler C, Edelstein-Singer M, Algoetti A, Eisenberg Z, Jaccard N, Weisman Y, Vitamin D deficiency in elderly patients in a general hospital. J Am Geriatr Soc 1989;37: 589–92.

Gorham ED, Mohr SB, Garland FC, Garland CF, Vitamin D for cancer prevention and survival. Clin Rev Bone Miner Metab 2009;7: 159–75.

Hagström E, Hellman P, Larsson TE, Ingelsson E, Berglund L, Sundström J, Melhus H, Held C, Lind L, Michaëlsson M, Ärnlöv J, Plasma parathyroid hormone and the risk of cardiovascular mortality in the community. Circulation 2009;119: 2765–71.

Heaney RP, Davies KM, Chen TC, Holick MF, Barger-Lux MJ, Human serum 25-hydroxycholecalciferol response to extended oral dosing with cholecalciferol. Am J Clin Nutr 2003;77: 204–10.

Helmer AC, Jansen CH, Vitamin D precursors removed from human skin by washing. Stud Institut Divi Thomae 1937;1: 207–16.

Hintzpeter B, Mensink GB, Thierfelder W, Müller MJ, Scheidt-Nave C, Vitamin D status and health correlates among German adults. Eur J Clin Nutr 2008;62: 1079–89.

Hirvonen T, Sinkho H, Valsta L, Hannila ML, Pietinen P, Development of a model for optimal food fortification: vitamin D among adults in Finland. Eur J Nutr 2007;46: 264–70.

History of vitamin D. http://vitamind.ucr.edu/history.html, accessed 01/24/2010.

Holick MF, Vitamin D deficiency. N Engl J Med 2007;357: 266–81.

Holick MF, Biancuzzo RM, Chen TC, Klein EK, Young A, Bibuld D, Reitz R, Salameh W, Ameri A, Tannenbaum AD, Vitamin D2 is as effective as vitamin D3 in maintaining circulating concentrations of 25-hydroxyvitamin D. J Clin Endocrinol Metab 2008;93: 677–81.

Hollis BW, Wagner CL, Randomized controlled trials to determine the safety of vitamin D supplementation during pregnancy and lactation. Fourteenth Workshop on Vitamin D, Brugge, Belgium, October 4–8, 2009, Abstracts volume. 2009; p. 134.

Holmes VA, Barnes MS, Alexander HD, McFaul P, Wallace JM, Vitamin D deficiency and insufficiency in pregnant women: a longitudinal study. Br J Nutr 2009;102: 876–81.

Horst RL, Reinhardt TA, Reddy GS, Vitamin D metabolism. In: Feldman D, Pike JW, Glorieux FH, editors. Vitamin D. 2nd ed. Amsterdam: Elsevier Academic Press, 2005. pp. 15–36.

Huh SY, Gordon CM, Vitamin D deficiency in children and adolescents: epidemiology, impact and treatment. Rev Endocr Metab Disord 2008;9: 161–70.

Kluthe B, Kassel P, Prodi 5.6.0.2 (Nbase 2.50). Stuttgart, Germany: Wissenschaftliche Verlagsgesellschaft mbH; 2009.

Konradsen S, Ag H, Lindberg F, Hexeberg S, Jorde R, Serum 1,25-dihydroxy vitamin D is inversely associated with body mass index. Eur J Nutr 2008;47: 87–91.

Krause R, Bohring M, Hopfenmhller W, Holick MF, Sharma AM, Ultraviolet B and blood pressure. Lancet 1998;352: 709–10.

Lehtonen-Veromaa M, Mottonen T, Nuotio I, Irjala K, Viikari J, The effect of conventional vitamin D(2) supplementation on serum 25(OH)D concentration is weak among peripubertal Finnish girls: a 3-year prospective study. Eur J Clin Nutr 2002;56: 431–7.

Liu PT, Stenger S, Li H, Wenzel L, Tan BH, Krutzik SR, Ochoa MT, Schauber J, Wu K, Meinken C, Kamen DL, Wagner M, Bals R, Steinmeyer A, Zügel U, Gallo RL, Eisenberg D, Hewison M, Hollis BW, Adams JS, Bloom BR, Modlin RL, Toll-like receptor triggering of a vitamin D mediated human antimicrobial response. Science 2006;311: 1770–3.

Meddeb N, Sahli H, Chahed M, Abdelmoula J, Feki M, Salah H, Frini S, Kaabachi N, Belkahia Ch, Mbazaa R, Zouari B, Sellami S, Vitamin D deficiency in Tunisia. Osteoporos Int 2005;16: 180–3.

Mithal A, Wahl DA, Bonjour JP, Burckhardt P, Dawson-Hughes B, Eisman JA, El-Hajj Fuleihan G, Josse RG, Lips P, Morales-Torres J; IOF Committee of Scientific Advisors (CSA) Nutrition Working Group, Global vitamin D status and determinants of hypovitaminosis D. Osteoporos Int 2009;20: 1807–20.

Nemere I, Farach-Carson MC, Membrane receptors for steroid hormones: a case for specific cell surface binding sites for vitamin D metabolites and estrogens. Biochem Biophys Res Commun 1998;248: 442–9.

Nesby-O'Dell S, Scanlon KS, Cogswell ME, Gillespie C, Hollis BW, Looker AC, Allen C, Doughertly C, Gunter EW, Bowman BA, Hypovitaminosis D prevalence and determinants among African American and white women of reproductive age: third National Health and Nutrition Examination Survey, 1988–1994. Am J Clin Nutr 2002;76: 187–92.

Norman AW, Receptors for 1a25(OH)2D3: past, present, and future. J Bone Miner Res 1998;13: 1360–9.

Norval M, Björn LO, de Gruijl FR, Is the action spectrum for the UV-induced production of previtamin D3 in human skin correct? Photochem Photobiol Sci 2010;9: 11–7.

Passeri G, Pini G, Troiano L, Vescovini R, Sansoni P, Passeri M, Gueresi P, Delsignore R, Pedrazzoni M, Franceschi C, Low vitamin D status, high bone turnover, and bone fractures in centenarians. J Clin Endocrinol Metab 2003;88: 5109–15.

Pietras SM, Obayan BK, Cai MH, Holick MF, Vitamin D2 treatment for vitamin D deficiency and insufficiency for up to 6 years. Arch Intern Med 2009;169: 1806–8.

Rajakumar K, Vitamin D, cod-liver oil, sunlight, and rickets: a historical perspective. Pediatrics 2003;112: e112–35.

Rao DS, Raghuramulu N, Is vitamin D redundant in an aquatic habitat? J Nutr Sci Vitaminol 1999;45: 1–8.

Sachan A, Gupta R, Das V, Agarwal A, Awasthi PK, Bhatia V, High prevalence of vitamin D deficiency among pregnant women and their newborns in northern India. Am J Clin Nutr 2005;81: 1060–4.

Schauber J, Dorschner RA, Coda AB, Büchau AS, Liu PT, Kiken D, Helfrich YR, Kang S, Elalieh HZ, Steinmeyer A, Zügel U, Bikle DD, Modlin RL, Gallo RL, Injury enhances TLR2 function and antimicrobial peptide expression through a vitamin D-dependent mechanism. J Clin Invest 2007;117: 803–11.

Schleithoff SS, Zittermann A, Tenderich G, Berthold HK, Stehle P, Koerfer R, Vitamin D supplementation improves cytokine profiles in patients with congestive heart failure: a double-blind, randomized, placebo-controlled trial. Am J Clin Nutr 2006;83: 754–9.

Schleithoff SS, Zittermann A, Tenderich G, Berthold HK, Stehle P, Koerfer R, Combined calcium and vitamin D supplementation is not superior to calcium supplementation alone in improving disturbed bone metabolism in patients with congestive heart failure. Eur J Clin Nutr 2007;62: 1388–94.

Stamp TC, Haddad JG, Twigg CA, Comparison of oral 25-hydroxycholecalciferol, vitamin D, and ultraviolet light as determinants of circulating 25-hydroxyvitamin D. Lancet 1977;8026: 1341–3.

Standing Committee on the Scientific Evaluation of Dietary Reference Intakes, Food and Nutrition Board and Institute of Medicine, Dietary reference intakes for calcium, phosphorus, magnesium, vitamin D and fluoride, Washington, DC: National Academy of Sciences; 1997. pp. 250–87.

Steingrimsdottir L, Gunnarsson O, Indridason OS, Franzson L, Sigurdsson G, Relationship between serum parathyroid hormone levels, vitamin D sufficiency, and calcium intake. J Am Med Assoc 2005;294: 2336–41.

Stubbs JR, Liu S, Tang W, Zhou J, Wang Y, Yao X, Quarles LD, Role of hyperphosphatemia and 1,25-dihydroxyvitamin D in vascular calcification and mortality in fibroblastic growth factor 23 null mice. J Am Soc Nephrol 2007;18: 2116–24.

The Scientific Committee for Food, Nutrient and energy intakes for the European Community (Opinion expressed on 11 December 1992). Reports of the Scientific Committee for Food, 31st series. Luxembourg: Office for Official Publications of the European Communities, 1993. pp. 1–248.

Thomas MK, Lloyd-Jones DM, Thadhani RI, Shaw AC, Deraska DJ, Kitch BT, Vamvakas EC, Dick IM, Prince RL, Finkelstein JS, Hypovitaminosis D in medical inpatients. N Engl J Med 1998;338: 777–83.

Trang HM, Cole DE, Rubin LA, Pierratos A, Siu S, Vieth R, Evidence that vitamin D3 increases serum 25-hydroxyvitamin D more efficiently than does vitamin D2. Am J Clin Nutr 1998;68: 854–8.

Tuohimaa P, Vitamin D and aging. J Steroid Biochem Mol Biol 2009;114: 78–84.

Vieth R, The pharmacology of vitamin D, including fortification strategies. In: Feldman D, Pike JW, Glorieux FH. Vitamin D. 2nd ed. Amsterdam: Elsevier Academic Press, 2005. pp. 995–1015.

Vieth R, Vitamin D and cancer mini-symposium: the risk of additional vitamin D. Ann Epidemiol 2009;19: 441–5.

Wagner CL, Howard C, Hulsey TC, Lawrence RA, Taylor SN, Will H, Ebeling M, Hutson J, Hollis BW, Circulating 25-hydroxyvitamin D levels in fully breastfed infants on oral vitamin D supplementation. Int J Endocrinol 2010;2010: 235035.

Wjst M, Is the increase in allergic asthma associated with an inborn Th1 maturation or with an environmental Th1 trigger defect? Allergy 2004;59: 148–50.

Wolf G, The discovery of vitamin D: the contribution of Adolf Windaus. J Nutr 2004;139: 1299–304.

Wortsman J, Matsuoka LY, Chen TC, Lu Z, Holick MF, Decreased bioavailability of vitamin D in obesity. Am J Clin Nutr 2000;72: 690–3.

Wulf Becker W, Lyhne N, Pedersen A, et al., Nordic Nutrition Recommendations 2004 – integrating nutrition and physical activity. Scand J Nutr 2004;48: 178–87.

Zittermann A, Serum 25-hydroxyvitamin D response to oral vitamin D intake in children. Am J Clin Nutr 2003a;78: 496–7.

Zittermann A, Vitamin D in preventive medicine – are we ignoring the evidence? Br J Nutr 2003b;89: 552–72.

Zittermann A, Vitamin D and disease prevention with special reference to cardiovascular disease. Prog Biophys Mol Biol 2006;92: 39–48.

Zittermann A, Koerfer R, Protective and toxic effects of vitamin D on vascular calcification: clinical implications. Mol Aspects Med 2008;29: 423–32.

Zittermann A, Heer M, Caillot-Augusso A, Rettberg P, Scheld K, Drummer C, Alexandre C, Horneck G, Vorobiev D, Stehle P, Microgravity inhibits intestinal calcium absorption as shown by a stable strontium test. Eur J Clin Invest 2000;30: 1036–43.

Zittermann A, Schleithoff SS, Gotting C, Dronow O, Fuchs U, Kuhn J, Kleesiek K, Tenderich G, Koerfer R, Poor outcome in end-stage heart failure patients with low circulating calcitriol levels. Eur J Heart Fail 2008;10: 321–7.

Zittermann A, Frisch S, Berthold HK, Götting C, Kuhn J, Kleesiek K, Stehle P, Koertke H, Koerfer R, Vitamin D supplementation enhances the beneficial effects of weight loss on cardiovascular disease risk markers. Am J Clin Nutr 2009a;89: 1321–7.

Zittermann A, Schleithoff SS, Götting C, Fuchs U, Kuhn J, Wlost S, Kleesiek K, Tenderich G, Koerfer R, Calcitriol deficiency and 1-year mortality in cardiac transplant recipients. Transplantation 2009b;87: 118–24.

10.2 Potential health effects of vitamin D

A. Zittermann

10.2.1 Introduction

Vitamin D is a steroid hormone that plays a pivotal role in regulating cellular metabolism: The vitamin D receptor is ubiquitously distributed in the human body. In addition, several tissues possess the ability to produce the active hormonal form of vitamin D, calcitriol, by themselves. Therefore, low availability of vitamin D could have profound consequences for cellular and overall health. The association of vitamin D with health outcomes can be investigated by the use of epidemiological and intervention studies in humans. Furthermore, experimental studies can give insights in vitamin D actions. During recent years, vitamin D receptor knockout (VDR) mice have been generated to study the metabolic and pathophysiological consequences of absent vitamin D actions in more detail (Bouillon et al., 2008). Because these mice usually develop severe hyperparathyroidism, hypocalcemia and osteomalacia, a rescue diet high in calcium has to be provided to guarantee survival. The VDR knockout mice and vitamin D-deficient mice show increased sensitivity to autoimmune diseases such as inflammatory bowel disease or type 1 diabetes after exposure to predisposing factors. VDR-deficient mice do not have a spontaneous increase in cancer, but are more prone to oncogene- or chemocarcinogen-induced tumors. They also develop high renin hypertension, cardiac hypertrophy and increased thrombogenicity (Bouillon et al., 2008), muscular and motor impairments (Burne et al., 2005), myopathy (Endo et al., 2003), impaired immune function (O'Kelly et al., 2002), and impaired insulin secretion (Zeitz et al., 2003). Additionally, they show increased anxiety (Kalueff et al., 2004), have ectopic calcification and a short life span (Tuohimaa, 2009). ▶Fig. 10.4 illustrates various

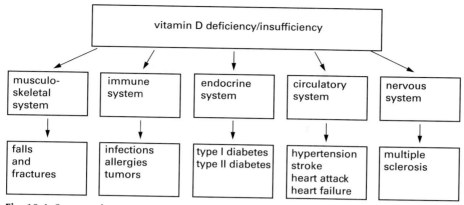

Fig. 10.4: Suggested association of vitamin D deficiency/insufficiency with chronic diseases.

metabolic impairments and subsequent diseases in humans that might result from vitamin D deficiency/insufficiency. Whether or not vitamin D deficiency/insufficiency in humans is associated with increased prevalence of diseases, as predicted by the VDR null phenotype, is outlined below. The association of vitamin D with bone health and cardiovascular health is summarized elsewhere in this book.

10.2.2 Vitamin D und muscle strengthening

Vitamin D deficiency causes reduced actomyosin content of myofibrils, low calcium content of mitochondria, reduced calcium uptake into the sarcoplasmic reticulum and low serum levels of muscle enzymes (Zittermann, 2003). Because skeletal muscles have a VDR, they might require vitamin D for maximum function. In line with this assumption, myopathy is a well known clinical symptom of severe vitamin D deficiency, e.g., osteomalacia. This disorder is not only characterized by bone-thinning, but also by proximal muscle weakness. The effects of osteomalacia are thought to contribute to chronic musculoskeletal pain. Performance speed and proximal muscle strength were markedly improved when circulating 25(OH)D concentrations increased from 10 to 40 nmol/l and continued to improve as the concentration increased to more than 100 nmol/l (Holick, 2007). The importance of vitamin D-repletion for adequate muscle function was underscored in a study on institutionalized people ≥60 years of age with insufficient vitamin D status (Moreira-Pfrimer et al., 2009). This randomized controlled trial (RCT) demonstrated that 6-month supplementation (December to May) of oral vitamin D (3750 μg once a month during the first 2 months, followed by 2250 μg once a month for the last 4 months) was able to improve lower limb muscle strength by 16–24%. Data support results of a meta-analysis of RCTs, demonstrating that daily doses of 17.5–20 μg supplemental vitamin D can prevent falls in elderly adults (Bischoff-Ferrari et al., 2009). The relative risk of falls was reduced by approximately 20% if the achieved serum 25(OH)D concentration is 60 nmol/l or more. In contrast to 'high dose' supplemental vitamin D, low dose daily supplemental vitamin D (5–15 μg) can not prevent falls (Bischoff-Ferrari et al., 2009). Thus, doses of supplemental vitamin D of less than 17.5 μg or serum 25-hydroxyvitamin D concentrations of less than 60 nmol/l might not reduce the risk of falling among older individuals. It is noteworthy that in elderly people the risk of falling predicts the risk of developing osteoporotic fractures. Therefore, the effects of vitamin D on muscle strength could contribute to the preventive effect of vitamin D on osteoporotic fractures. There is also evidence that adequate vitamin D supply is important for muscle function in children. Already more than 50 years ago, Ronge (1952) has demonstrated that children who have hands and face exposed to UVB radiation in their classroom at school for 3–5 h during wintertime show better endurance performance compared with a control group without UVB exposure. Endurance performance was assessed by bicycle ergometry. In that study, a similar positive effect on endurance performance was seen in children who received a single vitamin D bolus of 6.25 mg vitamin D in February.

10.2.3 Infections

There is mounting evidence for a pivotal role of vitamin D in the immune system. The immune system consists of the innate and the adaptive immune system (►Fig. 10.5). Calcitriol is able to induce the differentiation of monocytes into macrophages. In addition, calcitriol increases the activity of macrophages and facilitates their cytotoxic activity. Macrophages represent the first unspecific defense line of the immune system. It is well known that the prevalence of infections such as pneumonia is high in infants with rickets (Zittermann, 2003). The use of vitamin D (or cod liver oil) as a treatment for infections have been practiced for over 150 years. As early as 1903, Niels Finsen was awarded the Nobel Prize for Medicine and Physiology for his theory to cure lupus vulgaris (skin-tuberculosis) using phototherapy. In 2007, Schauber et al. (2007) published data demonstrating that vitamin D is able to stimulate synthesis of the antimicrobial peptide cathelicidin in human skin cells to enhance innate immunity. A meta-analysis of observational studies has demonstrated that patients with tuberculosis have lower circulating 25(OH)D concentrations compared with healthy controls (Nnoaham and Clarke, 2008). Ecological studies also support a preventive role of vitamin D in influenza: the seasonal and latitudinal distribution of outbreaks of influenza A in the world in 1967–1975, and weekly consultation rates for illnesses diagnosed clinically as

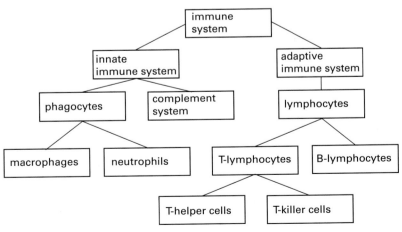

Fig. 10.5: Scheme of the human immune system.

influenza or influenza-like in England 1968–1970 were inversely associated with solar UVB radiation (Cannell et al., 2006). Supplementation with 30 μg vitamin D daily reduces the risk of wintertime influenza A in Japanese nursery-school children (Urashima et al., 2010). This amount was equivalent to 0.86 μg vitamin D/kg body weight per day. It is noteworthy that vitamin D is able to improve the activity of natural killer (NK) cells. These cells defend the body against viruses and other pathogens. Some viruses can suppress major histocompatibility complex (MHC) class I molecules on the surface of their host cell, thereby avoiding destruction by T lymphocytes. However, the loss of the MHC renders these cells vulnerable to NK cell-mediated apoptosis.

Some epidemiological data suggest that vitamin D could reduce the susceptibility to respiratory tract infections (Laaksi et al., 2007; Ginde et al., 2009). In line with these epidemiological results, vitamin D users of the RECORD trial (Avenell et al., 2007), an RCT with approximately 3500 participants who received 20 μg vitamin D or placebo, reported a lower tendency for infections and antibiotic use in March compared with vitamin D nonusers. In another RCT, compared with placebo, supplementation with 20 μg or 50 μg vitamin D daily for 3 years significantly reduced upper respiratory tract infections in individuals with baseline circulating concentrations below 50 nmol/l (Aloia et al., 2005). By contrast, a daily vitamin D supplement of 50 μg for 12 weeks did not prevent upper respiratory tract infections in individuals with baseline circulating 25(OH)D concentrations above 50 nmol/l (Li-Ng et al., 2009). Consequently, present data from RCTs do not consistently demonstrate that vitamin D supplementation can lower infections (Yamshchikov et al., 2009). One factor that has to be considered is baseline 25(OH)D concentration. Vitamin D is probably ineffective if baseline 25(OH)D concentrations lie already above the insufficiency range, e.g., >50 nmol/l. In addition, the relation between vitamin D supplementation, local calcitriol, local cathelicidin production and NK cell activity has to be investigated more detailed. Interestingly, oral intake of activated vitamin D in rickets patients for 4 weeks significantly increased human cathelicidin expression in neutrophils compared with age-matched healthy controls without administration of activated vitamin D (Misawa et al., 2009), indicating a crucial role of adequate calcitriol availability for regulation of the innate immune response.

10.2.4 Allergies

Allergic reactions represent a response of the adaptive immune system against generally harmless xenobiotics, mostly proteins. Activation of the adaptive immune system is complex. Generally, it is of importance that specific pathways of the specific immune system are adequately suppressed to avoid autoimmune diseases or allergic reactions. Regulatory T cells are crucial for the maintenance of immunological tolerance. Their major role is to shut down T cell-mediated immunity toward the end of an immune reaction and to suppress auto-reactive T cells. A strong T-helper (Th)2 predominance leads to pathologic conditions such as overproduction of IgE and allergic diseases, whereas a strong Th1 predominance leads to autoimmunity and severe allograft rejection. Of clinical importance is the fact that dendritic cells (DCs) might induce naïve T cells in an immunogenetic direction but also in a tolerogenic direction, depending on the state of their maturation and their cell surface receptor. Tolerogenic DCs generally are semimature. There is accumulating evidence that vitamin D modulates the adaptive immune system (Zittermann et al., 2009). Calcitriol appears to generate tolerogenic DCs *in vivo*, as demonstrated in models of transplantation and autoimmune disease. DCs appear to be key targets of calcitriol. Calcitriol arrests the differentiation and maturation of DCs, maintaining them in an immature state. Calcitriol can enhance the secretion by DCs of the anti-inflammatory and anti-allergic cytokine IL-10.

At present, the vitamin D hypothesis of allergies takes two forms: some argue that vitamin D deficiency could cause allergic reactions whereas others argue that vitamin D excess leads to an increased allergy risk. Wjst is a representative of the latter hypothesis. He argues that the increase in allergies in Bavaria after 1960 coincided with vitamin D supplementation intervention programs to prevent rickets in childhood. Moreover, both adherence to these programs and prevalence of allergies in children seem to be lower in farming communities in Bavaria (Wjst, 2005). The farm protection is observed mainly during the first year of life (Von Mutius, 2004), when vitamin D supplementation is also recommended. Wjst's hypothesis is based on the assumption that vitamin D could lead to Th2 predominance and increased IgE production. Generally, his hypothesis is supported by findings that maternal 25(OH)D in late pregnancy was inversely associated with asthma in their 9-year-old offspring (Gale et al., 2008), vitamin D supplementation during infancy was associated with a higher allergy risk (Hyppönen et al., 2004; Bäck et al., 2009), and the prevalence of allergic rhinitis increased across quartile groups of 25(OH)D serum levels in adults of NHANES III (Wjst and Hyppönen, 2007).

It is, however, noteworthy that several other epidemiological studies support the vitamin D deficiency hypothesis of allergic reactions (Zittermann et al., 2004; Camargo et al., 2007a,b; Oren et al., 2008; Erkkola et al., 2009). In addition, administration of calcitriol to blood cells of healthy persons and steroid-resistant asthmatic patients enhanced subsequent responsiveness to dexamethasone for induction of IL-10 (Oren et al., 2008). Very few intervention trials are available so far. In a small, randomized, double-blind, placebo-controlled trial, vitamin D_2 supplementation (25 µg/day) significantly improved skin symptoms in children with winter-related atopic dermatitis (Sidbury et al., 2008). In a study in heart failure patients, vitamin D_3 supplementation (50 µg/day) was able to increase blood levels of the anti-allergic cytokine IL-10 (Schleithoff et al., 2006). However, the effect on allergic reactions has not been elucidated in that earlier investigation.

In total, it cannot be ruled out that vitamin D deficiency as well as vitamin D excess might increase the risk of allergic reactions. This assumption is supported by recent findings. Hyppönen et al. (2009) observed a biphasic effect of vitamin D with both low and high 25(OH)D levels associated with elevated IgE concentrations in participants of the 1958 British birth cohort. Compared with the reference group with the lowest IgE concentrations [25(OH)D 100–125 nmol/l], adjusted IgE concentrations were 29% higher for participants with the 25(OH)D <25 nmol/l, and 56% higher for participants with 25(OH)D >135 nmol/l.

10.2.5 Cancer

Because vitamin D is a key regulator of various cellular metabolic pathways, it is important for cellular maturation, differentiation, and apoptosis (Zittermann, 2003). In the USA, colon cancer mortality shows a north-south gradient with highest mortality rates in the northeast (▶Fig. 10.6). In 2008, the WHO published a report from the International Agency for Research on Cancer (WHO/IARC, 2008) that came to the conclusion that

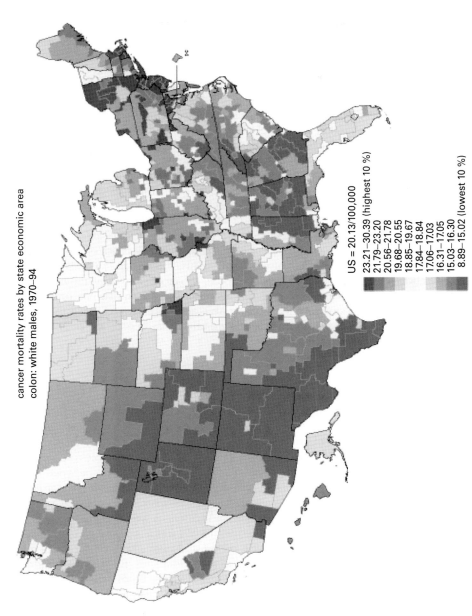

cancer mortality rates by state economic area
colon: white males, 1970–94

US = 20.13/100,000

23.21–30.39 (highest 10 %)
21.79–23.20
20.56–21.78
19.68–20.55
18.85–19.67
17.84–18.84
17.06–17.03
16.31–17.05
15.03–16.30
8.89–15.02 (lowest 10 %)

Fig. 10.6: Colon cancer mortality rates in white US males according to geographic latitude (available at www.sunarc.org).

there is: (i) consistent epidemiological evidence for an inverse association between 25(OH)D and colorectal cancer and colorectal adenomas; (ii) suggested epidemiological evidence for an inverse association between 25(OH)D and breast cancer; (iii) insufficient evidence for an inverse association between 25(OH)D and other types of cancer; and (iv) the need for new randomized controlled trials. One such RCT has already been published (Lappe et al., 2007). In a 4-year, population-based study, where the primary outcome was fracture incidence, and the principal secondary outcome was cancer incidence, 1179 community-dwelling women were randomly assigned to receive 1500 mg supplemental calcium/day alone (Ca-only), supplemental calcium plus 27.5 μg vitamin D/day (Ca+D), or placebo. Cancer incidence was 60–77% lower in the Ca+D women and 43% lower in the Ca-only group than in the control subjects ($p < 0.03$). Gorham et al. (2009) have estimated that in North America, Europe and East Asia approximately 32% of colon cancer and approximately 26% of breast cancer can be prevented with 50 μg vitamin D daily and 3–10 min daily of noon sunlight seasonality, when weather permits. Garland et al. (2009) estimated that raising the minimum year-around serum 25(OH)D level to 100–150 nmol/l would prevent approximately 58 000 new cases of breast cancer and 49 000 new cases of colorectal cancer each year, and three-fourths of deaths from these diseases in the USA and Canada. Such intakes also are expected to reduce case-fatality rates of patients who have breast, colorectal or prostate cancer by half. Nevertheless, there is also some concern that cancer risk is not only enhanced in individuals with deficient/insufficient vitamin D status, but also if 25(OH)D concentrations rise above 80 nmol/l (Tuohimaa et al., 2004), a concentration several vitamin D researchers consider adequate. However, this increase in cancer risk has only been observed in observational studies after multivariable adjustments have been made for confounding factors. This type of exploratory data analysis has been criticized by some researchers (Zittermann and Grant, 2009).

10.2.6 Diabetes mellitus

In vitro and *in vivo* studies suggest that vitamin D can prevent pancreatic beta-cell destruction and reduces the incidence of autoimmune diabetes. This could at least in part be owing to a suppression of proinflammatory cytokines such as tumor necrosis factor (TNF)-α. The immunomodulatory effects of vitamin D suggest a plausible role in autoimmune diseases, such as type 1 diabetes mellitus. Recently, the relation between UVB irradiance, the primary source of circulating vitamin D in humans, and age-standardized incidences of type 1 diabetes mellitus in children aged <14 years, was analyzed according to 51 regions of the world (Mohr et al., 2008). Incidences were generally higher at higher latitudes and were inversely associated with UVB irradiance. As early as 2001, Hyppönen et al. (2001) demonstrated in a birth cohort study that vitamin D supplementation was associated with a decreased frequency of type 1 diabetes. By contrast, children suspected of having rickets during the first year of life had a three times higher relative risk compared with those without such a suspicion. Meanwhile, a meta-analysis of four case-control studies has shown that the risk of type 1 diabetes is reduced by 29% in infants who are supplemented with vitamin D compared with those who are not supplemented (Zipitis and Akobeng, 2008). There is also some evidence of a dose-response effect, with those using higher amounts of vitamin D being at lower risk of developing type 1 diabetes. Finally, timing of supplementation might also be important for the subsequent development of type 1 diabetes. In a Chinese RCT (Li et al., 2009), the majority of adults with latent autoimmune diabetes increased their fasting state concentrations of plasma C-peptide levels after 1 year of treatment with activated vitamin D, whereas only a minority of patients treated with insulin alone maintained stable fasting C-peptide levels.

The pathogenesis of type 2 diabetes mellitus involves both beta-cell dysfunction and insulin resistance. In 2007, Pittas et al. (2007) conducted a systemic review and meta-analysis of observational studies and clinical trials in adults with outcomes related to glucose homeostasis in type 2 diabetes mellitus. Observational studies show a relatively consistent association between low vitamin D status and prevalent type 2 diabetes, with an odds ratio of 0.36 among non-blacks for highest versus lowest 25-hydroxyvitamin D. Evidence from RCTs with vitamin D and/or calcium supplementation suggests that combined vitamin D and calcium supplementation might have a role in the prevention of type 2 diabetes only in populations at high risk (i.e., glucose intolerance). Whereas vitamin D supplementation did not improve glycemic control in diabetic subjects with baseline serum 25(OH)D levels >50 nmol/l (Jorde and Figenschau, 2009), administration of 100 µg vitamin D_3 improved insulin sensitivity in insulin-resistant South Asian women with baseline 25(OH)D concentrations <50 nmol/l (von Hurst et al., 2010). Insulin resistance was most improved when endpoint serum 25(OH)D reached ≥80 nmol/l. Optimal vitamin D concentrations for reducing insulin resistance were shown to be 80–119 nmol/l. Again, data indicate that in particular, patients seem to benefit from vitamin D supplementation whose baseline 25(OH)D concentrations are in the insufficiency/deficiency range.

10.2.7 Multiple sclerosis

Multiple sclerosis (MS) is a demyelinating disease of the central nervous system that is debilitating and can be fatal. Manifestation of the disease is typically between the years of 20 and 40. In Europe and North America, regions with higher UVB radiation have low rates of MS and vice versa (Zitterman, 2003) (▶Fig. 10.7). Exceptions from this general north to south gradient in the MS prevalence of the Northern hemisphere are some Swiss districts at high altitude (2000 m), Greenland and the costal regions of Norway. In these regions a low MS prevalence was reported. Results are consistent with the hypothesis that an inadequate vitamin D status is an important pathogenetic factor in MS. Annual UVB irradiation is more intensive in Swiss districts of high altitude than in regions of low altitudes. In Greenland and at the costal regions of Norway there is a traditionally high consumption of vitamin D-rich fatty fish and cod liver oil. In Israel, MS prevalence depends on the country of origin. The prevalence is high in people who were born in a country with low UVB irradiance (Chaudhuri, 2005), indicating that vitamin D status during the period of early life is of importance for MS susceptibility. MS disease activity shows inverse fluctuations according to season and vitamin D status (Embry et al., 2000). In a prospective, nested case-control study among more than 7 million US military personnel (Munger et al., 2006), MS prevalence was lower in those people who had circulating 25-hydroxyvitamin D concentrations between 100 and 150 nmol/l compared with those who had 25-hydroxyvitamin D concentrations below 63 nmol/l. However, this association was only seen in Whites and not in Blacks, indicating that genetic factors play an important role in the pathogenesis of MS. Therefore, the recent finding is of importance that expression of the MS-associated MHC class II allele HLA-DRB1*1501 is regulated by vitamin D (Ramagopalan et al., 2009).

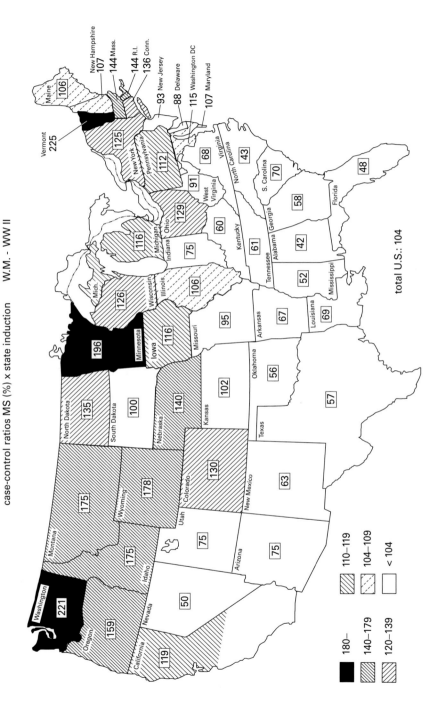

Fig. 10.7: Multiple Sclerosis in the United States. Case/cootrol/X100 for white male veterans according to place of residence prior to enlistment.

case-control ratios MS (%) x state induction   W.M. - WW II

total U.S.: 104

180–
140–179
120–139
110–119
104–109
< 104

New Hampshire 107
144 Mass.
144 R.I.
136 Conn.
93 New Jersey
88 Delaware
115 Washington DC
107 Maryland

Maine 106
Vermont 225
New York 125
Pennsylvania 112
West Virginia 91
Virginia 68
North Carolina 43
S. Carolina 70
Florida 48
Georgia 58
Alabama 42
Mississippi 52
Ohio 75
Indiana 60
Kentucky 61
Tennessee 67
Louisiana 69
Michigan 129
Mich. 116
Wisconsin 126
Illinois 106
Iowa 116
Missouri 95
Arkansas 102
Oklahoma 56
Texas 57
Minnesota 196
North Dakota 135
South Dakota 100
Nebraska 140
Kansas 102
Colorado 130
New Mexico 63
Montana 175
Wyoming 178
Utah 75
Arizona 75
Washington 221
Oregon 159
Idaho 175
Nevada 50
California 119

10.2.8 Other disorders

10.2.8.1 Pre-eclampsia

Pre-eclampsia is a medical condition where hypertension arises in pregnancy in association with significant amounts of protein in the urine. Pre-eclampsia could develop from 20 weeks gestation. Because calcium demands increase in the third trimester of pregnancy, vitamin D status becomes crucial for maternal health. The increased calcium demands are the reason for a rise in calcitriol concentrations from early to late pregnancy (Seki et al., 1991). By contrast, a decrease in 25(OH)D concentrations in pregnant women has been observed from early to late gestation, compared with non-pregnant women (Holmes et al., 2009). Low 25(OH)D concentrations are a risk factor for pre-eclampsia. A 50 nmol/l decline in 25(OH)D doubles the risk of pre-eclampsia (Bodnar et al., 2007). Intake of 15–20 µg vitamin D/day reduces the risk of pre-eclampsia compared with less than 5 µg/day by 24% (Haugen et al., 2009). Supplementation of pregnant women with 100 µg per day is not only able to increase 25(OH)D concentrations very effectively, but also results in a higher increase in calcitriol concentrations during pregnancy than under supplementation with 10 µg vitamin D daily (Hollis and Wagner, 2009). Obviously, the increased calcium and vitamin D demands during pregnancy lead to low 25(OH)D concentration in case of inadequate exogenous vitamin D supply, demonstrating the importance of vitamin D supplementation in this group of women.

10.2.8.2 Schizophrenia and depression

Vitamin D deficiency has been linked to an increased incidence of schizophrenia and depression. Maintaining vitamin D sufficiency *in utero* and during early life, to satisfy the vitamin D receptor transcriptional activity in the brain, could be important for brain development as well as for maintenance of mental function later in life (Holick, 2007).

10.2.8.3 Autoimmune diseases

Both, rheumatoid arthritis and inflammatory bowel disease are characterized by a chronic inflammatory state that involves overproduction of pro-inflammatory cytokines and a dysregulated T-helper cell type 1 response. In the USA, living at higher latitudes increases the risk of inflammatory bowel disease and rheumatoid arthritis (Sonnenberg and Wasserman, 1991; Costenbader et al., 2008). Patients with inflammatory bowel diseases and rheumatoid arthritis have high prevalence of 25(OH)D concentrations <50 nmol/l (Aguado et al., 2000; Jahnsen et al., 2002). At present, there is, however, only limited evidence that daily supplementation with high amounts of vitamin D or administration of active vitamin D might improve symptoms of rheumatoid arthritis (Zittermann, 2003).

10.2.8.4 Anemia

Owing to its pleiotropic effects, vitamin D might also influence erythropoiesis. An association between low vitamin D status and lower hemoglobin levels or iron deficiency has been observed in individuals with renal disease. In a large cross-sectional study in patients with chronic kidney disease (Patel et al., 2010), mean hemoglobin concentrations significantly decreased with decreasing tertiles of 25(OH)D and calcitriol. The lowest tertiles of 25(OH)D (<25 nmol/l) and calcitriol (<75 pmol/l) were independently associated with 2.8- and 2.0-fold increased prevalence of anemia compared with their respective highest tertiles (>75 nmol/l and >113 pmol/l). Patients with severe dual deficiency of 25(OH)D and calcitriol had a 5.4-fold prevalence of anemia compared with those replete in both. Administration of calcitriol is able to improve hemoglobin concentrations in patients with chronic kidney disease (Goicoechea et al., 1998; Neves et al., 2006). Low hemoglobin in combination with low 25(OH)D concentrations are also observed in children in minority communities in Britain (Grindulis et al., 1986; Lawson and Thomas, 1999). For example, in Asian immigrant children in England, one-fifth of children surveyed showed signs of both deficiencies; during the winter 50% of children with low vitamin D had low hemoglobin levels (versus 0% in children with normal vitamin D). In Tanzania, HIV infected women with 25(OH)D concentrations <80 nmol/l had 46% higher risk of developing severe anemia during follow-up, compared with women with adequate vitamin D levels (Mehta et al., 2010). In a Californian cross-sectional study, anemia was more prevalent in individuals with 25(OH)D concentrations below 75 nmol/l compared with normal 25-hydroxyvitamin D levels (49% versus 36%) (Sim et al., 2010).

Tab. 10.5: Evidence for association of circulating 25-hydroxyvitamin D level or vitamin D supplementation with all-cause mortality.

Study	Design	Number of individuals	Comparator	Hazard ratio (HR) or relative risk (RR) (95% CI)
Autier and Gandini (2007)	Meta-analysis of 18 vitamin D supplementation studies	57 311	Supplemented vs unsupplemented	RR 0.93 (0.87–0.99)
Dobnig et al. (2008)	Prospective cohort study with coronary angiography	3258	Median 25(OH)D 70 nmol/l vs 19 nmol/l	HR 0.48 (0.37–0.63)
Kuroda et al. (2009)	Prospective observational study in postmenopausal women	1232	≥50 nmol/l vs <50 nmol/l	HR 0.46 (0.27–0.79)
Ng et al. (2008)	Prospective cohort study in patients with colorectal cancer	304	Mean 41 nmol/l vs 100 nmol/l	HR 0.52 (0.29–0.94)
Ginde et al. (2009)	Prospective observational study in individuals >65 years	3408	25(OH)D >100 nmol/l vs <25 nmol/l	HR 0.55 (0.34–0.88)
Pilz et al. (2009)	Prospective observational study in individuals 50–75 years	614	Three highest quartiles vs lowest quartile	HR 0.51 (0.28–0.93)

Urashima M, Segawa T, Okazaki M, Kurihara M, Wada Y, Ida H, Randomized trial of vitamin D supplementation to prevent seasonal influenza A in schoolchildren. Am J Clin Nutr 2010;91: 1255–60.

von Hurst PR, Stonehouse W, Coad J, Vitamin D supplementation reduces insulin resistance in South Asian women living in New Zealand who are insulin resistant and vitamin D deficient – a randomised, placebo-controlled trial. Br J Nutr 2010;103: 549–55.

Von Mutius E, Influences in allergy: epidemiology and the environment. J Allergy Clin Immunol 2004;113: 373–9.

Wang AY, Lam CW, Sanderson JE, Wang M, Chan IH, Lui SF, Sea MM, Woo J, Serum 25-hydroxyvitamin D status and cardiovascular outcomes in chronic peritoneal dialysis patients: a 3-y prospective cohort study. Am J Clin Nutr 2008;87: 1631–8.

Wjst M, Another explanation for the low allergy rate in the rural Alpine foothills. Clin Mol Allergy 2005;3: 7.

Wjst M, Hyppönen E, Vitamin D serum levels and allergic rhinitis. Allergy 2007;62: 1085–6.

World Health Organization. International Agency for Research on Cancer. Vitamin D and cancer. IARC Working Group Reports, Vol. 5. Geneva, Switzerland: WHO Press; 2008. p. 148.

Yamshchikov AV, Desai NS, Blumberg HM, Ziegler TR, Tangpricha V, Vitamin D for treatment and prevention of infectious diseases: a systematic review of randomized controlled trials. Endocr Pract 2009;15: 438–49.

Zeitz U, Weber K, Soegiarto DW, Wolf E, Balling R, Erben RG, Impaired insulin secretory capacity in mice lacking a functional vitamin D receptor. FASEB J 2003;17: 509–11.

Zipitis CS, Akobeng AK, Vitamin D supplementation in early childhood and risk of type 1 diabetes: a systematic review and meta-analysis. Arch Dis Child 2008;93: 512–7.

Zittermann A, Vitamin D in preventive medicine – are we ignoring the evidence? Br J Nutr 2003;89: 552–72.

Zittermann A, Dembinski J, Stehle P, Low vitamin D status is associated with low cord blood levels of the immunosuppressive cytokine interleukin 10. Pediatr Allergy Immu 2004;15: 242–6.

Zittermann A, Grant WB. 25-hydroxyvitamin D levels and all-cause mortality. Arch Intern Med 2009;169: 1075–6.

Zittermann A, Tenderich G, Koerfer R, Vitamin D and the adaptive immune system with special emphasis to allergic reactions and allograft rejection. Inflamm Allergy Drug Targets 2009;8: 161–8.

10.3 Measurement of vitamin D

Markus Herrmann; Paul F. Williams

10.3.1 Introduction

Vitamin D is a group of fat-soluble prohormones, which are derived from cholesterol. The two major circulating forms of vitamin D are 25-hydroxy vitamin D_2 (synonym: ergocalciferol; abbreviation 25-OH D_2) and 25-hydroxy vitamin D_3 (synonym: cholecalciferol; abbreviation 25-OH D_3) with the latter being the predominant species under physiological circumstances (DeLuca, 2004). However, in some individuals significant amounts of 25-OH D_2 can be found and its low cross-reactivity in various assays for 25-hydroxy vitamin D (25-OHD) can mean some patients supplemented with 25-OH D_2 can be incorrectly diagnosed as vitamin D deficient. The variable cross-reactivity can interfere with the measurement of 25-OH D_3. Because 25-OH D is a prohormone it needs to be converted into its active form 1,25-dihydroxy vitamin D [1,25-(OH)$_2$D] (DeLuca, 2004). This conversion is catalysed by an enzyme named 1α-hydroxylase (synonym Cyp27b1), which is expressed in the kidney and other organs, such as bowel, prostate, breast, pancreas (pancreatic islets) and lungs. Under normal circumstances the majority of circulating 1,25-(OH)$_2$D is synthesized in the kidneys. However, during pregnancy, in individuals with chronic renal impairment, sarcoidosis, tuberculosis and rheumathoid arthritis significant amounts of 1,25-(OH)$_2$D can be derived from extra renal sources. Although renal 1,25-(OH)$_2$D synthesis is tightly regulated by serum levels of calcium, parathyroid hormone and 1,25-(OH)$_2$D itself there are other, mainly local factors that regulate 1,25-(OH)$_2$D synthesis in extra renal tissues.

For clinical purposes the 25-OH D concentration is considered the best measure of vitamin D status. The concentration of 25-OH D is approximately three orders of magnitude higher than that of 1,25-(OH)$_2$D and it has a long half-life in the circulation of 3 weeks (Hart et al., 2006). In addition, the conversion of 25-OH D into 1,25-(OH)$_2$D is tightly regulated with circulating calcium being one of the main determinants. Therefore, in patients with hypercalcaemia circulating 1,25-(OH)$_2$D levels not longer reflect the vitamin D supply of the organism.

Measurement of 1,25-(OH)$_2$D is only required in individuals with specific medical conditions, where 25-OH D is not longer a reliable surrogate of the supply of 1,25-(OH)$_2$D of the organism. Such conditions are, renal impairment, sarcoidosis, tuberculosis, 1α-hydroxylase deficiency and a defective vitamin D receptor causing vitamin D resistance.

10.3.2 Measurement of 25-OH vitamin D

Accurate and precise measurement of 25-OH D has been a challenge for many years. It is the strong lipophilic nature of vitamin D and the presence of vitamin D-binding protein, which complicates the quantification of 25-OH D. Traditionally, vitamin D is measured by high performance liquid chromatography (HPLC) and immunoassays [enzyme-linked immunoassay (ELISA) and radioimmunoassay (RIA)] (Hollis, 2004). Whereas HLPC assays are considered as reasonably accurate, immunoassays show very variable results (DeLuca, 2004). Results can differ up to 100% (►Fig. 10.8). Confounding problems are the presence of vitamin D-binding protein, which makes immunoassays difficult to control, and the extremely hydrophobic nature of vitamin D which means that matrix effects particularly lipids are difficult to control between standards and unknowns (Hollis and Horst, 2007). The older assays using vitamin D-binding protein and not antibodies were more susceptible to the matrix effects (Zerwekh, 2008). Therefore, many assays apply an extraction step using organic solvents (e.g., acetonitrile) to release protein-bound vitamin D and eliminate all proteins and minimise matrix effects from the sample. Unfortunately this extraction step makes an assay labour intensive and prevents automation. In fact, it is just recently that Roche Diagnostics has launched a first automated assay for the measurement of 25-OH D$_3$. This competitive chemiluminescence immunoassay does not use a protein extraction step. However, it appears that this assay has a limited accuracy. Individual results have been found to be 300% higher than with other assays.

In recent years liquid chromatography tandem mass spectrometry (LC Tandem MS) has been introduced for the measurements of 25-OH D. The main advantage of LC Tandem

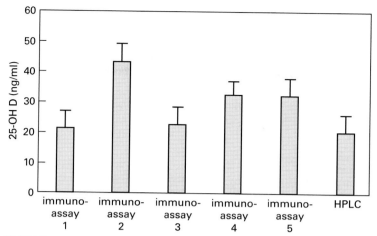

Fig. 10.8: 25-OH D concentrations in 20 serum samples, as measured with assay kits from five different commercial laboratories and with HPLC (modified from DeLuca et al., 2004).

MS is that 25-OH D_2 and 25-OH D_3 can be quantified separately with high accuracy and precision overcoming most technical problems of immunoassays and HPLC. For instance 25 OH D_2 can be associated with UV interfering peaks in HPLC assays using UV detection (Zerwekh, 2008). Because LC Tandem MS methods usually incorporate a protein extraction step, they are not affected by the presence of vitamin D binding protein. However, this protein extraction step is difficult to automate limiting the use of LC Tandem MS in high-throughput laboratories. Interference in infants of the inactive isomer 3-epi-25 OH D_3 can be a minor problem (Hollis and Horst, 2007). Another advantage of LC Tandem MS methods for the measurement of 25-OH D are minimal reagent costs. The only reagents required are calibrators, internal standards and some solvents, such as acetonitrile. Although calibrators are cheap internal standards cause significant costs. However, calibrators and internal standards can be used for an extended period of time. Disadvantages of LC Tandem MS methods for the measurement of 25-OH D are the requirement for expensive technical equipment and skilled staff to operate the system. In addition, there is no standard LC Tandem MS method that is generally recommended and, in fact, it is hard to find two laboratories applying exactly the same method. From a technical point of view LC Tandem MS methods can be subject to ion suppression affecting the reproducibility and accuracy of results particularly at low concentrations of analytes. Moreover, these methods require the measurement of recovery with deuterated internal standards (Hart et al., 2006).

10.3.2.1 Pre-analytical requirements

25-OH D should be measured in serum or plasma. Blood sampling should be done in a fasting state. In dialysis patients specimens should be collected before dialysis. Heparin injections increase circulating 25-OH D levels. In serum or plasma 25-OH D is stable and does not need to be frozen for transportation. At 4°C 25OH D is stable for weeks. For long-term storage, samples should be kept at –20°C. Samples need to be protected from direct exposure to sunlight.

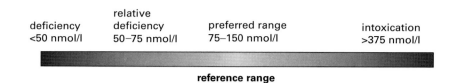

deficiency	relative deficiency	preferred range	intoxication
<50 nmol/l	50–75 nmol/l	75–150 nmol/l	>375 nmol/l

reference range
10–125 nmol/l

Fig. 10.9: Interpretation of 25-OH D serum concentrations. Conversion factor µg/l x 2.5 = nmol/l.

10.3.2.2 Reference ranges

The reference range of 25-OH D in apparently healthy individuals is 10–125 nmol/l. However, in regards to the high prevalence of vitamin D deficiency in the general population application of a traditional reference range is not useful to diagnose 25-OH D deficiencies. Most experts support the concept of a preferred range, which is based on circulating PTH (▶Fig. 10.9). 25-OH D levels are inversely related to PTH. At 25-OH D levels of 75 nmol/l this inverse relation levels off with serum PTH reaching a nadir. Therefore, the preferred range of 25-OH D starts at 75 nmol/l. There is general agreement that 25-OH D levels <50 nmol/l should be considered as deficient. Because intestinal calcium absorption has been shown to increase if 25-OH D levels rise from 50 to 75 nmol/l, this range has been classified as relative vitamin D deficiency. 25-OH D levels of ≥75 nmol/l indicate a sufficient vitamin D supply.

10.3.3 Measurement of 1,25-(OH)$_2$ vitamin D

Circulating 1,25-(OH)$_2$D levels are three orders of magnitude lower than 25-OH D precluding them from measurement with ELISA or chemiluminescence immunoassays. Only RIA or LC Tandem MS are sensitive enough to provide accurate and reliable measures of 1,25-(OH)$_2$D. Both methods are labour intensive and require extensive manual sample preparation. Sample preparation for RIA typically includes an extraction step with acetonitrile to remove proteins and lipids followed by chromatographic separation on a C18 silica cartridge. After several washing steps, 1,25-(OH)$_2$D is eluted from the columns and measured. Most commercial 1,25-(OH)$_2$D RIAs are competitive immunoassays using ^{125}I labelled 1,25-(OH)$_2$D, which competes with unlabelled 1,25-(OH)$_2$D in the sample. Although most RIAs detect 1,25-(OH)$_2$D$_3$ only some measure 1,25-(OH)$_2$D$_2$ and 1,25-(OH)$_2$D$_3$ (e.g., DIASORIN, ALPCO Diagnostics). As a result of increasing availability of LC Tandem MS technology in clinical laboratories and continuously improving sensitivity of these instruments it can be expected that 1,25-(OH)$_2$D testing will shift from RIA to LC Tandem MS. Laboratory scientists are currently working on LC Tandem MS methods combining 25-OH D with 1,25-(OH)$_2$D in one run, which would be a major advantage.

10.3.3.1 Pre-analytical requirements

1,25-(OH)$_2$D can be measured in serum or plasma. Blood sampling should be done in a fasting state. In serum or plasma 1,25-(OH)$_2$D is stable and does not need to be frozen for transportation. At 4°C 1,25-(OH)$_2$D is stable for weeks. For long-term storage, samples should be kept at –20°C. Samples need to be protected from direct exposure to sunlight.

Tab. 10.6: Serum or plasma concentration 1,25-(OH)$_2$D reference intervals.

Adults <50 years	75–200 pmol/l
Adults >50 years	63–125 pmol/l
Pregnant women	100–325 pmol/l
Children	100–250 pmol/l

Conversion factor: ng/l × 2.5 = pmol/l.

10.3.3.2 Reference ranges

The reference range of 1,25-(OH)$_2$D and 25-OH D varies with age (▶Tab. 10.6). Highest levels can be found in children and pregnant women.

References

DeLuca HF, Overview of general physiologic features and functions of vitamin D. Am J Clin Nutr 2004;80: 1689S–96S.
Hart GR, Furniss JL, Laurie D, Durham SK, Measurement of vitamin D status: background, clinical use, and methodologies. Clin Lab 2006;52: 335–43.
Hollis BW, Editorial: the determination of circulating 25-hydroxyvitamin D: no easy task. J Clin Endocrinol Metab 2004;89: 3149–51.
Hollis BW, Horst RL, The assessment of circulating 25(OH)D and 1,25(OH)2D: where we are and where we are going. J Steroid Biochem Mol Biol 2007;103: 473–6.
Zerwekh JE, Blood biomarkers of vitamin D status. Am J Clin Nutr 2008;87: 1087S–91S.

10.4 Using vitamin D for management of human diseases

Jörg Reichrath

10.4.1 Vitamin D-deficiency – a serious health problem

Vitamin D-deficiency/insufficiency is now an epidemic. It has been estimated that approximately 1 billion people worldwide are vitamin D-deficient or insufficient (Holick, 2007). This is a serious problem, because a connection between vitamin D-deficiency and a broad variety of independent diseases has been established. In particular various types of cancer (e.g., colon-, prostate- and breast cancer), bone disease, autoimmune disease, infectious disease, cardiovascular disease and hypertension have been confirmed in a large number of studies (Garland et al., 1989, 2007; Gorham et al., 1990, 2007; Garland and Gorham, 1991; Grant, 2002). Approximately 90% of all required vitamin D has to be formed within the skin through the action of the sun, resulting in a dilemma on how to balance between the positive and the negative effects of solar UV-radiation.

10.4.2 The vitamin D and cancer hypothesis

The hypothesis that links vitamin D and cancer is not new and presents the idea that sunlight exposure and vitamin D formed from this can inhibit the growth of human cancers (Schwartz et al., 1998). When Peller in 1936 found an apparent deficit of other cancer forms among US Navy personnel, who experienced an excess of skin cancer, he concluded that skin cancers induced a relative immunity to other types of cancer (Peller, 1936). Consequently, he advocated the deliberate induction of non-melanoma skin cancers, which were easily detected and treated, as a form of vaccination against more life-threatening and less treatable cancers. It was in 1941 when the American pathologist Frank Apperly published geographic data that demonstrated for the first time an inverse correlation between levels of UV-radiation in North America and mortality rates from cancers (Apperly, 1941). Apperly concluded that "the presence of skin cancer was really only an occasional accompaniment of relative cancer immunity, but the immunity was in some way related to exposure to ultraviolet radiation". He also concluded that "A closer study of the action of solar radiation on the body, might well reveal the nature of cancer immunity". Since Apperly's first report, an association has been confirmed between the increased risk of dying of various internal malignancies (e.g., breast, colon, prostate and ovarian cancer) and the decrease in latitude from the poles towards the equator (Grant, 2002). A correlation of cancer incidence with increasing altitude, lower sun exposure and vitamin D serum levels has been demonstrated (Garland et al., 1989; Grant, 2002). Moreover, it has been reported that sun exposure is associated with a relatively favorable prognosis and increased survival rate in various malignancies, including malignant melanoma (Berwick et al., 2005; Moan et al., 2005; Porojnicu et al., 2007). It has been speculated that these findings were related to UV-exposure-induced higher serum levels of vitamin D. Berwick et al. in a population-based study of cutaneous melanoma ($n = 528$) that were followed for an average of more than 5 years, found that sunburn, high intermittent solar UV-exposure, and solar elastosis were statistically significantly inversely associated with death from melanoma (Berwick et al., 2005). They concluded that exposure to sun was associated with increased survival from melanoma (Berwick et al., 2005).

In 2007, Gorham et al. reported a quantitative meta-analysis to derive an optimal vitamin D concentration for colorectal cancer prevention (Gorham et al., 2007). Although previous studies such as the Women's Health Initiative, have shown that a low dose of vitamin D did not protect against colorectal cancer, meta-analysis convincingly indicated that a higher dose might reduce the incidence. In attempting a quantitative meta-analysis, five studies of serum 25(OH)D in association with colorectal cancer risk were identified using PubMed. The results of all five serum studies were combined using standard methods for pooled analysis. The pooled results were divided into quintiles with median 25(OH)D values of 6, 16, 22, 27 and 37 ng/ml. Odds ratios for the pooled data were calculated by quintiles using Peto's Assumption-Free Method, with the lowest quintile of 25(OH)D used as the reference group. A dose-response curve for the pooled data was plotted for the odds of each quintile of 25 (OH)D values. Data were extracted and analyzed in 2006. They showed that odds ratios from lowest to highest quintile for the combined data on serum 25(OH)D levels were 1.00, 0.82, 0.66, 0.59 and 0.46 (p(trend) < 0.0001), respectively, for colorectal cancer. According to the Der Simonian-Laird test for homogeneity of pooled data, the studies were homogeneous (Chi^2 = 1.09, df = 4, $p = 0.90$). The pooled odds ratio for the highest quintile versus the lowest was 0.49 ($p < 0.0001$, 95% confidence interval, 0.35–0.68). A 50% lower risk of colorectal cancer was associated with serum 25(OH)D levels ≥33 ng/ml when compared with 25 (OH)D levels ≥12 ng/ml. They concluded that the evidence suggested that a daily intake of 1000–2000 IU of vitamin D_3 per day could reduce the incidence of colorectal with minimal other risk.

Lappe et al. performed a randomized placebo-controlled trial among 1179 healthy community-dwelling postmenopausal women (Lappe et al., 2007). This study included three treatment groups: placebo, calcium (1400–1500 mg) and calcium (1400–1500 mg) plus vitamin D (1100 IU). Fifty women developed cancer during the 4 years of the study including 13 cases during the first year of the study. Compared with the placebo group, the risk of cancer was reduced by 60% in the vitamin D plus calcium group (RR 0.40; 95% CI 0.20–0.82). This analysis was repeated in a 1-year follow-up in women free of cancer to reduce any possible bias for occult cancer that was already present but not diagnosed at baseline. In this analysis, the risk of cancer was reduced by 77% in the calcium plus vitamin D treatment group versus the placebo group (RR 0.23; 95% CI 0.09–0.60). In both of these analyses there were no significant difference in cancer incidence between the placebo and the calcium treatment group. The study of Lappe et al. was of great importance because it was the first randomized placebo-controlled trial that demonstrated that vitamin D supplementation significantly reduced cancer incidence. In addition, it should be noted that the International Agency for Research on Cancer (IARC) has released a report, questioning the relevance of vitamin D for cancer (IARC, 2008), that has been criticized by well-recognized experts in the field owing to its many deficiencies in the interpretation of the data (Grant, 2009; Holick, 2009).

Animal experiments as well as epidemiological data from some countries related the survival of various malignancies including colon- and lung cancer with exposure to solar UV, with latitude and with vitamin D_3-synthesis in the skin (Moan et al., 2005; Porojnicu et al., 2007). Moreover, laboratory investigations are showing the importance of the integrity of the vitamin D hormone and receptor systems for the pathogenesis and progression of cancer and are supporting the hypothesis that vitamin D is linked to cancer prevention. As an example, an increasing body of evidence now demonstrates an association between several vitamin D receptor (VDR) polymorphisms and the risk of cancer and cancer progression (Köstner et al., 2009; Raimondi et al., 2009).

It is interesting to note that the evolution of our understanding of the role of vitamin D in cancer and in various other diseases that are not related to bone and calcium metabolism including infectious and autoimmune diseases, parallels the evolution of our understanding of the importance of vitamin D for rickets (Holick, 2003). In both diseases, epidemiologic observations about consequences of solar UV-exposure preceeded but were subsequently supported by laboratory investigations. Apperly's enlightening observations on sunlight exposure and cancer, similarly to those of Theobold Palm on the protective effects of solar UV-radiation on rickets a half century earlier (Palm 1890), were almost unnoticed for many years, and were only to be rediscovered by epidemiologists decades later. During recent years, increasing progress has been made in laboratory investigations that searched for the 'missing link' in the connection between vitamin D and cancer. The discovery that earlier assumptions were incorrect and that skin, prostate, colon, breast and many other tissues expressed the enzyme to convert 25(OH)D to its biologically active form, $1,25(OH)_2D$ was very important (Schwartz et al., 1998; Lehmann et al., 2004; Mitschele et al., 2004). Therefore, $1,25(OH)_2D$ is now not considered to be exclusively a calciotropic hormone but it is also considered to be a locally produced potent regulator of cell growth (Holick, 2007).

10.4.3 Association of vitamin D deficiency with infectious diseases, cardiovascular diseases and autoimmune diseases

As already mentioned above, a lack of sunlight exposure leads to more than increased bone disease and an increased cancer risk; there are multiple other effects that include decreased protection against infectious disease. It has been shown that $1,25(OH)_2D$ is a direct regulator of the antimicrobial innate immune response (Wang et al., 2004; Gombard et al., 2005; Weber et al., 2005; Liu et al., 2006). The innate immune system of mammals provides a rapid response to repel assaults from numerous infectious agents including bacteria, viruses, fungi, and parasites. Major component of this system are a diverse combination of cationic antimicrobial peptides (CAMP) that include α- and β-defensins and the cathelicidins (Gombard et al., 2005). Because bacteria are quickly killed by CAMPs they have difficulty developing resistance against them. This class of peptide antibiotic antimicrobial agents is now being commercially developed (Gombard et al., 2005). Interestingly, the promoter regions of the human CAMP and defensin 2 (*defB2*) genes contain consensus vitamin D response elements (VDRE) that mediate $1,25(OH)_2D$-dependent gene expression (Wang et al., 2004). $1,25(OH)_2D$ induced antimicrobial peptide gene expression in isolated human keratinocytes, monocytes and neutrophils, and in cultured human cell lines. $1,25(OH)_2D$ along with LPS synergistically induced CAMP expression in neutrophils (Wang et al., 2004). Moreover, $1,25(OH)_2D$ induced a corresponding increase in the production and secretion of antimicrobial proteins providing antimicrobial activity against pathogens including *Pseudomonas aeruginosa* (Wang et al., 2004). In human keratinocytes, Weber et al. reported an up-regulation of *CAMP* by approximately one order of magnitude after treatment with 100 nM $1,25(OH)_2D$ or MC 903 (calcipotriol) (Weber et al., 2005). Surprisingly, $25(OH)D_3$, the precursor of biologically active $1,25(OH)_2D$, stimulated *CAMP* expression to the same extent that $1,25(OH)_2D$ or MC 903 did. All these compounds were active down to levels of 10 nM but the precursor of vitamin D biosynthesis, 7-dehydrocholesterol (7-DHC), was ineffective at all the concentrations tested (Weber et al., 2005). Western blot analysis in two independent investigations confirmed that the elevated transcription of CAMP genes was reflected by an increase in their protein levels (Gombard et al., 2005; Weber et al., 2005). The induction of *CAMP* gene expression occurred via a consensus VDRE in the promoter that bound the VDR. In conclusion, there is convincing evidence that $1,25(OH)_2D$ and analogues directly regulate antimicrobial peptide gene expression in humans, demonstrating the potential of these compounds for the treatment of opportunistic infections. It is well known that in innate immune responses, activation of Toll-like receptors (TLR) triggers direct antimicrobial activity against intracellular bacteria, which in murine, but not in human monocytes and macrophages is mediated principally by nitric oxide (Liu et al., 2006). It has recently been reported that TLR activation of human macrophages up-regulated expression of the VDR and the vitamin D-1α hydroxylase (1α OHase) (CYP27B1) genes, leading to the induction of cathelicidin and the consequent killing of intracellular *Mycobacterium tuberculosis*. In this study, it was observed that sera from African-American individuals, known to have increased susceptibility to tuberculosis, had low $25(OH)D_3$ and were inefficient in inducing cathelicidin messenger RNA production. These data support a link between TLRs and vitamin D-mediated innate immunity and suggests that differences in the ability of human populations to produce vitamin D could contribute to increased susceptibility to microbial infection (Liu et al., 2006). It has been reported that vitamin D deficiency predisposes children to respiratory infections and that volunteers inoculated with live attenuated influenza virus are more likely to develop fever and serological evidence of an immune response in the winter (Cannell et al., 2006). Ultraviolet radiation (either from artificial sources or from sunlight) reduces the incidence of viral respiratory infections, as does cod liver oil (which contains vitamin D).

An interventional study showed that vitamin D reduced the incidence of respiratory infections in children and it has been concluded that a lack of vitamin D might be of importance for the remarkable seasonality of epidemic influenza (Hope-Simpson's 'seasonal stimulus') (Cannell et al., 2006). Taken together, these data suggest the effects of solar UV radiation on the immune system are not exclusively immunosuppressive, but might even stimulate distinct immune responses.

10.4.4 Impact of vitamin D deficiency on all-cause mortality

In recent years, several large non-randomized prospective studies on the impact of vitamin D status on all-cause mortality have been reported. In 2007, Autier and Gandini published a meta-analysis of randomized controlled trials (RCTs) on vitamin D status and mortality that were not primarily designed to investigate mortality (Autier and Gandini, 2007). The authors concluded that vitamin D supplementation (daily doses ranged between 10 µg and 50 µg of vitamin D) was associated with lower all-cause mortality (risk reduction was 7% with a mean follow-up of 5.7 years) in middle-aged and elderly individuals with low 25(OH)D-serum levels, when compared with unsupplemented individuals. Ginde et al. in 2009 reported on a subgroup analysis of 3.408 NHANES III participants aged 65 and older (Ginde et al., 2009). They demonstrated that the adjusted mortality risk for individuals with 25(OH)D-serum levels of 25.0–49.9 nmol/l was 47% higher and 83% higher for individuals with 25(OH)D-serum levels less than 25.0 nmol/l when compared with individuals with 25(OH)D-serum levels at or in excess of 100.0 nmol/l (Ginde et al., 2009). In 2008 Dobnig et al. published an analysis of 3258 consecutive male and female participants in the LURIC (Ludwigshafen Risk and Cardiovascular Health) study, that were scheduled for coronary angiography (Dobnig et al., 2008). They reported that in the two lower 25(OH)D-serum level quartiles (median 19.0 and 33.3 nmol/l) multivariate adjusted all-cause mortality was 128% and 60% higher when compared with individuals in the highest 25(OH)D-serum quartile (median 71.0 nmol/l) (Dobnig et al., 2008). Median follow-up time for this study was 7.7 years and 737 participants (22.6%) died during that time. Pilz et al. recently published a study analyzing 614 older individuals from the Netherlands (Pilz et al., 2009). They reported that low 25(OH)D-serum levels were significantly associated with increased mortality rates. In the lowest 25(OH)D-serum quartile (median 30.6 nmol/l), the unadjusted and multivariate-adjusted all-cause mortality risks were 124% and 97% higher when compared with all other participants. Summarizing the present knowledge about the impact of vitamin D status on all cause mortality, it can be concluded that improving vitamin D status by either supplementation or by UV-exposure might be a promising public health strategy to reduce mortality rates. In the German population, according to conservative estimates, at least 2.2% of all deaths or 18 300 lives annually could probably be saved by raising 25(OH)D serum concentrations to at least 75 nmol/l (Zittermann et al., submitted).

10.4.5 Sun protection increases the risk of vitamin D-deficiency

We have investigated whether patients that need to protect themselves for medical reasons from solar and artificial UV-exposure are at an increased risk of becoming vitamin D-deficient. In this study we determined 25(OH)D-plasma levels in renal transplant patients with adequate renal function to an age- and gender-matched control group at the end of winter (Querings et al., 2006). Owing to their increased risk of developing UV-induced skin cancer, all renal transplant patients have been advised to protect themselves against solar and artificial UV-radiation after transplantation. We found that 25(OH)D-serum levels were significantly lower ($p = 0.007$) in renal transplant patients [$n = 31$, geometric mean 10.9 ng/ml (95% confidence interval 8.2–14.3)] when compared with age- and gender-matched controls [$n = 31$, vitamin D = 20.0 ng/ml (95% confidence interval 15.7–25.5)] (Querings et al., 2006). We have made similar findings in another pilot study, where we analyzed basal 25(OH)D-serum levels in a small group of patients with xeroderma pigmentosum (XP, $n = 3$) and basal cell nevus syndrome (BCNS, $n = 1$) (Querings and Reichrath, 2004). At the end of winter (February/March), 25(OH)D-levels were markedly decreased in all four patients (mean 9.5 ng/ml), when compared with the normal range (15.0–90.0 ng/ml) (Querings and Reichrath, 2004). In conclusion, we demonstrated in these two investigations that reduced 25(OH)D-serum levels were found in risk groups that protect themselves against artificial and solar UV-radiation (Querings and Reichrath, 2004; Querings et al., 2006).

10.4.6 How much vitamin D do we need?

At present, there is an ongoing debate on how much vitamin D we need to achieve a protective effect against cancer and other diseases. From an historical point of view, the US Recommended Dietary Allowance (RDA) of vitamin D from 1989 was 200 IU (Vieth, 1999). Despite this, investigations in the past decades have shown that taking 200 IU vitamin D orally daily has no effect on bone status (Dawson-Hughes et al., 1995). In consequence, it has been recommended by some authors that adults at a minimum might need, five times the RDA, or 1000 IU daily, to be adequately protected against bone fractures, some cancers and to derive the other broad-ranging health benefits from vitamin D (Vieth, 1999). In conclusion, the 1989 RDA of 200 IU is antiquated, and the newer 600 IU Daily Reference Intake (DRI) dose for adults older than 70 might still not be adequate (Vieth, 1999). It has been suggested that 2000 IU taken daily orally, [previously considered to represent the upper tolerable intake (the official safety limit)], does not deliver the optimal amounts of vitamin D (Vieth, 1999). To evaluate putative risks that could be associated with vitamin D-supplementation, one should first consider the physiological capacity of the human skin to synthesize vitamin D. On a sunny summer day, total body sun exposure of the skin can produce more than 10 000 IU vitamin D per day. Considering this fact, concerns about toxic overdose with dietary supplements that exceed 800 IU vitamin D are poorly founded. Moreover, it has been speculated that a person would have to consume almost 67 times more vitamin D than the previously recommended intake for older adults of 600 IU to experience symptoms of overdosage (Vieth, 1999). Vieth proposes that people need 4000–10 000 IU vitamin D daily and that the toxic side effects are not a concern until a dose/day exceeds 40000 IU (Vieth, 1999). Several other reports are in line with these findings and it has been suggested by several experts that older adults, sick adults and 'perhaps all adults' would need 800–1000 IU vitamin D daily. It was also indicated that a daily dose of 2400 IU (four times the recommended intake) could be consumed safely (Vieth, 1999). According to recent estimates an intake of 1000 IU daily would bring 25(OH)D serum levels in at least 50% of the population up to an advantageous range of 30 ng/ml (Bischoff-Ferrari, 2008). Thus, higher doses of vitamin D oral supplements are needed for those individuals who do not reach the desired ranges.

The vitamin D-cancer dose-response relation has been investigated in three studies. A meta-analysis of five observational studies of serum 25(OH)D found that it takes approximately 1500 IU of vitamin D_3 per day to reduce the risk of colorectal cancer by 50%, based on the assumption that 25(OH)D-levels of the population are generally low (Gorham et al., 2007). In a separate cohort study of male health professionals, it was found that taking 1500 IU daily of vitamin D_3 should reduce all-cancer mortality rates for males in the USA by approximately 30% (Giovannucci et al., 2006). Based on two studies of 25(OH)D-serum levels in breast cancer, it was concluded that it would take approximately 4000 IU/day for a 50% reduction in the risk for breast cancer (Garland et al., 2007).

However, account has to be taken of the fact that most of the studies outlined above are either epidemiological, ecological or observational. Although ecological studies have been criticized because of inconsistencies when compared with observational intervention studies, they have important advantages, as they incorporate the effects of diet and lifestyle over a long time period. It has to be noted that these advantages previously widely underestimated and are now being increasingly recognized. It is well known that cancer and other diseases can take several decades to develop and progress, the advantages outlined above are extremely important for the investigation of these diseases. Additionally, it should be noted that the primary criteria for causality in a biological system established by Hill (1965): strength of association, reproducibility in different populations, accounting for confounding factors, identification of the mechanisms and experimental confirmation, are fulfilled when analyzing the role of vitamin D as a risk reduction factor for several types of cancer (Grant, 2008).

10.4.7 Beneficial versus adverse effects of solar UV-exposure: time for a paradigm shift!

What conclusions can we draw from the findings reported above, most importantly the demonstration of an association between vitamin D-deficiency and the occurrence of numerous independent diseases, including cancer? The important take home message for dermatologists and other clinicians is that health campaigns promoting strict sun protection procedures to prevent skin cancer could induce a severe health risk of vitamin D-deficiency. There is no doubt that UV-radiation is mutagenic and is the main reason for the development of non-melanoma skin cancers. Therefore, excessive sun exposure has to be avoided, particularly in childhood. To reach this goal, the use of sunscreens as well as wearing of protective clothing and glasses is of paramount importance. An increase in solar UVB-radiation reaching the surface of the earth is an important consequence of stratospheric ozone depletion, and is a matter of concern (Grant et al., 2007; Norval et al., 2007). Recently however, it has been assumed that the net effects of solar UVB-radiation on human health are beneficial at or near current levels (Grant et al., 2007; Grant, 2008). It has to be emphasized that artificial UVB exposure could be an addition or an alternative to solar UV exposure. Artificial UVB exposure has the advantage that the wavelength spectrum and radiation intensity can be optimized for cutaneous vitamin D synthesis. Moreover, it can easily be performed. It has been noted that UVB doses needed to guarantee a sufficient vitamin D status are much lower when compared with the UV doses needed for the commonly used phototherapy of dermatologic diseases, including atopic dermatitis or psoriasis. In conclusion, clinicians including dermatologists have to recognize the convincing evidence of the protective effect of less intense solar radiation and that this outweighs its mutagenic effect. In agreement with this assumption, it has been concluded that many lives could be prolonged through careful exposure to sunlight or with vitamin D-supplementation, particularly in non-summer months (Grant, 2008). Therefore, it is time for a paradigm shift and the recommendations of health campaigns on sun protection to be moderated and present a more balanced view of positive and negative effects of solar UV-exposure. As Michael Holick reported previously (Holick, 2001, 2007), we have learned that at latitudes similar to Boston, USA, very short and limited solar UV-exposure is sufficient to obtain 'adequate' vitamin D-levels. Exposure of the body in a bathing suit to one minimal erythemal dose (MED) of sunlight is equivalent to ingesting at least approximately 10 000 IU of vitamin D and it has been reported that exposure of less than 18% of the body surface (hands, arms, and face) two to three times a week to a third to a half of an MED; (approx. 5 min for adult skin-type-II in Boston in July at noon) in the spring, summer and autumn is more than adequate to maintain vitamin D levels. Anyone intending to stay exposed to sunlight for longer times than recommended above should apply a sunscreen with a sufficient sun protection factor to prevent sunburn and the damaging effects of excessive exposure to sunlight. According to Holick's rule, exposure of 25% of the body's surface with 25% MED UVB provides the human body with approximately 25 µg of vitamin D_3. Although further work is needed to define the impact of vitamin D-deficiency on the occurrence of melanoma and non-melanoma skin cancer, it is at present very important that dermatologists particularly strengthen the message on the importance of adequate vitamin D-status if UV exposure is to be seriously curtailed for medical reasons. It has to be emphasized that in people that are at high risk of developing vitamin D-deficiency (e.g., nursing home residents; patients with skin type I or patients under immunosuppressive therapy that require protection from solar UV-exposure), need to have their vitamin D-status closely monitored. As a consequence of the severe health risks associated with vitamin D-deficiency, vitamin D-deficiency needs to be treated, e.g., by giving vitamin D orally as recommended previously (Vieth, 1999; Holick, 2001). It has been shown that a single dose of 50 000 IU vitamin D once a week for 8 weeks is a very efficient and safe way to treat vitamin D-deficiency (Vieth, 1999). An alternative means of ensuring vitamin D-sufficiency, particularly in nursing home residents, would be to give 50 000 IU of vitamin D once a month. A further alternative to prevent vitamin D-deficiency would be to use of vitamin D-containing ointments. However, it has to be mentioned that vitamin D-containing ointments are, at least in Europe, not allowed as cosmetics. These antiquated laws are a hangover from the fear of inducing vitamin D-intoxication that was evident in Europe in the 1950s (British Pediatric Association, 1956) and need to be re-evaluated, for they oppose our present scientific knowledge. If we carefully follow the guidelines discussed above, they will ensure an adequate vitamin D-status, in patients, thereby reducing the adverse effects of protecting against solar UV radiation, that are still recommended in many public health campaigns. Most importantly, these measures will protect us sufficiently against the influence of vitamin D-deficiency on the development of various malignancies and other diseases without increasing the risk of developing UV-radiation-induced skin cancer. To reach this goal it is important that this information is communicated to every clinician, particularly dermatologists. Otherwise dermatologists will not support the moderation of current recommendations for protection against artificial and solar UV-radiation. These modifications are necessary to protect the population from vitamin D-deficiency induced cancer and other diseases.

10.4.8 Conclusions

Epidemiological and laboratory data are generally consistently in favor of the hypothesis that sufficient vitamin D status protects against the initiation and progression of cancer and other severe diseases, including autoimmune, cardiovascular, neurological, metabolic and infectious diseases as well as fractures and falls. In recognition of the multiple health benefits of vitamin D, the high prevalence of vitamin D deficiency in the general population and the inexpensive, ease and safe way that vitamin D can be supplemented, it is of high importance to implement public health strategies for maintaining the vitamin D status in the general population at sufficient levels.

References

Apperly FL, The relation of solar radiation to cancer mortality in North America. Cancer Res 1941;1: 191–5.
Autier P, Gandini S, Vitamin D supplementation and total mortality: a meta-analysis of randomized controlled trials. Arch Intern Med 2007;167: 1730–7.
Berwick M, Armstrong BK, Ben-Porat L, Fine J, Kricker A, Eberle C, Barnhill R, Sun exposure and mortality from melanoma. J Natl Cancer Inst 2005;97: 195–9.
Bischoff-Ferrari HA, Optimal serum 25-hydroxyvitamin D levels for multiple health outcomes. Adv Exp Med Biol 2008;624: 55–71.
British Pediatric Association, Hypercalcemia in infants and vitamin D. Br Med J 1956;2: 149.
Cannell JJ, Vieth R, Umhau JC, Holick MF, Grant WB, Madronich S, Garland CF, Giovannucci E, Epidemic influenza and vitamin D. Epidemiol Infect 2006;7: 1–12.
Dawson-Hughes B et al., Rates of bone loss in post-menopausal women randomly assigned to one of two dosages of vitamin D. Am J Clin Nutr 1995;61: 1140–5.
Dobnig H, Pilz S, Scharnagl H, Renner W et al., Independent association of low serum 25-hydroxyvitamin D and 1,25-dihydroxyvitamin D levels with all-cause and cardiovascular mortality. Arch Intern Med 2008;168: 1340–9.
Garland CF, Comstock GW, Garland FC et al., Serum 25-hydroxyvitamin D and colon cancer: eight year prospective study. Lancet 1989;2: 1176–8.
Garland CF, Garland FC, Gorham ED, Can colon cancer incidence and death rates be reduced with calcium and vitamin D? Am J Clin Nutr 1991;54: 193S–201S.
Garland CF, Gorham ED, Mohr SB, Grant WB, Giovannucci EL, Lipkin M, Newmark H, Holick MF, Garland FC, Vitamin D and prevention of breast cancer: pooled analysis. J Steroid Biochem Mol Biol 2007;103: 708–11.

Ginde AA, Scragg R, Schwartz RS, Camargo CA, Prospective study of serum 25-hydroxyvitamin D level, cardiovascular disease mortality, and all cause mortality in older US adults. J Am Geriatr Soc 2009;57: 1595–603.

Giovannucci E, Liu Y, Rimm EB, Hollis BW, Fuchs CS, Stampfer MJ, Willett WH, Prospective study of predictors of vitamin D status and cancer incidence and mortality in men. J Natl Cancer Inst 2006;98: 451–459.

Gombard HF, Borregaard N, Koeffler HP, Human cathelicidin antimicrobial peptide (CAMP) gene is a direct target of the vitamin D receptor and is strongly up-regulated in myeloid cells by 1,25-dihydroxyvitamin D3. FASEB J 2005;19: 1067–77.

Gorham ED, Garland FC, Garland CF, Sunlight and breast cancer incidence in the USSR. Int J Epidemiol 1990;19: 614–22.

Gorham ED, Garland CF, Garland FC, Grant WB, Mohr SB, Lipkin M, Newmark HL, Giovannucci E, Wei M, Holick MF, Optimal vitamin d status for colorectal cancer prevention a quantitative meta analysis. Am J Prev Med 2007;32: 210–6.

Grant WB, An estimate of premature cancer mortality in the U.S. due to inadequate doses of solar ultraviolet-B radiation. Cancer 2002;94: 1867–75.

Grant WB, Solar ultraviolet irradiance and cancer incidence and mortality. Adv Exp Med Biol 2008; 624: 16–30.

Grant WB, A critical review of *Vitamin D and Cancer*. Dermato-Endocrinology 2009;1: 25–33.

Grant WB, Moan J, Reichrath J, Comment on "The effects on human health from stratospheric ozone depletion and its interactions with climate change" by M. Norval, A.P. Cullen, F.R. de Gruijl, J. Longstreth, Y. Takizawa, R.M. Lucas, F.P. Noonan and J.C. van der Leun, Photochem. Photobiol. Sci., 2007, 6, 232. Photochem Photobiol Sci 2007;6: 912–5.

Hill AB, The environment and disease: association or causation? Proc R Soc Med 1965;58: 295–300.

IARC, Vitamin D and cancer. IARC working group reports. Lyon, France: International Agency for Research on Cancer; 2008.

Köstner K, Denzer N, Müller CSL, Klein R, Tilgen W, Reichrath J, The relevance of vitamin D receptor (VDR) gene polymorphisms for cancer: a meta-analysis of the literature. Anticancer Res, in press.

Holick MF, Sunlight 'D' ilemma: risk of skin cancer or bone disease and muscle weakness. Lancet 2001;357: 961.

Holick MF, Evolution and function of vitamin D. Recent Results Cancer Res 2003;164: 3–28.

Holick MF, Vitamin D deficiency. N Engl J Med 2007;357: 266–81.

Holick MF, Shining light on the vitamin D. Dermato-Endocrinology 2009;1: 4–6.

Lappe JM, Travers-Gustavson D, Davies KM, Recker RR, Heaney RP, Vitamin D and calcium supplementation reduced cancer risk: results of a randomised trial. Am J Clin Nutr 2007;85: 6–18.

Lehmann B, Querings K, Reichrath J, Vitamin D and skin: new aspects for dermatology. Exp Dermatol 2004;13(s4): 11–15.

Liu PT, Stenger S, Li H, Wenzel L, Tan BH, Krutzik SR, Ochoa MT, Schauber J, Wu K, Meinken C, Kamen DL, Wagner M, Bals R, Steinmeyer A, Zugel U, Gallo RL, Eisenberg D, Hewison M, Hollis BW, Adams JS, Bloom BR, Modlin RL. Toll-like receptor triggering of a vitamin D-mediated human antimicrobial response. Science 2006;311: 1770–3.

Mitschele T, Diesel B, Friedrich M, Meineke V, Maas RM, Gärtner BC, Kamradt J, Meese E, Tilgen W, Reichrath J, Analysis of the vitamin D system in basal cell carcinomas (BCCs). Lab Invest 2004;84: 693–702.

Moan J, Porojnicu AC, Robsahm TE, Dahlback A, Juzeniene A, Tretli S, Grant W, Solar radiation, vitamin D and survival rate of colon cancer in Norway. J Photochem Photobiol B 2005;78: 189–93.

Norval M, Cullen AP, de Gruijl FR, Longstreth J, Takizawa Y, Lucas RM, Noonan FP, van der Leun JC, The effects on human health from stratospheric ozone depletion and its interactions with climate change. Photochem Photobiol Sci 2007;6: 232.

Palm TA, The geographical distribution and etiology of rickets. Practitioner 1890;45: 270–79.

Peller S, Carcinogenesis as a means of reducing cancer mortality. Lancet 1936;2: 552–6.

Pilz S, Dobnig H, Nijpels G, Heine G et al., Vitamin D and mortality in older men and women. Clin Endocrinol 2009;71: 666–72.

Porojnicu AC, Robsahm TE, Dahlback A, Berg JP, Christiani D, Bruland OS, Moan J, Seasonal and geographical variations in lung cancer prognosis in Norway. Does vitamin D from the sun play a role? Lung Cancer 2007;55: 263–70.

Querings K, Reichrath J, A plea for detection and treatment of vitamin D deficiency in patients under photoprotection, including patients with xeroderma pigmentosum and basal cell nevus syndrome. Cancer Causes Control 2004;15: 219.

Querings K, Girndt M, Geisel J, Georg T, Tilgen W, Reichrath J, 25-Hydroxyvitamin D-deficiency in renal transplant recipients: an underrecognized health problem. J Clin Endocrinol Metab 2006;91: 526–9.

Raimondi S, Johansson H, Maisonneuve P, Gandini S, Review and meta-analysis on vitamin D receptor polymorphisms and cancer risk. Carcinogenesis 2009;30: 1170–80.

Schwartz GG, Whitlatch LW, Chen TC, Lokeshwar BL, Holick MF, Human prostate cells synthesize 1,25-dihydroxyvitamin D_3 from 25-hydroxyvitamin D_3. Cancer Epidemiol Biomarkers Prev 1998;7: 391–5.

Vieth R, Vitamin D supplementation, 25-hydroxyvitamin D concentrations, and safety. Am J Clin Nutr 1999;69: 842–56.

Wang T-T, Nestel FP, Bourdeau V, Nagai Y, Wang Q, Liao J, Tavera-Mendoza L, Lin R, Hanrahan JH, Mader S, White JH, Cutting edge: 1,25-dihydroxyvitamin D_3 is a direct inducer of antimicrobial peptide gene expression. J Immunol 2004;173: 2909–12.

Weber G, Heilborn JD, Chamorro Jimenez CI, Hammarsjö A, Törmä H, Ståhle M, Vitamin D induces the antimicrobial protein hCAP18 in human skin. J Invest Dermatol 2005;124: 1080–2.

Zittermann A, von Helden R, Grant WB, Kipshofen C et al., An estimate of the survival benefit of improving vitamin D status in the adult German population, submitted.

10.5 Vitamin D and cardiovascular disease: a review of the epidemiological and clinical evidence

Robert Scragg

10.5.1 Introduction

Scientific opinion about the role of vitamin D in cardiovascular disease has done a complete U-turn since the 1970s. Until then, the predominant viewpoint held that vitamin D was a cause of cardiovascular disease. This arose from linking the rare condition of infantile hypercalcaemia, thought to caused by ingestion of too high doses of vitamin D (Fraser, 1967), with an even rarer condition characterised by supravalvular aortic stenosis, elfin facies and severe mental retardation (Anonymous, 1966; Friedman, 1967; Seelig, 1969; Taussig, 1966). Moreover, the vascular conditions seen in supravalvular aortic stenosis could be reproduced in animal experiments by giving very high doses of vitamin D (Garcia et al., 1964). The development of animal models of arteriosclerosis caused by hypervitaminosis D, using mega-doses of 5000–10 000 IU/kg/day (Eisenstein et al., 1964; Schenk et al., 1965), equivalent to daily doses of 350 000–700 000 IU for a 70 kg adult human, confirmed early belief in the dangers of vitamin D. Reviews in the 1970s consistently concluded that vitamin D was a cause of atherosclerosis and coronary heart disease (Taylor et al., 1972; Yogamundi Moon, 1972; Kummerow, 1979).

There are two limitations of this earlier research that allowed researchers at that time to come to conclusions that are opposite to recent research. Firstly, there was an over-reliance on case reports in coming to conclusions about causation, which did not have controls to act as a reference point for determining whether the level of vitamin D intake during pregnancy by the mothers of cases was high or low. Secondly, there was a lack of appreciation that the amounts of vitamin D used in animal models were orders of magnitude higher than normally consumed by humans.

10.5.2 Early epidemiological studies

Epidemiological studies carried out in the 1970s were strongly influenced by the results of animal studies showing that toxic doses of vitamin D caused cardiovascular disease. An ecological study of eight regions within England and Wales found positive associations between vitamin D intake and mortality from ischemic heart disease ($r = 0.58$) and cerebrovascular disease ($r = 0.49$) during 1964–1969 (Knox et al., 1973). This finding was confirmed shortly after by a Norwegian case-control study which reported significantly higher mean daily intakes of vitamin D in myocardial infarction cases compared with age- and sex-matched controls (Linden, 1974).

The limitations of studies which used dietary methods to determine vitamin D status were revealed in the 1970s with the development of competitive protein-binding assays to measure blood 25-hydroxyvitamin D (25(OH)D) (Hollis and Horst, 2007), the main marker of vitamin D status. This method showed that most vitamin D comes from sun exposure, and less than 20% from diet (Haddad and Hahn, 1973; Poskitt et al., 1979).

Surprisingly at the time, case-control studies which first used the new assay observed 25(OH)D levels that were the same or lower in cases compared with controls, not higher as was expected (►Tab. 10.7). The first was a small case-control study from

Tab. 10.7: Summary of case-control studies of the association between blood levels of 25-hydroxyvitamin D and cardiovascular disease.

Study	Sample	Results
Schmidt-Gayk et al. (1977)	Heidelberg, Germany.	25(OH)D (Mean, range) in cases (32, 8–87) nmol/l, similar to controls in January and to controls aged 40–60 years (42, 10–79) and 60–79 years (21, 3–45) nmol/l.
	15 MI cases, mean age 65 years (range 51–78 years) interviewed in winter. 10 controls aged 40–60 years, and 10 aged 60–89 years.	
Lund et al. (1978)	Copenhagen, Denmark.	Total sample: 25(OH)D (Mean ± SD) in cases – MI (24.0 ± 10.0 ng/ml), angina (23.5 ± 9.6) – was similar to controls (28.8 ± 12.3).

(Continued)

Tab. 10.7 (*Continued*)

	128 cases (53 with MI and 75 with angina) consecutively admitted to hospital. 409 controls.	Cases had lower 25(OH)D levels than controls in May–June (p < 0.01) and July-August (p < 0.05).
Scragg et al. (1990)	Auckland, New Zealand.	Odds ratio (95% CI) by quartile of 25(OH)D.
	179 MI cases aged 35–64 years from register, with blood sample collected within 12 h of onset of symptoms.	<25 ng/ml = 1.00 25–32 ng/ml = 0.56 (0.30, 1.03) 33–42 ng/ml = 0.33 (0.17, 0.64) ≥ 43 ng/ml = 0.30 (0.15, 0.61)
	179 controls from electoral roll matched for age, sex and date of blood collection.	
Rajasree et al. (2001)	Kerala, India.	Median 25(OH)D for both cases and controls = 222.5 nmol/l (89 ng/ml).
	143 IHD hospital male cases, 88 patients with previous IHD referred for coronary angiography, 55 patients with acute MI.	59.4% of cases and 22.1% of controls were above the median 25(OH)D.
	70 male controls free of IHD, registered at same institute, and in same age range, as angiography cases.	Odds ratio (95% CI) for 25(OH)D ≥ median = 3.18 (1.31, 7.73), adjusted for smoking, blood lipids, blood calcium and phosphate.
Poole et al. (2006)	Cambridge, England.	Mean (95% CI) Z score for 25(OH)D in stroke cases = −1.4 (−1.7, −1.1), $p < 0.0001$.
	44 stroke cases, mean age 73 years, no prior history of stroke, blood sample collected within 30 days of stroke.	No relation between 25(OH)D level and length of time between stroke onset and collection of blood to measure 25OHD ($p = 0.77$).
	96 healthy free-living volunteers, mean age 69 years, provided blood samples every 2 months for 1 year to establish normal range for 25(OH)D.	

MI, myocardial infarction; 25(OH)D, 25-hydroxyvitamin D; IHD, ischaemic heart disease.

Heidelberg, with only 15 myocardial infarction cases interviewed in winter who had a mean 25(OH)D level of 32 nmol/l, which was similar to that for controls interviewed at the same time of year (Schmidt-Gayk et al., 1977). The next was a much larger study from Copenhagen (128 cases of myocardial infarction and angina, 409 controls) which reported similar mean 25(OH)D levels for cases and controls in the total sample, although cases had lower vitamin D levels than controls during May–August (Lund et al., 1978).

The third study was from Tromso (Vik et al., 1979), by the same research group which had previously reported higher oral vitamin D intakes in cases (Linden, 1974). The blood results came from a nested case-control study, similar in design to a cohort study with vitamin D levels in blood samples collected and stored at baseline, and then measured in cases who had a myocardial infarction during the follow-up period and in matched controls free of this disease during follow-up (results shown in ▶Tab. 10.8 for cohort studies). Again, 25(OH)D levels were found to be slightly lower in cases than controls, particularly after adjusting for vitamin D-binding protein.

10.5.3 Hypothesis that vitamin D protects against cardiovascular disease

Shortly after, a synthesis of the geographical variations in cardiovascular disease mortality by season, latitude and altitude lead to the hypothesis published in 1981 (Scragg, 1981), and later expanded (Scragg, 1995), that solar ultraviolet (UV) radiation, by increasing vitamin D levels, could protect against cardiovascular disease. The hypothesis provided a plausible explanation for two well-documented observations from the descriptive epidemiology of cardiovascular disease that were inconsistent with the temperature hypothesis that cold temperatures in winter are responsible for the mortality excess in cardiovascular disease at that time of year (Kvaloy and Skogvoll, 2007).

Firstly, the winter excess in cardiovascular disease mortality occurs in warm climates, such as North Queensland where average day-time winter temperatures are in the mid-20s °C (Scragg, 1995), in Los Angeles (Kloner et al., 1999) and in Hawaii where there is only a small seasonal variation in temperature from 22.8° to 27.8°C (Seto et al., 1998). Cold temperature is a convincing explanation for the winter excess in cardiovascular disease mortality in very cold climates such as the UK and USA (Donaldson and Keatinge, 2002; Barnett, 2007), but not for populations close to the equator. Secondly, the temperature hypothesis is not consistent with the well-documented inverse association between altitude and mortality from both cardiovascular disease and all-causes (Mortimer et al., 1977; Buechley et al., 1979; Voors and Johnson, 1979; Weinberg et al., 1987; Baibas et al., 2005; Winkelmayer et al., 2009), because temperature decreases by approximately 6.5°C for each 1000 m elevation from sea level (Scragg, 1995). By contrast, UV radiation increases by approximately 15% per 1000 m because of decreasing ozone (Barton and Paltridge, 1979), so that it is inversely associated with mortality. Further, the photoconversion of 7-dehydrocholesterol to previtamin D_3 has been shown to increase with altitude, particularly above 2000 m (Holick et al., 2007). The data showing an inverse association between solar radiation and coronary heart disease mortality in western Europe have recently been updated (Wong, 2008a).

Tab. 10.8: Summary of cohort studies from community samples of the association between blood levels of 25-hydroxyvitamin D and cardiovascular disease.

Study	Sample	Results
Vik et al. (1979)	Tromso, Norway.	Data for 23 cases and 46 matched controls free of disease at baseline.
	Nested case-control study.	25(OH)D (mean+SD) in cases (59.0 + 24.1 nmol/l) was similar to controls (63.4 + 27.2 nmol/l).
	Blood sample to measure 25(OH)D collected at baseline in 1974.	Mean 25(OH)D was lower in cases after correcting for blood level of vitamin D-binding protein ($p = 0.024$).
	30 MI male cases over 4 years follow-up matched with two controls each of same age and sex (controls $n = 60$).	
Wang et al. (2008)	Framingham, USA.	Adjusted hazard ratio (95% CI) by category of 25(OH)D:
	1739 men and women, mean age 59 years, without CV or renal disease at time of blood collection (during 1996–2001) for 25(OH)D.	>15 ng/ml = 1.00 10 to <15 ng/ml = 1.53 (1.00, 2.36) <10 ng/ml = 1.80 (1.05, 3.08) p-value for linear trend = 0.01
	120 participants had a CV event during mean 5.4 years of follow-up.	Stronger inverse association seen in people with hypertension than without, although p-value for interaction borderline (= 0.08).
Giovannucci et al. (2008)	Male health professionals, USA.	Adjusted odds ratio (95% CI) by category of 25(OH)D:
	Nested case-control study.	>30 ng/ml = 1.00
	18 225 men provided blood samples during 1993–1995 which was stored.	22.6–29.9 ng/ml = 1.60 (1.10, 2.32) 15.1–22.5 ng/ml = 1.43 (0.96, 2.13) <15.0 ng/ml = 2.09 (1.24, 3.54).
	During 10 years follow-up, 25(OH)D was measured in blood samples from 454 cases with fatal and non-fatal MI, without history of CV disease, and 900 controls individually matched for age, month of blood collection and smoking.	P-value for linear trend = 0.02
Ginde et al. (2009)	Third National Health & Nutrition Examination Survey, USA.	Adjusted hazard ratio (95% CI) for CV disease mortality by category of 25(OH)D:

(Continued)

Tab. 10.8 (*Continued*)

	3,408 men and women, representative sample of US population aged >65 years, provided blood sample at interview during 1998–1994.	<25.0 nmol/l = 2.36 (1.17, 4.75) 25.0–49.9 nmol/l = 1.54 (1.01, 2.34) 50.0–74.9 nmol/l = 1.26 (0.85, 1.88) 75.0–99.9 nmol/l = 1.20 (0.79, 1.81) ≥100.0 nmol/l = 1.00
	767 CV deaths, during median 7.3 years of follow-up to end of 2000.	
Kilkkinen et al. (2009)	Mini-Finland Health Survey.	Adjusted hazard ratio (95% CI) for CV disease mortality by quintile (Q) of 25(OH)D:
	6,219 men and women, mean age 49 years, surveyed in 40 centres, with collection of blood, during 1978–1980.	Q1 (low) = 1.00 Q2 = 1.04 (0.86, 1.26) Q3 = 0.81 (0.66, 1.00) Q4 = 0.86 (0.70, 1.06) Q5 = 0.76 (0.61, 0.95)
	933 participants died from CV disease during median 27.1 years of follow-up to end of 2006.	p-value for linear trend = 0.005
Pilz et al. (2009a)	Hoorn Study, the Netherlands.	Adjusted hazard ratio (95% CI) for CV disease mortality by quartile (Q) of 25(OH)D:
	Original sample recruited in 1989–1992.	Q1 (low) = 5.02 (1.88, 13.42) Q2–4 = 1.00 p-value = 0.001
	614 men and women, mean age ≈ 70 years, provided blood sample during 2000–2001.	
	20 participants died from CV disease during median 6.2 years of follow-up to 01 July 2007.	

MI, myocardial infarction; 25(OH)D, 25-hydroxyvitamin D; CV, cardiovascular; BMI, body mass index (kg/m²). nmol/l = 2.5 x ng/ml.

The hypothesis is also consistent with the well-known associations that vitamin D has with demographic factors. Older people, who have increased rates of cardiovascular disease, have lower vitamin D blood levels owing to a decreased capacity of the skin to synthesise vitamin D from solar exposure (MacLaughlin and Holick, 1985); and people with increased skin pigmentation, who have high rates of cardiovascular disease (Ramaraj and Chellappa, 2008), also synthesise less vitamin D from sun exposure (Clemens et al., 1982).

Direct evidence that vitamin D could have a role in cardiovascular function came initially from animal studies in North America with the detection of the receptor to 1,25-dihydroxyvitamin D, the active metabolite of vitamin D, in both cardiac muscle (Simpson, 1983) and smooth muscle (Kawashima, 1987); whereas myocardial hypertrophy could be produced in vitamin D-deficient rats, independent of changes in serum calcium, suggesting a direct effect of vitamin D on cardiac function (Weishaar and Simpson, 1987).

10.5.4 Case-control studies

The first major test of the hypothesis was a population-based case-control study carried out in Auckland, New Zealand, in the mid-1980s and published in 1990 (Scragg et al., 1990). Incident myocardial infarction cases, restricted to those with a blood sample collected within 12 h of onset of symptoms, to avoid any acute-phase reaction from the coronary event (Scragg et al., 1989), were compared with controls selected randomly from the electoral roll and matched for age, sex and date of blood collection (►Tab. 10.7). The unit of measurement for 25(OH)D in this study was actually ng/ml, rather than nmol/l as reported, but the findings are unchanged because the case-control comparisons were internal to the study. There was a significant inverse association between plasma 25(OH)D and risk of myocardial infarction, with the odds ratio for those in the highest 25(OH)D quartile being 0.30 (95% CI: 0.15, 0.61) compared with the lowest quartile (Scragg et al., 1990). The results held after further adjustment for serum cholesterol, smoking, BMI, physical activity, treatment of hypertension and past history of coronary heart disease.

The next major test of the hypothesis from an epidemiological study with hard disease endpoints did not come until 2001 when a further case-control study from Kerala, India, was published, which did not support the hypothesis (Rajasree et al., 2001). This study reported a significantly higher proportion of cases (59.4%) than controls (22.1%) with serum 25(OH)D levels above 222.5 nmol/l, a median value that was unusually high (►Tab. 10.7). However, this study had some major limitations which are likely to have invalidated its results. These include the selection of prevalent cases of ischaemic heart disease who had blood samples collected for vitamin D measurements an indeterminate time after their coronary event, and a sampling frame for cases and controls that is not well-described and which was hospital-based.

The next epidemiological study with disease end-points was a case-control study of stroke from Cambridge, England, published in 2006 (Poole et al., 2006). Incident cases of stroke were recruited, who were found to have a significantly lower mean Z-score of 25(OH)D than matched controls, although blood samples for vitamin D measurements were collected up to 30 days after the onset of disease in cases (►Tab. 10.7). Thus, there were continuing doubts about the validity of the case-control studies because of the possibility of the acute-phase reaction arising from the disease event causing a decrease in blood 25(OH)D levels in cases.

10.5.5 Cohort studies

During the past decade, for the first time since the 1979 nested case-control study from Tromso (Vik et al., 1979), reports from cohort studies began to be published, which overcame the concerns about the validity of the findings from the case-control studies. Beginning in 2003, these studies were initially of US haemodialysis patients, comparing survival in patients who were or were not given active vitamin D (analogues of

1,25-dihydroxyvitamin D). These studies have consistently shown an approximately 20% reduction in total mortality among patients prescribed active vitamin D (Al-Aly, 2007), mainly owing to reductions in mortality from cardiovascular diseases but also from respiratory infections (Shoji et al., 2004; Teng et al., 2005; Wolf et al., 2007; Naves-Diaz et al., 2008).

Since the beginning of 2008, several cohort studies have been published from samples of healthy people, mainly from the US, greatly strengthening the body of evidence linking low vitamin D status with increased risk of cardiovascular disease and all-cause mortality in the general population. Researchers working on the Framingham Study Offspring cohort ($n = 1739$) were first to publish (Wang et al., 2008). They found that participants with baseline serum 25(OH)D levels <10 ng/ml (25 nmol/l) had a hazard ratio of 1.80 (95% CI: 1.05, 3.08) for cardiovascular disease (fatal or non-fatal) during the 5-year follow-up period, compared with those >15 ng/ml (37.4 nmol/l) adjusting for a wide range of variables including demographic, blood pressure, blood lipids, cigarette smoking and body mass index (BMI) (▶Tab. 10.8). Further adjustment for physical activity, another potential confounder, did not affect the findings.

The next publication was a nested case-control comparison from the US Health Professionals Follow-up Study ($n = 18\,225$) which found that men with baseline plasma 25(OH)D levels ≤15 ng/ml (37.4 nmol/l) had a relative risk of 2.09 (95% CI: 1.24, 3.54) for myocardial infarction (fatal plus non-fatal) over 10 years follow-up compared with those with 25OHD ≥30 ng/ml (74.9 nmol/l) (Giovannucci et al., 2008). These results were adjusted for demographic and cardiovascular variables including season of month of blood collection, history of hypertension and diabetes, blood lipids, smoking status, alcohol intake, physical activity and BMI (▶Tab. 10.8).

This was followed by a third report, which was from the follow-up cohort ($n = 13\,331$) of the Third National Health and Nutrition examination Survey (NHANES III), a representative sample of the US population surveyed during 1988–1994 (Melamed et al., 2008a). Participants in the lowest quartile of baseline serum 25(OH)D <17.8 ng/ml (44.4 nmol/l) had a 26% (95% CI: 8, 46) increased risk of all-cause mortality during a median 8.7 years follow-up, compared with those in the highest 25OHD quartile (>32.1 ng/ml or 80.1 nmol/l), adjusting for demographic and cardiovascular risk factors, including physical activity and BMI. A further analysis of the NHANES III follow-up cohort, restricted to those ≥65 years, found that people with baseline 25(OH)D levels <25 nmol/l had more than double the risk of cardiovascular disease (hazard ratio 2.36, 95% CI: 1.17, 4.75) during follow-up compared with those with baseline 25OHD ≥100 nmol/l (▶Tab. 10.8), adjusting for demographic variables and major cardiovascular risk factors (Ginde et al., 2009).

The most recent US cohort study, published in 2009, found in a sample of 714 community-dwelling women aged 70–79 years from Baltimore, that women in the lowest vitamin D quartile (serum 25(OH)D <15.3 ng/ml or 38.2 nmol/l) had 2.45 (95% CI: 1.12, 5.36) times the risk of death (from all causes) during 6 years follow-up, compared with women in the highest quartile (>27.0 ng/ml or 67.4 nmol/l), after adjusting for demographic and cardiovascular variables (Semba et al., 2009).

Two cohort studies of European community samples have been published in 2009. The first is from the Mini-Finland Health Survey, which followed 6219 men and women aged ≥30 years, free of cardiovascular disease at baseline interviews in 1978–1980 up to the end of 2006 (Kilkkinen et al., 2009). Participants in the highest vitamin D quintile (serum 25(OH)D >62 nmol/l for men and >56 nmol/l for women) had a 24% reduction in cardiovascular disease mortality compared with those in the lowest quintile (<28 nmol/l for men and <23 nmol/l for women), adjusting for all covariates (►Tab. 10.8). The second comes from the Hoorn study in the Netherlands, which followed 614 men and women from 2000 to 2001, when their mean age was approximately 70 years, for a mean of 6.2 years until 01 July 2007 (Pilz et al., 2009a). Participants in the lowest vitamin D quartile (mean 25(OH)D = 30.6 nmol/l) had a 5-fold increase in the risk of cardiovascular mortality, and nearly 2-fold increase in all-cause mortality (hazard ratio = 1.93; 95% CI: 1.06, 3.51), when compared with the other three vitamin D quartiles, adjusting for all covariates including physical activity (►Tab. 10.8).

A further European study from Ludwigshafen in Germany, although not from a population cohort but patients (n = 3258) referred for coronary angiography, is described here because it used a similar design to the above studies (Dobnig et al., 2008). After a median period of 7.7 years, patients with baseline serum 25OHD levels in the bottom quartile had a significantly increased relative risk of all-cause mortality (hazard ratio = 2.08; 95% CI: 1.60, 2.70) and cardiovascular mortality (hazard ratio = 2.22; 95% CI: 1.57, 3.13) compared with those in the highest baseline 25OHD quartile, after adjusting for demographic and cardiovascular risk factors including smoking, blood pressure, blood lipids, physical activity and BMI. This study also reported that low serum levels of 1,25-dihydroxyvitamin D predicted both cardiovascular and all-cause mortality. A recent cohort study of patients referred to a specialist heart centre in Bad Oeynhausen, Germany, found that low serum levels of 1,25-dihydroxyvitamin D, but not 25(OH)D, predicted 1-year all-cause mortality (Zittermann et al., 2009).

10.5.6 Cross-sectional surveys

Recently, results from several cross-sectional surveys have been published showing significant inverse associations between serum 25(OH)D levels and risk of cardiovascular disease. These include data from the US NHANES surveys for 1988–1994 (Kendrick et al., 2009) and 2001–2004 (Kim et al., 2008), and German national nutrition surveys (Hintzpeter et al., 2008). However, these studies do not add to the body of evidence regarding the possible aetiological role of low vitamin D in cardiovascular disease, because the people with prevalent disease in these surveys will have had their disease event a variable time before they were interviewed, and it is not possible to infer anything about their vitamin D status at that time. By contrast, these studies do document a greater risk of vitamin D deficiency in people with prior cardiovascular disease, and should future intervention studies confirm a protective effect from vitamin D, these patients would warrant treatment with vitamin D supplements, given their increased risk of further cardiovascular events.

10.5.7 Experimental studies

The strongest evidence for causation comes from clinical trials. However, to-date, there has only been one randomised clinical trial (RCT) with the power (by itself) to detect any beneficial effect from vitamin D supplementation on cardiovascular disease risk. This is the Women's Health Initiative study which recruited 36 282 women aged 50–79 years at 40 sites in the US, who were randomised to take either calcium carbonate 500 mg with vitamin D 200 IU twice daily or placebo (Hsia et al., 2007). The adjusted hazard ratios of cardiovascular disease (fatal and non-fatal) after 7 years follow-up in the treated group versus control were 1.04 (95% CI: 0.92, 1.18) for coronary heart disease and 0.95 (95% CI: 0.82, 1.10) for stroke.

The lack of an effect seen in the women in the intervention arm of this study could be due to a possible increased risk of cardiovascular disease from the calcium supplements, which has recently been observed in a New Zealand study (Bolland et al., 2008), nullifying any beneficial effect from vitamin D. Alternatively, other well-recognised limitations of this study might explain the null findings. These include: a dose of vitamin D (400 IU/day) that would have only raised 25(OH)D levels by approximately 10 nmol/l (Heaney, 2008); poor compliance with only 59% of participants taking >80% of study medication; and contamination because participants in the placebo arm were able to take vitamin D (Michos and Blumenthal, 2007).

10.5.8 Other cardiovascular diseases

The above discussion has focused on evidence showing that vitamin D is inversely associated with risk of coronary heart disease and stroke, which both have acute onsets that make them suitable for epidemiological studies of disease events. However, there is increasing research showing that vitamin D is also inversely associated with other medical conditions across the spectrum of cardiovascular diseases, including those that are chronic in nature.

10.5.8.1 Hypertension

There is a substantial body of research linking vitamin D status and blood pressure, which goes back to studies in the 1980s showing elevated parathyroid hormone (PTH) levels in hypertension cases (McCarron et al., 1980; Zachariah et al., 1988), along with research showing inverse associations between blood levels of both $1,25(OH)_2D$ and PTH with renin in hypertension patients (Resnick et al., 1986). This research coincided with the detection of the receptor of 1,25-dihydroxyvitamin D in smooth muscle, mentioned above (Kawashima, 1987). Given the inverse association between vitamin D status and PTH, these studies suggested that low vitamin D levels might be a risk factor for hypertension. Recent observational studies support this proposal. An analysis of the Third National Health and Nutrition Examination Survey (NHANES III), a representative sample of the US population, found an inverse association between serum 25(OH)D and systolic blood pressure, but not diastolic, after adjusting for BMI (Scragg et al., 2007). A cross-sectional survey of Hispanic and African-Americans observed inverse associations between plasma 25(OH)D and both systolic and diastolic blood pressure which were no longer significant after adjusting for BMI (Schmitz et al., 2009). In cohort studies of US health professionals, baseline plasma 25(OH)D levels were inversely associated with risk of incident hypertension in both men and women (Forman et al., 2007).

However, experimental studies provide conflicting evidence. A randomised trial of patients with hypertension, carried out in Berlin, found that exposure to UV-B radiation over 6 weeks, which increases vitamin D, lowered blood pressure by 6 mmHg compared with the UV-A control group ($p<0.05$) (Krause et al., 1998). A randomised trial in elderly women, conducted in Bad Pyrmont, Germany, found that 800 IU of vitamin D_3 per day (with 1200 mg of calcium) after 8 weeks significantly decreased systolic blood pressure by 5 mmHg, but not diastolic, compared with placebo (Pfeifer et al., 2001). By contrast, vitamin D supplementation (with calcium) did not lower blood pressure in the US Women's Health Initiative study (Margolis et al., 2008), probably because of the low vitamin D dose and poor compliance (Geleijnse, 2008). A single 100 000 IU dose of vitamin D also did not have any effect on blood pressure after 5 weeks follow-up in a study carried out in Cambridge, UK (Scragg et al., 1995). Given the inconsistent evidence, large clinical trials using a daily vitamin D dose of >2000 IU are required to determine with certainty whether vitamin D lowers blood pressure.

10.5.8.2 Congestive heart failure

Since the early 1980s, there have been case reports of congestive heart failure with vitamin D deficiency and hypocalcaemia, in both adults and children, being successfully treated by vitamin D (in combination with calcium) (Connor et al., 1982; Gillor et al., 1989; Brunvand et al., 1995). These studies are consistent with animal experiments showing that vitamin D deficiency causes cardiac hypertrophy (Weishaar and Simpson, 1987). Studies of heart failure patients support the above findings. A US case series of patients with severe congestive heart failure undergoing evaluation for cardiac transplantation, found that patients with more severe disease had significantly lower 25(OH)D levels than other patients (Shane et al., 1997). Congestive heart failure patients referred to a clinic in Bad Oeynhausen, Germany, were found to have lower 25(OH)D and 1,25-dihydroxyvitamin D levels than controls (Zittermann et al., 2003). A recent case-control study also reported lower 1,25-dihydroxyvitamin D levels in patients with congestive heart failure than controls (Abou-Raya and Abou-Raya, 2009). A limitation of these studies is that the low vitamin D levels in heart failure patients could have been a consequence from less outdoor sun exposure owing to feeling unwell from their disease.

10.5.9 Vitamin D and pathophysiology

Evidence has progressively accumulated over the past 2–3 decades, from animal and clinical studies, to identify a range of mechanisms which potentially explain the effects of vitamin D on cardiovascular disease (▶Fig. 10.10).

10.5.9.1 Arterial function

There is increasing evidence that vitamin D directly influences endothelial and arterial function. Serum 25(OH)D levels are inversely associated with pulse pressure in both the general population (Scragg et al., 2007) and renal patients (Matias

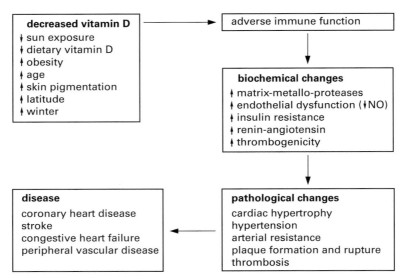

Fig. 10.10: Mechanisms by which low vitamin D status could increase the risk of cardiovascular disease.

et al., 2009), suggesting vitamin D might decrease vascular resistance. This possibility is supported by studies of vascular resistance, blood flow and flow-mediated dilatation in patients with hypertension and end-stage renal disease (Duprez et al., 1993; London et al., 2007) whereas vitamin D supplementation has been shown to increase flow-mediated brachial artery dilatation in type 2 diabetes patients who have 25(OH)D levels below 50 nmol/l (Sugden et al., 2008) and in young healthy volunteers with 25(OH)D levels below 25 nmol/l (Tarcin et al., 2009). Vitamin D could also affect the morphology of the arterial intima, with a study of type 2 diabetes patients observing an inverse association between serum 25(OH)D$_3$ and carotid artery intimal medial (Targher et al., 2006); although this has not been confirmed in studies of community samples (Michos et al., 2009; Pilz et al., 2009b). The inverse associations between serum 25(OH)D and flow-mediated dilatation suggest vitamin D could improve impaired endothelial function arising from reduced endothelial nitric oxide synthesis (Zieman et al., 2005), by reducing calcium influx into endothelial cells which decreases production of endothelium-derived contracting factors (Wong, 2008b); and leading ultimately to a reduced risk of coronary heart disease (Abrams, 1997; Monnink et al., 2004).

The above studies of arterial function also provide a potential explanation for recent evidence that vitamin D might be involved with micro-vascular disease. Analysis of data from the US NHANES survey (for 2001–2004) found that the prevalence ratio of peripheral arterial disease, as measured by the ratio of ankle to brachial artery blood pressures, increased by 35% for each 10 ng/ml (25 nmol/l) decrease in serum 25(OH)D (Melamed et al., 2008b); whereas an inverse association has been observed between serum 25(OH)D and micro-vascular complications in Japanese patients with type 2 diabetes (Suzuki et al., 2006).

10.5.9.2 Cardiac function

In humans, clinical trials have shown that vitamin D supplementation reduces heart rate (Scragg et al., 1995; Pfeifer et al., 2001); whereas a recent analysis of the US NHANES data shows that serum 25(OH)D levels are inversely associated with heart rate and also with the rate-pressure product (Scragg et al., 2010). The latter product (heart rate times systolic blood pressure) is a measure of cardiac work and cardiac oxygen demand, and is correlated with myocardial blood flow in healthy volunteers (Czernin et al., 1993; Chareonthaitawee et al., 2001). The inverse association between serum 25(OH)D and rate-pressure product suggests that low vitamin D status might increase cardiac work.

However, studies of direct measures of cardiac function provide inconsistent results. Studies of haemodialysis patients have found that vitamin D supplementation (with either 1-α-hydroxyvitamin D or 1,25-dihydroxyvitamin D) improves left ventricular cardiac function, as measured with echocardiography, by increasing fractional fibre shortening and decreasing end-systolic and end-diastolic diameter (McGonigle et al., 1981; Coratelli et al., 1984; Lemmila et al., 1998); and reduces measures of cardiac size (intraventricular wall thickness and left ventricle mass), without any change in blood pressure or cardiac output, in 15 haemodialysis patients compared with 10 control patients from Korea (Park et al., 1999). By contrast, a recent randomised controlled trial of 93 patients with congestive heart failure, from Bad Oeynhausen, Germany, did not observe an effect of vitamin D supplementation on echocardiographic measures of cardiac function (Schleithoff et al., 2006). Further trials, with larger sample sizes to ensure sufficient statistical power, are required.

10.5.9.3 Matrix-metalloproteinases

Recent animal studies, particularly with knock-out mice, have increased understanding of the effects of perturbations in vitamin D metabolism on the cardiovascular system. Mice lacking the receptor for 1,25-dihydroxyvitamin D have hypertension owing to up-regulation of the renin-angiotensin system (Li et al., 2002), and also cardiac hypertrophy and fibrosis from increased interstitial collagen deposition (Simpson et al., 2007), and up-regulation of matrix-metalloproteinases (MMP-2 and MMP-9) (Rahman et al., 2007). Mice without the enzyme that converts 25(OH)D to the active metabolite (1,25-dihydroxyvitamin D) also develop hypertension, cardiac hypertrophy and up-regulation of the renin-angiotensin system which are reversed by adding vitamin D to their food, through direct effects that are independent of changes in serum calcium and phosphorus (Zhou et al., 2008); whereas the 1-α hydroxylase enzyme has been detected in cardiac tissue providing evidence for the autocrine synthesis of 1,25-dihydroxyvitamin D locally within the heart (Chen et al., 2008).

This evidence is consistent with human studies which have shown that vitamin D supplementation lowers blood MMP-9 and MMP-2 (Timms et al., 2002); and observed raised plasma levels of MMP-9 in men who had increased left-ventricular end-diastolic dimensions and wall thickness from the Framingham study (Sundstrom et al., 2004). Vitamin D, in addition to cardiac tissue, could also influence remodelling of blood vessels by preventing MMP-induced intimal thickening of blood vessels and thereby reduce arterial stiffness (Yasmin et al., 2005).

10.5.9.4 Thrombosis

The seasonality of cardiovascular disease, with increased rates in winter when vitamin D levels are low (Scragg, 1981; Scragg, 1995), is consistent with an effect of vitamin D on thrombotic function. Recently, a cohort study of Swedish women found an inverse association between sun exposure and risk of venous thrombo-embolism (Lindqvist et al., 2009). A clinical trial of cancer patients has reported that high dose calcitriol decreased thrombotic events (Beer et al., 2006); whereas a Norwegian cross-sectional survey found a positive association between serum 25(OH)D and fibrinolytic activity (Jorde et al., 2007). Animal and laboratory studies have observed effects of vitamin D on thrombotic factors (Aihara et al., 2004; Wu-Wong et al., 2007).

10.5.9.5 Inflammatory factors

Vitamin D is now known to influence the innate immune system by stimulating the synthesis of the antimicrobial peptide cathelicidin (Liu et al., 2006). Cytokines are also influenced by vitamin D. *In vitro* studies have shown that calcitriol decreases production of pro-inflammatory cytokines such as the cytokine interleukin-6 (IL-6) and tumour-necrosis-factor-α (TNFα) by macrophages and lymphocytes (Muller et al., 1991; Willheim et al., 1999; Zhu et al., 2005) and up-regulates synthesis of anti-inflammatory IL-10 (Canning et al., 2001). However, results from human studies are not consistent. Vitamin D supplementation (2000 IU/day for 9 months) decreased TNFα and increased IL-10, with no effect on C-reactive protein, in German patients with congestive heart failure (Schleithoff et al., 2006). Calcitriol supplementation decreased blood levels of IL-1 and IL-6 in haemodialysis patients (Turk et al., 2002). Serum levels of 25(OH)D were inversely associated with C-reactive protein and IL-6 in German coronary angiography patients (Dobnig et al., 2008). By contrast, studies which gave lower doses of vitamin D ($\leq$800 IU/day) did not find any effect from it on IL-6, TNFα and C-reactive protein (Turk et al., 2002; Pittas et al., 2007).

Inflammatory factors are centrally involved in the process of atherosclerosis and plaque rupture (Ross et al., 1999; Hansson et al., 2002; Rao et al., 2006). Blood levels of inflammatory markers, such as C-reactive protein and IL-6, predict subsequent risk of cardiovascular disease (Rao et al., 2006; Tousoulis et al., 2006). Inflammatory cytokines also influence endothelial function (Cardaropoli et al., 2003; Tousoulis et al., 2006), which is an independent predictor of cardiovascular disease (Khoshdel et al., 2007), and synthesis of MMPs (Newby, 2005) which also have a role in cardiovascular disease (Loftus and Thompson, 2002; Perlstein and Lee, 2006); whereas positive associations have been reported between IL-6 and insulin resistance (Mohamed-Ali et al., 1997; Bastard et al., 2000; Turk et al., 2002). The emerging evidence suggests that alterations in inflammatory processes and immune function might underpin the effects of vitamin D on the cardiovascular system (▶Fig. 10.10).

10.5.10 Summary

Research on vitamin D and cardiovascular disease has reached a crucial point, where clinical trials are required to determine the safety of long-term high-dosage vitamin D supplementation (>2000 IU per day), and its effectiveness on cardiovascular disease rates. A recent meta-analysis of vitamin D supplementation trials, originally implemented to assess the effect on fracture rates of vitamin D, often in combination with calcium, has observed a 7% absolute reduction in all-cause mortality among those receiving vitamin D (Autier and Gandini, 2007). This effect was produced by a weighted vitamin D dose of 528 IU/day. Extrapolating this effect out to higher vitamin D doses, and assuming a linear effect, it is possible that higher doses could potentially result in greater reductions in mortality (e.g., relative risk for 2000 IU/day = $0.93^4 = 0.75$, or a 25% reduction in total mortality). If randomised trials do show that vitamin D reduces risk of cardiovascular disease, simple and cheap prevention strategies will lead to significant gains in public health.

References

Anonymous, Congenital supravalvular aortic stenosis, idiopathic hypercalcemia, and vitamin D. Nutr Rev 1966;24: 311–3.

Abou-Raya S, Abou-Raya A, Osteoporosis and congestive heart failure (CHF) in the elderly patient: double disease burden. Arch Gerontol Geriatr 2009;49: 250–4.

Abrams J, Role of endothelial dysfunction in coronary artery disease. Am J Cardiol 1997;79: 2–9.

Aihara K, Azuma H, Akaike M, Ikeda Y, Yamashita M, Sudo T, Hayashi H, Yamada Y, Endoh F, Fujimura M, Yoshida T, Yamaguchi H, Hashizume S, Kato M, Yoshimura K, Yamamoto Y, Kato S, Matsumoto T, Disruption of nuclear vitamin D receptor gene causes enhanced thrombogenicity in mice. J Biol Chem 2004;279: 35798–802.

Al-Aly Z, Vitamin D as a novel nontraditional risk factor for mortality in hemodialysis patients: the need for randomized trials. Kidney Int 2007;72: 909–11.

Autier P, Gandini S, Vitamin D supplementation and total mortality: a meta-analysis of randomized controlled trials. Arch Intern Med 2007;167: 1730–7.

Baibas N, Trichopoulou A, Voridis E, Trichopoulos D, Residence in mountainous compared with lowland areas in relation to total and coronary mortality. A study in rural Greece. J Epidemiol Community Health 2005;59: 274–8.

Barnett AG, Temperature and cardiovascular deaths in the US elderly: changes over time. Epidemiology 2007;18: 369–72.

Barton IJ, Paltridge GW, The Australian climatology of biologically effective ultraviolet radiation. Australas J Dermatol 1979;20: 68–74.

Bastard JP, Jardel C, Bruckert E, Blondy P, Capeau J, Laville M, Vidal H, Hainque B, Elevated levels of interleukin 6 are reduced in serum and subcutaneous adipose tissue of obese women after weight loss. J Clin Endocrinol Metab 2000;85: 3338–42.

Beer TM, Venner PM, Ryan CW, Petrylak DP, Chatta G, Dean Ruether J, Chi KN, Curd JG, De-Loughery TG, High dose calcitriol may reduce thrombosis in cancer patients. Br J Haematol 2006;135: 392–4.

Bolland MJ, Barber PA, Doughty RN, Mason B, Horne A, Ames R, Gamble GD, Grey A, Reid IR, Vascular events in healthy older women receiving calcium supplementation: randomised controlled trial. Br Med J 2008;336: 262–6.

Brunvand L, Haga P, Tangsrud SE, Haug E, Congestive heart failure caused by vitamin D deficiency? Acta Paediatr 1995;84: 106–8.

Buechley RW, Key CR, Morris DL, Morton WE, Morgan MV, Altitude and ischemic heart disease in tricultural New Mexico: an example of confounding. Am J Epidemiol 1979;109: 663–6.

Canning MO, Grotenhuis K, de Wit H, Ruwhof C, Drexhage HA, 1-alpha,25-Dihydroxyvitamin D3 (1,25(OH)(2)D(3)) hampers the maturation of fully active immature dendritic cells from monocytes. Eur J Endocrinol 2001;145: 351–7.

Cardaropoli S, Silvagno F, Morra E, Pescarmona GP, Todros T, Infectious and inflammatory stimuli decrease endothelial nitric oxide synthase activity in vitro. J Hypertens 2003;21: 2103–10.

Chareonthaitawee P, Kaufmann PA, Rimoldi O, Camici PG, Heterogeneity of resting and hyperemic myocardial blood flow in healthy humans. Cardiovasc Res 2001;5: 151–61.

Chen S, Glenn DJ, Ni W, Grigsby CL, Olsen K, Nishimoto M, Law CS, Gardner DG, Expression of the vitamin D receptor is increased in the hypertrophic heart. Hypertension 2008;52: 1106–12.

Clemens TL, Adams JS, Henderson SL, Holick MF, Increased skin pigment reduces the capacity of skin to synthesise vitamin D3. Lancet 1982;1: 74–76.

Connor TB, Rosen BL, Blaustein MP, Applefeld MM, Doyle LA, Hypocalcemia precipitating congestive heart failure. N Engl J Med 1982;307: 869–72.

Coratelli P, Petrarulo F, Buongiorno E, Giannattasio M, Antonelli G, Amerio A, Improvement in left ventricular function during treatment of hemodialysis patients with 25-OHD3. Contrib Nephrol 1984;41: 433–7.

Czernin J, Muller P, Chan S, Brunken RC, Porenta G, Krivokapich J, Chen K, Chan A, Phelps ME, Schelbert HR, Influence of age and hemodynamics on myocardial blood flow and flow reserve. Circulation 1993;88: 62–9.

Dobnig H, Pilz S, Scharnagl H, Renner W, Seelhorst U, Wellnitz B, Kinkeldei J, Boehm BO, Weihrauch G, Maerz W, Independent association of low serum 25-hydroxyvitamin D and 1,25-dihydroxyvitamin D levels with all-cause and cardiovascular mortality. Arch Intern Med 2008;168: 1340–9.

Donaldson GC, Keatinge WR, Excess winter mortality: influenza or cold stress? Observational study. Br Med J 2002;324: 89–90.

Duprez D, De Buyzere M, De Backer T, Clement D, Relationship between vitamin D and the regional blood flow and vascular resistance in moderate arterial hypertension. J Hypertens 1993;11(Suppl): S304–5.

Eisenstein R, Zeruolis L, Vitamin D-induced aortic calcification. Arch Pathol 1964;77: 27–35.

Forman JP, Giovannucci E, Holmes MD, Bischoff-Ferrari HA, Tworoger SS, Willett WC, Curhan GC, Plasma 25-hydroxyvitamin D levels and risk of incident hypertension. Hypertension 2007;49: 1063–9.

Fraser D, The relation between infantile hypercalcemia and vitamin D – public health implications in North America. Pediatrics 1967;40: 1050–61.

Friedman WF, Vitamin D as a cause of the supravalvular aortic stenosis syndrome. Am Heart J 1967;73: 718–20.

Garcia RE, Friedman WF, Kaback MM, Rowe RD, Idiopathic hypercalcemia and supravalvular aortic stenosis. Documentation of a new syndrome. N Engl J Med 1964;271: 117–20.

Geleijnse JM, Vitamin D and hypertension: does the women's health initiative solve the question? Hypertension 2008;52: 803–4.

Gillor A, Groneck P, Kaiser J, Schmitz-Stolbrink A, Congestive heart failure in rickets caused by vitamin D deficiency. Monatsschr Kinderheilkd 1989;137: 108–10.

Ginde AA, Scragg R, Schwartz RS, Camargo CA Jr, Prospective study of serum 25-hydroxyvitamin D Level, cardiovascular disease mortality, and all-cause mortality in older U.S. adults. J Am Geriatr Soc 2009;57: 1595–603.

Giovannucci E, Liu Y, Hollis BW, Rimm EB, 25-Hydroxyvitamin D and risk of myocardial infarction in men: a prospective study. Arch Intern Med 2008;168: 1174–80.

Haddad JG Jr, Hahn TJ, Natural and synthetic sources of circulating 25-hydroxyvitamin D in man. Nature 1973;244: 515–7.

Hansson GK, Libby P, Schonbeck U, Yan ZQ, Innate and adaptive immunity in the pathogenesis of atherosclerosis. Circ Res 2002;91: 281–91.

Heaney RP, Vitamin D in health and disease. Clin J Am Soc Nephrol 2008;3: 1535–41.

Hintzpeter B, Mensink GB, Thierfelder W, Muller MJ, Scheidt-Nave C, Vitamin D status and health correlates among German adults. Eur J Clin Nutr 2008;62: 1079–89.

Holick MF, Chen TC, Lu Z, Sauter E, Vitamin D and skin physiology: a D-lightful story. J Bone Miner Res 2007;22(Suppl 2): V28–33.

Hollis BW, Horst RL, The assessment of circulating 25(OH)D and 1,25(OH)2D: where we are and where we are going. J Steroid Biochem Mol Biol 2007;103: 473–6.

Hsia J, Heiss G, Ren H, Allison M, Dolan NC, Greenland P, Heckbert SR, Johnson KC, Manson JE, Sidney S, Trevisan M, Calcium/vitamin D supplementation and cardiovascular events. Circulation 2007;115: 846–54.

Jorde R, Haug E, Figenschau Y, Hansen JB, Serum levels of vitamin D and haemostatic factors in healthy subjects: the Tromso study. Acta Haematol 2007;117: 91–7.

Kawashima H, Receptor for 1,25-dihydroxyvitamin D in a vascular smooth muscle cell line derived from rat aorta. Biochem Biophys Res Commun 1987;146: 1–6.

Kendrick J, Targher G, Smits G, Chonchol M, 25-Hydroxyvitamin D deficiency is independently associated with cardiovascular disease in the Third National Health and Nutrition Examination Survey. Atherosclerosis 2009;205: 255–60.

Khoshdel AR, Carney SL, Nair BR, Gillies A, Better management of cardiovascular diseases by pulse wave velocity: combining clinical practice with clinical research using evidence-based medicine. Clin Med Res 2007;5: 45–52.

Kilkkinen A, Knekt P, Aro A, Rissanen H, Marniemi J, Heliovaara M, Impivaara O, Reunanen A, Vitamin D status and the risk of cardiovascular disease death. Am J Epidemiol 2009;170: 1032–9.

Kim DH, Sabour S, Sagar UN, Adams S, Whellan DJ, Prevalence of hypovitaminosis D in cardiovascular diseases (from the National Health and Nutrition Examination Survey 2001 to 2004). Am J Cardiol 2008;102: 1540–4.

Kloner RA, Poole WK, Perritt RL, When throughout the year is coronary death most likely to occur? A 12-year population-based analysis of more than 220,000 cases. Circulation 1999;100: 1630–4.

Knox EG, Ischaemic-heart-disease mortality and dietary intake of calcium. Lancet 1973;1: 1465–7.

Krause R, Buhring M, Hopfenmuller W, Holick MF, Sharma AM, Ultraviolet B and blood pressure. Lancet 1998;352: 709–10.

Kummerow FA, Nutrition imbalance and angiotoxins as dietary risk factors in coronary heart disease. Am J Clin Nutr 1979;32: 58–83.

Kvaloy JT, Skogvoll E, Modelling seasonal and weather dependency of cardiac arrests using the covariate order method. Stat Med 2007;26: 3315–29.

Lemmila S, Saha H, Virtanen V, Ala-Houhala I, Pasternack A, Effect of intravenous calcitriol on cardiac systolic and diastolic function in patients on hemodialysis. Am J Nephrol 1998;18: 404–10.

Li YC, Kong J, Wei M, Chen ZF, Liu SQ, Cao LP, 1,25-Dihydroxyvitamin D(3) is a negative endocrine regulator of the renin-angiotensin system. J Clin Invest 2002;110: 229–38.

Linden V, Vitamin D and myocardial infarction. Br Med J 1974;3: 647–50.

Lindqvist PG, Epstein E, Olsson H, Does an active sun exposure habit lower the risk of venous thrombotic events? A D-lightful hypothesis. J Thromb Haemost 2009;7: 605–10.

Liu PT, Stenger S, Li H, Wenzel L, Tan BH, Krutzik SR, Ochoa MT, Schauber J, Wu K, Meinken C, Kamen DL, Wagner M, Bals R, Steinmeyer A, Zugel U, Gallo RL, Eisenberg D, Hewison M, Hollis BW, Adams JS, Bloom BR, Modlin RL, Toll-like receptor triggering of a vitamin D-mediated human antimicrobial response. Science 2006;311: 1770–3.

Loftus IM, Thompson MM, The role of matrix metalloproteinases in vascular disease. Vasc Med 2002;7: 117–33.

London GM, Guerin AP, Verbeke FH, Pannier B, Boutouyrie P, Marchais SJ, Metivier F, Mineral metabolism and arterial functions in end-stage renal disease: potential role of 25-hydroxyvitamin D deficiency. J Am Soc Nephrol 2007;18: 613–20.

Lund B, Badskjaer J, Lund B, Soerensen OH, Vitamin D and ischaemic heart disease. Horm Metab Res 1978;10: 553–6.

MacLaughlin J, Holick MF, Aging decreases the capacity of human skin to produce vitamin D3. J Clin Invest 1985;76: 1536–8.

Margolis KL, Ray RM, Van Horn L, Manson JE, Allison MA, Black HR, Beresford SA, Connelly SA, Curb JD, Grimm RH Jr, Kotchen TA, Kuller LH, Wassertheil-Smoller S, Thomson CA, Torner JC, Effect of calcium and vitamin D supplementation on blood pressure: the Women's Health Initiative Randomized Trial. Hypertension 2008;52: 847–55.

Matias PJ, Ferreira C, Jorge C, Borges M, Aires I, Amaral T, Gil C, Cortez J, Ferreira A, 25-Hydroxyvitamin D3, arterial calcifications and cardiovascular risk markers in haemodialysis patients. Nephrol Dial Transplant 2009;24: 611–8.

McCarron DA, Pingree PA, Rubin RJ, Gaucher SM, Molitch M, Krutzik S, Enhanced parathyroid function in essential hypertension: a homeostatic response to a urinary calcium leak. Hypertension 1980;2: 162–8.

McGonigle RJ, Timmis AD, Keenan J, Jewitt DE, Weston MJ, Parsons V, The influence of 1 alpha-hydroxycholecalciferol on left ventricular function in end-stage renal failure. Proc Eur Dial Transplant Assoc 1981;18: 579–85.

Melamed ML, Michos ED, Post W, Astor B, 25-hydroxyvitamin D levels and the risk of mortality in the general population. Arch Intern Med 2008a;168: 1629–37.

Melamed ML, Muntner P, Michos ED, Uribarri J, Weber C, Sharma J, Raggi P, Serum 25-hydroxyvitamin D levels and the prevalence of peripheral arterial disease. Results from NHANES 2001 to 2004. Arterioscler Thromb Vasc Biol 2008b;28: 1179–85.

Michos ED, Blumenthal RS, Vitamin D supplementation and cardiovascular disease risk. Circulation 2007;115: 827–8.

Michos ED, Streeten EA, Ryan KA, Rampersaud E, Peyser PA, Bielak LF, Shuldiner AR, Mitchell BD, Post W, serum 25-hydroxyvitamin D levels are not associated with subclinical vascular disease or C-reactive protein in the Old Order Amish. Calcif Tissue Int 2009;84: 195–202.

Mohamed-Ali V, Goodrick S, Rawesh A, Katz DR, Miles JM, Yudkin JS, Klein S, Coppack SW, Subcutaneous adipose tissue releases interleukin-6, but not tumor necrosis factor-alpha, in vivo. J Clin Endocrinol Metab 1997;82: 4196–200.

Monnink SH, Tio RA, van Boven AJ, van Gilst WH, van Veldhuisen DJ, The role of coronary endothelial function testing in patients suspected for angina pectoris. Int J Cardiol 2004;96: 123–9.

Mortimer EA Jr, Monson RR, MacMahon B, Reduction in mortality from coronary heart disease in men residing at high altitude. N Engl J Med 1977;296: 581–5.

Muller K, Diamant M, Bendtzen K, Inhibition of production and function of interleukin-6 by 1,25-dihydroxyvitamin D3. Immunol Lett 1991;28: 115–20.

Naves-Diaz M, Alvarez-Hernandez D, Passlick-Deetjen J, Guinsburg A, Marelli C, Rodriguez-Puyol D, Cannata-Andia JB, Oral active vitamin D is associated with improved survival in hemodialysis patients. Kidney Int 2008;74: 1070–8.

Newby AC, Dual role of matrix metalloproteinases (matrixins) in intimal thickening and atherosclerotic plaque rupture. Physiol Rev 2005;85: 1–31.

Park CW, Oh YS, Shin YS, Kim CM, Kim YS, Kim SY, Choi EJ, Chang YS, Bang BK, Intravenous calcitriol regresses myocardial hypertrophy in hemodialysis patients with secondary hyperparathyroidism. Am J Kidney Dis 1999;33: 73–81.

Perlstein TS, Lee RT, Smoking, metalloproteinases, and vascular disease. Arterioscler Thromb Vasc Biol 2006;26: 250–6.

Pfeifer M, Begerow B, Minne HW, Nachtigall D, Hansen C, Effects of a short-term vitamin D(3) and calcium supplementation on blood pressure and parathyroid hormone levels in elderly women. J Clin Endocrinol Metab 2001;86: 1633–7.

Pilz S, Dobnig H, Nijpels G, Heine RJ, Stehouwer CD, Snijder MB, van Dam RM, Dekker JM, Vitamin D and mortality in older men and women. Clin Endocrinol (Oxf) 2009a;71: 666–72.

Pilz S, Henry RM, Snijder MB, van Dam RM, Nijpels G, Stehouwer CD, Tomaschitz A, Pieber TR, Dekker JM, 25-Hydroxyvitamin D is not associated with carotid intima-media thickness in older men and women. Calcif Tissue Int 2009b;84: 423–4.

Pittas AG, Harris SS, Stark PC, Dawson-Hughes B, The effects of calcium and vitamin D supplementation on blood glucose and markers of inflammation in nondiabetic adults. Diabetes Care 2007;30: 980–6.

Poole KE, Loveridge N, Barker PJ, Halsall DJ, Rose C, Reeve J, Warburton EA, Reduced vitamin D in acute stroke. Stroke 2006;37: 243–5.

Poskitt EM, Cole TJ, Lawson DE, Diet, sunlight, and 25-hydroxy vitamin D in healthy children and adults. Br Med J 1979;1: 221–3.

Rahman A, Hershey S, Ahmed S, Nibbelink K, Simpson RU, Heart extracellular matrix gene expression profile in the vitamin D receptor knockout mice. J Steroid Biochem Mol Biol 2007;103: 416–9.

Rajasree S, Rajpal K, Kartha CC, Sarma PS, Kutty VR, Iyer CS, Girija G, Serum 25-hydroxyvitamin D3 levels are elevated in South Indian patients with ischemic heart disease. Eur J Epidemiol 2001;17: 567–71.

Ramaraj R, Chellappa P, Cardiovascular risk in South Asians. Postgrad Med J 2008;84: 518–23.

Rao M, Jaber BL, Balakrishnan VS, Inflammatory biomarkers and cardiovascular risk: association or cause and effect? Semin Dial 2006;19: 129–35.

Resnick LM, Muller FB, Laragh JH, Calcium-regulating hormones in essential hypertension. Relation to plasma renin activity and sodium metabolism. Ann Intern Med 1986;105: 649–54.

Ross R, Atherosclerosis – an inflammatory disease. N Engl J Med 1999;340: 115–26.

Schenk EA, Penn I, Schwartz S, Experimental atherosclerosis in the dog: a morphologic evaluation. Arch Pathol 1965;80: 102–9.

Schleithoff SS, Zittermann A, Tenderich G, Berthold HK, Stehle P, Koerfer R, Vitamin D supplementation improves cytokine profiles in patients with congestive heart failure: a double-blind, randomized, placebo-controlled trial. Am J Clin Nutr 2006;83: 754–9.

Schmidt-Gayk H, Goossen J, Lendle F, Seidel D, Serum 25-hydroxycalciferol in myocardial infarction. Atherosclerosis 1977;26: 55–8.

Schmitz KJ, Skinner HG, Bautista LE, Fingerlin TE, Langefeld CD, Hicks PJ, Haffner SM, Bryer-Ash M, Wagenknecht LE, Bowden DW, Norris JM, Engelman CD, Association of 25-hydroxyvitamin D with blood pressure in predominantly 25-hydroxyvitamin D deficient Hispanic and African Americans. Am J Hypertens 2009;22: 867–70.

Scragg R, Seasonality of cardiovascular disease mortality and the possible protective effect of ultraviolet radiation. Int J Epidemiol 1981;10: 337–41.

Scragg R, Sunlight, vitamin D and cardiovascular disease. In: Crass MF, Avioloi LV, editors. Calcium-regulating hormones and cardiovascular function. Boca Raton: CRC Press; 1995. pp. 213–37.

Scragg R, Jackson R, Holdaway I, Woollard G, Woollard D, Changes in plasma vitamin levels in the first 48 hours after onset of acute myocardial infarction. Am J Cardiol 1989;64: 971–4.

Scragg R, Jackson R, Holdaway IM, Lim T, Beaglehole R, Myocardial infarction is inversely associated with plasma 25-hydroxyvitamin D3 levels: a community-based study. Int J Epidemiol 1990;19: 559–3.

Scragg R, Khaw KT, Murphy S, Effect of winter oral vitamin D3 supplementation on cardiovascular risk factors in elderly adults. Eur J Clin Nutr 1995;49: 640–6.

Scragg R, Sowers M, Bell C, Serum 25-hydroxyvitamin D, ethnicity, and blood pressure in the Third National Health and Nutrition Examination Survey. Am J Hypertens 2007;20: 713–9.

Scragg RK, Camargo CA, Simpson RU, Relation of Serum 25-Hydroxyvitamin D to Heart Rate and Cardiac Work (From the National Health and Nutrition Examination Surveys). Am J Cardiol 2010 (in press).

Seelig MS, Vitamin D and cardiovascular, renal, and brain damage in infancy and childhood. Ann NY Acad Sci 1969;147: 539–82.

Semba RD, Houston DK, Ferrucci L, Cappola AR, Sun K, Guralnik JM, Fried LP, Low serum 25-hydroxyvitamin D concentrations are associated with greater all-cause mortality in older community-dwelling women. Nutr Res 2009;29: 525–30.

Seto TB, Mittleman MA, Davis RB, Taira DA, Kawachi I, Seasonal variation in coronary artery disease mortality in Hawaii: observational study. Br Med J 1998;316: 1946–7.

Shane E, Mancini D, Aaronson K, Silverberg SJ, Seibel MJ, Addesso V, McMahon DJ, Bone mass, vitamin D deficiency, and hyperparathyroidism in congestive heart failure. Am J Med 1997;103: 197–207.

Shoji T, Shinohara K, Kimoto E, Emoto M, Tahara H, Koyama H, Inaba M, Fukumoto S, Ishimura E, Miki T, Tabata T, Nishizawa Y, Lower risk for cardiovascular mortality in oral 1alpha-hydroxy vitamin D3 users in a haemodialysis population. Nephrol Dial Transplant 2004;19: 179–84.

Simpson RU, Evidence for a specific 1,25-dihydroxyvitamin D3 receptor in rat heart. Circulation 1983;68: 239.

Simpson RU, Hershey SH, Nibbelink KA, Characterization of heart size and blood pressure in the vitamin D receptor knockout mouse. J Steroid Biochem Mol Biol 2007;103: 521–4.

Sugden JA, Davies JI, Witham MD, Morris AD, Struthers AD, Vitamin D improves endothelial function in patients with Type 2 diabetes mellitus and low vitamin D levels. Diabet Med 2008;25: 320–5.

Sundstrom J, Evans JC, Benjamin EJ, Levy D, Larson MG, Sawyer DB, Siwik DA, Colucci WS, Sutherland P, Wilson PW, Vasan RS, Relations of plasma matrix metalloproteinase-9 to clinical cardiovascular risk factors and echocardiographic left ventricular measures: the Framingham Heart Study. Circulation 2004;109: 2850–6.

Suzuki A, Kotake M, Ono Y, Kato T, Oda N, Hayakawa N, Hashimoto S, Itoh M, Hypovitaminosis D in type 2 diabetes mellitus: Association with microvascular complications and type of treatment. Endocr J 2006;53: 503–10.

Tarcin O, Yavuz DG, Ozben B, Telli A, Ogunc AV, Yuksel M, Toprak A, Yazici D, Sancak S, Deyneli O, Akalin S, Effect of vitamin D deficiency and replacement on endothelial function in asymptomatic subjects. J Clin Endocrinol Metab 2009;94: 4023–30.

Targher G, Bertolini L, Padovani R, Zenari L, Scala L, Cigolini M, Arcaro G, Serum 25-hydroxyvitamin D3 concentrations and carotid artery intima-media thickness among type 2 diabetic patients. Clin Endocrinol (Oxf) 2006;65: 593–7.

Taussig HB, Possible injury to the cardiovascular system from vitamin D. Ann Intern Med 1966;65: 1195–200.

Taylor CB, Hass GM, Ho KJ, Liu LB, Risk factors in the pathogenesis of atherosclerotic heart disease and generalized atherosclerosis. Ann Clin Lab Sci 1972;2: 239–43.

Teng M, Wolf M, Ofsthun MN, Lazarus JM, Hernan MA, Camargo CA Jr, Thadhani R, Activated injectable vitamin D and hemodialysis survival: a historical cohort study. J Am Soc Nephrol 2005;16: 1115–25.

Timms PM, Mannan N, Hitman GA, Noonan K, Mills PG, Syndercombe-Court D, Aganna E, Price CP, Boucher BJ, Circulating MMP9, vitamin D and variation in the TIMP-1 response with VDR genotype: mechanisms for inflammatory damage in chronic disorders? Q J Med 2002;95: 787–96.

Tousoulis D, Antoniades C, Koumallos N, Stefanadis C, Pro-inflammatory cytokines in acute coronary syndromes: from bench to bedside. Cytokine Growth Factor Rev 2006;17: 225–33.

Turk S, Akbulut M, Yildiz A, Gurbilek M, Gonen S, Tombul Z, Yeksan M, Comparative effect of oral pulse and intravenous calcitriol treatment in hemodialysis patients: the effect on serum IL-1 and IL-6 levels and bone mineral density. Nephron 2002;90: 188–94.

Vik T, Try K, Thelle DS, Forde OH, Tromso Heart Study: vitamin D metabolism and myocardial infarction. Br Med J 1979;2: 176.

Voors AW, Johnson WD, Altitude and arteriosclerotic heart disease mortality in white residents of 99 of the 100 largest cities in the United States. J Chronic Dis 1979;32: 157–62.

Wang TJ, Pencina MJ, Booth SL, Jacques PF, Ingelsson E, Lanier K, Benjamin EJ, D'Agostino RB, Wolf M, Vasan RS, Vitamin D deficiency and risk of cardiovascular disease. Circulation 2008;117: 503–11.

Weinberg CR, Brown KG, Hoel DG, Altitude, radiation, and mortality from cancer and heart disease. Radiat Res 1987;112: 381–90.

Weishaar RE, Simpson RU, Involvement of vitamin D3 with cardiovascular function. II. Direct and indirect effects. Am J Physiol 1987;253: E675–83.

Willheim M, Thien R, Schrattbauer K, Bajna E, Holub M, Gruber R, Baier K, Pietschmann P, Reinisch W, Scheiner O, Peterlik M, Regulatory effects of 1alpha,25-dihydroxyvitamin D3 on the cytokine production of human peripheral blood lymphocytes. J Clin Endocrinol Metab 1999;84: 3739–44.

Winkelmayer WC, Liu J, Brookhart MA, Altitude and all-cause mortality in incident dialysis patients. J Am Med Assoc 2009;301: 508–12.

Wolf M, Shah A, Gutierrez O, Ankers E, Monroy M, Tamez H, Steele D, Chang Y, Camargo CA Jr, Tonelli M, Thadhani R, Vitamin D levels and early mortality among incident hemodialysis patients. Kidney Int 2007;72: 1004–13.

Wong A, Incident solar radiation and coronary heart disease mortality rates in Europe. Eur J Epidemiol 2008a;23: 609–14.

Wong MS, Delansorne R, Man RY, Vanhoutte PM, Vitamin D derivatives acutely reduce endothelium-dependent contractions in the aorta of the spontaneously hypertensive rat. Am J Physiol 2008b;295: H289–96.

Wu-Wong JR, Nakane M, Ma J, Vitamin D analogs modulate the expression of plasminogen activator inhibitor-1, thrombospondin-1 and thrombomodulin in human aortic smooth muscle cells. J Vasc Res 2007;44: 11–8.

Yasmin, McEniery CM, Wallace S, Dakham Z, Pulsalkar P, Maki-Petaja K, Ashby MJ, Cockcroft JR, Wilkinson IB, Matrix metalloproteinase-9 (MMP-9), MMP-2, and serum elastase activity are associated with systolic hypertension and arterial stiffness. Arterioscler Thromb Vasc Biol 2005;25: 372–8.

Yogamundi Moon J, Factors affecting arterial calcification associated with atherosclerosis. A review. Atherosclerosis 1972;16: 119–26.

Zachariah PK, Schwartz GL, Strong CG, Ritter SG, Parathyroid hormone and calcium. A relationship in hypertension. Am J Hypertens 1988;1: 79S–82S.

Zhou C, Lu F, Cao K, Xu D, Goltzman D, Miao D, Calcium-independent and 1,25(OH)2D3-dependent regulation of the renin-angiotensin system in 1alpha-hydroxylase knockout mice. Kidney Int 2008;74: 170–9.

Zhu Y, Mahon BD, Froicu M, Cantorna MT, Calcium and 1 alpha,25-dihydroxyvitamin D3 target the TNF-alpha pathway to suppress experimental inflammatory bowel disease. Eur J Immunol 2005;35: 217–24.

Zieman SJ, Melenovsky V, Kass DA, Mechanisms, pathophysiology, and therapy of arterial stiffness. Arterioscler Thromb Vasc Biol 2005;25: 932–43.

Zittermann A, Schleithoff SS, Tenderich G, Berthold HK, Korfer R, Stehle P, Low vitamin D status: a contributing factor in the pathogenesis of congestive heart failure? J Am Coll Cardiol 2003;41: 105–12.

Zittermann A, Schleithoff SS, Frisch S, Gotting C, Kuhn J, Koertke H, Kleesiek K, Tenderich G, Koerfer R, Circulating calcitriol concentrations and total mortality. Clin Chem 2009;55: 1163–70.

10.6 Vitamin D and bone health

Markus Herrmann; Gustavo Duque

10.6.1 Introduction

A relation between vitamin D and bone health was first established approximately 90 years ago. In 1922 the chemist Verner McCollum and the paediatrician John Howland discovered a new vitamin in liver extract, which they found was involved in calcium deposition. The role of this vitamin in calcium metabolism was independent of vitamin A as shown by inactivation of vitamin A by pre-treatment of liver extract with oxidants. It was the fourth vitamin discovered, after vitamins A, B and C, and was therefore named 'vitamin D'.

Around the time of the discovery of vitamin D, rickets was a common childhood disease in industrialized countries. The condition manifested as impeded growth and development of long bones in children. In the period 1918–1920, Edward Mellanby was able to demonstrate that rickets was linked to a dietary deficiency and that cod liver oil was effective in preventing its development. It was only a few years later that deficiency of vitamin D was identified as the underlying cause of rickets.

In the ensuing years, more became known about rickets and its adult form, osteomalacia. Similar to rickets, osteomalacia is characterized by the softening of bones. Both these conditions are caused by a defect in the mineralization of the protein framework of bone known as osteoid. This defective mineralization is mainly caused by a lack of vitamin D or its faulty utilization. Fortification of milk with vitamin D in the 1930s led to a sharp decline in the number of rickets cases. Nowadays both diseases are rare in industrialized countries. However, in developing countries where poor nutrition remains a problem, rickets and osteomalacia still occur.

Although in modern societies extreme manifestations, such as rickets and osteomalacia, are rare vitamin D deficiency is increasingly becoming a common problem. This is the result of changing lifestyle patterns, including an increased amount of time spent indoors and use of sunscreen. Elderly individuals appear to be most commonly affected, which is probably explained by their lack of exposure to sunlight and a reduction in the capacity of their skin to activate vitamin D precursors. Even in countries where the potential for UV-light exposure is very high, the prevalence of vitamin D deficiency is surprising. For example, it is estimated that in Australia there are 2 million individuals with insufficient vitamin D levels, this corresponds to 10% of the total population.

Although extreme manifestations of vitamin D deficiency are rare in developed countries, the effects of suboptimal vitamin D levels are common. Osteoporosis is one such example that affects approximately 25 million individuals worldwide. Osteoporosis is a degenerative condition characterized by loss of bone mass, reduced biomechanical bone properties and an increased fracture risk. The effect of osteoporotic fractures is devastating. In fact, 20% of individuals who sustain a hip fracture die within 1 year and 50% do not recover full mobility. Suboptimal vitamin D status is thought to contribute to many cases of osteoporosis and the improvement of vitamin D levels in the developed world is considered to be of major importance for the prevention of degenerative bone disease.

10.6.2 Physiological role of vitamin D in bone metabolism

Vitamin D is integrally involved in the maintenance of calcium and phosphate homeostasis. Homeostasis is achieved physiologically via the interaction of vitamin D and parathyroid hormone (PTH), with these hormones being inversely related. The homeostasis of serum calcium concentration is crucial for the maintenance of bone health. Under normal conditions, the serum calcium is supersaturating with respect to bone mineral requirements. If plasma calcium falls below the saturation threshold bone mineralization fails (Underwood and DeLuca, 1984).

The predominant role of vitamin D in calcium homeostasis is the regulation of intestinal calcium absorption. Vitamin D is the only known hormone that can induce production of the proteins involved in active intestinal calcium absorption (DeLuca, 2004). Without vitamin D, only 10–15% of dietary calcium and approximately 60% of phosphorus is absorbed. The presence of sufficient amounts of vitamin D can increase the efficiency of intestinal calcium absorption to 30–40% and phosphorus absorption to approximately 80% (Heaney, 2003; Heaney et al., 2003; Holick, 2007). Vitamin D levels below 75 nmol/l have been shown to result in a significant decrease in calcium absorption and an increase in circulating PTH levels. PTH regulates tubular reabsorption of calcium and the conversion of 25-hydroxy-vitamin D (25(OH)D) into the active hormone 1,25-dihydroxy-vitamin D (1,25(OH)$_2$D) in the kidneys. Thereby PTH can compensate for low 25(OH)D levels. Other mechanisms by which vitamin D increases circulating calcium levels are mobilization of calcium from bone and reabsorption of filtered calcium from the distal tubule in the kidneys. Both these mechanisms require the simultaneous presence of PTH. Hence, circulating vitamin D levels should always be considered in conjunction with PTH.

In bone vitamin D and PTH stimulate resorption indirectly by activation of osteoblasts. The activity of bone forming osteoblasts and bone resorbing osteoclasts is tightly regulated and both cell types closely communicate with each other. Together vitamin D and PTH stimulate the synthesis of receptor activator of nuclear factor-B ligand (RANKL) by osteoblasts, which then binds to its receptor RANK. The binding of RANKL to RANK triggers the transformation of preosteoclasts into mature osteoclasts and activates resting osteoclasts. Subsequently, active osteoclasts dissolve the mineralized collagen matrix in bone and release calcium into the circulation. Therefore, vitamin D in conjunction with PTH enables the organism to mobilize calcium from bone when it is absent from the diet.

The classical view of the effect of vitamin D on bone has been that it acts entirely indirectly via modulation of calcium and phosphate homeostasis. However, recent data indicate that in certain medical conditions, such as osteoporosis, vitamin D can have direct actions on bone cells. This concept is supported by the fact that 25-hydroxyvitamin D-1α-hydroxylase (cyp27b1), and the vitamin D receptor (VDR) are expressed in osteoblasts, osteoclasts and chondrocytes. 1,25(OH)$_2$D$_3$ has been shown to suppress excessive bone resorption under pathological conditions such as osteoporosis (Takasu, 2008). This suppression can at least partly be ascribed to direct effects of vitamin D acting via the VDR on osteoclast precursor cells. c-Fos protein appears to be a key target molecule of VDR action in this process (Takasu et al., 2006). In addition, synthetic vitamin D analogues such as DD$_2$81 possess potent anti-resorptive activity.

Direct effects of vitamin D on osteoblasts have also been demonstrated. Similar to its effects on osteoclasts, vitamin D can exert both stimulatory and inhibitory effects on osteoblasts depending mainly from cell differentiation and maturation. In cell culture 1,25(OH)$_2$D has been shown to stimulate type I collagen and alkaline phosphatase expression in mature osteoblasts whereas the expression of both genes is inhibited in preosteoblasts (Owen et al., 1991). In addition, 1,25(OH)$_2$D vitamin D has shown to stimulate osteoblastogenesis and bone formation in a model of accelerated senescence with severe osteoporosis (Duque et al., 2005). Several in vitro and in vivo studies suggest that the VDR acts directly to inhibit the differentiation and function of osteoblasts. Cultured osteoblasts from VDR-deficient mice show an increased expression of alkaline phosphatase, bone sialoprotein and osteocalcin, as well as a sustained increase in mineralization (Sooy et al., 2005). Bones from VDR knockout mice appear to have increased bone mass and bone mineral density (Tanaka and Seino, 2004; St-Arnaud, 2008). By contrast, over-expression of VDR in mature osteoblasts was found to increase both cortical and trabecular bone (Gardiner et al., 2000; Misof et al., 2003; Baldock et al., 2006). Lastly, *in vitro* experiments have shown that vitamin D affects the osteoblastic expression of lysyl oxidases (LOX) and lysyl hydrolases and thus extracellular collagen cross-linking (Nagaoka et al., 2008). The cross-linking of collagen type I is a major determinant of biomechanical properties of bone.

Bone growth of long bones depends on the activity of chondrocytes in the growth plate. Recent molecular genetic studies have revealed direct effects of $1,25(OH)_2D$ on growth plate chondrocytes, which are mediated through the VDR. In mice $1,25(OH)_2D$ appears to reduced RANKL expression in growth plate chondrocytes and delaying osteoclastogenesis. This results in a transient increase in bone volume at the primary spongiosa. In addition, $1,25(OH)_2D$ has been shown to reduce circulating levels of FGF23 and thus increase serum phosphate concentrations.

Considering the diverse and even opposing calcium-independent effects of vitamin D on bone cells, the relevance of these results in humans needs to be clarified.

10.6.3 Regulation of calcium homoeostasis by PTH, vitamin D and calcitonin

Because of the many physiologic functions of calcium the human organism relies on the maintenance of a constant blood calcium concentration. Circulating calcium is monitored by the calcium sensing receptor (CaSR) located in the parathyroid glands. In the parathyroid glands the CaSR controls calcium homoeostasis by regulating the release of PTH. When the calcium concentration falls below normal (even slightly) this G-protein coupled transmembrane protein stimulates the secretion of PTH. Within seconds PTH arrives at its main target cells, osteoblasts and the cells of the proximal convoluted tubules in the kidneys. PTH activates the 1α-hydroxylase in the convoluted tubule cells and thereby promotes the conversion of the inactive pro-hormone 25(OH)D into the active hormone $1,25(OH)_2D$. At low concentrations $1,25(OH)_2D$ stimulates intestinal calcium absorption (►Fig. 10.11). The mobilization of calcium from bone and renal reabsorption requires a higher $1,25(OH)_2D$ concentration and the simultaneous presence of PTH. Once circulating calcium is back in the normal range PTH secretion is reduced. If calcium mobilization from bone is excessive, calcitonin released from the C-cells of the thyroid gland can counteract this process. Calcitonin also stimulates the renal 1α-hydroxylase to provide $1,25(OH)_2D$ for calcium-independent functions.

Of note, the regulation of 1,25(OH)2D and PTH is organized in a way that under normal conditions dietary calcium is the preferred source of calcium for the maintenance of calcium homoeostasis. Only when this source is insufficient the system requires calcium mobilization from bone and reabsorption in the kidney to satisfy the needs of the organism. This results in loss of calcium from the skeleton and can ultimately lead to osteoporosis.

10.6.4 Definition and prevalence of vitamin D deficiency

The prevalence of vitamin D deficiency strongly depends on the cut-off applied. The simple use of a reference interval as defined by the interval between 2.5th and

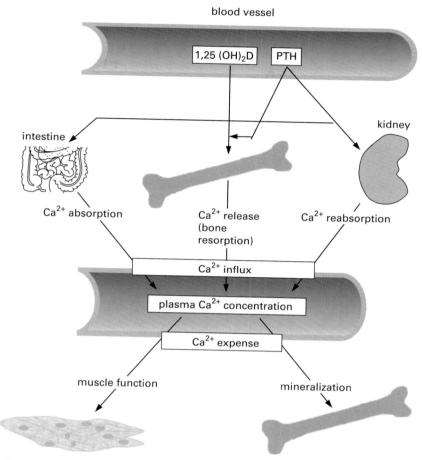

Fig. 10.11: Illustration of the role of vitamin D and PTH in calcium homoeostasis. Modified from DeLuca (2004).

97.5th percentile of values observed within an apparently healthy population has not been proven appropriate. According to this definition the reference interval ranges somewhere between 10 and 125 nmol/l depending on the population investigated and varies between winter and summer (Lips, 2001). One of the main objections to the use of a population-based reference range is that it has been demonstrated that fracture risk and BMD can be improved if 25(OH)D levels are increased above the reference range (Bischoff-Ferrari et al., 2005, 2009a). A reduction in fracture risk has been observed if 25(OH)D levels are ≥75 nmol/l. In other studies, 25(OH)D serum levels were directly related to BMD (Bischoff-Ferrari et al., 2006, 2009a). Maximum BMD was observed at 25(OH)D levels of ≥100 nmol/l. In addition, circulating 25(OH)D and PTH levels are inversely related until a 25(OH)D level between 70 and 100 nmol/l, at which point PTH reaches a nadir (▶Fig. 10.12) (Chapuy et al., 1997; Thomas et al., 1998; Heaney et al., 2003; Dawson-Hughes et al., 2005). These two

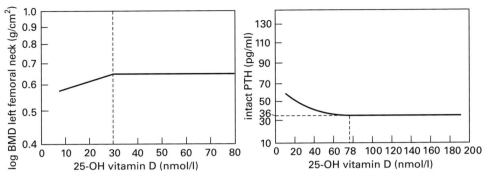

Fig. 10.12: Left: relation between serum 25(OH)D and BMD of the femoral neck in 300 elderly women. The best fit was obtained by a linear regression model with a threshold for serum 25(OH)D at 30 nmol/l; modified from Ooms et al. (1995). Right: relation between serum 25(OH)D and intact PTH levels.

facts illustrate that bone metabolism is not always ideal at vitamin D levels within the reference interval or, in other words, many individuals have a functional vitamin D deficiency at these levels. In the light of this situation most experts favour the concept of desirable or sufficient 25(OH)D levels. Based on existing data the following classification has been recommended (Holick, 2007):

- Preferred range: 75–150 nmol/l
- Relative or functional deficiency: 50–75 nmol/l
- Deficiency: <50 nmol/l

Based on this classification, it has been estimated that 1 billion people worldwide have vitamin D deficiency or insufficiency (Holick, 2007). Elderly individuals exhibit the highest prevalence of vitamin D deficiency. In industrialized western countries approximately 50% of elderly persons (65 years and older) have inadequate 25(OH)D levels (Norman et al., 2007) with figures varying between 40 and 100% in different study populations (Lips, 2001; Holick, 2007). Recent evidence indicates that children and young adults are also at high risk for vitamin D deficiency. Two studies from the USA reported 48–52% of preadolescents and adolescents having 25(OH)D levels below 50 nmol/l (Gordon et al., 2004; Sullivan et al., 2005). Other studies in young and middle-aged adults found 32 and 42% of individuals with deficient 25(OH)D levels below 50 nmol/l (Nesby-O'Dell et al., 2002; Tangpricha et al., 2002). Of note, the frequency of vitamin D deficiency varies between different geographic areas depending from nutritional habits and sunlight exposure (van der Wielen et al., 1995; Vieth et al., 2004). However, rather than geographic latitude and net sun exposure it is the ratio between skin surface and sun exposure determining 25(OH)D levels. In areas with the highest sun exposure worldwide, such as Australia, Arabic countries, and India, 30–50% of children and adults have 25(OH)D levels of less than 50 nmol/l owing to clothing covering most of the skin and the use of sun blocker (Sedrani, 1984; El-Hajj et al., 2001; McGrath et al., 2001; Marwaha et al., 2005). In agreement with these studies a recent meta-analysis was not able

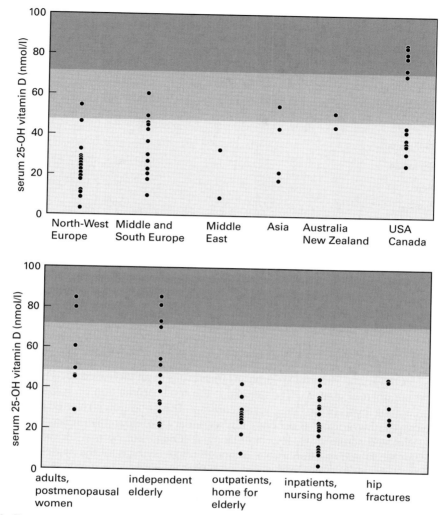

Fig. 10.13: Top: average serum 25(OH)D levels from various studies according to their geographic origin. Bottom: average serum 25(OH)D in elderly individuals according to residence status; modified from Lips (2001).

to establish a consistent relation between sunlight exposure and 25(OH)D levels (▶Fig. 10.13) (Hagenau et al., 2009).

Pregnant and lactating women are also at high risk for vitamin D deficiency. In an American study 73% of pregnant women and 80% of their infants were vitamin D deficient although they took a multivitamin containing 400 IU vitamin D during pregnancy. In addition, most of them ate fish and drank more than two glasses of milk per day (Hollis and Wagner, 2004; Bodnar et al., 2007; Lee et al., 2007). ▶Tab. 10.9 provides a comprehensive overview about average 25(OH)D levels in different categories.

Tab. 10.9: Average 25(OH)D levels in different categories (Hagenau et al., 2009).

Group	Number of studies	Mean 25(OH)D level (nmol/l)
All	394	55 ± 1.4
≤15 years	21	37 ± 5.7
15–65 years	214	57 ± 1.8
≥65 years	147	53 ± 2.1
66–75 years	95	57 ± 2.7
≥75 years	52	47 ± 3.6
Men	105	50 ± 2.6
Women	277	56 ± 1.6
Caucasians	96	68 ± 3.2
Non-Caucasians	55	47 ± 4.0

10.6.5 Clinical implications of vitamin D deficiency for bone health

10.6.5.1 Secondary hyperparathyroidism

Vitamin D and PTH are functionally related via circulating calcium. A low serum 25(OH)D concentration is usually associated with a small decrease of serum 1,25(OH)$_2$D and calcium absorption. This results in an increased secretion of PTH from the parathyroid glands. PTH stimulates the renal production of 1,25(OH)$_2$D keeping circulating levels of the latter nearly constant. This condition is referred to as 'secondary hyperparathyroidism'. Biochemically secondary hyperparathyroidism is characterized by elevated serum PTH, low circulating 25(OH)D but normal (or mildly decreased) 1,25(OH)$_2$D and calcium levels. Although relatively high for the associated serum calcium concentration in some cases serum PTH might even be within the reference interval. Owing to seasonal variability of 25(OH)D levels the disease is most marked at the end of winter and early spring (Woitge et al., 2000; Lips, 2001; Meier et al., 2004). In addition to the stimulation of renal 1,25(OH)$_2$D synthesis the elevated circulating PTH mobilizes bone calcium an thereby increases bone turnover. This results in bone loss, primarily affecting cortical bone. According to current concepts secondary hyperparathyroidism is the principal mechanism whereby vitamin D deficiency contributes to bone loss and fragility fractures (Lips, 2001). However, it is important to know that not all individuals with low 25(OH)D levels develop secondary hyperparathyroidism. In a recent study of 1280 frail elderly Australians Chen et al. found 53% of all individuals with a hypovitaminosis D and absence of secondary hyperparathyroidism (Chen et al., 2008). These 'non-responders' appear to have a longer survival, similar to vitamin D sufficient subjects.

Numerous studies have reported an association between increased serum PTH concentrations and vitamin D deficiency (Chapuy et al., 1987, 1997; Lips et al., 1987; Krall et al., 1989; Dawson-Hughes et al., 1991; Ooms et al., 1995; Bruce et al., 1999; Lips, 2001; Visser et al., 2003; Holick, 2007). Serum PTH correlates negatively with serum

25(OH)D (Chapuy et al., 1987, 1997; Lips et al., 1987, 1988; Ooms et al., 1995; Lips, 2001; Holick, 2007) with correlation coefficients usually ranging between 0.2 and 0.4. The type of PTH assay used is important for this correlation because many two-site intact PTH (1–84) assays also detect inactive fragments such as PTH (7–84). In patients with impaired renal function these fragments can account for more than 50% of the measured PTH (Lepage et al., 1998).

The seasonal variation of 25(OH)D levels results in a marked seasonal variation of bone turnover. A population-based German study including 580 adults showed higher values of the bone turnover markers bone alkaline phosphatase and urinary pyridi-noline in winter than in summer (Woitge et al., 2000). In addition, markers of bone resorption (urine hydroxyproline excretion) and bone formation (alkaline phosphatase activity, serum osteocalcin) are significantly increased in patients with osteomalacia compared with healthy controls (Demiaux et al., 1992). Below a 25(OH)D concentration of 30 nmol/l serum osteocalcin exhibits a negative correlation with serum 25(OH)D (Ooms et al., 1995). Another study measured serum levels of 25(OH)D and bone turnover markers in 119 active elderly women (Sahota et al., 1999) and found insufficient 25(OH)D concentrations in 27% of the participants. As expected, serum PTH correlated inversely with serum 25(OH)D ($r = -0.42$, $p = 0.01$). In this study vitamin D-insufficient subjects had lower bone mineral density in the hip than vitamin D-sufficient individuals. In approximately half of the patients with vitamin D insufficiency, one or more bone turnover markers were elevated above the upper reference limit. Therefore, biochemical markers of bone turnover might be helpful in diagnosing functional vitamin D deficiency.

10.6.5.2 Vitamin D deficiency, bone mineral density (BMD) and bone structure

Bone mineral density (BMD) is a strong predictor of fracture risk (Cummings et al., 1995, 2002). Considering the relation between vitamin D levels and fracture risk a significant association between vitamin D and BMD can be expected. At present the most compelling evidence for such an association is provided by the National Health and Nutrition Examination Survey III (NHANES III), including 13 432 younger (20–49 years) and older (>50 years) persons with different ethnic-racial backgrounds (Bischoff-Ferrari et al., 2004b). When subjects were divided in quintiles of their serum 25(OH)D level BMD was highest in the 5th quintile and lowest in the 1st quintile. The differences between the 1st and the 5th quintile ranged from 4.1% to 4.8% in white subjects, from 1.8% to 3.6% in Hispanic individuals and from 1.2% to 2.5% in blacks. Of note, higher serum 25(OH)D concentrations were associated with higher BMD throughout the reference range of 22.5–94 nmol/l in all subgroups (▶Fig. 10.14). In younger whites and younger Mexican Americans, higher serum 25(OH)D was associated with higher BMD, even at 25(OH)D levels >100 nmol/l.

Although the NHANES III study is by far the largest study addressing this issue there are several smaller cross-sectional studies supporting a positive relation between serum 25(OH)D and BMD (Woitge et al., 2000; Visser et al., 2003; Dawson-Hughes et al., 2005; Chen et al., 2008). A Dutch study in 330 elderly women found a significant positive correlation at serum 25(OH)D levels below 30 nmol/l (Ooms et al., 1995). However, the NHANES III study clearly shows that this threshold is much higher and depends on the ethnic and racial background. A positive relation between serum 25(OH)D and

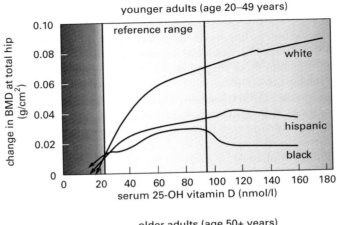

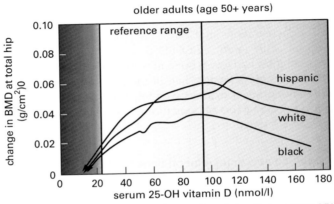

Fig. 10.14: Regression plot of difference in bone mineral density by serum 25(OH)D concentrations in younger and older adults after adjustment for sex, age, BMI, smoking, calcium intake, oestrogen use, month of vitamin D measurement, and poverty income ratio; modified after Bischoff-Ferrari et al. (2006).

BMD of the hip was also observed in middle-aged women in the UK (45–65 years) (Khaw et al., 1992) and in elderly women in New Zealand (McAuley et al., 1997). This relation appears to be stronger for cortical bone (femoral neck) than for trabecular bone (trochanter) (Ooms et al., 1995).

However, not all studies found significant relations between serum 25(OH)D and BMD (Garnero et al., 2007; Kremer et al., 2009). In the OFELY study 669 postmenopausal women were divided according to their serum 25(OH)D level. No significant difference in BMD was observed between individuals above and below any cut-off applied between 50 and 75nmol/l. This finding was consistent across all anatomical sites studies. Moreover, in young postpubertal females, aged 16–22 years, vitamin D appeared to have no role in regulating bone mass acquisition (Kremer et al., 2009).

The lower BMD in vitamin D deficient individuals is caused by bone mineral loss owing to several mechanisms including both reversible and an irreversible components

(Frame and Parfitt, 1978; Lips, 2001). The reversible component is characterized by (1) an increased formation and accumulation of (predominantly unmineralized) osteoid, (2) a lower mineralization degree of mineralized osteons, and (3) and increased remodelling space. Parfitt et al. showed that in patients who were treated with vitamin D and calcium the osteoid volume decreased by 80% in cortical (from 6% to 1.5%) and trabecular bone (from 30% to 6%) (Parfitt et al., 1985). Cortical porosity decreased from 10.3% to 7.8%. Mineralized bone volume increased by 7.5% in cortical and 40% in trabecular bone. The irreversible component of vitamin D deficiency-related bone loss is owing to a negative remodelling balance per osteon. In a state of high turnover, the negative remodelling balance is multiplied by the high number of remodelling osteons, whereas in low turnover states, bone loss owing to negative remodelling balance is much lower (Parfitt, 1980). The irreversible cortical bone loss appears to be owing to endosteal bone resorption and subsequent cortical thinning (Parfitt et al., 1985).

10.6.5.3 Vitamin D and fracture risk

Fragility fractures are the most common complications of osteoporosis with often devastating consequences for the affected individual. Approximately 50% of patients with a hip fracture do not recover full mobility and 20% die within the first year after the fracture. Therefore the relation between vitamin D status and fracture risk is of major importance. The highest level of evidence for a relation between serum 25(OH)D and fracture risk comes from prospective studies (Woo et al., 1990; Cummings et al., 1998; Gerdhem et al., 2005; Cauley et al., 2008; Looker and Mussolino, 2008). The quality of these studies ranges from poor (Catherwood et al., 1985) to good (Cummings et al., 1998). Duration of follow up ranges from 30 months to a maximum of 7.1 years. The early prospective studies failed to find a significant association between 25(OH)D and fracture because of small sample size and high drop out rate (Woo et al., 1990) or use of an older 25(OH)D assays (Cummings et al., 1998). Although these studies did not reach significance they showed clear trends. Recent large epidemiologic studies clearly show a significant association between serum 25(OH)D and hip fractures in elderly individuals (Cauley et al., 2008; Looker and Mussolino, 2008). For younger individuals and other fracture sites the relation between serum 25(OH)D and fracture has not yet been proven (Roddam et al., 2007). A role for low serum 25(OH)D as a risk factor for fractures is also supported by several case-control studies (▶Fig. 10.15) (Punnonen et al., 1986; Lips et al., 1987; Lau et al., 1989; Villareal et al., 1991; Boonen et al., 1997, 1999; Thiebaud et al., 1997; Diamond et al., 1998; LeBoff et al., 1999; Nuti et al., 2004; Bakhtiyarova et al., 2006; Bodnar et al., 2007). Only two case-control studies were unable to show a relation between serum 25(OH)D levels and fractures (Lund et al., 1975; Erem et al., 2002). However, with 21 (Erem et al., 2002) and 67 fracture cases (Lund et al., 1975), respectively, these studies were rather small. In one of these studies it was not mentioned if controls and cases were matched by age (Lund et al., 1975).

The five prospective studies available merit further consideration. The first prospective study was conducted in 1990 by Woo et al. and followed 427 independently living elderly Chinese subjects (mean age 69 years for men and 70 years for women) for 2.5 years (Woo et al., 1990). The relative fracture risk (RR) for subjects with low serum 25(OH)D levels (<79 nmol/l in males and <65.5 nmol/l in females) was 3.42

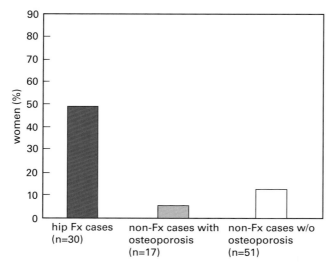

Fig. 10.15: Prevalence of vitamin D deficiency with serum 25(OH)D levels <30 nmol/l in women with and without hip fractures (Fx); modified from LeBoff et al. (1999).

(95%) confidence interval (CI), 0.79–14.9). Although the risk for individuals with low 25(OH)D levels appeared to be increased, the CI was wide and the result was not significant. In addition, this study had several limitations, including a high loss to follow up (34%), a low event rate (only nine subjects sustained fractures) and a lack of adjustment for confounders such as BMD and age. The next prospective cohort study was the Study of Osteoporotic Fractures, a study in four US centres (Cummings et al., 1998). This study employed a case-cohort approach. From a cohort of 9704 Caucasian community-dwelling women aged 65 years and older, a subset of 133 women with a first hip fracture and 138 women with a new vertebral fracture were selected randomly. All fractures occurred within 5.9 years after baseline assessment. In addition, 343 women without incident fractures were selected as controls. Although moderate 25(OH)D deficiency with serum 25(OH)D levels <47 nmol/l was not a predictor of hip or vertebral fracture risk a low serum 1,25(OH)$_2$D (<57 pmol/l) was associated with an increased risk for hip fracture. The age and weight adjusted relative risk was 2.1 (95% CI, 1.2–3.5) and 1.6 (95% CI, 0.9–2.8) for hip and vertebral fractures, respectively. In this study the prevalence of 25(OH)D deficiency with serum levels below 47.5 nmol/l was 22%. In 2005 Gerdhem et al. evaluated the association between 25(OH)D and fractures in a 3-year prospective cohort of 1044 ambulatory women in Sweden. In individuals with serum 25(OH)D levels <50 nmol/l the hazard ratio (HR) for fracture was 2.04 (95% CI, 1.04–4.04), Women with serum 25(OH)D levels <75 nmol/l had a hazard ratio of 1.01 (95% CI, 0.71–1.61). A major limitation of this study was that the average serum 25(OH)D level was very high (95 ± 30 nmol/l) and only 4.4% of subjects had serum 25(OH)D levels <50 nmol/l. Recent results from the Women's Health Initiative Study provide the most compelling evidence for an association between serum 25(OH)D and fracture risk (Cauley et al., 2008). Cauley et al. selected 400 cases of incident hip fractures and 400 matched controls from 39 795 postmenopausal women without previous hip fractures, not using estrogens or other bone-active therapies. The average follow-up time was 7.1 years. The mean serum

25(OH)D level was lower in cases than in controls (56.2 ± 20.3 nmol/l vs 59.7 ± 18 nmol/l, $p = 0.007$). A 25 nmol/l decrease in 25(OH)D was associated with a 33% increased risk of hip fracture (odds ratio = 1.33; 95% CI, 1.06–1.68). In women with a serum 25(OH)D level <47.5 nmol/l the odds ratio of hip fracture was 1.71; 95% CI, 1.05, 2.79) when compared with women having serum 25(OH)D levels of ≥70.7 nmol/l. Adjustment for falls, physical function, frailty, renal function, or sex steroid hormones had no effect on this association. Measurement of bone turnover markers showed that this association was, in part, mediated by bone resorption. These results are consistent with a recent report from the Third National Health and Nutrition Examination Survey (NHANES III), where 1917 white men and women ≥65 years were investigated. The relative risk of hip fracture was 0.64 (95% CI, 0.46–0.89) among subjects with 25(OH)D levels >62.5 nmol/l compared with those with lower levels. When grouped into quartiles of serum 25(OH)D, the multivariate-adjusted relative risk for the second, third and fourth versus the first quartile were 0.50 (95% CI, 0.25–1.00), 0.41 (95% CI, 0.24–0.70), and 0.50 (95% CI, 0.29–0.86), respectively.

By contrast, a nested case-control study of 730 incident fracture cases and 1445 controls found no evidence of an association between serum 25(OH)D and fracture (Roddam et al., 2007). However, this study investigated a relatively young population with an average age of only 50 years and included various fracture sites. However, in total there were only 22 hip fractures. It can be speculated that vitamin D might be more strongly linked to frailty related fractures such as hip fractures which tend to occur in much older women.

More prospective epidemiological studies on risk factors for osteoporotic fractures including vitamin D deficiency are underway, e.g., the European Prospective Osteoporosis Study, the Rotterdam Study and the Longitudinal Aging Study Amsterdam.

10.6.5.4 Vitamin D, myopathy and falls

Osteoporotic fractures usually occur during minor trauma, such as falls. Falls are directly related to sensorimotor coordination and proprioception. Therefore, muscle function is causally involved in the pathogenesis of fractures. Considering the relation between circulating vitamin D and fracture risk the question arises if this relation is entirely owing to direct osseous effects of vitamin D or not. In the light of many non-osseous functions of vitamin D (e.g., immune defence, cell proliferation and differentiation) numerous studies have investigated if there is an association between vitamin D status, muscle function and falls rate. Although not all prospective studies were able to find a significant relation between serum 25(OH)D and falls risk, there is convincing evidence that lower extremity function is related to the serum 25(OH)D concentration. In a recent study Bischoff-Ferrari et al. investigated lower extremity function in 4100 elderly Americans (≥60 years) according to serum 25(OH)D concentrations (Bischoff-Ferrari et al., 2004a). Lower extremity function was estimated by an 8-foot (2.4-m) walking-speed test and a timed test of five repetitions of rising from a chair and sitting down (sit-to-stand test). When subjects were stratified in quintiles of their serum 25(OH)D levels subjects in the highest quintile were able to perform both tests significantly faster than those in the lowest quartile: 8-foot walk test: −0.27 s (95% CI, −0.44 to −0.09 s, $p = 0.001$), sit-to-stand test: −0.67s (95% CI, −1.11 to −0.23 s, $p = 0.017$). When subjects were categorized in quintiles of their lower extremity function there was a linear increase in 25(OH)D levels with virtually no overlap of serum 25(OH)D ranges between individual quintiles. Most of the improvement occurred in subjects with 25(OH)D concentrations between 22.5 and 40 nmol/l, but further improvement was seen in the range of 40–94 nmol/l. A relation between serum vitamin D and muscle function is also supported by data from the Longitudinal Aging Study Amsterdam including 1351 Dutch men and women aged ≥65 years (▶Fig. 10.16). In this study Visser et al. analysed the loss of muscle strength and muscle mass according to serum 25(OH)D over a 3-year period (Visser et al., 2003). Individuals with 25(OH)D levels <25 nmol/l had a more than twice the risk of experiencing sarcopaenia (defined as 40% loss of grip strength and 3% loss of muscle mass). A later report from the same study showed that loss of muscle strength and muscle mass translates into a significantly elevated falls risk (Visser et al., 2003). In a multivariate model adjusting for age, sex, education level, region, season, physical activity, smoking, and alcohol intake, the odds ratios (95% CI) were 1.78 (1.06–2.99) for subjects who experienced two falls or more as compared with those who did not fall or fell once and 2.23 (1.17–4.25) for subjects who fell three or more times as compared with those who fell two times or less. An Australian study among 1719 elderly residential care women observed an independent association between serum 25(OH)D and the time to the first fall (Flicker et al., 2003). The authors calculated that doubling of the vitamin D level would result in a 20% reduction in the risk of falling. By contrast, in a relatively small prospective study in institutionalized subjects, serum 25(OH)D was associated with the time to first fall, but this association did not remain significant after adjustment for confounders (Sambrook et al., 2004). However, the latter two studies examined only the time to the first fall, which is deemed to be a less accurate measure of falls owing to impaired muscle function. A first fall is often owing to an extrinsic cause, however, recurrent falls are often associated with intrinsic causes.

In vivo and *in vitro* studies have shown that skeletal muscle cells possess nuclear and cell membrane-bound vitamin D receptors (VDR) and are therefore a target of 1,25-(OH)$_2$D. Vitamin D has been shown to affect skeletal muscle morphology, metabolism

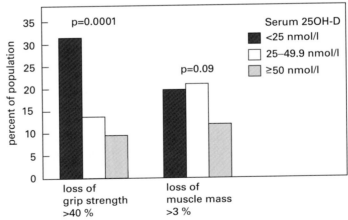

Fig. 10.16: Prevalence of grip strength loss and appendicular muscle mass loss during 3-year follow-up according to categories of baseline serum 25(OH)D concentration; modified from Visser et al. (2003).

and development (Pfeifer et al., 2002; Ceglia, 2008). Molecular mechanisms by which vitamin D acts on muscle tissue include genomic and non-genomic effects. Genomic effects are initiated by binding of $1,25(OH)_2D$ to its nuclear receptor, which results in changes in gene transcription of mRNA and subsequent protein synthesis. Non-genomic effects of vitamin D are rapid and mediated through membrane bound VDR on the cell surface. In rodents, vitamin D deficiency causes increased myofibrillar protein degradation, which might affect muscle protein turnover by inducing hypocalcaemia and decreasing insulin secretion (Wassner et al., 1983). Depletion of vitamin D stores also impairs muscle contraction kinetics in animals (Rodman and Baker, 1978; Pleasure et al., 1979). Moreover, treating humans with a vitamin D analogue has been shown to increase the relative number and cross-sectional area of fast-twitch fibres after a 3–6-month treatment period (Sorensen et al., 1979).

10.6.6 Modification of fracture risk and falls rate by vitamin D supplementation

10.6.6.1 Vitamin D supplementation and serum vitamin D levels

The high prevalence of vitamin D deficiency, its multiple implications for health and the fact that low levels can easily be corrected by vitamin D supplementation are the main reasons why vitamin D supplementation received broad attention. With regard to bone health, prevention of falls and fractures are the main goals. Numerous trials have assessed the effectiveness of vitamin D supplementation in humans. In general there are three questions to answer: (1) Does vitamin D supplementation increase the serum 25(OH)D level? (2) Can vitamin D supplementation improve bone health? (3) What doses are required and what serum 25(OH)D level should be achieved? Before going into detail it is important to mention that there are different types of vitamin D supplements available containing either vitamin D_2 or D_3. However, the market penetration of vitamin D_2 is constantly shrinking and in many countries, such as Germany and Australia vitamin D_2 supplements have almost completely disappeared. In addition, it appears that vitamin D_2 is less potent than vitamin D_3 (Cranney et al., 2007; Holick et al., 2008; Leventis and Kiely, 2009). Therefore most guidelines recommend using vitamin D_3 supplements. Thus, in the following discussion we focus on vitamin D_3 supplements and will only mention vitamin D_2 supplementation where relevant or no other data are available.

With regard to the first question, a recent meta-regression analysis provided convincing evidence that supplements can increase serum 25(OH)D in a dose dependent manner ($p = 0.04$) (Cranney et al., 2007). According to this meta-regression supplementation of 100 IU of vitamin D_3 will increase the serum 25(OH)D concentrations by 1–2 nmol/l (▶Fig. 10.17). This suggests that doses of 400–800 IU daily could be inadequate to prevent vitamin D deficiency in at-risk individuals.

There are only a few trials that examined the effect of vitamin D on 25(OH)D in children or adolescents with daily doses ranging from 200 to 2000 IU of vitamin D_3 and 400 IU of vitamin D_2. These studies showed similar treatment effects to those observed in adults. Treatment effects varied from increases in serum 25(OH)D of 8 nmol/l (200 IU), 6.5 (with 600 IU D_3) to 60 nmol/l (2000 IU of vitamin D_3) (Guillemant et al., 2001; Schou et al., 2003; El-Hajj et al., 2006). Although data are limited, 400 IU of vitamin D_2 appears to reliably correct vitamin D deficiency in infants (Greer and Marshall, 1989; Zeghoud et al., 1997; Pehlivan et al., 2003) whereas lower doses, such as 100 and

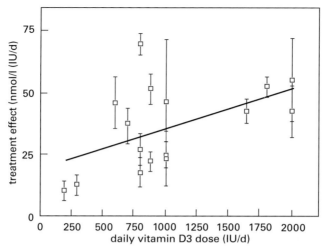

Fig. 10.17: Meta-regression analysis between the daily vitamin D3 dose and serum 25(OH)D level (Cranney et al., 2007).

200 IU per day failed to do so in some infants (Specker et al., 1992). Only a few small studies investigated vitamin D supplementation in pregnant women. These studies showed that 1000–3600 IU/day of vitamin D_2 and 1000 IU/day of vitamin D_3 increased serum 25(OH)D concentrations in mothers and in cord blood. However, in one study supplementation of lactating mothers with 1000 IU of vitamin D_2 during winter was not enough to increase serum 25(OH)D concentrations in the infants (Ala-Houhala, 1985).

10.6.6.2 Fracture prevention

The efficacy of vitamin D supplementation for the prevention of fractures is still a matter of ongoing discussion. The reason for this is the heterogeneity of existing studies in terms of vitamin D dosage and concomitant calcium supplementation. According to recent meta-analyses of double-blind randomized placebo controlled trials (RCT) fracture prevention depends from the vitamin D dose used, the achieved serum 25(OH)D level and the concomitant use of calcium. Oral supplementation with 700–800 IU/day of vitamin D_3 reduces hip and nonvertebral fractures by at least 20% in individuals aged 65 years or older. Supplementation with 400 IU/day is insufficient to prevent fractures. Although data are limited, existing studies suggest that a sufficient supply with calcium is permissive for the protective effect of vitamin D.

At present the largest individual study conducted is the Women's Health Initiative including 36 282 postmenopausal women, 50–79 years of age. Participants received 1000 mg of calcium plus 400 IU of vitamin D daily. Overall this treatment had no significant effect on fracture risk with the following hazard ratios: hip fractures: 0.88 (95% CI, 0.72–1.08), vertebral fractures: 0.90 (95% CI, 0.74–1.10), total fractures: 0.96 (95% CI, 0.91–1.02) (Jackson et al., 2006). However, excluding data from women when they ceased to adhere to the study medication reduced the hazard ratio for hip fracture to 0.71 (95% CI, 0.52–0.97). Moreover, this study also showed that repletion of the serum 25(OH)D level to 65 nmol/l is required to reduce fracture risk.

In the light of numerous studies with variable design and outcome, discussing all of them individually is of little use. However, three meta-analyses have been conducted which pool data from multiple studies into single analyses. The first meta-analysis, published in 2003, combined results from 13 RCTs of vitamin D_2 and D_3 supplementation with and without concomitant supplementation of calcium. This analysis showed a non-significant reduction in total fractures. However, this meta-analysis included studies employing low vitamin D doses down to 300 IU of vitamin D_3 per day. In addition, some of the studies involved concomitant supplementation with calcium whereas others did not. According to recent data it appears that vitamin D is only effective with a sufficient calcium supply (Grant et al., 2005). To account for this fact the authors then combined seven trials of vitamin D_3 (400–800 IU) supplementation plus calcium, which showed a significant reduction in hip and total fracture risk. However, in a subgroup analysis, this benefit was only evident when combining trials of institutionalized elderly subjects. The authors argue that the mean serum 25(OH)D level achieved in trials of institutionalized subjects was higher than in the trials on community dwellers. The combined estimate from trials with higher end-of-study serum 25(OH)D concentrations (>74 nmol/l) was consistent with a significant reduction in fractures.

A later meta-analysis by Bischoff-Ferrari et al. looked at double-blind RCTs examining hip and non-vertebral fractures in individuals >60 years (▶Figs. 10.18 and 10.19) (Bischoff-Ferrari et al., 2005) all supplemented vitamin D_3 orally with or without calcium. Five RCTs for hip fracture ($n = 9294$) and seven RCTs for nonvertebral fracture risk ($n = 9820$) met the inclusion criteria and entered in the analysis. Similar to the aforementioned meta-analysis the pooled RR for preventing hip fractures was not significant (RR 0.88, 95% CI, 0.69–1.13). However, testing for heterogeneity showed that outcomes were variable and differed according to the vitamin D dose employed. Heterogeneity among studies disappeared after separating RCTs with low (400 IU/day) and high (700–800 IU/day) doses of vitamin D. A vitamin D dose of 700–800 IU/day reduced the risk of hip fracture by 26% (three RCTs, 5572 persons; RR 0.74; 95% CI, 0.61–0.88) and nonvertebral fractures by 23% (five RCTs, 6098 persons; RR 0.77; 95% CI, 0.68–0.87) versus calcium alone or placebo. Low dose vitamin D supplementation with 400 IU did not prevent fractures independently of calcium use and fracture site (hip fractures: RR 1.15; 95% CI, 0.88–1.50; nonvertebral fracture: RR 1.03; 95% CI, 0.86–1.24).

In 2009 Bischoff-Ferrari et al. performed another meta-analysis including 12 RCTs for nonvertebral fractures ($n = 42\ 279$) and eight RCTs for hip fractures ($n = 40\ 886$). All studies were limited to individuals ≥65 years and oral vitamin D supplementation with or without concomitant calcium supplementation. This latest meta-analysis also accounted for adherence to treatment. The pooled relative risk (RR) was 0.86 (95% CI, 0.77–0.96) for prevention of nonvertebral fractures and 0.91 (95% CI, 0.78–1.05) for the prevention of hip fractures, but with significant heterogeneity for both end points. Anti-fracture efficacy increased with higher vitamin D doses and higher achieved serum 25(OH)D levels. Similar to their earlier meta-analysis heterogeneity between studies resolved when only studies with a daily dose >400 IU/day were included (nonvertebral fractures: RR 0.80; 95% CI, 0.72–0.89, $n = 33\ 265$ from nine trials; hip fractures: RR 0.82; 95% CI, 0.69–0.97; $n = 31\ 872$ from five trials). In contrast to the first meta-analysis from 2003 the risk-reduction for nonvertebral fractures was greatest in community-dwelling individuals (−29%) and smaller in institutionalized individuals (−15%). The effect was independent of additional calcium supplementation.

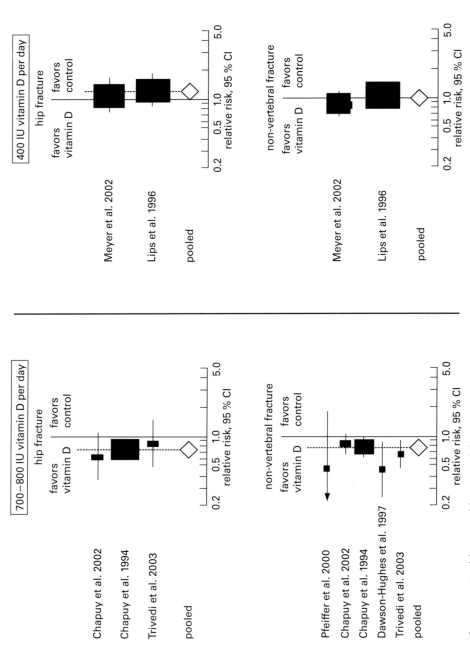

Fig. 10.18: Modification of fracture risk by vitamin D supplementation; modified from Bischoff-Ferrari et al. (2005).

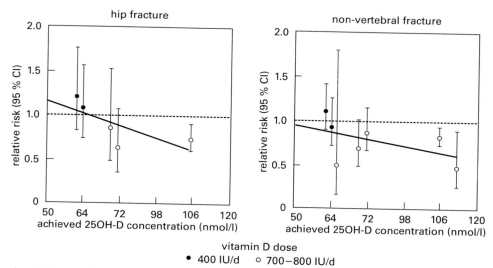

Fig. 10.19: Modification of fracture risk by vitamin D supplementation according to the achieved serum 25(OH)D level; modified from Bischoff-Ferrari et al. (2005).

The question of whether vitamin D needs to be supplemented together with calcium has been addressed by the RECORD trial. In this RCT 5292 people aged 70 years or older were randomly assigned to 800 IU daily oral vitamin D_3, 800 IU daily oral vitamin D_3 combined with 1000 mg of calcium, 1000 mg calcium, or placebo. Participants were followed up for between 24 and 62 months. Unfortunately, this trial failed to show any treatment effect for vitamin D independent of calcium intake. However, this study has several limitations, which might explain the negative outcome. Firstly, the RECORD trial investigated only patients with a previous low trauma fracture. Secondly, owing to small group sizes the statistical power was relatively low. Thirdly, vitamin D supplementation increased serum 25(OH)D from 38 to 62 nmol/l, which was below the threshold thought to provide anti-fracture efficacy. Because there are no more studies available addressing this matter, it remains unresolved for the moment.

A protective effect of vitamin D supplementation on bone health is also supported by studies looking at BMD. Overall, there is good evidence that supplementation of vitamin D_3 plus calcium results in a small beneficial effect on lumbar spine, femoral neck and total body BMD (Cranney et al., 2007). Vitamin D_3 alone appears to have no significant effect on BMD. However, it has to be mentioned that most trials had small sample sizes, were 2–3 years in duration and used vitamin D doses of ≤800 IU/day.

10.6.6.3 Falls prevention

Because vitamin deficiency is associated with impaired muscle function and an increased falls rate, the question arises if muscle function and falls rate can be improved by vitamin D supplementation.

Similar to the situation regarding fracture prevention, existing trials have heterogeneous outcomes (Bischoff-Ferrari et al., 2009b). In a relatively small RCT from Austria,

242 community-dwelling seniors were supplemented for up to 20 months with either 1000 mg of calcium or 1000 mg of calcium plus 800 IU vitamin D per day (Pfeifer et al., 2009). The number of first falls significantly decreased by 27% after 12 months and by 39% after 20 months in the vitamin D treatment group when compared with calcium only. The reduction in falls was accompanied by improved muscle function. Other studies were not able to confirm this finding although most of them showed at least a trend towards falls prevention. In contrast to work regarding fracture risk most studies investigating falls prevention are fairly small with 48–625 participants. To resolve this problem a recent meta-analysis has pooled eight RCTs ($n = 2426$, ►Fig. 10.20). Analysis of heterogeneity showed that falls prevention depends on the vitamin D dose and the achieved 25(OH)D serum level. High dose vitamin D supplementation with 700–1000 IU/day has been found to raise serum 25(OH)D to levels >60 nmol/l and reduces falls risk by 19% (RR 0.81; 95% CI, 0.71–0.92; $n = 1921$, seven trials). Low dose supplementation with vitamin D doses between 200–600 IU/day does not reduce the risk for falls (RR 1.10; 95% CI, 0.89–1.35; $n = 505$ from two trials) and results in serum 25(OH)D levels of less than 60 nmol/l. When active $1,25(OH)_2D$ was used fall risk was reduced by 22% (RR 0.78; 95% CI, 0.64–0.94). Although total numbers are still relatively small the existing data support the hypothesis that supplementation with 700–800 IU/day vitamin D can reduce fall risk.

10.6.6.4 Vitamin D supplementation and bone health in infants, children and adolescents

There is increasing evidence that infants, children and adolescents have a high prevalence of vitamin D deficiency. However, studies examining the effects of vitamin D supplementation on bone health in these individuals are limited and the results are inconsistent. There is no study that was able to demonstrate a consistent positive effect on BMD or fracture risk in infants. Two RCTs investigated the effect of vitamin D supplementation on BMD/BMC in children but were unable to find a beneficial effect across sites and age groups.

10.6.6.5 Vitamin D toxicity

Although vitamin D supplementation is generally considered to be safe, toxic effects can occur when circulating 25(OH)D levels exceed 350–400 nmol/l (Holick, 2007). This raises the question of whether intake of vitamin D above the recommended daily intake leads to toxicity. Overall, vitamin D intake above current reference intakes is well tolerated. A recent meta-analysis found only a non-significant increase in the risk of hypercalcaemia and hypercalciuria in vitamin D-supplemented individuals when compared with placebo (Cranney et al., 2007). In the large scale Womenís Health Initiative Trial the only significantly increased adverse event was renal stones (Jackson et al., 2006). The participants of this study were women between 50 and 79 years of age who received 400 IU of vitamin D_3 plus 1000 mg calcium per day. This vitamin D dose is similar to the recommended daily intake for individuals of this age group. Vitamin D supplemented individuals had a hazard ratio for the occurrence of renal stones of 1.17 (95% CI 1.02–1.34), corresponding to 5.7 events per 10 000 person-years of exposure. Caution is required when 'mega-doses' of vitamin D are used. One trial in infants administered

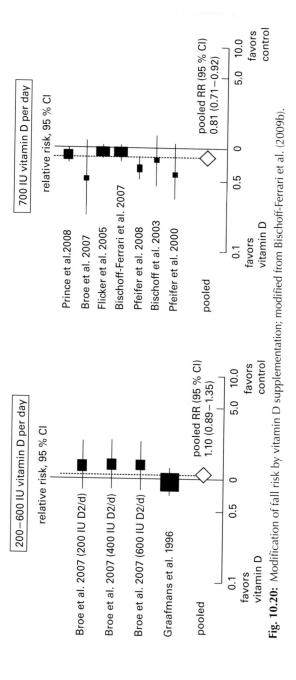

Fig. 10.20: Modification of fall risk by vitamin D supplementation; modified from Bischoff-Ferrari et al. (2009b).

a single dose of 600 000 IU of vitamin D_3 reported an increased risk of hypercalcaemia (Cesur et al., 2003).

Existing data about the potential toxicity of vitamin D are limited by the incomplete reporting of outcomes, variable exposure lengths, small sample sizes and the lack of long-term data. Furthermore, it is unclear whether vitamin D_2 and D_3 exhibit similar toxicity profiles.

10.6.7 Conclusion

There is a large body of evidence regarding vitamin D status and bone health in older adults with a lack of studies in premenopausal women and infants, children and adolescents. In older adults, there is reasonable evidence that serum 25(OH)D is positively association with BMD, falls and fracture risk. Owing to the lack of sufficient data no definite conclusions can be drawn for infants, adolescents, pregnant and lactating women. Serum 25(OH)D can be increased by supplementation of vitamin D_3 or vitamin D_2 in a dose-dependent manner. However, vitamin D_2 appears to be less effective than vitamin D_3. A dose of 100 IU/day have been estimated to increase serum 25(OH)D by 1–2 nmol/l. Supplementation of vitamin D_3 in combination with calcium results in small increases in BMD in older adults. Vitamin D_3 supplementation with daily doses of ≥700 IU/day is associated with a reduction of fracture and fall risk of approximately 20%. Lower doses are insufficient to modify fall and fracture risk. The question of whether co-treatment with calcium is permissive for the beneficial effects of vitamin D still needs to be answered.

There is little evidence that vitamin D above current reference intakes is harmful. In most trials, hypercalcaemia and hypercalciuria were not associated with clinically relevant events (Cranney et al., 2007). The Womenís Health Initiative study did report a small increase in kidney stones in postmenopausal women whose daily vitamin D_3 intake was 400 IU (the reference intake for 50–70 years, and below the reference intake for >70 years) combined with 1000 mg calcium. The increase in renal stones corresponded to 5.7 events per 10 000 person-years of exposure.

References

Ala-Houhala M, 25-Hydroxyvitamin D levels during breast-feeding with or without maternal or infantile supplementation of vitamin D. J Pediatr Gastroenterol Nutr 1985;4: 220–6.

Bakhtiyarova S, Lesnyak O, Kyznesova N, Blankenstein MA, Lips P, Vitamin D status among patients with hip fracture and elderly control subjects in Yekaterinburg, Russia. Osteoporos Int 2006;17: 441–6.

Baldock PA, Thomas GP, Hodge JM et al., Vitamin D action and regulation of bone remodeling: suppression of osteoclastogenesis by the mature osteoblast. J Bone Miner Res 2006;21: 1618–26.

Bischoff-Ferrari HA, Dietrich T, Orav EJ et al., Higher 25-hydroxyvitamin D concentrations are associated with better lower-extremity function in both active and inactive persons aged > or = 60 y. Am J Clin Nutr 2004a;80: 752–8.

Bischoff-Ferrari HA, Dietrich T, Orav EJ, Dawson-Hughes B, Positive association between 25-hydroxy vitamin D levels and bone mineral density: a population-based study of younger and older adults. Am J Med 2004b;116: 634–9.

Bischoff-Ferrari HA, Willett WC, Wong JB, Giovannucci E, Dietrich T, Dawson-Hughes B, Fracture prevention with vitamin D supplementation: a meta-analysis of randomized controlled trials. J Am Med Assoc 2005;293: 2257–64.

Bischoff-Ferrari HA, Giovannucci E, Willett WC, Dietrich T, Dawson-Hughes B, Estimation of optimal serum concentrations of 25-hydroxyvitamin D for multiple health outcomes. Am J Clin Nutr 2006;84: 18–28.

Bischoff-Ferrari HA, Kiel DP, Dawson-Hughes B et al., Dietary calcium and serum 25-hydroxyvitamin D status in relation to BMD among U.S. adults. J Bone Miner Res 2009a;24: 935–42.

Bischoff-Ferrari HA, Dawson-Hughes B, Staehelin HB et al., Fall prevention with supplemental and active forms of vitamin D: a meta-analysis of randomised controlled trials. B Med J 2009b;339: b3692.

Bodnar LM, Simhan HN, Powers RW, Frank MP, Cooperstein E, Roberts JM, High prevalence of vitamin D insufficiency in black and white pregnant women residing in the northern United States and their neonates. J Nutr 2007;137: 447–52.

Boonen S, Broos P, Verbeke G et al., Calciotropic hormones and markers of bone remodeling in age-related (type II) femoral neck osteoporosis: alterations consistent with secondary hyperparathyroidism-induced bone resorption. J Gerontol A Biol Sci Med Sci 1997;52: M286–93.

Boonen S, Mohan S, Dequeker J et al., Down-regulation of the serum stimulatory components of the insulin-like growth factor (IGF) system (IGF-I, IGF-II, IGF binding protein [BP]-3, and IGFBP-5) in age-related (type II) femoral neck osteoporosis. J Bone Miner Res 1999;14: 2150–8.

Bruce DG, St John A, Nicklason F, Goldswain PR, Secondary hyperparathyroidism in patients from Western Australia with hip fracture: relationship to type of hip fracture, renal function, and vitamin D deficiency. J Am Geriatr Soc 1999;47: 354–9.

Catherwood BD, Marcus R, Madvig P, Cheung AK, Determinants of bone gamma-carboxyglutamic acid-containing protein in plasma of healthy aging subjects. Bone 1985;6: 9–13.

Cauley JA, LaCroix AZ, Wu L et al., Serum 25-hydroxyvitamin D concentrations and risk for hip fractures. Ann Intern Med 2008;149: 242–50.

Ceglia L, Vitamin D and skeletal muscle tissue and function. Mol Aspects Med 2008;29: 407–14.

Cesur Y, Caksen H, Gundem A, Kirimi E, Odabas D, Comparison of low and high dose of vitamin D treatment in nutritional vitamin D deficiency rickets. J Pediatr Endocrinol Metab 2003;16: 1105–9.

Chapuy MC, Chapuy P, Meunier PJ, Calcium and vitamin D supplements: effects on calcium metabolism in elderly people. Am J Clin Nutr 1987;46: 324–8.

Chapuy MC, Preziosi P, Maamer M et al., Prevalence of vitamin D insufficiency in an adult normal population. Osteoporos Int 1997;7: 439–43.

Chen JS, Sambrook PN, March L et al., Hypovitaminosis D and parathyroid hormone response in the elderly: effects on bone turnover and mortality. Clin Endocrinol (Oxf) 2008;68: 290–8.

Cranney AH, Horsley T, OíDonnell S et al., Effectiveness and safety of vitamin D in relation to bone health. Evidence report/technology assessment no. 158 (Prepared by the University of Ottawa Evidence-based Practice Center (UO-EPC) under Contract No. 290-02-0021. AHRQ Publication 2007;No:07-E013. Rockville, MD: Agency for Healthcare Research and Quality. 2007.

Cummings SR, Nevitt MC, Browner WS et al., Risk factors for hip fracture in white women. Study of Osteoporotic Fractures Research Group. N Engl J Med 1995;332: 767–73.

Cummings SR, Browner WS, Bauer D et al., Endogenous hormones and the risk of hip and vertebral fractures among older women. Study of Osteoporotic Fractures Research Group. N Engl J Med 1998;339: 733–8.

Cummings SR, Karpf DB, Harris F et al., Improvement in spine bone density and reduction in risk of vertebral fractures during treatment with antiresorptive drugs. Am J Med 2002;112: 281–9.

Dawson-Hughes B, Dallal GE, Krall EA, Harris S, Sokoll LJ, Falconer G, Effect of vitamin D supplementation on wintertime and overall bone loss in healthy postmenopausal women. Ann Intern Med 1991;115: 505–12.

Dawson-Hughes B, Heaney RP, Holick MF, Lips P, Meunier PJ, Vieth R, Estimates of optimal vitamin D status. Osteoporos Int 2005;16: 713–6.

DeLuca HF, Overview of general physiologic features and functions of vitamin D, Am J Clin Nutr 2004;80: 1689S–96S.

Demiaux B, Arlot ME, Chapuy MC, Meunier PJ, Delmas PD, Serum osteocalcin is increased in patients with osteomalacia: correlations with biochemical and histomorphometric findings. J Clin Endocrinol Metab 1992;74: 1146–51.

Diamond T, Smerdely P, Kormas N, Sekel R, Vu T, Day P, Hip fracture in elderly men: the importance of subclinical vitamin D deficiency and hypogonadism. Med J Aust 1998;169: 138–41.

Duque G, Macoritto M, Dion N, Ste-Marie LG, Kremer R, 1,25(OH)2D$_3$ acts as a bone-forming agent in the hormone-independent senescence-accelerated mouse (SAM-P/6). Am J Physiol Endocrinol Metab 2005;288: E723–E730.

El-Hajj FG, Nabulsi M, Choucair M et al., Hypovitaminosis D in healthy schoolchildren. Pediatrics 2001;107: E53.

El-Hajj FG, Nabulsi M, Tamim H et al., Effect of vitamin D replacement on musculoskeletal parameters in school children: a randomized controlled trial. J Clin Endocrinol Metab 2006; 91: 405–12.

Erem C, Tanakol R, Alagol F, Omer B, Cetin O, Relationship of bone turnover parameters, endogenous hormones and vit D deficiency to hip fracture in elderly postmenopausal women. Int J Clin Pract 2002;56: 333–7.

Flicker L, Mead K, MacInnis RJ et al., Serum vitamin D and falls in older women in residential care in Australia. J Am Geriatr Soc 2003;51: 1533–8.

Frame B, Parfitt AM, Osteomalacia: current concepts. Ann Intern Med 1978;89: 966–82.

Gardiner EM, Baldock PA, Thomas GP et al., Increased formation and decreased resorption of bone in mice with elevated vitamin D receptor in mature cells of the osteoblastic lineage. FASEB J 2000;14: 1908–16.

Garnero P, Munoz F, Sornay-Rendu E, Delmas PD, Associations of vitamin D status with bone mineral density, bone turnover, bone loss and fracture risk in healthy postmenopausal women. The OFELY study. Bone 2007;40: 716–22.

Gerdhem P, Ringsberg KA, Obrant KJ, Akesson K, Association between 25-hydroxy vitamin D levels, physical activity, muscle strength and fractures in the prospective population-based OPRA Study of Elderly Women. Osteoporos Int 2005;16: 1425–31.

Gordon CM, DePeter KC, Feldman HA, Grace E, Emans SJ, Prevalence of vitamin D deficiency among healthy adolescents. Arch Pediatr Adolesc Med 2004;158: 531–7.

Grant AM, Avenell A, Campbell MK et al., Oral vitamin D3 and calcium for secondary prevention of low-trauma fractures in elderly people (Randomised Evaluation of Calcium Or vitamin D, RECORD): a randomised placebo-controlled trial. Lancet 2005;365: 1621–8.

Greer FR, Marshall S, Bone mineral content, serum vitamin D metabolite concentrations, and ultraviolet B light exposure in infants fed human milk with and without vitamin D2 supplements. J Pediatr 1989;114: 204–12.

Guillemant J, Le HT, Maria A, Allemandou A, Peres G, Guillemant S, Wintertime vitamin D deficiency in male adolescents: effect on parathyroid function and response to vitamin D3 supplements. Osteoporos Int 2001;12: 875–9.

Hagenau T, Vest R, Gissel TN et al., Global vitamin D levels in relation to age, gender, skin pigmentation and latitude: an ecologic meta-regression analysis. Osteoporos Int 2009;20: 133–40.

Heaney RP, Quantifying human calcium absorption using pharmacokinetic methods. J Nutr 2003;133: 1224–6.

Heaney RP, Dowell MS, Hale CA, Bendich A, Calcium absorption varies within the reference range for serum 25-hydroxyvitamin D. J Am Coll Nutr 2003;22: 142–6.

Holick MF, Vitamin D deficiency. N Engl J Med 2007;357: 266–81.

Holick MF, Biancuzzo RM, Chen TC et al., Vitamin D2 is as effective as vitamin D3 in maintaining circulating concentrations of 25-hydroxyvitamin D. J Clin Endocrinol Metab 2008;93: 677–81.

Hollis BW, Wagner CL, Assessment of dietary vitamin D requirements during pregnancy and lactation. Am J Clin Nutr 2004;79: 717–26.

Jackson RD, LaCroix AZ, Gass M et al., Calcium plus vitamin D supplementation and the risk of fractures. N Engl J Med 2006;354: 669–83.

Khaw KT, Sneyd MJ, Compston J, Bone density parathyroid hormone and 25-hydroxyvitamin D concentrations in middle aged women. B Med J 1992;305: 273–7.

Krall EA, Sahyoun N, Tannenbaum S, Dallal GE, Dawson-Hughes B, Effect of vitamin D intake on seasonal variations in parathyroid hormone secretion in postmenopausal women. N Engl J Med 1989;321: 1777–83.

Kremer R, Campbell PP, Reinhardt T, Gilsanz V, Vitamin D status and its relationship to body fat, final height, and peak bone mass in young women. J Clin Endocrinol Metab 2009;94: 67–73.

Lau EM, Woo J, Swaminathan R, MacDonald D, Donnan SP, Plasma 25-hydroxyvitamin D concentration in patients with hip fracture in Hong Kong. Gerontology 1989;35: 198–204.

LeBoff MS, Kohlmeier L, Hurwitz S, Franklin J, Wright J, Glowacki J, Occult vitamin D deficiency in postmenopausal US women with acute hip fracture. J Am Med Assoc 1999;281: 1505–11.

Lee JM, Smith JR, Philipp BL, Chen TC, Mathieu J, Holick MF, Vitamin D deficiency in a healthy group of mothers and newborn infants. Clin Pediatr (Phila) 2007;46: 42–4.

Lepage R, Roy L, Brossard JH et al., A non-(1–84) circulating parathyroid hormone (PTH) fragment interferes significantly with intact PTH commercial assay measurements in uremic samples. Clin Chem 1998;44: 805–9.

Leventis P, Kiely PD, The tolerability and biochemical effects of high-dose bolus vitamin D2 and D3 supplementation in patients with vitamin D insufficiency. Scand J Rheumatol 2009;38: 149–53.

Lips P, Vitamin D deficiency and secondary hyperparathyroidism in the elderly: consequences for bone loss and fractures and therapeutic implications. Endocr Rev 2001;22: 477–501.

Lips P, van Ginkel FC, Jongen MJ, Rubertus F, van der Vijgh WJ, Netelenbos JC, Determinants of vitamin D status in patients with hip fracture and in elderly control subjects. Am J Clin Nutr 1987;46: 1005–10.

Lips P, Wiersinga A, van Ginkel FC et al., The effect of vitamin D supplementation on vitamin D status and parathyroid function in elderly subjects. J Clin Endocrinol Metab 1988;67: 644–50.

Looker AC, Mussolino ME, Serum 25-hydroxyvitamin D and hip fracture risk in older U.S. white adults. J Bone Miner Res 2008;23: 143–50.

Lund B, Sorensen OH, Christensen AB, 25-Hydroxycholecaliferol and fractures of the proximal. Lancet 1975;2: 300–2.

Marwaha RK, Tandon N, Reddy DR et al., Vitamin D and bone mineral density status of healthy schoolchildren in northern India. Am J Clin Nutr 2005;82: 477–82.

McAuley KA, Jones S, Lewis-Barned NJ, Manning P, Goulding A, Low vitamin D status is common among elderly Dunedin women. NZ Med J 1997;110: 275–7.

McGrath JJ, Kimlin MG, Saha S, Eyles DW, Parisi AV, Vitamin D insufficiency in south-east Queensland. Med J Aust 2001;174: 150–1.

Meier C, Woitge HW, Witte K, Lemmer B, Seibel MJ, Supplementation with oral vitamin D3 and calcium during winter prevents seasonal bone loss: a randomized controlled open-label prospective trial. J Bone Miner Res 2004;19: 1221–30.

Misof BM, Roschger P, Tesch W et al., Targeted overexpression of vitamin D receptor in osteoblasts increases calcium concentration without affecting structural properties of bone mineral crystals. Calcif Tissue Int 2003;73: 251–7.

Nagaoka H, Mochida Y, Atsawasuwan P, Kaku M, Kondoh T, Yamauchi M, 1,25(OH)2D$_3$ regulates collagen quality in an osteoblastic cell culture system. Biochem Biophys Res Commun 2008;377: 674–8.

Nesby-OíDell S, Scanlon KS, Cogswell ME et al., Hypovitaminosis D prevalence and determinants among African American and white women of reproductive age: third National Health and Nutrition Examination Survey, 1988ñ1994. Am J Clin Nutr 2002;76: 187–92.

Norman AW, Bouillon R, Whiting SJ, Vieth R, Lips P, 13th Workshop consensus for vitamin D nutritional guidelines. J Steroid Biochem Mol Biol 2007;103: 204–5.

Nuti R, Martini G, Valenti R et al., Vitamin D status and bone turnover in women with acute hip fracture. Clin Orthop Relat Res 2004;422: 208–13.

Ooms ME, Lips P, Roos JC et al., Vitamin D status and sex hormone binding globulin: determinants of bone turnover and bone mineral density in elderly women. J Bone Miner Res 1995;10: 1177–84.

Owen TA, Aronow MS, Barone LM, Bettencourt B, Stein GS, Lian JB, Pleiotropic effects of vitamin D on osteoblast gene expression are related to the proliferative and differentiated state of the bone cell phenotype: dependency upon basal levels of gene expression, duration of exposure, and bone matrix competency in normal rat osteoblast cultures. Endocrinology 1991;128: 1496–504.

Parfitt AM, Morphologic basis of bone mineral measurements: transient and steady state effects of treatment in osteoporosis. Miner Electrolyte Metab 1980;4: 273–87.

Parfitt AM, Rao DS, Stanciu J, Villanueva AR, Kleerekoper M, Frame B, Irreversible bone loss in osteomalacia. Comparison of radial photon absorptiometry with iliac bone histomorphometry during treatment. J Clin Invest 1985;76: 2403–12.

Pehlivan I, Hatun S, Aydogan M, Babaoglu K, Gokalp AS, Maternal vitamin D deficiency and vitamin D supplementation in healthy infants. Turk J Pediatr 2003;45: 315–20.

Pfeifer M, Begerow B, Minne HW, Vitamin D and muscle function. Osteoporos Int 2002;13: 187–94.

Pfeifer M, Begerow B, Minne HW, Suppan K, Fahrleitner-Pammer A, Dobnig H, Effects of a long-term vitamin D and calcium supplementation on falls and parameters of muscle function in community-dwelling older individuals. Osteoporos Int 2009;20: 315–22.

Pleasure D, Wyszynski B, Sumner A et al., Skeletal muscle calcium metabolism and contractile force in vitamin D-deficient chicks. J Clin Invest 1979;64: 1157–67.

Punnonen R, Salmi J, Tuimala R, Jarvinen M, Pystynen P, Vitamin D deficiency in women with femoral neck fracture. Maturitas 1986;8: 291–5.

Roddam AW, Neale R, Appleby P, Allen NE, Tipper S, Key TJ, Association between plasma 25-hydroxyvitamin D levels and fracture risk: the EPIC-Oxford study. Am J Epidemiol 2007; 166: 1327–36.

Rodman JS, Baker T, Changes in the kinetics of muscle contraction in vitamin D-depleted rats. Kidney Int 1978;13: 189–93.

Sahota O, Masud T, San P, Hosking DJ, Vitamin D insufficiency increases bone turnover markers and enhances bone loss at the hip in patients with established vertebral osteoporosis. Clin Endocrinol (Oxf) 1999;51: 217–21.

Sambrook PN, Chen JS, March LM et al., Serum parathyroid hormone predicts time to fall independent of vitamin D status in a frail elderly population. J Clin Endocrinol Metab 2004; 89: 1572–6.

Schou AJ, Heuck C, Wolthers OD, Vitamin D supplementation to healthy children does not affect serum osteocalcin or markers of type I collagen turnover. Acta Paediatr 2003;92: 797–801.

Sedrani SH, Low 25-hydroxyvitamin D and normal serum calcium concentrations in Saudi Arabia: Riyadh region. Ann Nutr Metab 1984;28: 181–5.

Sooy K, Sabbagh Y, Demay MB, Osteoblasts lacking the vitamin D receptor display enhanced osteogenic potential in vitro. J Cell Biochem 2005;94: 81–7.

Sorensen OH, Lund B, Saltin B et al., Myopathy in bone loss of ageing: improvement by treatment with 1 alpha-hydroxycholecalciferol and calcium. Clin Sci (Lond) 1979;56: 157–61.

Specker BL, Ho ML, Oestreich A et al., Prospective study of vitamin D supplementation and rickets in China. J Pediatr 1992;120: 733–9.

St-Arnaud R, The direct role of vitamin D on bone homeostasis. Arch Biochem Biophys 2008;473: 225–30.

Sullivan SS, Rosen CJ, Halteman WA, Chen TC, Holick MF, Adolescent girls in Maine are at risk for vitamin D insufficiency. J Am Diet Assoc 2005;105: 971–4.

Takasu H, Anti-osteoclastogenic action of active vitamin D, Nutr Rev 2008;66: S113–5.

Takasu H, Sugita A, Uchiyama Y et al., c-Fos protein as a target of anti-osteoclastogenic action of vitamin D, and synthesis of new analogs. J Clin Invest 2006;116: 528–35.

Tanaka H, Seino Y, Direct action of 1,25-dihydroxyvitamin D on bone: VDRKO bone shows excessive bone formation in normal mineral condition. J Steroid Biochem Mol Biol 2004;89–90: 343–5.

Tangpricha V, Pearce EN, Chen TC, Holick MF, Vitamin D insufficiency among free-living healthy young adults. Am J Med 2002;112: 659–62.

Thiebaud D, Burckhardt P, Costanza M et al., Importance of albumin, 25(OH)-vitamin D and IGFBP-3 as risk factors in elderly women and men with hip fracture. Osteoporos Int 1997;7: 457–62.

Thomas MK, Lloyd-Jones DM, Thadhani RI et al., Hypovitaminosis D in medical inpatients. N Engl J Med 1998;338: 777–83.

Underwood JL, DeLuca HF, Vitamin D is not directly necessary for bone growth and mineralization. Am J Physiol 1984;246: E493–8.

van der Wielen RP, Lowik MR, van den BH et al., Serum vitamin D concentrations among elderly people in Europe. Lancet 1995;346: 207–10.

Vieth R, Why the optimal requirement for Vitamin D3 is probably much higher than what is officially recommended for adults. J Steroid Biochem Mol Biol 2004;89–90: 575–9.

Villareal DT, Civitelli R, Chines A, Avioli LV, Subclinical vitamin D deficiency in postmenopausal women with low vertebral bone mass. J Clin Endocrinol Metab 1991;72: 628–34.

Visser M, Deeg DJ, Lips P, Low vitamin D and high parathyroid hormone levels as determinants of loss of muscle strength and muscle mass (sarcopenia): the Longitudinal Aging Study Amsterdam. J Clin Endocrinol Metab 2003;88: 5766–72.

Wassner SJ, Li JB, Sperduto A, Norman ME, Vitamin D Deficiency, hypocalcemia, and increased skeletal muscle degradation in rats. J Clin Invest 1983;72: 102–12.

Woitge HW, Knothe A, Witte K et al., Circaannual rhythms and interactions of vitamin D metabolites, parathyroid hormone, and biochemical markers of skeletal homeostasis: a prospective study. J Bone Miner Res 2000;15: 2443–50.

Woo J, Lau E, Swaminathan R, Pang CP, MacDonald D, Biochemical predictors for osteoporotic fractures in elderly Chinese – a longitudinal study. Gerontology 1990;36: 55–8.

Zeghoud F, Vervel C, Guillozo H, Walrant-Debray O, Boutignon H, Garabedian M, Subclinical vitamin D deficiency in neonates: definition and response to vitamin D supplements. Am J Clin Nutr 1997;65: 771–8.

11 Vitamin E – Alpha-tocopherol

11.1 Vitamin E in human nutrition: importance of its antioxidant function

Maret G. Traber

11.1.1 Introduction

The molecular mechanisms of action of vitamin E, a potent lipid soluble antioxidant that is necessary for reproduction, are unknown (Traber and Atkinson, 2007). A dichotomy exists between the antioxidant and biologic activities of vitamin E. Plants synthesize eight different molecules with vitamin E antioxidant activity, yet only one of these, α-tocopherol, is a nutrient required by animals and humans.

We believe that the lack of success in determining the molecular function of α-tocopherol results from some major obstacles. First, α-tocopherol requires special transport mechanisms for delivery to tissues; these mechanisms make outcomes from cell culture studies largely misleading. Secondly, α-tocopherol is involved in complex interactions between various oxidizing and antioxidant systems; these interactions make outcomes from cell culture studies largely misleading because antioxidants are often depleted in culture medium. Thirdly, it is difficult using experimental animals to obtain tissues (particularly embryos) that are sufficiently α-tocopherol-depleted to be useful to identify α-tocopherol-sensitive functions. This chapter will address these issues, define the gaps in our knowledge, and emphasize the importance of vitamin E in human nutrition.

11.1.2 Forms and functions

Vitamin E is a lipid-soluble antioxidant that halts lipid peroxidation (Traber and Atkinson, 2007). Traber and Atkinson (2007) reviewed the data that the antioxidant function of α-tocopherol is its only vitamin function. α-Tocopherol prevents the chain reaction that occurs when a peroxyl radical (ROO$^\bullet$) attacks polyunsaturated fatty acids. When α-tocopherol intercepts a ROO$^\bullet$, an α-tocopheroxyl radical (α-TO$^\bullet$) is formed; its most probable fate is to be reduced back to α-tocopherol by ascorbic acid (Buettner, 1993). An adequate supply of ascorbic acid will ensure recycling of the α-tocopheroxyl radical to its unoxidized form and thus prolong the α-tocopherol lifetime. Importantly, ascorbic acid does not directly inhibit lipid peroxidation, but it can react with various reactive oxygen species that could initiate lipid peroxidation.

Dietary components with vitamin E antioxidant activity include α-, β-, γ-, and δ-tocopherols and tocotrienols (▶Fig. 11.1). They all have a chromanol ring with varying numbers of methyl groups and either have a phytyl tail (tocopherols) or an unsaturated tail (tocotrienols). Differences in the biologic activities of the eight different naturally occurring forms of vitamin E were first recognized over 80 years ago (Emerson et al., 1937). Although differences in antioxidant activity might have explained those differences,

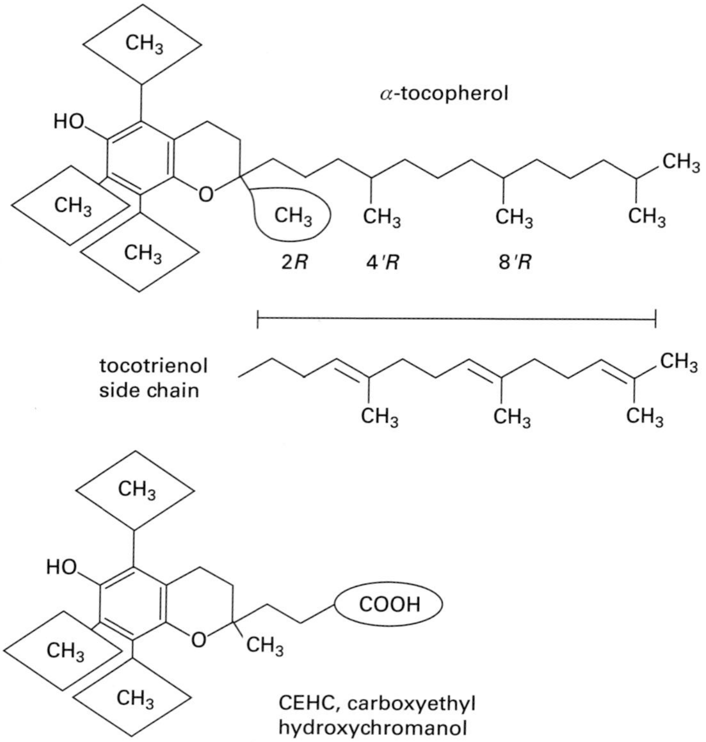

Fig. 11.1: Structures. *RRR*-α-tocopherol [2,5,7,8-tetramethyl-2*R*-(4′*R*,8′*R*,12-trimethyltridecyl)-6-chromanol] has three methyl groups on the chromanol ring shown in diamonds; three of the methyl groups (at 2, 4′ and 8′) on the phytyl tail have *R*-stereochemistry, not *S*. Importantly, the 2 position methyl group (shown encircled) must have *R*-stereochemistry for α-tocopherol to be recognized by α-TTP. Other antioxidants with vitamin E antioxidant activity have fewer methyl groups; β- and γ- have two, and δ-tocopherol has one. Tocotrienols have the same head groups but an unsaturated side chain. Shown also is α-CEHC, the water-soluble metabolite of α-tocopherol and α-tocotrienol; similar metabolites are formed from the other tocopherols and tocotrienols.

they did not, as reviewed (Traber, 2007). For example, the antioxidant activities of natural and synthetic α-tocopherols are identical, but because the synthetic is composed of eight different stereoisomeric forms, the natural and synthetic α-tocopherols have different biologic activities. Differences between natural and synthetic α-tocopherols were first described over 50 years ago (Harris and Ludwig, 1949).

11.1.3 Transport, delivery and metabolism

11.1.3.1 Vitamin E absorption

In humans, all vitamin E forms are absorbed and transported by chylomicrons from the intestine to the liver (Traber and Kayden, 1989; Traber et al., 1990a). There are no definitive studies quantitating α-tocopherol absorption in humans. Studies from 1960–70 using radioactive α-tocopherol in humans reported fractional vitamin E absorption in normal subjects ranging from 55 to 79% (Kelleher and Losowsky, 1968; MacMahon and Neale, 1970). These were balance studies and depended upon the complete collection of fecal material; any loss of labeled material resulted in increased apparent absorption. By contrast, more recent studies using deuterium-labeled α-tocopherol suggested that vitamin E absorption in humans was only 33% (Bruno et al., 2006b). However, these estimates were based observed plasma labeled α-tocopherol concentrations and thus are probably underestimations. Clifford et al. (2006) reported 77% vitamin E absorption in studies conducted in one person using ^{14}C-labeled α-tocopherol and accelerator mass spectrometry for measurements of fecal radioactivity. These data emphasize our lack of knowledge concerning quantitation of vitamin E absorption.

11.1.3.2 Vitamin E and dietary fat intakes

The amount of fat in the accompanying meal could alter vitamin E absorption. Using deuterium-labeled vitamin E, Leonard et al. (2004) showed plasma-labeled α-tocopherol concentrations were higher following consumption of a fortified breakfast cereal (30 IU) as compared with a vitamin E pill (400 IU) consumed with a glass of water! Probably, the emulsifier used to solubilize vitamin E for spraying it onto the cereal surface also aided its absorption.

A follow-up trial using only food was then implemented to assess the importance of the fat content of the meal given with the labeled vitamin E dose (Bruno et al., 2006b). Apples were fortified with deuterated α-tocopherol (22 mg d_6-α-tocopherol) and were consumed: (1) alone; (2) with bagels and fat-free cream cheese; or (3) with bagels and full fat cream cheese (Bruno et al., 2006b). Increasing d_6-α-tocopherol bioavailability was observed with increasing amounts of fat consumed (▶Fig. 11.2). It should be noted that the vitamin E-fortified apples were consumed with breakfast, and in each trial lunch containing 36% fat was eaten ~5 h later, yet had no apparent effect on d_6-α-tocopherol absorption. These findings highlight the importance of fat absorption in the role of vitamin E absorption.

11.1.3.3 Mechanism for vitamin E absorption

The mechanism for vitamin E absorption from the intestinal lumen into the enterocyte is not understood, but advances have been made. Cholesterol absorption from mixed micelles is mediated by Niemann-Pick C1-Like 1 (NPC1L1), a protein that facilitates cholesterol transfer into endocytic vesicles for intracellular trafficking (Ge et al., 2008; Wang et al., 2009). Importantly, this protein also facilitates vitamin E absorption (Narushima et al., 2008). Hypothetically, drugs, such as ezetemibe, which inhibit cholesterol absorption by targeting NPC1L1, will also decrease vitamin E absorption in humans.

11.1.3.4 Vitamin E transport

Progress in defining the mechanisms for differences in biologic activity came with the discovery of the hepatic α-tocopherol transfer protein (α-TTP) (Sato et al., 1991, 1993) and its cloning (Meier et al., 2003; Min et al., 2003). In studies of normal subjects

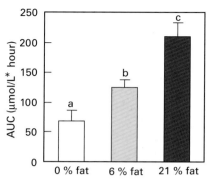

Fig. 11.2: Effect of fat on vitamin E absorption. Five healthy participants consumed apples fortified with deuterium-labeled α-tocopheryl acetate (22 mg d_6-*RRR*-α-tocopherol/serving) in three sequential trials with a breakfast containing increasing fat (0, 6, 21% kcal, e.g., 0, 2.4, 11 g) (Bruno, 2006b). Blood samples were obtained up to 72 h following isotope administration; plasma labeled and unlabeled α-tocopherol concentrations were measured and the area under the curve (AUC) was used as a measure of bioavailability. The time (T_{max}, 9 ± 2 h) of peak plasma d_6-α-tocopherol and the fractional disappearance rates (FDRs, 0.022 ± 0.003 pools/day) did not differ significantly between the three trials. Additionally, the FDRs were not correlated with fat intake. Given the lack of change in T_{max} and FDRs between trials, the increase in bioavailability with increased fat intake resulted from increased vitamin E absorption. Bars not bearing the same letter are significantly different ($p < 0.05$).

consuming deuterium-labeled vitamin E, the liver was found to preferentially secrete α-tocopherol into plasma lipoproteins (Traber et al., 1990a). Subsequently, studies were conducted in patients who were vitamin E deficient (Traber et al., 1990b, 1993), and were later described to have genetic defects in α-TTP (Ben Hamida et al., 1993; Doerflinger et al., 1995). The patients not only developed vitamin E deficiency symptoms, but were unable to discriminate between various forms of vitamin E and were unable to secrete α-tocopherol from the liver (Traber et al., 1990b, 1993), suggesting that α-TTP was crucial for discrimination between vitamin E forms.

Various mechanisms for lipid and lipoprotein trafficking serve to deliver α-tocopherol to tissues and return it to the liver, as reviewed (Traber, 1999, 2007). Importantly, no tissue serves as a vitamin E store, releasing α-tocopherol on demand. Nonetheless, adipose tissue and nerves both become depleted in humans experiencing vitamin E deficiency (Traber et al., 1987).

11.1.3.5 α-Tocopherol pharmacokinetics

Vitamin E because it is fat soluble, transported by lipoproteins, and dependent upon mechanisms of lipid and lipoprotein metabolism for delivery to tissues has complex pharmacokinetics (Traber, 2007). Some information is known about vitamin E pharmacokinetics using orally administered deuterium-labeled vitamin E(s). The plasma half-life of *RRR*-α-tocopherol is ~48–60 h (Traber et al., 1994; Leonard et al., 2005), whereas that of *SRR*-α-tocopherol (synthetic form) is ~15 h (Traber et al., 1994). α-Tocopherol recirculation from the liver to the plasma is crucial for this long half-life (Traber et al., 1994). The rapid recirculation results in the daily replacement of nearly all of the circulating α-tocopherol (Traber et al., 1994).

11.1.3.6 Vitamin E metabolism and excretion

Metabolism has an important role in defining the preference for α-tocopherol, for limiting α-tocopherol accumulation, and for determining the circulating levels of various vitamin E forms. The vitamin E metabolite derived from α-tocopherol and from α-tocotrienol (α-CEHC, carboxyethyl hydroxychroman), is tail-shortened, but has an unoxidized head group (▶Fig. 11.1) (Brigelius-Flohé and Traber, 1999). Similar products are synthesized from the other tocopherols and tocotrienols (Sontag and Parker, 2002, 2007). Studies using deuterium-labeled α- and γ-tocopherols demonstrated that the preference for α-tocopherol depended upon the rapid metabolism of γ-tocopherol to γ-CEHC (Leonard et al., 2005). This conclusion is emphasized by studies in *Drosophila*, which documented that the flies lack the α-tocopherol transfer protein, but were capable of metabolizing both δ- and γ-tocopherols to their respective CEHCs (Parker and McCormick, 2005). Importantly, the flies preferentially retained α-tocopherol. Thus, the metabolic rates of α-tocopherol are relatively low compared with those other vitamin E forms, thereby explaining the α-tocopherol accumulation.

11.1.4 Human vitamin E deficiency signs and symptoms

11.1.4.1 Causes of vitamin E deficiency in humans

Overt α-tocopherol deficiency occurs rarely in humans and usually only as a result of genetic abnormalities in α-TTP or various fat malabsorption syndromes (Traber, 1999). Genetic defects in human α-TTP are associated with a characteristic syndrome, ataxia with vitamin E deficiency (AVED) (Cavalier et al., 1998). Friedreich's ataxia shares many similar symptoms, and α-TTP gene deletions in experimental models are commonly referred to as creating 'Friedreich-like ataxia with vitamin E deficiency'.

Human α-tocopherol deficiency symptoms include a progressive peripheral neuropathy with a specific 'dying back' of the large caliber axons of the sensory neurons, which results in ataxia (Sokol et al., 1988). The primary manifestations include spinocerebellar ataxia and skeletal myopathy (Sokol, 1993). However, severe α-tocopherol deficiency in rodents causes fetal resorption (Food and Nutrition Board, 2000). Thus, adequate vitamin E levels are probably necessary for successful reproduction in humans.

11.1.4.2 Vitamin E and α-TTP in pregnancy and fetal development

Vitamin E was discovered in 1922 when rats fed rancid fat failed to carry their offspring to term (Evans and Bishop, 1922). This 'fetal resorption test' remains in use today as an assay of biologic activities of various vitamin E forms (Traber, 1999). To prevent fetal resorption, vitamin E must be administered to the rodent mother on post-fertilization days 5–9 (Leth et al., 1977; Ames, 1979). Interestingly, this is the same crucial period where the 12/15-LOX pathway appears to mediate implantation (Li et al., 2004). Similarly, GPx4 expression increases at day 7.5 and is the same time at which GPx4-knockout mice embryos are resorbed (Imai et al., 2003). These findings suggest that during days 5–9 of rodent embryogenesis, lipid peroxidation can be particularly damaging.

Both low fetal and maternal α-tocopherol concentrations could be important factors during fetal resorption. Retention of uterine α-tocopherol by the mother appears essential to maintain pregnancy because α-TTP is increased at the site of implantation (Jishage et al., 2001; Kaempf-Rotzoll et al., 2002) and is also expressed in the syncytiotrophoblast of the human placenta (Kaempf-Rotzoll et al., 2003). Early failure of pregnancy is associated with lipid peroxidation with resultant damage to the syncytiotrophoblast (Hempstock et al., 2003). Thus, it is probable that α-tocopherol is needed by the mother to protect her from the oxidative stress of the rapidly growing fetus. Although α-TTP is described as a liver protein in adult rodents and humans, Jauniaux et al. (2004) showed that human yolk sac, placenta and uterus express α-TTP. They further suggest that during very early human fetal development, the human embryo obtains α-tocopherol from the yolk sac. Taken together, these data suggest that both the mother and the fetus need α-tocopherol, yet we do not know the molecular mechanisms as to why α-tocopherol is necessary.

11.1.4.3 Interactions of oxidants and antioxidants during development

Apoptosis is a key function during embryologic development that must be closely regulated. For example, cavitation is dependent upon apoptosis (Coucouvanis and Martin, 1995). An imbalance between oxidant production and removal causes increased oxidative stress and apoptosis in chorion trophoblast cells from human fetal tissues (Yuan et al., 2008); thus, inappropriate increases in oxidative stress can cause abnormal cell death. Frequently, α-tocopherol is reported to decrease apoptosis. For example, buthionine-sulfoximine (BSO) causes increased oxidative stress by inhibiting glutathione (GSH) synthesis, thereby depleting intracellular GSH and subsequently inducing cell death. In a model of BSO-induced cytotoxicity in rat striatal cultures, α-tocopherol prevented the cytotoxicity caused by GSH-depletion (Osakada et al., 2003). Furthermore, α-tocopherol reversed staurosporine-induced apoptosis (Osakada et al., 2003); staurosporine both inhibits kinases and prevents apoptosis-inducing factor (AIF)-mediated apoptosis (Zhang et al., 2004). Thus, similar functions appear to be performed by GSH (a water-soluble, thiol antioxidant) and α-tocopherol (a lipid-soluble antioxidant). Clearly, α-tocopherol provides antioxidant protection during lipid peroxidation, but it has been nearly impossible to identify specific oxidized lipids, leading some to suggest that α-tocopherol has 'non-antioxidant', signaling functions (Azzi, 2007). However, most of these 'non-antioxidant' functions can be implemented by other antioxidants, or are increased by oxidative stress (Traber and Atkinson, 2007); therefore, it seems probable that α-tocopherol is protecting some key lipid mediator.

A clue to the role of α-tocopherol during apoptosis comes from a study that linked α-tocopherol, GSH, oxidative stress, lipid peroxidation and AIF-mediated cell death (Seiler et al., 2008). GPx4 (also known as phospholipid glutathione peroxidase, PHGPx) was reported to sense and translate oxidative stress into cell death that was dependent upon both 12/15-LOX and AIF (Seiler et al., 2008). GPx4 is a member of the glutathione peroxidase family that uses GSH to detoxify hydroperoxides (Brigelius-Flohé, 2006), and is also a recognized anti-apoptotic factor (Nakagawa, 2004), whereas 12/15 LOX generates lipid peroxyl radicals (Jacquot et al., 2008). Importantly, both α-tocopherol and GSH, but not other water-soluble antioxidants, efficiently prevented cell death. These findings begin to give a molecular basis for the requirement for vitamin E, but their specificity for α-tocopherol is not yet apparent.

11.1.5 Human vitamin E requirements

11.1.5.1 Recommended intakes

Only α-tocopherol meets human vitamin E requirements (Food and Nutrition Board, 2000). The recommended dietary allowance (RDA) for vitamin E (15 mg (22 IU) *RRR*-α-tocopherol) was described in the 2000 Dietary Reference Intakes (DRIs) (Food and Nutrition Board, 2000). Importantly, 96% of American women and 93% of men do not meet the current vitamin E recommendations (Moshfegh et al., 2005); the mean dietary intakes in the US are only ~6 mg α-tocopherol (Gao et al., 2006).

11.1.5.2 Optimal α-tocopherol intakes

Are recommendations too high or is dietary vitamin E consumption by most people too low? In general, to set an estimated dietary requirement (EAR), the amount of a nutrient needed to fulfill a specific biochemical function is estimated. Then, the amount needed from the diet is estimated based on the fractional absorption. Given that the biochemical function of vitamin E is its antioxidant activity, and the fractional absorption is not known, the 2000 vitamin E RDAs had to be set by correlation of antioxidant activity with dietary intakes. The only relevant data available were from studies conducted more than 50 years ago (Food and Nutrition Board, 2000). Those studies assumed that vitamin E protects membrane lipids and that increased erythrocyte fragility is a vitamin E deficiency symptom (Food and Nutrition Board, 2000). Erythrocytes were obtained from seven male psychiatric state hospital patients who had consumed a vitamin E-deficient diet for more than 6 years, and then each man was repleted with a different dose of vitamin E for at least 100 days (Horwitt et al., 1956). The lowest dose necessary to prevent *in vitro* peroxide-induced erythrocyte hemolysis was chosen as the EAR. No women were studied. The RDA was based on these measures because these were the only available data despite the general agreement that the hemolysis assay is highly dependent on assay conditions, and that no lipid peroxidation measures have been described that are specific solely for vitamin E (Food and Nutrition Board, 2000).

11.1.5.3 Is there a health benefit associated with optimal α-tocopherol intakes?

The Alpha-Tocopherol, Beta-Carotene Cancer Prevention (ATBC) study tested in Finnish smokers whether supplementation for 5 years with vitamin E (50 IU DL-α-tocopheryl acetate) and/or β-carotene (20 mg) would decrease cancer incidence (Albanes et al., 1996). Although supplementation had no effect on mortality, a follow-up report (Wright et al., 2006) described baseline vitamin E status of the 29 092 Finnish men, who were followed for 19 years during which time 13 380 deaths ensued. The men at baseline in the highest compared with the lowest quintiles of serum α-tocopherol had significantly lower incidences of total mortality [relative risk (RR) = 0.82 (95% CI: 0.78, 0.86)] and cause-specific mortality [cancer RR = 0.79 (0.72, 0.86), cardiovascular disease RR = 0.81 (0.75, 0.88), and other causes RR = 0.70 (0.63, 0.79); p for trend for each <0.0001]. A reduction in mortality occurred at serum α-tocopherol concentrations (30 μmol/l) associated with dietary intakes of ~13 mg α-tocopherol (Wright et al., 2006), consistent with the vitamin E RDA in the 2000 DRIs (Food and Nutrition Board, 2000).

Thus, a generous dietary intake of vitamin E over a lifetime apparently can decrease chronic disease incidence.

The Women's Health Study (Lee et al., 2005) tested the efficacy of vitamin E supplements to prevent heart disease or cancer in normal healthy women. They evaluated 600 IU vitamin E or placebo taken every other day for 10 years by ~40 000 healthy women aged 45 years and older. Overall, vitamin E supplements had no effect on the incidence of cancer, cardiovascular events or on total mortality. However, deaths from cardiovascular disease were reduced 24% (RR = 0.76; 95% CI, 0.59–0.98; p = 0.03). The decrease in cardiovascular death was attributed to a decrease in sudden death (Lee et al., 2005). Given that the incidence of cardiovascular disease is low in women until they are over 65 years and that women lag behind men by 20 years with respect to sudden death (http://www.americanheart.org), these findings suggest that vitamin E supplements are effective in decreasing death from cardiovascular disease. It is not clear if supplements just ensure that women consume 'optimal amounts' of vitamin E (15 mg, as discussed above) or if other mechanisms are involved.

11.1.6 Vitamin E antioxidant effects *in vivo*

The evidence in humans that α-tocopherol functions as a lipid soluble antioxidant is limited. Because cigarette smoking generates free radicals (Pryor, 1992), we investigated α-tocopherol kinetics in smokers compared with non-smokers.

11.1.6.1 Vitamin E kinetics during oxidative stress as studied in cigarette smokers

Vitamin E kinetics in smokers and nonsmokers following six d deuterium-labeled α-tocopheryl acetate supplementation (75 mg each d_3-*RRR*- and d_6-*all rac*-α-tocopheryl acetates) (Bruno et al., 2005a,b). Supplementation (six d) was sufficient for both groups to achieve similar plasma-deuterated α-tocopherol concentrations (data not shown). Plasma labeled and unlabeled α-tocopherol concentrations were measured up to 3 weeks post-dosing. Plasma α-tocopherol concentrations for each isotope (d_3, d_6 and d_0), for each subject, at each time point were used to calculate the percentage of d_3-α-tocopherol, which was fitted by a two-compartment model, as described (Traber et al., 2001). The two compartments were assumed to have reached the same deuterated α-tocopherol concentrations in the two groups. α-Tocopherol fractional disappearance rates (FDRs) were ~13% greater and half-lives were ~11% shorter in the smokers compared with nonsmokers. With respect to vitamin C and E interactions, the smokers with the lowest ascorbic acid concentrations had the fastest plasma α-tocopherol disappearance (Bruno et al., 2005b).

11.1.6.2 Interaction of vitamins E and C in humans

The most important finding from the vitamin E studies in cigarette smokers was the inverse association between vitamin C status and α-tocopherol fractional disappearance rates (FDRs) (Bruno et al., 2005b). This finding led to the hypothesis that vitamin C supplements in smokers could normalize their vitamin E pharmacokinetics. We conducted this study using a double-blind, placebo-controlled randomized crossover design in which the participants served as their own controls (Bruno et al., 2006a). Smokers ($n = 11$) and nonsmokers ($n = 13$) ingested deuterium-labeled α- and γ-tocopherols (50 mg each d_6-α-*RRR*- and d_2-γ-*RRR*-tocopheryl acetates) with a breakfast following 2 weeks daily supplementation with placebo or 1 g ascorbic acid (Bruno et al., 2006a). During the placebo trial, both smokers and nonsmokers had low plasma ascorbic acid concentrations (~45 μmol/l), but only smokers' plasma α-and γ-tocopherols disappeared faster relative to the vitamin C supplemented state. We previously attributed this phenomenon to the higher oxidative stress level observed in smokers (Bruno et al., 2005b). Because it is well known that ascorbate regenerates α-tocopherol from an α-tocopheroxyl radical *in vitro* (Buettner, 1993), the purpose of this study was to test the extent to which increased plasma ascorbic acid concentrations in humans would slow the disappearance of α- and γ-tocopherols. Remarkably, ascorbic acid supplementation for 2 weeks did not decrease lipid peroxidation (as measured by F_2-isoprostanes) (Taylor et al., 2008), but rather normalized smokers' α- and γ-tocopherol FDRs (Bruno et al., 2006a). This is the first *in vivo* demonstration that ascorbate maintains tocopherols through 'recycling'. Moreover, the lack of change in nonsmokers' disappearance rates suggests that the efflux of tocopherols from the body is generally not dependent on oxidative stress, but rather is a measure of the constant flux of tocopherols.

11.1.6.3 Implications of *in vivo* oxidative stress on vitamin E requirements

Our studies in smokers suggest that vitamin E requirements are dependent upon both oxidative stress status and vitamin C status. It is unclear whether the oxidative stress caused by cigarette smoking is equivalent to other forms of oxidative stress. Obesity has been recognized to be an inflammatory disease associated with increased oxidative stress (Keaney et al., 2003). Presumably, obese subjects with diabetes have an even greater degree of oxidative stress, because type II diabetics have higher levels of circulating F_2-isoprostanes than do normal subjects (Gopaul et al., 1995) and these lipid peroxidation biomarkers further increase during bouts of hyperglycemia (Sampson et al., 2002). Consistent with our observations in smokers (Bruno et al., 2006a, Taylor et al., 2006), vitamin C supplementation (1.5 g daily) in type II diabetics for 3 weeks did not improve lipid peroxidation biomarkers (Darko et al., 2002).

11.1.7 Conclusions

Vitamin E remains an enigma because its molecular function, other than its antioxidant function as a peroxyl radical scavenger, is unknown. In this chapter, the role of vitamin E in protecting the fetus, in maintaining normal membrane function, in preventing nerve degeneration, and the possibility that it functions to protect against various chronic diseases is discussed. These various functions are well described, but the mechanisms of action remain elusive. It is clear that α-tocopherol is required for human health, we just have to determine why!

References

Albanes D, Heinonen OP, Taylor PR, Virtamo J, Edwards BK, Rautalahti M, Hartman AM, Palmgren J, Freedman LS, Haapakoski J, Barrett MJ, Pietinen P, Malila N, Tala E, Liippo K, Salomaa ER,

Tangrea JA, Teppo L, Askin FB, Taskinen E, Erozan Y, Greenwald P, Huttunen JK, Alpha-Tocopherol and beta-carotene supplements and lung cancer incidence in the alpha-tocopherol, beta-carotene cancer prevention study: effects of base-line characteristics and study compliance. J Natl Cancer Inst 1996;88: 1560–70.

Ames SR, Biopotencies in rats of several forms of alpha-tocopherol. J Nutr 1979;109: 2198–204.

Azzi A, Molecular mechanism of alpha-tocopherol action. Free Radic Biol Med 2007;43: 16–21.

Ben Hamida M, Sirugo G, Ben Hamida C, Panayides K, Ionannou P, Beckmann J, Mandel JL, Hentati F, Koenig M, et al. Friedreich's ataxia phenotype not linked to chromosome 9 and associated with selective autosomal recessive vitamin E deficiency in two inbred Tunisian families. Neurology 1993;43: 2179–83.

Brigelius-Flohé R, Glutathione peroxidases and redox-regulated transcription factors. Biol Chem 2006;387: 1329–35.

Brigelius-Flohé R, Traber MG, Vitamin E: function and metabolism. FASEB J 1999;13: 1145–55.

Bruno RS, Leonard SW, Li J, Bray TM, Traber MG, Lower plasma α-carboxyethyl-hydroxychroman after deuterium labeled α-tocopherol supplementation suggests decreased vitamin E metabolism in smokers. Am J Clin Nutr 2005a;81: 1052–9.

Bruno RS, Ramakrishnan R, Montine TJ, Bray TM, Traber MG, α-Tocopherol disappearance is faster in cigarette smokers and is inversely related to their ascorbic acid status. Am J Clin Nutr 2005b;81: 95–103.

Bruno RS, Leonard SW, Atkinson JK, Montine TJ, Ramakrishnan R, Bray TM, Traber MG, Faster vitamin E disappearance in smokers is normalized by vitamin C supplementation. Free Radic Biol Med 2006a;40: 689–97.

Bruno RS, Leonard SW, Park S-I, Zhao Y, Traber MG, Human vitamin E requirements assessed with the use of apples fortified with deuterium-labeled α-tocopheryl acetate. Am J Clin Nutr 2006b;83: 299–304.

Buettner GR, The pecking order of free radicals and antioxidants: lipid peroxidation, alpha-tocopherol, and ascorbate. Arch Biochem Biophys 1993;300: 535–43.

Cavalier L, Ouahchi K, Kayden HJ, Di Donato S, Reutenauer L, Mandel JL, Koenig M, Ataxia with isolated vitamin E deficiency: heterogeneity of mutations and phenotypic variability in a large number of families. Am J Hum Genet 1998;62: 301–10.

Clifford AJ, de Moura FF, Ho CC, Chuang JC, Follett J, Fadel JG, Novotny JA, A feasibility study quantifying in vivo human alpha-tocopherol metabolism. Am J Clin Nutr 2006;84: 1430–41.

Coucouvanis E, Martin GR, Signals for death and survival: a two-step mechanism for cavitation in the vertebrate embryo. Cell 1995;83: 279–87.

Darko D, Dornhorst A, Kelly FJ, Ritter JM, Chowienczyk PJ, Lack of effect of oral vitamin C on blood pressure, oxidative stress and endothelial function in Type II diabetes. Clin Sci (Lond) 2002;103: 339–44.

Doerflinger N, Linder C, Ouahchi K, Gyapay G, Weissenbach J, Le Paslier D, Rigault P, Belal S, Ben Hamida C, Hentati F, Ben Hamida M, Pandolfo M, DiDonato S, Sokol R, Kayden H, Landrieu P, Durr A, Brice A, Goutières F, Kohlschütter A, Sabouraud P, Benomar A, Yahyaoui M, Mandel J-L, Koenig M, Ataxia with vitamin E deficiency: refinement of genetic localization and analysis of linkage disequilibrium by using new markers in 14 families. Am J Hum Genet 1995;56: 1116–24.

Emerson OH, Emerson GA, Mohammad A, Evans HM, The chemistry of vitamin E. Tocopherols from natural sources. J Biol Chem 1937;22: 99–107.

Evans HM, Bishop KS, On the existence of a hitherto unrecognized dietary factor essential for reproduction. Science 1922;56: 650–1.

Food and Nutrition Board, Institute of Medicine. Dietary reference intakes for vitamin C, vitamin E, selenium, and carotenoids. Washington: National Academy Press; 2000.

Gao X, Martin A, Lin H, Bermudez OI, Tucker KL, alpha-Tocopherol intake and plasma concentration of Hispanic and non-Hispanic white elders is associated with dietary intake pattern. J Nutr 2006;136: 2574–9.

Ge L, Wang J, Qi W, Miao HH, Cao J, Qu YX, Li BL, Song BL, The cholesterol absorption inhibitor ezetimibe acts by blocking the sterol-induced internalization of NPC1L1. Cell Metab 2008;7: 508–19.

Gopaul NK, Anggard EE, Mallet AI, Betteridge DJ, Wolff SP, Nourooz-Zadeh J, Plasma 8-epi-PGF2 alpha levels are elevated in individuals with non-insulin dependent diabetes mellitus. FEBS Lett 1995;368: 225–9.

Harris PL, Ludwig MI, Relative vitamin E potency of natural and of synthetic α-tocopherol. J Biol Chem 1949;179: 1111–5.

Hempstock J, Jauniaux E, Greenwold N, Burton GJ, The contribution of placental oxidative stress to early pregnancy failure. Hum Pathol 2003;34: 1265–75.

Horwitt MK, Harvey CC, Duncan GD, Wilson WC, Effects of limited tocopherol intake in man with relationships to erythrocyte hemolysis and lipid oxidations. Am J Clin Nutr 1956;4: 408–19.

Imai H, Hirao F, Sakamoto T, Sekine K, Mizukura Y, Saito M, Kitamoto T, Hayasaka M, Hanaoka K, Nakagawa Y, Early embryonic lethality caused by targeted disruption of the mouse PHGPx gene. Biochem Biophys Res Commun 2003;305: 278–86.

Jacquot C, Wecksler AT, McGinley CM, Segraves EN, Holman TR, van der Donk WA, Isotope sensitive branching and kinetic isotope effects in the reaction of deuterated arachidonic acids with human 12- and 15-lipoxygenases. Biochemistry 2008;47: 7295–303.

Jauniaux E, Cindrova-Davies T, Johns J, Dunster C, Hempstock J, Kelly FJ, Burton GJ, Distribution and transfer pathways of antioxidant molecules inside the first trimester human gestational sac. J Clin Endocrinol Metab 2004;89: 1452–8.

Jishage K, Arita M, Igarashi K, Iwata T, Watanabe M, Ogawa M, Ueda O, Kamada N, Inoue K, Arai H, Suzuki H, Alpha-tocopherol transfer protein is important for the normal development of placental labyrinthine trophoblasts in mice. J Biol Chem 2001;273: 1669–72.

Kaempf-Rotzoll DE, Igarashi K, Aoki J, Jishage K, Suzuki H, Tamai H, Linderkamp O, Arai H, Alpha-tocopherol transfer protein is specifically localized at the implantation site of pregnant mouse uterus. Biol Reprod 2002;67: 599–604.

Kaempf-Rotzoll DE, Horiguchi M, Hashiguchi K, Aoki J, Tamai H, Linderkamp O, Arai H, Human placental trophoblast cells express alpha-tocopherol transfer protein. Placenta 2003;24: 439–44.

Keaney JF Jr, Larson MG, Vasan RS, Wilson PW, Lipinska I, Corey D, Massaro JM, Sutherland P, Vita JA, Benjamin EJ, Obesity and systemic oxidative stress: clinical correlates of oxidative stress in the Framingham Study. Arterioscler Thromb Vasc Biol 2003;23: 434–9.

Kelleher J, Losowsky MS, The absorption of vitamin E in man. Biochem J 1968;110: 20P–1P.

Lee IM, Cook NR, Gaziano JM, Gordon D, Ridker PM, Manson JE, Hennekens CH, Buring JE, Vitamin E in the primary prevention of cardiovascular disease and cancer: the Women's Health Study: a randomized controlled trial. J Am Med Assoc 2005;294: 56–65.

Leonard SW, Good CK, Gugger ET, Traber MG, Vitamin E bioavailability from fortified breakfast cereal is greater than that from encapsulated supplements. Am J Clin Nutr 2004;79: 86–92.

Leonard SW, Paterson E, Atkinson JK, Ramakrishnan R, Cross CE, Traber MG, Studies in humans using deuterium-labeled α- and γ-tocopherol demonstrate faster plasma γ-tocopherol disappearance and greater γ-metabolite production. Free Radic Biol Med 2005;38: 857–66.

Leth T, Sondergaard H, Biological activity of vitamin E compounds and natural materials by the resorption-gestation test, and chemical determination of the vitamin E activity in foods and feeds. J Nutr 1977;107: 2236–43.

Li Q, Cheon YP, Kannan A, Shanker S, Bagchi IC, Bagchi MK, A novel pathway involving progesterone receptor, 12/15-lipoxygenase-derived eicosanoids, and peroxisome proliferator-activated receptor gamma regulates implantation in mice. J Biol Chem 2004;279: 11570–81.

MacMahon MT, Neale G, The absorption of alpha-tocopherol in control subjects and in patients with intestinal malabsorption. Clin Sci 1970;38: 197–210.

Meier R, Tomizaki T, Schulze-Briese C, Baumann U, Stocker A, The molecular basis of vitamin E retention: structure of human alpha-tocopherol transfer protein. J Mol Biol 2003;331: 725–34.

Min KC, Kovall RA, Hendrickson WA, Crystal structure of human α-tocopherol transfer protein bound to its ligand: Implications for ataxia with vitamin E deficiency. Proc Natl Acad Sci USA 2003;100: 14713–8.

Moshfegh A, Goldman J, Cleveland L, What we eat in America, NHANES 2001–2002: usual nutrient intakes from food compared to dietary reference intakes 2005, United States Department of Agriculture, Agricultural Research Service. http://www.ars.usda.gov/ba/bhnrc/fsrg.

Nakagawa Y, Role of mitochondrial phospholipid hydroperoxide glutathione peroxidase (PHGPx) as an antiapoptotic factor. Biol Pharm Bull 2004;27: 956–60.

Narushima K, Takada T, Yamanashi Y, Suzuki H, Niemann-pick C1-like 1 mediates alpha-tocopherol transport. Mol Pharmacol 2008;74: 42–9.

Osakada F, Hashino A, Kume T, Katsuki H, Kaneko S, Akaike A, Neuroprotective effects of alpha-tocopherol on oxidative stress in rat striatal cultures. Eur J Pharmacol 2003;465: 15–22.

Parker RS, McCormick CC, Selective accumulation of alpha-tocopherol in *Drosophila* is associated with cytochrome P450 tocopherol-omega-hydroxylase activity but not alpha-tocopherol transfer protein. Biochem Biophys Res Commun 2005;338: 1537–41.

Pryor WA, Biological effects of cigarette smoke, wood smoke, and the smoke from plastics: the use of electron spin resonance. Free Radic Biol Med 1992;13: 659–76.

Sampson MJ, Gopaul N, Davies IR, Hughes DA, Carrier MJ, Plasma F2 isoprostanes: direct evidence of increased free radical damage during acute hyperglycemia in type 2 diabetes. Diabetes Care 2002;25: 537–41.

Sato Y, Hagiwara K, Arai H, Inoue K, Purification and characterization of the alpha-tocopherol transfer protein from rat liver. FEBS Lett 1991;288: 41–5.

Sato Y, Arai H, Miyata A, Tokita S, Yamamoto K, Tanabe T, Inoue K, Primary structure of alpha-tocopherol transfer protein from rat liver. Homology with cellular retinaldehyde-binding protein. J Biol Chem 1993;268: 17705–10.

Seiler A, Schneider M, Forster H, Roth S, Wirth EK, Culmsee C, Plesnila N, Kremmer E, Radmark O, Wurst W, Bornkamm GW, Schweizer U, Conrad M, Glutathione peroxidase 4 senses and translates oxidative stress into 12/15-lipoxygenase dependent- and AIF-mediated cell death. Cell Metab 2008;8: 237–48.

Sokol RJ, Vitamin E deficiency and neurological disorders., In: Packer L, Fuchs J, editors. Vitamin E in health and disease. New York: Marcel Dekker; 1993. pp. 815–49.

Sokol RJ, Kayden HJ, Bettis DB, Traber MG, Neville H, Ringel S, Wilson WB, Stumpf DA, Isolated vitamin E deficiency in the absence of fat malabsorption – familial and sporadic cases: characterization and investigation of causes. J Lab Clin Med 1988;111: 548–59.

Sontag TJ, Parker RS, Cytochrome P450 omega-hydroxylase pathway of tocopherol catabolism: Novel mechanism of regulation of vitamin E status. J Biol Chem 2002;277: 25290–6.

Sontag TJ, Parker RS, Influence of major structural features of tocopherols and tocotrienols on their omega-oxidation by tocopherol-omega-hydroxylase. J Lipid Res 2007;48: 1090–8.

Taylor AW, Bruno RS, Frei B, Traber MG, Benefits of prolonged gradient separation for high-performance liquid chromatography-tandem mass spectrometry quantitation of plasma total 15-Series F2-isoprostanes. Anal Biochem 2006;350: 41–51.

Taylor AW, Bruno RS, Traber MG, Women and smokers have elevated urinary F(2)-isoprostane metabolites: a novel extraction and LC-MS methodology. Lipids 2008;43: 925–36.

Traber MG, Vitamin E, In: Shils ME, Olson JA, Shike M, Ross AC, editors. Modern nutrition in health and disease. Baltimore: Williams & Wilkins; 1999. pp. 347–62.

Traber MG, Vitamin E regulatory mechanisms. Annu Rev Nutr 2007a;27: 347–62.

Traber MG, Atkinson J, Vitamin E, antioxidant and nothing more. Free Radic Biol Med 2007b;43: 4–15.

Traber MG, Kayden HJ, Preferential incorporation of alpha-tocopherol vs gamma-tocopherol in human lipoproteins. Am J Clin Nutr 1989;49: 517–26.

Traber MG, Sokol RJ, Ringel SP, Neville HE, Thellman CA, Kayden HJ, Lack of tocopherol in peripheral nerves of vitamin E-deficient patients with peripheral neuropathy. N Engl J Med 1987;317: 262–5.

Traber MG, Burton GW, Ingold KU, Kayden HJ, RRR- and SRR-alpha-tocopherols are secreted without discrimination in human chylomicrons, but RRR-alpha-tocopherol is preferentially secreted in very low density lipoproteins. J Lipid Res 1990a;31: 675–85.

Traber MG, Sokol RJ, Burton GW, Ingold KU, Papas AM, Huffaker JE, Kayden HJ, Impaired ability of patients with familial isolated vitamin E deficiency to incorporate alpha-tocopherol into lipoproteins secreted by the liver. J Clin Invest 1990b;85: 397–407.

Traber MG, Sokol RJ, Kohlschütter A, Yokota T, Muller DPR, Dufour R, Kayden HJ, Impaired discrimination between stereoisomers of α-tocopherol in patients with familial isolated vitamin E deficiency. J Lipid Res 1993;34: 201–10.

Traber MG, Ramakrishnan R, Kayden HJ, Human plasma vitamin E kinetics demonstrate rapid recycling of plasma RRR-α-tocopherol. Proc Natl Acad Sci USA 1994;91: 10005–8.

Traber MG, Winklhofer-Roob BM, Roob JM, Khoschsorur G, Aigner R, Cross C, Ramakrishnan R, Brigelius-Flohé R, Vitamin E kinetics in smokers and non-smokers. Free Radic Biol Med 2001;31: 1368–74.

Wang J, Chu BB, Ge L, Li BL, Yan Y, Song BL, Membrane topology of human NPC1L1, a key protein in enterohepatic cholesterol absorption. J Lipid Res 2009;50: 1653–62.

Wright ME, Lawson KA, Weinstein SJ, Pietinen P, Taylor PR, Virtamo J, Albanes D, Higher baseline serum concentrations of vitamin E are associated with lower total and cause-specific mortality in the Alpha-Tocopherol, Beta-Carotene Cancer Prevention Study. Am J Clin Nutr 2006;84: 1200–7.

Yuan B, Ohyama K, Bessho T, Uchide N, Toyoda H, Imbalance between ROS production and elimination results in apoptosis induction in primary smooth chorion trophoblast cells prepared from human fetal membrane tissues. Life Sci 2008;82: 623–30.

Zhang XD, Gillespie SK, Hersey P, Staurosporine induces apoptosis of melanoma by both caspase-dependent and -independent apoptotic pathways. Mol Cancer Ther 2004;3: 187–97.

11.2 Vitamin E and cardiovascular disease

Ian S. Young; Jayne V. Woodside

11.2.1 Introduction

Cardiovascular disease remains the most important cause of morbidity and mortality across the developed world. Although there has been a decline in coronary artery disease in many countries, it is anticipated that the increasing burden of obesity and type 2 diabetes will reverse this trend over the next decade. It is now recognised that atherosclerosis develops as a consequence of two fundamental pathological processes, lipid deposition in the arterial wall and inflammation, and that these processes might be linked by lipid peroxidation (Van Gaal et al., 2006). Nutritional antioxidants represent a key component of the antioxidant defence systems. Therefore, there has been considerable interest in the link between antioxidant status and cardiovascular disease, and in the potential of antioxidant supplementation to reduce cardiovascular events. This chapter will focus on the relation between vitamin E and cardiovascular disease, and will discuss the potential role of vitamin E within the arterial wall in preventing atherosclerosis, the epidemiological evidence that high vitamin E intakes are associated with a reduced risk of cardiovascular disease, and the results of clinical trials of vitamin E supplementation.

11.2.2 Oxidative stress and atherosclerosis

A wealth of evidence indicates that oxidation of low-density lipoprotein (LDL) and triglyceride rich lipoproteins plays an important role in the initiation and propagation

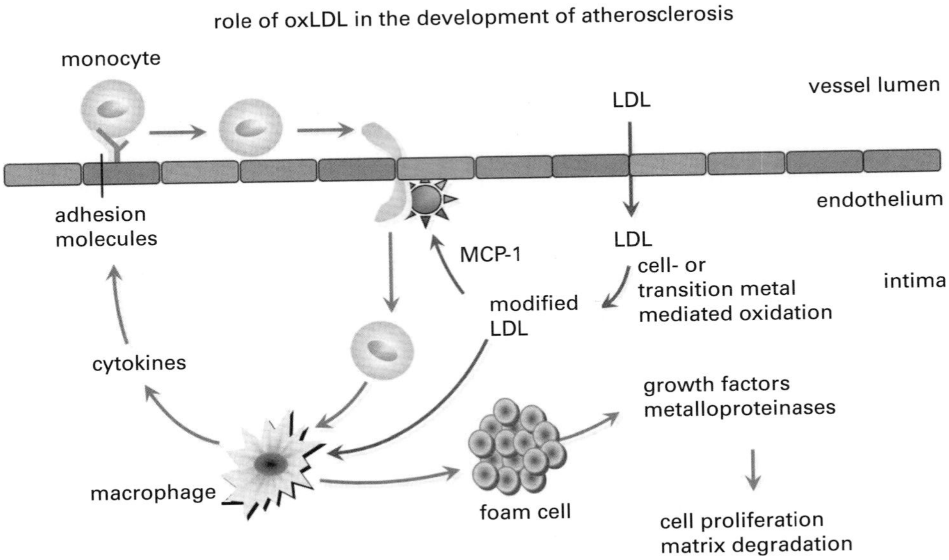

Fig. 11.3: The role of oxidized LDL in the development of atherosclerosis.

of the atherosclerotic process (Steinberg, 2009). In brief, LDL entering the arterial wall by transcytosis becomes exposed to a microenvironment where oxidation of poly-unsaturated fatty acids can take place as a result of interactions with reactive oxygen species generated by cells within the arterial wall (►Fig. 11.3). This might lead to modification of key amino acids within the apoB protein, as a result of which modified LDL (oxLDL) is taken up in an uncontrolled way via the scavenger pathway by mono-cytes or vascular smooth muscle cells, leading to foam cell formation. oxLDL also promotes the secretion of a range of inflammatory intermediates, including cytokines, adhesion molecules and matrix metalloproteinases, which attract inflammatory cells from the circulation into the growing atherosclerotic plaque (Niessner et al., 2007). Endothelial function becomes impaired (Chouinard et al., 2008), partly as a result of reduced availability of nitric oxide, and the balance between thrombotic and anti-thrombotic factors is altered in a way which favours thrombus formation (Bai et al., 2006). As the plaque matures, the presence of significant numbers of inflammatory cells is associated with thinning of the fibrous cap and an increased risk of plaque rupture (Meuwissen et al., 2006).

High density lipoproteins (HDL) protect against the development of atherosclerosis. Traditionally, the main role of HDL has been considered to be promotion of reverse cholesterol transport, whereby cholesterol is transported from the arterial wall to the liver for catabolism and excretion. More recently, it has been recognised that HDL has multiple other anti-atherogenic effects, particularly through inhibiting lipid peroxidation and inflammation (Petraki et al., 2009). Oxidation of lipids within HDL leads to a loss of these anti-atherogenic actions (Deakin et al., 2007).

Given the key role of lipid peroxidation and oxidative stress in the processes described above, it is not surprising that antioxidants have the potential to protect against the development of atherosclerosis. Numerous studies have shown that alpha-tocopherol can protect LDL and other lipoproteins against oxidation (Jialal and Grundy, 1993; Chang et al., 2005). Alpha-tocopherol behaves as a chain-breaking antioxidant, preventing lipid peroxidation within LDL and the subsequent series of events described above. For instance, alpha-tocopherol supplementation has been shown to preserve endothelial function both in animal studies (Koga et al., 2004) and short-term clinical trials in humans (Skyrme-Jones et al., 2000). Expression of adhesion molecules by endothelial cells is reduced, as is synthesis of monocyte chemotactic factor. Vitamin E also has a range of anti-atherogenic effects on vascular smooth muscle cells (Munteanu and Zingg, 2007). In particular, uptake of oxLDL by the scavenger pathway and subsequent formation of foam cells is inhibited, as is vascular smooth muscle cell proliferation and migration, leading to a reduction in vascular narrowing. The secretion of a range of cytokines and vascular and matrix is reduced, with a subsequent reduction in monocyte infiltration and an increase in plaque stability. Vascular smooth muscle cell apoptosis and contraction are inhibited, as is signal transduction and aberrant gene expression within vascular smooth muscle cells in response to toxic stimuli.

In vitro, alpha-tocopherol has also been shown to inhibit platelet aggregation and other pro-thrombotic activities (Murohara et al., 2004). In addition, alpha-tocopherol has direct effects on monocytes and other inflammatory cells which are involved in the atherosclerotic process, in general decreasing inflammatory factors (Zingg and Azzi, 2004). Alpha-tocopherol can also protect HDL against oxidation (Schnell et al., 2001), potentially preserving its anti-atherogenic properties, although some studies have also suggested that alpha-tocopherol could promote pro-atherogenic changes in HDL (Garner et al., 1998). Given the important role of ascorbate in recycling alpha-tocopherol, the anti-atherosclerotic effects of vitamin E might be augmented in the presence of vitamin C.

The sequence of events outlined above provides a strong justification for an anti-atherogenic role of vitamin E and is supported by a wealth of *in vitro* experiments. However, it has also been suggested that alpha-tocopherol might paradoxically promote lipid peroxidation both *in vitro* and *in vivo* (Thomas and Stocker, 2000). This process, which has been referred to as tocopherol-mediated peroxidation, has been demonstrated when lipid peroxidation occurs within LDL in the absence of another antioxidant (such as ascorbate) which can reduce the tocopheryl radical. In these circumstances, the tocopheryl radical could propagate the lipid peroxidation chain reaction. Although this paradoxical pro-oxidant effect of alpha-tocopherol has been convincingly demonstrated *in vitro*, the evidence that it takes place *in vivo* is less compelling. Nonetheless, the potential for alpha-tocopherol to promote lipid peroxidation, albeit in limited circumstances, is a factor which needs to be considered when interpreting the results of the clinical trials outlined below.

11.2.3 Epidemiological evidence that vitamin E protects against cardiovascular disease

Epidemiological evidence suggests that a high intake of fruit and vegetables is strongly protective against cardiovascular disease (He et al., 2007). This has been cited by many as supporting a key role for antioxidants in protection against atherosclerosis, in keeping with the mechanisms outlined above. Studies which have looked at intake or baseline status for individual antioxidants have generally found a stronger relation between vitamin E intake and reduced risk than for other antioxidants. Because alpha-tocopherol is the main chain-breaking antioxidant within LDL and therefore the chief defence against lipid peroxidation, this is not surprising.

A large number of prospective observational studies have assessed vitamin E intake or serum alpha-tocopherol levels at baseline in healthy subjects with follow-up extending up to 15 years. Although there is some inconsistency, the majority of such studies have shown that individuals with either high vitamin E intakes or high serum levels are protected against subsequent cardiovascular events. In some studies, it appears that individuals with the highest intakes (which were achieved as a result of the use of supplements) are particularly protected. The results of some of these keys studies are summarised in ▶Tab. 11.1. A recent meta-analysis described all cohort studies providing a relative risk and corresponding 95% confidence interval of for coronary heart disease in relation to

Tab. 11.1: Major epidemiological studies assessing the relation between vitamin E status and cardiovascular endpoints.

Study		Population	Follow-up period	Vitamin E protective against cardiovascular disease
Basel Protective Study	Stahelin et al. (2002)	2974 European men	12 years	Negative
Nurses Health Study	Stampfer et al. (1993)	87 245 American nurses, women aged 34–59 years	8 years	Positive
Health Professionals Follow-Up	Rimm et al. (1993)	39 910 male American health professionals	4 years	Positive
Finland Social Insurance Study	Knekt et al. (1994)	5133 Finns, aged 30–69 years	14 years	Positive
Atherosclerosis Risk in Communities study	Kritchevsky et al. (1995)	11 307 Americans, aged 45–64 years		Positive in women
EPESE	Losonczy et al. (1996)	11 178 Americans, aged 67–105 years	6 years	Positive
Iowa Women's Health Study	Kushi et al. (1996)	34 486 post-menopausal American women, aged 55–69 years	7 years	Positive
Rotterdam Study	Klipstein-Grobusch et al. (1999)	4802 Dutch adults, 1856 men and 2946 women, aged 55–95 years	4 years	Negative

antioxidant vitamin intake from diet or supplement (Ye and Song, 2008). Fifteen cohort studies were identified involving a total of 7415 incident coronary heart disease (CHD) cases and 374 488 participants with a median follow-up of approximately 10, 8.5 and 15 years for vitamins C, E and beta-carotene, respectively. For vitamins C, E and beta-carotene, a comparison of individuals in the top third with those in the bottom third of baseline value yielded a combined relative risk of 0.84 (95% CI, 0.73–0.95), 0.76 (95% CI, 0.63–0.89) and 0.78 (95% CI, 0.53–1.04), respectively. Subgroup analyses show that dietary intake of vitamins C and E and supplement use of vitamin E have an inverse association with CHD risk, but supplement use of vitamin C has no significant association with CHD risk. In the dose-response meta-analysis, each 30 IU/day increase in vitamin E yielded the estimated overall relative risk for CHD of 0.96 (95% CI, 0.94–0.99).

Overall, there is little dispute that in epidemiological studies vitamin E appears to be protective against cardiovascular disease, in support of mechanistic and *in vitro* studies. However, at best epidemiology can demonstrate only associations and not causality. It remains possible that within the epidemiological studies there is residual confounding which cannot be adequately corrected through statistical analysis. Thus, it might be that individuals with the highest intakes of vitamin E, particularly those who routinely use supplements, tend to adopt more healthy lifestyles in other ways. It could be these other aspects of their lifestyles which convey protection against cardiovascular disease, rather than the high intake of vitamin E itself. The same argument could be put forward in relation to high fruit and vegetable intake, where individuals with a healthy diet are also likely to adopt other healthy behaviours.

11.2.4 Effects of vitamin E supplementation

11.2.4.1 Animal studies

Overall, animal studies of vitamin E supplementation have given somewhat inconsistent results, although this might reflect the difficulty in developing suitable animal models. Several studies in the cholesterol-fed rabbit model have suggested that alpha-tocopherol supplementation will significantly reduce formation of atherosclerotic lesions (Prasad and Kalra, 1993; Schwenke et al., 2002). Similar findings have been reported in some studies using an apoE knockout mouse with a high-cholesterol diet (Peluzio et al., 2003). Interestingly, studies in which animals are fed a standard diet and are then supplemented with additional alpha-tocopherol have tended to show no benefit. This could be because the vitamin E content of standard rat chow is relatively high, and that supplementation is only of benefit against the background of the vitamin E-deficient diet (Robinson et al., 2006). This might be relevant when we come to consider the interpretation of the nature clinical trials in humans.

11.2.4.2 Short-term studies in humans with intermediate endpoints

Numerous short-term studies have demonstrated that supplementation with vitamin E can improve intermediate endpoints which might be associated with reduced cardiovascular risk. One commonly used endpoint has been the resistance of LDL to oxidation *in vitro*. Supplementation with vitamin E, at doses of 100 mg/day of alpha-tocopherol or greater, leads to LDL which is more resistant to copper-mediated oxidation as assessed by the measurement of the lag time before the onset of the propagation phase of the peroxidation reaction (Islam et al., 2000). Vitamin E supplementation has also been shown to improve a range of other intermediate endpoints over a relatively short period which might be anticipated to convey protection against the development of cardiovascular disease. These include other markers of oxidative stress (Devaraj et al., 2007), serum adhesion molecule levels (Woollard et al., 2006), arterial endothelial function (Duffy et al., 2001) and platelet aggregation (Liu et al., 2003). However, results are not entirely consistent and adverse effects of vitamin E supplements on intermediate endpoints have also been shown.

11.2.4.3 Long-term trials with clinical endpoints

The evidence summarised above from *in vitro* experiments and biological studies, epidemiology and short-term clinical trials provided a strong justification for large-scale clinical trials of vitamin E supplementation in humans with clinical endpoints. A significant number of such trials have now been completed, and a clear view has emerged of the effects of vitamin E supplementation on cardiovascular disease. The main findings are summarised in ▶Tab. 11.2.

In general, the major clinical trials have been placebo-controlled and lasted for up to 10 years. Studies have used a range of doses of vitamin E, usually in combination with other antioxidants. This makes the interpretation of the results more difficult, particularly because it is now accepted that some of the other antioxidants which have been used are likely to have predominantly adverse effects (for instance, beta-carotene, particularly in smokers) (Tanvetyanon and Bepler, 2008). The rationale for using combinations of antioxidants in clinical trials derived from *in vitro* observations of the interactions between alpha-tocopherol and other antioxidants, and in addition, from the epidemiological evidence that high intakes of several antioxidants were likely to be beneficial. The dose of vitamin E also varied from 50 mg/day to over 1000 IU/day. In addition, some studies used vitamin E from natural sources, which contains a range of isoforms, whereas others used synthetic alpha-tocopherol. At the time of study design this was considered not to be an important issue. However, there is now recognition that different forms of vitamin E might have different biological effects (Ogawa et al., 2008).

In contrast to the positive findings from the epidemiological studies and short-term supplementation, the long-term trials with clinical endpoints have generally shown little or no benefit. Indeed, in recent letter analysis it has been suggested that supplementation with vitamin E at doses above 400 IU/day could be associated with an increase in total mortality (Bjelakovic et al., 2008). What are the possible reasons for the discrepancy between the long-term clinical trials and the other evidence?

11.2.4.3.1 Vitamin E might not protect against cardiovascular disease

The first possible explanation for the negative outcomes of clinical trials is that vitamin E does not protect against cardiovascular disease. If this is the case, then the clinical trials are correct, and the hypothesis that vitamin E protects against cardiovascular disease should be rejected. This implies that the basic biology and epidemiology have been

Tab. 11.2: Selected clinical trials of vitamin E supplementation with cardiovascular endpoints.

Trial		History	Subjects	Vitamin E dose and type	Follow-up (years)	Parameters	Relative risk
Primary prevention							
ATBC	Virtamo et al. (1998)	Male smokers; 50–69 years	29 133	50 mg *all rac*-tocopheryl-acetate	6.1	MI, stroke deaths	Negative
Primary Prevention Project	Sacco et al. (2003)	High risk for CVD; mean age 64.4 years	4495	300 mg *all rac*-α-tocopherol	3.6	CVD mortality, MI	Negative
SUVIMAX	Hercberg et al. (2004)	Healthy	13 017	30 mg/day vitamin E	7.5	CVD	Negative
Physicians' Health Study	Sesso et al. (2008)	Male physicians, >55 years	15 000	400 IU synthetic α-tocopherol on alternate days	8.0	CVD	Negative
ASAP	Salonen et al. (2003)	Plasma cholesterol >5 mM; 45–69 years	458	136 IU, 2× per day *RRR*-α-tocopheryl-acetate	3.0	IMT progression	Positive
VEAPS	Hodis et al. (2002)	Plasma cholesterol >3.4 mM; over 40 years old	350	400 IU/day DL-α-tocopherol	3.0	IMT progression	Negative

(Continued)

Tab. 11.2 (*Continued*)

Trial		History	Subjects	Vitamin E dose and type	Follow-up (years)	Parameters	Relative risk
Secondary prevention							
CHAOS	Stephens et al. (1996)	CAD patients; mean age 62 years	2002	400–800 IU *RRR-α*-tocopherol	1.4	CVD and total mortality	Negative
						Non-fatal MI	Positive
SPACE	Boaz et al. (2000)	Haemodialysis and known CVD; 40–75 years	196	800 IU *RRR-α*-tocopherol	1.4	MI, CVD mortality	Positive
GISSI	GISSI (1999)	Recent MI (<3 months); 50–80 years	11 324	300 mg *all rac-α*-tocopherol	3.5	CVD mortality, non-fatal MI	Negative (but borderline)
HOPE	Lonn et al. (2002)	CVD or diabetes patients; mean age 66	9541	400 IU/day RRR-α-tocopheryl-acetate	4.5	CVD mortality	Negative
Heart Protection Study	Heart Protection Study Collaborative Group (2002)	High risk for CVD or established CVD	20 536	600 mg/day RRR-α-tocopheryl-acetate	5.0	CVD	Negative

CAD, coronary artery disease; CVD, cardiovascular disease; MI, myocardial infarction; IMT, intima-to-media thickness.

misinterpreted. In support of this view, it could be suggested that *in vitro* studies have often used unrealistic concentrations of alpha-tocopherol and in addition have used alpha-tocopherol in solution rather than incorporating it into lipoproteins, which is the form in which the majority of alpha-tocopherol is present in serum. As discussed above, positive results from epidemiological studies could be a consequence of residual confounding owing to the generally more healthy lifestyles of those individuals with high intakes of vitamin E. Although it is possible that this is the case, the strength of the other evidence is such that it seems very unlikely that high intakes of vitamin E are without benefit. It is therefore worth considering other potential explanations for the negative clinical trials.

11.2.4.3.2 The duration of supplementation in clinical trials has been too short

Atherosclerosis is a disease of the whole life course, commencing in childhood and developing throughout adult life, with clinical manifestations in middle or advanced age. Fatty streaks, the earliest stage of the atherosclerotic plaque, can be detected in children from the age of 7 or 8 years (Nakashima et al., 2007). Many asymptomatic middle-aged adults have extensive atherosclerosis as a consequence of lifetime exposure to cardiovascular risk factors. In general, clinical trials of vitamin E supplementation have recruited middle-aged or older individuals at high risk of cardiovascular disease or with established cardiovascular disease. Even when apparently healthy, it is probable that atherosclerosis is well advanced in many subjects. Therefore, the hypothesis which has been tested to date is whether supplementation with vitamin E for up to 5 years in individuals with established atherosclerosis can prevent clinical events. It appears from the trials that this is not the case, but it remains plausible that high intakes of vitamin E from early in life would prevent the development of atherosclerosis and cardiovascular events if sustained over many years. This would certainly fit with the biological and epidemiological evidence, and in addition it is possible that the early stages of atherosclerosis can be prevented with vitamin E supplementation, whereas impact on established atherosclerosis might be less significant. If this perspective is accepted, then to properly test whether vitamin E supplementation can prevent cardiovascular disease would require a placebo-controlled intervention trial commencing in childhood and continuing for 50–60 years. Unfortunately, it is unlikely that such a trial would ever be conducted and therefore the benefit of very long-term supplementation with vitamin E is unlikely to ever be formally tested in humans.

11.2.4.3.3 The dose or form of alpha-tocopherol used in clinical trials might have been inappropriate

As summarised in ▶Tab. 11.2, the majority of clinical trials have used approximately 400 IU/day of alpha-tocopherol, either as the synthetic or natural form. This level of intake is much greater than that which would be achieved from dietary sources, and is likely to exert pharmacological as well as antioxidant effects. For instance, it has been demonstrated that intakes of alpha-tocopherol at this level results in reduced serum concentrations of gamma-tocopherol (Deveraj, 2005). Knowledge about the differential biological effects of alpha-tocopherol and other forms of tocopherol is still limited, so it is at least possible that very high doses such of alpha-tocopherol might have unanticipated deleterious effects, impacting on the availability of other forms of vitamin E or increasing the likelihood of unanticipated paradoxical pro-oxidant actions. Meta-analysis suggests that there could be some benefit of lower intakes of alpha tocopherol, with an overall likelihood of harm at levels greater or equal to 400 units/day. It is therefore unfortunate (although understandable) that such high doses have been used in the majority of clinical trials; supplementation at lower levels might be more likely to have benefit. It has also been suggested that the mixture of isoforms found in natural tocopherol could be more likely to have benefit, in contrast to the synthetic alpha-tocopherol used in many trials.

11.2.4.3.4 Benefit from alpha-tocopherol might be restricted to subgroups of the population

A wide range of individuals have participated in clinical trials to date, and results have been reported for unselected populations. This is particularly the case in relation to meta-analysis, where individuals have been included regardless of underlying disease. It is possible that the majority of the population might not benefit from high-dose alpha-tocopherol supplementation, whereas there is benefit to subgroups of the population such as those with low baseline vitamin E status. In general, trials completed to date have not included pre-specified secondary analyses of those with low vitamin E at baseline. In addition, some of the studies which have suggested benefit have been conducted in groups of patients (such as advanced renal failure) where there is substantial evidence of increased oxidative stress beyond that observed in healthy individuals, even those at high risk of cardiovascular disease (Boaz et al., 2000). It has also been proposed that there could be genotypic variance (for instance, at the haptoglobin gene), which might influence likelihood of response to vitamin E supplementation (Zingg et al., 2008). Further work is required to test the hypothesis that certain disease groups could benefit from relatively short-term vitamin E supplementation in adult life.

11.2.4.3.5 A diet high in vitamin E might be beneficial even though supplements are not

Supplementation with vitamin E is convenient and relatively cheap. However, when natural source vitamin E is ingested as part of a mixed diet a wide range of other antioxidant micronutrients are taken at the same time, and benefit might result as a consequence of the interaction of these micronutrients or as a result of other characteristics of the diet which they contain. Supplementation with vitamin E will achieve higher intakes than can be obtained from diet alone, but fail to replicate the other features of a diet high in natural source vitamin E. Therefore, even if antioxidant supplementation is accepted to be without benefit, it is likely to remain important to promote a diet high in antioxidants as part of a healthy lifestyle to prevent a range of chronic diseases, including cardiovascular disease and cancers.

11.2.5 Conclusions

There is very strong evidence from basic biology and epidemiological studies that a high intake of vitamin E is likely to protect against cardiovascular disease. However, when this hypothesis has been tested in clinical trials results have been mainly negative. There are several potential explanations for this, and overall it remains prudent to promote a fruit- and vegetable-rich diet which will include relatively high intakes of vitamin E to prevent cardiovascular disease. It remains possible that there are subgroups of the population who would benefit from vitamin E supplementation; future studies should focus on identification of such subgroups and testing the possibility of benefit in targeted clinical trials.

References

Bai H, Liu BW, Deng ZY, Shen T, Fang DZ, Zhao YH, et al., Plasma very-low-density lipoprotein, low-density lipoprotein, and high-density lipoprotein oxidative modification induces procoagulant profiles in endogenous hypertriglyceridemia. Free Radic Biol Med 2006;40: 1796–803.

Bjelakovic G, Nikolova D, Gluud LL, Simonetti RG, Gluud C, Antioxidant supplements for prevention of mortality in healthy participants and patients with various diseases. Cochrane Database Syst Rev 2008;2: CD007176.

Boaz M, Smetana S, Weinstein T, Matas Z, Gafter U, Iaina A, et al., Secondary prevention with antioxidants of cardiovascular disease in endstage renal disease (SPACE): randomised placebo-controlled trial. Lancet 2000;356: 1213–8.

Chang CJ, Hsieh RH, Wang HF, Chin MY, Huang SY, Effects of glucose and alpha-tocopherol on low-density lipoprotein oxidation and glycation. Ann N Y Acad Sci 2005;1042: 294–302.

Chouinard JA, Grenier G, Khalil A, Vermette P, Oxidized-LDL induce morphological changes and increase stiffness of endothelial cells. Exp Cell Res 2008;314: 3007–16.

Deakin S, Moren X, James RW, HDL oxidation compromises its influence on paraoxonase-1 secretion and its capacity to modulate enzyme activity. Arterioscler Thromb Vasc Biol 2007;27: 1146–52.

Devaraj S, Tang R, Adams-Huet B, Harris A, Seenivasan T, de Lemos JA, et al., Effect of high-dose alpha-tocopherol supplementation on biomarkers of oxidative stress and inflammation and carotid atherosclerosis in patients with coronary artery disease. Am J Clin Nutr 2007;86: 1392–8.

Duffy SJ, O'Brien RC, New G, Harper RW, Meredith IT, Effect of anti-oxidant treatment and cholesterol lowering on resting arterial tone, metabolic vasodilation and endothelial function in the human forearm: a randomized, placebo-controlled study. Clin Exp Pharmacol Physiol 2001;28: 409–18.

Garner B, Witting PK, Waldeck AR, Christison JK, Raftery M, Stocker R, Oxidation of high density lipoproteins. I. Formation of methionine sulfoxide in apolipoproteins AI and AII is an early event that accompanies lipid peroxidation and can be enhanced by alpha-tocopherol. J Biol Chem 1998;273: 6080–7.

GISSI. Dietary supplementation with n-3 polyunsaturated fatty acids and vitamin E after myocardial infarction: results of the GISSI-Prevenzione trial. Gruppo Italiano per lo Studio della Sopravvivenza nell'Infarto miocardico. Lancet 1999;354: 447–55.

He FJ, Nowson CA, Lucas M, MacGregor GA, Increased consumption of fruit and vegetables is related to a reduced risk of coronary heart disease: meta-analysis of cohort studies. J Hum Hypertens 2007;21: 717–28.

Heart Protection Study Collaborative Group. MRC/BHF Heart Protection Study of antioxidant vitamin supplementation in 20,536 high-risk individuals: a randomised placebo-controlled trial. Lancet 2002;360: 23–33.

Hercberg S, Galan P, Preziosi P, Bertrais S, Mennen L, Malvy D, et al., The SUVIMAX Study: a randomized, placebo-controlled trial of the health effects of antioxidant vitamins and minerals. Arch Intern Med 2004;164: 2335–42.

Hodis HN, Mack WJ, LaBree L, Mahrer PR, Sevanian A, Liu CR, et al., Alpha-tocopherol supplementation in healthy individuals reduces low-density lipoprotein oxidation but not atherosclerosis: the Vitamin E Atherosclerosis Prevention Study (VEAPS). Circulation 2002;106: 1453–9.

Islam KN, O'Byrne D, Devaraj S, Palmer B, Grundy SM, Jialal I, Alpha-tocopherol supplementation decreases the oxidative susceptibility of LDL in renal failure patients on dialysis therapy. Atherosclerosis 2000;150: 217–24.

Jialal I, Grundy SM, Effect of combined supplementation with alpha-tocopherol, ascorbate, and beta carotene on low-density lipoprotein oxidation. Circulation 1993;88: 2780–6.

Klipstein-Grobusch K, Geleijnse JM, den Breeijen JH, Boeing H, Hofman A, Grobbee DE, et al., Dietary antioxidants and risk of myocardial infarction in the elderly: the Rotterdam Study. Am J Clin Nutr 1999;69: 261–6.

Knekt P, Reunanen A, Jarvinen R, Seppanen R, Heliovaara M, Aromaa A, Antioxidant vitamin intake and coronary mortality in a longitudinal population study. Am J Epidemiol 1994;139: 1180–9.

Koga T, Kwan P, Zubik L, Ameho C, Smith D, Meydani M, Vitamin E supplementation suppresses macrophage accumulation and endothelial cell expression of adhesion molecules in the aorta of hypercholesterolemic rabbits. Atherosclerosis 2004;176: 265–72.

Kritchevsky SB, Shimakawa T, Tell GS, Dennis B, Carpenter M, Eckfeldt JH, et al., Dietary antioxidants and carotid artery wall thickness. The ARIC Study. Atherosclerosis Risk in Communities Study. Circulation 1995;92: 2142–50.

Kushi LH, Folsom AR, Prineas RJ, Mink PJ, Wu Y, Bostick RM, Dietary antioxidant vitamins and death from coronary heart disease in postmenopausal women. N Engl J Med 1996;334: 1156–62.

Liu M, Wallmon A, Olsson-Mortlock C, Wallin R, Saldeen T, Mixed tocopherols inhibit platelet aggregation in humans: potential mechanisms. Am J Clin Nutr 2003;77: 700–6.

Lonn E, Yusuf S, Hoogwerf B, Pogue J, Yi Q, Zinman B, et al., Effects of vitamin E on cardiovascular and microvascular outcomes in high-risk patients with diabetes: results of the HOPE study and MICRO-HOPE substudy. Diabetes Care 2002;25: 1919–27.

Losonczy KG, Harris TB, Havlik RJ, Vitamin E and vitamin C supplement use and risk of all-cause and coronary heart disease mortality in older persons: the Established Populations for Epidemiologic Studies of the Elderly. Am J Clin Nutr 1996;64:190–6.

Meuwissen M, van der Wal AC, Niessen HW, Koch KT, de Winter RJ, van der Loos CM, et al., Colocalisation of intraplaque C reactive protein, complement, oxidised low density lipoprotein, and macrophages in stable and unstable angina and acute myocardial infarction. J Clin Pathol 2006;59: 196–201.

Munteanu A, Zingg JM, Cellular, molecular and clinical aspects of vitamin E on atherosclerosis prevention. Mol Aspects Med 2007;28: 538–90.

Murohara T, Ikeda H, Otsuka Y, Aoki M, Haramaki N, Katoh A, et al., Inhibition of platelet adherence to mononuclear cells by alpha-tocopherol: role of P-selectin. Circulation 2004;110: 141–8.

Nakashima Y, Fujii H, Sumiyoshi S, Wight TN, Sueishi K, Early human atherosclerosis: accumulation of lipid and proteoglycans in intimal thickenings followed by macrophage infiltration. Arterioscler Thromb Vasc Biol 2007;27: 1159–65.

Niessner A, Goronzy JJ, Weyand CM, Immune-mediated mechanisms in atherosclerosis: prevention and treatment of clinical manifestations. Curr Pharm Des 2007;13: 3701–10.

Ogawa Y, Saito Y, Nishio K, Yoshida Y, Ashida H, Niki E, Gamma-tocopheryl quinone, not alpha-tocopheryl quinone, induces adaptive response through up-regulation of cellular glutathione and cysteine availability via activation of ATF4. Free Radic Res 2008;42: 674–87.

Peluzio MC, Miguel E Jr, Drumond TC, Cesar GC, Santiago HC, Teixeira MM, et al., Monocyte chemoattractant protein-1 involvement in the alpha-tocopherol-induced reduction of atherosclerotic lesions in apolipoprotein E knockout mice. Br J Nutr 2003;90: 3–11.

Petraki MP, Mantani PT, Tselepis AD, Recent advances on the antiatherogenic effects of HDL-derived proteins and mimetic peptides. Curr Pharm Des 2009;15: 3146–3166.

Prasad K, Kalra J, Oxygen free radicals and hypercholesterolemic atherosclerosis: effect of vitamin E. Am Heart J 1993;125: 958–73.

Rimm EB, Stampfer MJ, Ascherio A, Giovannucci E, Colditz GA, Willett WC, Vitamin E consumption and the risk of coronary heart disease in men. N Engl J Med 1993;328: 1450–6.

Robinson I, de Serna DG, Gutierrez A, Schade DS, Vitamin E in humans: an explanation of clinical trial failure. Endocr Pract 2006;12: 576–82.

Sacco M, Pellegrini F, Roncaglioni MC, Avanzini F, Tognoni G, Nicolucci A, et al., Primary prevention of cardiovascular events with low-dose aspirin and vitamin E in type 2 diabetic patients: results of the Primary Prevention Project (PPP) trial. Diabetes Care 2003;26: 3264–72.

Salonen RM, Nyyssonen K, Kaikkonen J, Porkkala-Sarataho E, Voutilainen S, Rissanen TH, et al., Six-year effect of combined vitamin C and E supplementation on atherosclerotic progression: the Antioxidant Supplementation in Atherosclerosis Prevention (ASAP) Study. Circulation 2003;107: 947–53.

Schnell JW, Anderson RA, Stegner JE, Schindler SP, Weinberg RB, Effects of a high polyunsaturated fat diet and vitamin E supplementation on high-density lipoprotein oxidation in humans. Atherosclerosis 2001;159: 459–66.

Schwenke DC, Rudel LL, Sorci-Thomas MG, Thomas MJ, Alpha-tocopherol protects against diet induced atherosclerosis in New Zealand white rabbits. J Lipid Res 2002;43: 1927–38.

Sesso HD, Buring JE, Christen WG, Kurth T, Belanger C, MacFadyen J, et al., Vitamins E and C in the prevention of cardiovascular disease in men: the Physicians' Health Study II randomized controlled trial. J Am Med Assoc 2008;300: 2123–33.

Skyrme-Jones RA, O'Brien RC, Berry KL, Meredith IT, Vitamin E supplementation improves endothelial function in type I diabetes mellitus: a randomized, placebo-controlled study. J Am Coll Cardiol 2000;36: 94–102.

Stahelin HB, Eichholzer M, Gey KF, Nutritional factors correlating with cardiovascular disease: results of the Basel Study. Bibl Nutr Dieta 1992;49: 24–35.

Stampfer MJ, Hennekens CH, Manson JE, Colditz GA, Rosner B, Willett WC, Vitamin E consumption and the risk of coronary disease in women. N Engl J Med 1993;328: 1444–9.

Steinberg D, The LDL modification hypothesis of atherogenesis: an update. J Lipid Res 2009; 50(Suppl): S376–81.

Stephens NG, Parsons A, Schofield PM, Kelly F, Cheeseman K, Mitchinson MJ, Randomised controlled trial of vitamin E in patients with coronary disease: Cambridge Heart Antioxidant Study (CHAOS). Lancet 1996;347: 781–6.

Tanvetyanon T, Bepler G, Beta-carotene in multivitamins and the possible risk of lung cancer among smokers versus former smokers: a meta-analysis and evaluation of national brands. Cancer 2008;113: 150–7.

Thomas SR, Stocker R, Molecular action of vitamin E in lipoprotein oxidation: implications for atherosclerosis. Free Radic Biol Med 2000;28: 1795–805.

Van Gaal LF, Mertens IL, De Block CE, Mechanisms linking obesity with cardiovascular disease. Nature 2006;444: 875–80.

Virtamo J, Rapola JM, Ripatti S, Heinonen OP, Taylor PR, Albanes D, et al., Effect of vitamin E and beta carotene on the incidence of primary nonfatal myocardial infarction and fatal coronary heart disease. Arch Intern Med 1998;158: 668–75.

Woollard KJ, Rayment SJ, Bevan R, Shaw JA, Lunec J, Griffiths HR, Alpha-tocopherol supplementation does not affect monocyte endothelial adhesion or C-reactive protein levels but reduces soluble vascular adhesion molecule-1 in the plasma of healthy subjects. Redox Rep 2006;11: 214–22.

Ye Z, Song H, Antioxidant vitamins intake and the risk of coronary heart disease: meta-analysis of cohort studies. Eur J Cardiovasc Prev Rehabil 2008;15: 26–34.

Zingg JM, Azzi A, Non-antioxidant activities of vitamin E. Curr Med Chem 2004;11: 1113–33.

Zingg JM, Azzi A, Meydani M, Genetic polymorphisms as determinants for disease-preventive effects of vitamin E. Nutr Rev 2008;66: 406–14.

11.3 Vitamin E and neuroinflammation

Kanwaljit Chopra; Anurag Kuhad; Vinod Tiwari

11.3.1 Introduction

Vitamin E is an essential, fat-soluble nutrient that functions as an antioxidant in the human body. Vitamin E represents a generic term for all tocopherols and their derivatives having the biological activity of *RRR*-α-tocopherols, the naturally occurring stereoisomer compounds (Traber and Packer, 1995; Traber and Sies, 1996). The term vitamin E covers mainly eight fat-soluble compounds found in nature. Four of them are called tocopherols and the other four tocotrienols. They are identified by the prefixes α, β, γ and δ. α-Tocopherol is the most common and biologically the most active of these naturally occurring forms of vitamin E. Natural tocopherols occur in *RRR*-configuration only (*RRR*-α-tocopherol was formerly designated as D-α-tocopherol). The chemical synthesis of α-tocopherol results in a mixture of eight different stereoisomeric forms which is called *all-rac*-α-tocopherol (or DL-α-tocopherol). The biological activity of the synthetic form is lower than that of the natural form. The name tocopherol derives from the Greek words *tocos*, meaning childbirth, and *pherein*, meaning to bring forth. The name was coined to highlight its essential role in the reproduction of various animal species. The ending *-ol* identifies the substance as being an alcohol (Sen et al., 2006). The importance of vitamin E in humans was not accepted until fairly recently. For decades, vitamin E pioneers Drs Wilfred and Evan Shute were deprived of much-deserved recognition. Because its deficiency is not manifested by a well-recognized, widespread vitamin deficiency disease such as scurvy (vitamin C deficiency) or rickets (vitamin D deficiency), science only began to recognize the importance of vitamin E at a relatively late stage.

11.3.2 Unique functional activities shared by vitamin E family members

Vitamin E refers to a family of eight molecules having a chromanol ring (chroman ring with an alcoholic hydroxyl group) and a 12-carbon aliphatic side chain containing two methyl groups in the middle and two more methyl groups at the end. For the four tocopherols, the side chain is saturated, whereas for the four tocotrienols the side chain contains three double-bonds, all of which adjoin a methyl group. The four tocopherols and the four tocotrienols have an alpha, beta, gamma and delta form – named on the basis of the number and position of the methyl groups on the chromanol ring. The alpha form has three methyl groups, the beta and gamma forms have two methyl groups and the delta form has only one methyl group (Theriault et al., 1999).

The alpha form of tocopherol constitutes approximately 90% of the tocopherol in animal tissue, originally designated D-alpha-tocopherol on the basis of optical activity. There are actually three asymmetric carbon atoms in tocopherol, one at the 2-position of the chromanol ring, and the other two on the aliphatic chain, at the 4′ and 8′ positions – all being locations of methyl groups. The International Union of Pure and Applied Chemistry (IUPAC) advocate an *R* and *S* system of stereoisomer designation, rather than the 'D-' & 'L-' prefixes (which indicate optical activity. Therefore, the common natural form of alpha tocopherol has the IUPAC name 2*R*,4′*R*,8′*R*-alpha-tocopherol (*RRR*-alpha-tocopherol, for short) – 'D-alpha-tocopherol' is now obsolete.

Experimental evidence suggesting that α-tocopherol might have functions independent of its antioxidant property came from the study of platelet adhesion. α-Tocopherol strongly inhibits platelet adhesion. Doses of 400 IU/day provide greater than 75% inhibition of platelet adhesion to a variety of adhesive proteins when tested at low shear rate in a laminar flow chamber (Steiner, 1993). At the post-translational level, α-tocopherol inhibits protein kinase C, 5-lipoxygenase and phospholipase A2 and activates protein phosphatase 2A and diacylglycerol kinase. Some genes (e.g., scavenger receptors, α-TTP, α-tropomyosin, matrix metalloproteinase-19 and collagenase) are specifically modulated by α-tocopherol at the transcriptional level. α-Tocopherol also inhibits cell proliferation, platelet aggregation and monocyte adhesion. These effects have been characterized to be unrelated to the antioxidant activity of vitamin E, and possibly reflect specific interactions of α-tocopherol with enzymes, structural proteins, lipids and transcription factors (Zingg and Azzi, 2004). γ-Tocopherol represents the major form of vitamin E in the diet in the USA, but not in Europe. Desmethyl tocopherols, such as γ-tocopherol and specific tocopherol metabolites, most notably the carboxyethyl-hydroxychroman (CEHC) products, exhibit functions that are not shared by α-tocopherol. The activities of these other tocopherols do not map directly to their chemical antioxidant behavior but rather reflect anti-inflammatory, antineoplastic and natriuretic functions possibly mediated through specific binding interactions (Hensley et al., 2004).

Further evidence supporting the unique biological significance of vitamin E family members is provided by current results derived from α-tocotrienol research. α-Tocotrienol possesses numerous functions that are not shared by α-tocopherol. For example, nanomolar concentrations of α-tocotrienol uniquely prevent inducible neurodegeneration by regulating specific mediators of cell death (Sen et al., 2000; Khanna et al., 2003). In addition, tocopherols do not seem to share the cholesterol-lowering properties of tocotrienol (Qureshi et al., 1986, 2002). Tocotrienol, not tocopherol, administration reduces oxidative protein damage and extends the mean life span of *Caenorhabditis elegans* (Adachi and Ishii, 2000).

11.3.3 Neuroinflammation

The central nervous system (CNS) was previously considered to be 'immune privileged', neither susceptible to, nor contributing to, inflammation. It is now appreciated that the CNS does exhibit features of inflammation, and in response to injury, infection or disease, resident CNS cells generate inflammatory mediators, including proinflammatory cytokines, prostaglandins, free radicals and complement, which, in turn, induce chemokines and adhesion molecules, recruit immune cells and activate glial cells. Much of the key evidence demonstrates that inflammation and inflammatory mediators contribute to acute, chronic and psychiatric CNS disorders (Farooqui et al., 2007).

Neuroinflammation is a host defense mechanism associated with neutralization of an insult and restoration of normal structure and function of brain. Neuroinflammation is a hallmark of all major CNS diseases. Glial cells, the microglia, astrocytes and oligodendrocytes, constitute more than 70% of the total cell population in the brain tissue (Diamond et al., 1999). Oligodendrocytes are responsible for myelination, astrocytes participate in a wide variety of physiological and pathophysiological processes, and microglial cells in collaboration with astrocytes monitor and maintain the physiological homeostasis and microenvironment for the survival of neurons. Residential microglia, which represent 20% of the total glial cell population, also sense changes in the periphery and respond quickly to pathogenic stimuli to protect the brain.

An active, coordinated program of inflammatory resolution is initiated in the first few hours after an inflammatory response begins. Histologically, the neuroinflammatory response requires the activation of microglia and recruitment of polymorphonuclear leukocytes (PMN) from the blood stream into brain tissue. This PMN migration is a coordinated multistep process involving chemotaxis, adhesion of PMN to endothelial cells in the area of inflammation, and diapedesis, the penetration of tight junctions and migration through the endothelial monolayer and into the interstitium (Diamond et al., 1999). These PMN eliminate invading antigens by phagocytosis and release free radicals and lytic enzymes into phagolysosomes. This is followed by a process called resolution, a turning off mechanism by neural cells to limit tissue injury. After entering tissues, granulocytes promote the switch off arachidonic acid-derived prostaglandins and leukotrienes to lipoxins, which initiate the termination sequence. This process prevents recruitment of neutrophils. The onset of cellular apoptosis occurs. These events coincide with the biosynthesis of resolvins and protectins, which critically shorten the period of neutrophil infiltration by initiating apoptosis. Consequently, apoptotic neutrophils undergo phagocytosis by macrophages, leading to neutrophil clearance and release of anti-inflammatory and reparative cytokines such as transforming growth factor-β. The anti-inflammatory program ends with the departure of macrophages through the lymphatics.

A variety of immune system modulators including complement proteins, adhesion molecules, inflammatory cytokines such as interleukin-1 alpha (IL-1α), interleukin-1 beta (IL-1β), interleukin-3 (IL-3), interleukin-6 (IL-6), tumor necrosis factor-alpha (TNF-α), colony-stimulating factor-1, and tumor growth factors (TGF-α and β), are made and secreted by both microglia and astrocytes. These factors propagate and maintain neuroinflammation by several mechanisms, including the activation of multiple forms of PLA2, cyclooxygenases (COX) and lipoxygenases (LOX), causing the release of non-esterified AA from neural membrane phospholipids and generating lyso-glycerophospholipids, platelet-activating factor (PAF), proinflammatory prostaglandins, and reactive oxygen species (ROS) perception. Furthermore, microglia, astrocytes, neurons, endothelial cells and oligodendrocytes also produce complement proteins. Cytokines such as TNF-α and IL-1β are usually the first cytokines to be up-regulated after neural trauma and infection. Transcription factors such as nuclear factor kappa B (NFκB) controls the expression of a large array of genes involved in immune function and cell survival whereas peroxisome proliferator-activated receptors (PPARs), elicit anti-neoplastic and anti-inflammatory activities in neural cells. Toll-like receptors (TLRs) play a key role in the recognition of products from virtually all classes of pathogenic organisms. Production of these cytokines also initiates signaling through TLRs that recognize host-derived molecules released from injured tissues and cells.

However, inflammatory mediators could have dual roles, with detrimental acute effects but beneficial effects in long-term repair and recovery, leading to complications in their application as novel therapies. However, these complications are avoided in acute diseases in which treatment duration might be relatively short-term. Targeting IL-1 is a promising novel therapy for stroke and traumatic brain injury, the naturally occurring antagonist (IL-1ra) being well tolerated by rheumatoid arthritis patients. Chronic disorders represent a greater therapeutic challenge, a problem highlighted in Alzheimer's disease (AD); significant data suggested that anti-inflammatory agents might reduce the probability of developing AD, or slow its progression, but prospective clinical trials of nonsteroidal anti-inflammatory drugs or cyclooxygenase inhibitors have been disappointing. The complex interplay between inflammatory mediators, aging, genetic background, and environmental factors might ultimately regulate the outcome of acute CNS injury and progression of chronic neurodegeneration, and be crucial for development of effective therapies for CNS diseases.

11.3.4 Neuroinflammation and neurodegenerative disorders

Currently, neurodegenerative disorders are responsible for 27% of all years lived with disability (YLDs) in developing countries and, with the exception of Sub-Saharan Africa, they are the leading contributors to YLDs in all regions of the world. Although cost-effective treatments to reduce the burden of certain brain disorders, including AD, diabetic and alcoholic encephalopathy, tardive dyskinesia, amylotropic lateral sclerosis, and neuropathic pain, are available in the developed world, this is not the case in the developing world. According to a World Health Organization 2004 report, in India, for a population of nearly one billion people, there are an estimated four million people with neuropsychiatric disorders, with different degrees of impact on some twenty-five million family members.

Neurodegenerative disorders, such as AD, are more common in the elderly with an incidence of 0.7% in India. Owing to the prevalence, morbidity and mortality of the neurodegenerative diseases, they represent significant medical, social and financial burden on the society; more so, because the average life expectancy is also increasing towards a greater proportion of elderly in our population. AD is the most prevalent neurodegenerative disease affecting the aging population, and is characterized by memory loss and decline in cognitive functions. The presence of activated glial cells and the increase in inflammation-associated proteins in the brain of AD patients support the neuroinflammatory nature of this disease. Although the underlying mechanism(s) for neuroinflammation in the AD brain is not clearly understood, there is considerable evidence supporting a role for specific forms of amyloid beta peptide (Aβ) in inducing production of pro-inflammatory cytokines by microglia and astrocytes (Moses et al., 2006).

Chronic hyperglycemia is associated with a high incidence of progressive dementia in humans (Ryan et al., 2003). The potential mechanisms for this not only include direct effects of hypo- or hyperglycemia and hypo- or hyperinsulinemia, but also indirect effects via cerebrovascular alterations (Brands et al., 2004; Lobnig et al., 2005). Under chronic hyperglycemia, endogenous TNF-α production is accelerated in microvascular and neural tissues, which could cause increased microvascular permeability, hypercoagulability and nerve damage, thus initiating and promoting the development of characteristic lesions of diabetic microangiopathy, polyneuropathy and encephalopathy (▶Fig. 11.4) (Satoh et al., 2003; Brands et al., 2004).

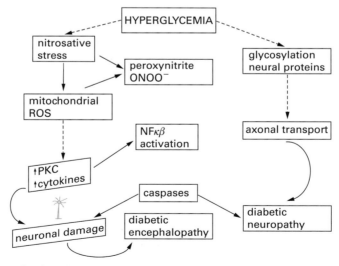

Fig. 11.4: Pathophysiology of diabetic encephalopathy and neuropathy depicting neuroinflammation as a major contributor.

Peripheral neuropathy is a frequent complication of diabetes that ultimately accounts for significant morbidity. Pathogenetic mechanisms underlying the progressive nerve fiber loss seem to be multifactorial, including polyol pathway, glycation, reactive oxygen species and altered protein kinase C activity (Brownlee, 2001). Hyperglycemia and inflammation unleash a cascade of events that affects cellular proteins, gene expression and cell surface receptor expression, ultimately resulting in progressive pathologic changes and subsequent diabetic complications (▶Fig. 11.4) (Pop-Busui et al., 2006).

Chronic alcohol intake is also known to induce the selective neuronal damage associated with increase oxidative-nitrosative stress and activation of inflammatory cascade finally resulting in neuronal apoptosis and thus dementia (alcoholic encephalopathy). Alcohol-induced brain damage produces some of the most insidious effects of alcoholism, including cognitive deficits such as learning and memory impairment (Pfefferbaum et al., 1998; White, 2003). The mechanism behind ethanol-induced selective neuronal damage is not well understood, but several explanations have been proposed. These include excitotoxicity associated with excessive neurotransmitter release, oxidative stress leading to free radical damage (Crews et al., 2004) and edema caused by alterations in cellular control of ion transport (Collins et al., 1998). Crews et al. (2006) suggested that alcohol-induced neurodegeneration involves NFκB activation, microglial activation and increased COX2 immunoreactivity, all of which are indicative of an enhanced neuro-inflammatory response (▶Fig. 11.5).

The peripheral neuropathy is a potentially incapacitating complication of chronic consumption of ethanol, characterized by pain and dysesthesias, primarily in the lower extremities, and is poorly relieved by available therapies (Monforte et al., 1995). Ethanol is oxidized to acetaldehyde by cytochrome P450, which increases reactive oxygen

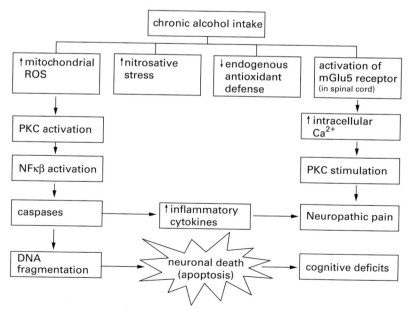

Fig. 11.5: Involvement of neuroinflammation in alcohol-induced behavioral deficits.

species, with concomitant changes in redox balance (Mantle et al., 1999). Studies have suggested that chronic ethanol increases oxidative damage to proteins, lipids and DNA (Mansouri et al., 2001; McDonough, 2003). In our study, we also found that chronic alcohol intake is known to decrease the nociceptive threshold with increased oxidative-nitrosative stress and release of proinflammatory cytokines (►Fig. 11.5; Tiwari et al., 2009).

Tardive dyskinesia (TD) is a syndrome of late-onset, abnormal, choreoathetoid involuntary movements that develops in some patients who receive chronic neuroleptic medications. The neurodegenerative hypothesis, which was proposed in the mid-1980s suggests that persistent TD might be associated with, or induced by, neuronal damage somewhere in the basal ganglia. Cadet and Lohr (1989) proposed that the damage, which could affect the neuronal membrane function and, if unchecked, could lead to cell death, might involve the presynaptic catecholaminergic fibers as well as other neurotransmitter systems. They also proposed that these neuronal changes were secondary to free radical generation from increased dopamine metabolism and turnover, a consequence of neuroleptic medication.

Amylotrophic lateral sclerosis (ALS) is the most frequent adult onset motor neuron disease (Gonzalez de Aguilar et al., 2007). Approximately 85–90% of cases are sporadic (SALS), the remaining 10–15% categorized as familial (FALS). SALS and FALS are clinically and pathologically similar (Bruijn et al., 2004). The pathological hallmarks of the disease are the selective and progressive atrophy of neurons in the corticospinal tract, swelling of perikarya and proximal axons and the presence of Bunina bodies, axonal spheroids and inclusions. Disease pathogenesis in ALS involves several interconnected mechanisms all resulting in the rapid deterioration of motor neurons. The main mechanisms include enhanced free radical production (Bogdanov et al., 1998), protein misfolding (Takamiya et al., 2005), aberrant protein aggregation, excitotoxicity, mitochondrial dysfunction (Higgins et al., 2003), neuroinflammation (Hensley et al., 2006) and apoptosis (Sathasivam and Shaw, 2005).

Parkinson's disease is characterized by a slow and progressive degeneration of dopaminergic neurons in the substantia nigra. Despite intensive research, the cause of the neuronal loss in Parkinson's disease is poorly understood. Neuroinflammatory mechanisms might contribute to the cascade of events leading to neuronal degeneration. As with ALS and AD, there is well-documented increase in oxidative damage to Parkinson's disease-affected human brain (Hald and Lotharius, 2005) and brains of animals exposed to toxins that selectively target the nigrostriatal brain circuitry (Dauer and Przedborski, 2003).

Huntington's disease (HD) is an autosomal dominant neurodegenerative disease with an average onset between the fourth and fifth decade of life; it leads to death 15–20 years after the onset of symptoms. HD is characterized by the inhibition of complex II of respiratory chain and increase in ROS-mediated neuroinflammation (Gomez-Lazaro et al., 2007). Although several drugs seem effective in controlling the incapacitating manifestations of HD, no specific therapy is known.

Stroke is widely considered to have an oxidative stress component originating directly from the physical biochemistry of the ischemia/reperfusion event, and later from secondary events such as excitotoxicity and neuroinflammation (Alexandrova et al., 2003). In the early stages of ischemia, oxygen tension drops leading to an effective blockade of mitochondrial electron transport and an accumulation of reducing equivalents. Upon reperfusion, these can rapidly promote incomplete reduction of molecular oxygen yielding free radicals and peroxides (Kutala et al., 2007). Conversion of xanthine dehydrogenase to the superoxide-generating xanthine oxidase (XO) has also been implicated as an early source of free radicals during reperfusion (Margaill et al., 2005).

Aging leads to change in microenvironment of brain, thus making it more susceptible to insults and genetic predisposition of various neurodegenerative diseases. Although the etiology of brain aging is not well understood, the free radical theory of aging describes a compelling mechanistic rationale for the age-related decline in function of many biological systems. This oxidative stress-based theory describes a redox imbalance, whereby the production of free radicals overtakes endogenous antioxidant capacity, leading to oxidative damage to crucial cellular elements (Harman, 1993). The free radical theory of aging might be particularly relevant for the brain, because the brain utilizes relatively high levels of oxygen but has relatively low levels of endogenous antioxidants. Indeed, oxidative stress has been repeatedly implicated in brain aging and in neurodegenerative disorders such as AD (Markesbery and Lovell, 1998).

11.3.5 Vitamin E as a neuroinflammatory agent

The majority of the available research on the role of antioxidant nutrients in neurological function and disease has focused on vitamin E. Vitamin E is the major lipid-soluble, chain-breaking antioxidant in the body, protecting the integrity of membranes by inhibiting lipid peroxidation. Mostly on the basis of symptoms of primary vitamin E deficiency, it has been demonstrated that vitamin E has a central role in maintaining neurological structure and function (Muller and Goss-Sampson, 1990). Orally supplemented vitamin E reaches the cerebrospinal fluid and brain (Vatassery et al., 1998). One of the most extensively studied aspects of vitamin E is its antioxidant property. Most of the vitamin E-sensitive neurological disorders are associated with elevated levels of oxidative damage markers. This has led to a popular hypothesis stating that the neuroprotective effects of vitamin E are wholly mediated by its antioxidant property (Vatassery, 1998).

Vitamin E is a natural, highly tolerable and cost-effective molecule. Beyond the nonspecific antioxidant effect specific effects of Vitamin E, which includes gene regulation, have been revealing, and non-antioxidant properties of tocopherols are current topics of interest (Azzi and Stocker, 2000). Protein kinase C (PKC) is one of the pathways used by α-tocopherol (Boscoboinik et al., 1991). Sharma et al. (1994) reported that tocopherol inhibits not only free radical formation but also tyrosine kinase activity in tissue plasminogen activator (TPA)-induced primary human fibroblasts or HL-60 cells. Lipoxygenase activity is sensitive to vitamin E. α-Tocopherol strongly inhibits purified 5-LOX with IC50 of 5 lM. The inhibition is independent of the antioxidant property of tocopherol.

The hepatic α-tocopherol transfer protein (α-TTP), together with the tocopherol-associated proteins (TAP) is responsible for the endogenous accumulation of natural α-tocopherol. Although these systems have a much lower affinity to transport tocotrienols, it has been evident that orally supplemented tocotrienol results in plasma tocotrienol concentration in the range of 1 μM (O'Byrne et al., 2000). Of note, such circulating levels of α-tocotrienol are almost an order of magnitude higher than that required to protect neurons against a range of neurotoxic insults (Sen et al., 2000; Khanna et al., 2003). Despite such promising potential, tocotrienol research accounts for less than 1% of all vitamin E research published in PubMed. The unique vitamin action of α-tocopherol, combined with its prevalence in the human body and the similar efficiency of tocopherols as chain-breaking antioxidants, led biologists to almost completely discount the 'minor' vitamin E molecules as topics for basic and clinical research. Recent discoveries have forced a serious reconsideration of this conventional wisdom (Hensley et al., 2004).

A possible neuroprotective property of tocotrienols was indicated in a study testing the efficacy of the tocotrienol-rich fraction from palm oil to protect against oxidative damage of rat brain mitochondria. The tocotrienol-rich fraction from palm oil was significantly more effective than α-tocopherol in protecting the brain against damage caused by exposure to ascorbate-Fe21, the free radical initiator azobis (2-amidopropane) dihydrochloride, or photosensitization (Kamat and Devasagayam, 1995). At concentrations of 25–50 µM, α-tocopherol is known to regulate signal transduction pathways by mechanisms that are independent of its antioxidant properties. α-Tocopherol, but not β-tocopherol having comparable antioxidant properties, inhibited inducible protein kinase C activity in smooth muscle cells (Boscoboinik et al., 1994; Azzi et al., 1995). The signal transduction regulatory properties of tocotrienols, however, are yet unknown. At nanomolar concentrations α-tocotrienol, in contrast to α-tocopherol, protects against glutamate-induced neuronal death by suppressing inducible pp60 c-src kinase activation. α-Tocotrienol provided the most potent neuroprotection among all vitamin E analogs (Sen et al., 2000). Oral tocotrienol crosses the blood-brain barrier to reach brain tissue; more so for the fetal brain when pregnant rats are supplemented with tocotrienol (Roy et al., 2002). At nanomolar concentrations α-tocotrienol, in contrast to α-tocopherol, protects against glutamate-induced neuronal death by suppressing inducible 12-lipoxygenase activation in mice (Khanna et al., 2003). Injected α-tocotrienol decreased the size of the cerebral infarcts 1 day after stroke in mice; γ-tocotrienol and delta-tocotrienol did not protect (Mishima et al., 2003). α-Tocotrienol provided the most potent neuroprotection among vitamin E analogs on cultured striatal neurons of rats (Osakada et al., 2004).

11.3.5.1 Alzheimer's disease

In an animal model of AD (intracerebroventricular streptozotocin, ICV STZ) cognitive impairment is associated with increased oxidative-nitrosative stress and inflammatory cascade (Lannert and Hoyer, 1998). In our findings, we also found that the antioxidant property of both the isoforms of vitamin E (α-tocopherol and tocotrienol) could be responsible for protecting against the oxidative stress, possibly by increasing the endogenous defensive capacity of the brain to combat oxidative stress induced by ICV STZ (▶Fig. 11.6A). In addition to potent antioxidant activity the suppression of nitrosative stress (▶Fig. 11.6B) and acetylcholinesterase activity also contributes significantly in preventing the cognitive impairment in the ICV STZ model in rats (Tiwari et al., 2009a).

In an another study from our laboratory, after 10 weeks of steptozotocin injection, the rats produced significant increase in transfer latency which was coupled with enhanced acetylcholinestrease activity, increased oxidative-nitrosative stress, TNF-α, IL-1β, caspase-3 activity and active p65 subunit of NFκB in different regions of diabetic rat brain (▶Fig. 11.7A,B). Interestingly, co-administration of tocotrienol significantly and dose-dependently prevented behavioral, biochemical and molecular changes associated with diabetes (Kuhad et al., 2009).

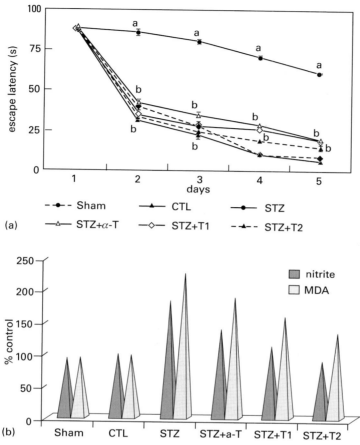

Fig. 11.6: (A) Effect of α-tocopherol and tocotrienol treatment on the performance of spatial memory acquisition phase in intracerebroventricular streptozotocin-treated rats. (a) Different from control group; (b) different from intracerebroventricular streptozotocin-treated group; (c) different from one another. CTL, control; STZ, intracerebroventricular streptozotocin (3 mg/kg); α-T, α-tocopherol (100 mg/kg); T1, tocotrienol (50 mg/kg); T2, tocotrienol (100 mg/kg); (adapted from Tiwari et al., 2009a). (B) Effect of α-tocopherol and tocotrienol treatment on brain nitrite and MDA levels of intracerebroventricular streptozotocin treated rats. (a) Different from control group; (b) different from intracerebroventricular streptozotocin-treated group; (c) different from one another. CTL, control; STZ, intracerebroventricular streptozotocin (3 mg/kg); α-T, α-tocopherol (100 mg/kg); T1, tocotrienol (50 mg/kg); T2, tocotrienol (100 mg/kg); (adapted from Tiwari et al., 2009a).

11.3.5.2 Diabetic neuropathy and encephalopathy

Sharma et al. (2006) found that 2 weeks of treatment with Trolox (a water-soluble derivative of vitamin E) in the dose of 10 and 30 mg/kg, i.p. initiated at the 6th week of STZ injection significantly improved motor nerve conduction velocity (MNCV), nerve blood flow (NBF) and inhibited thermal hyperalgesia. Trolox treatment also improved

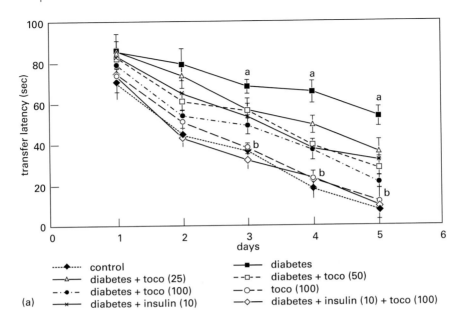

(a)

----◆---- control
—△— diabetes + toco (25)
—•— diabetes + toco (100)
—×— diabetes + insulin (10)

—■— diabetes
--□-- diabetes + toco (50)
—○-- toco (100)
—◇— diabetes + insulin (10) + toco (100)

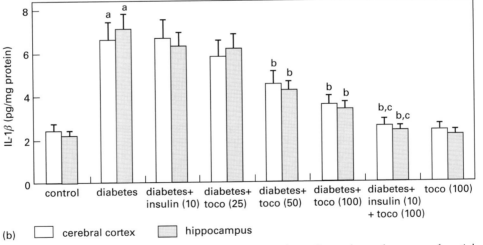

(b)   ☐ cerebral cortex   ▨ hippocampus

Fig. 11.7: (A) Effect of tocotrienol and its combination with insulin on the performance of spatial memory acquisition phase in control and diabetic rats. (a) Different from control group; (b) different from diabetic group; (c) different from *per se* group. Toco (25), tocotrienol (25 mg/kg); Toco (50), tocotrienol (50 mg/kg); Toco (100), tocotrienol (100 mg/kg); (adapted from Kuhad et al., 2009). (B) Effect of tocotrienol and its combination with insulin on IL-1β levels in cerebral cortex and hippocampus of diabetic rats. (a) Different from control; (b) different from diabetic group; (c) different from *per se* group. Toco (25), tocotrienol (25 mg/kg); Toco (50), tocotrienol (50 mg/kg); Toco (100), tocotrienol (100 mg/kg); (adapted from Kuhad et al., 2009).

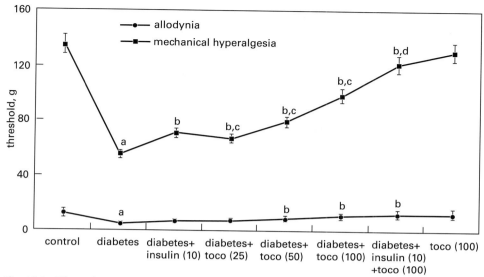

Fig. 11.8: Effect of tocotrienol and its combination with insulin on mechanical hyperalgesia and allodynia in the diabetic rats. (a) Different from control; (b) different from diabetic group; (c) different from one another; (d) different from tocotrienol and insulin *per se* groups. Toco (25), tocotrienol (25 mg/kg); Toco (50), tocotrienol (50 mg/kg); Toco (100), tocotrienol (100 mg/kg); (adapted from Kuhad and Chopra, 2009).

the activity of antioxidant enzymes and inhibited lipid peroxidation in sciatic nerves of diabetic rats suggesting its potential in diabetic neuropathy. In our study, we also found that diabetic rats developed neuropathy which was evident from a marked hyperalgesia and allodynia (▶Fig. 11.8) associated with enhanced nitrosative stress, release of inflammatory mediators (TNF-α, IL-1β, TGF-1β) and caspase-3 (▶Fig. 11.9A,B). Chronic treatment with tocotrienol (25, 50 and 100 mg/kg body weight; p.o.) for 4 weeks starting from the 4th week of streptozotocin injection significantly attenuated behavioral, biochemical and molecular changes associated with diabetic neuropathy (Kuhad and Chopra, 2009).

In our recent study (Tiwari et al., 2009b), from the 6th week onwards, ethanol-treated rats showed significant increase in transfer latency (▶Fig. 11.10) in the Morris water maze which was coupled with enhanced acetylcholinesterase activity, increased oxidative-nitrosative stress, TNF-α and IL-1β levels in the cerebral cortex and hippocampus of ethanol-treated rats which is indicative of enhanced neuroinflammation in the two main regions of brain involved in learning and memory (▶Fig. 11.11). Chronic treatment with tocopherol and tocotrienol significantly and dose-dependently reduced both the cytokines (TNF-α and IL-1β) in different brain regions of ethanol-administered rats.

11.3.5.3 Alcoholic neuropathy and encephalopathy

Chronic alcohol consumption produces a painful peripheral neuropathy for which there is no reliable successful therapy. Alcoholic neuropathy is characterized by spontaneous burning pain, hyperalgesia (an exaggerated pain in response to painful stimuli) and allodynia (a pain evoked by normally innocuous stimuli). Chronic alcohol intake is

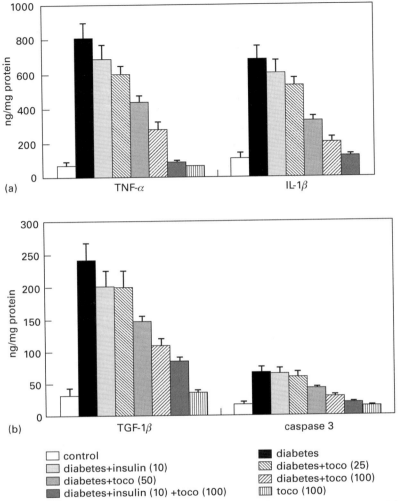

Fig. 11.9: (A) Effect of tocotrienol and its combination with insulin on TNF-α and IL-1β levels in the sciatic nerve of diabetic rats. (a) Different from control; (b) different from diabetic group; (c) different from one another; (d) different from tocotrienol and insulin *per se* groups. Toco (25), tocotrienol (25 mg/kg); Toco (50), tocotrienol (50 mg/kg); Toco (100), tocotrienol (100 mg/kg); (adapted from Kuhad and Chopra, 2009). (B) Effect of tocotrienol and its combination with insulin on TGF-1β and caspase 3 levels in the sciatic nerve diabetic rats. (a) Different from control; (b) different from diabetic group; (c) different from one another; (d) different from tocotrienol and insulin *per se* groups. Toco (25), tocotrienol (25 mg/kg); Toco (50), tocotrienol (50 mg/kg); Toco (100), tocotrienol (100 mg/kg); (adapted from Kuhad and Chopra, 2009).

known to decrease the nociceptive threshold with increased oxidative-nitrosative stress and release of proinflammatory cytokines coupled with activation of protein kinase C. In one of our studies, we also found that ethanol-treated animals (10 weeks) showed a significant decrease in nociceptive threshold as evident from decreased tail flick

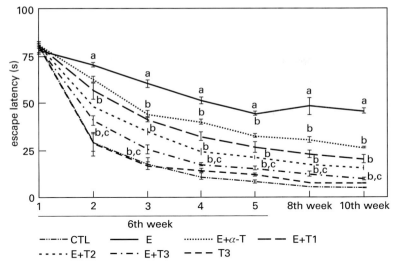

Fig. 11.10: Effect of α-tocopherol and tocotrienol treatment on escape latency in Morris water maze in ethanol-administered rats. (a) Different from control group ($p < 0.05$); (b) different from ethanol-administered group ($p < 0.05$); (c) different from one another ($p < 0.05$). CTL, control; E, ethanol (10 g/kg); α-T, tocopherol (100 mg/kg); T1, tocotrienol (50 mg/kg); T2, tocotrienol (100 mg/kg); T3, tocotrienol (200 mg/kg); (adapted from Tiwari et al., 2009b).

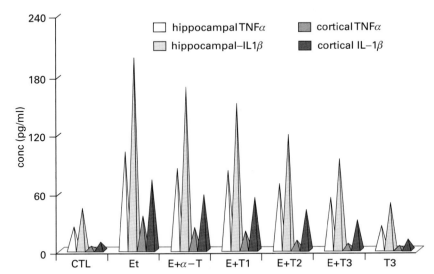

Fig. 11.11: Effect of α-tocopherol and tocotrienol treatment on hippocampal and cortical TNF-α and IL-1β levels in ethanol-administered rats. CTL, control; E, ethanol (10 g/kg); α-T, tocopherol (100 mg/kg); T1, tocotrienol (50 mg/kg); T2, tocotrienol (100 mg/kg); T3, tocotrienol (200 mg/kg); (adapted from Tiwari et al., 2009b).

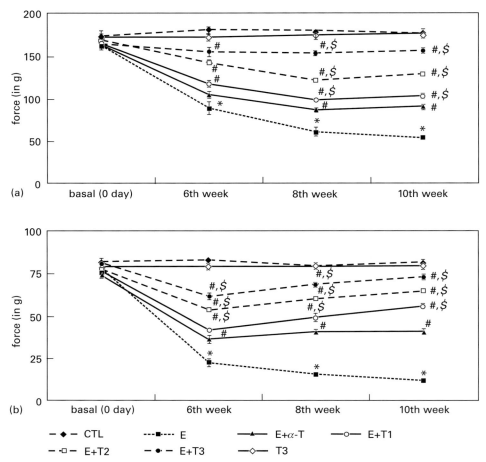

Fig. 11.12: (A) Effect of chronic treatment with α-tocopherol and tocotrienol on mechanical hyperalgesia in Randall-Sellito test. (*) Different from control group (p < 0.05); (#) different from ethanol-administered group (p < 0.05); ($) different from one another (p < 0.05). CTL, control; E, ethanol (10 g/kg), α-T, tocopherol (100 mg/kg); T1, tocotrienol (50 mg/kg); T2, tocotrienol (100 mg/kg); T3, tocotrienol (200 mg/kg); (adapted from Tiwari et al., 2009c). (B) Effect of chronic treatment with α-tocopherol and tocotrienol mechanical allodynia in von-Frey hair test. (*) Different from control group (p < 0.05); (#) different from ethanol-administered group (p < 0.05); ($) different from one another (p < 0.05). CTL, control; E, ethanol (10 g/kg); α-T, tocopherol (100 mg/kg); T1, tocotrienol (50 mg/kg); T2, tocotrienol (100 mg/kg); T3, tocotrienol (200 mg/kg); (adapted from Tiwari et al., 2009c).

latency (thermal hyperalgesia) and decreased paw-withdrawal threshold in the Randall-Sellito test (mechanical hyperalgesia, ▶Fig. 11.12A) and von-Frey hair test (mechanical allodynia, ▶Fig. 11.12B) along with the reduction in nerve glutathione and superoxide dismutase levels. TNF-α and IL-1β levels were also significantly increased in both serum and sciatic nerves of ethanol-treated rats (▶Fig. 11.13). Treatment with α-tocopherol and tocotrienol for 10 weeks significantly improved all the above-stated functional and

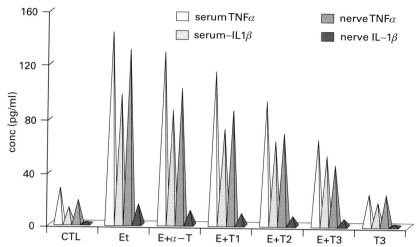

Fig. 11.13: Effect of α-tocopherol and tocotrienol treatment on serum and nerve TNF-α and IL-1β levels in ethanol-administered rats. CTL, control; E, ethanol (10 g/kg), α-T, tocopherol (100 mg/kg); T1, tocotrienol (50 mg/kg); T2, tocotrienol (100 mg/kg); T3, tocotrienol (200 mg/kg); (adapted from Tiwari et al., 2009c).

biochemical deficits in a dose-dependent manner with more potent effects observed with tocotrienol (Tiwari et al., 2009c).

11.3.5.4 Tardive dyskinesia

In a study of 128 schizophrenia patients, McCreadie et al. (1995) measured plasma lipid peroxide, a by-product of free radical damage to lipids, and serum vitamin E levels in patients with and without tardive dyskinesia (TD) and in normal controls. They reported that patients with schizophrenia have a higher level of lipid peroxide and lower serum vitamin E levels than normal subjects. In another study, by Lohr et al. (1987), 15 patients with persistent TD of relatively short duration were treated with a total of 1200 IU/day of vitamin E for 6 weeks in a double-blind, placebo-controlled fashion. There was significant improvement in TD following vitamin E treatment, with a mean reduction in movements of 43%. Seven patients improved more than 50%. This finding was replicated by Elkashef et al. (1990) in another placebo controlled, double-blind study of eight patients with TD. Patients showed significant improvement after receiving 1200 IU/day of vitamin E for 4 weeks compared with placebo. Of a total of 11 published studies investigating the effect of vitamin E on TD, seven reported significantly positive effects, three were negative, and one lent support to the idea that a subgroup of patients with TD, specifically those with mild TD of relatively short duration, could benefit from vitamin E.

11.3.5.5 Amylotropic lateral sclerosis

In amylotropic lateral sclerosis (ALS) patients, vitamin E and Riluzole had no effect on the rate of motor function deterioration and survival versus patients supplemented with placebo and Riluzole (Desnuelle et al., 2001). Another ALS clinical study found that a high dose of vitamin E plus Riluzole showed a trend for a lower vital capacity versus placebo-supplemented patients, despite less patients on vitamin E requiring intermittent assisted ventilation (Graf et al., 2005). Despite these negative results, one epidemiological study analyzing individuals who regularly consume vitamin E showed that habitual use was associated with a lower risk of ALS (Ascherio et al., 2005).

11.3.5.6 Parkinsonism

Antioxidant trials have achieved variable success in non-human models of Parkinson's disease. Most studies suggest that vitamin E (defined solely as α-tocopherol) does not protect in the most common animal models of PD including the MPTP model. Very early work by Perry's group found that four different antioxidants (α-tocopherol, β-carotene, N-acetyl cysteine or ascorbic acid) partially protected C57-black mice against the acute neurotoxicity of MPTP (Perry et al., 1985). More sophisticated approaches have been recently designed to compare α- or γ-tocopherol as anti-Parkinsonian agents. Itoh et al. (2006) used α-tocopherol transfer protein (TTP)-knockout mice and found that only γ-tocopherol significantly protected against dopaminergic toxicity. γ-Tocopherol might be able to protect neurons differently from α-tocopherol owing to the inherent ability of the former tocopherol to absorb nitration equivalents in a way that the latter cannot.

11.3.5.7 Huntington's disease

Malonate-induced ROS production and subsequent p38 MAP kinase activation mediates the activation of the pro-apoptotic Bax protein to induce mitochondrial membrane permeabilization, neuronal apoptosis and Huntington-like symptoms in rats (Gomez-Lazaro et al., 2007).Treatment with vitamin E diminished ROS production, reduced the activation status of p38 MAP kinase, inhibited Bax translocation, and protected against malonate-induced apoptosis. Peyser et al. (1995) performed a prospective, double-blind, placebo-controlled study of high-dose α-tocopherol on a cohort of 73 HD patients. Vitamin E had no effect on neurologic or psychiatric symptoms, but *post hoc* analysis revealed a significant effect of intervention on neurological symptoms in early stage patients. More recent work suggests that vitamin E plus coenzyme Q10 provides some mitigation of 3-nitro propionic acid-induced striatal energy deficits in aged rats (Kasparova et al., 2006).

11.3.5.8 Cerebral ischemia

In an animal model of cerebral ischemia, α-tocopherol scavenges reactive oxygen species and reduces lipid peroxidation and protein oxidation, as evidenced by the decreased levels of malondialdehyde and protein carbonyl following α-tocopherol treatment in ischemia/reperfusion-induced oxidative brain damage (Chaudhary et al., 2003; Jhoo et al., 2004). α-Tocopherol also reduces the infarct volume after middle cerebral artery occlusion in mice (Mishima et al., 2003), and prevents deterioration of the infarct-related neurological functions (e.g., muscle coordination and locomotor activity) in the middle cerebral artery occlusion model of stroke (Chaudhary et al., 2003). In another study by Annaházi et al. (2007), 2 weeks of treatment with α-tocopherol prevents learning deficits, prevents neuronal cell loss, preserves dendritic arborizations and attenuates microglial activation in a rat model of chronic cerebral hypoperfusion.

11.3.5.9 Aging

In a prospective study (Morris et al., 2002) the relation between vitamin E intake (assessed by a food frequency questionnaire) and the rate of cognitive decline in adults aged 65 years and over has been considered. During a 3-year period, a 36% reduction in cognitive decline was observed between those individuals categorized as 'high' compared with 'low' vitamin E consumers. In another recent study, it has been shown that higher cognitive function and a slower rate of cognitive decline were associated with vitamin E intake in older adults (aged 65 years or over) during a 7-year period (Wengreen et al., 2007). Recently, Takatsu et al., (2009) showed that vitamin E-supplementation to aged rats resulted in marked retention of their maximum memory function suggesting neuroprotective potential of vitamin E in aging-associated cognitive decline.

11.3.6 Future implications and conclusions

Vitamin E represents one of the most fascinating natural resources that have the potential to influence a broad range of mechanisms underlying human health and disease. Vitamin E is essential for normal neurological function. The crucial significance of vitamin E in neurological health and disease was recognized several decades ago. Since then, vitamin E research has developed in a highly asymmetric fashion, with emphasis on α-tocopherol in particular, and with the least studied natural vitamin E being the tocotrienols. Tocotrienols are naturally occurring and are routinely consumed by humans with no documented adverse effects. However, in the recent past, evidence has started building up regarding potent neuroprotective properties of tocotrienol. As a general trend, nutrients are required at high micromolar or millimolar levels to influence biological responses. The neuroprotective ability of 100 nM (1/10th of the concentration achieved in the plasma of humans receiving supplement) tocotrienol could be viewed as the most potent of all properties of vitamin E characterized so far.

   The current state of knowledge warrants strategic investment into the lesser known forms of vitamin E with emphasis on uncovering the specific conditions that govern the function of vitamin E molecules *in vivo*. Outcomes studies designed in light of such information would yield lucrative returns.

References

Adachi H, Ishii N, Effects of tocotrienols on life span and protein carbonylation in *Caenorhabditis elegans*. J Gerontol A Biol Sci Med Sci 2000;55: B280–5.

Alexandrova ML, Bochev PG, Markova VI, Bechev BG, Popova MA, Danovska MP, Simeonova VK, Oxidative stress in the chronic phase after stroke. Redox Rep 2003;8: 169–76.

Annaházi A, Mracskó E, Süle Z, Karg E, Penke B, Bari F, Farkas E, Pre-treatment and post-treatment with alpha-tocopherol attenuates hippocampal neuronal damage in experimental cerebral hypoperfusion. Eur J Pharmacol 2007;571: 120–8.

Ascherio A, Weisskopf MG, O'Reilly EJ, Jacobs EJ, McCullough ML, Calle EE, Cudkowicz M, Thun MJ, Vitamin E intake and risk of amyotrophic lateral sclerosis. Ann Neurol 2005;57: 104–10.

Azzi A, Stocker A, Vitamin E: non-antioxidant roles. Prog Lipid Res 2000;39: 231–55.

Azzi A, Boscoboinik D, Marilley D, Ozer NK, Stäuble B, Tasinato A, Vitamin E: a sensor and an information transducer of the cell oxidation state. Am J Clin Nutr 1995;62(6 Suppl): 1337S–46S.

Bogdanov MB, Ramos LE, Xu Z, Beal MF, Elevated 'hydroxyl radical' generation in vivo in an animal model of amyotrophic lateral sclerosis. J Neurochem 1998;71: 1321–34.

Boscoboinik D, Szewczyk A, Hensey C, Azzi A, Inhibition of cell proliferation by α-tocopherol. Role of protein kinase. J Biol Chem 1991;266: 6188–94.

Boscoboinik DO, Chatelain E, Bartoli GM, Stäuble B, Azzi A, Inhibition of protein kinase C activity and vascular smooth muscle cell growth by d-alpha-tocopherol. Biochim Biophys Acta 1994;1224: 418–26.

Brands AM, Kessels RP, de Haan EH, Kappelle LJ, Biessels GJ, Cerebral dysfunction in type 1 diabetes: effects of insulin, vascular risk factors and blood-glucose levels. Eur J Pharmacol 2004;490: 159–68.

Brownlee M, Biochemistry and molecular cell biology of diabetic complications. Nature 2001;414: 813–20.

Bruijn LI, Miller TM, Cleveland DW, Unraveling the mechanisms involved in motor neuron degeneration in ALS. Annu Rev Neurosci 2004;27: 723–49.

Cadet JL, Lohr JB, Possible involvement of free radicals in neuroleptic-induced movement disorders: Evidence from treatment of tardive dyskinesia with vitamin E. Ann N Y Acad Sci 1989;570: 176–85.

Chaudhary G, Sinha K, Gupta YK, Protective effect of exogenous administration of alpha-tocopherol in middle cerebral artery occlusion model of cerebral ischemia in rats. Fundam Clin Pharmacol 2003;17: 703–7.

Collins MA, Zou JY, Neafsey EJ, Brain damage due to episodic alcohol exposure in vivo and in vitro: furosemide neuroprotection implicates edema-based mechanism. FASEB J 1998;12: 221–30.

Crews F, Nixon K, Kim D, Joseph J, Shukitt-Hale B, Qin L, Zou J, BHT blocks NF-kB activation and ethanol-induced brain damage. Alcohol Clin Exp Res 2006;30: 1938–49.

Crews FT, Collins MA, Dlugos C, Littleton J, Wilkins L, Neafsey EJ, Pentney R, Snell LD, Tabakoff B, Zou J, Noronha A, Alcohol induced neurodegeneration: when, where and why? Alcohol Clin Exp Res 2004;28: 350–64.

Dauer W, Przedborski S, Parkinson's disease: mechanisms and models. Neuron 2003;39: 889–909.

Desnuelle C, Dib M, Garrel C, Favier A, A double-blind, placebo-controlled randomized clinical trial of alpha-tocopherol (vitamin E) in the treatment of amyotrophic lateral sclerosis. ALS riluzole-tocopherol Study Group. Amyotroph Lateral Scler Other Motor Neuron Disord 2001;2: 9–18.

Diamond P, McGinty A, Sugrue D, Brady HR, Godson C, Regulation of leukocyte trafficking by lipoxins. Clin Chem Lab Med 1999;37, 293–7.

Elkashef AM, Ruskin PE, Bacher N, Barrett D, Vitamin E in the treatment of tardive dyskinesia. Am J Psychiatry 1990;147: 505–6.

Farooqui AA, Horrocks LA, Farooqui T, Modulation of inflammation in brain: a matter of fat. J Neurochem 2007;101, 577–99.

Gomez-Lazaro M, Galindo MF, Melero-Fernandez de Mera RM, Fernandez-Gómez FJ, Concannon CG, Segura MF, Comella JX, Prehn JH, Jordan J, Reactive oxygen species and p38 mitogen-activated protein kinase activate Bax to induce mitochondrial cytochrome c release and apoptosis in response to malonate. Mol Pharmacol 2007;71: 736–43.

Gonzalez de Aguilar JL, Echaniz-Laguna A, Fergani A, René F, Meininger V, Loeffler JP, Dupuis L, Amyotrophic lateral sclerosis: all roads lead to Rome. J Neurochem 2007;101: 1153–60.

Graf M, Ecker D, Horowski R, Kramer B, Riederer P, Gerlach M, Hager C, Ludolph AC, Becker G, Osterhage J, Jost WH, Schrank B, Stein C, Kostopulos P, Lubik S, Wekwerth K, Dengler R, Troeger M, Wuerz A, Hoge A, Schrader C, Schimke N, Krampfl K, Petri S, Zierz S, Eger K, Neudecker S, Traufeller K, Sievert M, Neundörfer B, Hecht M; German vitamin E/ALS Study Group, High dose vitamin E therapy in amyotrophic lateral sclerosis as add-on therapy to riluzole: results of a placebo-controlled double-blind study. J Neural Transm 2005;112: 649–60.

Hald A, Lotharius J, Oxidative stress and inflammation in Parkinson's disease: is there a causal link? Exp Neurol 2005;193: 279–90.

Harman D, Free radical involvement in aging. Pathophysiology and therapeutic implications. Drugs Aging 1993;3: 60–80.

Hensley K, Benaksas EJ, Bolli R, Comp P, Grammas P, Hamdheydari L, Mou S, Pye QN, Stoddard MF, Wallis G, Williamson KS, West M, Wechter WJ, Floyd RA, New perspectives on vitamin E: gammatocopherol and carboxyelthylhydroxychroman metabolites in biology and medicine. Free Radic Biol Med 2004;36: 1–15.

Hensley K, Mhatre M, Mou S, Pye QN, Stewart C, West M, Williamson KS, On the relation of oxidative stress to neuroinflammation: lessons learned from the G93ASOD1 mouse model of amyotrophic lateral sclerosis. Antioxid Redox Signal 2006;8: 2075–87.

Higgins CM, Jung C, Xu Z, ALS-associated mutant SOD1G93A causes mitochondrial vacuolation by expansion of the intermembrane space and by involvement of SOD1 aggregation and peroxisomes. BMC Neurosci 2003;4: 16.

Itoh N, Masuo Y, Yoshida Y, Cynshi O, Jishage K, Niki E, gamma-Tocopherol attenuates MPTP induced dopamine loss more efficiently than alpha-tocopherol in mouse brain. Neurosci Lett 2006;403: 136–40.

Jhoo JH, Kim HC, Nabeshima T, Yamada K, Shin EJ, Jhoo WK, Kim W, Kang KS, Jo SA, Woo JI, Beta-amyloid (1-42)-induced learning and memory deficits in mice: involvement of oxidative burdens in the hippocampus and cerebral cortex. Behav Brain Res 2004;155: 185–96.

Kamat JP, Devasagayam TP, Tocotrienols from palm oil as potent inhibitors of lipid peroxidation and protein oxidation in rat brain mitochondria. Neurosci Lett 1995;195: 179–82.

Kasparova S, Sumbalova Z, Bystricky P, Kucharska J, Liptaj T, Mlynarik V, Gvozdjakova A, Effect of coenzyme Q10 and vitamin E on brain energy metabolism in the animal model of Huntington's disease. Neurochem Int 2006;48: 93–9.

Khanna S, Roy S, Ryu H, Bahadduri P, Swaan PW, Ratan RR, Sen CK, Molecular basis of vitamin E action: tocotrienol modulates 12-lipoxygenase, a key mediator of glutamate-induced neurodegeneration. J Biol Chem 2003;278: 43508–15.

Kuhad A, Bishnoi M, Tiwari V, Chopra K, Suppression of NF-κβ signaling pathway by tocotrienol can prevent diabetes associated cognitive deficits. Pharmacol Biochem Behav 2009;92: 251–9.

Kuhad A, Chopra K, Tocotrienol attenuates oxidative–nitrosative stress and inflammatory cascade in experimental model of diabetic neuropathy. Neuropharmacology 2009;57: 456–62.

Kutala VK, Khan M, Angelos MG, Kuppusamy P, Role of oxygen in postischemic myocardial injury. Antioxid Redox Signal 2007;9: 1193–206.

Lannert H, Hoyer S, Intracerebroventricular administration of streptozotocin causes long-term diminutions in learning and memory abilities and in cerebral energy metabolism in adult rats. Behav Neurosci 1998;112: 1199–208.

Lobnig BM, Kromeke O, Optenhostert-Porst C, Wolf OT, Hippocampal volume and cognitive performance in long-standing Type 1 diabetic patients without macrovascular complications. Diabetic Med 2005;23: 32–9.

Lohr JB, Cadet JI, Lohr MA, Jeste DV, Wyatt RJ, Alpha-tocopherol in tardive dyskinesia. Lancet 1987;1: 913–4.

Mansouri A, Demeilliers C, Amsellem S, Pessayre D, Fromenty B, Acute ethanol administration oxidatively damages and depletes mitochondrial DNA in mouse liver, brain, heart, and skeletal muscles: protective effects of antioxidants. J Pharmacol Exp Ther 2001;298: 737–43.

Mantle D, Preedy VR, Free radicals as mediators of alcohol toxicity. Adverse Drug React Toxicol Rev 1999;18: 235–52.

Margaill I, Plotkine M, Lerouet D, Antioxidant strategies in the treatment of stroke. Free Radic Biol Med 2005;39: 429–43.

Markesbery WR, Lovell MA, Four-hydroxynonenal, a product of lipid peroxidation, is increased in the brain in Alzheimer's disease. Neurobiol Aging 1998;19: 33–6.

McCreadie RG, MacDonald E, Wiles D, Campbell G, Paterson JR, The Nithsdale scizophrenia surveys. XIV: Plasma lipid peroxide and serum vitamin E levels in patients with and without tardive dyskinesia, and in normal subjects. Br J Psychiatry 1995;167: 610–7.

McDonough KH, Antioxidant nutrients and alcohol. Toxicology 2003;189: 89–97.

Mishima K, Tanaka T, Pu F, Egashira N, Iwasaki K, Hidaka R, Matsunaga K, Takata J, Karube Y, Fujiwara M, Vitamin E isoforms alpha-tocotrienol and gamma-tocopherol prevent cerebral infarction in mice. Neurosci Lett 2003;337: 56–60.

Monforte R, Estruch R, Valls-Sole J, Nicolas J, Villalta J, Urbano-Marquez A, Autonomic and peripheral neuropathies in patients with chronic alcoholism. A dose-related toxic effect of alcohol. Arch Neurol 1995;52: 45–51.

Morris MC, Evans DA, Bienias JL, Tangney CC, Wilson RS, Vitamin E and cognitive decline in older persons. Arch Neurol 2002;59: 1125–32.

Moses GS, Jensen MD, Lue LF, Walker DG, Sun AY, Simonyi A, Sun GY, Secretory PLA2-IIA: a new inflammatory factor for Alzheimer's disease. J Neuroinflammation 2006;3: 28.

Muller DP, Goss-Sampson MA, Neurochemical, neurophysiological, and neuropathological studies in vitamin E deficiency. Crit Rev Neurobiol 1990;5: 239–63.

O'Byrne D, Grundy S, Packer L, Devaraj S, Baldenius K, Hoppe PP, Kraemer K, Jialal I, Traber MG, Studies of LDL oxidation following alpha-, gamma-, or delta-tocotrienyl acetate supplementation of hypercholesterolemic humans. Free Radic Biol Med 2000;29: 834–45.

Osakada F, Hashino A, Kume T, Katsuki H, Kaneko S, Akaike A, Alpha-tocotrienol provides the most potent neuroprotection among vitamin E analogs on cultured striatal neurons. Neuropharmacology 2004;47: 904–15.

Perry TL, Yong VW, Clavier RM, Jones K, Wright JM, Foulks JG, Wall RA, Partial protection from the dopaminergic neurotoxin N-methyl-4-phenyl-1,2,3,6-tetrahydropyridine by four different antioxidants in the mouse. Neurosci Lett 1985;60: 109–14.

Peyser CE, Folstein M, Chase GA, Starkstein S, Brandt J, Cockrell JR, Bylsma F, Coyle JT, McHugh PR, Folstein SE, Trial of d-alpha-tocopherol in Huntington's disease. Am J Psychiatry 1995;152: 1771–5.

Pfefferbaum A, Sullivan EV, Rosenbloom MJ, Mathalon DH, Lim KO, A controlled study of cortical gray matter and ventricular changes in alcoholic men over a 5-year interval. Arch Gen Psychiatry 1998;55: 905–12.

Pop-Busui R, Sima A, Stevens M, Diabetic neuropathy and oxidative stress. Diabetes Metab Res Rev 2006;22: 257–73.

Qureshi AA, Burger WC, Peterson DM, Elson CE, The structure of an inhibitor of cholesterol biosynthesis isolated from barley. J Biol Chem 1986;261: 10544–50.

Qureshi AA, Sami SA, Salser WA, Khan FA, Dose-dependent suppression of serum cholesterol by tocotrienol-rich fraction (TRF25) of rice bran in hypercholesterolemic humans. Atherosclerosis 2002;161: 199–207.

Roy S, Lado BH, Khanna S, Sen CK, Vitamin E sensitive genes in the developing rat fetal brain: a high density oligonucleotide microarray analysis. FEBS Lett 2002;530: 17–23.

Ryan CM, Geckle MO, Orchard TJ, Cognitive efficiency declines over time in adults with type 1 diabetes: effects of micro-and macrovascular complications. Diabetologia 2003;46: 940–8.

Sathasivam S, Shaw PJ, Apoptosis in amyotrophic lateral sclerosis – what is the evidence? Lancet Neurol 2005;4: 500–9.

Satoh J, Yagihashi S, Toyota T, The possible role of tumor necrosis factor-alpha in diabetic polyneuropathy. Exp Diabesity Res 2003;4: 65–71.

Sen CK, Khanna S, Roy S, Packer L, Molecular basis of vitamin E action. Tocotrienol potently inhibits glutamate-induced pp60(c-Src) kinase activation and death of HT4 neuronal cells. J Biol Chem 2000;275: 13049–55.

Sen CK, Khanna S, Roy S, Tocotrienols: Vitamin E beyond tocopherols. Life Sci 2006;78: 2088–98.

Sharma S, Stutzman JD, Kelloff GJ, Steele VE, Screening of potential chemopreventive agents using biochemical markers of carcinogenesis. Cancer Res 1994;54: 5848–55.

its biological onset or against dementia risk factors, whereas secondary prevention refers to the early detection of asymptomatic disease with associated opportunities for intervention before symptoms are evident. However, the US Preventive Services Task Force suggests there is insufficient evidence to support instituting a universal dementia screening program (US Preventive Services Task Force, 2003). Syndromes of cognitive impairment in non-demented older adults have been the focus of studies aiming to identify subjects at high risk to develop dementia. Mild cognitive impairment (MCI) is characterized by isolated memory deficits in non-demented persons with subjective memory problems, normal general cognitive functioning, and intact activities of daily living (Burns and Morris, 2008). MCI has been estimated to affect 10–17% of the elderly population (Burns and Morris, 2008).

The attempts of identifying MCI subjects have the main aim of allowing the earliest symptomatic stages of dementia to be better recognized and treated. In the attempt of avoiding dementia development, there are several risk factors to be taken into account, some of which are non-modifiable and include age with age-influencing early-life deleterious conditions, gender and genetic influence. As mentioned before, a great deal of attention is being dedicated to the identification and modulation of those factors which have a large potential to be managed before the onset or during the early asymptomatic course of the disease. These include vascular and lifestyle factors. Among vascular risk factors, considerable evidence from randomized controlled trials and longitudinal cohort studies has established the relation between hypertension and dementia as well as between hyperlipidemia and dementia. Both systolic hypertension above 160 mmHg and serum cholesterol above 6.5 mmol/l (240 mg/dl) are known to be associated with an increased RR of 1.5 and 2.1 to develop AD (Patterson et al., 2008). Based on the recommendations of the Third Canadian Consensus Conference on Diagnosis and Treatment of Dementia held in March 2006 (Patterson et al., 2008), statin therapy, acetylsalicylic acid and carotid artery stenosis reopening on a first level of evidence and control of type 2 diabetes mellitus, hyperlipidemia and hyperhomocysteinemia on a second level of evidence should not be recommended with the single specific purpose of reducing the risk of dementia.

As far as the modulation of lifestyle factors against dementia onset and progression is concerned, the research efforts of the past recent years have been based mainly upon the consistent observation and the strong epidemiologic evidence that a poor diet and physical inactivity are among the leading causes of death for Americans (Mangialasche et al., 2009). Diet plays a crucial role in prevention of age-related chronic diseases including dementia, and its determinant influence is mediated by bioactive compounds such as antioxidants mostly contained in fruits and vegetables.

11.4.6.2 Antioxidant vitamins, cognition and dementia

Oxidative stress, which occurs owing to an imbalance between oxidants and antioxidants and causes loss of function in oxidized biomolecules (Sies and Cadenas, 1985), is well documented as a pathogenic factor in neurodegenerative disorders with dementia and AD in particular. Indeed, several biomarkers of oxidative damage against proteins, lipids and DNA have been found in AD brains and peripheral tissues in elevated levels (Guérin et al., 2005). Independently of the cause of oxidative stress in AD, however, several antioxidant strategies have been tried in the past recent decades to assess the potentially beneficial effects against AD development or progression. A huge amount of epidemiological evidence derives in first instance from natural nutrition studies, because decreased food intakes, eating behavior disturbances and loss of body weight are particularly significant problems among patients with AD and as because malnutrition has been shown to be associated with a more rapid AD worsening of AD (Anlasik et al., 2005). Fruits and vegetables are thought to represent the best source of antioxidant micronutrients owing to synergisms of their components, because they might allow a better bioavailability of protective compounds than single vitamins, and owing to their low content in saturated fats. The effects of dietary counseling on fruit and vegetable intake as well as of improved fruit and vegetable intake on the levels of circulating antioxidants, biomarkers of oxidative stress and cognitive performance in healthy subjects are positive and beneficial (Shatenstein et al., 2008; Polidori et al., 2009). This suggests that a nutritional counseling program can lead to an improvement of cognition and plasma antioxidant status even in healthy populations.

In patients with a typical age-related disease such as AD, showing increased circulating levels of biomarkers of oxidative stress, a targeted nutritional intervention aimed at increasing plasma antioxidant levels and at decreasing the ongoing condition of oxidative stress might prove beneficial in addition to standard therapeutic options. To follow the natural evolution of dietary and nutrition status among elderly community-dwelling adults with AD, Shatenstein et al. prospectively studied 36 community-dwelling patients in early stages of AD and 58 age-matched cognitively intact community-based controls over an 18-month period (Morris et al., 2006). In this study, nutrient intakes from diet and supplements were higher in control subjects, with significant differences in energy, the micronutrients calcium, iron, zinc, vitamin K, vitamin A, and dietary fiber as well as n-3 and n-6 fatty acids (Morris et al., 2006). The authors suggested that suboptimal micronutrient status is an early feature during disease development and that AD patients would benefit from systematic dietary assessment and intervention to prevent further deterioration in food consumption and increased nutritional risk.

In a prospective cohort study of over 3700 older participants of the Chicago Health and Age Project, high vegetable consumption was associated with a slower rate of cognitive decline over 6 years after adjusting for age, gender, race, education, cardiovascular-related conditions and risk factors (Scarmeas et al., 2006). In this study the consumption of green leafy vegetables, rich in antioxidant micronutrients, showed the strongest inverse linear association with the rate of cognitive decline. The specific protection shown by vegetables and particularly by the green leafy ones appears to be in disagreement with the concept that fruit and vegetable consumption might be beneficial in the frame of a generally healthy lifestyle, as health-conscious individuals tend to consume both fruits and vegetables.

Healthy diet in general and the Mediterranean regimen in particular have been recently shown to affect risk for and mortality from AD (Scarmeas et al., 2006; Barberger-Gateau et al., 2007; Scarmeas et al., 2007; Burgener et al., 2008). The existing evidence does not support the recommendation of specific supplements, foods, or diets for the prevention of AD. However, a review of 34 studies in the areas of dietary restriction, antioxidants and Mediterranean diet provided evidence that nutritional interventions against dementia and AD have a great potential of influencing dementia development (Serra-Majem et al., 2009).

11.4.6.3 Vitamin E and AD

Most recently, the association between a higher quintile of adherence to a Mediterranean dietary pattern and a lower inadequacy for the intake of vitamin E among other micronutrients was shown (Galbusera et al., 2004). Vitamin E, which is known to reach therapeutic levels in the brain of AD patients, has been shown to decrease lipid peroxidation susceptibility by 60% in AD patients as compared with controls (Morris et al., 2005). Most of the studies on vitamin E have focused so far on α-tocopherol levels, both in its absolute levels and as the ratio of the serum tocopherol concentration to the sum of the serum concentrations of cholesterol and triglycerides. However, the contribution of γ-tocopherol as a source of antioxidant activity needs to be considered further. The richest sources of vitamin E in many diets are vegetable oils such as soybean oil and corn oil which interestingly contain more γ-tocopherol than α-tocopherol, but the biological activity of γ-tocopherol is only 15% of that of *all-rac*-α-tocopheryl acetate. None of the commercial preparations contain γ-tocopherol, despite animal studies have shown that giving α-tocopherol to rats increases the γ-tocopherol forebrain content, and despite several tocopherol forms ingested with food rather than α-tocopherol alone have been suggested to be important in the vitamin E protective association with AD (Hill, 1971; Ravaglia et al., 2008).

Based upon the hypothesis that if vitamin E enhances neuronal survival there would be a positive relation between serum concentrations and cognitive function, vitamin E plasma levels have been measured in several recent human studies, and a vitamin E deficiency has been consistently found in patients with AD and MCI. Five causal criteria have been established to evaluate the strength of evidence linking the availability of a micronutrient to cognitive or behavioral function which include: (1) a plausible biological rationale, (2) a consistent association, (3) specificity of cause and effect, (4) a dose-response relation and (5) the ability to experimentally manipulate the effect (McCann and Ames, 2005). These criteria have been already evaluated for docosahexaenoic acid (McCann et al., 2006), choline (McCann and Ames, 2008) and vitamin D (Martin et al., 1999), and, as far as vitamin E is concerned, it appears that those criteria most convincingly satisfied are the biological rationale and the associations between vitamin E intake/levels found so far (Sano et al., 1977; Grundman, 2000; Masaki et al., 2000; Martin et al., 2002; Morris et al., 2002; Grodstein et al., 2003; Helmer et al., 2003; Zandi et al., 2004; Cherubini et al., 2005).

On the basis of the biological rationale, a seminal multicenter clinical trial from Sano et al. in 1997 showed that AD patients randomly assigned to receive α-tocopherol (2000 IU/day) had a slow functional decline; despite this, it was also found to be true for the patients assigned to receive selegiline or selegiline plus vitamin E and no effect of any treatment was seen at cognitive tests (Isaac et al., 2008). Further trials of vitamin E supplementation have demonstrated no major benefit against cognitive impairment or the progression to AD in MCI subjects (Isaac et al., 2008; Mecocci et al., 2008; Mangialasche et al., 2010). There are several reasons explaining this discrepancy. One key point for it is the largely unexplored relation between intake of fruits and vegetables, antioxidant micronutrient status, a condition of oxidative stress and cognitive performance in healthy subjects. There are, however, some hints of biological interactions between these components after evaluation of independent measurements in healthy subjects, and it is also probable that when the clinical symptoms of AD appear a large proportion of neuronal cells might already be destroyed and therefore the intervention with vitamin E, particularly when a single form is used instead of a network, could come too late.

In randomized controlled trials usually high doses of α-tocopherol have been used, whereas a balanced intake of different vitamin E congeners can be more effective in terms of neuroprotection. Indeed, epidemiological evidence suggests that the protective effect of vitamin E against AD can be owing to the contribution of its different forms (Ravaglia et al., 2008; Gutierrez et al., 2009), whereas intake of high doses of α-tocopherol can decrease the bioavailability of the other congeners (Khanna et al., 2005; Bjelakovic et al., 2007), and it has been related to increased mortality risk (Bjelakovic et al., 2007). More information are needed to clarify the biological effects and interactions of all vitamin E family members in humans, to better refine their potential therapeutic effects in preventing cognitive decline and dementia in older adults.

11.4.7 Conclusions and future directions

It has been almost a century since the discovery of vitamin E, but its functional role(s) remain not fully elucidated. However, during these years the isolation and identification of the various types of tocopherols and tocotrienols, their chemical synthesis and availability has helped enormously the field in establishing some of the biological effects for each of them. All the available evidence accumulated so far supports a primary role as antioxidant, but new roles have also emerged: modulator of specific signaling pathways and genes involved in metabolic, inflammatory events.

Most of the human observational epidemiological studies are, in general, consistent with the hypothesis that there is an inverse correlation between vitamin E levels and intake, cognitive function and ultimately the risk to develop AD. By contrast, randomized clinical trials with vitamin E do not fully support this evidence. However, a closer look to these studies reveals their inconclusive nature owing to several old and more recent unresolved issues, some of which are related to the complex biochemistry of this vitamin.

In general, within the human body vitamin E levels are under tight control, with mainly α-tocopherol and, to a lesser extent, γ-tocopherol retained and delivered to different tissues. However, it is now more and more evident that other forms of vitamin E, which are typically not found in significant concentrations, are involved in some biological effects different from those of α-tocopherol such as apoptosis and cell death. Considering these novel aspects of vitamin E biochemistry, and the significant differences in metabolism and biological properties of the individual congeners, it should not be surprising that many of the clinical studies, both epidemiological and interventional, which did not take into consideration those aspects are inconclusive. More research aimed at defining the uses and the dosage of different tocopherols and tocotrienols in prospective interventional studies is warranted before a final conclusion can be reached.

References

Anlasik T, Sies H, Griffiths HR, Mecocci P, Stahl W, Polidori MC, Dietary habits are major determinants of the plasma antioxidant status in healthy elderly subjects. Br J Nutr 2005;94: 639–42.

Azzi A, Aratri E, Boscoboinik D, Clement S, Ozer NK, Ricciarelli R, Spycher S, Molecular basis of α-tocopherol control of smooth muscle cell proliferation. Biofactors 1998;7: 3–14.

Barberger-Gateau P, Raffaitin C, Letenneur L, Berr C, Tzourio C, Dartigues JF, Alperovitch A, Dietary patterns and risk of dementia. Neurology 2007;69: 1921–30.

Berr C, Wancata J, Ritchie K, Prevalence of dementia in the elderly in Europe. Eur Neuropsychopharm 15: 463–471, 2005.

Bjelakovic G, Nikolova D, Gluud LL, Simonetti RG, Gluud C, Mortality in randomized trials of antioxidant supplements for primary and secondary prevention: systematic review and meta-analysis. J Am Med Assoc 2007;297: 842–57.

Brigelius-Flohé R, Vitamin E: the shrew waiting to be tamed. Free Radic Biol Med 2009;46: 543–54.

Brigelius-Flohé R, Traber MG, Vitamin E: function and metabolism. FASEB J 1999;13: 1145–55.

Burgener SC, Buettner L, Coen Buckwalter K, Beattie E, Bossen AL, Fick DM, Fitzsimmons S, Kolanowski A, Richeson NE, Rose K, Schreiner A, Pringle Specht JK, Testad I, Yu F, McKenzie S, Evidence supporting nutritional interventions for persons in early stage Alzheimer's disease. J Nutr Health Aging 2008;12: 18–21.

Burns JM, Morris JC, Mild cognitive impairment and early Alzheimer's disease. Chichester: Wiley; 2008.

Burton GW, Traber MG, Vitamin E: antioxidant activity, biokinetics, and bioavailability. Annu Rev Nutr 1990;10: 357–82.

Cherubini A, Martin A, Andres-Lacueva C, Di Iorio A, Lamponi M, Mecocci P, Bartali B, Corsi A, Senin U, Ferrucci L, Vitamin E levels, cognitive impairment and dementia in older persons: the In CHIANTI Study. Neurobiol Aging 2005;26: 987–94.

Corrada MM, Brookmeyer R, Berlau D, Paganini-Hill A, Kawas CH, Prevalence of dementia after age 90: results from The 90+ Study. Neurology 2008;71: 337–43.

Drachman DA, If we live long enough, will we all be demented? Neurology 2004;44: 1563–5.

Essink-Bot ML, Periera J, Packer C, Schwarzinger M, Burstrom K, Cross-national comparability of burden of disease estimates: the European Disability Weights Project. Bull World Health Org 2002;80: 644–52.

Evans HM, Bishop KS, On the existence of a hitherto unrecognized dietary factor essential for reproduction. Science 1922;56: 650–1.

Galbusera C, Facheris M, Magni F, Galimberti G, Sala G, Tremolada L, Isella V, Guerini FR, Apollonio I, Galli-Kienle M, Ferrarese C, Increased susceptibility to plasma lipid peroxidation in Alzheimer disease patients. Curr Alzheimers Res 2004;1: 103–9.

Gavrilov LA, Heuveline P, Aging of population. In: Demeny P, McNicoll G, editors. The encyclopedia of population. New York: Macmillan USA; 2003. pp. 32–7.

Granados H, Dam H, On the histochemical relationship between peroxidation and the yellow-brown pigment in the adipose tissue of vitamin E-deficient rats. Acta Pathol Microbiol Scand 1950;27: 591–8.

Grodstein F, Chen J, Willet WC, High-dose antioxidant supplements and cognitive function in community-dwelling elderly women. Am J Clin Nutr 2003;77: 975–84.

Grundman M, Vitamin E and Alzheimer disease: the basis for additional clinical trials. Am J Clin Nutr 2000;71: S630–66.

Guérin O, Andrieu S, Schneider SM, Milano M, Boulahssass R, Brocker P, Vellas B, Different modes of weight loss in Alzheimer disease: a prospective study of 395 participants. Am J Clin Nutr 2005; 82: 435–41.

Gutierrez AD, de Serna DG, Robinson I, Schade DS, The response of gamma vitamin E to varying dosages of alpha vitamin E plus vitamin C, Metabolism 2009;58: 469–78.

Haan MN, Wallace R, Can dementia be prevented? Brain aging in a population-based context. Annu Rev Public Health 2004;25: 1–24.

Hacquebard M, Carpentier YA, Vitamin E: absorption, plasma transport and cell uptake. Curr Opin Clin Nutr Metab Care 2005;8: 133–8.

Harris PL, Embree ND, Quantitative consideration of the effect of polyunsaturated fatty acid content of the diet upon the requirements for vitamin E. Am J Clin Nutr 1963;13: 385–92.

Helmer C, Peuchant E, Letenneur L, Bourdel-Marchasson I, Larrieu S, Dartigues JF, Dubourg L, Thomas MJ, Barberger-Gateau P, Association between antioxidant nutritional indicators and the incidence of dementia: results from the PAQUID prospective cohort study. Eur J Clin Nutr 2003;57: 1555–61.

Hill A, Principles of medical statistics, 9th ed. New York: Oxford University Press, 1971.

Hogan DB, Bailey P, Black S, Carswell A, Chertkow H, Clarke B, Cohen C, Fisk JD, Forbes D, Man-Son-Hing M, Lanctot K, Morgan D, Thorpe L, Diagnosis and treatment of dementia: 5. Nonpharmacologic and pharmacologic therapy for mild to moderate dementia. Can Med Ass J 2008;179: 1019–26.

Hogan DB, If we live long enough, will we all be demented? Redux Neurol 2008;71: 310–1.

Horiguchi M, Arita M, Kaempf-Rotzoll DE, Tsujimoto M, Inoue K, Arai H, pH-dependent translocation of alpha-tocopherol transfer protein (alpha-TTP) between hepatic cytosol and late endosomes. Genes Cells 2003;8: 789–800.

Isaac MG, Quinn R, Tabet N, Vitamin E for Alzheimer's disease and mild cognitive impairment. Cochrane Database Syst Rev 2008;16: CD002854.

IUPAC-IUB Joint Commission on Biochemical Nomenclature. Nomenclature of tocopherols and related compounds. Recommendations 1982. Eur J Biochem 1982;123: 473–5.

Khanna S, Patel V, Rink C, Roy S, Sen CK, Delivery of orally supplemented alpha-tocotrienol to vital organs of rats and tocopherol-transport protein deficient mice. Free Radic Biol Med 2005;39: 1310–9.

Khanna S, Parinandi NL, Kotha SR, Roy S, Rink C, Bibus D, Sen CK, Nanomolar vitamin E alpha-tocotrienol inhibits glutamate-induced activation of phospholipase A2 and causes neuroprotection. J Neurochem 2010;112: 1249–60.

Kolosova NG, Shcheglova TV, Sergeeva SV, Loskutova LV, Long-term antioxidant supplementation attenuates oxidative stress markers and cognitive deficits in senescent-accelerated OXYS rats. Neurobiol Aging 2006;27: 1289–97.

Mangialasche F, Polidori MC, Monastero R, Ercolani S, Cecchetti R, Mecocci P, Biomarkers of oxidative and nitrosative damage in Alzheimer's disease and mild cognitive impairment. Ageing Res Rev 2009;8: 285–305.

Mangialasche F, Kivipelto M, Mecocci P, Rizzuto D, Palmer K, Winblad B, Fratiglioni L, High plasma levels of vitamin E forms and reduced Alzheimer's disease risk in advanced age. J Alzheimers Dis 2010;20: 1029–37.

Martin A, Janigian D, Shukitt-Hale B, Prior RL, Joseph JA, Effect of vitamin E intake on levels of vitamins E and C in the central nervous system and peripheral tissues: implications for health recommendations. Brain Res 1999;845: 50–9.

Martin A, Youdim K, Szprengiel A, Shukitt-Hale B, Joseph JA, Roles of vitamins C and E on neuro-degenerative diseases and cognitive performance. Nutr Rev 2002;60: 308–34.

Masaki KH, Losonczy KG, Izmirlian G, Folcy DJ, Ross GW, Petrovitch H, Haulik R, White LR, Association of vitamin C and E supplement use with cognitive function and dementia in elderly men. Neurology 2000;54: 1265–72.

McCann JC, Ames BN, Is docosahexaenoic acid, an n-3 long chain polyunsaturated fatty acid, required for the development of normal brain function? An overview of evidence from cognitive and behavioural tests in humans and animals. Am J Clin Nutr 2005;82: 281–95.

McCann JC, Ames BN, Is there convincing biological or behavioural evidence linking vitamin D deficiency to brain dysfunction? FASEB J. 2008;22: 982–1001.

McCann JC, Hudes M, Ames BN, An overview of evidence for a causal relationship between dietary availability of choline during development and cognitive function in offspring. Neurosci Biobehav Rev 2006;30: 697–712.

Mecocci P, Mariani E, Polidori MC, Hensley K, Butterfield DA, Antioxidant agents in Alzheimer's disease. Cent Nerv Syst Agents Med Chem 2008;8: 48–63.

Morris MC, Evans DA, Biennas JL, Tangney CC, Wilson RS, Vitamin E and cognitive decline in older persons. Arch Neurol 2002;59: 1125–32.

Morris MC, Evans DA, Tangney CC, Bienias JL, Wilson RS, Aggarwal NT, Scherr PA, Relation of the tocopherol forms to incident Alzheimer disease and to cognitive change. Am J Clin Nutr 2005;81: 508–14.

Morris MC, Evans DA, Tangney CC, Bienias JL, Wilson RS, Associations of vegetable and fruit consumption with age-related cognitive change. Neurology 2006;67: 1370–6.

Naito Y, Shimozawa M, Kuroda M, Nakabe N, Manabe H, Katada K, Kokura S, Ichikawa H, Yoshida N, Noguchi N, Yoshikawa T, Tocotrienols reduce 25-hydroxycholesterol-induced monocyte-endothelial cell interaction by inhibiting the surface expression of adhesion molecules. Atherosclerosis 2005;180: 19–25.

O'Byrne D, Grundy S, Packer L, Devaraj S, Baldenius K, et al., Studies of LDL oxidation following alpha-, gamma-, or delta-tocotrienyl acetate supplementation of hypercholesterolemic humans. Free Rad Biol Med 2000;29: 834–45.

Patterson C, Feightner GW, Garcia A, Hsiung GYR, MacKnight C, Sadovnick AD, Diagnosis and treatment of dementia: 1. Risk assessment and primary prevention of Alzheimer disease. Can Med Ass J 2008;178: 548–56.

Polidori MC, Carrillo JC, Verde PE, Sies H, Siegrist J, Stahl W, Plasma micronutrient status is improved after a 3-month dietary intervention with 5 daily portions of fruits and vegetables: implications for optimal antioxidant levels. Nutr J 2009;8: 10.

Polidori MC, Praticó D, Mangialasche Mariani E, Aust O, Anlasik T, Mang N, Pientka L, Stahl W, Sies H, Mecocci P, Nelles G, High fruit and vegetable intake, high antioxidant status and good cognitive performance are associated in healthy subjects. J Alzheimers Dis 2009;17: 921–7.

Ravaglia G, Forti P, Lucicesare A, Pisacane N, Rietti E, Mangialasche F, Cecchetti R, Patterson C, Mecocci P, Plasma tocopherols and risk of cognitive impairment in an elderly Italian cohort. Am J Clin Nutr 2008;87: 1306–13.

Reiter E, Jiang Q, Christen S, Anti-inflammatory properties of alpha- and gamma-tocopherol. Mol Aspects Med 2007;28: 668–91.

Rimbach G, Minihane AM, Majewicz J, Fisher A, Pallauf J, Virgili F, Weinberg PD, Regulation of cell signaling by vitamin E. Proc Nutr Soc 2002;61: 415–25.

Roy S, Lado BH, Khanna S, Sen CK, Vitamin E sensitive genes in the developing rat fetal brain: a high–density oligonucleotide microarray analysis. FEBS Lett 2002;530: 17–23.

Sano M, Ernesto C, Thomas RG, Klauber MR, Schafer K, Grundman M, Woodbury P, Growdon J, Cotman CW, Pfeiffer E, Schneider LS, Thal LJ, A controlled trial of selegiline, alpha-tocopherol, or both as treatment for Alzheimer's disease. The Alzheimer's Disease Cooperative Study. N Engl J Med 1977;336: 1216–22.

Scarmeas N, Stern Y, Mayeaux R, Luchsinger GA, Mediterranean diet, Alzheimer disease, and vascular mediation. Arch Neurol 2006;63: 1709–17.

Scarmeas N, Stern Y, Tang MX, Mayeux R, Luchsinger JA, Mediterranean diet and the risk for Alzheimer's disease. Ann Neurol 2006;59: 912–21.

Scarmeas N, Luchsinger JA, Mayeux R, Stern Y, Mediterranean diet and Alzheimer's disease mortality. Neurology 2007;69: 1084–93.

Sen CK, Khanna S, Rink C, Roy S, Tocotrienols: the emerging face of natural vitamin E. Vitam Horm 2007;76: 203–61.

Serra-Majem L, Bes-Rastrollo M, Román-Viñas B, Pfrimer K, Sánchez-Villegas A, Martínez-González MA, Dietary patterns and nutritional adequacy in a Mediterranean country. Br J Nutr 2009;101(Suppl 2): S21–8.

Shatenstein B, Kergoat MJ, Reid I, Chicoine ME, Dietary intervention in older adults with early-stage Alzheimer dementia: early lessons learned. J Nutr Health Aging 2008;12: 461–9.

Sheppard AJ, Pennington JAT, Weihrauch JL, Analysis and distribution of vitamin E in vegetable oils and foods. In: Packer L, Fuchs J, editors. Vitamin E in health and disease. New York: Marcel Dekker, Inc.; 1993. pp. 9–31.

Sies H, Murphy ME, Role of tocopherols in the protection of biological systems against oxidative damage. J Photochem Photobiol 1991;8: 211–8.

Sies H, Cadenas E, Oxidative stress: damage to intact cells and organs. Phil Trans R Soc Lond B Biol Sci 1985;311: 617–31.

Sondergaad E, Dam H, Influence of the level of dietary linoleic acid on the amount of d-alpha-tocopherol acetate required for protection against encephalomalcia. Z Ernahrungswiss 1966;6: 253–8.

Traber MG, Elsner A, Brigelius-Flohé R, Synthetic as compared with natural vitamin E is preferentially excreted as alpha-CEHC in human urine: studies using deuterated alpha-tocopheryl acetates. FEBS Lett 1998;437: 145–8.

Traber MG, Burton GW, Hamilton RL, Vitamin E trafficking. Ann N Y Acad Sci 2005;1031: 1–12.

Traber MG, Atkinson J, Vitamin E, antioxidant and nothing more. Free Radic Biol Med 2007;43: 3–15.

US Preventive Services Task Force. Guide to clinical preventive services, 3rd ed. Periodic updates. Screen for dementia, 2003. Recommendations and rationale and summary of the evidence. www. ahcpr.gov/clinic/uspstf/uspsdeme.htm

Wolf G, The discovery of the antioxidant function of vitamin E: the contribution of Henry A. Matill. J Nutr 2005;135: 363–6.

Yap SP, Yuen KH, Wong JW, Pharmacokinetics and bioavailability of alpha-, gamma-, and delta-tocotrienols under different food status. J Pharm Pharmacol 2001;53: 67–71.

Yeo LH, Horan MA, Jones M, Pendleton N, Perceptions of risk and prevention of dementia in the healthy elderly. Dement Geriatr Cogn Disord 2007;23: 368–71.

Zandi PP, Anthony JC, Khachaturian AS, Stone SV, Gustafson D, Tschanz JT, Norton MC, Welsch-Bohmer KA, Breitner JCS for the Cache County Study Group. Reduced risk of Alzheimer disease in users of antioxidant vitamin supplements. Arch Neurol 2004;61: 82–8.

Zhu X, Lee HG, Perry G, Smith MA, Alzheimer disease, the two-hit hypothesis: an update. Biochim Biophys Acta 2007;1772: 494–502.

Zingg JM, Modulation of signal transduction by vitamin E. Mol Aspects Med 2007;28: 481–506.

Zingg JM, Azzi A, Non antioxidant activities of vitamin E. Curr Med Chem 2004;11: 1113–33.

12 Vitamin K

Vitamins and vitamin-like nutrients for prevention of human diseases

Martin J. Shearer; Renata Gorska; Dominic J. Harrington; Leon J. Schurgers; Paul Newman

12.1 Introduction

At one time regarded as the 'Cinderella' of fat-soluble vitamins, vitamin K has emerged in the past 3 decades from a single-function 'haemostasis vitamin' to a 'multifunction vitamin' and arguably the most fascinating of all of the vitamins. This fascination largely stems from the growing number of vitamin K-dependent (Gla) proteins that have been discovered and found to have a variety of metabolic functions. Allied to this is a growing appreciation that these non-coagulation Gla proteins play important roles in various areas of human health. Importantly, the evidence suggests that, as with the vitamin K-dependent coagulation proteins, the γ-carboxyglutamic acid residues of these proteins are essential for their activity. This means that a deficiency of vitamin K could have multiple health consequences outside of its classical coagulation role. Although the cofactor role through γ-carboxylation of these specialised Gla proteins is central to the mechanism of action of vitamin K, there is also evidence that K vitamins could play a direct role in several cellular pathways. Particularly interesting is the modulation of cellular systems, including gene regulation, by menaquinone-4, a member of the vitamin K2 series that can be uniquely synthesised *in vivo* (from the major dietary form phylloquinone) and which has a distinctive tissue distribution. The role of vitamin K supplementation in human health continues to expand from its well-established use in the prevention of vitamin K deficiency bleeding to modern investigations of the potential benefits to bone and vascular health and even in the treatment of certain cancers. Again, the potential benefits of giving vitamin K compounds to promote health or to prevent age-related disease can be divided into either ensuring optimal γ-carboxylation of extrahepatic Gla-proteins (some of which are known to have higher requirements for vitamin K than hepatic coagulation proteins) or modulating biochemical pathways that do not depend on γ-glutamyl carboxylation.

Within this chapter we identify and discuss some key areas in which vitamin K might impact on human health with special emphasis on the extrahepatic roles of vitamin K. We begin with a short overview covering the 'Chemistry, Nutritional Sources and Biological Function of Vitamin K' (RG and MJS) with respect to the synthesis of Gla proteins followed by a short overview of the 'Classical Role of Vitamin K in Haemostasis' (RG and MJS). The theme of haemostasis is continued with a discussion of 'Vitamin K Deficiency in the Hospital Setting' (DJH). In keeping with the theme of this book we have devoted major sections to three modern areas in which recent evidence gives promise that preventing local vitamin K deficiency or promoting therapeutic strategies with vitamin K compounds might affect health outcomes. These sections review current knowledge of 'Vitamin K and Bone Health' (MJS), 'Vitamin K and Vascular Calcification' (LJS) and 'Vitamin K and Cancer' (PN). We end with a section 'Miscellaneous effects of Vitamin K' (PN) that highlights some intriguing and unusual roles of vitamin K.

12.2 Chemistry, nutritional sources and biological function of vitamin K

12.2.1 Chemistry

Vitamin K is the generic term for a series of isoprenoid compounds derived from the parent structure 2-methyl-1,4-naphthoquinone. The various naturally occurring isoprenologues of vitamin K differ in the length and saturation of the poly-isoprenoid side-chain at the 3-position (▶Fig. 12.1). Phylloquinone (2-methyl-3-phytyl-1,4-naphthoquinone), is

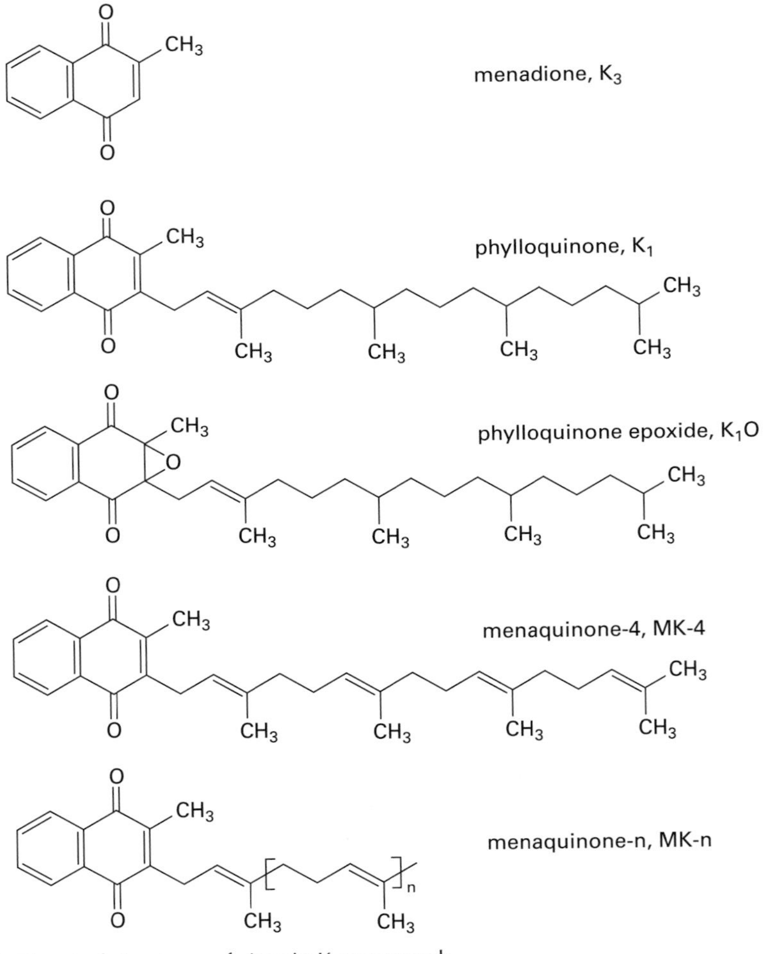

Fig. 12.1: Chemical structures of vitamin K compounds.

the form synthesised by plants which in older nomenclature (still common in medicine) is called vitamin K1. The menaquinones, also collectively known as vitamin K2 in the original nomenclature are a series of compounds, mainly of bacterial origin, comprising an unsaturated side-chain with differing numbers of prenyl units. In the systematic nomenclature of menaquinones the number of prenyl groups is assigned as a suffix, e.g., a menaquinone with n prenyl units is called menaquinone-n, abbreviated MK-n. Some bacterially synthesised menaquinones can also contain a partially saturated side-chain, in which the position of saturation of the dihydro (H2), tetrahydro (H4), etc., side-chains are described by a roman numeral system (counting from the ring system); in this system a menaquinone with the second double bond saturated would be named MK-n (II-H2), and one which had the sixth and seventh double bonds saturated as MK-n (VI,VII-H4), etc.

The naphthoquinonoid ring structure, 2-methyl-1,4-naphthoquinone, (trivial name menadione and historically called vitamin K3) is common to all K vitamins but without a side-chain at the 3 position this compound does not possess intrinsic biological activity as a cofactor for the γ-glutamyl carboxylase. However, menadione does possess *in vivo* cofactor activity in vertebrates because of their ability to add on a geranylgeranyl side-chain at the 3 position to produce menaquinone-4 (MK-4): in this sense menadione might be regarded as a provitamin K. Synthetic menadione, as water-soluble salts, is widely used as a feed supplement in animal husbandry and therefore can enter the human food chain indirectly, either unchanged or as preformed MK-4.

Among the naturally occurring K-vitamins, substantial differences might be expected, and have been reported, with respect to physiological processes such as their intestinal absorption, cellular uptake, tissue distribution and turnover. These differences are largely the result of the different lipophilicity of K vitamins that is determined by the length and degree of saturation of their side-chains. One notable exception to the above rules (particularly with respect to tissue distribution) is MK-4 for which there is a body of evidence relating to its unique synthesis from phylloquinone in certain tissues and to biological actions not shared by other K vitamins that seem to be determined by the geranylgeranyl side-chain (Shearer and Newman, 2008).

12.2.2 Nutritional sources (dietary and non-dietary)

The major dietary source of vitamin K for most populations is phylloquinone from plant sources. In dietary surveys conducted in Europe and the USA, 60%, or more, of total intakes of phylloquinone are provided by vegetables (Booth and Suttie, 1998; Thane et al., 2002, 2006). In general, the phylloquinone content of vegetables correlates with its known association with photosynthetic tissues, with the highest values (normally in the range 400–700 µg/100 g) being found in green-leafy vegetables. The next best sources are certain vegetable oils (e.g., soybean, rapeseed and olive oils) which contain 50–200 µg/100 g and are also important contributors to dietary vitamin K intakes. Other vegetable oils, such as peanut, corn, sunflower and safflower oils, have much lower contents of phylloquinone (1–10 µg/100 g). Lower amounts of phylloquinone are found in many other foods such as fruits, grains and dairy products.

Dietary intakes of menaquinones have been less well studied but have a more restricted distribution in the diet than does phylloquinone. A dietary survey in The

Netherlands suggested that menaquinones accounted for only 10% of total vitamin K intakes (Schurgers et al., 1999). Apart from animal livers, the richest dietary sources of long-chain menaquinones are fermented foods, typically represented by cheeses (MK-8, MK-9) in Western diets and natto (MK-7) in Japan. The relative concentrations of MK-8 and MK-9 in cheeses range from 10 to 20 µg/100 g for MK-8 and 35 to 55 µg/100 g for MK-9 (Schurgers and Vermeer, 2000). Lower contents of MK-8 and MK-9 are found in yogurts. Although MK-4 is synthesised *in vivo* by the human body from menadione and phylloquinone, the concentrations of MK-4 in the diet are fairly low being mainly found in egg yolk (~30 µg/100 g), butter (~15 µg/100 g), cheeses (~5 µg/100 g), and meats (~1–10 µg/100 g). Yeasts do not synthesise menaquinones and menaquinone-rich foods are those with a bacterial fermentation stage. The Japanese food natto (fermented soybeans) has a very high content of menaquinone-7 (MK-7) of approximately 1000 µg/100 g in a highly bioavailable form (Schurgers and Vermeer, 2000).

The human intestinal microflora synthesise large amounts of menaquinones, which at least in theory could serve as a potential source of vitamin K for human requirements. By far the largest reservoir of intestinal bacteria is found in the large intestine. Quantitatively, the *Bacteroides* and *Bifidobacterium* genera together account for over half of the total anaerobic bacterial population of which only *Bacteroides* synthesise menaquinones. The major bacterial menaquinones present in the human large intestine are MK-10 and MK-11 synthesised by *Bacteroides*, MK-8 by *Enterobacteria*, MK-7 by *Veillonella*, and MK-6 by *Eubacterium lentum* (Conly and Stein, 1992).

The longstanding question of whether the menaquinones synthesised by the colonic microbiota provide a quantitatively significant source of menaquinones that can be absorbed and utilised has still not been satisfactorily answered and has been reviewed in detail elsewhere (Shearer, 1992; Suttie, 1995). Overall, the weight of evidence suggests that although gut menaquinones might make some nutritional contribution, their importance is much less than previously thought (Shearer, 1992; Suttie, 1995). Recent evidence that intestinal menaquinones alone cannot maintain Gla protein synthesis comes from studies in healthy human subjects that demonstrate that relatively mild, short-term, dietary restriction of vitamin K results in increased concentrations of circulating species of undercarboxylated hepatic Gla proteins (prothrombin) and bone Gla proteins (osteocalcin) (Shearer, 1992; Suttie, 1995; Booth and Al Rajabi, 2008). The reason for their poor bioavailability from bacteria is that menaquinones are highly lipophilic molecules that are tightly bound to the bacterial cytoplasmic membrane, and remain locked in the membrane even after cell death. Even if low concentrations of free menaquinones are present in the colon, the bile salts that are obligatory for their absorption are lacking in this region. Menaquinone-producing bacteria are also present in the distal terminal ileum, albeit at vastly lower concentrations than the colon, and this site represents a more promising site of absorption given sufficient intraluminal concentrations of bile salts (Conley and Stein, 1992).

12.2.3 Biological function of vitamin K in Gla-protein synthesis

A detailed historical review of the pioneering studies that led to the discovery of the molecular function of vitamin K has recently been published by John Suttie, who himself played a leading role in these events (Suttie, 2009). In brief, in the late 1960s, the isolation of an abnormal form of prothrombin from the plasma of patients treated with the vitamin K antagonist warfarin, provided investigators with a tool to try and locate the structural differences between abnormal and native prothrombin and hence the nature of the vitamin K-dependent modification. Based on these studies it was concluded that vitamin K was needed for the attachment of some type of calcium-binding prosthetic group. Then in 1974 Johan Stenflo and co-workers published their studies in which they analysed a peptide from the calcium-binding region of native prothrombin by NMR and mass spectroscopy and found that it contained a structure that was identified as a new amino-acid called γ-carboxyglutamic acid (Stenflo et al., 1974). Stenflo has recently recounted the story of the discovery of this vitamin K-dependent modification (Stenflo, 2006).

We now know that vitamin K is required as an essential cofactor for a carboxylation reaction that transforms selective glutamic acid (Glu) residues in a peptide precursor into γ-carboxyglutamic acid (abbreviated Gla). The reaction is catalysed by a microsomal enzyme called γ-glutamyl or vitamin K-dependent carboxylase and requires molecular oxygen and carbon dioxide (Furie et al., 1999).

An unusual feature of γ-glutamyl carboxylation is that the reaction has been shown to be intimately linked to a metabolic sequence known as the vitamin K-epoxide cycle. This cycle and the associated enzyme activities [(1) γ-glutamyl carboxylase, (2) vitamin K epoxide reductase and (3) NAD(P)H-dependent quinone reductase] are shown in ▶Fig. 12.2a. In all tissues and cells that synthesise Gla proteins, the active cofactor form of vitamin K required by the γ-glutamyl carboxylase is not the stable quinone structure found in the diet but the intermittently reduced quinol (or hydroquinone) structure (KH_2). One mechanistic hypothesis by Dowd et al. (1995) is that the oxidation of vitamin KH_2 to vitamin K 2,3 epoxide provides the energy for the abstraction of a proton from the γ-carbon of the Glu residue to generate a carbanion that then undergoes carboxylation to yield the final Gla product. The epoxide produced during γ-glutamyl carboxylation is recycled back to vitamin KH_2 via vitamin K quinone. Only the enzyme vitamin K epoxide reductase is able to carry out the reduction of vitamin K epoxide to the quinone, whereas several reductases can carry out the reduction of the quinone to vitamin KH_2. Efforts to purify and determine the structure of the thiol-dependent vitamin K epoxide reductase are incomplete but the identification of the human and rat genes for vitamin K epoxide (Li et al., 2004; Rost et al., 2004) have lead to a greater understanding of its physiological role (Suttie, 2009). The available evidence suggests that the small 18-kDa protein expressed by the vitamin K epoxide reductase gene carries out both the reduction of the epoxide to the quinone form of vitamin K as well as the reduction of the quinone to the quinol (Chu et al., 2006).

An important property of the dithiol-dependent vitamin K epoxide reductase is its sensitivity to certain antagonists; particularly those based on 4-hydroxycoumarin (e.g., warfarin) or indandione structures (▶Fig. 12.2b). Vitamin K antagonist drugs based on these structures have long been used as oral anticoagulants and it is now clear that their anticoagulant action is based on their ability to inhibit the epoxide reductase activity and block the recycling of the vitamin. Because it is well known that vitamin K can overcome this inhibition, the question arises as to how vitamin K is reduced to vitamin KH_2 if the vitamin K epoxide is completely blocked, as it

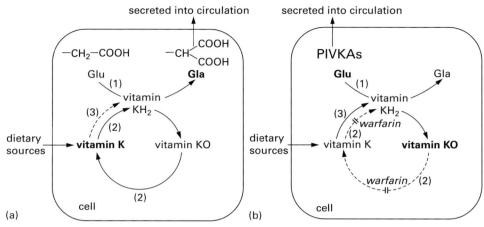

Fig. 12.2: Scheme showing the vitamin K epoxide cycle in the absence (a) and presence (b) of warfarin. (a) shows the linkage of the post-translational conversion of peptide-bound glutamic acid (Glu) to γ-carboxy glutamic acid (Gla) residues to the metabolic recycling of vitamin K by a pathway known as the vitamin K-epoxide cycle. Enzyme activities shown are (1) γ-glutamyl carboxylase; (2) vitamin K epoxide reductase (VKOR) and (3) NAD(P)H-dependent quinone reductase(s). The active cofactor form of vitamin K required by the γ-glutamyl carboxylase is the reduced form vitamin K quinol (KH_2). During γ-glutamyl carboxylation KH2 becomes oxidised to vitamin K epoxide (KO) which in turn undergoes reductive recycling, first to the vitamin K quinone (K) and then to KH_2. Only the VKOR enzyme can carry out the reduction of KO to K and under usual physiological conditions (▶Fig. 12.2a) the VKOR also probably carries out the reduction of K to KH_2. (b) shows the metabolic inhibition and consequences of a vitamin K antagonist such as warfarin. These drugs block the activity of the VKOR (2) leading to an accumulation of KO in the cell. Given a sufficient supply of vitamin K (e.g. from the diet) an alternative hepatic quinone reductase activity (3) can bypass the warfarin inhibition of the VKOR to provide the KH_2 substrate for the carboxylase enzyme and overcome the inhibitory action of warfarin, even under extreme blockade. The scheme also shows that in the absence of warfarin, the carboxylated substrates (Gla proteins) are secreted into the circulation (▶Fig. 12.2a) whereas in the presence of warfarin, species of undercarboxylated forms called PIVKAS are also secreted into the circulation (▶Fig. 12.2b).

might be in anticoagulant overdose. The answer seems to be that the liver contains other NAD(P)H-dependent quinone reductases that are less sensitive to warfarin and which provide an alternative pathway for the reduction of vitamin K to vitamin KH_2. This quinone reductase activity equates to enzyme activity (3) shown in ▶Fig. 12.2a,b. It follows that stable therapeutic anticoagulation is dependent on a balance being achieved between the inhibition of the recycling enzymes and the amount of dietary vitamin K that can enter the cycle to support carboxylation at a reduced efficiency.

12.2.4 Discovery of new Gla-proteins, characteristics and metabolic functions

From the early 1950s until the mid 1970s there were only four known vitamin K-dependent proteins, namely prothrombin (factor II) and factors VII, IX and X. They were all procoagulants synthesised in the liver and released into the circulation where they were already known to play a central role as the 'vitamin K-dependent clotting factors' in the so-called coagulation cascade that ultimately leads to the generation of thrombin and the formation of a fibrin clot. After the demonstration that vitamin K was needed for the enzymic transformation of specific Glu residues to Gla in prothrombin it was quickly shown that factors VII, IX and X also contained Gla residues thus unifying the concept that vitamin K played the same cofactor role in the post-translational modification of all these proteins.

With this discovery the way became open to search for other vitamin K-dependent proteins, either by assaying for the carboxylase enzyme responsible for γ-glutamyl carboxylation, or by isolating the product of action of vitamin K, namely Gla. Within a short time, γ-glutamyl carboxylase activity had been detected in a wide variety of extra-hepatic tissues such as bone, kidney, placenta, spleen, lung, testis and the vessel wall. Meanwhile Stenflo had discovered a fifth Gla-containing coagulation protein (protein C) that turned out to play a feedback anticoagulant role in haemostasis by reducing thrombin generation and procoagulant activity (Stenflo, 2006). New Gla-proteins continue to be discovered; a list of the major Gla-proteins that could have relevance to human health is shown in ▶Tab. 12.1. Some of these

Tab. 12.1: The major vitamin K-dependent (Gla) proteins and their putative health roles.

Gla protein	Tissue	Known and putative roles
Factors II, VII, IX and X	Liver (then blood plasma)	Blood coagulation (procoagulants)
Protein C	Liver (then blood plasma)	Blood coagulation (anticoagulant)
		Immune response
Protein S	Liver (then blood plasma)	Cofactor for protein C
	Bone	Role in bone unknown
Osteocalcin (bone Gla protein)	Bone and dentin	Bone remodelling and mineralization
		New role proposed as hormone that regulates glucose metabolism and fat mass
Matrix Gla protein	Most tissues, highest expression by chondrocytes and VSMCs	Inhibitor of calcium precipitation and crystallization (inhibitor of vascular calcification)
Periostin	Bone marrow mesenchymal stromal cells	Implicated in bone development
		Maintenance and repair of bone and heart

(Continued)

Tab. 12.1 (*Continued*)

Gla protein	Tissue	Known and putative roles
Gas6	Most tissues	Ligand for Axl, Sky, Mer receptor tyrosine kinases
		Cell growth, cell survival, platelet signalling, immune response
Gla-rich protein	Most tissues, highest expression by chondrocytes	Implicated as regulator of mineral formation (potential inhibitor of vascular and skin calcifications)
	Accumulates at sites of mineral deposition	

Gla-proteins are found in only one major tissue (e.g., procoagulant factors in liver and osteocalcin in bone) whereas some (e.g., matrix Gla protein and protein S) are more widely distributed. The structure and function of these new Gla proteins, particularly osteocalcin and MGP, will be considered in greater depth in the sections 'Vitamin K and bone health' and 'Vitamin K and vascular health': both osteocalcin and MGP are attracting major interest with respect to their health roles in these two areas.

All Gla-containing proteins are secretory proteins and are characterised by an intracellular precursor form possessing a leader sequence that facilitates specific post-translational events and is then normally cleaved before secretion (Furie et al., 1999). Within the leader sequence, a hydrophobic pre-sequence facilitates the translocation of the precursor Gla-proteins across the endoplasmic reticulum, and a second pro-sequence serves as a recognition signal for the vitamin K-dependent carboxylase. With the exception of matrix-Gla protein, the pro-sequence of currently characterised Gla-proteins is located immediately before the N-terminal of the mature protein. In matrix-Gla protein the carboxylation recognition site is internal and is retained in the mature protein. The number of Gla residues varies: the four classical vitamin K-dependent clotting factors contain 10–12 Gla residues whereas the much smaller MGP and osteocalcin contain 5 and 3 Gla residues, respectively.

12.3 Classical role of vitamin K in haemostasis

12.3.1 Role of Gla-proteins in haemostasis

The only unequivocal biochemical role for vitamin K is as a cofactor for the γ-glutamyl carboxylase and apart from a rare embryonic skeletal defect the only well proven human deficiency syndromes relate to its long established role in blood coagulation (Suttie, 2009).

The vitamin K-dependent coagulation proteins comprise four plasma procoagulants (factors II, VII, IX and X) and two feedback anticoagulants (proteins C and S). The physiological function of a seventh plasma protein (protein Z) is less established but seems to play a role in dampening coagulation by acting as a cofactor for the inhibition of factor Xa. The four vitamin K-dependent procoagulants have long been known to play a central role in the blood clotting cascade leading to the formation of a fibrin clot. Circulating as inactive forms (or zymogens) of serine proteases their biological activity is dependent on their ability to bind to anionic phospholipid surfaces where cleavage of the zymogens yields the active protease clotting factors. The Gla residues of these clotting factors provide an efficient chelating site for calcium ions that enables ion bridges to be made between the factor and the surface phospholipids of platelets and endothelial cells where, together with other cofactors, they form membrane-bound enzyme complexes. The intricate control of coagulation is illustrated by the fact that protein C, once activated, performs an inhibitory role by specifically degrading phospholipid-bound activated factors V and VIII in the presence of calcium. This anticoagulant activity of activated protein C is dependent on protein S that acts as a synergistic cofactor by enhancing the binding of activated protein C to negatively-charged phospholipids.

Although vitamin K is needed for the synthesis of haemostatic proteins with both procoagulant and anticoagulant functions, the consequence of an acquired deficiency of vitamin K is always to promote a bleeding tendency. Thus the consequences of vitamin K deficiency for haemostasis are an inability to synthesise functional molecules of factors II, VII, IX and X resulting in a hypocoagulable state. The haemostatic system has a considerable capacity to function adequately at low-factor concentrations but as vitamin K deficiency progresses, a point will be reached when the procoagulatory mechanisms fail and bleeding occurs. This point is highly individual and unpredictable.

12.3.2 Laboratory diagnosis of vitamin K deficiency

12.3.2.1 Coagulation tests

Overt vitamin K deficiency is often initially detected by so called global coagulation assays such as the prothrombin time (PT) and the activated partial thromboplastin time. A lengthening in these coagulation times is sensitive to a diminution of certain biologically active γ-carboxylated forms of vitamin K-dependent clotting factors (depending on the coagulation test used) but are not specific to these factors. For instance further evidence that a lengthening of the PT is owing to vitamin K deficiency can be obtained by demonstrating that two or more of the four vitamin K-dependent procoagulants are specifically reduced and, even more pertinently, by showing that the prolonged PT (and individual factors) can be corrected by vitamin K administration. Inherent to the PT is its insensitivity which although allowing the diagnosis of an imminent bleeding tendency, is not useful for picking up subclinical deficiency (Suttie, 1992).

12.3.2.2 Serum vitamin K concentrations

In most people the major dietary and circulating form of vitamin K is phylloquinone and its measurement in serum is a useful status indicator of tissue stores. The majority of circulating phylloquinone is carried by triglyceride-rich lipoproteins (Shearer and Newman, 2008). To minimise interpretive errors arising from recent dietary intakes, measurements of phylloquinone should ideally be made in fasting individuals.

Fasting phylloquinone reference values in healthy adults range from 0.15 to 1.0 µg/l with a median of approximately 0.5 µg/l. Well-controlled metabolic studies have shown that fasting phylloquinone reflects both dietary depletion and repletion (Booth and Al Rajabi, 2008). Infants are born with very low and usually undetectable concentrations (<0.05 µg/l) but thereafter, until weaning, circulating concentrations might be either lower or higher than in adults depending on whether they are predominately breast-fed or formula-fed, respectively (Shearer, 2009).

There are several studies showing a high prevalence of low phylloquinone levels in hospitalised patients, particularly in intensive care (O'Shaughnessy et al., 2003), in advanced cancer (Harrington et al., 2008) or after surgery (Usui et al., 1990) (see also section on 'Populations at risk of bleeding').

12.3.2.3 Undercarboxylated vitamin K-dependent proteins in serum

In states of vitamin K insufficiency, undercarboxylated functionally defective molecules of vitamin K-dependent proteins are produced at their site of synthesis and released into the bloodstream (▶Fig. 12.2b). These abnormal molecules comprise a heterogeneous spectrum of uncarboxylated or partially carboxylated molecules. The historical collective term for these undercarboxylated species is PIVKA (Proteins Induced by Vitamin K Absence or Antagonism). Other names in common use are 'undercarboxylated' proteins or 'des-γ-carboxy' proteins. Thus, undercarboxylated species of prothrombin (factor II) are called PIVKA-II or des-γ-carboxyprothrombin (abbreviated DCP); for consistency in this chapter the abbreviation PIVKA-II will be used to denote undercarboxylated prothrombin. Undercarboxylated species of osteocalcin (OC) and MGP are usually called undercarboxylated osteocalcin (ucOC) and undercarboxylated MGP (ucMGP), respectively.

Methods are available to measure PIVKA for prothrombin, osteocalcin and MGP. Potentially these assays offer true functional assays of the γ-glutamyl carboxylation status of individual Gla-proteins. Because the synthesis of some Gla-proteins is tissue-specific (e.g., prothrombin PIVKA-II in liver and osteocalcin in bone) PIVKA assays also offer a way of determining local vitamin K status (Vermeer et al., 2004).

Assays for undercarboxylated factor II (PIVKA-II) have proved to be extremely useful to monitor subclinical vitamin K deficiency (Suttie, 1992), particularly for at-risk groups such as young infants (Shearer, 2009) and patients with malabsorption from various causes (Conway et al., 2005). The most sensitive assays are enzyme immunoassays with antibodies that recognise PIVKA-II but do not cross-react with native factor II.

In addition to PIVKA-II as a biomarker for hepatic vitamin K status, the measurement of ucOC is widely used as a surrogate marker of the vitamin K reserves of bone. Its advantages are that osteocalcin is expressed only by osteoblasts (and odontoblasts) and has been well studied as a marker of bone formation. Its disadvantages include variability of different methodologies and the fact that serum osteocalcin levels, including the ucOC fraction, also reflect bone turnover. For this reason, ucOC levels are usually expressed as a percentage of total osteocalcin.

12.3.2.4 Miscellaneous status indicators

Other biomarkers that that have been used to assess vitamin K status are urinary measurements of free Gla and vitamin K metabolites reflecting the whole body turnover of

Gla-proteins and vitamin K, respectively. The rationale for measuring urinary Gla is that this amino acid represents the final catabolic product of all Gla-containing proteins and will be diminished in states of vitamin K insufficiency (Topp et al., 1998). The rationale for measuring vitamin K metabolite excretion is that the side-chains of phylloquinone and menaquinones are catabolised by a common degradative pathway so that the measurement of the two major urinary metabolites reflects the turnover and excretion of all K vitamins (Harrington et al., 2005). It was recently shown that urinary vitamin K excretion responds to both vitamin K depletion and repletion (Harrington et al., 2007).

12.3.2.5 Practical detection of subclinical vitamin K deficiency

A useful way to assess vitamin K status in patients is to measure both serum phylloquinone and PIVKA-II combining a marker of tissue reserves with a functional marker of coagulation, respectively. We use a sensitive immunoassay for PIVKA-II that can detect undercarboxylated species of factor II when their circulating concentration is as low as 0.2% of that of total native factor II. This threshold is well below the reduction of approximately 50% in circulating levels of active total factor II that is needed to trigger a detectable change in the PT (Suttie, 1992). The finding of a low serum phylloquinone (<0.15 µg/l) alone often serves as a warning of low tissue stores. The combination of a low phylloquinone combined with a raised PIVKA-II usually indicates a subclinical vitamin K-deficient state that can be confirmed by the disappearance of PIVKA-II when vitamin K is given. The half-life of clearance of PIVKA-II is similar to native factor II (~60 h) so that PIVKA-II could remain detectable for several days after the correction of vitamin K deficiency. This slow clearance is often useful for the retrospective diagnosis of vitamin K deficiency after vitamin K has been administered. The major caveat to interpretation is that PIVKA-II is occasionally raised in certain liver disorders, although high levels are usually only found in hepatocellular carcinoma (Liebman et al., 1984).

12.3.3 Populations at risk of bleeding

12.3.3.1 Vitamin K deficiency bleeding in infants

As recently reviewed (Shearer, 2009), vitamin K deficiency bleeding in early infancy represents a rare but significant public health problem throughout the world. The window of risk is the first 6 months of life and the major risk factors are exclusive breast feeding and undiagnosed hepatobiliary disease. The deficiency syndrome was previously known as 'haemorrhagic disease of the newborn' (HDN) but is now renamed vitamin K deficiency bleeding (VKDB) to give a better description that the cause of bleeding is due to vitamin K deficiency. There is now a convincing body of evidence that without vitamin K prophylaxis, breast-fed infants have a small but real risk of bleeding from this vitamin K deficiency syndrome. Worryingly, from the public health point of view, VKDB often has no warning symptoms and after the first week of life the most common site of bleeding is the brain (Shearer, 2009).

The time of onset of VKDB is more unpredictable than previously supposed and it is now useful to recognise three syndromes according to the age of onset: early, classical, and late (▶Tab. 12.2). Until the 1960s, VKDB was considered to be solely a problem of the first week of life. Then, in 1966, came the first reports from Thailand of a new vitamin K

Tab. 12.2: Classification of vitamin K deficiency in the newborn (VKDB).

VKDB syndrome	Time of presentation	Common bleeding sites	Etiological factors
Early	First 24 h	Scalp subperiosteal or skin, intracranial, intrathoracic, intra-abdominal	Maternal drugs (e.g., warfarin, anticonvulsants, rifampicin)
Classical	Days 1–7	Gastrointestinal, umbilical, skin, nose, post-circumcision	Mainly idiopathic, breast-feeding (low milk intakes in first week of life)
Late	Day 8 to 6 months (peak 3–8 weeks)	Intracranial, skin, gastrointestinal	Idiopathic or secondary, breast-feeding, undiagnosed cholestasis often present
			Secondary case from malabsorption owing to underlying disease (e.g., biliary atresia, α-1-antitrypsin deficiency, cystic fibrosis) or to chronic diarrhoea
			Antibiotic therapy sometimes implicated

deficiency syndrome that typically presented between 1 and 2 months of life and is now termed late VKDB. In 1977, Bhanchet and colleagues (Bhanchet, 1977), who had first described this syndrome, summarised their studies of 93 affected Thai infants, establishing the idiopathic history, preponderance of breast-fed infants (98%), and high incidence of intracranial bleeding (63%). More reports from South-East Asia and Australia followed, and in 1983 McNinch et al. (1983) reported the return of VKDB in the UK. This increased incidence was ascribed to a decrease in the practice of vitamin K prophylaxis and to an increased trend towards exclusive human milk feeding (McNinch et al., 1983). Human milk has lower concentrations of vitamin K than commercial milk formulas (Haroon et al., 1982).

Without vitamin K prophylaxis, the incidence of late VKDB (per 100 000 births), based on acceptable surveillance data, has been estimated to be 4.4 in the UK, 7.2 in Germany, and as high as 72 in Thailand (see review by Shearer, 2009). The earlier high incidence of late VKDB in Thailand has been brought down to European levels by a national prophylaxis program (Chuansumrit et al., 1998) but incidences of VKDB as high as 100 per 100 000 births still exist in low-income, rural areas of some Asian countries such as China and Vietnam (Shearer, 2009). Of real concern is that late VKDB, unlike the classic form, has a high incidence of death or severe and permanent brain damage resulting from intracranial haemorrhage (Shearer, 2009).

The major form of vitamin K in breast milk is phylloquinone and typical concentrations are approximately 1 µg/l compared with 50 µg/l in a typical formula milk (Shearer, 2009). The resulting large disparity in dietary intakes of phylloquinone between breast- and formula-fed infants is reflected in plasma concentrations that in exclusively breast-fed infants can be an order of magnitude lower than in their formula-fed counterparts. Thus, Greer et al. (1991) found that average plasma concentrations at 6, 12 and 26 weeks ranged from 0.13 to 0.24 µg/l compared with 4.4 to 6.0 µg/l in formula-fed infants.

One question is how low intakes of vitamin K in individual breast-fed infants might translate to an increased risk of classical and late VKDB. With respect to classical VKDB, von Kries et al. (1987) showed that in the first week of life it is the cumulative intake of human milk rather than an abnormally low milk concentration *per se* that is of greater importance in determining the vitamin K status of breast-fed infants (von Kries et al., 1987; Shearer, 2009). This and other studies have shown that low intakes of milk in the first five days of life were associated with lower activities of vitamin K-dependent coagulation factors and higher prevalence of a raised PIVKA-II (see Shearer, 2009). Thus, classical VKDB might be related, at least in part, to a failure to establish early breastfeeding practices. For late VKDB other factors seem to be important because the deficiency syndrome occurs when breastfeeding is well established and as reviewed by von Kries et al. (1988), mothers of affected infants appear to have normal concentrations of vitamin K in their milk. For instance, some (although not all) infants who develop late VKDB are later found to have abnormalities of liver function that might affect their bile acid production and result in a degree of malabsorption of vitamin K. The degree of cholestasis can be mild and its course transient and self-correcting, but affected infants will have an increased dietary requirement for vitamin K because of reduced absorption efficiency (Shearer, 2009).

12.3.3.2 Vitamin K prophylaxis in infants

Because bleeding can occur spontaneously and because no screening test is available, it is now common paediatric practice to protect all infants by giving vitamin K supplements in the immediate perinatal period. Vitamin K prophylaxis has had a chequered history but in recent years surveillance studies implemented in several countries have convincingly demonstrated that VKDB in early infancy can be virtually eliminated by adopting appropriate prophylactic policies. However, there is still ongoing debate as to the route and formulation of vitamin K that should be used. In the early 1990s a reported epidemiological association from the UK between vitamin K given intramuscularly and the later development of childhood cancer led to a greater use of multiple oral supplements (see Shearer, 2009). However, the failure to substantiate any link with cancer together with findings that have shown that some oral regimes fail, has led to an increase in the use of the traditional single intramuscular injection (usually of 1 mg phylloquinone) given at birth. This intramuscular route is considered the gold standard for protection against which other regimes should be compared.

12.3.3.3 Vitamin K deficiency in adults

In adults, primary vitamin K-deficient states that manifest as bleeding are almost unknown except when the absorption of the vitamin is impaired as a result of an underlying pathology (Suttie, 2009). Therefore this topic of vitamin K deficiency will be considered in a separate section below which describes the etiology and treatment of vitamin K deficiency in a hospital setting.

12.4 Vitamin K deficiency in the hospital setting

12.4.1 Body stores and tissue distribution of K vitamins

The human liver contains phylloquinone and is the main storage organ for the long chain menaquinones (MKs 6–12) (Shearer et al., 1988; Thijssen and Drittij-Reijnders, 1996). Shearer et al. (1988) reported that on a molar basis, menaquinones account for 75–91% of total hepatic vitamin K stores. The same investigators reported that menaquinones were undetectable in the livers from foetuses and neonates up to 7 days suggesting that the newborn are largely dependent on phylloquinone for clotting factor synthesis (Shearer et al., 1988).

Fat tissue taken from human bone biopsies was reported to contain significant concentrations of phylloquinone and MK-6, MK-7 and MK-8 (Hodges et al., 1993a). Subsequent unpublished data (see Shearer and Newman, 2008) suggest a very different profile of menaquinones in bone compared with liver, with phylloquinone and MK-4 accounting for 60% and 22% of the vitamin K content of bone lipid, respectively, and the remaining 18% being equally distributed between MK-5, MK-6 and MK-7; menaquinones with longer side-chains were undetectable. Recent work reviewed by Shearer and Newman (2008) suggests that lipoprotein-borne vitamin K is taken up by osteoblasts in a similar way that fat soluble vitamins carried by chylomicron remnants are delivered to the liver.

As already discussed under the laboratory diagnosis of vitamin K deficiency, the major circulating form of vitamin K is phylloquinone. In the fasting state, typical endogenous serum concentrations for phylloquinone are 0.17–0.68 µg/l (Shearer et al., 1988). Menaquinone 4, MK-7 and MK-8 are also sometimes detectable in serum, with MK-7 most often predominating (Shearer et al., 1988; Hodges et al., 1990). Circulating levels of phylloquinone and menaquinones rapidly respond to dietary intake or supplementation, but the plasma concentration-time profiles differ. A comparative study in human volunteers given equimolar oral doses of phylloquinone, MK-4 and MK-9 showed considerable differences of the plasma appearance and disappearance kinetics that could be accounted for by differences in their lipoprotein distribution (Schurgers and Vermeer, 2002).

Thijssen and Drittij-Reijnders (1994) examined the tissue distribution of phylloquinone and MK-4 after first feeding rats with a vitamin K-free diet (resulting in a prolonged prothrombin time) and again after dietary resupplementation with phylloquinone. After the resupplementation phase, phylloquinone was widely distributed in all tissues with the highest levels found in liver, heart, bone and cartilaginous tissue (sternum) but low levels in the brain (Thijssen and Drittij-Reijnders, 1994). After the vitamin K-depletion phase relatively high levels of phylloquinone remained in the heart, pancreas, bone and sternum. These results did not follow the expected association with γ-glutamyl carboxylase activities because the heart, brain and muscle are low in this enzyme. Another unexpected finding was that MK-4 was also detected in all tissues, with low levels in plasma and liver, and much higher levels (exceeding those of phylloquinone) in the brain, pancreas, salivary gland and sternum (Thijssen and Drittij-Reijnders, 1994). The results indicated that there is a tissue-selective distribution of phylloquinone and MK-4. Supplementation with phylloquinone caused levels of MK-4 to rise, suggesting that MK-4 could be derived from dietary phylloquinone. It seems unlikely that the specific accumulation of MK-4 in tissues such as heart, pancreas and salivary gland are related to demands for γ-glutamyl carboxylation and more probable that this accumulation reflects another biochemical role yet to be elucidated (Thijssen and Drittij-Reijnders, 1994). Human tissues also display a similar tissue-specific distribution of phylloquinone and MK-4 as found in the rat (Thijssen and Drittij-Reijnders, 1996). It has now been definitively shown that the conversion of phylloquinone to MK-4 does not involve bacterial metabolism in the gut and that animal cells can carry out this conversion of phylloquinone to MK-4 (for review see Shearer and Newman, 2008).

12.4.2 Absorption and turnover of vitamin K

Studies using oral (Shearer et al., 1970) or injected (Shearer et al., 1974; Bjornsson et al., 1979; Olson et al., 2002) doses of tritium-labelled phylloquinone showed that phylloquinone is absorbed from the proximal intestine and is dependent on bile and pancreatic juice secretions (Shearer et al., 1974). Phylloquinone is subsequently incorporated into nascent chylomicron particles within the intestine before direct secretion into the lymph and circulation, transformation into chylomicron remnants in the capillaries and uptake by the liver. In rats given a tracer dose of radioactive phylloquinone, approximately 40% of the dose was present in the liver 3 h later, falling to 10% within 24 h, suggesting a rapid turnover of phylloquinone (Thierry and Suttie, 1971). Circulatory vitamin K is primarily transported by triglyceride-rich lipoproteins and to a lesser extent by low-density lipoproteins and high-density lipoproteins (Kohlmeier et al., 1996; Lamon-Fava et al., 1998; Schurgers and Vermeer, 2002). The absorption of a physiological dose of deuterium-labelled phylloquinone incorporated into collard greens showed peak plasma concentrations 6–9 h after ingestion with a return to baseline levels within 24 h, and confirmed the triglyceride fraction as a major carrier of phylloquinone (Erkkilä et al., 2004). In contrast to phylloquinone and menaquinones, menadione does not require bile salts for absorption and can be absorbed in the distal small intestine (Hollander and Truscott, 1974a) and colon (Hollander and Truscott, 1974b) by a process of passive diffusion.

12.4.3 Risk factors for vitamin K deficiency

Vitamin K deficiency can develop rapidly, with hepatic stores of phylloquinone depleted within 3 days of dietary restriction (Usui et al., 1990). In the hospital setting, primary vitamin K deficiency has been identified as an unexpected cause of bleeding (Pineo et al., 1973; Ansell et al., 1977). Vitamin K deficiency can develop in patients for several reasons. These include: poor dietary intake, intestinal malabsorption, hepatic dysfunction, diarrhoea or frequent antibiotic therapy. It is important to rule out exposure to vitamin K antagonists (e.g., warfarin, superwarfarins) as a cause of vitamin K deficiency.

12.4.4 Prevalence of deficiency in different diseases

Dietary vitamin K, mainly as phylloquinone, is absorbed chemically unchanged from the proximal intestine after solubilisation into mixed micelles composed of bile salts and the products of pancreatic lipolysis (Shearer et al., 1974). Therefore, any condition causing the prolonged intestinal malabsorption of fat (e.g., obstructive jaundice, pancreatic insufficiency, cystic fibrosis, coeliac disease, Crohn's disease, etc.) might lead to a secondary acquired deficiency of vitamin K. In patients with severe malabsorption the majority of phylloquinone is excreted in the faeces, compared with approximately 20% in healthy subjects (Shearer et al., 1970; Shearer et al., 1974). Deficient states lead to the depletion of tissue stores and are indicated by a decrease in circulating phylloquinone or increase in PIVKA long before pathological changes develop. In a study of 93 children with cystic fibrosis (median age 11 years) living in the north of England, Conway and co-workers measured serum concentrations of phylloquinone and PIVKA-II to demonstrate that vitamin K status was suboptimal in 70% of study participants (Conway et al., 2005).

Many patients with advanced cancer have a poor dietary intake (Rimmer, 1998), and the use of chemotherapy could cause epithelial damage to the gastrointestinal tract resulting in fat and fat-soluble vitamin malabsorption. The susceptibility of these patients to vitamin K deficiency has been highlighted by two studies. In one study, autologous bone marrow transplantation was linked with a rapid fall in circulating phylloquinone and PIVKA-II was detectable within a few days (Elston et al., 1995). In a second study, very low serum phylloquinone concentrations were present in a fifth of palliative care patients (Harrington et al., 2008). A precarious vitamin K status was confirmed by elevated levels of PIVKA-II in 78% of patients.

12.4.5 Prevention of deficiency

Recommendations on the adequate nutritional intake of vitamin K have not been precisely established, partly because of the unquantifiable contribution made by the intestinal bacteria but also because of insufficient population studies relating vitamin K intakes with biomarkers of vitamin K status that indicate a health risk. At the present time most countries including the USA, have concluded that there is insufficient evidence to make any recommendation with respect to vitamin K intakes and bone health and therefore most recommendations only relate to the prevention of vitamin K deficiency bleeding (Food and Nutrition Board, 2001). In the UK, the current Dietary Reference Value set in 1991 is 1 μg/kg per day, an intake that was considered adequate for the coagulation function of vitamin K (COMA, 1991). In 2001 the US Food and Nutrition Board set an Adequate Intake of 120 and 90 μg/day for men and women, respectively; these values were based on representative dietary intake data from healthy individuals (Food and Nutrition Board, 2001). Data from 11 studies indicate that the mean (range) intake of phylloquinone in young adults (<45 years) is 80 (60–110) μg/d and that older adults (>55 years) consume 150 (80–210) μg/day, a finding that has been attributed to the higher intake of vegetables by the elderly (Booth and Suttie, 1998).

There are few reports of human toxicity following vitamin K ingestion. Menadione formulations that were used for vitamin K prophylaxis in the newborn until the early 1960s were shown to cause kernicterus and haemolytic anaemia when given in high doses to premature infants (Allison, 1955). This toxicity is not found with phylloquinone formulations. In rats, mice and chicks acute doses of phylloquinone up to 25 000 mg/kg caused no fatalities. By contrast, oral administration of 200 mg/kg of menadione to rats caused anaemia and 100% mortality in mice (Molitor and Robinson, 1940).

12.5 Vitamin K and bone health

12.5.1 Gla-containing proteins in bone: historical perspective and putative roles

There are now known to be at least five vitamin K-dependent proteins synthesised in bone or cartilage. The isolation of the first of these, osteocalcin (also called bone Gla protein), was reported in 1975 soon after the discovery a year earlier of the molecular function of vitamin K as an essential cofactor in the synthesis of the coagulation factor prothrombin (Shearer, 1995; Suttie, 2009). Thus, once it was known that vitamin K was needed for the synthesis of γ-carboxyglutamate (Gla) in prothrombin, the search began for other vitamin K-dependent proteins. This search resulted in the independent discoveries by groups in Harvard and the University of California, San Diego that bone contained both free Gla and a gamma-carboxylated protein substrate (Hauschka et al., 1975; Price et al., 1976). Furthermore, bone microsomes could carry out the conversion of Glu to Gla (Lian and Friedman, 1978) by an enzyme now known to be the same vitamin K-dependent γ-glutamyl carboxylase as found in the liver.

Osteocalcin is a small protein of 49–50 (human 49) residues with a central Gla-domain comprising three Gla residues situated at residues 17, 21 and 24 (▶Fig. 12.3). The primary structure and position of these three Gla residues has been highly conserved in vertebrates suggesting that the Gla amino acids are essential to its biological function(s), as is known for the vitamin K-dependent proteins of the coagulation system. It is the most abundant noncollagenous protein of the bone extracellular matrix (accounting for 10–20% of non-collagen proteins), and is synthesised by osteoblasts and odontoblasts. An important physicochemical property that the three Gla residues confer on osteocalcin is the high-affinity binding to the hydroxyapatite mineral component of bone (Hoang et al., 2003). The precise molecular role of osteocalcin is unclear, but there is evidence to support a role of osteocalcin in the regulation of bone remodelling and mineralisation (Boskey et al., 1998; Lian et al., 1999; Atkins et al., 2009).

During the extraction of osteocalcin from bone it was found that a proportion of bone Gla was not extracted by the usual extraction agents. This mysterious insoluble Gla fraction was later explained by the isolation and sequencing from bovine bone of a second Gla-containing protein termed matrix Gla protein (MGP) that was firmly associated with the organic phase of bone and cartilage. It is now known that MGP is found in a variety of tissues such as heart, lung, kidney and the arterial vessel wall. The structure of MGP and the impressive series of experiments that have clearly established MGP as a key inhibitor of vascular calcification *in vivo* (Price et al., 1998; Shearer, 2000; Schurgers et al., 2008) are described in detail in the section 'Vitamin K and Vascular Calcification'. This section also considers the potential pathological consequences of vitamin K deficient states to vascular health in humans and the potential value of novel MGP assays as biomarkers of vascular calcification.

The first direct evidence that Gla proteins (and by implication vitamin K) play an important role in bone health comes from skeletal abnormalities that can occur in the developing bone of animals and humans exposed *in utero* to maternal vitamin K antagonists such as warfarin. In the human foetus such exposure to oral anticoagulants might result in a condition variously called the warfarin embryopathy or chondrodysplasia punctata, which is characterised by pathological skeletal calcification, including that

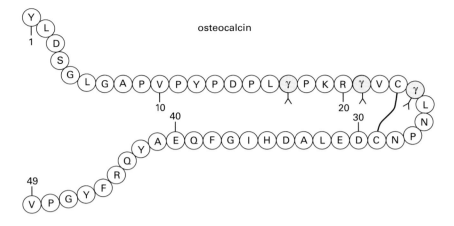

osteocalcin

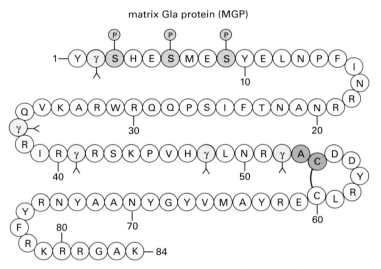

matrix Gla protein (MGP)

Fig. 12.3: Molecular structures of osteocalcin and matrix Gla protein. The positions of Gla-residues in both proteins are denoted by "γ" and the phosphorylation of three serine residues in MGP by "P".

of the growth plate (Shearer, 2000). Chondrodysplasia punctata is a heterogeneous condition with a variable phenotype that includes a disorder of mineralisation known as Keutel syndrome characterised by abnormal calcification of the cartilage of the auricles, nose, larynx, trachea and ribs. Further evidence for a specific role of MGP in chondrodysplasia punctata comes from the finding that Keutel syndrome is associated with certain congenital mutations in MGP (Shearer, 2000). Finally, evidence that MGP (and perhaps other Gla proteins) need to be γ-carboxylated comes from reported cases of chondrodysplasia punctata in maternal dietary deficiency of vitamin K (for review see Shearer, 2000).

Other Gla proteins present in bone or cartilage are protein S and Gas6 and the recently discovered periostin (Coutu et al., 2008) and Gla-rich protein (Viegas et al., 2008).

Protein S has long been known to play a central role in haemostasis as a cofactor for the anticoagulant protein C but is also synthesised by osteoblasts. Its role in bone is unknown but could be connected with its known properties as a ligand and activator of TAM (Tyro, Axl, Mer) tyrosine kinase receptors. Hereditary protein S deficiency has been associated with osteopaenia.

Gas6 shares 40% homology to protein S (Manfioletti et al., 1993) and is also a ligand of TAM tyrosine kinase receptors that when bound triggers signal transduction within cells. Through such signalling pathways Gas6 has been reported to be associated with a wide range of cellular responses including the stimulation of osteoclastic bone resorption that could have a key role in bone loss through oestrogen deficiency (Katagiri et al., 2001).

Periostin is secreted by bone marrow-derived mesenchymal stromal cells and, unusually for a Gla-protein, contains four consensus γ-carboxylase recognition sites (Coutu et al., 2008). Confocal microscopy analysis demonstrated extensive deposition of γ-carboxylated periostin only in the mineralised matrix of bone nodules produced *in vitro* suggesting a role of periostin in extracellular matrix mineralisation (Coutu et al., 2008).

Gla-rich protein (GRP) is a 10.2-kDa secreted protein isolated in 2008 from the calcified cartilage of sturgeon (Viegas et al., 2008). A remarkable feature of this protein is that it contains 16 Gla residues, which on the basis of protein size is the highest ratio of Gla residues found in any vitamin K-dependent protein identified to date. Furthermore, although GRP has no significant sequence homology with the Gla region of other vitamin K-dependent proteins the number and position of the precursor Glu residues appears to have been conserved over more than 450 million years of vertebrate evolution. GRP is not uniquely expressed by cartilage being also expressed in rat trabecular bone by both osteoblasts and osteocytes (Viegas et al., 2008).

12.5.2 Relation of bone health to dietary intakes and biochemical markers of vitamin K status

One of the first indications suggesting a possible connection between an impaired vitamin K status and osteoporosis were a series of investigations by the group of Joe Chayen in London who in collaboration with one of the authors (MJS) conducted the first plasma measurements of phylloquinone in patients with osteoporosis. These small observational studies consistently showed dramatically reduced levels of phylloquinone and sometimes menaquinones in patients who had sustained femoral neck or spinal crush fractures (Hart et al., 1985; Hodges et al., 1991, 1993b). This association between low plasma phylloquinone concentrations and an increased incidence of vertebral fracture was recently reproduced in a much larger prospective study in Japanese women followed up for 3–4 years (Tsugawa et al., 2008). However, it has not been possible to clarify whether low plasma phylloquinone is causally related to skeletal fragility or an unintentional marker linked to other lifestyle factors that predispose to fracture risk.

Several population studies have now been published linking skeletal health to either dietary consumption of vitamin K or biochemical markers of vitamin K status. Examples include reported associations of low dietary intakes of vitamin K (phylloquinone) with increased fracture risk (Feskanich et al., 1999; Booth et al., 2000) or a lower bone mass (Booth et al., 2003; MacDonald et al., 2008), and associations of impaired vitamin K status with low bone mass (Booth et al., 2004) or increased bone turnover (Kalkwarf et al., 2004). One note of caution is that the studies do not consistently show this association with fractures or bone mineral density (BMD) across different age groups or between men and women. This could reflect a weak association between vitamin K intakes and bone health, or indicate that certain population groups are more vulnerable to vitamin K insufficiency than others. Another explanation is that low dietary intakes of phylloquinone could reflect a poor diet in general, and might merely reflect deficiencies of other nutrients or a combination of nutrients important to bone health. Among the negative studies is a population-based study in a cohort of over 2000 Danish perimenopausal women that showed no association of vitamin K intakes with BMD or fracture risk or with changes in BMD over a 10-year follow up; moreover a nested case-control study showed no effect of vitamin K intakes on fracture prevalence (Rejnmark et al., 2006).

Apart from associations with vitamin K intakes, several epidemiological studies have found that high circulating concentrations of ucOC constitute an independent risk factor for bone fracture (Szulc et al., 1996; Vergnaud et al., 1997; Luukinen et al., 2000) and low BMD (Szulc et al., 1994; Knapen et al., 1998). The strength of these studies is that ucOC is an accepted functional marker of the vitamin K status of the bone matrix and that this association has been found in more than one country with different methodologies for measuring ucOC. Their weakness is a lack of understanding of the molecular function of osteocalcin and again that ucOC might be a surrogate marker of a poor diet.

12.5.3 Vitamin K intervention trials and bone health

Most of the vitamin K intervention studies published to date have been conducted in Japan with high pharmacological doses (generally 45 mg/day) of MK-4 (menatetrenone). In Japan high-dose MK-4 is often used as a second-line treatment for osteoporosis in combination with bisphosphonates as the first-line treatment (Nawata et al., 2005). Most of the published trials with MK-4 have been implemented in patients with pre-existing involutional or secondary osteoporosis or osteopaenia. A recent meta-analysis of published randomised controlled intervention trials with vitamin K suggested a strong association of menatetrenone supplementation with reduced fracture incidence, as well as an effect in reducing bone loss (Cockayne et al., 2006). This meta-analysis also included two positive Dutch trials using phylloquinone at doses of either 10 mg/day phylloquinone in endurance athletes or 1 mg/day in postmenopausal women. The latter 3-year intervention study did not have a vitamin K group alone, but compared a group taking combined vitamins K and D (with calcium and additional minerals) with a group receiving vitamin D with calcium and additional minerals and a group taking a placebo (Braum et al., 2003). Only participants taking combined phylloquinone (1 mg), vitamin D (320 IU; 8 μg) and minerals showed a slowing of bone loss at the site of the femoral neck, but not at the lumbar spine.

There are two published randomised controlled supplementation trials in healthy elderly subjects from the UK and USA that have employed the major dietary form of vitamin K, phylloquinone at fairly modest doses of 200 μg/day (Bolton-Smith et al., 2007) and 500 μg/day, (Booth et al., 2008) respectively. Such daily amounts are potentially achievable from the diet although this would be difficult for a dose of 500 μg/day given the poor bioavailability from green-leafy vegetables which represent the richest sources of vitamin K and generally account for approximately 50% of habitual intakes. In the first UK 'dietary phylloquinone' trial over 2 years, healthy, older Scottish women were randomised to four groups as follows: (i) placebo; (ii) 200 μg phylloquinone; (iii) 400 IU (10 μg) vitamin D3 plus 1 g calcium; or (iv) combined 200 μg phylloquinone and 400 IU (10 μg) vitamin D3 plus 1 g calcium (Bolton-Smith et al., 2007). This study showed no significant intervention effect on bone loss between groups, but did show a significant increase in BMD and BMC in group (iv) at the site of the ultradistal radius, but not at other sites in the hip or radius (Bolton-Smith et al., 2007). It is of interest that a meta-analysis of studies examining the effects of vitamin K antagonists also showed that the ultradistal site was the bone site that was most responsive to loss of bone after exposure to oral anticoagulants (Caraballo et al., 1999). This effect of vitamin K antagonists seems to mirror the findings of vitamin K supplementation in the Scottish women, albeit in reverse. Overall, the opposing effects of phylloquinone in this Scottish study and the effects of vitamin K antagonists on BMD were both modest. In the USA 'dietary phylloquinone' trial over 3 years, healthy elderly North American men and women were randomised to two groups to receive daily amounts of either (i) 500 μg phylloquinone, 400 IU (10 μg) vitamin D3 plus 600 mg calcium or (ii) 400 IU (10 μg) vitamin D3 plus 600 mg calcium (Booth et al., 2008). This study showed no effect of the extra 500 μg phylloquinone (taken in addition to recommended amounts of calcium and vitamin D) on bone health as assessed by changes in BMD (femoral neck, spine, or total body) or biochemical markers of bone turnover either in men or women (Booth et al., 2008).

A recently published randomised, placebo-controlled trial from Canada tested the effect of a much larger pharmacological 5 mg daily dose of phylloquinone in postmenopausal women over 2 years and found no significant changes in BMD at any site. In a subset followed for up to 4 years, significantly fewer women in the vitamin K group had fractures than in the placebo group although numbers were small and it could not be excluded that this was a chance finding (Cheung et al., 2008).

12.5.4 Interpretation of vitamin K supplementation trials: mechanistic feasibility

It is difficult to interpret the results of the vitamin K and bone health trials that have been published to date. In part this is because of the disparity in formulations used (mainly phylloquinone or MK-4), the doses (ranging from nutritional to pharmacological) and the different populations (healthy, osteopaenic or osteoporotic). Nevertheless, the available evidence suggests that although most studies show no effect of phylloquinone or MK-4 on BMD, some studies suggest a reduction in fractures. A consistent finding of all studies is that the concentrations of circulating ucOC are markedly reduced but inter-study comparisons are restricted by the lack of method standardisation for measuring ucOC and by the finding that significant concentrations of ucOC are found in ostensibly very healthy individuals (Vermeer et al., 2004). The finding that a fraction of osteocalcin is undercarboxylated in healthy people contrasts to the finding that vitamin K-dependent coagulation proteins (synthesised in the liver) are completely carboxylated. This has led to the concept of tissue-specific requirements for vitamin K with greater intakes being required to maintain carboxylation of osteocalcin in bone compared with Gla coagulation proteins in the liver (Vermeer et al., 2004). Therefore, a key question is whether the epidemiological associations shown for high circulating ucOC and fracture risk can be explained on a mechanistic basis. We are hampered in this regard by a lack of knowledge of the molecular function(s) of osteocalcin. For example, osteocalcin-knockout mice have an increased bone formation, and seemingly stronger bones (Ducy et al., 1996). However, Fourier transform infrared microspectroscopy of osteocalcin-deficient mice suggested that osteocalcin regulates the maturation of bone mineral crystals (Boskey et al., 1998). Such changes in the mineralisation process are subtle and would not show up in conventional assessments of bone mineralisation (Boskey et al., 1998). A very recent study using human primary osteoblasts supports the concept that vitamin K is needed to promote mineralisation, and to promote osteoblast-to-osteocyte transition, at the same time deceasing the osteoclastogenic potential of these cells (Atkins et al., 2009). Although both phylloquinone and MK-4 promoted mineralisation of primary osteoblasts, that induced by MK-4 was greater and resistant to warfarin inhibition. This implied that the positive effect of vitamin K compounds on mineralisation was partly dependent on γ-carboxylation (i.e., the γ-carboxylation of proteins such as osteocalcin) and was partly γ-carboxylation-independent (Atkins et al., 2009). By contrast, the changes in cellular morphology and gene regulation induced by MK-4 were not inhibited by warfarin implying that this form can directly influence cellular events as discussed more fully in the next section ('Direct effects of menaquinone-4 in bone').

Experiments such as those by Boskey et al. (1998) and Atkins et al. (2009) suggest that vitamin K has a greater effect on bone quality than density, implying that BMD measurements alone might not reflect the real benefits of vitamin K on the skeleton (Liu and Peacock, 1998). This view is supported by recent reports that vitamin K improves hip bone geometry and bone strength indices (Kaptoge et al., 2005; Knapen et al., 2007).

If undercarboxylation of osteocalcin were very harmful, we might expect to see pronounced effects on the skeleton in patients on long-term therapy with vitamin K antagonists such as warfarin. There have now been many studies of various designs to try and answer this question but as summarised by Suttie (2009) the results have been mixed and the weight of evidence does not suggest that warfarin therapy is a significant additive risk factor for an increase in fracture rate. Whether or not ucOC is detrimental to bone health, a substantial and sustained increase in the γ-carboxylation status of osteocalcin is readily achievable by dietary supplementation with nutritionally relevant amounts of phylloquinone. This was clearly seen in the UK (Bolton-Smith et al., 2007) and USA (Booth et al., 2008) intervention studies in which daily supplementation with 200 μg and 500 μg phylloquinone, respectively, resulted in an approximate average 50% reduction in the fraction of total osteocalcin that was undercarboxylated. The vitamin K2 member, MK-7, has a longer half-life of circulation than phylloquinone and was shown to be more effective than phylloquinone in carboxylating osteocalcin when the same molar dose of 0.22 mol/day (100 μg phylloquinone; 142 μg MK-7) was given to healthy adults for 40 days (Schurgers et al., 2007c). However, without a generally accepted explanation for the role of carboxylated osteocalcin in preserving skeletal health, it is not yet possible to judge what degree of osteocalcin carboxylation is optimal; this problem is compounded by the lack of consensus on how to measure the carboxylated and undercarboxylated fractions of osteocalcin.

12.5.5 Direct effects of menaquinone-4 in bone

Although many of the effects of naturally occurring vitamin K compounds on bone can be explained by their cofactor activity in the γ-carboxylation of Gla proteins such as osteocalcin, MGP, periostin, or Gla-rich protein (thus conferring presumed biological functionality on these proteins) there is evidence that some effects are mediated by direct mechanisms that are independent of γ-carboxylation. Particular attention has focussed on one molecular form, MK-4 that appears to display unique biological actions not shared by other isoprenologues. MK-4 is also unusual in that it can be synthesised in the body from phylloquinone (and possibly other K vitamins) and has a highly specific tissue distribution suggestive of local synthesis (for review see Shearer and Newman, 2008).

The molecular biological effects of MK-4 on bone are complex and have recently been reviewed by two of the authors (Shearer and Newman, 2008). As discussed in that review many of the studies of the possible effects of MK-4 have centred on its effect on the NF-κB pathway whereby a trio of peptides called the OPG/RANKL/RANK system regulate the generation of osteoclasts. In brief, the original cloning and characterisation of osteoprotegerin (OPG) as a soluble, decoy receptor belonging to the TNF receptor super-family was the first step that led to the identification of its ligand RANKL (Receptor Activator of NF-κB Ligand) and its receptor RANK. RANKL is the cytokine essential for the differentiation of osteoclasts expressed by osteoblasts and stromal cells of bone marrow whereas its receptor RANK is expressed by osteoclasts and their precursors. OPG serves as a regulating molecule for the system by interfering with the interaction between RANKL and RANK.

One interesting feature of MK-4 is that its 3′-polyprenyl side-chain comprises the structure geranylgeranyl which is a major functional group in many isoprenylated proteins responsible for protein-protein binding. In fact Hara et al. (1995) found that both geranylgeraniol and MK-4 were able to inhibit the release of calcium from mouse calvariae induced by either $1,25(OH)_2D3$ or PGE2. A related compound, geranylgeranylacetone inhibited osteoclastogenesis from monocytes treated with RANKL and also prevented bone loss in two different animal models, ovariectomy and hindlimb unloading (Nanke et al., 2005). There are several other studies that have attributed anti-bone-resorptive effects of MK-4 to the inhibition of osteoclastogenesis mediated via control of RANKL (for review see Shearer and Newman, 2008).

Osteoclasts are short-lived cells and their activity is often terminated by apoptosis. Kameda et al. (1996) reported that MK-4, but not phylloquinone, is capable of inducing apoptosis of isolated osteoclasts cultured on dentin slices. The mechanism whereby MK-4 induced apoptosis was not addressed and this finding does not seem to have been supported by further reports. However, there is much literature concerning the apoptotic effects of MK-4 and related compounds on leukaemia cells (see section on 'Vitamin K and Cancer') so it is plausible that the monocytic progenitors of osteoclasts could be sensitive to micromolar concentrations of MK-4.

Another hypothesis that has been proposed to explain the direct actions of MK-4 on bone cells originated from the finding that MK-4 was a ligand for the steroid and xenobiotic receptor (SXR), also known as the pregnane X receptor (PXR). In brief, Tabb et al. (2003) first showed that both MK-4 and rifampicin, a prototypic SXR ligand, up-regulated the expression of several osteoblastic marker genes in several human osteosarcoma-derived cell lines and calvarial bone cells. A subsequent study by Ichikawa et al. (2006) using DNA microarray technology identified three genes with increased expression in human osteosarcoma-derived cells treated with MK-4 and rifampicin and found that one of the MK-4-responsive genes resulted in enhanced collagen accumulation. The problem of proving specificity of MK-4 versus other SXR ligands in controlling extracellular matrix-related genes appears to have been solved by further microarray analysis in which Ichikawa et al. (2007) showed that at least two genes, GDF15 and STC2, are up-regulated by MK-4 but not by phylloquinone, other menaquinones, geranylgeraniol or rifampicin. Furthermore, the regulation of these two genes was independent of γ-carboxylation with evidence that gene expression is modulated through a protein kinase A-dependent mechanism (Ichikawa et al. 2007). The potential of MK-4 regulating through SXR/PXR-mediated mechanisms, reviewed by Shearer and Newman (2008), also has relevance to some of the effects of MK-4 on cancer cells (see also section on 'Vitamin K and Cancer')

In conclusion, the way in which vitamin K compounds, particularly MK-4, exert direct biological effects on bone *in vitro* shows an almost bewildering complexity and multiplicity of possible mechanisms that still need to be resolved. Perhaps the most promising lines of enquiry are those based on the modulation of the OPG/RANKL/RANK system and gene regulation via the SXR/PXR pathways. Such pathways seem to be independent of vitamin K-dependent γ-carboxylation but might work in synergy with the measurable increase in γ-carboxylation of osteocalcin (and presumably other bone Gla-proteins) seen *in vivo*, including human trials. At present there have been too few human trials with fracture as the main outcome measure and although such trials would be costly, a recent review commissioned by the UK Health Technology Assessment programme suggested that an appropriately designed vitamin K trial would be a cost effective use of resources (Stevenson et al., 2009).

12.6 Vitamin K and vascular calcification

12.6.1 Historical perspective

As already outlined in the section on 'Vitamin K and Bone Health', the vitamin K-dependent protein MGP was purified from bone in the mid-1980s and originally believed only to play a role in bone metabolism, particularly in the prevention of inappropriate calcification of the growth plate. It was not until 1997 that the creation of the MGP-knockout mouse by the group of Karsenty revealed a hitherto unsuspected extension of the anti-mineralisation properties seen in growing bone to its role as a crucial inhibitor of calcification in vessel walls (Luo et al., 1997). MGP-deficient animals all died before reaching the age of 8 weeks owing to ruptures of the calcified vascular system. Elastic fibres in the vascular media were all calcified and some vascular smooth muscle cells (VSMCs) trans-differentiated into chondrocyte-like and osteoblast-like cells, supporting further calcification. In a follow up study the same group elegantly showed that the anti-mineralisation property of MGP was only functional when the protein was synthesised locally (Murshed et al., 2004). Thus, to inhibit vascular calcification, MGP needs to be synthesised by the VSMCs. No protection against calcification was seen in knockout mice in which hepatic synthesis had been restored and, with this systemic presence, plasma concentrations raised (Murshed et al., 2004). Substitution of MGP by the vitamin K-dependent protein osteocalcin did not rescue the calcification phenotype of knockout mice. Moreover, mutagenesis of glutamate residues that normally undergo γ-carboxylation into aspartate residues completely blocked the function of MGP providing evidence that the Gla residues are essential for the anti-mineralisation properties of MGP. The crucial role of vitamin K in the inhibition of vascular calcification *in vivo* became clear from experiments in a rat model developed by Paul Price to study the effect of the vitamin K antagonist warfarin on arterial calcification (Price et al., 1998). This model draws on knowledge that when high doses of warfarin are administered to rats the concomitant administration of vitamin K can overcome the antagonism of warfarin in liver but not in extrahepatic tissues such as bone and the vasculature. Thus the effects of warfarin on extrahepatic tissues can be studied without the animals succumbing to bleeding. Using this rat model Price and co-workers showed that warfarin caused calcification of the elastic lamellae in arteries and heart valves within 2–4 weeks (Price et al., 1998). An explanation for the lack of antidotal effect of vitamin K in inhibiting vascular calcification was provided by Reidar Wallin who showed that the warfarin-insensitive, vitamin K reductase activity in VSMCs was 100-fold less active than that in the liver (Wallin et al., 1999). By contrast, using the same warfarin/vitamin K model, Spronk et al. (2003) showed that substituting phylloquinone with MK-4 resulted in complete inhibition of vascular calcification with evidence of a preferential uptake and utilisation of MK-4 by aortic tissue; the authors also suggested that the anti-mineralisation properties of MK-4 might be due to the atypical actions shown by MK-4 on cells as described elsewhere in this chapter.

12.6.2 Matrix Gla-protein: structure and properties

Matrix Gla-protein (MGP) is a 10 kDa protein which is expressed by many cells, but mainly by chondrocytes and VSMCs. In addition to the vitamin K-dependent carboxylation, MGP undergoes a second post-translational modification, namely serine-phosphorylation. To date, the best studied modification is γ-glutamyl carboxylation in which five of the originally synthesised nine glutamate residues are converted into Gla residues (▶Fig. 12.3). Phosphorylation of serine residues can occur at positions 3, 6 and 9 of MGP. It has been shown that the motif in MGP that serves as a signal to enable serine phosphorylation is the tandemly repeated Ser-X-Glu sequence (Price et al., 1983). By analogy to other proteins with the same motif, MGP is probably phosphorylated by Golgi casein kinase, a membrane kinase located in the Golgi apparatus (Price et al., 1983; Wajih et al., 2004). The function of MGP phosphorylation is not precisely known, but could play a role in regulating the secretion of proteins into the extracellular environment. This is supported by the finding that phosphorylated MGP exits VSMCs via the secretory pathway, whereas the non-phosphorylated MGP appears in the cytosol (Wajih et al., 2004).

12.6.3 Brief overview of molecular concepts of vascular calcification

It is well known that human arteries are prone to calcification and that this process increases with age and is also associated with a wide range of diseases. It can occur independently at two sites; firstly the tunica media which when calcified is known as medial elastocalcinosis and secondly the intima in association with atherosclerosis.

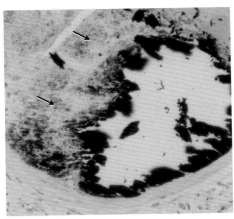

Fig. 12.4: Disease-induced calcification of the tunica media of human arteries. Section of a peripheral artery obtained from a patient with diabetes mellitus and end stage renal disease. The section was stained with von Kossa stain which shows areas of mineralization as dark brown or black from the deposition of silver. The medial layer of the artery can be seen to be completely calcified. The arrows indicate vesicular structures that are characteristic of the onset of calcification.

Vascular calcification was once considered to be a passive, clinically irrelevant process, resulting from a high calcium–phosphate product, inflammation, lipid accumulation or diabetes. However, recent studies clearly demonstrate that vascular calcification is an actively regulated process. Apoptosis is thought to precede vascular calcification (Proudfoot et al., 2002). The formation of matrix vesicles and apoptotic bodies in the vessel wall is thought to be crucial in the process of vascular calcification (Reynolds et al., 2004). VSMCs undergoing apoptosis generate phosphatidyl serine positive membrane particles which, if not properly phagocytosed, promote the initiation of calcification by serving as the initial starting point for calcium salt precipitation (Proudfoot et al., 2002; Reynolds et al., 2004; Shroff et al., 2008). Matrix vesicles and apoptotic bodies have been shown to be present in atherosclerotic plaques and in medial elastocalcinosis. These small calcium crystals are the next trigger for the differentiation of VSMCc into chondrocyte- and osteoblast-like cells. Medial arterial calcification is highly prevalent in certain diseases such as type II diabetes and chronic kidney disease and also portends cardiovascular morbidity and mortality risk. ▶Fig. 12.4 illustrates the complete calcification of the medial layer of a peripheral artery taken from a patient with diabetes and end-stage renal disease.

12.6.4 How does MGP prevent vascular calcification?

One of the characteristics of Gla-containing proteins is their negative charge, enabling them to bind to negatively charged phospholipids via calcium. The inhibitory effect of MGP on calcium precipitation and crystallisation could be achieved in a similar direct way (Schurgers et al., 2005; Schurgers et al., 2007a). Another putative mechanism whereby MGP prevents calcification is through the inhibition of bone morphogenetic protein-2 (BMP-2) (Wallin et al., 2000; Bostrom et al., 2001). BMP-2 belongs to the TGF-beta family. BMP-2 serves as an osteogenic growth factor, causing VSMCs to trans-differentiate into bone-like cells. MGP is found concentrated in so-called matrix vesicles and apoptotic bodies (Reynolds et al., 2004). These vesicular structures are thought to be the nidus for vascular calcification. VSMCs could respond to stress signals by shed-ding off these vesicles. These vesicular structures, when not phagocytosed efficiently can nucleate calcium and phosphate intravesicularly, the same action as observed in hypertrophic chondrocytes. One hypothesis is that MGP counterbalances potentially harmful high intracellular or intravesicular calcium concentrations.

The development of conformation-specific antibodies against MGP by one of the authors (LJS) and co-workers in Maastricht (Schurgers et al., 2005) has enabled the differential detection and localisation of undercarboxylated MGP (ucMGP) from car-boxylated MGP (cMGP) in tissues (Schurgers et al., 2005; Shroff et al., 2008). Using these antibodies, immunohistochemical analysis of healthy and sclerotic human arter-ies has revealed that sites of vascular calcification are associated with high amounts of ucMGP whereas healthy arteries largely contain cMGP located around elastin fibres in the tunica media (Schurgers et al., 2005; Shroff et al., 2008). Several studies have dem-onstrated that ucMGP accumulates in and around the calcified vascular areas, whereas cMGP is absent from calcified regions. Presently the relations between these findings with respect to cause and effect are unclear. On the one hand, it could be argued that a chronic local vitamin K insufficiency is the initiating event leading to impaired γ-carboxylation and increased synthesis of ucMGP, which is unable to prevent vascular calcification. On the other hand, local vascular calcification comes first (e.g., induced by inflammation and oxidative stress) leading to exhaustion of local vitamin K stores, again preventing the γ-carboxylation of MGP, which itself would lead to accelerated and enhanced vascular calcifications. However, in both scenarios, ucMGP and cMGP might serve as discriminating biomarkers for vascular calcification. Moreover, the use of these antibodies in ELISA-based techniques could result in the measurement of circulating MGP, serving as biomarkers for vascular disease.

12.6.5 Measurement of serum MGP in different disease states

The use of circulating biomarkers such as MGP for detecting or screening cardiovas-cular disease and/or vascular calcification is an attractive possibility. One use in the diagnostic area might be to pre-screen patients before subjecting them to electron beam or X-ray multislice computed tomography (CT) scanning. Such imaging techniques are already widely used to screen patients for coronary calcifications (Raggi et al., 2004) but have the disadvantages of causing an increased cancer risk owing to the radiation load (Brenner et al., 2007). Radiation exposure is particularly important for regular follow-up during treatment.

Currently, markers for vascular calcification include osteoprotegerin, fetuin-A, under carboxylated osteocalcin, fibroblast growth factor-23 and MGP. The advantage of MGP is that it represents a locally synthesised vascular protein and its functional activity can be modified by vitamin K or vitamin K-antagonists (coumarin or indanedione oral anticoagulants) (Schurgers et al., 2008). The concentrations of MGP reaching the cir-culation will depend on the rate of MGP synthesis and MGP activity in vascular tissue and subsequent binding of MGP to calcified vascular areas. Early assays for serum MGP measured only the total circulating protein independently of the phosphorylation and carboxylation post-translational modifications. Using such an assay O'Donnell et al. (2006) measured total MGP in two separate populations of Americans free of clinically apparent cardiovascular disease and found that MGP concentrations were associated with individual coronary heart disease risk factors.

Potentially, MGP can be secreted or released into the circulation as different species according to the degree to which they possess the phosphorylated and γ-carboxylated post-translational modifications (i.e., combinations of phosphorylated, desphosphory-lated, carboxylated, undercarboxylated, fragments) (Schurgers et al., 2008). Therefore, both basic and clinical research is needed to try and correlate each MGP species with local vascular events. The effect of phosphorylation and γ-carboxylation is to confer an extra negative charge to the MGP protein, thereby increasing the affinity for calcifica-tion sites (Schurgers et al., 2007a). The fully functional form of MGP would be both phosphorylated and carboxylated but the extent to which this form can escape from the vasculature into the circulation is presently unknown because assays that can de-tect serum concentrations of the fully active protein are presently lacking. By contrast, desphosphorylated or undercarboxylated species of MGP have less affinity for calcifi-cation sites, and therefore might be expected to be released into the bloodstream. The Maastricht group have developed conformation specific MGP immunoassays for mea-suring desphosphorylated and undercarboxylated MGP (Schurgers et al., 2008) and the results using these assays support the concept of their greater discriminating power in clinical studies (Cranenburg et al., 2008; Schurgers et al., 2010). Thus far, the use of dif-ferent assays for MGP appears to offer a valuable tool for predicting vascular and aortic calcification (Cranenburg et al., 2009; Koos et al., 2009) or even mortality (Schurgers et al., 2010).

The serum ucMGP competitive immunoassay developed in Maastricht has been used to investigate the usefulness of this assay as a marker for vascular disease in a wide range of patient populations prone to develop arterial calcification, including patients with atherosclerosis and renal disease (Cranenburg et al., 2008). This ucMGP assay was found to be particularly successful in identifying vascular mineralisation pathologies in patients with end-stage renal disease (haemodialysis patients). The very low serum ucMGP levels found in haemodialysis patients might be explained by the known ac-cumulation of ucMGP at sites of arterial calcification (Schurgers et al., 2005; Shroff et al., 2008), suggesting that ucMGP is not easily set free into the circulation . This could indicate that low ucMGP levels are a marker of active calcification. This is supported by the findings in a well-characterised cohort of haemodialysis patients that showed an inverse correlation between circulating ucMGP levels and coronary artery calcium scores as measured by multislice CT (Cranenburg et al., 2009; Koos et al., 2009). Unfor-tunately, the serum assay for ucMGP was not influenced by vitamin K supplementation or coumarin therapy and so could not be used to predict the vascular vitamin K-status; this is in contrast to analogous assays for osteocalcin (ucOC) that are sensitive to vita-min K status. The further development by the Maastricht group of an immunoassay that could detect the MGP antigen that was both desphosphorylated and uncarboxylated (dp-ucMGP) was expected to be more informative because it is known that this inactive protein has low affinity for calcium-salts and matrix vesicles (Schurgers et al., 2007a) and should be readily set free into the circulation. High serum concentrations of dp-ucMGP might thus reflect an impaired vascular vitamin K-status. In a recent study in

109 haemodialysis patients, it was found that high serum dp-ucMGP concentrations significantly correlated with both vascular calcification (as measured by multislice CT scan) and mortality (Schurgers et al., 2010). In a second study in which dp-ucMGP was measured in aortic stenosis patients it was confirmed that high dp-ucMGP was correlated with mortality and heart failure (Ueland et al., 2010). Thus the measurement of biomarkers such as MGP, which reflect early signs of vascular disease, could be of great importance to decision-making in clinical practice. Most results to date have been obtained in chronic kidney disease, diabetes mellitus or aortic stenosis patients. Currently data are lacking in atherosclerotic patients. More research is needed to link each circulating MGP fraction to specific vascular events.

12.6.6 Vitamin K status and vascular health: Epidemiological studies and intervention trials

In an analysis among 4500 subjects of the so-called Rotterdam Study cohort the dietary intake of menaquinones (vitamin K2) was inversely associated with vascular calcification and cardiovascular mortality (Geleijnse et al., 2004). The cardiovascular mortality in the highest tertile for menaquinone intake was some 50% lower compared with the lowest tertile of menaquinone intake. No such association was found for phylloquinone intakes. In another recent epidemiological study from the Netherlands, it was found that menaquinone intakes were associated with cardio-protective activity (Gast et al., 2009). This study examined data from 16 000 women aged 49–70 years, enrolled to the Dutch Prospect–EPIC study who were free of cardiovascular disease at baseline and who were followed up for an average of 8 years. The results suggested a reduction of incidence of coronary heart disease of 9% for every 10 µg increase in adjusted dietary intake of menaquinones. The first clinical trial investigating vitamin K intake and vascular properties was done in postmenopausal women (Braam et al., 2004). In this randomised controlled trial, a daily supplement of 1 mg phylloquinone (also containing vitamin D and other minerals) taken for 3 years improved vascular compliance, distensibility and intima-media thickness as compared with the placebo group. Recently, an intervention trial in apparently healthy older men and women provided further evidence for an important function of vitamin K in vascular health (Shea et al., 2009). In this randomised controlled trial the daily intake of an extra 0.5 mg phylloquinone contained in a multi-vitamin formulation for 3 years significantly halted the progression of coronary artery calcification as measured by multislice CT imaging. Furthermore, phylloquinone-associated decreases in coronary artery calcium progression were independent of changes in total serum MGP antigen or changes in proinflammatory cytokine markers (Shea et al., 2009).

12.6.7 Warfarin and vitamin K interactions: effects on vascular calcification

As previously discussed in the 'Historical perspective' section, vitamin K-antagonists such as warfarin block vitamin K-metabolism, leading to impaired MGP synthesis. Schurgers et al. (2007b) showed that warfarin-induced calcification in rats could be reversed after stopping warfarin therapy by administering high-dose phylloquinone or MK-4; the degree of calcification reversal was estimated to be approximately 40% within 6 weeks of stopping warfarin. In addition to reversing calcification, high-dose phylloquinone and MK-4 treatment also restored measures of vascular elasticity. In the same study, it had been shown that control rats accumulated MK-4 in their aortas at higher concentrations than phylloquinone (Schurgers et al., 2007b); this finding is in keeping with the known ability of cells to convert phylloquinone to MK-4 as discussed elsewhere in this chapter. However in the warfarin-treated rats, MK-4 was undetectable in aortas and the only detectable molecular forms of vitamin K were phylloquinone and phylloquinone epoxide. The accumulation of the epoxide-form of vitamin K suggests that the VKOR cycle was active but could not prevent calcification. The same absence of aortal MK-4 in the Price warfarin/phylloquinone rat model had been previously found in an earlier study from this group although in that study MK-4 had been shown to be superior in preventing arterial calcification (Spronk et al., 2003). The absence of MK-4 in the arteries of the warfarin-treated rats given phylloquinone can be explained by previous data showing that prenylation of menadione to MK-4 is inhibited by vitamin K-antagonists (Taggart et al., 1969). This, together with evidence that menadione is an intermediate in the conversion of phylloquinone to MK-4 (i.e., produced by side-chain cleavage) (Shearer and Newman, 2008), gives an explanation for the lack of efficacy of phylloquinone when warfarin is being given as well as an explanation of why phylloquinone can be effective once warfarin is stopped.

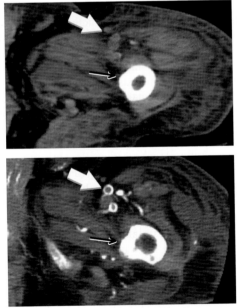

Fig. 12.5: Coumarin anticoagulants promote vascular calcification. CT scans of the leg of a patient diagnosed with atrial fibrillation taken before (**top**) and after (**bottom**) a 9-month course of therapy with a coumarin anticoagulant. In these scans mineralized tissue can be seen as white areas with the small arrows denoting the femur bone. In the pre-treatment scan (**top**) no calcification of the femoral arteries was evident. However, after coumarin treatment (**bottom**) the patient had developed massive calcification of all medium-sized and larger arterial vessels (large arrows).

There is now evidence that an unintended consequence of oral anticoagulant therapy in humans is to accelerate vascular calcification (Schurgers et al., 2004). This is illustrated by the CT scan in ▶Fig. 12.5 showing the development of arterial calcification within 9 months of a patient starting oral anticoagulant therapy.

12.6.8 Patient population studies

The finding that vitamin K-deficiency induced by warfarin is strongly linked to vascular calcification is leading to new investigations of vitamin K status in patient groups prone to vascular calcification, particularly those with chronic kidney disease. A recent study of vitamin K status in stages 3–5 of chronic kidney disease found that subclinical vitamin K deficiency was common with an elevated PIVKA-II (a marker of suboptimal liver stores of vitamin K) seen in 95% of the patients studied (Holden et al., 2010). In another study using the newly developed dp-ucMGP assay, high circulating levels were found in all dialysis patients suggesting severe local vitamin K deficiency in the vasculature (Schurgers et al., 2010). The first dose-finding pilot study in which daily oral supplements of a long-chain vitamin K2 (MK-7) were given to haemodialysis patients was recently published in abstract form and resulted in significant improvements in γ-carboxylation of MGP, osteocalcin and prothrombin (Westenfeld et al., 2008). The perceived advantage of using MK-7 (rather than phylloquinone or MK-4) is that MK-7 has a longer half-life in the circulation (Shearer and Newman, 2008) and has a greater efficacy for carboxylating both hepatic and extrahepatic Gla-proteins (Schurgers et al., 2007c).

12.6.9 MGP and vascular health: conclusions

It is now well established that MGP has an important biological function as a potent inhibitor of vascular calcification. MGP functional activity is reduced by vitamin K-absence or antagonism, and a dysfunctional protein becomes a significant contributor to vascular calcification. Further investigations of the value of MGP measurements as a biomarker of calcification and local vascular vitamin K status, as well as clinical trials to investigate the potential benefit of vitamin K supplementation, will result in a better understanding of the role of MGP. Further research is needed to evaluate the relations between dietary intakes of vitamin K or measures of local vascular vitamin K status with vessel wall calcification and elasticity outcome measures. The potential deleterious effects of oral anticoagulant therapy on vascular health also need to be further evaluated.

12.7 Vitamin K and cancer

Within the past 20 years several studies have provided evidence that in some cancer cell types certain forms of vitamin K can restrict growth or induce apoptotic cell death or differentiation. Some studies have compared the effects of different forms of vitamin K, or the effects on different cell types, or both and the results are not entirely consistent. Most work has been done on either cells or cell lines isolated from patients with leukaemia or hepatocellular carcinoma (HCC). There is also some epidemiologic evidence linking menaquinone intake with cancer risk.

12.7.1 Studies on leukaemia cells

One of the earliest of these studies tested the effects of menadione, phylloquinone and warfarin on cultured murine leukaemia cell lines (Chlebowski et al., 1985) and found that menadione inhibited growth of L1210 cells. This growth inhibition was enhanced when combined with warfarin. When the same cells were cultured in soft agar to measure colony formation, the same drugs inhibited this effect as well. A variety of human tumour explants from ovary, colon, stomach, kidney, lung and breast tumours were also grown in soft agar and they responded to menadione in the same concentration range. Another study showed that MK-4, but not phylloquinone, induced several human myeloid cell lines including ML1, HL-60 and U937 to differentiate (Sakai et al., 1994). The effect was enhanced when MK-4 was combined with another inducer of differentiation such as retinoic acid, interferon-gamma or campothecin, implying that MK-4 could have potential as a non-toxic therapeutic for some forms of leukaemia. The fact that phylloquinone did not have this effect suggested that the geranylgeranyl side-chain of the molecule might be responsible.

In a separate study Ohizumi et al., (1995) found that geranylgeraniol, the alcohol derivative of the side-chain of MK-4 could induce apoptosis in one of the same cell lines, HL-60, in addition to two other leukaemia-derived cell lines and one from a colonic adenocarcinoma. A later study (Yaguchi et al., 1997) compared the effects of three menaquinones MKs-3, -4 and -5 on leukaemia cell lines with their corresponding 3'-side-chain polyprenyl alcohols and phylloquinone. They found that all three MKs and geranylfarnesol, the alcohol derivative of the side-chain of MK-3, can induce apoptosis in all freshly isolated leukaemia cells tested and on two leukaemia cell lines whereas phylloquinone had no effect. The induction of apoptosis was enhanced by the addition of all-trans-retinoic acid. Subsequent flow-cytometric analysis showed that the cells being targeted were mainly poorly differentiated blastic cells rather than mature myeloid cells (Yaguchi et al., 1998).

12.7.2 Apoptosis versus differentiation

The literature mentioned above showed evidence for vitamins K causing either apoptosis or differentiation in leukaemia cells and two studies have addressed the issue of why vitamin K should cause one effect or the other. When HL-60 cells were treated with MK-4 they underwent apoptosis but when they were first transfected with bcl-2, a gene which protects cells against apoptosis, they predictably became less apoptotic but upon MK-4 treatment they instead underwent cell cycle arrest and differentiation (Miyazawa et al., 2001). However, when HL-60 cells were induced to undergo differentiation by the addition of a novel synthetic vitamin D derivative, the combination of this compound and MK-4 caused cell cycle arrest, greatly enhanced differentiation and suppressed apoptotic responses such as caspase-3 expression suggesting that differentiation and apoptosis are inversely regulated (Funato et al., 2002).

12.7.3 Studies on hepatocellular carcinoma

A common feature of HCC, which is often used as a diagnostic test for the disease, is the appearance of high concentrations of PIVKA-II in the circulation (Liebman et al., 1984).

At one time it was thought that PIVKA-II could be a cause of neoplasia rather than an effect that results from it. This explains why early investigators sought to reduce PIVKA-II synthesis in HCC cells by supplementing them with vitamin K and thereby discovered that some forms of vitamin K were themselves growth inhibitory agents. It has since been proposed that PIVKA-II becomes synthesised by hepatocytes when they undergo epithelial to mesenchymal transition because of cytoskeletal changes which compromise their ability to take in lipoproteins, and therefore vitamin K, by clathrin-mediated endocytosis (Murata and Sakamoto, 2008).

As found in leukaemia cell lines, MK-4 and menadione appear to have growth suppressive effects on HCC cells but phylloquinone does not. Early studies found that vitamins K suppressed growth of HCC cell lines in culture and that this growth inhibition was accompanied by different alterations in gene expression to those found in response to TGF-beta, a known inhibitor of hepatocyte proliferation (Bouzahzah et al., 1995; Wang et al., 1995). Wang et al. (1995) demonstrated that menadione, MK-4 and phylloquinone all suppressed the secretion of PIVKA-II in an HCC line and additionally MK-4 and menadione, but not phylloquinone, inhibited cell growth in a reversible fashion. The mechanism of action of the two compounds was clearly not the same because the menadione-induced inhibition was blocked by the addition of the enzyme catalase which suggested that menadione was working by inducing oxidative stress in the cells. MK-4 effects were not blocked by catalase implying that it had a different means of retarding cell growth which has been the subject of extensive studies. MK-4 suppressed HCC tumour growth in athymic nude mice (Hitomi et al., 2005) and was observed to induce cell cycle arrest in HCC cells *in vitro* (Matsumoto et al., 2006; Liu et al., 2007). This corresponded with a decrease in the mRNA and protein levels of cyclin D1 and in some cell lines with an increase in the mRNA levels of the cdk inhibitors p21 and p27 (Ozaki et al., 2007). Furthermore, the expression of cyclin D1 was shown to be due to suppression of the NF-κB pathway via the inhibition of IκB kinase and a reduction in the phosphorylation and degradation of IκBα. Other cell cycle molecules have also been found to be regulated by vitamins K such as cdk4 which was reduced in experimental tumours when the animals were treated with MK-4, menadione or vitamin K5, a synthetic derivative of menadione, whereas the cell cycle-suppressing molecules p16INK4a and Rb were elevated (Kuriyama et al., 2005). MK-4 has also been reported to inhibit the invasiveness of HCC and appears to do so by activation of AP-2, USF-1 and CREB dependent transcription, possibly by activation of protein kinase A (Otsuka et al., 2004). MK-4 has also been shown to inhibit the proliferation of endothelial cells in culture and suppress the formation of endothelial cell tubules (Yoshiji et al., 2005) which has implications for angiogenesis. There is also a report that MK-4 inhibits expression of metalloproteinases 1, 3 and 7 which again, appears to be mediated through suppression of the NF-κB pathway (Ide et al., 2009).

The means by which vitamins K mediate their effects in cells are still poorly understood, however MK-4 is a known ligand of the nuclear receptor SXR (Ichikawa et al., 2006) (see section on 'Vitamin K and Bone Health'). Recent work has shown that MK-4 can suppress the proliferation of HCC cell lines when they were made to overexpress SXR and exposed to MK-4 (Azuma et al., 2009). The SXR-transfected cells also became less motile when challenged with MK-4 in a cell migration assay. This does suggest that at least some of the cellular effects of MK-4 could be mediated through SXR although it would seem that there are multiple mechanisms at work in the actions of MK-4 on HCC cells.

12.7.4 Clinical cancer studies and combination therapies

MK-4 has been used clinically to reduce the incidence of HCC in high-risk groups. An early trial involved giving 45 mg/day to women with viral liver cirrhosis which often predisposes individuals to HCC (Habu et al., 2004). Although only a small study, the incidence of HCC was lower in the treated group with only two out of 21 patients compared with nine out of 19 in the control group. Another trial tested the effect of MK-4 on the recurrence of HCC in remission patients following the removal of primary tumours by either surgical resection or by ablation therapy (Mizuta et al., 2006). The MK-4 group experienced less HCC recurrence after 1, 2 or 3 years with a survival rate of 87% after 3 years compared with 64% in the control group although some further studies have failed to confirm this finding using MK-4 as a single agent.

For over 20 years vitamin K compounds have been tested for the ability to potentiate the effects of several chemotherapeutic drugs. Initially menadione was used in conjunction with various drugs in a mouse model of transplanted liver tumours and generally increased the mean survival time when it was administered before the drug rather than after it (Taper et al., 1987). Menadione is rather toxic to humans so more recent efforts have been directed to menaquinones and phylloquinone. Using an animal model in which hepatocarcinogenesis was induced in rats using diethylnitrosamine, Yoshiji et al. (2005) reported that a combination of MK-4 and the angiotensin converting enzyme-inhibitor perindopril reduced both the number and size of pre-neoplastic hepatic lesions to a greater extent than either agent alone (Yoshiji et al., 2005). A similar effect was seen on the expression of CD31, a marker of neovascularisation which was elevated by carcinogenesis but reduced by treatment with MK-4 and perindopril. The same group have recently published a small clinical study in which the same two drugs were administered for 36–48 months to patients following curative therapy for HCC (Yoshiji et al., 2009). The results showed that the combination significantly reduced the recurrence of HCC but that either drug alone was unable to do so. Yoshiji's clinical study also reported that serum VEGF levels were significantly reduced by MK-4/perindopril after 12 months of treatment which taken together with the previous findings that MK-4 was anti-proliferative for endothelial cells suggest that the reduction in HCC recurrence was at least in part, caused by an inhibition of angiogenesis.

Most investigations have been done on HCC but one recent study tested the combined effects of vitamins K and sorafenib on three pancreatic adenocarcinoma cell lines (Wei et al., 2010). The combination of vitamin K and sorafenib, which is a multikinase inhibitor, reduced cell growth more than either agent alone and induced caspase-mediated apoptosis. This study was unusual in that it reported a growth inhibitory effect using phylloquinone whereas virtually all other studies, mainly on cancer cell lines derived from HCC or leukaemia, reported effects with menaquinones such as MK-4, or menadione but no effect with phylloquinone. This might be unique to pancreatic cancer cells. Finally, the effects of several vitamin K compounds were compared in an *in vivo* tumour model using colorectal cancer cells injected subcutaneously into mice (Ogawa et al., 2007). The compounds were tested on cultured cells first and menadione and K5 were found to reduce cell viability far more than MK-4 whereas phylloquinone had no effect. When tested on tumours *in vivo*, menadione, K5 and MK-4 all induced apoptotic cell death in the tumours. Phylloquinone was not tested *in vivo*.

12.7.5 Epidemiological studies of vitamin K and cancer

There are a few epidemiological studies which attempted to evaluate any association between dietary intake of vitamin K and prostate cancer. Nimptsch et al. (2008) assessed the intake of phylloquinone and menaquinones 4–14 of over 11 000 men and recorded the incidence of prostate cancer over a mean follow-up period of 8.6 years. No association was found for phylloquinone and prostate cancer but a non-significant inverse association was found between menaquinones and relative risk of prostate cancer. This association was stronger when restricted only to cases of advanced prostate cancer and even stronger when limited only to MKs 5–9 which are mainly derived from dairy sources rather than other menaquinones which are mostly derived from dietary meat or offal. More recently, this study has been extended to investigate possible associations between vitamin K intake and the incidence and mortality of other common cancers including lung, breast and colorectal in addition to prostate (Nimptsch et al., 2010). The findings show a non-significant inverse association between menaquinone intake and overall cancer incidence and a stronger inverse association with cancer mortality. A significant effect was seen in men but not in women and this was related to particularly strong inverse associations for prostate and lung cancers, which were the first and third most frequent cancer sites in men in this study, but not breast cancer which was the most common cancer site among women. As before, no association was found between phylloquinone intake and cancer. Finally, an attempt was made to use a biomarker of vitamin K status, namely ucOC, to investigate the association between vitamin K and prostate cancer to overcome the errors associated with food-frequency questionnaires which were used in the studies mentioned above (Nimptsch et al., 2009). The problem here is that the ratio of ucOC to intact total OC (ucOC/iOC) only gives an indication of overall vitamin K status but does not distinguish between phylloquinone or menaquinone status. The authors try to overcome this by combining data on menaquinone intake and ucOC/OC ratios into a 'vitamin K supply score' which was non-significantly inversely associated with total prostate cancer. However, a comparison of the highest and lowest quartiles of vitamin K supply score showed a significant decreased risk for advanced stage prostate cancer in the highest quartile.

12.8 Miscellaneous effects of vitamin K

12.8.1 Anti-inflammatory effects of vitamin K

Vitamin K has been linked to anti-inflammatory effects in certain cell and animal models and, to some extent in a population study. When fibroblasts were treated with lipopolysaccharide (LPS) they secreted interleukin-6 (IL-6), a potent inflammatory mediator but the response was reduced when the cells were treated first with vitamin K as either MK-4, phylloquinone or various synthetic forms (Reddi et al., 1995). A further study on rats using a DNA microarray technique demonstrated that when the animals were fed on a diet depleted in vitamin K the expression of genes involved in the acute inflammatory response was elevated (Ohsaki et al., 2006). Animals fed with a diet supplemented with phylloquinone had decreased expression levels of some inflammatory markers in blood plasma and liver when compared with the control group. The authors also showed that

LPS-induced stimulation of IL-6 expression in human THP-1 macrophages is suppressed when the cells were pre-incubated with phylloquinone before exposure to LPS. This is interesting because the effect of LPS on IL-6 expression is known to be mediated by the NF-κB pathway which appears to be a target of vitamin K action in HCC although in that case only MK-4 was reported to be active.

A publication from the Framingham Offspring Study cohort has reported associations between the status and intake of vitamins K and D and a series of proinflammatory markers. The results showed an inverse relation between phylloquinone, either measured in blood plasma or estimated from dietary intake, and the expression of inflammatory markers (Shea et al., 2008).

12.8.2 Vitamin K can prevent oxidative damage to oligodendrocytes

Vitamin K has shown potential as a means of protecting developing oligodendrocytes from oxidative cell death which might be of use in preventing ischaemic brain injury in premature infants. When primary cultures of rat oligodendrocytes were exposed to oxidative stress by changing the cells to a cysteine-free medium, the resulting glutathione deficiency led to cell death. This was prevented by the addition of either phylloquinone or MK-4 to the culture medium at normal physiological concentrations in the nanomolar range (Li et al., 2003). This protective effect required the entire naphthoquinone molecules, not just the 3-side-chains and did not require γ-glutamyl carboxylase activity. The compounds did not appear to be working by a simple antioxidant mechanism because no such activity attributable to vitamin K could be detected in the experimental system used.

The most recent report on this topic focused on oxidative damage caused by arachidonic acid which is released by the action of phospholipase A2 on membrane phospholipids during brain ischaemia and then metabolised to free radicals and peroxides. In these experiments both phylloquinone and MK-4 were found to reduce the activity of 12-lipoxygenase, and the subsequent formation of reactive oxygen species and cell death (Li et al., 2009). This was found not to be due to direct binding of vitamin K molecules to the enzyme itself and therefore more probably due to inhibition of pathways upstream of the lipoxygenase itself or to inhibition by vitamin K metabolites. The exact mechanism of action is still not known but the low toxicity of vitamin K means it has potential as a therapeutic agent in preventing ischaemic injury to oligodendrocytes.

12.8.3 Vitamin K secretion by the pancreas

The ratio of phylloquinone to menaquinones varies between different tissues, however, the pancreas has been found to secrete MK-4 when stimulated with either cholecystokinin-8 or secretin which are both known to be active on pancreatic acinar cells (Thomas et al., 2004). The purpose of this MK-4 secretion is not known but occurs concurrently with the release of phospholipase enzymes and caveolin-1, a membrane trafficking protein so it could have some exocrine function in these cells. Immunohistochemical staining with anti-Gla antibodies showed staining in the α-cells of the pancreas which secrete glucagon, but very little staining in the acinar cells which means that the function of MK-4 is unlikely to be related to carboxylation (Stenberg et al., 2001).

12.8.4 Vitamin K and sphingolipid biosynthesis

Sphingolipids are a group of lipids abundant in the brain which are derived from the amino alcohol sphingosine. Vitamin K has been known to be involved in the biosynthesis of sphingolipids since the early 1970s when it was discovered that a vitamin K-dependent bacteria developed defective cell envelopes when grown in a vitamin K-depleted medium (Lev and Milford, 1972). This was due to the reduced activity of the first enzyme of the sphingolipid synthetic pathway, 3-ketodihydrosphingosine synthase. The mammalian equivalent of this enzyme was also found to be depleted in microsomal preparations from warfarin-treated mouse brain which resulted in a significant reduction in brain sulfatides (Sundaram and Lev, 1988). This was restored to normal by the administration of phylloquinone to the mice. A further enzyme in the brain, galactocerebroside sulfotransferase was also found to be sensitive to vitamin K depletion and was restored by either phylloquinone or MK-4 (Sundaram and Lev, 1990; Sundaram et al., 1996). MK-4 is the principal form of vitamin K found in mammalian brain (Thijssen and Drittij-Reijnders, 1994; Thijssen and Drittij-Reijnders, 1996) and its distribution in the brain correlates with areas of high sphingolipid concentrations (Carrie et al., 2004) although it is still not known by which mechanism vitamin K exerts its effects on these enzymes. Sphingolipids are important components of myelinated cells and it is possible that their depletion might explain behavioural disorders related to warfarin treatment or vitamin K deficiency in animal studies (Cocchetto et al., 1985).

12.8.5 Summary of cellular mechanisms of vitamin K action

In summary, cancer cell growth was generally inhibited by menadione and MK-4, and in some cases other menaquinones but not by phylloquinone. The notable exception was the study on pancreatic cancer cells which showed that phylloquinone in combination with sorafenib inhibited their growth but that phylloquinone had little or no effect alone (Wei et al., 2010).

Menadione is active at lower concentrations than menaquinones typically at approximately 10–50 μM depending on the cell line and seems to work by imposing oxidative stress on the cells. Menaquinones do not affect oxidative stress and appear to be nontoxic but only inhibit growth at higher concentrations, typically at approximately the 100 μM range in cell culture. Most of the work on menaquinones and cancer cells has been done using MK-4, probably because this is widely used clinically in Japan (brand-name Menatetrenone), as a treatment for osteoporosis. It is therefore known to be safe when administered for long periods at a high dose, typically 45 mg/day in Japan.

Some of the cellular effects of menaquinones, including the induction of apoptosis in some leukaemia cells, are mimicked by the alcohol or aldehyde derivatives of their 3'-side-chains such as geranylgeraniol or geranylfarnesol, the alcohol derivatives of the side-chains of MK-4 and MK-3, respectively. These compounds could be acting through different mechanisms to the menaquinones and, indeed, this has been suggested to be the case in bone where osteoclast formation is inhibited by both MK-4 and geranylgeraniol but by different means (Hiruma et al., 2004). By contrast, the protective effects of both phylloquinone and MK-4 on oligodendrocytes require the entire molecule and probably work by an entirely different mechanism.

MK-4 can exert some of its effects through the SXR/PXR receptor which does not bind either phylloquinone or menadione and this explains at least some of its effects on HCC proliferation and invasion. The general lack of an effect of phylloquinone on most cancer cell types could mean that this is an important mode of action of MK-4 which merits further investigation. MK-4 also mediates actions via suppression of the NF-κB pathway by inhibiting IκB kinase and thereby reducing the phosphorylation and degradation of IκB although the way in which this happens is still unclear and the molecular target of MK-4 is unknown.

References

Allison AC, Danger of vitamin K to newborn. Lancet 1955;265: 669.

Ansell JE, Kumar R, Deykin D, The spectrum of vitamin K deficiency. J Am Med Assoc 1977;238: 40–2.

Atkins GJ, Welldon KJ, Wijenayaka AR, Bonewald LF, Findlay DM, Vitamin K promotes mineralization, osteoblast-to-osteocyte transition, and an anticatabolic phenotype by γ-carboxylation-dependent and -independent mechanisms. Am J Physiol Cell Physiol 2009;297: C1358–67.

Azuma K, Urano T, Ouchi Y, et al., Vitamin K2 suppresses proliferation and motility of hepatocellular carcinoma cells by activating steroid and xenobiotic receptor. Endocr J 2009;56: 843–9.

Bhanchet P, Tuchinda S, Hathirat P, Visudhiphan P, Bhamaraphavati N, Bukkavesa S, A bleeding syndrome in infants due to acquired prothrombin complex deficiency: a survey of 93 affected infants. Clin Pediatr (Phila) 1977;16: 992–8.

Bjornsson TD, Meffin PJ, Swezey SE, Blaschke TF, Effects of clofibrate and warfarin alone and in combination on the disposition of vitamin K_1. J Pharmacol Exp Ther 1979;210: 322–6.

Bolton-Smith C, McMurdo ME, Paterson CR, Mole PA, Harvey JM, Fenton ST, Prynne CJ, Mishra GD, Shearer MJ, Two-year randomized controlled trial of vitamin K1 (phylloquinone) and vitamin D3 plus calcium on the bone health of older women. J Bone Miner Res 2007;22: 509–19.

Booth SL, Al Rajabi A, Determinants of vitamin K status in humans. Vitam Horm 2008;78: 1–22.

Booth SL, Suttie JW, Dietary intake and adequacy of vitamin K. J Nutr 1998;128: 785–8.

Booth SL, Tucker KL, Chen H et al., Dietary vitamin K intakes are associated with hip fracture but not with bone mineral density in elderly men and women. Am J Clin Nutr 2000;71: 1201–8.

Booth SL, Broe KE, Gagnon DR et al., Vitamin K intake and bone mineral density in women and men. Am J Clin Nutr 2003;77: 512–6.

Booth SL, Broe KE, Peterson JW, Cheng DM, Dawson-Hughes B, Gundberg CM, Cupples LA, Wilson PW, Kiel DP, Associations between vitamin K biochemical measures and bone mineral density in men and women. J Clin Endocrinol Metab 2004;89: 4904–9.

Booth SL, Dallal G, Shea MK, Gundberg C, Peterson JW, Dawson-Hughes B, Effect of vitamin K supplementation on bone loss in elderly men and women. J Clin Endocrinol Metab 2008;93: 1217–23.

Boskey AL, Gadaleta S, Gundberg C, Doty SB, Ducy P, Karsenty G, Fourier transform infrared microspectroscopic analysis of bones of osteocalcin-deficient mice provides insight into the function of osteocalcin. Bone 1998;23: 187–96.

Bostrom K, Tsao D, Shen S, Wang Y, Demer LL, Matrix GLA protein modulates differentiation induced by bone morphogenetic protein-2 in C3H10T1/2 cells. J Biol Chem 2001;276: 14044–52.

Bouzahzah B, Nishikawa Y, Simon D, et al., Growth control and gene expression in a new hepatocellular carcinoma cell line, Hep40: Inhibitory actions of vitamin K. J Cell Physiol 1995;165: 459–67.

Braam LA, Knapen MH, Geusens P, Brouns F, Hamulyak K, Gerichhausen MJ, Vermeer C, Vitamin K1 supplementation retards bone loss in postmenopausal women between 50 and 60 years of age. Calcif Tissue Int 2003;73: 21–6.

Braam LA, Hoeks AP, Brouns F, Hamulyak K, Gerichhausen MJ, Vermeer C, Beneficial effects of vitamins D and K on the elastic properties of the vessel wall in postmenopausal women: a follow-up study. Thromb Haemost 2004;91: 373–80.

Brenner DJ, Hall EJ, Computed tomography – an increasing source of radiation exposure. N Engl J Med 2007;357: 2277–84.

Caraballo PJ, Gabriel SE, Castro MR, Atkinson EJ, Melton LJ 3rd, Changes in bone density after exposure to oral anticoagulants: a meta-analysis. Osteoporos Int 1999;9: 441–8.

Carrie I, Portoukalian J, Vicaretti R, et al., Menaquinone-4 concentration is correlated with sphingolipid concentrations in rat brain. J Nutr 2004;134: 167–72.

Cheung AM, Tile L, Lee Y, et al., Vitamin K supplementation in postmenopausal women with osteopenia (ECKO trial): a randomized controlled trial. PLoS Med 2008;5: e196.

Chlebowski RT, Dietrich M, Akman S, et al., Vitamin K3 inhibition of malignant murine cell growth and human tumor colony formation. Cancer Treat Rep 1985;69: 527–32.

Chu PH, Huang TW, Williams J, Stafford DW, Purified vitamin K epoxide reductase alone is sufficient for conversion of vitamin K epoxide to vitamin K and vitamin K to vitamin KH2. Proc Natl Acad Sci USA 2006;103: 19308–13.

Chuansumrit A, Isarangkura P, Hathirat P, Vitamin K Study Group, Vitamin K deficiency bleeding in Thailand: a 32-year history. Southeast Asian J Trop Med Public Health 1998;29: 649–54.

Cocchetto DM, Miller DB, Miller LL, et al., Behavioral perturbations in the vitamin K-deficient rat. Physiol Behav 1985;34: 727–34.

Cockayne S, Adamson J, Lanham-New S, Shearer MJ, Gilbody S, Torgerson DJ, Vitamin K and the prevention of fractures: systematic review and meta-analysis of randomized controlled trials. Arch Intern Med 2006;166: 1256–61.

COMA, Dietary reference values for food energy and nutrients for the United Kingdom. Report of the panel on dietary reference values, committee on medical aspects of food and nutrition policy. London: HMSO; 1991.

Conly JM, Stein K, Quantitative and qualitative measurements of K vitamins in human intestinal contents. Am J Gastroenterol 1992;87: 311–6.

Conway SP, Wolfe SP, Brownlee KG, White H, Oldroyd B, Truscott JG, Harvey JM, Shearer MJ, Vitamin K status among children with cystic fibrosis and its relationship to bone mineral density and bone turnover. Pediatrics 2005;115: 1325–31.

Coutu DL, Wu JH, Monette A, Rivard GE, Blostein MD, Galipeau J, Periostin, a member of a novel family of vitamin K-dependent proteins, is expressed by mesenchymal stromal cells. J Biol Chem 2008;283: 17991–8001.

Cranenburg EC, Vermeer C, Koos R, Boumans ML, Hackeng TM, Bouwman FG, Kwaijtaal M, Brandenburg VM, Ketteler M, Schurgers LJ, The circulating inactive form of matrix Gla protein (ucMGP) as a biomarker for cardiovascular calcification. J Vasc Res 2008;45: 427–36.

Cranenburg EC, Brandenburg VM, Vermeer C, Stenger M, Muhlenbruch G, Mahnken AH, Gladziwa U, Ketteler M, Schurgers LJ, Uncarboxylated matrix Gla protein (ucMGP) is associated with coronary artery calcification in haemodialysis patients. Thromb Haemost 2009;101: 359–66.

Dowd P, Hershline R, Ham SW, Naganathan S, Vitamin K and energy transduction: a base strength amplification mechanism. Science 1995;269: 1684–91.

Ducy P, Desbois C, Boyce B, et al., Increased bone formation in osteocalcin-deficient mice. Nature 1996;382: 448–52.

Elston TN, Dudley JM, Shearer MJ, Schey SA, Vitamin K prophylaxis in high-dose chemotherapy. Lancet 1995;345: 1245.

Erkkilä AT, Lichtenstein AH, Dolnikowski GG, Grusak MA, Jalbert SM, Aquino KA, Peterson JW, Booth SL, Plasma transport of vitamin K in men using deuterium-labeled Collard greens. Metabolism 2004;53: 215–21.

Feskanich D, Weber P, Willett WC, Rockett H, Booth SL, Colditz GA, Vitamin K intake and hip fractures in women: a prospective study. Am J Clin Nutr 1999;69: 74–9.

Food and Nutrition Board, Institute of Medicine. Dietary Reference Intakes for vitamin A, vitamin K, arsenic, boron, chromium, copper, iodine, manganese, molybdenum, nickel, silicon, vanadium and zinc. Washington, DC: National Academy Press; 2001.

Funato K, Miyazawa K, Yaguchi M, et al., Combination of 22-oxa-1, 25-dihydroxyvitamin D(3), a vitamin D(3) derivative, with vitamin K(2) (VK2) synergistically enhances cell differentiation but suppresses VK2-inducing apoptosis in HL-60 cells. Leukemia 2002;16: 1519–27.

Furie B, Bouchard BA, Furie BC, Vitamin K-dependent biosynthesis of γ-carboxyglutamic acid. Blood 1999;93: 1798–808.

Gast GC, de Roos NM, Sluijs I, Bots ML, Beulens JW, Geleijnse JM, Witteman JC, Grobbee DE, Peeters PH, van der Schouw YT, A high menaquinone intake reduces the incidence of coronary heart disease in women. Nutr Metab Cardiovasc Dis 2009;19: 504–10.

Geleijnse JM, Vermeer C, Grobbee DE, Schurgers LJ, Knapen MH, van der Meer IM, Hofman A, Witteman JC, Dietary intake of menaquinone is associated with a reduced risk of coronary heart disease: the Rotterdam Study. J Nutr 2004;134: 3100–5.

Greer FR, Marshall S, Cherry J, Suttie, JW, Vitamin K status of lactating mothers, human milk, and breast-feeding infants. Pediatrics 1991;88: 751–6.

Habu D, Shiomi S, Tamori A, et al., Role of vitamin K2 in the development of hepatocellular carcinoma in women with viral cirrhosis of the liver. J Am Med Assoc 2004;292: 358–61.

Hara K, Akiyama Y, Nakamura T, et al., The inhibitory effect of vitamin K_2 (menatetrenone) on bone resorption may be related to its side chain. Bone 1995;16: 179–84.

Haroon Y, Shearer MJ, Rahim S, Gunn WG, McEnery G, Barkhan P, The content of phylloquinone (vitamin K_1) in human milk, cows' milk and infant formula foods determined by high-performance liquid chromatography. J Nutr 1982;112: 1105–17.

Harrington DJ, Soper R, Edwards C, Savidge GF, Hodges SJ, Shearer MJ, Determination of the urinary aglycone metabolites of vitamin K by HPLC with redox-mode electrochemical detection. J Lipid Res 2005;46: 1053–60.

Harrington DJ, Booth SL, Card DJ, Shearer MJ, Excretion of the urinary 5C- and 7C-aglycone metabolites of vitamin K by young adults responds to changes in dietary phylloquinone and dihydrophylloquinone intakes. J Nutr 2007;137: 1763–8.

Harrington DJ, Western H, Seton-Jones C, Rangarajan S, Beynon T, Shearer MJ, A study of the prevalence of vitamin K deficiency in patients with cancer referred to a hospital palliative care team and its association with abnormal haemostasis. J Clin Pathol 2008;61: 537–40.

Hart JP, Shearer MJ, Klenerman L, Catterall A, Reeve J, Sambrook PN, Dodds RA, Bitensky L, Chayen J, Electrochemical detection of depressed circulating levels of vitamin K_1 in osteoporosis. J Clin Endocrinol Metab 1985;60: 1268–9.

Hauschka PV, Lian JB, Gallop PM, Direct identification of the calcium-binding amino acid, γ-carboxyglutamate, in mineralized tissue. Proc Natl Acad Sci USA 1975;72: 3925–3929.

Hiruma Y, Nakahama K, Fujita H, et al., Vitamin K2 and geranylgeraniol, its side chain component, inhibited osteoclast formation in a different manner. Biochem Biophys Res Commun 2004;314: 24–30.

Hitomi M, Yokoyama F, Kita Y, et al., Antitumor effects of vitamins K1, K2 and K3 on hepatocellular carcinoma in vitro and in vivo. Int J Oncol 2005;26: 713–20.

Hoang QQ, Sicheri F, Howard AJ, Yang DSC, Bone recognition mechanism of porcine osteocalcin from crystal structure. Nature 2003;425: 977–80.

Hodges SJ, Pilkington MJ, Shearer MJ, Bitensky L, Chayen J, Age-related changes in the circulating levels of congeners of vitamin K2, menaquinone-7 and menaquinone-8. Clin Sci (Lond) 1990;78: 63–6.

Hodges SJ, Pilkington MJ, Stamp TCB, Catterall A, Shearer MJ, Bitensky L, Chayen J, Depressed levels of circulating menaquinones in patients with osteoporotic fractures of the spine and femoral neck. Bone 1991;12: 387–9.

Hodges SJ, Akesson K, Vergnaud P, Obrant K, Delmas PD, Circulating levels of vitamins K_1 and K_2 decreased in elderly women with hip fracture. J Bone Miner Res 1993b;8: 1241–5.

Hodges SJ, Bejui J, Leclercq M, Delmas PD, Detection and measurement of vitamins K_1 and K_2 in human cortical and trabecular bone. J Bone Min Res 1993a;8: 1005–8.

Holden RM, Morton AR, Garland JS, Pavlov A, Day AG, Booth SL, Vitamins K and D status in stages 3–5 chronic kidney disease. Clin J Am Soc Nephrol 2010;5: 590–7.

Hollander D, Truscott TC, Colonic absorption of vitamin K_3. J Lab Clin Med 1974b;83: 648–56.

Hollander D, Truscott TC, Mechanism and site of vitamin K_3 small intestinal transport. Am J Physiol 1974a;226: 1516–22.

Ichikawa T, Horie-Inoue K, Ikeda K, et al., Steroid and xenobiotic receptor SXR mediates vitamin K2-activated transcription of extracellular matrix-related genes and collagen accumulation in osteoblastic cells. J Biol Chem 2006;281: 16927–34.

Ichikawa T, Horie-Inoue K, Ikeda K, et al., Vitamin K_2 induces phosphorylation of protein kinase A and expression of novel target genes in osteoblastic cells. J Mol Endocrinol 2007;39: 239–47.

Ide Y, Zhang H, Hamajima H, et al., Inhibition of matrix metalloproteinase expression by menetetrenone, a vitamin K2 analogue. Oncol Rep 2009;22: 599–604.

Kalkwarf HJ, Khoury JC, Bean J, Elliot JG, Vitamin K, bone turnover, and bone mass in girls. Am J Clin Nutr 2004;80: 1075–80.

Kameda T, Miyazawa K, Mori Y, et al., Vitamin K_2 inhibits osteoclastic bone resorption by inducing osteoclast apoptosis. Biochem Biophys Res Commun 1996;220: 515–9.

Kaptoge S, Dalzell N, Welch A, Shearer MJ, Khaw KT, Reeve J, Vitamin K and fracture risk: an effect on bone width not BMD? J Bone Miner Res 2005;20: 1293.

Katagiri M, Hakeda Y, Chikazu D, et al., Mechanism of stimulation of osteoclastic bone resorption through Gas6/Tyro 3, a receptor tyrosine kinase signaling, in mouse osteoclasts. J Biol Chem 2001;276: 7376–82.

Knapen MH, Nieuwenhuijzen Kruseman AC, Wouters RS, Vermeer C, Correlation of serum osteocalcin fractions with bone mineral density in women during the first 10 years after menopause. Calcif Tissue Int 1998;63: 375–9.

Knapen MH, Schurgers LJ, Vermeer C, Vitamin K2 supplementation improves hip bone geometry and bone strength indices in postmenopausal women. Osteoporos Int 2007;18: 963–72.

Kohlmeier M, Salomon A, Saupe J, Shearer MJ, Transport of vitamin K to bone in humans. J Nutr 1996;126(4 Suppl): 1192S–6S.

Koos R, Krueger T, Westenfeld R, Kuhl HP, Brandenburg V, Mahnken AH, Stanzel S, Vermeer C, Cranenburg EC, Floege J, Kelm M, Schurgers LJ, Relation of circulating Matrix Gla-Protein and anticoagulation status in patients with aortic valve calcification. Thromb Haemost 2009;101: 706–13.

Kuriyama S, Hitomi M, Yoshiji H, et al., Vitamins K2, K3 and K5 exert in vivo antitumor effects on hepatocellular carcinoma by regulating the expression of G1 phase-related cell cycle molecules. Int J Oncol 2005;27: 505–11.

Lamon-Fava S, Sadowski JA, Davidson KW, O'Brien ME, McNamara JR, Schaefer EJ, Plasma lipoproteins as carriers of phylloquinone (vitamin K_1) in humans. Am J Clin Nutr 1998;67: 1226–31.

Lev M, Milford AF, Effect of vitamin K depletion and restoration on sphingolipid metabolism in *Bacteroides melaninogenicus*. J Lipid Res 1972;13: 364–70.

Li J, Lin JC, Wang H, et al., Novel role of vitamin K in preventing oxidative injury to developing oligodendrocytes and neurons. J Neurosci 2003;23: 5816–26.

Li T, Chang CY, Jin DY, Lin PJ, Khvorova A, Stafford DW, Identification of the gene for vitamin K epoxide reductase. Nature 2004;427: 521–44.

Li J, Wang H, Rosenberg PA, Vitamin K prevents oxidative cell death by inhibiting activation of 12-lipoxygenase in developing oligodendrocytes. J Neurosci Res 2009;87: 1987–2005.

Lian JB, Friedman PA, The vitamin K-dependent synthesis of γ-carboxyglutamic acid by bone microsomes. J Biol Chem 1978;253: 6623–6.

Lian JB, Stein GS, Stein JL, van Wijnen AJ, Regulated expression of the bone-specific osteocalcin gene by vitamins and hormones. Vitam Horm 1999;55: 443–509.

Liebman HA, Furie BC, Tong MJ, et al., Des-gamma-carboxy (abnormal) prothrombin as a serum marker of primary hepatocellular carcinoma. N Engl J Med 1984;310: 1427–31.

Liu G, Peacock M, Age-related changes in serum undercarboxylated osteocalcin and its relationships with bone density, bone quality, and hip fracture. Calcif Tissue Int 1998;62: 286–9.

Liu W, Nakamura H, Yamamoto T, et al., Vitamin K2 inhibits the proliferation of HepG2 cells by up-regulating the transcription of p21 gene. Hepatol Res 2007;37: 360–5.

Luo G, Ducy P, McKee MD, Pinero GJ, Loyer E, Behringer RR, Karsenty G, Spontaneous calcification of arteries and cartilage in mice lacking matrix GLA protein. Nature 1997;386: 78–81.

Luukinen H, Kakonen SM, Pettersson K, Koski K, Laippala P, Lovgren T, Kivela SL, Vaananen HK, Strong prediction of fractures among older adults by the ratio of carboxylated to total serum osteocalcin. J Bone Miner Res 2000;15: 2473–8.

MacDonald HM, McGuigan FE, Lanham-New SA, Fraser WD, Ralston SH, Reid DM, Vitamin K_1 intake is associated with higher bone mineral density and reduced bone resorption in early postmenopausal Scottish women: no evidence of gene-nutrient interaction with apolipoprotein E polymorphisms. Am J Clin Nutr 2008;87: 1513–20.

Manfioletti G, Brancolini C, Avanzi G, Schneider C, The protein encoded by a growth arrest-specific gene (gas6) is a new member of the vitamin K-dependent proteins related to protein S, a negative coregulator in the blood coagulation cascade. Mol Cell Biol 1993;13: 4976–85.

Matsumoto K, Okano J, Nagahara T, et al., Apoptosis of liver cancer cells by vitamin K2 and enhancement by MEK inhibition. Int J Oncol 2006;29: 1501–8.

McNinch AW, Orme RL, Tripp JH, Haemorrhagic disease of the newborn returns. Lancet 1983;1: 1089–90.

Miyazawa K, Yaguchi M, Funato K, et al., Apoptosis/differentiation-inducing effects of vitamin K2 on HL-60 cells: dichotomous nature of vitamin K2 in leukaemia cells. Leukemia 2001;15: 1111–7.

Mizuta T, Ozaki I, Eguchi Y, et al., The effect of menatetrenone, a vitamin K2 analog, on disease recurrence and survival in patients with hepatocellular carcinoma after curative treatment: a pilot study. Cancer 2006;106: 867–72.

Molitor LG, Robinson HJ, Oral and parenteral toxicity of vitamin K_1, phthiocol and 2-methyl-1, 4-naphthoquinone. Proc Soc Exp Biol Med 1940;43: 125–8.

Murata K, Sakamoto A, Impairment of clathrin-mediated endocytosis via cytoskeletal change by epithelial to fibroblastoid conversion in HepG2 cells: a possible mechanism of des-gamma-carboxy prothrombin production in hepatocellular carcinoma. Int J Oncol 2008;33: 1149–55.

Murshed M, Schinke T, McKee MD, Karsenty G, Extracellular matrix mineralization is regulated locally; different roles of two gla-containing proteins. J Cell Biol 2004;165: 625–30.

Nanke Y, Kotake S, Ninomiya T, et al., Geranylgeranylacetone inhibits formation and function of human osteoclasts and prevents bone loss in tail-suspended rats and ovariectomized rats. Calcif Tissue Int 2005;77: 376–85.

Nawata H, Soen S, Takayanagi R, et al., Guidelines on the management and treatment of glucocorticoid-induced osteoporosis of the Japanese Society for Bone and Mineral Research (2004). J Bone Miner Metab 2005;23: 105–9.

Nimptsch K, Rohrmann S, Linseisen J, Dietary intake of vitamin K and risk of prostate cancer in the Heidelberg cohort of the European Prospective Investigation into Cancer and Nutrition (EPIC-Heidelberg). Am J Clin Nutr 2008;87: 985–92.

Nimptsch K, Rohrmann S, Nieters A, et al., Serum undercarboxylated osteocalcin as biomarker of vitamin K intake and risk of prostate cancer: A nested case-control study in the Heidelberg cohort of the European prospective investigation into cancer and nutrition. Cancer Epidemiol Biomarkers Prev 2009;18: 49–56.

Nimptsch K, Rohrmann S, Kaaks R, et al., Dietary vitamin K intake in relation to cancer incidence and mortality: results from the Heidelberg cohort of the European Prospective Investigation into Cancer and Nutrition (EPIC-Heidelberg). Am J Clin Nutr 2010;91: 1348–58.

O'Donnell C J, Shea MK, Price PA, Gagnon DR, Wilson PW, Larson MG, Kiel DP, Hoffmann U, Ferencik M, Clouse ME, Williamson LM, Cupples LA, Dawson-Hughes B, Booth SL, Matrix Gla protein is associated with risk factors for atherosclerosis but not with coronary artery calcification. Arterioscler Thromb Vasc Biol 2006;26: 2769–74.

Ogawa M, Nakai S, Deguchi A, et al., Vitamins K2, K3 and K5 exert antitumor effects on established colorectal cancer in mice by inducing apoptotic death of tumor cells. Int J Oncol 2007;31: 323–31.

Ohizumi H, Masuda Y, Nakajo S, et al., Geranylgeraniol is a potent inducer of apoptosis in tumor cells. J Biochem 1995;117: 11–3.

Ohsaki Y, Shirakawa H, Hiwatashi K, et al., Vitamin K suppresses lipopolysaccharide-induced inflammation in the rat. Biosci Biotechnol Biochem 2006;70: 926–32.

Olson RE, Chao J, Graham D, Bates MW, Lewis JH, Total body phylloquinone and its turnover in human subjects at two levels of vitamin K intake. Br J Nutr 2002;87: 543–53.

O'Shaughnessy D, Allen C, Woodcock T, Pearce K, Harvey J, Shearer M, Echis time, under-carboxylated prothrombin and vitamin K status in intensive care patients. Clin Lab Haematol 2003;25: 397–404.

Otsuka M, Kato N, Shao RX, et al., Vitamin K2 inhibits the growth and invasiveness of hepatocellular carcinoma cells via protein kinase A activation. Hepatology 2004;40: 243–51.

Ozaki I, Zhang H, Mizuta T, et al., Menatetrenone, a vitamin K2 analogue, inhibits hepatocellular carcinoma cell growth by suppressing cyclin D1 expression through inhibition of nuclear factor κB activation. Clin Cancer Res 2007;13: 2236–45.

Pineo GF, Gallus AS, Hirsh J, Unexpected vitamin K deficiency in hospitalized patients. Can Med Assoc J 1973;109: 880–3.

Price PA, Otsuka AS, Poser JW, Kristaponis J, Raman N, Characterization of a γ-carboxyglutamic acid-containing protein from bone. Proc Natl Acad Sci USA 1976;73: 1447–51.

Price PA, Urist MR, Otawara Y, Matrix Gla protein, a new gamma-carboxyglutamic acid-containing protein which is associated with the organic matrix of bone. Biochem Biophys Res Commun 1983;117: 765–71.

Price PA, Faus SA, Williamson MK, Warfarin causes rapid calcification of the elastic lamellae in rat arteries and heart valves. Arterioscler Thromb Vasc Biol 1998;18: 1400–7.

Proudfoot D, Davies JD, Skepper JN, Weissberg PL, Shanahan CM, Acetylated low-density lipoprotein stimulates human vascular smooth muscle cell calcification by promoting osteoblastic differentiation and inhibiting phagocytosis. Circulation 2002;106: 3044–50.

Raggi P, Shaw LJ, Berman DS, Callister TQ, Prognostic value of coronary artery calcium screening in subjects with and without diabetes. J Am Coll Cardiol 2004;43: 1663–69.

Reddi K, Henderson B, Meghji S, et al., Interleukin 6 production by lipopolysaccharide-stimulated human fibroblasts is potently inhibited by naphthoquinone (vitamin K) compounds. Cytokine 1995;7: 287–90.

Rejnmark L, Vestergaard P, Charles P, Hermann AP, Brot C, Eiken P, Mosekilde L, No effect of vitamin K_1 intake on bone mineral density and fracture risk in perimenopausal women. Osteoporos Int 2006;17: 1122–32.

Reynolds JL, Joannides AJ, Skepper JN, McNair R, Schurgers LJ, Proudfoot D, Jahnen-Dechent W, Weissberg PL, Shanahan CM, Human vascular smooth muscle cells undergo vesicle-mediated calcification in response to changes in extracellular calcium and phosphate concentrations: a potential mechanism for accelerated vascular calcification in ESRD. J Am Soc Nephrol 2004;15: 2857–67.

Rimmer T, Treating the anorexia of cancer. Eur J Palliat Care 1998;5: 179–81.

Rost S, Fregin A, Ivaskevicius V, et al., Mutations in VKORC1 cause warfarin resistance and multiple coagulation factor deficiency type 2. Nature 2004;427: 537–41.

Sakai I, Hashimoto S, Yoda M, et al., Novel role of vitamin K2: A potent inducer of differentiation of various human myeloid leukaemia cell lines. Biochem Biophys Res Commun 1994;205: 1305–10.

Schurgers LJ, Vermeer C, Determination of phylloquinone and menaquinones in food. Effect of food matrix on circulating vitamin K concentrations. Haemostasis 2000;30: 298–307.

Schurgers LJ, Vermeer C, Differential lipoprotein transport pathways of K-vitamins in healthy adults. Biochim Biophys Acta 2002;1570: 27–32.

Schurgers LJ, Geleijnse JM, Grobbee DE, Pols HAP, Hofman A, Witteman JCM, Vermeer C, Nutritional intake of vitamin K1 (Phylloquinone) and K2 (Menaquinone) in The Netherlands. J Nutr Environ Med 1999;9: 115–22.

Schurgers LJ, Aebert H, Vermeer C, Bültmann B, Janzen J, Oral anticoagulant treatment: friend or foe in cardiovascular disease? Blood 2004;104: 3231–2.

Schurgers LJ, Teunissen KJ, Knapen MH, Kwaijtaal M, van Diest R, Appels A, Reutelingsperger CP, Cleutjens JP, Vermeer C, Novel conformation-specific antibodies against matrix gamma-carboxyglutamic acid (Gla) protein: undercarboxylated matrix Gla protein as marker for vascular calcification. Arterioscler Thromb Vasc Biol 2005;25: 1629–33.

Schurgers LJ, Spronk HM, Skepper JN, Hackeng TM, Shanahan CM, Vermeer C, Weissberg PL, Proudfoot D, Post-translational modifications regulate matrix Gla protein function: importance for inhibition of vascular smooth muscle cell calcification. J Thromb Haemost 2007a;5: 2503–11.

Schurgers LJ, Spronk HM, Soute BA, Schiffers PM, DeMey JG, Vermeer C, Regression of warfarin-induced medial elastocalcinosis by high intake of vitamin K in rats. Blood 2007b;109: 2823–31.

Schurgers LJ, Teunissen KJ, Hamulyak K, Knapen MH, Vik H, Vermeer C Vitamin K-containing dietary supplements: comparison of synthetic vitamin K_1 and natto-derived menaquinone-7. Blood 2007c;109: 3279–83.

Schurgers LJ, Cranenburg EC, Vermeer C, Matrix Gla-protein: the calcification inhibitor in need of vitamin K, Thromb Haemost 2008;100: 593–603.

Schurgers LJ, Barreto DV, Barreto FC, Liabeuf S, Renard C, Magdeleyns EJ, Vermeer C, Choukroun G, Massy ZA, The circulating inactive form of matrix Gla protein is a surrogate marker for vascular calcification in chronic kidney disease: A preliminary report. Clin J Am Soc Nephrol 2010;5: 568–75.

Shea MK, Booth SL, Massaro JM, et al., Vitamin K and vitamin D status: associations with inflammatory markers in the Framingham Offspring study. Am J Epidemiol 2008;167: 313–20.

Shea MK, O'Donnell CJ, Hoffmann U, Dallal GE, Dawson-Hughes B, Ordovas JM, Price PA, Williamson MK, Booth SL, Vitamin K supplementation and progression of coronary artery calcium in older men and women. Am J Clin Nutr 2009;89: 1799–807.

Shearer MJ, Vitamin K metabolism and nutriture. Blood Rev 1992;6: 92–104.

Shearer MJ, Vitamin K. Lancet 1995;345: 229–234.

Shearer MJ, Role of vitamin K and Gla proteins in the pathophysiology of osteoporosis and vascular calcification. Curr Opin Clin Nutr Metab Care 2000;3: 433–8.

Shearer MJ, Vitamin K deficiency bleeding (VKDB) in early infancy. Blood Rev 2009;23: 49–59.

Shearer MJ, Newman P, Metabolism and cell biology of vitamin K, Thromb Haemost 2008;100: 530–47.

Shearer MJ, Barkhan P, Webster GR, Absorption and excretion of an oral dose of tritiated vitamin K1 in man, Br J Haematol 1970;18: 297–308.

Shearer MJ, McBurney A, Barkhan P, Studies on the absorption and metabolism of phylloquinone (vitamin K_1) in man. Vitam Horm 1974;32: 513–42.

Shearer MJ, McCarthy PT, Crampton OE, Mattock MB, The assessment of human vitamin K status from tissue measurements. In: Suttie J, editor. Current advances in vitamin K research. New York: Elsevier Science; 1988. pp. 438–52.

Shroff RC, McNair R, Figg N, Skepper JN, Schurgers L, Gupta A, Hiorns M, Donald AE, Deanfield J, Rees L, Shanahan CM, Dialysis accelerates medial vascular calcification in part by triggering smooth muscle cell apoptosis. Circulation 2008;118: 1748–57.

Spronk HM, Soute BA, Schurgers LJ, Thijssen HH, De Mey JG, Vermeer C, Tissue-specific utilization of menaquinone-4 results in the prevention of arterial calcification in warfarin-treated rats. J Vasc Res 2003;40: 531–7.

Stenberg LM, Nilsson E, Ljungberg O, et al., Synthesis of gamma-carboxylated polypeptides by alpha-cells of the pancreatic islets. Biochem Biophys Res Commun 2001;283: 454–9.

Stenflo J, From γ-carboxy-glutamate to protein C. J Thromb Haemost 2006;4: 2521–6.

Stenflo J, Fernlund P, Egan W, Roepstorff P, Vitamin K dependent modifications of glutamic acid residues in prothrombin. Proc Natl Acad Sci USA 1974;71: 2730–3.

Stevenson M, Lloyd-Jones M, Papaioannou D, Vitamin K to prevent fractures in older women: systematic review and economic evaluation. Health Technol Assess 2009;13: iii–xi, 1–134.

Sundaram KS, Lev M, Warfarin administration reduces synthesis of sulfatides and other sphingolipids in mouse brain. J Lipid Res 1988;29: 1475–9.

Sundaram KS, Lev M, Regulation of sulfotransferase activity by vitamin K in mouse brain. Arch Biochem Biophys 1990;277: 109–13.

Sundaram KS, Fan JH, Engelke JA, et al., Vitamin K status influences brain sulfatide metabolism in young mice and rats. J Nutr 1996;126: 2746–51.

Suttie JW, Vitamin K and human nutrition. J Am Diet Assoc 1992;92: 585–90.

Suttie JW, The importance of menaquinones in human nutrition. Annu Rev Nutr 1995;15: 399–417.

Suttie JW, Vitamin K in health and disease. Boca Raton: CRC Press; 2009. 224 pp.

Szulc P, Arlot M, Chapuy MC, Duboeuf F, Meunier PJ, Delmas PD, Serum undercarboxylated osteocalcin correlates with hip bone mineral density in elderly women. J Bone Miner Res 1994;9: 1591–5.

Szulc P, Chapuy MC, Meunier PJ, Delmas PD, Serum undercarboxylated osteocalcin is a marker of the risk of hip fracture: a three year follow-up study. Bone 1996;18: 487–8.

Tabb MM, Sun A, Zhou C, et al., Vitamin K_2 regulation of bone homeostasis is mediated by the steroid and xenobiotic receptor SXR. J Biol Chem 2003;278: 43919–27.

Taggart WV, Matschiner JT, Metabolism of menadione-6,7–3H in the rat. Biochemistry 1969;8: 1141–6.

Taper HS, de Gerlache J, Lans M, et al., Non-toxic potentiation of cancer chemotherapy by combined C and K3 vitamin pre-treatment. Int J Cancer 1987;40: 575–9.

Thane CW, Bolton-Smith C, Coward WA, Comparative dietary intake and sources of phylloquinone (vitamin K1) among British adults in 1986–7 and 2000–1. Br J Nutr 2006;96: 1105–15.

Thane CW, Paul AA, Bates CJ, Bolton-Smith C, Prentice A, Shearer MJ, Intake and sources of phylloquinone (vitamin K1): variation with socio-demographic and lifestyle factors in a national sample of British elderly people. Br J Nutr 2002;87: 605–13.

Thierry MJ, Suttie JW, Effect of warfarin and the chloro analog of vitamin K on phylloquinone metabolism. Arch Biochem Biophys 1971;147: 430–5.

Thijssen HHW, Drittij-Reijnders MJ, Vitamin K distribution in rat tissues: dietary phylloquinone is a source of tissue menaquinone-4. Br J Nutr 1994;72: 415–25.

Thijssen HHW, Drittij-Reijnders MJ, Vitamin K status in human tissues: tissue-specific accumulation of phylloquinone and menaquinone-4. Br J Nutr 1996;75: 121–7.

Thomas DD, Krzykowski KJ, Engelke JA, et al., Exocrine pancreatic secretion of phospholipid, menaquinone-4, and caveolin-1 in vivo. Biochem Biophys Res Commun 2004;319: 974–9.

Topp H, Iontcheva V, Schoch G, Renal excretion of -carboxyglutamic acid and metabolic rate in 3–18 year old humans. Amino Acids 1998;14: 371–7.

Tsugawa N, Shiraki M, Suhara Y, Kamao M, Ozaki R, Tanaka K, Okano T, Low plasma phylloquinone concentration is associated with high incidence of vertebral fracture in Japanese women. J Bone Miner Metab 2008;26: 79–85.

Ueland T, Gullestad L, Dahl CP, et al., Undercarboxylated matrix Gla protein is associated with indices of heart failure and mortality in symptomatic aortic stenosis. J Intern. Med. "Accepted Article": doi:10.1111/j.1365-2796.2010.02264.x.

Usui Y, Tanimura H, Nishimura N, Kobayashi N, Okanoue T, Ozawa K, Vitamin K concentrations in the plasma and liver of surgical patients. Am J Clin Nutr 1990;51: 846–52.

Vergnaud P, Garnero P, Meunier PJ, Breart G, Kamihagi K, Delmas PD, Undercarboxylated osteocalcin measured with a specific immunoassay predicts hip fracture in elderly women: the EPIDOS Study. J Clin Endocrinol Metab 1997;82: 719–24.

Vermeer C, Shearer MJ, Zittermann A, et al., Beyond deficiency: potential benefits of increased intakes of vitamin K for bone and vascular health. Eur J Nutr 2004;43: 325–35.

Viegas CSB, Simes DC, Laize V, Williamson MK, Price PA, Cancela ML, Gla-rich protein (GRP), a new vitamin K-dependent protein identified from sturgeon cartilage and highly conserved in vertebrates. J Biol Chem 2008;283: 36655–64.

von Kries R, Becker A, Göbel U, Vitamin K in the newborn: influence of nutritional factors on acarboxyprothrombin detectability and factor II and VII clotting activity. Eur J Pediatr 1987;146: 123–7.

von Kries R, Shearer MJ, Göbel U, Vitamin K in infancy. Eur J Pediatr 1988;147: 106–12.

Wajih N, Borras T, Xue W, Hutson SM, Wallin R, Processing and transport of matrix gamma-carboxyglutamic acid protein and bone morphogenetic protein-2 in cultured human vascular smooth muscle cells: evidence for an uptake mechanism for serum fetuin. J Biol Chem 2004;279: 43052–60.

Wallin R, Cain D, Sane DC, Matrix Gla protein synthesis and gamma-carboxylation in the aortic vessel wall and proliferating vascular smooth muscle cells – a cell system which resembles the system in bone cells. Thromb Haemost 1999;82: 1764–7.

Wallin R, Cain D, Hutson SM, Sane DC, Loeser R, Modulation of the binding of matrix Gla protein (MGP) to bone morphogenetic protein-2 (BMP-2). Thromb Haemost 2000;84: 1039–44.

Wang Z, Wang M, Finn F, et al., The growth inhibitory effects of vitamins K and their actions on gene expression. Hepatology 1995;22: 876–82.

Wei G, Wang M, Carr BI, Sorafenib combined vitamin K induces apoptosis in human pancreatic cancer cell lines through RAF/MEK/ERK and c-jun NH-2-terminal kinase pathways. J Cell Physiol 2010;224: 112–9.

Westenfeld R, Krüger T, Schlieper G, Cranenburg E, Heidenreich S, Holzmann S, Vermeer C, Ketteler M, Floege J, Schurgers LJ, Vitamin K2 supplementation reduces the elevated inactive form of the calcification inhibitor matrix Gla protein in hemodialysis patients. American Society of Nephrology (ASN). 2008; TH-FC044 (Abstract).

Yaguchi M, Miyazawa K, Katagiri T, et al., Vitamin K2 and its derivatives induce apoptosis in leukaemia cells and enhance the effect of all-trans retinoic acid. Leukemia 1997;11: 779–87.

Yaguchi M, Miyazawa K, Otawa M, et al., Vitamin K2 selectively induces apoptosis of blastic cells in myelodysplastic syndrome: flow cytometric detection of apoptotic cells using APO2.7 monoclonal antibody. Leukemia 1998;12: 1392–7.

Yoshiji H, Kuriyama S, Noguchi R, et al., Combination of vitamin K2 and the angiotensin-converting enzyme inhibitor, perindopril, attenuates the liver enzyme-altered preneoplastic lesions in rats via angiogenesis suppression. J Hepatol 2005;42: 687–93.

Yoshiji H, Noguchi R, Toyohara M, et al., Combination of vitamin K2 and angiotensin-converting enzyme inhibitor ameliorates cumulative recurrence of hepatocellular carcinoma. J Hepatol 2009;51: 315–21.

B-Vitamin like Nutrients

13 Betaine

Betaine: osmolyte and methyl donor

Michael Lever; Sandy Slow; Per M. Ueland

13.1 What is betaine?

In the 1860s, Scheibler isolated an organic base from sugar beet (*Beta vulgaris*) which he named 'betaine' (Scheibler, 1869, 1870), and he showed that it was N,N,N-trimethylglycine (▶Fig. 13.1). Betaine is a highly polar but neutral zwitterionic compound that is very soluble in water. As its isolation shows, betaine is a natural product, and now commercially produced betaine is a by-product of the sugar beet industry. Subsequently other natural products have been isolated which are chemically related to betaine, and these are generically called 'betaines'; some examples are shown in ▶Fig. 13.1. For this reason the compound Scheibler described is often called 'glycine betaine'. Although several betaines are found in the human diet (de Zwart et al., 2003), the only other betaine that has a known metabolic role in mammals is carnitine.

Retail outlets selling dietary supplements are likely to have betaine, usually called 'trimethylglycine' or 'TMG', on their shelves with claims that it gives health benefits ranging from preventing vascular disease to correcting autism. These claims are not justified by the available evidence, and one of the aims of this chapter is to present a realistic assessment of what role betaine might have in health, and the limitations on our current understanding.

13.2 Sources and availability of betaine

Betaine either comes from our food, or we convert dietary choline into betaine. The relative importance of these sources has not been well documented, but it could be expected to vary with dietary patterns. Both choline and betaine are essential for human well-being, but although dietary choline can, in principle, supply all the requirements for both choline and betaine, the converse is not true. Nevertheless when the dietary supply of choline is limiting, the choline-sparing effect of dietary betaine (Dilger et al., 2007) could become nutritionally important.

In western style diets, betaine is mostly obtained from cereals, particularly wheat (Sakamoto et al., 2002; Zeisel et al., 2003; de Zwart et al., 2003). Another important source is the beet family, which includes popular vegetables such as spinach, chard and beetroot. Several estimates of daily intake have given essentially concordant results (Slow et al., 2005; Cho et al., 2006; Chiuve et al., 2007; Bidulescu et al., 2007; Detopoulou et al., 2008), and most people in the various population groups that were studied had intakes between 100 and 300 mg/day. The actual value will not be the same in different

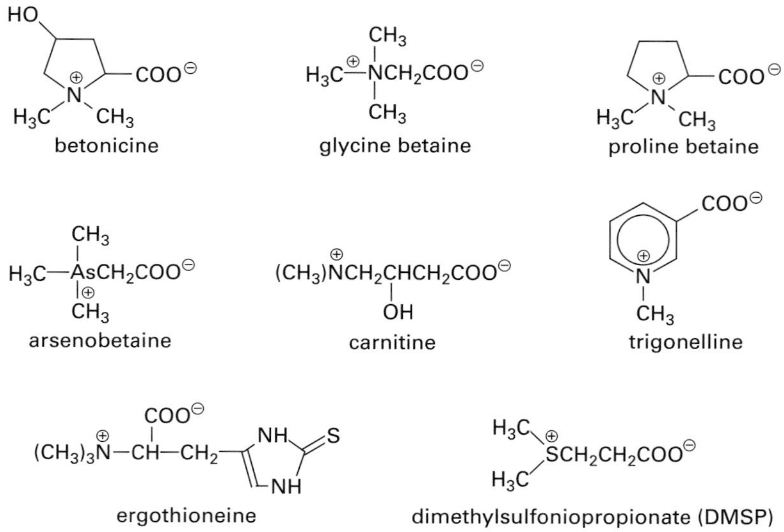

Fig. 13.1: Structures of betaine (glycine betaine) and analogues that are found in the diet.

populations, because it depends both on the diet and on the growing conditions of food plants; this latter is because many plants use betaine as an osmolyte, and accumulate more of it when grown on saline soils or when water deprived (Slow et al., 2008). In some of the earlier literature there were suggestions that the daily intake of betaine might be commonly over a gram a day (Craig, 2004; Olthof and Verhoef, 2005), but more recent estimates support a lower intake, and we have found (Elmslie, unpublished) that it is difficult to design an acceptable diet to supply more than approximately 800 mg/day long-term without supplementation. A factor which affects the actual betaine content of the diet, is food preparation. Betaine is highly water soluble, and boiled vegetables lose most of their betaine in the cooking water. By contrast, betaine is stable to oven cooking (de Zwart et al., 2003).

Because betaine occurs entirely as a simple solute, which is highly water soluble and is not protein bound, it would be expected that the bioavailability of dietary betaine and of betaine supplements would be similar, and this is the case (Atkinson et al., 2008). The details of betaine uptake are not well documented, but this uptake is efficient. There are at least three betaine transport systems in the mammalian gut (Thwaites and Anderson, 2007). In chickens (Kettunen et al., 2001c), as in rats (Slow et al., 2009), betaine is actively accumulated in the intestinal linings where this accumulation appears to be osmoregulated (Kettunen et al., 2001a) and stabilizes the mucosal structure (Kettunen et al., 2001c). Labeled betaine supplied orally to chickens is rapidly distributed through the body into various tissues and the methyl groups used to form tissue methionine (Kettunen et al., 2001b). Betaine absorption is obviously similarly rapid in humans (Schwahn et al., 2003; Atkinson et al., 2008) and there is no reason to believe that the mechanisms are not similar. Of the other betaines in the diet (de Zwart et al., 2003; Slow et al., 2005) only proline betaine (present in large amounts in citrus foods, including orange juice, and in legume sprouts) needs to be considered, because it inhibits the renal resorption of glycine betaine (Lever et al., 2004; Atkinson et al., 2007) and can lead to an apparently abnormal excretion of betaine by healthy subjects. The effect is not sufficient to acutely affect plasma homocysteine concentrations (Atkinson et al., 2007), although it suggests that we need to be cautious about using orange juice in experimental protocols involving one-carbon metabolism. Trigonelline (found in coffee and legume sprouts) does not have a similar effect and trigonelline does not explain the homocysteine-raising effect of coffee (Slow et al., 2004b).

13.3 Betaine functions and metabolism

13.3.1 Physiological roles of betaine

Betaine has two important roles in mammalian physiology. One is as a major osmolyte, accumulated in most tissues to assist cell volume regulation (Feng et al., 2001; Schliess and Häussinger, 2002; Lang, 2007). The other role is as a methyl donor for the remethylation of homocysteine to methionine. Tissue betaine concentrations are higher than plasma concentrations in almost all rat organs (Slow et al., 2009), and often reach millimolar concentrations (exceptional concentrations, >100 mM, are possible in the renal medulla). The osmoregulated betaine transporter BGT-1 was originally identified in the kidney (Yamauchi et al., 1992; Kempson and Montrose, 2004) and it has since been shown that it is expressed in many tissues (Warskulat et al., 1995, 2004, 2009; Zhang et al., 1996; Denkert et al., 1998; Weik et al., 1998; Petronini et al., 2000; Olsen et al., 2005; Rainesalo et al., 2005). There are several other mammalian betaine transporters (Thwaites and Anderson, 2007), including the carnitine transporter OCTN2 (Pochini et al., 2004) and betaine transport by these other systems could be osmoregulated in some cells (Petronini et al., 2000; Alfieri et al., 2002, 2004; Anas et al., 2007): none of the transporters are specific for betaine. Osmolyte-mediated volume regulation is under tight control (Häussinger, 2004) and its disruption has serious consequences, including apoptosis (Häussinger, 1996; Dmitrieva and Burg, 2005; Reinehr and Häussinger, 2006). Thus an adequate supply of betaine is needed for tissue integrity. As with most osmolytes, betaine is also a 'compensatory' or 'counteracting' solute (Gilles, 1997) that enhances the stability of proteins, and it is (along with other chemically related osmolytes containing a trimethylamine functional group) particularly effective at countering the denaturing effect of urea (Yancey and Somero, 1979; Yancey and Burg, 1990; Burg et al., 1996; Venkatesu et al., 2009), a function that is particularly important in the renal medulla (Burg et al., 1996).

The second function for tissue betaine is a supply of methyl groups for the remethylation of homocysteine to methionine by the enzyme betaine-homocysteine methyltransferase (BHMT). The two functions of betaine interact, because BHMT is osmoregulated (Delgado-Reyes and Garrow, 2005; Schäfer et al., 2007), with high tonicity reducing its expression, so that betaine metabolism (and hence the mobilization of methyl groups) decreases when osmolyte concentrations need to be maintained.

13.3.2 Metabolic pathways involving betaine

A claim that humans cannot convert choline to the betaine (Barak et al., 2002; Sparks et al., 2006) is an error and dietary choline is undoubtedly an important source of betaine, and hence methyl groups. Betaine is an intermediate in the metabolism of choline, and dietary choline is an important source of betaine, and hence methyl groups, for humans. Choline is converted to betaine in two steps involving the enzymes choline dehydrogenase and betaine aldehyde dehydrogenase (▶Fig. 13.2). Choline dehydrogenase and betaine aldehyde dehydrogenase are often grouped together as the 'choline oxidase' system, which can cause confusion (Olthof et al., 2005a; Li et al., 2007; Mato et al., 2008; Batra and Devasagayam, 2009). Choline oxidase (EC 1.1.3.17) is correctly a bacterial enzyme that catalyzes the conversion of choline to betaine by molecular oxygen (Rozwadowski et al., 1991; Fan and Gadda, 2005). In mammals choline dehydrogenase (EC 1.1.99.1) converts choline to betaine aldehyde (▶Fig. 13.2), which is then oxidized to betaine by a separate enzyme (Zhang et al., 1992), betaine aldehyde dehydrogenase (EC 1.2.1.8), the two enzymes being co-localized in mitochondria (Chern and Pietruszko, 1999). Betaine synthesis from choline probably occurs only in the liver and kidney as the enzymes necessary for its oxidation have not been found outside these tissues, although there is an early report of choline oxidation to betaine in the hamster intestinal mucosa (Flower et al., 1972). The primary control point of this process is the transport of choline into the mitochondria (Porter et al., 1992; Kaplan et al., 1993; O'Donoghue et al., 2009). Choline can enter the mitochondria via a high capacity non-saturable diffusion process, dependent on a high membrane potential, or it can be transported via a low-capacity high affinity choline transporter, which has been identified in the inner membrane in isolated rat liver and kidney mitochondria (Porter et al., 1992; Kaplan et al., 1993; O'Donoghue et al., 2009). It has been estimated that at physiological choline concentrations the transport-mediated process is dominant in both liver and kidney (90% and 96%, respectively) (Kaplan et al., 1993; O'Donoghue et al., 2009). The choline transport rate in the kidney is estimated to be approximately five to six times that of the liver, possibly reflecting a higher synthesis of betaine from choline in the kidney where betaine is accumulated to high levels and functions as an osmolyte (O'Donoghue et al., 2009). The uptake of choline into both liver and kidney mitochondria is not coupled to betaine efflux, which is believed to be by passive diffusion as no active transport process has been identified.

In the reaction mediated by betaine homocysteine methyltransferase (BHMT) a methyl group is transferred from betaine to homocysteine, forming dimethylglycine (DMG) and methionine (▶Fig. 13.2). The BHMT remethylation pathway contributes as much as 50% of the homocysteine methylation capacity of the liver (Finkelstein and Martin, 1984), implying an important role for betaine in the generation and maintenance of methionine and S-adenosylmethionine (SAM) concentrations. BHMT is a zinc metalloprotein (Garrow, 1996; Millian and Garrow, 1998), accounting for most of the bound zinc in the liver. It is cytosolic, makes up 0.5–2% of the soluble liver protein and is associated with the microtubules (Sandu et al., 2000). It has been highly conserved in chordate evolution and no metabolic abnormalities associated with low or absent BHMT are known, implying an essential role. In humans, BHMT is expressed in the liver, renal cortex and lens (Sunden et al., 1997), but although BHMT is thought to be primarily a liver and kidney enzyme, it is expressed in other cells and in early embryonic development (Anas et al., 2008). Disruption of BHMT should cause disturbed homocysteine metabolism, which in turn will lower SAM concentrations and reduce methylation capacity, and this is shown in mice when BHMT activity is inhibited by the potent and specific inhibitor S-(δ-carboxybutyl)-DL-homocysteine. This causes significant increases

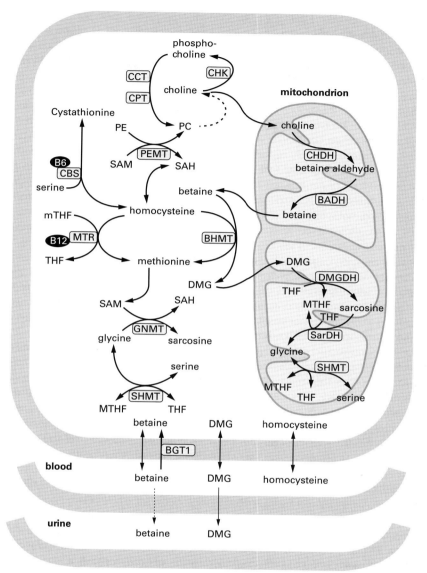

Fig. 13.2: Paths for betaine metabolism. *Metabolite abbreviations:* PE, phosphatidylethanolamine; PC, phosphatidylcholine; THF, tetrahydrofolate; mTHF, 5,10-methylenetetrahydrofolate; MTHF, 5-methyltetrahydrofolate; DMG, *N,N*-dimethylglycine; SAM, *S*-adenosylmethionine; SAH, *S*-adenosylhomocysteine. *Enzyme abbreviations:* CCT, CTP:phosphocholine cytidyltransferase; CPT, CDP-choline:diacylglycerol cholinephosphotransferase; CHK, choline kinase; CBS, cystathionine β-synthase; PEMT, phoshoethanolamine methyltransferase; CHDH, choline dehydrogenase; BADH, betaine aldehyde dehydrogenase; MTR, methionine synthase; BHMT, betaine-homocysteine methyltransferase; DMGDH, dimethylglycine dehydrogenase; GNMT, glycine *N*-methyltransferase; SarDH, sarcosine dehydrogenase; SHMT, serine hydroxymethyltransferase; BGT1, an osmoregulated betaine transporter.

(up to 7-fold) of both fasting and post-methionine load (which mimics the fed-state) plasma total homocysteine and reduces SAM concentrations (Collinsova et al., 2006). To date, 25 single nucleotide polymorphisms (SNPs) have been identified in the *BHMT* gene, of which only four encode non-synonymous changes that alter the amino acid sequence, none of the amino acid substitutions are near the active site or at intermolecular protein-protein contacts (Li et al., 2008). Of the *BHMT* SNPs, only one, the 742 G>A (c.716G>A), R239Q, is relatively common with a minor allele frequency of >10% (Li et al., 2008). There seems to be no difference in the stability or enzymatic activity of the Q isoform when compared with the R isoform (Weisburg et al., 2003). However, Li et al. (2008) have recently reported that *in vitro* the K_m for homocysteine and betaine is lower for the Q isoform. In humans, *BHMT* 742G>A was found not to be related to plasma tHcy concentration (Heil et al., 2000; Morin et al., 2003; Weisberg et al., 2003; Fredriksen et al., 2007), but a recent large epidemiological study demonstrated a decrease in dimethylglycine (the product of the BHMT reaction) according to the number of 742A alleles (Fredriksen et al., 2007), suggesting that this polymorphism could have metabolic effects *in vivo*.

As well as BHMT, mammals express another gene product called BHMT2. This name was coined when a gene was identified that encoded a putative protein with a 73% amino acid identity to BHMT (Chadwick et al., 2000). The gene product has proven not to be stable but might co-oligomerize with BHMT (Li et al., 2008), and it appears that its name is a misnomer because it does not use betaine as a substrate; instead it transfers methyl groups from *S*-methylmethionine (Szegedi et al., 2008).

Plasma betaine and urinary betaine excretion are determinants of plasma homocysteine, and this presumably reflects the importance of BHMT in one-carbon metabolism. Betaine becomes the major determinant of fasting homocysteine during pregnancy (Velzing-Arts et al., 2005), and is almost certainly the main determinant in the non-fasting state. It is particularly important when the supply of folate is limiting as the BHMT pathway appears to compensate for the lower homocysteine remethylation via the folate/vitamin B_{12}-dependent methionine synthase pathway (Holm et al., 2007). BHMT gene expression and activity can be increased when methyl donor availability (betaine, choline or various betaine analogues) is increased, particularly when dietary methionine is limiting (Emmert et al., 1996; Finkelstein et al., 1982a,b, 1983; Park et al., 1997; Park and Garrow, 1999; Slow et al., 2004a; Slow and Garrow, 2006). BHMT activity is subject to feedback inhibition, strongly by DMG and weakly by methionine (Allen et al., 1993). It is also regulated by osmotic stress (Delgado-Reyes and Garrow, 2005; Schäfer et al., 2007) and its expression is influenced by various hormones, including corticosteroids, insulin, estradiol, thyroid hormones and testosterone (Finkelstein et al., 1971; Park and Garrow, 1999; Shibata et al., 2003; Wijekoon et al., 2005; Ratnam et al., 2006). In an elderly cohort we found that the strongest predictors of plasma betaine were estradiol and cortisol (Storer et al., unpublished), which is consistent with the control of BHMT in rat liver (Finkelstein et al., 1971).

Aside from methionine, the other product of the BHMT-catalyzed reaction is *N,N*-dimethylglycine (DMG; ►Fig. 13.2). This is the only known route in mammals to this metabolite, so the presence of DMG is evidence that homocysteine has been methylated to methionine by BHMT. DMG is a potent feed-back inhibitor of BHMT (Finkelstein et al., 1972) and is further metabolized by the mitochondrial enzyme dimethylglycine dehydrogenase; this is an oxidative demethylation, coupled to the electron-transport chain. Dimethylglycine dehydrogenase is a flavoprotein and converts the methyl group into a one-carbon unit attached to tetrahydrofolate (forming 5,10-methylene THF). The other product is monomethyl glycine, sarcosine, which, in turn, can be demethylated by sarcosine dehydrogenase, a very similar (indeed, highly homologous) enzyme to dimethylglycine dehydrogenase, with glycine as the final product. Sarcosine is not an unambiguous marker of this pathway because it is also the product of the methylation of glycine by SAM, catalyzed by glycine N-methyltransferase. Glycine methylation by glycine N-methyltransferase controls methionine and SAM concentrations, and hence the distribution of methyl groups. Elevated methionine leads to increased expression of glycine N-methyltransferase (Rowling et al., 2002) and thus causes an increased consumption of S-adenosylmethionine, and consequently homocysteine. Because much of the homocysteine so produced is remethylated to methionine the carbon skeleton of homocysteine is not lost. As a result of this cyclic process, a large dose of betaine makes only a small difference to the plasma homocysteine concentration; plasma homocysteine is not an equilibrium concentration but a steady-state concentration (Hoffer, 2004; Mudd et al., 2007), and increasing the supply of methyl groups only results in a small shift in the steady state concentrations of methionine and homocysteine.

13.3.3 Plasma and urine betaine

Plasma betaine concentrations are usually much lower than tissue concentrations (Slow et al., 2009). Despite the importance of betaine as an osmolyte, plasma concentrations are little affected by osmotic stress, and appear to remain stable for years (Lever et al., 2004). Concentrations are higher in men than in women (Lever et al., 1994a; Konstantinova et al., 2008a), and this sex difference is also seen in rats (Slow et al., 2009). Thus it would seem that plasma betaine is an inherent and presumably genetically controlled individual characteristic, however, plasma betaine concentrations are affected by the dietary intake of betaine (Alfan et al., 2004; Schwab et al., 2006; Atkinson et al., 2008, 2009). Plasma betaine increases in a dose-related manner with increased betaine intake (Schwab et al., 2006), but when subjects change their daily betaine intake the fasting plasma concentrations appear to reach a new steady state within a few days (Alfan et al., 2004; Atkinson et al., 2009) (▶Fig. 13.3). This observation explains why there appears to be long-term stability despite the dietary effects on plasma concentrations, and individual subjects maintain similar plasma betaine concentrations for years (▶Fig. 13.4). Plasma betaine is probably mainly controlled by liver betaine concentrations (Slow et al., 2009), which, in turn, are controlled by the activity of BHMT. Given the control of BHMT, the overall effect is that plasma betaine concentrations are highly individual (Lever et al., 2004, 2009a), but plasma concentrations of the betaine metabolite, dimethylglycine, do not show similar control (Lever et al., 2009a); plasma dimethylglycine does increase slightly after a betaine load, but the effect is small and transitory. The supply of folate (necessary for the *de novo* generation of methyl groups) also affects plasma betaine concentrations (Melse-Boonstra et al., 2005) and they are lowered by folate deficiency in some patients (Allen et al., 1993). Folate-deficient patients had elevated serum dimethylglycine, which is consistent with an increased use of betaine as a source of methyl groups (Allen et al., 1993).

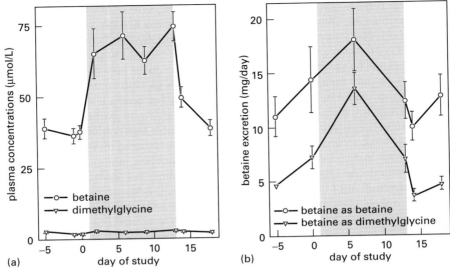

Fig. 13.3: Effect of a betaine supplement (1 g/day), taken during the shaded period, on 8 healthy young male subjects. Data are given as means and standard errors of the means. (a) Plasma betaine and *N,N*-dimethylglycine concentrations. (b) Urinary excretion of betaine and *N,N*-dimethylglycine (expressed as mg betaine lost). Data from Atkinson et al. (2009).

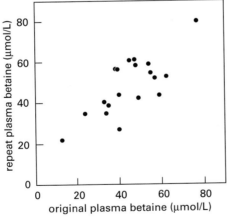

Fig. 13.4: Reproducibility of plasma betaine concentrations in normal adult subjects, samples taken 3 years apart; $r = 0.80$. Data from Lever et al. (2004).

Minimal betaine is excreted in the urine. Normally, the fractional clearance is less than 1.5% (Lever et al., 1994a) and the urinary excretion does not correlate with plasma concentrations. When normal subjects receive a betaine supplement there is at most a small and transient increase in the urine excretion (Schwab et al., 2006; Atkinson et al., 2008, 2009), and after two weeks on a supplement normal subjects are not excreting significantly more betaine than before the supplementation period

(▶Fig. 13.3) even though plasma betaine concentrations remain higher. Similarly, urinary betaine excretion is not significantly affected by osmotic stress (Lever et al., 2007c), and instead, individual subjects appear to excrete an approximately constant amount of betaine for weeks and possibly years. The urinary betaine excretion, as measured by the ratio to creatinine, is stable through a day, and collecting 24-hour urine samples does not seem to add to the information given by the creatinine ratio (Lever et al., 2007c, 2009a). Therefore, random urine samples are sufficient for assessing betaine excretion, because the betaine:creatinine ratio is not significantly affected by either food intake or hydration status. Urinary dimethylglycine increases after a betaine load, although this only accounts for a small proportion of the betaine supplied and appears to be transitory (Atkinson et al., 2009). Although the fractional clearance of dimethylglycine is not as low as that of betaine (Lever et al., 2005) the predominant route for its clearance is probably mitochondrial by dimethylglycine dehydrogenase rather than urinary clearance.

Some ingested betaine could be stored in tissues, and plasma concentrations do not change significantly under conditions that would be expected to affect tissue concentrations. However, in the longer supplementation studies (Alfthan et al., 2004; Atkinson et al., 2009) most of the betaine in the supplements appears to have been metabolized, and this must have involved the conversion of homocysteine to methionine. The small (sometimes undetectable) changes in plasma homocysteine show the limitation of this approach for lowering homocysteine, because the methionine produced will be metabolized to produce homocysteine. Studies of the fate of methyl-labeled betaine fed to chickens supports the concept of rapid distribution to tissues and the transfer of the methyl groups (Kettunen et al., 2001b).

13.3.4 Effect of a methionine load

When a load of methionine is supplied to humans or other mammals, plasma homocysteine increases. This is expected because excess methionine is metabolized by glycine N-methyltransferase, an enzyme controlled by the methionine supply, thus generating homocysteine. The catabolism of the carbon skeleton of methionine almost entirely proceeds through cystathionine β-synthase (▶Fig. 13.2), but this step is limiting and controlled by methionine and S-adenosylmethionine; most of the homocysteine is remethylated, completing a cycle. Thus supplying a methionine load predictably increases the steady-state concentration of homocysteine, and the steady-state ratio of methionine to homocysteine will depend on the supply of methyl groups for remethylation (Hoffer, 2004; Mudd et al., 2007). Tissue betaine is the major reserve of preformed methyl groups: this means that the supply of betaine is the major determinant of the post-methionine load increase in homocysteine (Holm et al., 2004). The methionine load test could be regarded as a test for betaine sufficiency.

13.4 Betaine in development

Maternal nutrition is important for normal human development, and in particular the supply of methyl groups is vital at all stages from conception to early infancy (Zeisel, 2009a,b). The role of different sources of methyl groups changes during development.

13.4.1 Early embryogenesis

In the mouse early pre-implantation embryo betaine is transported via a single saturable transporter, SIT1 (encoded by *Slc6a20a*) that is different from the osmoregulated betaine transporter BGT1 (Hammer and Baltz, 2002; Anas et al., 2007, 2008). SIT1 betaine transport is Na^+ and Cl^- dependent, and it is active a few hours after fertilization. It is present only in the fertilized egg and at lower levels at the two-cell stage, and is completely absent by the four-cell stage (Anas et al., 2007, 2008). SIT1 also transports proline and it is inhibited by several methylamino acids and proline derivatives *in vitro* (Anas et al., 2007), however, it has been suggested that its primary function *in vivo* is to mediate betaine accumulation and retention (Anas et al., 2008). One- and two-cell mouse pre-implantation embryos cultured in the presence of betaine have ≈4-fold higher betaine levels than those cultured without. Similarly, betaine appears to accumulate to relatively high levels *in vivo*, with intracellular concentrations corresponding to ≈6–7 mM (Anas et al., 2008) and is comparable to the average concentration of ≈4 mM in rat liver (Slow et al., 2009). The accumulated betaine remains present until the blastocyst stage (Lee et al., 2009).

Developing embryos depend on obtaining betaine from the mother, and the earliest stages of embryogenesis takes place in the oviduct. Mouse oviducts contain significant amounts of betaine (≈0.5 millimolar) averaged over the whole organ (Anas et al., 2007), and it is possible that this tissue store is an important supply of betaine that can be transferred via SIT1 to the pre-implantation embryo. The activation of betaine transport via SIT1 after fertilization and its transient presence during a short period of development implies that betaine has an important function during pre-implantation embryo development, however, the mechanism by which betaine exerts a beneficial effect is not known. It has been shown *in vitro* that betaine protects pre-implantation embryo development against increased osmolarity (Biggers et al., 1993; Dawson and Baltz, 1997; Hammer and Baltz, 2002) but it is yet to be established that it performs this role *in vivo*. The accumulated betaine could be important for methylation reactions including the maintenance of the methylation profile of DNA, which is an important control mechanism that regulates gene expression. The methylation profile of DNA (whether the gene is 'imprinted' or 'non-imprinted') depends on the stage of pregnancy (Delaval and Feil, 2004; Swales and Spears, 2005; Trasler, 2006; Zeisel, 2009a). However, for betaine to be utilized as a methyl donor, BHMT must be expressed and active in the pre-implantation embryo. BHMT mRNA transcript has been found to be expressed from the four-cell stage to the blastocyst. High levels of transcript, comparable to that found within the maternal liver, is found at the morula stage, which then decreases sharply in the blastocyst (Lee et al., 2009). Active BHMT protein is found in the inner cell mass of the blastocyst, but not the morula and it is only detectable for 48 h after blastocyst hatching, indicating that BHMT activity is transient and restricted to the blastocyst (Lee et al., 2009). This suggests that the betaine accumulated by the two-cell stage might be stored in the pre-implantation embryo and subsequently utilized as a supply of methyl groups via BHMT in the blastocyst, and thus betaine could have an important role as a source of methyl groups in the pre-implantation embryo. However, the consequences for pre-implantation embryo development should the betaine supply or BHMT activity be disrupted is as yet unknown. Notably, folate does not appear to be taken up by the mouse pre-implantation embryo at any stage (Baltz, personal communication), suggesting that the BHMT pathway might be the only means of maintaining methylation capacity, thus having a supply of betaine might be crucial at these early developmental stages.

Choline is also actively transported in the pre-implantation embryo via a Na^+-independent transporter, whose activity can be detected from the one-cell stage and increases 100-fold in the conceptus between the two-cell and blastocyst stages of development (Van Winkle et al., 1993). The primary role of choline in the pre-implantation embryo is thought to be for phospholipid synthesis (Van Winkle et al., 1993), which is required by blastocysts for morphological changes and growth. It has been shown that choline is incorporated into phosphatidylcholine and lysolecithin in mouse pre-implantation embryos, whereas the omission of choline from culture media inhibits the hatching of hamster blastocysts (Van Winkle et al., 1993). It is not known whether any of the transported choline is oxidized to betaine or if the oxidation pathway is active in the pre-implantation embryo.

13.4.2 Pregnancy and fetal development

The near-term rat fetus has been reported to have a betaine content of <2 mM whereas the placenta has >4 mM (Zeisel et al., 1995). In humans, maternal plasma betaine and dimethylglycine concentrations decline until gestational week 20 and thereafter remain constant, whereas plasma choline concentrations increase continuously during pregnancy (Molloy et al., 2005; Ueland et al., 2005; Velzing-Aarts et al., 2005). Maternal plasma homocysteine concentrations are reduced during gestation (Molloy et al., 2005; Wallace et al., 2008) with the lowest concentrations occurring in the second trimester (Velzing-Aarts et al., 2005). Plasma choline is a positive predictor of homocysteine, whereas from gestational week 20 onward maternal plasma betaine is a strong negative predictor of homocysteine (Molloy et al., 2005; Velzing-Aarts, 2005). It is believed that these changes during pregnancy are important to ensure choline availability for placental transfer, with subsequent use by the growing fetus. Choline is actively transported across the placenta and is ≈3-fold higher in the fetal circulation compared with those of the mother (Molloy et al., 2005; Velzing-Aarts et al., 2005; Friesen et al., 2007). Similarly, betaine and dimethylglycine are elevated 1- to 2-fold higher in the fetal circulation as assessed from umbilical cord blood at birth (Molloy et al., 2005; Friesen et al., 2007).

The inverse relation between maternal plasma betaine and homocysteine reflects the role of betaine in one-carbon metabolism during normal pregnancy. This suggests that a low betaine status during pregnancy might predispose to pregnancy complications associated with high homocysteine (Velzing-Aarts et al., 2005). In contrast to the pre-implantation embryo, BHMT expression has not been detected in the mouse fetus until gestational day 10 (Fisher et al., 2002), suggesting that expression is switched off in the post-implantation embryo only to be switched on again in the early fetus: thus the BHMT expression profile appears to be biphasic and dependent on the stage of pregnancy. It is also probable that fetal betaine is important for osmoregulation: however, the importance and partitioning of betaine between these two important competing functions (methyl donor and osmolyte) during human pregnancy has not been elucidated.

13.4.3 The relevance of choline versus betaine during pregnancy

Choline is an essential nutrient and is particularly crucial during fetal and neonatal life to ensure optimal neurodevelopment in rodents (Zeisel, 2000, 2009a). Normally, most of the betaine needs of the body can be met by choline oxidation. During pregnancy, the majority of choline is utilized for the production of phospholipids, including phosphatidylcholine and sphingomyelin, which are involved in membrane synthesis, and are crucial for normal spinal cord and brain development. The embryo/fetus develops in a high choline environment where the concentration in amniotic fluid is up to 10-fold higher than in maternal blood (Zeisel, 2006a, 2009a,b). In rats fed a diet considered to be adequate in choline, demands are so high during pregnancy that maternal liver choline concentrations are significantly depleted (Zeisel et al., 1995). The *de novo* synthesis of phosphatidylcholine, catalyzed by phosphatidylethanolamine methyltransferase (PEMT), is also up-regulated. This reaction requires the sequential addition of three methyl groups, provided by SAM, to phosphatidylethanolamine to form one molecule of phosphatidylcholine, thus utilizing a significant portion of SAM, and a supply of methyl groups other than choline is required (Zeisel, 2006a). As stated above, in humans, there is a negative association between betaine and homocysteine whereas maternal plasma choline concentrations positively correlate with homocysteine concentrations, suggesting there is also substantial phosphatidylcholine synthesis via PEMT during pregnancy (Molloy et al., 2005).

Choline oxidation is irreversible and diminishes the availability of choline for its other vital functions. Dietary betaine therefore spares choline and might be essential during pregnancy to ensure adequate choline for phospholipid and neurotransmitter synthesis. In addition, adequate dietary betaine can reduce maternal plasma homocysteine, which can have a direct deleterious effect on the developing embryo. Maternal flux through the choline oxidation pathway is thought to be increased during pregnancy providing betaine for homocysteine remethylation, thus supplying adequate methionine and methyl donors to the fetus for protein synthesis and methylation reactions (Molloy et al., 2005; Wallace et al., 2008) which could also explain the strong inverse association observed in human pregnancy between maternal plasma betaine and homocysteine concentrations. Similarly, maternal choline oxidation and dietary betaine intake are thought to be even more important for normal fetal development when the mother's supply of methionine or folate is limited or deficient, because it appears that the BHMT remethylation pathway compensates for the inadequate flux through the methionine synthase pathway (Molloy et al., 2005; Wallace et al., 2008).

13.4.4 Clinical significance of methylation in pregnancy

Failure to re-establish the methylation profile of non-imprinted genes or to maintain the methylation of imprinted genes during embryogenesis is associated with embryo loss, fetal abnormalities (Wolff et al., 1998; Paulsen and Ferguson-Smith, 2001; Wu et al., 2004; Niculescu et al., 2006; Waterland et al., 2006), perturbations in growth and placental formation/function *in utero* (Mann et al., 2004; Coan et al., 2005) as well as cancer (Feinburg and Vogelstein, 1983; Jones and Laird, 1999; Davis and Uthus, 2004), disturbed neurobehavioral processes (Robertson, 2005), obesity (Garfinkel and Ruden, 2004; Waterland et al., 2008), diabetes (Brownlee, 1995) and vascular disease

(Roher et al., 1993; Brownlee, 1995; Stadtman and Levine, 2000) in the newborn and adult progeny. Thus it is essential that the maternal dietary intake of methyl groups, both periconceptually and throughout gestation, is adequate to meet the requirements of the developing progeny. This is clearly illustrated by dietary manipulation in the *agouti* and *axin fused* mice, where maternal supplementation of folate, vitamin B12, methionine, choline and betaine before and during pregnancy permanently increased DNA methylation at the viable *yellow agouti (Avy)* (Wolff et al., 1998) and *AxinFU* (Waterland et al., 2006) metastable alleles affecting gene expression in the offspring as well as their health and longevity (Wolff et al., 1998). Similarly in humans, folate supplementation before and in early pregnancy reduces the recurrence and occurrence of neural tube defects (spina bifida, anencephaly and encephalocele).

The periconceptual maternal dietary intake of choline and to a lesser extent betaine has been associated with neural tube defects, where the risk was lowest in women whose diets were rich in choline, betaine and methionine (Shaw et al., 2004). However, the association for betaine was weaker and disappeared when folate status was high, suggesting that the stronger association with choline might be more related to its other functions rather than as a source of methyl groups via its oxidation to betaine. This is not surprising given that the BHMT pathway does not appear to be active in the post-implantation embryo and is only found in the early fetus at a time when neural tube closure is nearly complete (Fisher et al., 2002). However, because betaine is a requirement, the observed association could illustrate the choline-sparing effect of dietary betaine; women with high dietary betaine intakes can supply more choline to the developing embryo at time when it might be a more crucial nutrient for neural tube development. Similarly, a low periconceptual maternal betaine status or dietary intake might cause epigenetic disturbances during pre-implantation embryo development, a time when the betaine/BHMT pathway appears to be active, which could subsequently cause aberrant gene expression in the post-implantation embryo and, in turn, lead to an increased risk of neural tube defect.

It has been suggested that homocysteine metabolism via the BHMT pathway might be more important than metabolism via the folate-dependent methionine synthase pathway in late pregnancy (Ueland et al., 2005; Velzing-Aarts et al., 2005). In pre-eclampsia, homocysteine concentrations are elevated in both the maternal and fetal circulation and one hypothesis was that the high homocysteine concentrations might have been caused by a choline and betaine insufficiency. However, compared with uncomplicated pregnancies, maternal and fetal choline and betaine concentrations were higher in pre-eclampsia and the association between maternal plasma choline and homocysteine previously documented (Molloy et al., 2005) was not found (Braekke et al., 2007). These findings do not necessarily mean that the BHMT pathway is any less important in late pregnancy, or that too much betaine or choline increases the risk of pre-eclampsia. It could be that the elevations in both choline and betaine indicate that the BHMT pathway might be down-regulated in pre-eclampsia and the increase in choline and betaine is a consequence of the condition rather than a cause.

BHMT genotype could also contribute to the risk of adverse pregnancy outcomes and birth defects, but the number of studies that have investigated this are limited and the findings have been inconsistent. The BHMT A allele (742G>A; R239Q) has been associated with a decreased risk of neural tube defect, where the AA genotype in either the mother or the child was associated with decreased risk, albeit non-significantly

(Morin et al., 2003), whereas another study found no association with spina bifida and the A genotype (Zhu et al., 2005).The risk of orofacial clefts (cleft lip with or without cleft palate) has been found to be significantly lower in children with the AA genotype (Mostowska et al., in press), and by contrast, mothers homozygous for the A allele have an increased risk of placental abruption (Ananth et al., 2007). The sometimes seemingly contradictory findings have been attributed to possible differences in BHMT expression at different life stages. In adults BHMT functions predominantly in the liver, but little is known regarding the expression pattern in the developing embryo and it could be markedly different compared with the adult (Boyles et al., 2006). The mechanism by which the BHMT A allele affects risk is unknown although a recent *in vitro* study has shown that the apparent K_m values for homocysteine and betaine are considerably lower for the Q enzyme when compared to the wild-type R enzyme (Li et al., 2008) and it has been suggested that the A genotype could create a highly efficient enzyme variant *in vivo* (Mostowska et al., in press).

13.4.5 Neonatal development

Plasma, liver and kidney betaine concentrations change substantially between neonatal and adult life in rats (Wijekoon et al., 2005), all transiently increasing several-fold post-weaning, and remaining high, peaking at 28 days of age (1 week post-weaning) until day 42, before declining by day 56 (Rafter et al., 1991; Clow et al., 2008). The increases in plasma and tissue betaine appear to be a response to dietary intake, with the accumulation occurring because liver clearance is lower than intake (Clow et al., 2008). Choline oxidation to betaine is still occurring because rat pups fed a betaine-free diet still show a substantial transient increase in total liver betaine content, but animals fed a diet containing betaine have larger increases in plasma and tissue betaine, although the osmotic stresses on the animals, a major determinant of tissue betaine content, does not appear to have been controlled. Liver BHMT activity is high pre-weaning (day 14–21) before declining to remain constant from day 21 to 27. Choline dehydrogenase activity gradually increases to a plateau between 35 and 42 days of age. Pup dietary betaine intake post-weaning has little effect on either BHMT or choline dehydrogenase activity, neither does maternal dietary intake pre-weaning (Clow et al., 2008).

Neonatal rats and humans both excrete remarkable amounts of betaine (Davies et al., 1988), and this high excretion does not appear to occur *in utero* (Davies et al., 1992) but commences at birth (Trump et al., 2006). Excretion might increase for a short time after birth (Davies et al., 1992), but this is probably an artifact of expressing excretion as a ratio to creatinine, which is not reliable in the neonatal period (Trump et al., 2006). Certainly betaine excretion declines during human infancy and childhood (▶Fig. 13.5) although it does not reach the lower adult levels until the early teenage years (Lever et al., 2009a), and the neonatal betaine excretion might reflect the immaturity of the neonatal kidney. Because most of this betaine is presumably derived from choline it might compromise the supply of choline and consequently methyl groups (Davies et al., 1992; Holmes et al., 2000), and it is probable that the loss is of the same order as the supply, although the increase in the choline content of breast milk in the first few days should give a margin of safety (Holmes et al., 2000). However, this is probably not true if milk formulas are used (Holmes et al., 2000), and including additional betaine or choline in these formulas might be advisable.

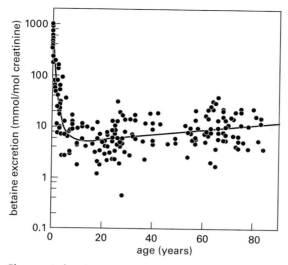

Fig. 13.5: Changes in betaine excretion with age (Lever et al. 2009a). Minimum at approximately 13 years.

13.5 Clinical importance

The possibility that disturbances in betaine intake, metabolism or excretion have clinical consequences has been canvassed for some years. Because betaine has important roles in normal physiology we would predict that a betaine insufficiency would have adverse consequences.

13.5.1 Betaine, obesity and fat metabolism

A major part of the world's betaine production is used by the animal industries. It has been known for many years that including betaine in animal feeds leads to better meat, more lean muscle mass and less fat (Eklund et al., 2005). Although this is best documented in pigs, similar effects are well known in poultry (Wang et al., 2004; Zhan et al., 2006), and can also be shown in lambs before rumen development (Fernández et al., 2000). How betaine affects body fat is not clear, and many mechanisms have been proposed (Eklund et al., 2005). Betaine is an osmolyte in intestinal cells and probably affects nutrient digestibility and partitioning, and increasing the availability of methionine has been invoked to explain increased protein production. Small animal studies also support a role for betaine, e.g., in the agouti mouse model the transgenerational amplification of obesity is prevented when animals are fed a diet high in betaine and its precursor choline (Waterland et al., 2008), and these results suggest that epigenetic methylation is involved. There is evidence in finishing pigs that betaine decreases lipogenesis by decreasing the mRNA expression of the relevant enzymes (Huang et al., 2008), and although it is suggested that this effect is mediated by growth hormone (which is elevated by betaine treatment), an epigenetic effect is possible. Despite the effects of betaine supplements on other mammals and on poultry, they have not been observed in humans. When otherwise healthy obese adult subjects were supplied a betaine supplement for 12 weeks no effect was seen on body fat as assessed by bio-electrical impedance or body mass index (BMI) (Schwab et al., 2002). By contrast, cross-sectional data (Konstantinova et al., 2008a) show a highly significant negative association between markers of obesity (BMI, percent body fat and waist circumference) and plasma betaine concentrations.

The effect on obesity implies an interaction between betaine and lipid metabolism. In several human cross-sectional studies (Lever et al., 2005, 2007b; Konstantinova et al., 2008a) plasma betaine is inversely related to lipid markers (triglycerides, apolipoprotein B, LDL-cholesterol), suggesting that low plasma betaine is associated with a greater vascular risk; however, betaine supplementation of healthy subjects, which raises plasma betaine concentrations, increases plasma cholesterol (Schwab et al., 2002). Indeed, Olthof et al. (2005b) questioned the safety of betaine supplementation on the basis of a small elevation in plasma triglycerides and LDL cholesterol in subjects receiving betaine supplements, although the significance of these results has been questioned (Zeisel, 2006b). Animal studies suggest a possible resolution of this apparent contradiction by suggesting that betaine affects the partitioning of lipid in the body, and in particular increases the export of tissue triglycerides. In normal rats, betaine supplementation (particularly when methionine is restricted) leads to increased hepatic production of apolipoprotein B (Sparks et al., 2006) and increased plasma LDL and triglycerides, and these changes are associated with a large decrease in tissue lipid, which has been confirmed in other studies (Hayes et al., 2003). When the water-soluble components of lean and obese Zucker rat livers were compared (Serkova et al., 2006), the largest differences were in betaine (approx. 4-fold lower in the obese animals) and methionine (more than 10-fold higher in the obese animals), which is consistent with what is seen in human cross-sectional studies because liver concentrations determine plasma concentrations. Other mechanisms, however, might be involved; betaine has also been shown to decrease fatty acid synthesis, in pigs (Huang et al., 2008), by decreasing the expression of the enzymes involved in lipogenesis. In an apolipoprotein E-deficient mouse model, which develops atherosclerotic lesions (Lv et al., 2009), betaine supplementation increased plasma cholesterol (but not triglycerides) but at the same time decreased atherosclerotic lesion areas. The difference was attributed to lowered TNF-α expression in the supplemented animals and hence less inflammation. Another mouse model, with a disruption of the methylenetetrahydrofolate reductase gene (with the result that the animals tend to have elevated plasma homocysteine) was given a diet supplemented with betaine, and in this model the plasma triglycerides decreased on long-term (1 year) supplementation whereas HDL-cholesterol increased; other improvements in the atherogenic risk factor profile were also observed (Schwahn et al., 2007). Another relevant observation on the connection between betaine and obesity is that making rats obese by supplying them with a high-fat diet more than doubles their betaine excretion (Kim et al., 2009).

The diverse effects of betaine supplementation on plasma lipids implies that the outcome also depends on other clinical conditions, and additionally in rats there is some evidence that diet also affects the results (Hayes et al., 2003). In the human cross-sectional studies low plasma betaine concentrations are associated with elevated plasma lipids and other components of the metabolic syndrome (Konstantinova et al., 2008a). Similarly, in a population that was being treated for dyslipidemia (Lever et al., 2005,

2007b) the plasma betaine concentrations were particularly low and consistent with the results reported by Konstantinova et al. (2008a). It is possible that in these studies many of the subjects, with elevated plasma lipids, had a betaine deficiency and that there is an association between betaine deficiency and the lipid abnormalities. A possible connecting theme is an association with mitochondrial function. The protective effect of betaine on the electron transport system has been attested in plant root mitochondria (Hamilton and Heckathorn, 2001), and suggested in rats (Ganesan et al., 2007). Mitochondrial dysfunction could be involved in many of the diseases where abnormalities of betaine homeostasis occur, and such an indirect connection would also explain the correlations between betaine and carnitine (Lever et al., 2005, 2007b) and a correlation between plasma betaine and coenzyme Q in acute coronary syndrome patients (unpublished data). Causal connections are not necessary because they could all be consequences of a common underlying pathology.

It is interesting that the reported studies of betaine supplementation in rats, mice and domestic animals are often longer-term than any reported in a human population. The overall impression is that long-term betaine supplementation is unlikely to be harmful and could be beneficial. The small increases in plasma lipids reported in some studies are not clinically significant, they might only apply to betaine-replete subjects and might not persist. By contrast, the loss of tissue lipid could be a long-term gain.

13.5.2 Betaine, diabetes and the metabolic syndrome

It has been known for years that more than 20% of patients with diabetes mellitus excrete abnormal amounts of betaine in their urine (Lever et al., 1994b; Dellow et al., 1999) while maintaining near-normal plasma concentrations, and the fractional clearance in some of these patients exceeds 100% (normal <1.5%), which suggests that there is an active process exporting the betaine. Abnormal betaine excretion is also frequent in other patient groups, e.g., in chronic renal failure patients (Lever et al., 1994b), in patients attending a lipid disorders clinic (Lever et al., 2005, 2007b) and in patients being treated with fibrates (Lever et al., 2009b). In patients with diabetes there is a positive correlation between the urinary excretion of betaine and of another renal osmolyte, sorbitol, and this has not been seen in other groups, which suggests that in at least some of the patients with diabetes a different mechanism is involved, possibly involving an overproduction of sorbitol.

As already noted, in the metabolic syndrome there is a tendency for plasma betaine to be lower than in a healthy population (Konstantinova et al., 2008a). The divergent associations of the substrate (choline) and product (betaine) of mitochondrial choline dehydrogenase could reflect disruption of this pathway as part of the mitochondrial dysfunction that prevails in metabolic syndrome. Elevated urinary betaine loss is common in metabolic syndrome patients (Lever et al., 2009a), so abnormal loss of betaine might be a factor in causing betaine insufficiency, which could be a common feature of the metabolic syndrome. Similarly, because some of the lipid disorders patients were persistently excreting abnormal amounts of betaine for years (Lever et al., 2007a) there must be some stress on the tissue betaine supply in these patients (tissue betaine is variable and much higher than the controlled circulating betaine concentrations). These are the population groups that are most likely to benefit from betaine supplementation.

13.5.3 Betaine, homocysteine and vascular disease

High doses (6 g/day or more) of betaine, alone or in combination with B-vitamins, have been used for years to treat patients with genetic disorders that cause homocystinuria (Wilcken et al., 1983, 1985; Ogier de Baulny et al., 1998; Yap, 2003). Because the betaine supply is the main determinant of plasma homocysteine under non-fasting conditions, several investigators have studied the consequences of more modest supplementation on plasma homocysteine, and it has been confirmed that there is a dose-related reduction of fasting homocysteine (by 20%) and post methionine load homocysteine (by 29–40%) sustained as long as betaine is administered (Schwab et al., 2002; Olthof et al., 2003; Steenge et al., 2003; Olthof and Verhoef, 2005). The methionine produced by methylating homocysteine can only be metabolized by conversion to homocysteine and in this cyclic process the steady-state concentrations of plasma homocysteine only change by a small amount compared with the large amount of betaine being processed (Hoffer, 2004; Mudd et al., 2007). This is a different effect from that of folate supplementation because folate provides a recyclable cofactor for the *de novo* synthesis of methyl groups, and reduces only fasting homocysteine, whereas betaine directly supplies the methyl groups and is consumed in the process of forming methionine (►Fig. 13.2).

That total plasma total homocysteine is a vascular risk factor is well-attested and recently reaffirmed (Loscalzo, 2006; Herrmann et al., 2007; Ueland and Clarke, 2007), but the results of prospective, secondary trials have thrown doubt on whether homocysteine is causal (Bønaa et al., 2006; HOPE, 2006). A significant reduction (by B-vitamin supplementation) in mean plasma total homocysteine concentrations did not significantly reduce the incidence of subsequent events. If the supply of methyl groups is crucial then betaine should be immediately and directly effective because the methyl groups of dietary betaine rapidly appear in tissue methionine, and similarly if the betaine supply is restricted then its function as an osmolyte is compromised. The groups where betaine deficiency is most likely to be found are patients with diabetes or metabolic syndrome, and it is possible that elevated homocysteine in some of these patients is an indicator of betaine status. There are few studies that directly test a connection between betaine supply and vascular disease. Short or medium-term betaine supplementation does not improve flow-mediated vasodilation, a marker of endothelial function, despite reduced homocysteine (Olthof and Verhoef, 2005; Olthof et al., 2006). One study demonstrated impaired vasodilation in subjects given betaine, no effect from low doses of folic acid and enhanced vasodilation in subject given folic acid at doses exceeding those required to obtain maximal homocysteine reduction, suggesting improved endothelial function by mechanisms independent of homocysteine (Moat et al., 2006).

A recent study on 3000 healthy Greek men and women demonstrated low plasma levels of inflammatory markers, such as C-reactive protein, interleukin-6 and TNF-α, in subjects with high intake of choline and betaine (Detopoulou et al., 2008). Because inflammation plays a role in atherogenesis, high intake of choline and betaine could protect against cardiovascular disease. However, two recent large prospective studies, based on the participants in the Dutch PROSPECT-EPIC cohort (Dalmeijer et al., 2007) and in the Atherosclerosis Risk in Communities (ARIC) study (Bidulescu et al., 2007), respectively, found no association between intake of choline and betaine and cardiovascular disease. These negative or contradictory findings could be related to the large measurement error of intake estimates for micronutrients such as choline and betaine (Bidulescu et al., 2009), or they might result from the selection of the study populations, and for clarification we must wait for the results of future studies.

13.5.4 Betaine and liver disease

Betaine is known to ameliorate the adverse effects of alcohol on the liver, in particular, fatty liver (Barak and Tuma, 1983; Barak et al., 1996, 1997), and this has been attributed to maintaining SAM levels and minimizing the accumulation of S-adenosylhomocysteine, SAH (Barak et al., 2003; Kharbanda et al., 2005). Alcohol is reported to inhibit methionine synthase, increasing the requirement for betaine to sustain methylation (Kharbanda, 2009). Methylation is particularly important in the liver for the *de novo* synthesis of phosphatidylcholine, which is essential for normal VLDL assembly and secretion, and thereby minimizes fatty accumulations (Kharbanda et al., 2007; 2009). Betaine can also improve liver health in non-alcoholic fatty liver diseases, and in liver disease induced by xenobiotics (Oliva et al., 2009) or bile salts (Graf et al., 2002). The proposed mechanism, involving the supply of methyl groups for phosphatidylcholine synthesis, is plausible, but other mechanisms have been suggested, including reduced endoplasmic reticulum stress (Ji and Kaplowitz, 2003; Ji, 2008) and epigenetic effects (Graf et al., 2002), and also betaine is a major liver osmolyte. The use of betaine in treating these conditions was reviewed by Craig (2004).

13.5.5 Betaine and other diseases

The first clinical role attributed to betaine was a negative one, as an osmoprotectant that enables bacteria (particularly *Escherichia coli*) to grow in urine that has enough salt and urea to normally preclude growth (Chambers and Kunin, 1985, 1987). This is important in urinary tract infections. The common invasive bacteria do not synthesize betaine (except from choline) but have betaine transport systems that are highly efficient, and to enable growth they accumulate betaine against concentration gradients greater than 10^7, so the actual betaine concentration in urine is not a clinically significant factor affecting growth, and patients with high betaine excretion might not be at a higher risk of developing infections.

Claims that betaine (TMG) alleviates autism do not appear to be supported by any controlled clinical studies, only by the suggestion that there is an impaired methylation capacity in autism (James et al., 2004). There might be an association between betaine and cognitive function, based on a study in which an elderly group (>70 years) was supplemented with folate and cobalamin (Eussen et al., 2007), which raised the plasma betaine concentrations, interestingly, there appeared to be an association between this increase in betaine and memory performance. Betaine supplementation has been suggested for other disorders involving disturbed methyl metabolism but few have been investigated (Craig, 2004).

13.6 Clinical laboratory aspects of betaine

13.6.1 Laboratory measurement

Measuring the concentration of betaine poses a challenge for the analyst. As a consequence of its high water solubility, and low solubility in organic solvents, it is not easily extracted from an aqueous solution. Its absorbance spectrum has no peaks in the visible or near-UV regions, and it has only a weak absorbance close to 200 nm where most metabolites absorb light, further, the quaternary amine group is unreactive, and the carboxyl group is highly deactivated and thus harder to derivatize than most carboxylates. An early approach exploited the low solubility of quaternary ammonium tri-iodides (Barak and Tuma, 1979, 1981), which enabled tissue concentrations to be measured; another approach was to use betaine homocysteine methyltransferase in enzymatic assays (Martin and Finkelstein, 1981), and when combined with derivatization of the product and mass spectroscopic detection this led to a method with sufficient sensitivity to measure blood concentrations (Allen et al., 1993). These methods were insensitive and time-consuming.

Nuclear magnetic resonance (NMR) has been extensively used to measure betaine, and has the advantages of being non-destructive, needing minimal sample preparation and rapidly providing a large amount of data. Almost all have used proton NMR, although ^{13}C-NMR has been used to measure betaine in bacteria (Ko et al., 1994), and the possibility of using ^{14}N-NMR has been explored (Balaban and Knepper, 1983; Bell et al., 1991). Proton NMR is attractive because of the strong singlet resonance from the nine identical protons on the three methyl groups, making for a relatively sensitive assay (Davies et al., 1988; Bell et al., 1991; Lundberg et al., 1995). It is possible to measure betaine directly in water after suppressing the water signal and techniques are available to suppress the protein resonances. The main limitation on the use of NMR is sensitivity. It has been shown to be a rapid and convenient technique for measuring betaine in urine (Lee et al., 2006) and tissues (Bedford et al., 1998), and recently NMR has been widely adopted in metabolomic studies (Beckonert et al., 2007; Martin et al., 2009; Bollard et al., 2010). A problem with measuring betaine in biological samples by proton NMR is the near co-resonance, at neutral pH, of the methyl protons of betaine and of trimethylamine N-oxide (TMAO); the choline signal is also close enough to interfere. The signals can be separated by changing the pH of the solution so that TMAO, and possibly betaine also, are protonated (Bell et al., 1991; Bedford et al., 1998; Lee et al., 2006). Overlooking this has led to mis-identifications in the past (Bell et al., 1991). It is probable that this confusion continues, e.g., the signals reported by Martin et al. (2009) as 'TMAO' are probably betaine, and the protocol recommended by Beckonert et al. (2007) will confuse these metabolites. These problems can be avoided, and because of its advantages NMR is likely to become increasingly popular for measuring betaine as more sensitive instruments become widely available, and probe technology improves.

High-performance liquid chromatography (HPLC) is widely used to measure betaine, although detection is a problem. Underivatized betaine has been chromatographed and detected by refractive index changes (Wolff et al., 1989) and this had sufficient sensitivity for measuring the high concentrations of tissue betaine, but lacks the sensitivity needed to measure the betaine in plasma or serum, and for these samples the betaine needs to be derivatized first. Most derivatization methods depend on alkylating the carboxyl group to add a UV-absorbing or fluorescent functional group, and the commonest derivatizing agents are 2'-bromophenacyl bromide (Laryea et al., 1998; Clow et al., 2008), 2'-bromophenacyl triflate (Lever et al., 1992; Mar et al., 1995) and 2-naphthacyl triflate (Storer and Lever, 2006); others can be used (Sakamoto et al., 2002; Happer et al., 2004; Storer and Lever, 2006). Preparing derivatives that have a higher UV absorbance, or are fluorescent, makes possible a simple method using a 10 µl or smaller plasma sample (Storer and Lever, 2006). The betaine derivatives are quaternary ammonium cations and can be separated by ion-exchange based chromatography systems (Sakamoto, 2002; Storer et al., 2006). Derivatization often leads to the derivatization of the betaine metabolite, N,N-dimethylglycine (Laryea et al., 1998; Storer et al., 2006), but this derivative is a double derivative, alkylated both on the nitrogen and the carboxyl to give a quaternary amine with two chromophores (Storer et al., 2006) which elutes too early on silica columns for reliable quantification. The alumina columns that made the separation possible (Storer et al., 2006) are no longer available, but similar separations can be made on titania or zirconia columns (unpublished data). Capillary electrophoresis (Zhang et al., 2002) is not sufficiently sensitive for measuring blood concentrations (Storer et al., 2006).

Betaine determination using mass spectrometry has a long history, being implemented directly on ester derivatives (Rhodes et al., 1987) or in combination with gas chromatography after conversion to volatile derivatives (Allen et al., 1993). However, mass spectrometry is now used in conjunction with liquid chromatography, which avoids the need for extraction and derivatization steps. Liquid chromatography-tandem mass spectrometry (LC-MS/MS) has become the method by which most betaine assays are conducted (Koc et al., 2002; Holm et al., 2003; Ueland et al., 2007). The detection is made highly selective by using multiple-reaction monitoring (MRM), and because high resolution is not necessary in the chromatography this can be made more rapid than with UV or fluorescence detection; e.g., betaine and related compounds can be separated and simultaneously quantified in under 5 min using less than 5 µl of sample (Holm et al., 2003). By these means, plasma betaine, choline and dimethylglycine can be measured simultaneously on over 300 samples in a day (Ueland et al., 2007) using one analytical system. This is the way that recent large epidemiological studies of betaine metabolism have become possible (Ueland et al., 2005; Fredriksen et al., 2007; Ueland et al., 2007; Konstantinova et al., 2008a,b; Johansson et al., 2009).

13.6.2 Clinical biochemistry of betaine

Formal reference ranges for plasma and urine concentrations of betaine and its metabolite, N,N-dimethylglycine are not available, and reports from different countries either include a small number of subjects or they focus on subsets of the populations. Fortunately these reports are consistent (▶Tab. 13.1) despite the variety of analytical methods used and the differences in the population groups that have been selected. Serum or plasma betaine tends to be higher in adult males than in females, and is usually in the 20–70 µmol/l range; less is known about serum or plasma dimethylglycine concentrations, but they are usually below 10 µmol/l. Urine betaine excretion is less well documented, but adults normally excrete between 2 and 35 mmol betaine per mole creatinine (▶Tab. 13.1).

Tab. 13.1: Reference range data for betaine and dimethylglycine.

Literature reference	n	Blood (µmol/l)		Urine (mmol/mole creatinine)	
		Betaine	DMG	Betaine	DMG
Allen et al. (1993)					
serum and urine	60	18–73[a]	1.4–5.3[a]	2–56[a]	1.2–12.2[a]
Lever et al. (1994)					
Plasma ♀	35	12–56[a]			
Plasma ♂	37	11–83[a]			
Urine	76			1.5–32.5[a]	
Holm et al. (2003)					
Serum fasting	59	28–42[b]	1.4–2.2[b]		
Plasma fasting	60	27–41[b]	1.3–2.0[b]		
Serum non-fasting	46	37–48[b]	1.6–2.5[b]		
Plasma non-fasting	60	36–47[b]	1.6–2.5[b]		
Schwab et al. (2006)					
Serum	10	27–67[a]			
Holm et al. (2007)					
Plasma 50–64 years ♀	5381	14.9–58.6[a]			
Plasma 50–64 years ♂	5221	23.2–71.1[a]			

(Continued)

Tab. 13.1: (*Continued*)

Literature reference	n	Blood (μmol/l)		Urine (mmol/mole creatinine)	
		Betaine	DMG	Betaine	DMG
Konstantinova et al. (2008)					
Plasma 47–49 years ♀	2062	16.9–56.2[a]			
Plasma 47–49 years ♂	1657	26.3–72.1[a]			
Plasma 71–74 years ♀	1860	20.4–62.3[a]			
Plasma 71–74 years ♂	1466	26.5–73.8[a]			
Lever et al. (2009a)					
Plasma ♀	74	17–60[a]			
Plasma ♂	81	21–78[a]			
Plasma ♀	37		0.4–12.3[a]		
Plasma ♂	43		0.8–9.6[a]		
Urine	160			1.8–35.9[a]	
Urine	52				0.4–30.5[a]

DMG, *N,N*-dimethylglycine. [a]95% range; [b]interquartile range. The two Lever et al. studies are not independent, and the later estimates differ slightly because more elderly subjects were recruited after the earlier report.

What is the clinical value of measuring betaine or dimethylglycine? Because there is no correlation between betaine excretion and plasma betaine concentration in either cross-sectional studies or within individual subjects (Lever et al., 2009a), these are potentially separate tests. Despite its high individuality, plasma betaine concentrations do not appear to have significant diagnostic value, being remarkably stable despite significant changes in tissue betaine (Lever et al., 2004). Although plasma betaine concentrations tend to be lower in the metabolic syndrome and in response to stress, the difference is not likely to have a diagnostic application. It is affected by dietary betaine intake, but the large changes seen in supplementation studies are not typical, and the small changes on a normal diet would not confound interpretation (Holm et al., 2003; Lever et al., 2004, 2005). Urine betaine excretion, measured as the ratio to creatinine, is potentially more useful; as well as the abnormally high betaine excretion in diabetes and the metabolic syndrome, high excretion is common in chronic renal failure patients without diabetes, and interestingly, an abnormally low betaine excretion is also found in some patients with diabetes or with chronic renal failure, although no clinical significance has yet been attached to this. Elevated excretion is also associated with fibrate therapy (Lever et al., 2009b), with particularly high excretions in patients with features of the metabolic syndrome who are being treated with a fibrate. Elevated betaine excretions also show individual persistence (Lever et al., 2007a). Random urine samples are adequate to identify abnormal urine excretion, because the betaine to creatinine ratio is at least as reliable as the 24-h excretion (Lever et al., 2009a), and is not significantly affected by food intake. This test could identify potential betaine deficient patients. As previously noted, urine betaine excretion might be elevated as a result of consuming foods containing proline betaine (Atkinson et al., 2007), and supplying betaine supplements in orange juice probably accounts for the different (although both low) estimates of urinary loss made by Schwab et al. (2006) and Atkinson et al. (2009), making it advisable to avoid using orange juice in investigations of one-carbon metabolism.

Although it has low individuality, plasma dimethylglycine concentrations could have diagnostic value (Lever et al., 2009a) as a marker of abnormal one-carbon metabolism because it is only produced via the betaine-homocysteine methyltransferase catalyzed reaction, and the plasma dimethylglycine to betaine ratio might be the preferred test (McGregor et al., 2001), but more work is needed to establish that these measures would add to the information available from more accessible tests. No clinical information has so far been identified in measures of urine dimethylglycine excretion, which correlate with both plasma dimethylglycine and with urine betaine excretion.

13.7 Summary

Betaine is an essential metabolite with important roles as a tissue osmolyte and as a reserve of metabolically available methyl groups. It is not an essential component of the diet because the requirements for betaine can be met by the metabolism of dietary choline, assuming that the supply of choline is sufficient. However, dietary betaine is efficiently absorbed and readily used, and this reduces the demand for choline, which is an essential nutrient with different roles in mammalian physiology. Betaine cannot be readily converted into choline and can only partly replace dietary choline.

The betaine supply could be inadequate in some patients with diabetes mellitus or with features of metabolic syndrome, one reason being that many of these patients lose excessive amounts of betaine in their urine. These patients typically present with dyslipidemia and elevated plasma homocysteine. It is possible that the betaine deficiency contributes to the health problems of this increasing section of the population, and that a modest level of betaine supplementation will be beneficial, however, long-term prospective studies on appropriate human populations have not been conducted to establish this. Betaine also has important roles in human development, in the period immediately before and after conception as well as later in pregnancy, and in the first few weeks after birth. The recent improvements in analytical methods and the availability of food composition data for choline and betaine have motivated clinical and epidemiological studies on the relation between choline and betaine status and disease risk, mainly for conditions previously investigated in relation to folate status. Human data are sparse, the number of studies is limited and no large placebo-controlled intervention trials on betaine or choline supplementation have been published; the claims of those marketing 'TMG' as a panacea are not based on reliable evidence. Betaine and human health is a research area in its infancy, but with the potential to generate data leading to rational strategies for disease prevention.

References

Alfieri RR, Cavazzoni A, Petronini PG, Bonelli MA, Caccamo AE, Borghetti AF, Wheeler KP, Compatible osmolytes modulate the response of porcine endothelial cells to hypertonicity and protect them from apoptosis. J Physiol 2002;540: 499–508.

Alfieri RR, Petronini PG, Bonelli MA, Desenzani S, Cavazzoni A, Borghetti AF, Wheeler KP, Roles of compatible osmolytes and heat shock protein 70 in the induction of tolerance to stresses in porcine endothelial cells. J Physiol 2004;555: 757–67.

Alfthan G, Tapani K, Nissinen K, Saarela J, Aro A, The effect of low doses of betaine on plasma homocysteine in healthy volunteers. Br J Nutr 2004;92: 665–9.

Allen RH, Stabler SP, Lindenbaum J, Serum betaine, N,N-dimethylglycine and N-methylglycine levels in patients with cobalamin and folate deficiency and related inborn errors of metabolism. Metabolism 1993;42: 1448–60.

Anas M, Hammer M, Lever M, Stanton JL, Baltz JM, The organic osmolytes betaine and proline are transported by a shared system in early preimplantation mouse embryos. J Cell Physiol 2007;210: 266–77.

Anas MI, Lee MB, Zhou C, Hammer M, Slow S, Karmouch J, Liu XJ, Bröer S, Lever M, Baltz JM, SIT1 is a betaine/proline transporter that is activated in mouse eggs after fertilization and functions until the 2-cell stage. Development 2008;135: 4123–30.

Ananth CV, Elsasser DA, Kinzler WL, Peltier MR, Getahun D, Leclerc D, Rozen RR, for the New Jersey-Placental Abruption Study Investigators, Polymorphisms in methionine synthase reductase and betaine-homocysteine S-methyltransferase genes: risk of placental abruption. Mol Genet Metab 2007;91: 104–10.

Atkinson W, Downer P, Lever M, Chambers ST, George PM, Effects of orange juice and proline betaine on glycine betaine and homocysteine in healthy male subjects. Eur J Nutr 2007;46: 446–52.

Atkinson W, Elmslie J, Lever M, Chambers ST, George PM, Dietary and supplementary betaine: acute effects on plasma betaine and homocysteine concentrations under standard and post methionine load conditions in healthy male subjects. Am J Clin Nutr 2008;87: 577–85.

Atkinson A, Slow S, Elmslie J, Lever M, Chambers ST, George PM, Dietary and supplementary betaine: effects on betaine and homocysteine concentrations in males. Nutr Metab Cardiovasc Dis 2009;19: 767–73.

Balaban RS, Knepper MA, Nitrogen-14 nuclear magnetic resonance spectroscopy of mammalian tissues. Am J Physiol 1983;245: C439–44.

Barak AJ, Tuma DJ, A simplified procedure for the determination of betaine in liver. Lipids 1979;14: 860–3.

Barak AJ, Tuma DJ, Determination of choline, phosphorylcholine and betaine. Methods Enzymol 1981;72: 287–92.

Barak AJ, Tuma DJ, Betaine, metabolic by-product or vital methylating agent? Life Sci 1983; 32: 771–4.

Barak AJ, Beckenhauer HC, Tuma DJ, Betaine, ethanol, and the liver: a review. Alcohol 1996;13: 395–8.

Barak AJ, Beckenhauer HC, Badakhsh S, Tuma DJ, The effect of betaine in reversing alcoholic steatosis. Alcohol Clin Exp Res 1997;21: 1100–2.

Barak AJ, Beckenhauer HC, Tuma DJ, Methionine synthase: a possible prime site of the ethanolic lesion in liver. Alcohol 2002;26: 65–7.

Barak AJ, Beckenhauer HC, Mailliard ME, Kharbanda KK, Tuma DJ, Betaine lowers elevated S-adenosylhomocysteine levels in hepatocytes from ethanol-fed rats. J Nutr 2003;33: 2845–8 .

Batra V, Devasagayama TPA, Interaction between cytotoxic effects of γ-radiation and folate deficiency in relation to choline reserves. Toxicology 2009;255: 91–9.

Beckonert O, Keun HC, Ebbels TMD, Bundy J, Holmes E, Lindon JC, Nicholson JK, Metabolic profiling, metabolomic and metabonomic procedures for NMR spectroscopy of urine, plasma, serum and tissue extracts. Nature Protocols 2007;2: 2692–703.

Bedford JJ, Harper JL, Leader JP, Smith RAJ, Identification and measurement of methylamines in elasmobranch tissues using proton nuclear magnetic resonance (^{1}H-NMR) spectroscopy. J Comp Physiol B 1998;168: 123–31.

Bell JD, Lee JA, Lee HA, Sadler PJ, Wilkie D R, Woodham RH, Nuclear magnetic resonance studies of blood plasma and urine from subjects with chronic renal failure: identification of trimethylamine-N-oxide. Biochim Biophys Acta 1991;1096: 101–7.

Bidulescu A, Chambless LE, Siega-Riz AM, Zeisel SH, Heiss G, Usual choline and betaine dietary intake and incident coronary heart disease: the Atherosclerosis Risk in Communities (ARIC) Study. BMC Cardiovasc Disord 2007;7: 20.

Bidulescu A, Chambless LE, Siega-Riz AM, Zeisel SH, Heiss G, Repeatability and measurement error in the assessment of choline and betaine dietary intake: the Atherosclerosis Risk in Communities (ARIC) Study. Nutr J 2009;8: 14.

Biggers JD, Lawitts JA, Lechene CP, The protective action of betaine on the deleterious effects of NaCl on preimplantation mouse embryos in vitro. Mol Reprod Dev 1993;34: 380–90.

Bollard ME, Contel N, Ebbels T, Smith L, Beckonert O, Cantor G, Lehman-McKeeman LD, Holmes E, Lindon JC, Nicholson JK, Keun HC, NMR-based metabolic profiling identifies biomarkers of liver regeneration following partial hepatectomy in the rat. J Proteome Res 2010;9: 59–69.

Bønaa KH, Njølstad I, Ueland PM, Schirmer H, Tverdal A, Steigen T, et al., Homocysteine lowering and cardiovascular events after acute myocardial infarction. New Engl J Med 2006;354: 1578–88.

Boyles AL, Billups AV, Deak KL, Siegel DG, Mehltretter L, Slifer SH, Bassuk AG, Kessler JA, Reed MC, Nijhout HF, George TM, Enterline DS, Gilber JR, Speer MC, NTD Collaborative Group, Neural tube defects and folate pathway genes: family based association tests of gene-gene and gene-environment interactions. Environ Health Perspect 2006;114: 1547–52.

Braekke K, Ueland PM, Harsem NK, Karlsen A, Blomhoff R, Staff AC, Homocysteine, cysteine and related metabolites in maternal and fetal plasma in preeclampsia. Pediatr Res 2007;62: 319–24.

Brownlee M, Advanced protein glycosylation in diabetes and aging. Annu Rev Med 1995;46: 223–4.

Burg MB, Kwon ED, Peters EM, Glycerophosphocholine and betaine counteract the effect of urea on pyruvate kinase. Kidney Int Suppl 1996;57: S100–4.

Chadwick LH, McCandless SE, Silverman GL, Schwartz S, Westaway D, Nadeau JH, Betaine-homocysteine methyltransferase-2: cDNA cloning, gene sequence, physical mapping, and expression of the human and mouse genes. Genomics 2000;70: 66–73.

Chambers ST, Kunin CM, Osmoprotective properties of urine for bacteria: the protective effect of betaine and human urine against low pH and high concentrations of electrolytes, sugars and urea. J Infect Dis 1985;152: 1308–15.

Chambers ST, Kunin CM, Osmoprotective activity for *Escherichia coli* in mammalian renal inner medulla and urine. Correlation of glycine and proline betaines and sorbitol with response to osmotic loads. J Clin Invest 1987;80: 1255–60.

Chern M, Pietruszko R, Evidence for mitochondrial localization of betaine aldehyde dehydrogenase in rat liver: purification, characterization, and comparison with human cytoplasmic E3 isozyme. Biochem Cell Biol 1999;77: 179–87.

Chiuve SE, Giovannucci EL, Hankinson SE, Zeisel SH, Dougherty LW, Willett WC, Rimm EB, The association between betaine and choline intakes and the plasma concentrations of homocysteine in women. Am J Clin Nutr 2007;86: 1073– 81.

Cho E, Zeisel H, Jacques P, Selhub J, Dougherty L, Colditz GA, Willett WC, Dietary choline and betaine assessed by food-frequency questionnaire in relation to plasma total homocysteine concentration in the Framingham Offspring Study. Am J Clin Nutr 2006;83: 905–11.

Clow KA, Treberg JR, Brosnan ME, Brosnan JT, Elevated tissue betaine contents in developing rats are due to dietary betaine, not to synthesis. J Nutr 2008;138: 1641–6.

Coan PM, Burton GJ, Ferguson-Smith AC, Imprinted genes in the placenta – a review. Placenta 2005;26: S11–20.

Collinsova M, Strakova J, Jiracek J, Garrow TA, Inhibition of betaine-homocysteine S-methyltransferase causes hyperhomocysteinemia in mice. J Nutr 2006;136: 1493–7.

Craig SAS, Betaine in human nutrition. Am J Clin Nutr 2004;80: 539–49.

Dalmeijer GW, Olthof MR, Verhoef P, Bots ML, van der Schouw YT, Prospective study on dietary intakes of folate, betaine, and choline and cardiovascular disease risk in women. Eur J Clin Nutr 2008;62: 386–94.

Davies SEC, Chalmers RA, Randall EW, Iles RA, Betaine metabolism in human neonates and developing rats. Clin Chim Acta 1988;178: 241–50.

Davies SEC, Woolf DA, Chalmers RA, Rafter JEM, Iles RA, Proton NMR studies of betaine excretion in the human neonate: consequences for choline and methyl group supply. J Nutr Biochem 1992;3: 523–30.

Davis CD, Uthus EO, DNA methylation, cancer susceptibility, and nutrient interactions. Exp Biol Med 2004;229: 988–95.

Dawson KM, Baltz JM, Organic osmolytes and embryos: substrates of the Gly and beta transport systems protect mouse zygotes against the effects of raised osmolarity. Biol Reprod 1997;56: 1550–8.

Delaval K, Feil R, Epigenetic regulation of mammalian genomic imprinting. Curr Opin Genet Develop 2004;14:188–95.

Delgado-Reyes CV, Garrow TA, High sodium chloride intake decreases betaine-homocysteine S-methyltransferase expression in guinea pig liver and kidney. Am J Physiol 2005;288: R182–7.

Dellow WJ, Chambers ST, Lever M, Lunt H, Robson RA, Elevated glycine betaine excretion in diabetes mellitus patients is associated with proximal tubular dysfunction and hyperglycemia. Diab Res Clin Pract 1999;43: 91–9.

Denkert C, Warskulat U, Hensel F, Haussinger D, Osmolyte strategy in human monocytes and macrophages: involvement of p38MAPK in hyperosmotic induction of betaine and myoinositol transporters. Arch Biochem Biophys 1998;354: 172–80.

Detopoulou P, Panagiotakos DB, Antonopoulou S, Pitsavos C, Stefanadis C, Dietary choline and betaine intakes in relation to concentrations of inflammatory markers in healthy adults: the ATTICA study. Am J Clin Nutr 2008;87: 424–30.

de Zwart FJ, Slow S, Payne RJ, Lever M, George PM, Gerrard JA, Chambers ST, Glycine betaine and glycine betaine analogues in common foods. Food Chem 2003;83: 197–204.

Dilger RN, Garrow TA, Baker DH, Betaine can partially spare choline in chicks but only when added to diets containing a minimal level of choline. J Nutr 2007;137: 2224–8.

Dmitrieva NI, Burg MB, Hypertonic stress response. Mutation Res 2005;569: 65–74.

Eklund M, Bauer E, Wamatu J, Mosenthin R, Potential nutritional and physiological functions of betaine in livestock. Nutr Res Rev 2005;18: 31–48.

Emmert JL, Garrow TA, Baker DH, Hepatic betaine-homocysteine methyltransferase activity in the chicken is influenced by dietary intake of sulfur amino acids, choline and betaine. J Nutr 1996; 126: 2050–8.

Eussen SJPM, Ueland PM, Clarke R, Blom HJ, Hoefnagels WHL, van Staveren WA, de Groot LCPGM, The association of betaine, homocysteine and related metabolites with cognitive function in Dutch elderly people. Br J Nutr 2007;98: 960–8.

Fan F, Gadda G, On the catalytic mechanism of choline oxidase. J Am Chem Soc 2005;127: 2067–74.

Feng YX, Muller V, Friedrich B, Risler T, Lang F, Clinical significance of cell volume regulation. Wiener Klinische Wochenscrift 2001;113: 477–84.

Fernández C, Lóez-Saez A, Gallego L, de la Fuente JM, Effect of source of betaine on growth performance and carcass traits in lambs. Animal Feed Sci Technol 2000;86: 71–82.

Feinburg AP, Vogelstein B, Hypomethylation distinguishes genes of some human cancers from their normal counterparts. Nature 1983;301: 89–91.

Finkelstein JD, Martin JJ, Methionine metabolism in mammals-distribution of homocysteine between competing pathways. J Biol Chem 1984; 259: 9508–13.

Finkelstein JD, Kyle WE, Harris BJ, Methionine metabolism in mammals. Regulation of homocysteine methyltransferases in rat tissue. Arch Biochem Biophys 1971;146: 84–92.

Finkelstein JD, Harris BJ, Kyle WE, Methionine metabolism in mammals: kinetic study of betaine-homocysteine methyltransferase. Arch Biochem Biophys 1972;153: 320–4.

Finkelstein JD, Harris BJ, Martin JJ, Kyle WE, Regulation of hepatic betaine-homocysteine methyltransferase by dietary methionine. Biochem Biophys Res Commun 1982a;108: 344–8.

Finkelstein JD, Martin JJ, Harris BJ, Kyle WE, Regulation of the betaine content of rat liver. Arch Biochem Biophys 1982b;218: 169–73.

Finkelstein JD, Martin JJ, Harris BJ, Kyle WE, Regulation of hepatic betaine-homocysteine methyltransferase by dietary betaine. J Nutr 1983;113: 519–21.

Fisher MC, Zeisel SH, Mar M-H, Sadler TW, Perturbations in choline cause neural tube defects in mouse embryos in vitro. FASEB J 2002;16: 619–21.

Flower RJ, Pollitt RJ, Sanford PA, Smyth DH, Metabolism and transfer of choline in hamster small intestine. J Physiol 1972;226: 473–89.

Fredriksen Å, Meyer K, Ueland PM, Vollset SE, Grotmol T, Schneede J, Large-scale population-based metabolic phenotyping of thirteen genetic polymorphisms related to one-carbon metabolism. Human Mutat 2007;28: 856–65.

Friesen RW, Novak EM, Hasman D, Innis SM, Relationship of dimethylglycine, choline and betaine with oxyproline in plasma of pregnant women and their newborn infants. J Nutr 2007;137: 2641–6.

Ganesan B, Rajesh R, Anandan R, Dhandapani N, Biochemical studies on the protective effect of betaine on mitochondrial function in experimentally induced myocardial infarction in rats. J Health Sci 2007;53: 671–81.

Garfinkel MD, Ruden DM, Chromatin effects in nutrition, cancer and obesity. Nutrition 2004;20: 56–62.

Garrow T, Purification, kinetic properties, and cDNA cloning of mammalian betaine-homocysteine methyltransferase. J Biol Chem 1996;271: 22831–8.

Gilles R, 'Compensatory' organic osmolytes in high osmolarity and dehydration stresses: history and perspectives. Comp Biochem Physiol 1997;117A: 279–90.

Graf D, Kurz AK, Reinehr R, Fischer R, Kircheis G, Häussinger D, Prevention of bile acid-induced apoptosis by betaine in rat liver. Hepatology 2002;36: 829–39.

Hamilton EW, Heckathorn SA, Mitochondrial adaptations to NaCl. Complex I is protected by anti-oxidants and small heat shock proteins, whereas complex II is protected by proline and betaine. Plant Physiol 2001;126: 1266–74.

Hammer MA, Baltz J, Betaine is a highly effective organic osmolyte but does not appear to be transported by established organic osmolyte transporters in mouse embryos. Mol Reprod Dev 2002;62: 195–202.

Happer DAR, Hayman CM, Storer MK, Lever M, Aracyl triflates as derivatising agents for betaines. Austr J Chem 2004;57: 467–72.

Häussinger D, The role of cellular hydration in the regulation of cell function. Biochem J 1996;313: 697–710.

Häussinger D, Neural control of hepatic osmolytes and parenchymal cell hydration. Anat Rec A Discov Mol Cell Evol Biol 2004;280A: 893–900.

Hayes KC, Pronczuk A, Cook, MW, Robbins MC, Betaine in sub-acute and sub-chronic rat studies. Food Chem Toxicol 2003;41: 1685–700.

Heil SG, Lievers KJA, Boers GH, Verhoef P, den Heijer M, Trijbels FJM, Blom HJ, Betaine-homocysteine methyltransferase (BHMT): genomic sequencing and relevance to hyperhomocysteinemia and vascular disease in humans. Mol Genet Metabol 2000;71: 511–9.

Herrmann W, Herrmann M, Obeid R, Hyperhomocysteinaemia: a critical review of old and new aspects. Curr Drug Metab 2007; 8: 17–31.

Hoffer LJ, Homocysteine remethylation and trans-sulfuration. Metabolism 2004;53: 1480–3.

Holm PI, Bleie Ø, Ueland PM, Lien EA, Refsum H, Nordrehaug JE, Nygård O, Betaine as a determinant of postmethionine load total plasma homocysteine before and after B-vitamin supplementation. Arterioscler Thromb Vasc Biol 2004;24: 301–7.

Holm PI, Ueland PM, Kvalheim G, Lien EA, Determination of choline, betaine, and dimethylglycine in plasma by a high-throughput method based on normal-phase chromatography-tandem mass spectrometry. Clin Chem 2003;49: 286–94.

Holm PI, Hustad S, Ueland PM, Vollset SE, Grotmol T, Schneede J, Modulation of the homocysteine-betaine relationship by methylenetetrahydrofolate reductase 677 C->T genotypes and B-vitamin status in a large-scale epidemiological study. J Clin Endocrinol Metab 2007;92: 1535–41.

Holmes HC, Snodgrass GJAI, Iles RA, Changes in the choline content of human breast milk in the first 3 weeks after birth. Eur J Pediatr 2000;159: 198–204.

HOPE: The Heart Outcomes Prevention Evaluation (HOPE) 2 Investigators, Homocysteine lowering with folic acid and B vitamins in vascular disease. New Engl J Med 2006;354: 1567–77.

Huang QC, Xu ZR, Han XY, Han XY, Li WF, Effect of dietary betaine supplementation on lipogenic enzyme activities and fatty acid synthase mRNA expression in finishing pigs. Animal Feed Sci Technol 2008;140: 365–75.

James SJ, Cutler P, Melnyk S, Jernigan S, Janak L, Gaylor DW, Neubrander JA, Metabolic biomarkers of increased oxidative stress and impaired methylation capacity in children with autism. Am J Clin Nutr 2004;80: 1611–7.

Ji C, Dissection of endoplasmic reticulum stress signaling in alcoholic and non-alcoholic liver injury. J Gastroenterol Hepatol 2008;23: S16–24.

Ji C, Kaplowitz N, Betaine decreases hyperhomocysteineimia, endoplasmic reticulum stress, and liver injury in alcohol-fed mice. Gastroenterol 2003;124: 1488–99.

Johansson M, Van Guelpen B, Vollset SE, Hultdin J, Bergh A, Key T, Midttun Ø, Hallmans G, Ueland PM, Stattin P, One-carbon metabolism and prostate cancer risk: prospective investigation of seven circulating B vitamins and metabolites. Cancer Epidemiol Biomarkers Prev 2009;18: 1538–43.

Jones PA, Laird PW, Cancer epigenetics comes of age. Nature Genet 1999;21: 163–7.

Kaplan CP, Porter RK, Brand MD, The choline transporter is the major site of control of choline oxidation in isolated rat liver mitochondria. FEBS Lett 1993; 321: 24–6.

Kempson SA, Montrose MH, Osmotic regulation of renal betaine transport: transcription and beyond. Pflugers Arch Eur J Physiol 2004;449: 227–34.

Kettunen H, Peuranen S, Tiihonen K, Betaine aids in the osmoregulation of duodenal epithelium of broiler chicks, and affects the movement of water across the small intestinal epithelium *in vitro*. Comp Biochem Physiol A 2001a;129: 595–603.

Kettunen H, Tiihonen K, Peuranen S, Saarinen MT, Intestinal uptake of betaine in vitro and the distribution of methyl groups from betaine, choline, and methionine in the body of broiler chicks. Comp Biochem Physiol A 2001b;128: 269–78.

Kettunen H, Tiihonen K, Peuranen S, Saarinen MT, Remus JC, Dietary betaine accumulates in the liver and intestinal tissue and stabilizes the intestinal epithelial structure in healthy and coccidia-infected broiler chicks. Comp Biochem Physiol A 2001c;130: 759–69.

Kharbanda KK, Alcoholic liver disease and methionine metabolism. Semin Liver Dis 2009; 29: 155–65.

Kharbanda KK, Rogers DD, Mailliard ME, Siford GI, Barak AJ, Beckenhauer HC, Sorrell MF, Tuma DJ, Role of elevated S-adenosylhomocysteine in rat hepatocyte apoptosis: Protection by betaine. Biochem Pharmacol 2005;70: 1883–90.

Kharbanda KK, Mailliard ME, Baldwin CR, Beckenhauer HC, Sorrell MF, Tuma DJ, Betaine attenuates alcoholic steatosis by restoring phosphatidylcholine generation via the phosphatidyl-ethanolamine methyltransferase pathway. J Hepatol 2007;46: 314–21.

Kharbanda KK, Todero SL, Ward BW, Cannella JJ, Tuma DJ, Betaine administration corrects ethanol-induced defective VLDL secretion. Mol Cell Biochem 2009;327: 75–8.

Kim S, Yang S, Kim H, Kim Y, Park T, Choi H, ^{1}H-nuclear magnetic resonance spectroscopy-based metabolic assessment in a rat model of obesity induced by a high-fat diet. Anal Bioanal Chem 2009;395: 1117–24.

Ko R, Smith LT, Smith M, Glycine betaine confers enhanced osmotolerance and cryotolerance on *Listeria monocytogenes*. J Bacteriol 1994;176: 426–31.

Koc H, Mar M-H, Ranasinghe A, Swenberg JA, Zeisel SH, Quantitation of choline and its metabolites in tissues and foods by liquid chromatography/electrospray ionization-isotope dilution mass spectrometry. Anal Chem 2002;74: 4734–40.

Konstantinova SV, Tell GS, Vollset SE, Nygård O, Bleie Ø, Ueland PM, Divergent associations of plasma choline and betaine with components of metabolic syndrome in middle age and elderly men and women. J Nutr 2008a;138: 914–20.

Konstantinova SV, Tell GS, Vollset SE, Ulvik A, Drevon CA, Ueland PM, Dietary patterns, food groups, and nutrients as predictors of plasma choline and betaine in middle-aged and elderly men and women. Am J Clin Nutr 2008b;88: 1663–9.

Lang F, Mechanisms and significance of cell volume regulation. J Am Coll Nutr 2007;26: 613S–23S.

Laryea MD, Steinhagen F, Pawliczek S, Wendel U, Simple method for the routine determination of betaine and *N,N*-dimethylglycine in blood and urine. Clin Chem 1998;44: 1937–41.

Lee M, Slow S, Fortier A, Lever M, Garrow T, Trasler J, Baltz JM, A major source of methyl groups in blastocysts may be betaine stored by pre-implantation embryos until betaine homocysteine methyltransferase (BHMT) is transiently expressed at high levels in the inner cell mass. Biol Reprod 2009;141: Abst 81.

Lee MB, Storer MK, Blunt JW, Lever M, Validation of ^{1}H NMR spectroscopy as an analytical tool for methylamine metabolites in urine. Clin Chim Acta 2006;365: 264–9.

Lever M, Bason L, Leaver C, Hayman CM, Chambers ST, Same day batch measurement of glycine betaine, carnitine and other betaines in biological material. Anal Biochem 1992;205: 14–21.

Lever M, Sizeland PCB, Bason LM, Hayman CM, Chambers ST, Glycine betaine and proline betaine in human blood and urine. Biochim Biophys Acta 1994a;1200: 259–64.

Lever M, Sizeland PC, Bason LM, Hayman CM, Robson RA, Chambers ST, Abnormal glycine betaine content of the blood and urine of diabetic and renal patients. Clin Chim Acta 1994b;230: 69–79.

Lever M, Sizeland PC, Frampton CM, Chambers ST, Short and long-term variation of plasma glycine betaine concentrations in humans. Clin Biochem 2004;37: 184–90.

Lever M, George PM, Dellow WJ, Scott RS, Chambers ST, Homocysteine, glycine betaine, and N,N-dimethylglycine in patients attending a lipid clinic. Metabolism 2005;54: 1–14.

Lever M, Atkinson W, Chambers ST, George PM, An abnormal urinary excretion of glycine betaine may persist for years. Clin Biochem 2007a;40: 798–801.

Lever M, Atkinson W, George PM, Chambers ST, Sex differences in the control of plasma concentrations and urinary excretion of glycine betaine in patients attending a lipid disorders clinic. Clin Biochem 2007b;40: 1225–31.

Lever M, Atkinson W, Sizeland, PCB, Chambers ST, George PM, Inter- and intra-individual variations in normal urinary glycine betaine excretion. Clin Biochem 2007c;40: 447–53.

Lever M, Atkinson W, Slow S, Chambers ST, George PM, Plasma and urine betaine and dimethylglycine variation in healthy young male subjects. Clin Biochem 2009a;42: 706–12.

Lever M, George PM, Slow S, Elmslie JL, Scott RS, Richards AM, Fink JN, Chambers ST, Fibrates may cause an abnormal urinary betaine loss which is associated with elevations in plasma homocysteine. Cardiovasc Drugs Ther 2009b;23: 395–401.

Li F, Feng Q, Lee C, Wang S, Pelleymounter LL, Moon I, Eckloff BW, Wieben ED, Schaid DJ, Yee V, Weinshilboum RM, Human betaine-homocysteine methyltransferase (BHMT) and BHMT2: Common gene sequence variation and functional characterization. Mol Genet Metab 2008;94: 326–35.

Li Z, Agellon LB, Vance DE, Choline redistribution during adaptation to choline deprivation. J Biol Chem 2007;282: 10283–9.

Loscalzo J, Homocysteine trials – clear outcomes for complex reasons. New Engl J Med 2006;354: 1629–32.

Lundberg P, Dudman NPB, Kuchel PW, Wilcken DEL, ^{1}H NMR determination of urinary betaine in patients with premature vascular disease and mild homocysteinemia. Clin Chem 1995;41: 275–83.

Lv S, Hou M, Tang Z, Ling W, Zhu H, Betaine supplementation attenuates atherosclerotic lesion in apolipoprotein E-deficient mice. Eur J Nutr 2009;48: 205–12.

McGregor DO, Dellow WJ, Lever M, George PM, Robson RA, Chambers ST, Dimethylglycine accumulates in uremia and predicts elevated plasma homocysteine concentrations. Kidney Int 2001;59: 2267–72.

Mann MR, Lee SS, Doherty AS, Verona RI, Nolen LD, Schultz RM, Bartolomei MS, Selective loss of imprinting in the placenta following preimplantation development in culture. Development 2004;131: 3727–35.

Mar MH, Ridky TW, Garner SC, Zeisel SH, A method for the determination of betaine in tissues using high performance liquid chromatography. J Nutr Biochem 1995;6: 392–8.

Martin FJ, Sprenger N, Yap IKS, Wang Y, Bibiloni R, Rochat F, Rezzi S, Cherbut C, Kochhar S, Lindon JC, Holmes E, Nicholson JK, Panorganismal gut microbiome-host metabolic crosstalk. J Proteome Res 2009;8: 2090–105.

Martin JJ, Finkelstein JD, Enzymatic determination of betaine in rat tissue. Anal Biochem 1981;111: 72–6.

Mato JM, Martínez-Chantar ML, Lu SC, Methionine metabolism and liver disease. Annu Rev Nutr 2008;28: 273–93.

Melse-Boonstra A, Holm PI, Ueland P, Olthof M, Clarke R, Verhoef P, Betaine concentration as a determinant of fasting total homocysteine concentrations and the effect of folic acid supplementation. Am J Clin Nutr 2005;81: 1378–82.

Millian NS, Garrow TA, Human betaine-homocysteine methyltransferase is a zinc metalloenzyme. Arch Biochem Biophys 1998; 356: 93–8.

Moat SJ, Madhavan A, Taylor SY, Payne N, Allen RH, Stabler SP, Goodfellow J, McDowell IF, Lewis MJ, Lang D, High- but not low-dose folic acid improves endothelial function in coronary artery disease. Eur J Clin Invest. 2006;36: 850–9.

Molloy AM, Mills JL, Cox C, Daly SF, Conley M, Brody LC, Kirke PN, Scott JM, Ueland PM, Choline and homocysteine interrelations in umbilical cord and maternal plasma at delivery. Am J Clin Nutr 2005;82: 836–42.

Morin I, Platt R, Weisburg I, Sabbaghian N, Wu Q, Garrow TA, Rozen R, Common variant in betaine-homocysteine methyltransferase (BHMT) and risk for spina bifida. Am J Med Genet 2003;119: 172–6.

Mostowska A, Hozyasz KK, Wojcicki P, Dziegelewska M, Jagodzinski PP, Associations of folate and choline metabolism gene polymorphisms with orofacial clefts. J Med Genet 2009; doi:10.1136/jmg.2009.070029.

Mudd SH, Brosnan JT, Brosnan ME, Jacobs RL, Stabler SP, Allen RH, Vance DE, Wagner C, Methyl balance and transmethylation fluxes in humans. Am J Clin Nutr 2007;85: 19–25.

Niculescu MD, Craciunescu CN, Zeisel SH, Dietary choline deficiency alters global and gene-specific DNA methylation in the developing hippocampus of mouse fetal brains. FASEB J 2006;20: 43–9.

O'Donoghue N, Sweeney T, Donagh R, Clarke KJ, Porter RK, Control of choline oxidation in rat kidney mitochondria. Biochim Biophys Acta 2009;1787: 1135–9.

Ogier de Baulny H, Gerard M, Saudubray JM, Zittoun J, Remethylation defects: guidelines for clinical diagnosis and treatment. Eur J Pediatr 1998;157: S77–83.

Oliva J, Bardag-Gorce F, Li J, French BA, Nguyen SK, Lu SC, French SW, Betaine prevents Mallory-Denk body formation in drug-primed mice by epigenetic mechanisms. Exp Mol Pathol 2009;86: 77–86.

Olsen M, Sarup A, Larsson OM, Schousboe A, Effect of hyperosmotic conditions on the expression of the betaine-GABA-transporter (BGT-1) in cultured mouse astrocytes. Neurochem Res 2005;30: 855–65.

Olthof MR, Verhoef P, Effect of betaine intake on plasma homocysteine concentrations and consequences for health. Current Drug Metabolism 2005;6: 15–22.

Olthof MR, van Vliet T, Boelsma E, Verhoef P, Low dose betaine supplementation leads to immediate and long term lowering of plasma homocysteine in healthy men and women. J Nutr 2003;133: 4135–8.

Olthof MR, Brink EJ, Katan MB, Verhoef P, Choline supplemented as phosphatidylcholine decreases fasting and postmethionine-loading plasma homocysteine concentrations in healthy men. Am J Clin Nutr 2005a;82: 111–7.

Olthof MR, van Vliet T, Verhoef P, Zock PL, Katan MB, Effect of homocysteine-lowering nutrients on blood lipids: results from four randomised, placebo-controlled studies in healthy humans. PLoS Med 2005b;2: e135.

Olthof MR, Bots ML, Katan MB, Verhoef P, Acute effect of folic acid, betaine, and serine supplements on flow-mediated dilation after methionine loading: a randomized trial. PLoS Clin Trials 2006;1: e4.

Park EI, Garrow TA, Interaction between dietary methionine and methyl donor intake on rat liver betaine-homocysteine methyltransferase gene expression and organization of the human gene. J Biol Chem 1999;274: 7816–24.

Park EI, Renduchintala MS, Garrow TA, Diet-induced changes in hepatic betaine homocysteine methyltransferase activity are mediated by changes in the steady-state level mRNA. J Nutr Biochem 1997; 8: 541–5.

Paulsen M, Ferguson-Smith AC, DNA methylation in genomic imprinting, development, and disease. J Pathol 2001;195: 97–110.

Petronini PG, Alfieri RR, Losio MN, Caccamo AE, Cavazzoni A, Bonelli MA, Borghetti AF, Wheeler KP, Induction of BGT-1 and amino acid system A transport activities in endothelial cells exposed to hyperosmolarity. Am J Physiol 2000;279: R1580–9.

Pochini L, Oppedisano F, Indiveri C, Reconstitution into liposomes and functional characterization of the carnitine transporter from renal cell plasma membrane. Biochim Biophys Acta 2004;1661: 78–86.

Porter RK, Scott JM, Brand MD, Choline transport into rat liver mitochondria. J Biol Chem 1992; 267: 14637–46.

Rafter JE, Bates TE, Bell JD, Iles RA, Metabolites in the developing rat liver – a proton nuclear magnetic resonance spectroscopic study. Biochim Biophys Acta 1991;1074: 263–9.

Rainesalo S, Keränen T, Saransaari P, Honkaniemi J, GABA and glutamate transporters are expressed in human platelets. Mol Brain Res 2005;141: 161–5.

Ratnam S, Wijekoon EP, Hall B, Garrow TA, Brosnan ME, Brosnan JT, Effects of diabetes and insulin on betaine-homocysteine S-methyltransferase expression in rat liver. Am J Physiol 2006;290: E933–9.

Reinehr R, Häussinger D, Hyperosmotic activation of the CD95 death receptor system. Acta Physiol 2006;187: 199–203.

Rhodes D, Rich PJ, Myers AC, Reuter CC, Jamieson GC, Determination of betaines by fast atom bombardment mass spectrometry. Plant Physiol 1987;84: 781–8.

Roher AE, Lowenson JD, Clarke S, Wolkow C, Wang R, Cotter RJ, Reardon IM, Zurcher-Neely HA, Heinrikson RL, Ball MJ, Greenburg BD, Structural alterations in the peptide backbone of beta-amyloid core protein may account for its deposition and stability in Alzheimer's disease. J Biol Chem 1993;268: 3072–83.

Robertson KD, DNA methylation and human disease. Nature Gene 2005; 6: 597–610.

Rowling MJ, McMullen MH, Chipman DC, Schalinske KL, Hepatic glycine N-methyltransferase is up-regulated by excess dietary methionine in rats. J Nutr 2002;132: 2545–50.

Rozwadowski KL, Khachatourians GG, Selvaraj G, Choline oxidase, a catabolic enzyme in *Arthrobacter pascens*, facilitates adaptation to osmotic stress in *Escherichia coli*. J Bacteriol 1991;173: 472–8.

Sakamoto A, Nishimura Y, Ono H, Sakura N, Betaine and homocysteine concentrations in foods. Pediatrics Int 2002;44: 409–13.

Sandu C, Nick P, Hess D, Schiltz E, Garrow TA, Brandsch R, Association of betaine-homocysteine S-methyltransferase with microtubules. Biol Chem 2000;381: 619–22.

Schäfer C, Hoffmann L, Heldt K, Lornejad-Schäfer MR, Brauers G, Gehrmann T, Garrow TA, Häussinger D, Mayatepek E, Schwahn BC, Schliess F, Osmotic regulation of betaine homocysteine-S-methyltransferase expression in H4IIE rat hepatoma cells. Am J Physiol 2007;292: G1089–98.

Scheibler C, Ueber das Betain, eine im Safte der Zuckerrüben (*Beta vulgaris*) vorkommende Pflanzenbase. Berichte Deutsch Chemisch Gesellschaft 1869;2: 292–5.

Scheibler C, Ueber das Betaïn und seine Constitution. Berichte Deutsch Chemisch Gesellschaft 1870;3: 155–61.

Schliess F, Häussinger D, The cellular hydration state: a critical determinant for cell death and survival. Biol Chem 2002;383: 577–83.

Schwab U, Törrönen A, Toppinen L, Alfthan G, Saarinen M, Aro A, Uusitupa M, Betaine supplementation decreases plasma homocysteine concentrations but does not affect body weight, body composition, or resting energy expenditure in human subjects. Am J Clin Nutr 2002;76: 961–7.

Schwab U, Törrönen A, Meririnne E, Saarinen M, Alfthan G, Aro A, Uusitupa M, Orally administered betaine has an acute and dose-dependent effect on serum betaine and plasma homocysteine concentrations in healthy humans. J Nutr 2006;136: 34–8.

Schwahn BC, Hafner D, Hohlfeld T, Balkenhol N, Laryea MD, Wendel U, Pharmacokinetics of oral betaine in healthy subjects and patients with homocystinuria. Br J Clin Pharmacol 2003;55: 6–13.

Schwahn BC, Wang X-L, Mikael LG, Wua Q, Cohn J, Jiang H, Maclean KN, Rozen R, Betaine supplementation improves the atherogenic risk factor profile in a transgenic mouse model of hyperhomocysteinemia. Atherosclerosis 2007;195: e100–7.

Serkova NJ, Jackman M, Brown JL, Liu T, Hirose R, Roberts JP, Maher JJ, Niemann CU, Metabolic profiling of livers and blood from obese Zucker rats. J Hepatol 2006;44: 956–2.

Shaw GM, Carmichael SL, Yang W, Selvin S, Schaffer D, Periconceptional dietary intake of choline and betaine and neural tube defects in offspring. Am J Epidemiol 2004;160: 102–9.

Shibata T, Akamine T, Nikki T, Yamashita H, Nobukuni K, Synthesis of betaine-homocysteine S-methyltransferase is continuously enhanced in fatty livers of thyroidectomized chickens. Poultry Sci 2003;82: 207–13.

Slow S, Garrow T, Liver choline dehydrogenase and kidney betaine homocysteine methyl transferase expression are not affected by methionine or choline intake in growing rats. J Nutr 2006;136: 2279–83.

Slow S, Lever M, Lee MB, George PM, Chambers ST, Betaine analogues alter homocysteine metabolism in rats. Int J Biochem Cell Biol 2004a;36: 870–80.

Slow S, Miller WE, McGregor DO, Lee MB, Lever M, George PM, Chambers ST, Trigonelline is not responsible for the acute increase in plasma homocysteine following ingestion of instant coffee. Eur J Clin Nutr 2004b;58: 1253–6.

Slow S, Donnaggio M, Cressey PJ, Lever M, George PM, Chambers ST, The betaine content of New Zealand foods and estimated intake in the New Zealand diet. J Food Comp Anal 2005;18: 473–5.

Slow S, Elmslie J, Lever M, Dietary betaine and inflammation. Am J Clin Nutr 2008;88: 247–8.

Slow S, Lever M, Chambers ST, George PM, Plasma dependent and independent accumulation of betaine in male and female rat tissues. Physiol Res 2009;58: 403–10.

Sparks JD, Collins HL, Chirieac DV, Cianci J, Jokinen J, Sowden MP, Galloway CA, Sparks CE, Hepatic very-low-density lipoprotein and apolipoprotein B production are increased following in vivo induction of betaine-homocysteine S-methyltransferase. Biochem J 2006;395: 363–71.

Stadtman ER, Levine RL, Protein oxidation. Ann NY Acad Sci 2000; 899: 191–208.

Steenge GR, Verhoef P, Katan MB, Betaine supplementation lowers plasma homocysteine in healthy men and women. J Nutr 2003;133: 1291–5.

Storer MK, Lever M, Aracyl triflates for preparing fluorescent and UV absorbing derivatives of unreactive carboxylates, amines and other metabolites. Anal Chim Acta 2006;558: 319–25.

Storer MK, McEntyre CJ, Lever M, Separation of cationic aracyl derivatives of betaines and related compounds. J Chromatog A 2006;1104: 263–71.

Sunden SLF, Renduchintala MS, Park EI, Miklasz SD, Garrow TA, Betaine-homocysteine methyltransferase expression in porcine and human tissues and chromosomal localization of the human gene. Arch Biochem Biophys 1997;345: 171–4.

Swales AKE, Spears N, Genomic imprinting and reproduction. Reproduction 2005;130:389–99.

Szegedi SS, Castro CC, Koutmos M, Garrow TA, Betaine-homocysteine S-methyltransferase-2 is an S-methylmethionine-homocysteine methyltransferase. J Biol Chem 2008;283: 8939–45.

Thwaites DT, Anderson CMH, Deciphering the mechanisms of intestinal imino (and amino) acid transport: the redemption of SLC36A1. Biochim Biophys Acta 2007;1768: 179–97.

Trasler JM, Gamete imprinting: setting epigenetic patterns for the next generation. Reprod Fertil Dev 2006;18: 63–9.

Trump S, Laudi S, Unruh N, Goelz R, Leibfritz D, ^{1}H-NMR metabolic profiling of human neonatal urine. Magn Reson Mater Phy 2006;19: 305–12.

Ueland PM, Clarke R, Homocysteine and cardiovascular risk: considering the evidence in the context of study design, folate fortification, and statistical power. Clin Chem 2007;53: 807–9.

Ueland PM, Holm PI, Hustad S, Betaine: a key modulator of one-carbon metabolism and homocysteine status. Clin Chem Lab Med 2005;43: 1069–75.

Ueland PM, Midttun Ø, Windelberg A, Svardal A, Rita Skålevik R, Hustad S, Quantitative profiling of folate and one-carbon metabolism in large-scale epidemiological studies by mass spectrometry. Clin Chem Lab Med 2007;45: 1737–45.

Van Winkle LJ, Campione AL, Mann DF, Wasserlauf HG, The cation receptor subsite of the choline transporter in preimplantation mouse conceptuses resembles a cation receptor subsite of several amino acid transporters. Biochim Biophys Acta 1993;1146: 38–44.

Velzing-Aarts FV, Holm P, Fokkema MR, van der Dijs FP, Ueland PM, Muskiet FA, Plasma choline and betaine and their relation to plasma homocysteine in normal pregnancy. Am J Clin Nutr 2005;81: 1383–9.

Venkatesu P, Lee M-J, Lin H-M, Osmolyte counteracts urea-induced denaturation of α-chymotrypsin. J Phys Chem B 2009;113: 5327–38.

Wallace JMW, Bonham MP, Strain JJ, Duffy EM, Robson PJ, Ward M, McNulty H, Davidson PW, Myers GJ, Shamlaye CF, Clarkson TW, Molloy AM, Scott JM, Ueland PM, Homocysteine concentration, related B vitamins, and betaine in pregnant women recruited to the Seychelles Child Development study. Am J Clin Nutr 2008;87: 391–7.

Wang YZ, Xu ZR, Feng J, The effect of betaine and DL-methionine on growth performance and carcass characteristics in meat ducks. Anim Feed Sci Technol 2004;116: 151–9.

Warskulat U, Wettstein M, Häussinger D, Betaine is an osmolyte in RAW 264.7 mouse macrophages. FEBS Letters 1995;377: 47–50.

Warskulat U, Reinen A, Grether-Beck S, Krutmann J, Häussinger D, The osmolyte strategy of normal human keratinocytes in maintaining cell homeostasis. J Invest Dermatol 2004;123: 516–21.

Warskulat U, Brookmann S, Felsner I, Brenden H, Grether-Beck S, Häussinger D, Ultraviolet A induces transport of compatible organic osmolytes in human dermal fibroblasts. Exp Dermatol 2009;17: 1031–6.

Waterland RA, Dolinoy DC, Lin J-R, Smith CA, Shi X, Tahiliani, KG, Maternal methyl supplements increase offspring DNA methylation at *Axin Fused*. Genesis 2006;44: 401–6.

Waterland RA, Travisano M, Tahiliani KG, Rached MT, Mirza S, Methyl donor supplementation prevents transgenerational amplification of obesity. Int J Obesity 2008;32: 1373–9.

Weik C, Warskulat U, Bode J, Peters-Regehr T, Haussinger D, Compatible osmolytes in rat liver sinusoidal endothelial cells. Hepatology 1998;27: 569–75.

Weisburg, IS, Park E, Ballman KV, Berger P, Nunn M, Suh DS, Breksa AP, Garrow TA, Rozen R, Investigations of a common genetic variant in betaine-homocysteine methyltransferase (BHMT) in coronary artery disease. Atherosclerosis 2003;167: 205–14.

Wijekoon EP, Hall B, Ratnam S, Brosnan ME, Zeisel SH, Brosnan JT, Homocysteine metabolism in ZDF (type 2) diabetic rats. Diabetes 2005;54: 3245–51.

Wilcken DEL, Wilcken B, Dudman NPB, Tyrrell PA, Homocystinuria – the effects of betaine in the treatment of patients not responsive to pyridoxine. New Engl J Med 1983;309: 448–53.

Wilcken DEL, Dudman NPB, Tyrrell PA, Homocystinuria due to cystathionine β-synthase deficiency – the effects of betaine treatment in pyridoxine-responsive patients. Metabolism 1985;34: 1115–21.

Wolff GL, Kodell RL, Moore SR, Cooney CA, Maternal epigenetics and methyl supplements affect *agouti* gene expression in A^{vy}/a mice. FASEB J 1998;12: 949–57.

Wolff SD, Yancey PH, Stanton TS, Balaban RS, A simple HPLC method for quantitating major organic solutes of renal medulla. Am J Physiol 1989;256: F954–6.

Wu G, Bazer FW, Cudd TA, Meininger CJ, Spencer TE, Maternal nutrition and fetal development. J Nutr 2004;134: 2169–72.

Yamauchi A, Uchida S, Kwon HM, Preston AS, Robey RB, Garcia-Perez A, Burg MB, Handler JS, Cloning of a Na(+)- and Cl(–)-dependent betaine transporter that is regulated by hypertonicity. J Biol Chem 1992;267: 649–52.

Yancey PH, Burg MB, Counteracting effects of urea and betaine in mammalian-cells in culture. Am J Physiol 1990;258: R198–204.

Yancey PH, Somero GN, Counteraction of urea destabilization by methylamine osmoregulatory compounds of elasmobranch fishes. Biochem J 1979;183: 317–23.

Yap S, Classical homocystinuria: vascular risk and its prevention. J Inherited Metab Dis 2003;26: 259–65.

Zeisel SH, Choline: an essential nutrient for humans. Nutrition 2000;16: 669–71.

Zeisel SH, Choline: critical role during fetal development and dietary requirements in adults. Ann Rev Nutr 2006a;26: 229–50.

Zeisel SH, Betaine supplementation and blood lipids: fact or artifact? Nutrition Rev 2006b;64: 77–9.

Zeisel SH, Importance of methyl donors during reproduction. Am J Clin Nutr 2009a;89(Suppl): 673S–7S.

Zeisel SH, Epigenetic mechanisms for nutrition determinants of later health outcomes. Am J Clin Nutr 2009b;89(Suppl): 1488S–93S.

Zeisel SH, Mar MH, Zhou Z, Costa KA, Pregnancy and lactation are associated with diminished concentrations of choline and its metabolites in rat liver. J Nutr 1995;125: 3049–54.

Zeisel SH, Mar MH, Howe JC, Holden JM, Concentrations of choline-containing compounds and betaine in common foods. J Nutr 2003;133: 1302–7.

Zhan XA, Li JX, Xu ZR, Zhao RQ, Effects of methionine and betaine supplementation on growth performance, carcase composition and metabolism of lipids in male broilers. Br Poultry Sci 2006;47: 576–80.

Zhang F, Warskulat U, Wettstein M, Häussinger D, Identification of betaine as an osmolyte in rat liver macrophages (Kupffer cells). Gastroenterology 1996;110: 1543–52.

Zhang J, Blusztajn JK, Zeisel SH, Measurement of the formation of betaine aldehyde and betaine in rat liver mitochondria by a high pressure liquid chromatography-radioenzymatic assay. Biochim Biophys Acta 1992;1117: 333–9.

Zhang J, Nishimura N, Okubo A, Yamazaki S, Development of an analytical method for the determination of betaines in higher plants by capillary electrophoresis at low pH. Phytochem Anal 2002;13: 189–94.

Zhu H, Curry S, Wen S, Wicker NJ, Shaw GM, Lammer EJ, Yang W, Jafarov T, Finnell RH, Are betaine-homocysteine methylatransferase (BHMT and BHMT2) genes risk factors for spina bifida and orofacial clefts? Am J Med Genet 2005;135: 274–7.

14 Choline

14.1 Choline in health and disease

Ya-Wen Teng; Steven H. Zeisel

14.1.1 Introduction

Choline is a water-soluble nutrient that is often grouped with the vitamin B complex. However, its functions suggest it is more than just another vitamin. Choline is crucial for the normal function of all cells (Zeisel and Blusztajn, 1994). It is needed for the structural integrity and signaling functions of cell membranes; it directly affects cholinergic neurotransmission; it is the major source of methyl groups in the diet; and it is required for lipid transport from liver and for normal muscle function (Zeisel and Blusztajn, 1994; Zeisel, 2006b). In early life, choline is crucial for fetal brain development; in later life, prolonged ingestion of a choline-deficient diet leads to fatty liver, and liver and muscle damage in humans (Zeisel, 2006b). Choline deficiency also reduces an individual's ability to handle a methionine (Met) load, resulting in elevated homocysteine (Hcy), a risk factor for cardiovascular diseases (CVDs) (da Costa et al., 2005). Conversely, choline supplementation in animal models might mitigate or ameliorate the symptoms of fetal alcohol syndrome (Thomas et al., 2009), traumatic brain injury (Guseva et al., 2008), brain abnormalities in mouse models of Rett syndrome (Nag et al., 2008; Ward et al., 2009) and schizophrenia (Stevens et al., 2008). In this chapter, we focus on the new observations that enhance our understanding of the roles of choline in human health and disease.

14.1.2 Dietary and endogenous sources of choline

Foods contain several choline-containing compounds as well as betaine, a choline-metabolite which spares some choline requirements (Zeisel et al., 2003). Excellent sources of dietary choline are foods that contain membranes, such as eggs and liver. Recently, the US Department of Agriculture (USDA) developed the first database of choline content in foods (http://www.ars.usda.gov/SP2UserFiles/Place/12354500/Data/Choline/Choln02.pdf last accessed 8-11-10). Average dietary choline intake on *ad libitum* diets for males and females are 8.4 mg/kg and 6.7 mg/kg choline per day, respectively (Fischer et al., 2005).

Also, choline can be formed endogenously (mainly in the liver) by the enzyme phosphatidylethanolamine-*N*-methyltransferase (PEMT) (▶Fig. 14.1). PEMT uses *S*-adenosylmethionine (SAM) converting phosphatidylethanolamine (PtdEtn) to phosphatidylcholine (PtdCho). This phospholipid is either incorporated into cell membranes or degraded to regenerate choline (Blusztajn et al., 1985). Mice that lack the PEMT gene rapidly develop fatty liver and severe liver damage, and die after 3 days of a choline-deficient diet; choline supplementation prevents this (Walkey et al., 1998).

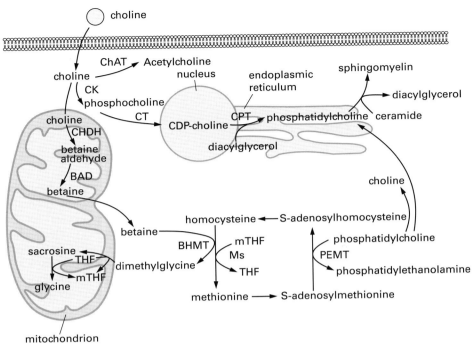

Fig. 14.1: Choline metabolism. CHDH, choline dehydrogenase; BADH betaine aldehyde dehydrogenase; BHMT, betaine homocysteine methyltransferase; MS, methionine synthase; PEMT, phosphatidylethanolamine-*N*-methyltransferase; CK, choline kinase; ChAT, choline acetyltransferase; CT, CTP:phosphocholine cytidylytransferase; CPT, choline phosphotransferase; THF, tetrahydrofolate; mTHF, methyl tetrahydrofolate.

PEMT-/- mice have lower choline pools in liver despite being fed sufficient or supplemental choline, suggesting that choline production by PEMT in the liver is a significant source of choline relative to dietary intake (Zhu et al., 2003).

14.1.3 Choline absorption and metabolism

Choline is found in foods as choline or choline esters, from which choline is freed by pancreatic enzymes. These choline esters include phosphocholine (PCho), glycerophosphocholine (GPCho), phosphatidylcholine (PtdCho) and sphingomyelin (SM) (Zeisel and Blusztajn, 1994). Choline is absorbed in the small intestine; free choline enters the portal circulation and is mostly taken up by liver (Lekim and Betzing, 1976), whereas lipid-soluble PtdCho and SM enter via lymph and bypass the liver. Therefore, different forms of choline could have different bioavailability (Cheng et al., 1996). All tissues accumulate choline, but uptake by liver, kidney, mammary gland, placenta and brain is of special importance. Kidney accumulates choline and uses it to form betaine and GPCho, both of which are organic osmolytes that allow kidney to reabsorb water from the renal tubule (Burg and Ferraris, 2008).

A small portion of choline is acetylated to ACho by choline acetyltransferase, an enzyme that is highly concentrated in cholinergic nerve terminals, but also in non-nervous tissues such as placenta (Blusztajn and Wurtman, 1983). In brain, the availability of choline limits the rate of ACho synthesis (Cohen and Wurtman, 1975; Blusztajn and Wurtman, 1983; Ulus et al., 1989; Wecker, 1991). Choline taken up by brain might first enter a storage pool, perhaps as the PtdCho in membranes, before being converted to ACho (Blusztajn et al., 1986). This reservoir is important when particular cholinergic neurons fire frequently or when the uptake of choline from the extracellular fluid is in-adequate (Cohen et al., 1995). Autopsy of individuals with Alzheimer's disease showed abnormal phospholipid metabolism (Nitsch et al., 1992), suggesting the importance of phospholipid turnover to brain function.

A major role for choline is the synthesis of membrane phospholipids. The predomi-nant membrane phospholipid is PtdCho, from which SM, another phospholipid, is formed. Both PtdCho and SM play important roles in signal transduction because they are sources of lipid second messengers (Zeisel and Blusztajn, 1994). PtdCho is also required for the formation of lipoproteins, which deliver the triacylglycerol produced by liver to other tissues. Biosynthesis of PtdCho occurs by two pathways (Vance, 1990). First, choline is phosphorylated to PCho, which is then converted to cytidine diphos-phocholine (CDP-choline). CDP-choline combines with diacylglycerol to form PtdCho. Alternatively, PtdCho can be synthesized from the PEMT pathway via three sequential methylation events using SAM as the methyl donor. As noted earlier, the PEMT pathway is most active in the liver, but has been identified in many other tissues, including brain and mammary gland (Blusztajn et al., 1985; Yang et al., 1988; Vance et al., 1997). Ap-proximately 70% of the PtdCho in liver derives from the CDP-choline pathway, with the remainder from the PEMT pathway (DeLong et al., 1999). These two pathways pro-duce different species of PtdCho, which have different physical properties and generate different signaling molecules (DeLong et al., 1999).

Choline contributes methyl groups after conversion to betaine (Niculescu and Zeisel, 2002). Choline is oxidized to betaine aldehyde and then to betaine by choline dehydro-genase (CHDH) and betaine aldehyde dehydrogenase (BADH), respectively, in the inner mitochondrial membrane (Lin and Wu, 1986). Liver and kidney are the major sites for choline oxidation. Because betaine cannot be reduced back to choline, the oxidation pathway commits choline to use for methylation pathway and diminishes the availabil-ity of choline for the alternative PtdCho synthesis pathway.

14.1.4 Choline, folate and methionine metabolism are inter-related

The methylation pathway of choline interacts with folate pathway at the step when Hcy is converted to Met (Finkelstein, 2000). Betaine:homocysteine methyltransferase (BHMT) uses betaine as the methyl donor, converting Hcy to Met. Alternatively, methio-nine synthase (MS) uses methyl-folate and vitamin B12 to convert Hcy to Met. Although little is known of its function, a novel enzyme BHMT-2 has been identified that uses S-methylmethionine (SMM), a derivative of Met, as a methyl donor to regenerate Met from Hcy (Szegedi et al., 2008). Methionine is the precursor for SAM, a methyl donor for various cellular events, including DNA and histone methylation. Perturbation of either MS or BHMT pathway, by nutrient deficiency or by mutations in genes involved in these pathways, results in elevated plasma Hcy concentration (Varela-Moreiras et al., 1995) and in compensatory changes in the other methyl donor pathway (Selhub et al., 1991; Varela-Moreiras et al., 1992). It also results in a reduction of tissue concentration of SAM (Zeisel et al., 1989), which could have potential epigenetic effects (discussed later). That several parallel pathways are evolutionarily conserved to regulate the level of Hcy and to ensure an adequate supply of SAM demonstrates the importance of these compounds.

14.1.5 Choline deficiency

Choline deficient humans develop fatty liver (Zeisel, 2000) owing to a lack of PtdCho limiting export of excess triglyceride from liver via very low density lipoprotein (VLDL) (Yao and Vance, 1988). Choline deficiency in humans is also associated with liver damage, characterized by elevated serum aminotransferases (Zeisel, 2000), enzyme that is released into blood stream when liver cells die. Choline deficiency in human can also present with muscle damage, characterized by elevated serum creatine phosphokinase (da Costa et al., 2004), or present with DNA damage and death in peripheral lymphocytes (da Costa et al., 2006b). Choline deficient humans are likely to accumulate Hcy, a risk factor for heart diseases, after a methionine rich diet (da Costa et al., 2005). In addition, women who have lower choline intakes during pregnancy have significantly increased risk of giving birth to a child with a neural tube defect (Velzing-Aarts et al., 2005). Women who have lower dietary intakes of choline could have an increased risk and mortality from breast cancer (Xu et al., 2008, 2009).

In animals, choline deficiency results in liver cell proliferation, apoptosis, and transformation into cancer cells (Newberne and Rogers, 1986). Choline deficiency compromises renal function, with abnormal concentrating ability, free water reabsorption, sodium excretion, glomerular filtration rate, renal plasma flow, and gross renal hemorrhage (Zeisel and Blusztajn, 1994). These signs appear to be owing to the lack of betaine, a choline derivative and an organic osmolyte crucial for normal renal function. Finally, choline deficiency during fetal development has been shown to affect learning and attentional processes throughout the lifespan (Meck et al., 1988, 1989; Meck and Williams, 1997abc).

14.1.6 Factors influencing choline requirement

There are not sufficient data to set an Estimated Average Requirement (EAR), and thus no calculation for a Recommendation Dietary Allowance (RDA) for choline. Instead, in 1998, the Food and Nutrition Board of the US Institute of Medicine established an adequate intake (AI) for choline of 550 mg/day for men and 425 mg/day for women and a tolerable upper intake limit (UL) for adults at 3.5 g/day (Institute of Medicine and National Academy of Sciences USA, 1998). The requirement increases to 450 mg/day and 500 mg/day for pregnancy and lactation, respectively. The main criterion for establishing the AI for choline is to prevent liver damage, whereas the UL is to prevent effects of excess choline such as hypotension and fish body odor. Factors such as gender, menopausal status, pregnancy, lactation and genetic mutation can affect choline requirement. As more information becomes available, we expect that these recommendations could be revised upwards, because approximately 10% of subjects in a human study needed approximately 850 mg choline/day (2× as much as the requirement) to avoid fatty liver, liver and muscle damage (Fischer et al., 2007).

14.1.6.1 Gender, menopausal status, pregnancy and lactation

Fifty-six percent of premenopausal women did not develop signs of choline deficiency when deprived of dietary choline for up to 42 days, whereas most adult men and post-menopausal women did (da Costa et al., 2004, 2005; Fischer et al., 2007). Premeno-pausal women require less dietary choline because estrogen induces the *PEMT* gene, thereby enhancing the *de novo* biosynthesis of choline moiety (see earlier discussion of PEMT). Estrogen binds to its receptors, ERα and ERβ, which bind to estrogen response elements (EREs) in the promoters of the *PEMT* gene, resulting in an up-regulation in PEMT mRNA expression and increased hepatic enzyme activity (Resseguie et al., 2007). Estrogen as the mediator of increasing PEMT activity in women is important, particu-larly during pregnancy when the fetus develops; estrogen concentration rises from 1 to 60 nM during pregnancy (Sarda and Gorwill, 1976; Adeyemo and Jeyakumar, 1993), suggesting that capacity for endogenous synthesis of choline should be highest at the end of pregnancy when choline is most needed by the fetus.

Pregnancy and lactation are stages that demand high dietary choline intake and leave mothers extremely vulnerable to choline deficiency. During pregnancy, placenta stores choline as ACho and delivers large amounts of choline to the fetus (Leventer and Rowell, 1984). *In utero*, the fetus is exposed to very high choline concentrations, with a progressive decline in blood choline concentration in the offspring until adult levels are achieved after the first weeks of life (McMahon and Farrell, 1985). Plasma or serum choline concentrations are 6–7× higher in the fetus and newborn than they are in adults (Zeisel and Wurtman, 1981; Ozarda Ilcol et al., 2002). High circulating choline in the neonate ensures the availability of choline to tissues. The neonate has a particularly high capacity for choline transport across the blood-brain barrier to the brain (Cornford and Cornford, 1986). There is also a novel form of PEMT in neonatal brain (not in adult brain) (Blusztajn et al., 1985), accompanied by sufficient SAM to enable PEMT to main-tain high rates of activity (Hoffman et al., 1979). These multiple mechanisms for provid-ing choline to fetal brain suggest the importance of choline during fetal development.

14.1.6.2 Gene polymorphism and choline requirement

Although premenopausal women are more resistant to choline deficiency, a significant portion of them (44%) still develop organ dysfunction when deprived of choline, suggest-ing individual differences in susceptibility to choline deficiency. In fact, some men and women require more than 850 mg/70 kg per day choline in their diet, whereas others require less than 550 mg/kg per day (Fischer et al., 2007). Genetic variation probably underlies the differences in dietary requirements. Choline is involved in several metabolic pathways, and mutations of genes (single-nucleotide polymorphism; SNP) in these path-ways can influence the metabolism choline and an individual's choline requirement.

Only a few reports investigate whether SNPs in the genes involved in one-carbon metabolism have roles in choline requirements (Kohlmeier et al., 2005; da Costa et al., 2006a). Premenopausal women with 5,10-methylenetetrahydrofolate dehydro-genase (MTHFD1 rs2236225) SNP were 15× more susceptible to choline deficiency than non-carriers (Kohlmeier et al., 2005). This variant increases the use of choline perhaps by limiting the availability of methyl-folate for Hcy remethylation and increasing the demand for choline as a methyl-group donor. In addition, individuals with PEMT rs12325817 or CHDH rs12676 SNPs were much more susceptible to choline deficiency, and women harboring these SNPs were affected more than were men (da Costa et al., 2006a). Conversely, CHDH rs9001 had a protective effect (da Costa et al., 2006a). SNPs in the PEMT gene might alter endogenous synthesis of choline, and SNPs in CHDH could change the utilization of the choline moiety.

Genetic variance can influence the efficiencies of choline pathways and have effects on choline requirement. It is important to take genetic variation into consideration when setting a dietary choline requirement.

14.1.7 Choline and developing brain

In early pregnancy, choline is needed for normal neural tube closure. Inhibition of choline uptake and metabolism is associated with the development of neural tube defects (NTDs) in mice (Fisher et al., 2001, 2002). This might also be true in humans. In California, women with low dietary folate intake, those who consumed the lowest amount of periconceptional dietary intake of choline had 4× the risk of having a baby with a NTD than did women who consumed the highest amount (Shaw et al., 2004). It is further shown in folate fortified population that low intake of choline is a risk factor, whereas high intake of choline is a protective factor for NTDs (Shaw et al., 2009).

Although no human studies are available, animal studies have shown that choline is crucial for the development of the hippocampus, the memory center of brain. Choline supplementation to pregnant rodent dams during later pregnancy and in the early postnatal period (the periods when neurogenesis and synaptogenesis occur) results in memory changes that extend throughout the life-span of the offspring pups, and prevents the memory decline normally observed in aged rats (Meck et al., 1988; Meck and Williams, 1997a,b,c, 1999, 2003; Williams et al., 1998). Interestingly, offspring of rat dams treated with supplemental choline during late pregnancy had greater improvement in memory (compared with controls) than did offspring of mothers supplemented during the early postnatal period (Meck et al., 1988), suggesting that late pregnancy might be a more sensible window for the effect of choline supplementation. Rats born of choline supplemented dams also had enhanced memory precision (less interference of new memory in current tests by the memory from previous tests) and were able to process memory more efficiently (Meck and Williams, 1997a,b,c; Meck and Williams, 1999). Also, supplemental choline *in utero* enhanced electrical properties of brain such as long-term potentiation (LTP) in the offspring (Pyapali et al., 1998). Remarkably, the memory enhancement by choline supplementation during these crucial periods lasted throughout the life-span. Adult rodents have a decrement in memory as they age; however, offspring exposed to extra choline *in utero* did not show this decline in cognitive function (Meck and Williams, 1997a,b,c; Meck and Williams, 2003). Also, choline exposure, *in utero*, attenuated age-related declines in exploratory behavior (Glenn et al., 2008).

The association between pre- and postnatal choline supplementation and brain function in humans has not yet been studied. However, the evidence from the animal studies could provide insights to how choline supplementation during these critical windows (pre- and early postnatal) can affect brain development and memory function. Moreover, prenatal or postnatal choline supplementation has also been explored as a potential therapeutic agent for several cognitive diseases using rodent models (see below).

14.1.8 Choline and other cognitive diseases

Fetal alcohol syndrome (FAS) occurs in 1 in every 750 infants born each year in the USA (Clarren et al., 2001). Rats exposed to alcohol neonatally had poor performance on memory tasks, and this was ameliorated by either prenatal or postnatal choline supplementation (Thomas et al., 2004, 2009). Rett syndrome is a neurodevelopmental disorder in the autism spectrum of disease, and is sometimes associated with mutations in the *methyl-CpG-Binding protein 2 (MeCP2)* gene (Nag et al., 2008; Ward et al., 2009). It is the second leading cause of mental retardation in girls (Nag et al., 2008; Ward et al., 2009). In mouse models of Rett syndrome (where the gene *MeCP2* has been deleted), prenatal or postnatal choline supplementation attenuated the motor coordination deficits and improved neuronal integrity, proliferation and survival (Nag et al., 2008; Ward et al., 2009). Choline supplementation might ameliorate the symptoms of traumatic brain injury (TBI) (Guseva et al., 2008), status epilepticus (Yang et al., 2000; Holmes et al., 2002; Wong-Goodrich et al., 2008) and schizophrenia (Stevens et al., 2008) in rodent model systems. Again, no equal experiments in humans are found.

14.1.9 Choline and epigenetics

The mechanism whereby choline manipulation during pregnancy results in permanent changes in memory of the fetus remains unknown. In adults, it is thought that increased dietary choline intake results in increased the synthesis and release of ACho. However, this is not likely to be the case in fetuses, because choline supplementation to dams resulted in the accumulation of PCho and betaine in the fetal brain rather than choline and ACho (Garner et al., 1995).

The term 'epigenetics' defines heritable changes in gene expression that are not coded in the DNA sequence itself. Epigenetic mechanisms can be mediated by DNA methylation and histone modifications that are read as signals that change gene expression. DNA methylation occurs predominantly at the cytosine bases followed by a guanosine (CpG) and when it occurs in the promoter regions (regions that regulate DNA expression) the expression of the associated gene is altered (Bird, 1986; Jeltsch, 2002). Although there are exceptions, increased DNA methylation is usually associated with gene silencing, whereas decreased methylation is associated with increased gene expression (Fuks, 2005). Histones are proteins around which DNA is tightly wound, forming the dynamic structure called chromatin. Chromatin can either be in an inactive state or in an active state in which transcription factors can pass through histones and bind to DNA (Quina et al., 2006). Histone acetylation predominantly promotes active chromatin, whereas histone methylation can be associated with both transcriptionally active and inactive chromatin (Kim et al., 2009). Furthermore, the degree of methylation (mono-, di- or tri-methylation) results in different effects on chromatin state (Rice et al., 2003).

Methylation of DNA and histones requires SAM as the methyl-donor for the methylation of cytosines in DNA and lysine and arginine residues in histones, respectively.

The availability of SAM is directly influenced by dietary choline. In rodents, choline deficiency or disturbance of choline pathways results in depletion of SAM and elevation of S-adenosylhomocysteine (SAH) (Zeisel et al., 1989). The SAM:SAH ratio modulates methylation enzyme activity; low SAM:SAH ratio inhibits the activities of DNA and histone methyltransferases. In cell and rodent models, methylation of genes that inhibit cell cycling is decreased during choline deficiency, resulting in over-expression of the inhibitory genes causing decreased progenitor cell proliferation and increased apoptosis in the fetal hippocampus (Niculescu et al., 2004, 2005). Gestational choline availability also affects histone methylation in the developing embryo, resulting in changes in gene expressions, primarily genes that regulate methylation and neuronal cell differentiation (Davison et al., 2009).

There are other examples where methyl groups in maternal diets have permanent effects on their offspring via epigenetic effects. Feeding pregnant Psudoagouti Avy/a mouse dams a methyl-supplemented diet altered epigenetic regulation of agouti expression in their offspring, as indicated by increased agouti/black mottling of their coats (Wolff et al., 1998; Cooney et al., 2002). In another example, methyl donor supplementation to dams increased DNA methylation of the fetal gene *axin fused* [*Axin(Fu)*] and reduced the incidence of tail kinking in offspring by 50% (Waterland et al., 2006). It is clear that the dietary manipulation of methyl donors (either deficiency or supplementation) can have a profound impact upon gene expression and, consequently an impact on normal physiological processes and on human diseases.

14.1.10 Choline and cancer

Choline is the only nutritional deficiency that causes liver cancer without any known carcinogen (Newberne and Rogers, 1986). In rodents, choline deficiency results in a higher incidence of spontaneous hepatocarcinomas (liver cancer) (Newberne and Rogers, 1986). Several mechanisms are suggested for its carcinogenic effects. Choline deficiency increases lipid peroxidation in the liver (Rushmore et al., 1984), which is a source of free radicals in the nucleus that could modify DNA and cause carcinogenesis. Choline deficiency perturbs protein kinase C (PKC) signaling, resulting in altered cell proliferation signals and cell apoptosis and eventually in carcinogenesis (da Costa et al., 1993). Epigenetic alterations also might mediate the mechanisms that underlie the etiology of cancers. Methyl deficiency results in hypomethylation of some genes but also paradoxically hypermethylation of CpG islands in specific genes (e.g., tumor suppressor genes) that are associated with gene silencing (Jones and Baylin, 2002; Feinberg and Tycko, 2004), leading to tumor development. Histone modifications also occur in methyl deficiency in various models of cancer (Pogribny et al., 2007; Dobosy et al., 2008; Davison et al., 2009).

Only a handful of epidemiologic studies explore how choline and betaine intakes alter cancer risk at the population level. The Long Island Breast Cancer Study Project found that high choline consumption reduced breast cancer risk (Xu et al., 2008), and high choline and betaine consumption reduced breast cancer mortality (Xu et al., 2009). Moreover, individuals with single nucleotide polymorphisms in genes of choline metabolism (*PEMT* rs12325817 SNP) had higher risk of developing breast cancer, whereas people with a polymorphism in choline metabolism gene *BHMT* rs3733890 had lower breast cancer mortality. These data suggest the importance of nutrients and genetic interactions in the etiology of cancer. Alternatively, the Nurse's Health Study II found no association between choline intake and breast cancer risk (Cho et al., 2007a), but a positive association between choline intake and colorectal cancer risk (Cho et al., 2007b), suggesting different etiologies between breast and colorectal cancer. More research is warranted.

14.1.11 Choline and heart disease

Choline and betaine might benefit heart health by reducing plasma Hcy, a risk factor for heart disease (Zeisel, 1981). Dietary choline intake was inversely related to circulating Hcy concentrations in the Framingham Heart Study (Cho et al., 2006) and in the Nurse's Health Study (Chiuve et al., 2007), suggesting a protective effect of choline intake. However, when looking at the association between dietary choline intake and heart disease incidence, no association was found in the European Prospective Investigation into Cancer and Nutrition (EPIC) study (Dalmeijer et al., 2008), and a marginal positive association was found in the Atherosclerosis Risk in Communities (ARIC) study (Bidulescu et al., 2007). It is important to note that in the ARIC study, the majority of individuals in the cohort had choline intake below the AI (Bidulescu et al., 2009). Hence, the effects of choline supplementation on heart disease risk remains unclear. Some human studies suggested that betaine supplementation increases plasma low-density lipoprotein (LDL)-cholesterol and triacylglycerol concentrations (McGregor et al., 2002; Schwab et al., 2002; Olthof et al., 2005), effects that might counterbalance its Hcy lowering effects. However, the changes in serum lipid concentrations were not associated with higher risk of heart disease. Moreover, the rise in LDL concentration could be an artifact of increasing VLDL and triacylglycerol excretion from fatty liver to plasma, which is not an adverse outcome (for a critical review see Zeisel, 2006b). The relation between choline and heart health warrants more study.

References

Adeyemo O, Jeyakumar H, Plasma progesterone, estradiol-17 beta and testosterone in maternal and cord blood, and maternal human chorionic gonadotropin at parturition. Afr J Med Sci 1993;22: 55–60.

Bidulescu A, Chambless LE, et al., Usual choline and betaine dietary intake and incident coronary heart disease: the Atherosclerosis Risk in Communities (ARIC) study. BMC Cardiovasc Disord 2007;7: 20.

Bidulescu A, Chambless LE, et al., Repeatability and measurement error in the assessment of choline and betaine dietary intake: the Atherosclerosis Risk in Communities (ARIC) study. Nutr J 2009;8: 14.

Bird AP, CpG-rich islands and the function of DNA methylation. Nature 1986;321: 209–13.

Blusztajn JK, Wurtman RJ, Choline and cholinergic neurons. Science 1983;221: 614–20.

Blusztajn JK, Zeisel SH, et al., Developmental changes in the activity of phosphatidylethanolamine N-methyltransferases in rat brain. Biochem J 1985;232: 505–11.

Blusztajn JK, Holbrook PG, et al., Autocannibalism of membrane choline-phospholipids: physiology and pathology. Psychopharmacol Bull 1986;22: 781–6.

Burg MB, Ferraris JD, Intracellular organic osmolytes: function and regulation. J Biol Chem 2008;283: 7309–13.

Cheng W-L, Holmes-McNary MQ, et al., Bioavailability of choline and choline esters from milk in rat pups. J Nutr Biochem 1996;7: 457–64.

Chiuve SE, Giovannucci EL, et al., The association between betaine and choline intakes and the plasma concentrations of homocysteine in women. Am J Clin Nutr 2007;86: 1073–81.

Cho E, Zeisel SH, et al., Dietary choline and betaine assessed by food-frequency questionnaire in relation to plasma total homocysteine concentration in the Framingham Offspring Study. Am J Clin Nutr 2006;83: 905–11.

Cho E, Holmes M, et al., Nutrients involved in one-carbon metabolism and risk of breast cancer among premenopausal women. Cancer Epidemiol Biomarkers Prev 2007a;16: 2787–90.

Cho E, Willett WC, et al., Dietary choline and betaine and the risk of distal colorectal adenoma in women. J Natl Cancer Inst 2007b;99: 1224–31.

Clarren SK, Randels SP, et al., Screening for fetal alcohol syndrome in primary schools: a feasibility study. Teratology 2001;63: 3–10.

Cohen BM, Renshaw PF, et al., Decreased brain choline uptake in older adults. An in vivo proton magnetic resonance spectroscopy study. J Am Med Assoc 1995;274: 902–7.

Cohen EL, Wurtman RJ, Brain acetylcholine: increase after systemic choline administration. Life Sci 1975;16: 1095–102.

Cooney CA, Dave AA, et al,. Maternal methyl supplements in mice affect epigenetic variation and DNA methylation of offspring. J Nutr 2002;132(8 Suppl): 2393S–400S.

Cornford EM, Cornford ME, Nutrient transport and the blood-brain barrier in developing animals. Fed Proc 1986;45: 2065–72.

da Costa K, Cochary EF, et al., Accumulation of 1,2-sn-diradylglycerol with increased membrane-associated protein kinase C may be the mechanism for spontaneous hepatocarcinogenesis in choline deficient rats. J Biol Chem 1993;268: 2100–5.

da Costa KA, Badea M, et al., Elevated serum creatine phosphokinase in choline-deficient humans: mechanistic studies in C2C12 mouse myoblasts. Am J Clin Nutr 2004;80: 163–70.

da Costa KA, Gaffney CE, et al., Choline deficiency in mice and humans is associated with increased plasma homocysteine concentration after a methionine load. Am J Clin Nutr 2005;81: 440–4.

da Costa KA, Kozyreva OG, et al., Common genetic polymorphisms affect the human requirement for the nutrient choline. FASEB J 2006a;20: 1336–44.

da Costa KA, Niculescu MD, et al., Choline deficiency increases lymphocyte apoptosis and DNA damage in humans. Am J Clin Nutr 2006;84: 88–94.

Dalmeijer GW, Olthof MR, et al., Prospective study on dietary intakes of folate, betaine, and choline and cardiovascular disease risk in women. Eur J Clin Nutr 2008;62: 386–94.

Davison JM, Mellott TJ, et al., Gestational choline supply regulates methylation of histone H3, expression of histone methyltransferases G9a (Kmt1c) and Suv39h1 (Kmt1a), and DNA methylation of their genes in rat fetal liver and brain. J Biol Chem 2009;284: 1982–9.

DeLong CJ, Shen YJ, et al., Molecular distinction of phosphatidylcholine synthesis between the CDP- choline pathway and phosphatidylethanolamine methylation pathway. J Biol Chem 1999;274: 29683–8.

Dobosy JR, Fu VX, et al., A methyl-deficient diet modifies histone methylation and alters Igf2 and H19 repression in the prostate. Prostate 2008;68: 1187–95.

Feinberg AP, Tycko B, The history of cancer epigenetics. Nat Rev Cancer 2004;4: 143–53.

Finkelstein JD, Pathways and regulation of homocysteine metabolism in mammals. Semin Thromb Hemost 2000;26: 219–25.

Fisher MC, Zeisel SH, et al., Inhibitors of choline uptake and metabolism cause developmental abnormalities in neurulating mouse embryos. Teratology 2001;64: 114–22.

Fisher MC, Zeisel SH, et al., Perturbations in choline metabolism cause neural tube defects in mouse embryos in vitro. FASEB J 2002;16: 619–21.

Fischer LM, Scearce JA, et al., Ad libitum choline intake in healthy individuals meets or exceeds the proposed adequate intake level. J Nutr 2005;135: 826–9.

Fischer LM, da Costa KA, et al., Sex and menopausal status influence human dietary requirements for the nutrient choline. Am J Clin Nutr 2007;85: 1275–85.

Fuks F, DNA methylation and histone modifications: teaming up to silence genes. Curr Opin Genet Dev 2005;15: 490–5.

Garner SC, Mar M-H, et al., Choline distribution and metabolism in pregnant rats and fetuses are influenced by the choline content of the maternal diet. J Nutr 1995;125: 2851–8.

Glenn MJ, Kirby ED, et al., Age-related declines in exploratory behavior and markers of hippocampal plasticity are attenuated by prenatal choline supplementation in rats. Brain Res 2008;1237: 110–23.

Guseva MV, Hopkins DM, et al., Dietary choline supplementation improves behavioral, histological, and neurochemical outcomes in a rat model of traumatic brain injury. J Neurotrauma 2008;25: 975–83.

Hoffman DR, Cornatzer WE, et al., Relationship between tissue levels of S-adenosylmethionine, S-adenosylhomocysteine, and transmethylation reactions. Can J Biochem 1979;57: 56–65.

Holmes GL, Yang Y, et al., Seizure-induced memory impairment is reduced by choline supplementation before or after status epilepticus. Epilepsy Res 2002;48: 3–13.

Institute of Medicine and National Academy of Sciences USA, Choline. Dietary reference intakes for folate, thiamin, riboflavin, niacin, vitamin B12, panthothenic acid, biotin, and choline. Vol. 1. Washington DC: National Academy Press; 1: 1998; pp. 390–422.

Jeltsch A, Beyond Watson and Crick: DNA methylation and molecular enzymology of DNA methyltransferases. Chembiochem 2002;3: 382.

Jones PA, Baylin SB, The fundamental role of epigenetic events in cancer. Nat Rev Genet 2002;3: 415–28.

Kim JK, Samaranayake M, et al., Epigenetic mechanisms in mammals. Cell Mol Life Sci 2009;66: 596–612.

Kohlmeier M, da Costa KA, et al., Genetic variation of folate-mediated one-carbon transfer pathway predicts susceptibility to choline deficiency in humans. Proc Natl Acad Sci USA 2005;102: 16025–30.

Lekim D, Betzing H, Intestinal absorption of polyunsaturated phosphatidylcholine in the rat. Hoppe Seylers Z Physiol Chem 1976;357: 1321–31.

Leventer SM, Rowell PP, Investigation of the rate-limiting step in the synthesis of acetylcholine by the human placenta. Placenta 1984;5: 261–70.

Lin CS, Wu RD, Choline oxidation and choline dehydrogenase. J Prot Chem 1986;5: 193–200.

McGregor DO, Dellow WJ, et al., Betaine supplementation decreases post-methionine hyperhomocysteinemia in chronic renal failure. Kidney Int 2002;61: 1040–6.

McMahon KE, Farrell PM, Measurement of free choline concentrations in maternal and neonatal blood by micropyrolysis gas chromatography. Clin Chim Acta 1985;149: 1–12.

Meck W, Williams C, Characterization of the facilitative effects of perinatal choline supplementation on timing and temporal memory. Neuroreport 1997a;8: 2831–5.

Meck W, Williams C, Perinatal choline supplementation increases the threshold for chunking in spatial memory. Neuroreport 1997b;8: 3053–9.

Meck W, Williams C, Simultaneous temporal processing is sensitive to prenatal choline availability in mature and aged rats. Neuroreport 1997c;8: 3045–51.

Meck WH, Williams CL, Choline supplementation during prenatal development reduces proactive interference in spatial memory. Brain Res Dev Brain Res 1999;118: 51–9.

Meck WH, Williams CL, Metabolic imprinting of choline by its availability during gestation: implications for memory and attentional processing across the lifespan. Neurosci Biobehav Rev 2003;27: 385–99.

Meck WH, Smith RA, et al., Pre- and postnatal choline supplementation produces long-term facilitation of spatial memory. Dev Psychobiol 1988;21: 339–53.

Meck WH, Smith RA, et al., Organizational changes in cholinergic activity and enhanced visuo-spatial memory as a function of choline administered prenatally or postnatally or both. Behav Neurosci 1989;103: 1234–41.

Nag N, Mellott TJ, et al., Effects of postnatal dietary choline supplementation on motor regional brain volume and growth factor expression in a mouse model of Rett syndrome. Brain Res 2008;1237: 101–9.

Newberne PM, Rogers AE, Labile methyl groups and the promotion of cancer. Ann Rev Nutr 1986;6: 407–32.

Niculescu MD, Zeisel SH, Diet, methyl donors and DNA methylation: interactions between dietary folate, methionine and choline. J Nutr 2002;132(8 Suppl): 2333S–5S.

Niculescu MD, Yamamuro Y, et al., Choline availability modulates human neuroblastoma cell proliferation and alters the methylation of the promoter region of the cyclin-dependent kinase inhibitor 3 gene. J Neurochem 2004;89: 1252–9.

Niculescu MD, Craciunescu CN, et al., Gene expression profiling of choline-deprived neural precursor cells isolated from mouse brain. Brain Res Mol Brain Res 2005;134: 309–22.

Nitsch RM, Blusztajn JK, et al., Evidence for a membrane defect in Alzheimer disease brain. Proc Natl Acad Sci USA 1992;89: 1671–5.

Olthof MR, van Vliet T, et al., Effect of homocysteine-lowering nutrients on blood lipids: results from four randomised, placebo-controlled studies in healthy humans. PLoS Med 2005;2: e135.

Ozarda Ilcol Y, Uncu G, et al., Free and phospholipid-bound choline concentrations in serum during pregnancy, after delivery and in newborns. Arch Physiol Biochem 2002;110: 393–9.

Pogribny IP, Tryndyak VP, et al., Methyl deficiency, alterations in global histone modifications, and carcinogenesis. J Nutr 2007;137(1 Suppl): 216S–22S.

Pyapali G, Turner D, et al., Prenatal choline supplementation decreases the threshold for induction of long-term potentiation in young adult rats. J Neurophysiol 1998;79: 1790–6.

Quina AS, Buschbeck M, et al., Chromatin structure and epigenetics. Biochem Pharmacol 2006;72: 1563–9.

Resseguie M, Song J, et al., Phosphatidylethanolamine n-methyltransferase (PEMT) gene expression is induced by estrogen in human and mouse primary hepatocytes. FASEB J 2007;21: 2622–32.

Rice JC, Briggs SD, et al., Histone methyltransferases direct different degrees of methylation to define distinct chromatin domains. Mol Cell 2003;12: 1591–8.

Rushmore T, Lim Y, et al., Rapid lipid peroxidation in the nuclear fraction of rat liver induced by a diet deficient in choline and methionine. Cancer Lett 1984;24: 251–5.

Sarda IR, Gorwill RH, Hormonal studies in pregnancy. I. Total unconjugated estrogens in maternal peripheral vein, cord vein, and cord artery serum at delivery. Am J Obstet Gynecol 1976;124: 234–8.

Schwab U, Torronen A, et al., Betaine supplementation decreases plasma homocysteine concentrations but does not affect body weight, body composition, or resting energy expenditure in human subjects. Am J Clin Nutr 2002;76: 961–7.

Selhub J, Seyoum E, et al., Effects of choline deficiency and methotrexate treatment upon liver folate content and distribution. Cancer Res 1991;51: 16–21.

Shaw GM, Carmichael SL, et al., Periconceptional dietary intake of choline and betaine and neural tube defects in offspring. Am J Epidemiol 2004;160: 102–9.

Shaw GM, RH Finnell, et al., Choline and risk of neural tube defects in a folate-fortified population. Epidemiology 2009;20: 714–9.

Stevens KE, Adams CE, et al., Permanent improvement in deficient sensory inhibition in DBA/2 mice with increased perinatal choline. Psychopharmacology (Berl) 2008;198: 413–20.

Szegedi SS, Castro CC, et al., Betaine-homocysteine S-methyltransferase-2 is an S-methylmethionine-homocysteine methyltransferase. J Biol Chem 2008;283: 8939–45.

Thomas JD, Garrison M, et al., Perinatal choline supplementation attenuates behavioral alterations associated with neonatal alcohol exposure in rats. Neurotoxicol Teratol 2004;26: 35–45.

Thomas JD, Abou EJ, et al., Prenatal choline supplementation mitigates the adverse effects of prenatal alcohol exposure on development in rats. Neurotoxicol Teratol 2009;31: 303–11.

Ulus IH, Wurtman RJ, et al., Choline increases acetylcholine release and protects against the stimulation-induced decrease in phosphatide levels within membranes of rat corpus striatum. Brain Res 1989;484: 217–27.

Vance DE, Boehringer Mannheim Award lecture. Phosphatidylcholine metabolism: masochistic enzymology, metabolic regulation, and lipoprotein assembly. Biochem Cell Biol 1990;68: 1151–65.

Vance DE, Walkey CJ, et al., Phosphatidylethanolamine N-methyltransferase from liver. Biochim Biophys Acta 1997;1348: 142–50.

Varela-Moreiras G, Selhub J, et al., Effect of chronic choline deficiency in rats on liver folate content and distribution. J Nutr Biochem 1992;3: 519–22.

Varela-Moreiras G, Ragel C, et al., Choline deficiency and methotrexate treatment induces marked but reversible changes in hepatic folate concentrations, serum homocysteine and DNA methylation rates in rats. J Am Coll Nutr 1995;14: 480–5.

Velzing-Aarts FV, Holm PI, et al., Plasma choline and betaine and their relation to plasma homocysteine in normal pregnancy. Am J Clin Nutr 2005;81: 1383–9.

Walkey CJ, Yu L, et al., Biochemical and evolutionary significance of phospholipid methylation. J Biol Chem 1998;273: 27043–6.

Ward BC, Kolodny NH, et al., Neurochemical changes in a mouse model of Rett syndrome: changes over time and in response to perinatal choline nutritional supplementation. J Neurochem 2009;108: 361–71.

Waterland RA, Dolinoy DC, et al., Maternal methyl supplements increase offspring DNA methylation at Axin fused. Genesis 2006;44: 401–6.

Wecker L, The synthesis and release of acetylcholine by depolorized hippocampal slices is increased by increased choline available in vitro prior to stimulation. J Neurochem 1991;57: 1119–27.

Williams CL, Meck WH, et al., Hypertrophy of basal forebrain neurons and enhanced visuospatial memory in perinatally choline-supplemented rats. Brain Res 1998;794: 225–38.

Wolff GL, Kodell RL, et al., Maternal epigenetics and methyl supplements affect agouti gene expression in Avy/a mice. FASEB J 1998;12: 949–57.

Wong-Goodrich SJ, Mellott TJ, et al., Prenatal choline supplementation attenuates neuropathological response to status epilepticus in the adult rat hippocampus. Neurobiol Dis 2008;30: 255–69.

Xu X, Gammon MD, et al., Choline metabolism and risk of breast cancer in a population-based study. FASEB J 2008;22: 2045–52.

Xu X, Gammon MD, et al., High intakes of choline and betaine reduce breast cancer mortality in a population-based study. FASEB J 2009;23: 4022–8.

Yang EK, Blusztajn JK, et al., Rat and human mammary tissue can synthesize choline moiety via the methylation of phosphatidylethanolamine. Biochem J 1988;256: 821–8.

Yang Y, Liu Z, et al., Protective effects of prenatal choline supplementation on seizure-induced memory impairment. J Neurosci 2000;20: RC109.

Yao ZM, Vance DE, The active synthesis of phosphatidylcholine is required for very low density lipoprotein secretion from rat hepatocytes. J Biol Chem 1988;263: 2998–3004.

Zeisel SH, Dietary choline: biochemistry, physiology, and pharmacology. Ann Rev Nutr 1981;1: 95–121.

Zeisel SH, Choline: an essential nutrient for humans. Nutrition 2000;16: 669–71.

Zeisel SH, Betaine supplementation and blood lipids: fact or artifact? Nutr Rev 2006a;64: 77–9.

Zeisel SH, Choline: critical role during fetal development and dietary requirements in adults. Annu Rev Nutr 2006b;26: 229–50.

Zeisel SH, Blusztajn JK, Choline and human nutrition. Ann. Rev. Nutr. 1994;14: 269–96.

Zeisel SH, Wurtman RJ, Developmental changes in rat blood choline concentration. Biochem J 1981;198: 565–70.

Zeisel SH, Zola T, et al., Effect of choline deficiency on S-adenosylmethionine and methionine concentrations in rat liver. Biochem J 1989;259: 725–9.

Zeisel SH, Mar M-H, et al., Erratum: Concentrations of choline-containing compounds and betaine in common foods J Nutr 133: 1302–1307. J Nutr 2003;133: 2918–9.

Zhu X, Song J, et al., Phosphatidylethanolamine N-methyltransferase (PEMT) knockout mice have hepatic steatosis and abnormal hepatic choline metabolite concentrations despite ingesting a recommended dietary intake of choline. Biochem J 2003;370: 987–93.

14.2 Choline in fetal programming

Jan Krzysztof Blusztajn

14.2.1 Introduction

The fields of basic and applied nutritional sciences have evolved from a traditional focus on deficiency states to a broader interest in improving health and quality of life. There are several challenges and novel concepts associated with this paradigm. These include: (1) nutrigenetics – how the genome of an organism governs its response to a nutrient; (2) nutrigenomics – how the nutrient interacts with the genome to modulate gene expression patterns; and (3) nutriepigenomics – how a nutrient influences the epigenome and thus modulates gene expression patterns. This chapter aims to illustrate some of these concepts using the nutrient, choline, as an example. With the recent advances in the studies of human genome and the possibility of correlating gene polymorphisms (particularly single nucleotide polymorphisms, SNPs) with phenotype, considerable progress in the field of human choline nutrigenetics is being made. This information is summarized here. In many other areas, the only available data derive from studies in animal models. In particular, this chapter will: (1) present information on how dietary choline during pregnancy in rodents influences ('programs') the phenotype of offspring; and (2) propose that a nutriepigenomic mechanism is probable.

14.2.2 Choline, an essential nutrient for humans

Choline was added to the list of essential nutrients recently. It was only in 1998 that the Food and Nutrition Board (FNB) of the Institute of Medicine of the National Academy of Sciences of the United States of America recognized that for the maintenance of normal health, humans needed to obtain choline from the diet and issued guidelines on its daily intake (FNB, 1998). Because at that time, and perhaps to this day, there were insufficient data to generate Reference Daily Intake (RDI) values, the FNB issued Adequate Intake (AI) recommendations (▶Tab. 14.1). The AI calls for the average intake of 7.5 mg of choline daily per kg of body weight. Notably, the AI is increased for pregnant and breast-feeding women to satisfy the needs of the fetus and baby whose choline is supplied via placenta (Garner et al., 1995) and milk (Zeisel et al., 1986; Holmes-McNary et al., 1996), respectively. The AI values were established primarily to ensure that dietary choline is sufficient to prevent liver dysfunction associated with low choline consumption

Tab. 14.1: Choline adequate intake.

Life stage	Age	Choline adequate intake (AI) (mg/day)	
		Females	Males
Infants	0–6 months	125	125
Infants	7–12 months	150	150
Children	1–3 years	200	200
Children	4–8 years	250	250
Children	9–13 years	375	375
Adolescents	14–18 years	400	550
Adults	19 years and older	425	550
Pregnancy	All ages	450	–
Breast-feeding	All ages	550	–

observed in adult men (Zeisel et al., 1991). Subsequent studies have shown that choline deficiency also leads to muscle damage (da Costa et al., 2004) and induces apoptotic death of lymphocytes (da Costa et al., 2006a).

14.2.3 Nutrigenetics and nutrigenomics of choline in humans

Since the publication of the FNB report much new research data have accumulated that indicate that even in an affluent country such as the USA, choline nutrition could be marginal among large segments of population (Jensen et al., 2007) and that there are previously understudied factors including gender, age and genotype that influence the individual's requirements for choline. In particular, it has become clear that non-pregnant, non-nursing, women of child-bearing age are relatively resistant to choline deficiency as compared with men and older, postmenopausal women (Fischer et al., 2007). This is explained by the apparently up-regulated endogenous biosynthesis of choline (in the form of phosphatidylcholine) in younger women catalyzed by the hepatic enzyme phosphatidylethanolamine N-methyltransferase (PEMT). PEMT activity constitutes the sole mechanism whereby mammals can synthesize choline *de novo* (▶Fig. 14.2). Interestingly, expression of the *PEMT* gene is increased by estrogens. In younger women, high levels of circulating estrogen are responsible for inducing high PEMT activity, and thus rendering the women relatively insensitive to low-choline diets (da Costa et al., 2006b; Resseguie et al., 2007). This, apparently adaptive genomic mechanism, could buffer both the mother and her offspring during gestation and lactation from the detrimental effects of a short supply of dietary choline. By contrast, postmenopausal women deplete their choline pools in a similar fashion to men. There are also several polymorphic genes that affect humans' requirement for choline, including certain alleles of *PEMT* (da Costa et al., 2006b; Caudill et al., 2009), 5,10-methylenetetrahydrofolate dehydrogenase (*MTHFD1*) (Kohlmeier et al., 2005), methyltetrahydrofolate reductase (*MTHFR*) (Holm et al., 2007; Abratte et al., 2008) and choline dehydrogenase (*CHDH*) (da Costa et al., 2006b). Taken together, these findings point to a significant heterogeneity of choline metabolism among

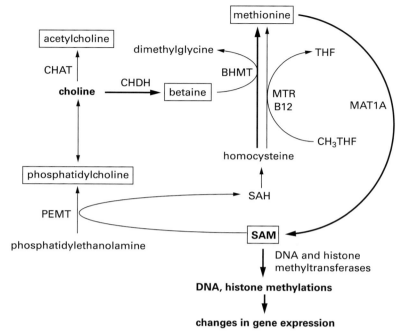

Fig. 14.2: Simplified pathways of choline and methyl group metabolism and its influence on regulation of gene expression. Choline is used as a precursor of phosphatidylcholine, acetylcholine [in a reaction catalyzed by choline acetyltransferase (CHAT)], or betaine [in a reaction catalyzed by choline dehydrogenase (CHDH)]. The methyl groups of betaine are used by betaine:homocysteine *S*-methyltransferase (BHMT) to regenerate methionine from homocysteine. In an alternative pathway catalyzed by vitamin B12-requiring 5-methyltetrahydrofolate-homocysteine *S*-methyltransferase (MTR), methyltetrahydrofolate (CH_3THF) is used as a methyl donor. Methionine is used as a precursor of *S*-adenosylmethionine (SAM) in a reaction catalyzed by methionine adenosyltransferase (MAT1A). Phosphatidylethanolamine *N*-methyltransferase (PEMT) uses SAM to synthesize phosphatidylcholine. The second product of this reaction, *S*-adenosylhomocysteine (SAH) is degraded to free homocysteine. SAM is also the methyl donor for DNA and histone methylations. The pathway linking choline to epigenetic mechanisms regulating gene expression, DNA and histone methylation is indicated by the thick arrows.

people and are helpful in setting the grounds for calculating the RDI values for choline that will probably take place in the near future.

One of the most valuable resources for this purpose and for general epidemiological studies on choline nutrition has been the establishment of the USDA Database for Choline Content of Common Foods (Patterson et al., 2008) that has already been used by investigators interested in the relationships between choline nutrition and disease. Recent studies using this tool found that high intake of choline and its metabolite, betaine (see below), during pregnancy was associated with lowered risk of orofacial clefts in infants (Shaw et al., 2006). Moreover, polymorphisms in genes encoding betaine:homocysteine methyltransferase (*BHMT*) (►Fig. 14.2) and CTP:phosphocholine cytidylytransferase (*PCYT1*) (the rate-limiting enzyme in phosphatidylcholine synthesis) were associated with altered risk of orofacial clefts (Mostowska et al., 2009), further supporting the role of choline metabolism and nutrition in this developmental disorder. The use of the USDA database also revealed that women in the highest quintile of choline and betaine consumption as adults had reduced risk of breast cancer (Xu et al., 2008) and high choline intake during pregnancy reduced the risk of neural tube defects in offspring (Shaw et al., 2004, 2009). These studies are the first to provide evidence for a preventive action of choline in human carcinogenesis and for the significance of choline nutrition during pregnancy for normal development of the fetal human central nervous system. The latter conclusion is supported by the findings that polymorphisms in genes encoding two enzymes of phosphatidylcholine synthesis, *PCYT1A* and choline kinase A (*CHKA*) modify the risk of neural tube defects (Enaw et al., 2006).

14.2.4 Fetal programming of brain development and cognitive function by choline: animal models

In rodent models, maternal choline consumption has profound and long-term effects on brain development and cognition in offspring. Choline deficiency during pregnancy inhibits fetal cell proliferation and stimulates apoptosis in subregions of the hippocampus (Albright et al., 1999a,b). By contrast, gestational choline supplementation stimulates hippocampal cell division (Craciunescu et al., 2003). Moreover, in a commonly-used model that employs the offspring of pregnant mice or rats consuming diets of varying choline content during only a 1-week period of the second half of gestation (embryonic days 11–17; pregnancy in these species lasts 19–21 and 20–22 days, respectively), choline deficiency causes impairments in certain memory tasks (Meck and Williams, 1997a), whereas choline supplementation improves memory and attention (Meck et al., 1988, 1989, 2008; Meck and Williams, 1997a,b,c, 1999; Mellott et al., 2004) and, remarkably, prevents age-related memory decline (Meck and Williams, 1997a; Meck et al., 2008). There are two central conclusions from these studies: (1) choline nutrition during gestation programs brain development and cognitive ability; and (2) cognitive decline is not an inevitable outcome of old age, but rather can be prevented by increased supply of choline during a crucial period of prenatal development.

The above-noted structural changes in prenatal brain subsequently translate into neuroanatomical, neurochemical, electrophysiological and molecular differences in the adult and aged animal. Certain aspects of learning and memory require continual production of new neurons that occurs in the dentate gyrus of the hippocampus throughout lifetime (Clelland et al., 2009; Kitamura et al., 2009). Prenatal choline supplementation enhances adult neurogenesis in the dentate gyrus whereas prenatal choline deficiency impairs this process (Glenn et al., 2007, 2008; Wong-Goodrich et al., 2008b). Moreover, the effect of choline supplementation was seen even in aged rats and correlated with a highly trophic microenvironment within the hippocampus of the prenatally choline supplemented rats that included elevated concentrations of brain-derived neurotrophic factor (BDNF), nerve growth factor (NGF), insulin-like growth factor I (IGF1), and vascular endothelial growth factor (VEGF) in these animals as compared with controls (Glenn et al., 2007, 2008; Wong-Goodrich et al., 2008a,b). Prenatal choline supplementation increases the size of the basal forebrain cholinergic neurons (Williams et al., 1998) that are crucial for the processes of learning and memory (Fibiger, 1991; Sarter and Parikh, 2005), and augments acetylcholine synthesis and release from these neurons

(Cermak et al., 1998; Meck et al., 2008). In addition, prenatal choline availability alters the activation levels of essential molecular components of memory processing (Sweatt, 2001), such that phosphorylation of hippocampal mitogen-activated protein kinase (MAPK) and cAMP response element binding protein (CREB) in response to stimulation by glutamate, N-methyl-D-aspartate (NMDA), or depolarizing concentrations of potassium is increased by prenatal choline supplementation and reduced by prenatal choline deficiency (Mellott et al., 2004). Concordant changes were observed in hippocampal electrophysiological synaptic plasticity measures termed long-term potentiation (LTP). Prenatal choline supplementation enhanced hippocampal LTP in the CA1 region by decreasing the stimulus intensity required for LTP induction (Pyapali et al., 1998; Jones et al., 1999), possibly as a result of an augmented NMDA receptor-mediated neurotransmission (Montoya and Swartzwelder, 2000). Mellott et al. analyzed gene expression patterns in brain of prenatally choline-deficient, choline-supplemented, and control rats using microarrays and found 530 hippocampal and 815 cerebral cortical mRNA species whose levels were modulated by prenatal choline status (Mellott et al., 2007). The protein products of several of these genes are known to participate in signaling pathways implicated in memory processes and thus might mediate the observed choline-induced changes in LTP and behavior. The list of these genes includes insulin-like growth factor II (IGF2), protein kinases PKCβ2, CaMKI and CaMKIIβ, a receptor for the neurotransmitter γ-aminobutyric acid (GABA$_B$R1), and a transcription factor Zif268 (EGR1) (Mellott et al., 2007).

14.2.5 Fetal programming by choline: an example of nutriepigenomics?

The molecular mechanisms that mediate this dramatic long-term programming of brain development by prenatal choline nutrition remain inadequately understood. Within the body choline subserves several functions (►Fig. 14.2): (1) it is the precursor of the neurotransmitter, acetylcholine in cholinergic neurons; (2) it is the precursor of certain phospholipids [phosphatidylcholine, sphingomyelin, plasmenylcholine] that constitute the bulk of phospholipids in all biological membranes; (3) it is the precursor of two signaling molecules, platelet-activating factor, and sphingosylphosphorylcholine; and (4) it can be enzymatically oxidized to betaine (mostly in peripheral tissues). The latter compound can be used for the conversion of homocysteine to methionine (in a reaction catalyzed by BHMT), and subsequently S-adenosylmethionine (SAM) (Finkelstein et al., 1983) that, in turn, is the methyl group donor for most biological methylation reactions including DNA methylation that involves the addition of a methyl group to the 5 position of cytosine in the context of CpG dinucleotide sequences, and the methylation of lysine and arginine residues of histones (Chiang et al., 1996).

14.2.5.1 DNA methylation

Methylation of DNA is a major epigenetic modification of mammalian genomes that participates in the regulation of cell-specific gene expression (Bird and Wolffe, 1999) (►Fig. 14.3). DNA methylation is also important for such regulatory mechanisms of gene expression as genomic imprinting, X chromosome inactivation, cell differentiation and chromatin structure, tumorigenesis and the expression changes that occur during aging (Razin, 1998; Bird and Wolffe, 1999; Robertson and Jones, 2000; Bird, 2002;

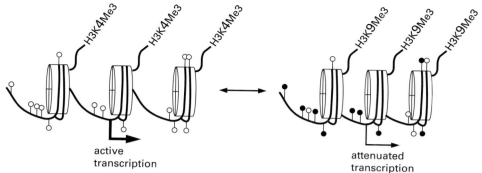

active

attenuated

Fig. 14.3: Methylation of DNA and histone H3 modifies chromatin state and regulates transcription. DNA is wrapped around nucleosomes that are composed of a histone octamer containing two molecules of H3. On the left, cytosines within CpGs of DNA are unmethylated (white lollipops) and H3 is methylated on lysine 4 (H3K4Me3). Under these conditions transcription tends to be active (thick arrow). On the right, DNA has become more methylated (black lollipops); initially owing to the *de novo* process catalyzed by the DNMT3 enzymes and subsequently maintained in the cell lineage by DNMT1, and H3 is methylated on lysine 9 (H3K9Me3). Under these conditions transcription is attenuated (thin arrow). Additional processes, including histone deacetylation, attachment of methylated DNA binding proteins (e.g., MECP2) also contribute to this transcriptional repression and chromatin compaction (illustrated on the right by closer packing of the nucleosomes). The two states are reversible: there are multiple histone demethylating enzymes, although direct (rather than passive, following mitosis) DNA demethylation remains controversial.

Bernstein et al., 2007). In general, CpG methylation causes transcriptional repression (Eden et al., 1998; Jones et al., 1998; Nan et al., 1998; Robertson and Wolffe, 2000; Paulsen and Ferguson-Smith, 2001; Takizawa et al., 2001; Tucker, 2001; Li, 2002; Reinhart et al., 2002) by recruiting specific proteins (MECP2, MBD1, MBD2, and MBD3) that bind to the methylated DNA via their methylated-CpG binding domains (MBD). Upon binding to methylated CpG sites, they further recruit transcriptional corepressors and histone deacetylases. Deacetylated nucleosomes are tightly packed which prevents the access of transcriptional activators to their binding sites in the DNA [reviewed in (Robertson and Wolffe, 2000; Li, 2002; Barrett and Wood, 2008)]. CpG methylation also contributes to transcriptional repression by specifically preventing transcriptional regulators from binding to their target gene promoters. For example, cMyb (Klempnauer, 1993), E2F (Campanero et al., 2000), CREB (Weih et al., 1991), AP2 (Comb and Goodman, 1990), NF-κB (Kirillov et al., 1996) and STAT3 (Takizawa et al., 2001), cannot bind to methylated forms of their DNA recognition sequences. However, DNA methylation could also up-regulate transcription by preventing the binding of a transcriptional repressor to a genomic silencer element, as is the case for *Igf2* gene (Eden et al., 2001; Murrell et al., 2001). DNA methylation is catalyzed by a family of DNA methyltransferase enzymes. The mammalian brain has high levels of expression of DNA methyltransferase 1 (DNMT1) both during development and in adulthood (Goto et al., 1994; Brooks et al., 1996; Trasler et al., 1996; Inano et al., 2000) and the degree of DNA methylation is higher in adult brain than in other tissues (Wilson et al., 1987; Tawa et al., 1990; Ono et al., 1993). Moreover, DNA methylation levels in brain undergo dynamic changes perinatally (Tawa et al., 1990), suggesting that DNA methylation is necessary for the differentiation process of the brain and there is evidence that neuronal activity regulates methylation of promoters of critically important brain genes, e.g., *Bdnf* and *reelin* (Martinowich et al., 2003; Levenson et al., 2006; Miller and Sweatt, 2007; Lubin et al., 2008; Nelson et al., 2008; Yossifoff et al., 2008). DNA methylation patterns acquired during development could be inherited through the cell divisions in a process catalyzed by DNMT1 that methylates hemimethylated CpG sites and thus restores the parental methylation pattern on the daughter DNA strand following DNA replication (Hsu et al., 1999). In addition, DNMT3A and DNMT3B generate the DNA methylation patterns *de novo* during development and in adulthood (Singal and vanWert, 2001; Okano and Li, 2002). The reported effects of choline- or methyl group deficiency on global DNA methylation in multiple models vary: several authors observed hypomethylation (Wilson et al., 1984; Bhave et al., 1988; Wainfan et al., 1989; Christman et al., 1993; Alonso-Aperte and Varela-Moreiras, 1996; Kim et al., 1997; James et al., 2003; Niculescu et al., 2006), some no change (Kim et al., 1995) and some hypermethylation (Song et al., 2000; Sohn et al., 2003; Pogribny et al., 2008), suggesting that DNA methylation might respond to the supply of methyl groups in a complex fashion that includes alterations in the activities of DNA methylating and/or demethylating enzymes. Indeed, diet can influence the expression of DNMTs. Fischer male rats fed a methyl group-deficient diet for at least 3 weeks display global DNA hypomethylation and increased expression and activity of cellular DNMTs, (DNMT1 and DNMT3A) possibly as a compensatory mechanism (Ghoshal et al., 2006). The hypothesis that choline intake by pregnant rats might alter DNA methylation and DNMT expression in the fetus was tested in a study by Kovacheva et al. (2007) who studied these parameters in liver and cerebral cortex on embryonic day 17 in rats following altered dietary supply of choline that had commenced on gestational day 11. The investigators focused on the differentially methylated region 2 (DMR2) of the *Igf2* gene because the DMR2 methylation signature changes dramatically during development (Lopes et al., 2003). Surprisingly, choline-deficient embryos had higher degree of methylation as compared with the control and choline-supplemented rats. One possible mechanism that leads to changes in the global, as well as gene-specific, DNA methylation is via alteration in the activity of DNMTs. It has been shown that DNMT1 is important for maintaining the methylation pattern of the *Igf2* gene and *Dnmt1* knockout mice have abnormal expression of *Igf2* (Li et al., 1993). In liver of choline-deficient embryos, *Dnmt1* mRNA, was overexpressed by more than 50% as compared with control and choline-supplemented embryos. The data suggested that maternal choline deficiency causes an apparently compensatory induction of *Dnmt1* expression in the fetus that prevents the loss of DNA methylation when choline (and possibly other sources of metabolic methyl groups) is in short supply.

14.2.5.2 Histone methylation

The methylation of histone tails at specific lysine and arginine residues is essential for the epigenetic regulation of transcription, cell division, and the formation of heterochromatin (Strahl and Allis, 2000; Jenuwein and Allis, 2001; Jenuwein, 2006) (▶Fig. 14.3). The addition of methyl groups to histones exerts different effects depending on which residue is methylated. Methylation of lysine 4 on histone 3 (H3K4) is associated with transcriptionally active genes (Strahl et al., 1999; Noma et al., 2001; Schneider et al., 2004) whereas methylation of lysine 9 and lysine 27 on histone 3 (H3K9 and H3K27, respectively) correlates with transcriptional repression (Rea et al., 2000; Cao et al., 2002). Furthermore, the degree of methylation at certain residues results in distinct effects on chromatin state. The addition of two methyl groups to the ε-amino group of H3K9 is a hallmark of transcriptional repression in euchromatic regions during development (Tachibana et al., 2001) whereas tri-methylation of the same residue is associated with pericentric heterochromatin (Rea et al., 2000; Nakayama et al., 2001). The enzymes that catalyze these modifications also differ, with the histone methyltransferase G9a (KMT1C, EHMT2) responsible for di-methylation of H3K9 to H3K9Me2 and for tri-methylation of H3K27 to H3K27Me3 (Tachibana et al., 2002), and histone methyltransferase Suv39h1 (KMT1A) responsible for tri-methylation at H3K9 to H3K9Me3 (Aagaard et al., 1999). Therefore, in addition to modulating DNA methylation, choline supply could affect the methylation of amino acid residues on histone tails (Zhu et al., 2004; Dobosy et al., 2008) leading to alterations in the expression of genes involved in growth and development. Davison et al. (2009) examined several components of the histone 3 methylating machinery in rat liver and cerebral cortex on embryonic day 17 of rat fetuses derived from mothers consuming varying amounts of choline. The methylation of H3K9 and H3K27 and expression of G9a and Suv39h1 were directly related to the availability of choline. Consistent with the studies of Kovacheva et al. (2007), DNA methylation of the *G9a* and *Suv39h1* genes was dramatically up-regulated by choline deficiency (Davison et al., 2009). The latter finding points to the possibility that the expression of these histone methyltransferase is under negative control of methylation of their genes.

14.2.6 Fetal programming by choline: mammary cancer in animal models

The mammary gland formation in humans commences prenatally (Russo and Russo, 1987). In rodents it begins on embryonic days 10–11 and a small ductal tree is seen by birth (Hennighausen and Robinson, 2001), i.e., the time when maternal choline nutrition influences the development of other organs such as brain and liver (see above). Therefore, the prenatal period could render the gland vulnerable to the conditions in its milieu, including availability of essential nutrients (e.g., choline), that might influence the risk of breast cancer in adulthood (Trichopoulos, 1990). Indeed in a female rat model of mammary carcinogenesis that employs administration of a single dose of the carcinogen 7,12-dimethylbenz[α]anthracene, mammary tumor growth rate was inversely related to the prenatal choline supply, resulting in 50% longer survival of the prenatally choline-supplemented as compared with the prenatally choline-deficient rats (Kovacheva et al., 2008). This was accompanied by distinct expression patterns of approximately 70 genes in tumors derived from the three dietary groups. Tumors from the prenatally choline-supplemented rats overexpressed genes that confer favorable prognosis in human cancers (*Klf6, Klf9, Nid2, Ntn4, Per1*, and *Txnip*) and underexpressed those associated with aggressive disease (*Bcar3, Cldn12, Csf1, Jag1, Lgals3, Lypd3, Nme1, Ptges2, Ptgs1*, and *Smarcb1*) (Kovacheva et al., 2008). DNA methylation within the tumor suppressor gene, stratifin (*Sfn*, 14-3-3σ), was proportional to the prenatal choline intake and correlated inversely with the expression of its mRNA and protein in tumors, suggesting that an epigenetic mechanism might underlie the altered molecular phenotype and tumor growth (Kovacheva et al., 2008). These results suggest a role for adequate maternal choline nutrition during pregnancy in prevention/alleviation of breast cancer in daughters.

14.2.7 Conclusions and future directions

Since the classification of choline as an essential nutrient for humans a decade ago, much progress has been made in our understanding of choline nutrition in people that will probably lead to the establishment of additional dietary guidelines on choline including calculating of the RDI. This progress has been made possible by advances in genetics and genomics and increased appreciation of the role of gender, physiological state and gene polymorphisms in human requirements for this nutrient. In addition to the studies reviewed above, a large body of evidence indicates that perinatal administration of choline in rats and mice causes long-lasting cognitive enhancement and is neuroprotective in a variety of models of neuronal damage, including that evoked by seizures, alcohol and genetic mutations (Schenk and Brandner, 1995; Ricceri and Berger-Sweeney, 1998; Tees, 1999a,b; Tees and Mohammadi, 1999; Thomas et al., 2000; Yang et al., 2000; Brandner, 2002; Holmes et al., 2002; Nag and Berger-Sweeney, 2007; Thomas et al., 2007; Nag et al., 2008; Ryan et al., 2008; Stevens et al., 2008; Ward et al., 2008, 2009). Thus, adequate supply of choline in early life is central for optimal development, adult cognitive performance and successful aging. This assertion is probably applicable to humans; however, no direct data exist to support it and more studies on humans are needed. Current data are consistent with the idea that choline intake during fetal development modulates patterns of gene expression via an epigenetic mechanism. However, this concept remains to be formally proven.

Acknowledgments

National Institute on Aging grant AG009525.

References

Aagaard L, Laible G, Selenko P, Schmid M, Dorn R, Schotta G, Kuhfittig S, Wolf A, Lebersorger A, Singh PB, Reuter G, Jenuwein T, Functional mammalian homologues of the *Drosophila* PEV-modifier Su(var)3-9 encode centromere-associated proteins which complex with the heterochromatin component M31. EMBO J 1999;18: 1923–38.

Abratte CM, Wang W, Li R, Moriarty DJ, Caudill MA, Folate intake and the MTHFR C677T genotype influence choline status in young Mexican American women. J Nutr Biochem 2008;19: 158–65.

Albright CD, Tsai AY, Friedrich CB, Mar MH, Zeisel SH, Choline availability alters embryonic development of the hippocampus and septum in the rat. Dev Brain Res 1999a;113: 13–20.

Albright CD, Friedrich CB, Brown EC, Mar MH, Zeisel SH, Maternal dietary choline availability alters mitosis, apoptosis and the localization of TOAD-64 protein in the developing fetal rat septum. Dev Brain Res 1999b;115: 123–9.

Alonso-Aperte E, Varela-Moreiras G, Brain folates and DNA methylation in rats fed a choline deficient diet or treated with low doses of methotrexate. Int J Vitam Nutr Res 1996;66: 232–6.

Barrett RM, Wood MA, Beyond transcription factors: the role of chromatin modifying enzymes in regulating transcription required for memory. Learn Mem 2008;15: 460–7.

Bernstein BE, Meissner A, Lander ES, The mammalian epigenome. Cell 2007;128: 669–81.

Bhave MR, Wilson MJ, Poirier LA, c-H-ras and c-K-ras gene hypomethylation in the livers and hepatomas of rats fed methyl-deficient, amino acid-defined diets. Carcinogenesis 1988;9: 343–8.

Bird A, DNA methylation patterns and epigenetic memory. Genes Dev 2002;16: 6–21.

Bird AP, Wolffe AP, Methylation-induced repression – belts, braces, and chromatin. Cell 1999;99: 451–4.

Brandner C, Perinatal choline treatment modifies the effects of a visuo-spatial attractive cue upon spatial memory in naive adult rats. Brain Res 2002;928: 85–95.

Brooks PJ, Marietta C, Goldman D, DNA mismatch repair and DNA methylation in adult brain neurons. J Neurosci 1996;16: 939–45.

Campanero MR, Armstrong MI, Flemington EK, CpG methylation as a mechanism for the regulation of E2F activity. Proc Natl Acad Sci USA 2000;97: 6481–6.

Cao R, Wang LJ, Wang HB, Xia L, Erdjument-Bromage H, Tempst P, Jones RS, Zhang Y, Role of histone H3 lysine 27 methylation in polycomb-group silencing. Science 2002;298: 1039–43.

Caudill MA, Dellschaft N, Solis C, Hinkis S, Ivanov AA, Nash-Barboza S, Randall KE, Jackson B, Solomita GN, Vermeylen F, Choline intake, plasma riboflavin, and the phosphatidylethanolamine N-methyltransferase G5465A genotype predict plasma homocysteine in folate-deplete Mexican-American men with the methylenetetrahydrofolate reductase 677TT genotype. J Nutr 2009;139: 727–33.

Cermak JM, Holler T, Jackson DA, Blusztajn JK, Prenatal availability of choline modifies development of the hippocampal cholinergic system. FASEB J 1998;12: 349–57.

Chiang PK, Gordon RK, Tal J, Zeng GC, Doctor BP, Pardhasaradhi K, McCann PP, S-adenosylmethionine and methylation. FASEB J 1996;10: 471–80.

Christman JK, Sheikhnejad G, Dizik M, Abileah S, Wainfan E, Reversibility of changes in nucleic acid methylation and gene expression induced in rat liver by severe dietary methyl deficiency. Carcinogenesis 1993;14: 551–7.

Clelland CD, Choi M, Romberg C, Clemenson GD Jr, Fragniere A, Tyers P, Jessberger S, Saksida LM, Barker RA, Gage FH, Bussey TJ, A functional role for adult hippocampal neurogenesis in spatial pattern separation. Science 2009;325: 210–3.

Comb M, Goodman HM, CpG methylation inhibits proenkephalin gene expression and binding of the transcription factor AP-2. Nucleic Acids Res 1990;18: 3975–82.

Craciunescu CN, Albright CD, Mar MH, Song J, Zeisel SH, Choline availability during embryonic development alters progenitor cell mitosis in developing mouse hippocampus. J Nutr 2003;133: 3614–8.

da Costa KA, Badea M, Fischer LM, Zeisel SH, Elevated serum creatine phosphokinase in choline-deficient humans: mechanistic studies in C2C12 mouse myoblasts. Am J Clin Nutr 2004;80: 163–70.

da Costa KA, Niculescu MD, Craciunescu CN, Fischer LM, Zeisel SH, Choline deficiency increases lymphocyte apoptosis and DNA damage in humans. Am J Clin Nutr 2006a;84: 88–94.

da Costa KA, Kozyreva OG, Song J, Galanko JA, Fischer LM, Zeisel SH, Common genetic polymorphisms affect the human requirement for the nutrient choline. FASEB J 2006b;20: 1336–44.

Davison JM, Mellott TJ, Kovacheva VP, Blusztajn JK, Gestational choline supply regulates methylation of histone H3, expression of histone methyltransferases G9a (Kmt1c) and Suv39h1 (Kmt1a) and DNA methylation of their genes in rat fetal liver and brain. J Biol Chem 2009;284: 1982–9.

Dobosy JR, Fu VX, Desotelle JA, Srinivasan R, Kenowski ML, Almassi N, Weindruch R, Svaren J, Jarrard DF, A methyl-deficient diet modifies histone methylation and alters Igf2 and H19 repression in the prostate. Prostate 2008;68: 1187–95.

Eden S, Hashimshony T, Keshet I, Cedar H, Thorne AW, DNA methylation models histone acetylation. Nature 1998;394: 842.

Eden S, Constancia M, Hashimshony T, Dean W, Goldstein B, Johnson AC, Keshet I, Reik W, Cedar H, An upstream repressor element plays a role in Igf2 imprinting. EMBO J 2001;20: 3518–25.

Enaw JO, Zhu H, Yang W, Lu W, Shaw GM, Lammer EJ, Finnell RH, CHKA and PCYT1A gene polymorphisms, choline intake and spina bifida risk in a California population. BMC Med 2006; 4: 36.

Fibiger HC, Cholinergic mechanisms in learning, memory and dementia: a review of recent evidence. Trends Neurosci 1991;14: 220–3.

Finkelstein JD, Martin JJ, Harris BJ, Kyle WE, Regulation of hepatic betaine-homocysteine methyltransferase by dietary betaine. J Nutr 1983;113: 519–21.

Fischer LM, daCosta KA, Kwock L, Stewart PW, Lu TS, Stabler SP, Allen RH, Zeisel SH, Sex and menopausal status influence human dietary requirements for the nutrient choline. Am J Clin Nutr 2007;85: 1275–85.

FNB, Dietary reference intakes for thiamin, riboflavin, niacin, vitamin B6, folate, vitamin B12, panthotenic acid, biotin, and choline. Washington, DC: National Academy Press;1998.

Garner SC, Mar MH, Zeisel SH, Choline distribution and metabolism in pregnant rats and fetuses are influenced by the choline content of the maternal diet. J Nutr 1995;125: 2851–8.

Ghoshal K, Li X, Datta J, Bai S, Pogribny I, Pogribny M, Huang Y, Young D, Jacob ST, A folate- and methyl-deficient diet alters the expression of DNA methyltransferases and methyl CpG binding proteins involved in epigenetic gene silencing in livers of F344 rats. J Nutr 2006;136: 1522–7.

Glenn MJ, Gibson EM, Kirby ED, Mellott TJ, Blusztajn JK, Williams CL, Prenatal choline availability modulates hippocampal neurogenesis and neurogenic responses to enriching experiences in adult female rats. Eur J Neurosci 2007;25: 2473–82.

Glenn MJ, Kirby ED, Gibson EM, Wong-Goodrich SJ, Mellott TJ, Blusztajn JK, Williams CL, Age-related declines in exploratory behavior and markers of hippocampal plasticity are attenuated by prenatal choline supplementation in rats. Brain Res 2008;1237: 110–23.

Goto K, Numata M, Komura JI, Ono T, Bestor TH, Kondo H, Expression of DNA methyltransferase gene in mature and immature neurons as well as proliferating cells in mice. Differentiation 1994;56: 39–44.

Hennighausen L, Robinson GW, Signaling pathways in mammary gland development. Dev Cell 2001;1: 467–75.

Holm PI, Hustad S, Ueland PM, Vollset SE, Grotmol T, Schneede J, Modulation of the homocysteine-betaine relationship by methylenetetrahydrofolate reductase 677 C->T genotypes and B-vitamin status in a large scale epidemiological study. J Clin Endocrinol Metab 2007;92: 1535–41.

Holmes GL, Yang Y, Liu Z, Cermak JM, Sarkisian MR, Stafstrom CE, Neill JC, Blusztajn JK, Seizure-induced memory impairment is reduced by choline supplementation before or after status epilepticus. Epilepsy Res 2002;48: 3–13.

Holmes-McNary MQ, Cheng WL, Mar MH, Fussell S, Zeisel SH, Choline and choline esters in human and rat milk and in infant formulas. Am J Clin Nutr 1996;64: 572–6.

Hsu DW, Lin MJ, Lee TL, Wen SC, Chen X, Shen CK, Two major forms of DNA (cytosine-5) methyltransferase in human somatic tissues. Proc Natl Acad Sci USA 1999;96: 9751–6.

Inano K, Suetake I, Ueda T, Miyake Y, Nakamura M, Okada M, Tajima S, Maintenance-type DNA methyltransferase is highly expressed in post- mitotic neurons and localized in the cytoplasmic compartment. J Biochem (Tokyo) 2000;128: 315–21.

James SJ, Pogribny IP, Pogribna M, Miller BJ, Jernigan S, Melnyk S, Mechanisms of DNA damage, DNA hypomethylation, and tumor progression in the folate/methyl-deficient rat model of hepatocarcinogenesis. J Nutr 2003;133: 3740S–7S.

Jensen HH, Batres-Marquez SP, Carriquiry A, Schalinske KL, Choline in the diets of the US population: NHANES, 2003–2004. FASEB J 2007;21: LB219.

Jenuwein T, The epigenetic magic of histone lysine methylation. FEBS J 2006;273: 3121–35.

Jenuwein T, Allis CD, Translating the histone code. Science 2001;293: 1074–80.

Jones JP, H Meck W, Williams CL, Wilson WA, Swartzwelder HS, Choline availability to the developing rat fetus alters adult hippocampal long-term potentiation. Dev Brain Res 1999;118: 159–67.

Jones PL, Veenstra GJ, Wade PA, Vermaak D, Kass SU, Landsberger N, Strouboulis J, Wolffe AP, Methylated DNA and MeCP2 recruit histone deacetylase to repress transcription. Nat Genet 1998;19: 187–91.

Kim YI, Pogribny IP, Basnakian AG, Miller JW, Selhub J, James SJ, Mason JB, Folate deficiency in rats induces DNA strand breaks and hypomethylation within the p53 tumor suppressor gene. Am J Clin Nutr 1997;65: 46–52.

Kim YI, Christman JK, Fleet JC, Cravo ML, Salomon RN, Smith D, Ordovas J, Selhub J, Mason JB, Moderate folate deficiency does not cause global hypomethylation of hepatic and colonic DNA or c-myc-specific hypomethylation of colonic DNA in rats. Am J Clin Nutr 1995;61: 1083–90.

Kirillov A, Kistler B, Mostoslavsky R, Cedar H, Wirth T, Bergman Y, A role for nuclear NF-kappaB in B-cell-specific demethylation of the Igkappa locus. Nat Genet 1996;13: 435–41.

Kitamura T, Saitoh Y, Takashima N, Murayama A, Niibori Y, Ageta H, Sekiguchi M, Sugiyama H, Inokuchi K, Adult neurogenesis modulates the hippocampus-dependent period of associative fear memory. Cell 2009;139: 814–27.

Klempnauer KH, Methylation-sensitive DNA binding by v-myb and c-myb proteins. Oncogene 1993;8: 111–5.

Kohlmeier M, da Costa KA, Fischer LM, Zeisel SH, Genetic variation of folate-mediated one-carbon transfer pathway predicts susceptibility to choline deficiency in humans. Proc Natl Acad Sci USA 2005;102: 16025–30.

Kovacheva VP, Mellott TJ, Davison JM, Wagner N, Lopez-Coviella I, Schnitzler AC, Blusztajn JK, Gestational choline deficiency causes global and Igf2 gene DNA hypermethylation by up-regulation of Dnmt1 expression. J Biol Chem 2007;282: 31777–88.

Kovacheva VP, Davison JM, Mellott TJ, Rogers AE, Yang S, O'Brien MJ, Blusztajn JK, Raising gestational choline intake alters gene expression in DMBA-evoked mammary tumors and prolongs survival. FASEB J 2008;23: 1054–63.

Levenson JM, Roth TL, Lubin FD, Miller CA, Huang IC, Desai P, Malone LM, Sweatt JD, Evidence that DNA (cytosine-5) methyltransferase regulates synaptic plasticity in the hippocampus. J Biol Chem 2006;281: 15763–73.

Li E, Chromatin modification and epigenetic reprogramming in mammalian development. Nat Rev Genet 2002;3: 662–73.

Li E, Beard C, Jaenisch R, Role for DNA methylation in genomic imprinting. Nature 1993;366: 362–5.

Lopes S, Lewis A, Hajkova P, Dean W, Oswald J, Forne T, Murrell A, Constancia M, Bartolomei M, Walter J, Reik W, Epigenetic modifications in an imprinting cluster are controlled by a hierarchy of DMRs suggesting long-range chromatin interactions. Hum Mol Genet 2003;12: 295–305.

Lubin FD, Roth TL, Sweatt JD, Epigenetic regulation of BDNF gene transcription in the consolidation of fear memory. J Neurosci 2008;28: 10576–86.

Martinowich K, Hattori D, Wu H, Fouse S, He F, Hu Y, Fan GP, Sun YE, DNA methylation-related chromatin remodeling in activity-dependent Bdnf gene regulation. Science 2003;302: 890–3.

Meck WH, Williams CL, Simultaneous temporal processing is sensitive to prenatal choline availability in mature and aged rats. Neuroreport 1997a;8: 3045–51.

Meck WH, Williams CL, Perinatal choline supplementation increases the threshold for chunking in spatial memory. Neuroreport 1997b;8: 3053–59.

Meck WH, Williams CL, Characterization of the facilitative effects of perinatal choline supplementation on timing and temporal memory. Neuroreport 1997c;8: 2831–5.

Meck WH, Williams CL, Choline supplementation during prenatal development reduces proactive interference in spatial memory. Dev Brain Res 1999;118: 51–9.

Meck WH, Smith RA, Williams CL, Pre- and postnatal choline supplementation produces long-term facilitation of spatial memory. Dev Psychobiol 1988;21: 339–53.

Meck WH, Smith RA, Williams CL, Organizational changes in cholinergic activity and enhanced visuospatial memory as a function of choline administered prenatally or postnatally or both. Behav Neurosci 1989;103: 1234–41.

Meck WH, Williams CL, Cermak JM, Blusztajn JK, Developmental periods of choline sensitivity provide an ontogenetic mechanism for regulating memory capacity and age-related dementia. Front Integr Neurosci 2008;1: 7.

Mellott TJ, Williams CL, Meck WH, Blusztajn JK, Prenatal choline supplementation advances hippocampal development and enhances MAPK and CREB activation. FASEB J 2004;18: 545–7.

Mellott TJ, Follettie MT, Diesl V, Hill AA, Lopez-Coviella I, Blusztajn JK, Prenatal choline availability modulates hippocampal and cerebral cortical gene expression. FASEB J 2007;21: 1311–23.

Miller CA, Sweatt JD, Covalent modification of DNA regulates memory formation. Neuron 2007;53: 857–69.

Montoya D, Swartzwelder HS, Prenatal choline supplementation alters hippocampal N-methyl-D-aspartate receptor-mediated neurotransmission in adult rats. Neurosci Lett 2000;296: 85–8.

Mostowska A, Hozyasz KK, Wojcicki P, Dziegelewska M, Jagodzinski PP, Associations of folate and choline metabolism gene polymorphisms with orofacial clefts. J Med Genet 2009. [E-pub ahead of print]

Murrell A, Heeson S, Bowden L, Constancia M, Dean W, Kelsey G, Reik W, An intragenic methylated region in the imprinted Igf2 gene augments transcription. EMBO Rep 2001;2: 1101–6.

Nag N, Berger-Sweeney JE, Postnatal dietary choline supplementation alters behavior in a mouse model of Rett syndrome. Neurobiol Dis 2007;26: 473–80.

Nag N, Mellott TJ, Berger-Sweeney JE, Effects of postnatal dietary choline supplementation on motor regional brain volume and growth factor expression in a mouse model of Rett syndrome. Brain Res 2008;1237: 101–9.

Nakayama T, Watanabe M, Yamanaka M, Hirokawa Y, Suzuki H, Ito H, Yatani R, Shiraishi T, The role of epigenetic modifications in retinoic acid receptor 2 gene expression in human prostate cancers. LabInvest 2001;81: 1049–57.

Nan X, Ng HH, Johnson CA, Laherty CD, Turner BM, Eisenman RN, Bird A, Transcriptional repression by the methyl-CpG-binding protein MeCP2 involves a histone deacetylase complex. Nature 1998;393: 386–9.

Nelson ED, Kavalali ET, Monteggia LM, Activity-dependent suppression of miniature neurotransmission through the regulation of DNA methylation. J Neurosci 2008;28: 395–406.

Niculescu MD, Craciunescu CN, Zeisel SH, Dietary choline deficiency alters global and gene-specific DNA methylation in the developing hippocampus of mouse fetal brains. FASEB J 2006;20: 43–9.

Noma K, Allis CD, Grewal SI, Transitions in distinct histone H3 methylation patterns at the heterochromatin domain boundaries. Science 2001;293: 1150–55.

Okano M, Li E, Genetic analyses of DNA methyltransferase genes in mouse model system. J Nutr 2002;132: 2462S–5S.

Ono T, Uehara Y, Kurishita A, Tawa R, Sakurai H, Biological significance of DNA methylation in the ageing process. Age Ageing 1993;22: S34–43.

Patterson KY, Bhagwat AS, Williams JR, Howe JC, Holden JM, Zeisel SH, Da Costa CA, Mar H, USDA database for the choline content of common foods. Release two. http://www.ars.usda.gov/Services/docs.htm?docid=6232, 2008

Paulsen M, Ferguson-Smith AC, DNA methylation in genomic imprinting, development, and disease. J Pathol 2001;195: 97–110.

Pogribny IP, Karpf AR, James SR, Melnyk S, Han T, Tryndyak VP, Epigenetic alterations in the brains of Fisher 344 rats induced by long-term administration of folate/methyl-deficient diet. Brain Res 2008;1237: 25–34.

Pyapali GK, Turner DA, Williams CL, Meck WH, Swartzwelder HS, Prenatal dietary choline supplementation decreases the threshold for induction of long-term potentiation in young adult rats. J Neurophysiol 1998;79: 1790–6.

Razin A, CpG methylation, chromatin structure and gene silencing-a three-way connection. EMBO J 1998;17: 4905–8.

Rea S, Eisenhaber F, O'Carroll D, Strahl BD, Sun ZW, Schmid M, Opravil S, Mechtler K, Ponting CP, Allis CD, Jenuwein T, Regulation of chromatin structure by site-specific histone H3 methyltransferases. Nature 2000;406: 593–9.

Reinhart B, Eljanne M, Chaillet JR, Shared role for differentially methylated domains of imprinted genes. Mol Cell Biol 2002;22: 2089–98.

Resseguie M, Song J, Niculescu MD, da Costa KA, Randall TA, Zeisel SH, Phosphatidylethanolamine N-methyltransferase (PEMT) gene expression is induced by estrogen in human and mouse primary hepatocytes. FASEB J 2007;21: 2622–32.

Ricceri L, Berger-Sweeney J, Postnatal choline supplementation in preweanling mice: sexually dimorphic behavioral and neurochemical effects. Behav Neurosci 1998;112: 1387–92.

Robertson KD, Jones PA, DNA methylation: past, present and future directions. Carcinogenesis 2000;21: 461–7.

Robertson KD, Wolffe AP, DNA methylation in health and disease. Nat Rev Genet 2000;1: 11–9.

Russo J, Russo IH, Development of the human mammary gland. In: Neville MC, Daniel CW, editors. The mammary gland: development, regulation and function. New York: Plenum; 1987. pp. 67–93.

Ryan SH, Williams JK, Thomas JD, Choline supplementation attenuates learning deficits associated with neonatal alcohol exposure in the rat: effects of varying the timing of choline administration. Brain Res 2008;1237: 91–100.

Sarter M, Parikh V, Choline transporters, cholinergic transmission and cognition. Nat Rev Neurosci 2005;6: 48–56.

Schenk F, Brandner C, Indirect effect of peri- and postnatal choline treatment on place-learning abilities in rat. Psychobiology 1995;23: 302–13.

Schneider R, Bannister AJ, Myers FA, Thorne AW, Crane-Robinson C, Kouzarides T, Histone H3 lysine 4 methylation patterns in higher eukaryotic genes. Nat Cell Biol 2004;6: 73–7.

Shaw GM, Carmichael SL, Yang W, Selvin S, Schaffer DM, Periconceptional dietary intake of choline and betaine and neural tube defects in offspring. Am J Epidemiol 2004;160: 102–9.

Shaw GM, Carmichael SL, Laurent C, Rasmussen SA, Maternal nutrient intakes and risk of orofacial clefts. Epidemiology 2006;17: 285–91.

Shaw GM, Finnell RH, Blom HJ, Carmichael SL, Vollset SE, Yang W, Ueland PM, Choline and risk of neural tube defects in a folate-fortified population. Epidemiology 2009;20: 714–9.

Singal R, vanWert JM, De novo methylation of an embryonic globin gene during normal development is strand specific and spreads from the proximal transcribed region. Blood 2001;98: 3441–6.

Sohn KJ, Stempak JM, Reid S, Shirwadkar S, Mason JB, Kim YI, The effect of dietary folate on genomic and p53-specific DNA methylation in rat colon. Carcinogenesis 2003;24: 81–90.

Song J, Sohn KJ, Medline A, Ash C, Gallinger S, Kim YI, Chemopreventive effects of dietary folate on intestinal polyps in Apc+/-Msh2-/- mice. Cancer Res 2000;60: 3191–9.

Stevens KE, Adams CE, Yonchek J, Hickel C, Danielson J, Kisley MA, Permanent improvement in deficient sensory inhibition in DBA/2 mice with increased perinatal choline. Psychopharmacology (Berl) 2008;198: 413–20.

Strahl BD, Allis CD, The language of covalent histone modifications. Nature 2000;403: 41–5.

Strahl BD, Ohba R, Cook RG, Allis CD, Methylation of histone H3 at lysine 4 is highly conserved and correlates with transcriptionally active nuclei in Tetrahymena. Proc Natl Acad Sci USA 1999;96: 14967–72.

Sweatt JD, The neuronal MAP kinase cascade: a biochemical signal integration system subserving synaptic plasticity and memory. J Neurochem 2001;76: 1–10.

Tachibana M, Sugimoto K, Fukushima T, Shinkai Y, Set domain-containing protein, G9a, is a novel lysine-preferring mammalian histone methyltransferase with hyperactivity and specific selectivity to lysines 9 and 27 of histone H3. J Biol Chem 2001;276: 25309–17.

Tachibana M, Sugimoto K, Nozaki M, Ueda J, Ohta T, Ohki M, Fukuda M, Takeda N, Niida H, Kato H, Shinkai Y, G9a histone methyltransferase plays a dominant role in euchromatic histone H3 lysine 9 methylation and is essential for early embryogenesis. Genes Dev 2002;16: 1779–91.

Takizawa T, Nakashima K, Namihira M, Ochiai W, Uemura A, Yanagisawa M, Fujita N, Nakao M, Taga T, DNA methylation is a critical cell-intrinsic determinant of astrocyte differentiation in the fetal brain. Dev Cell 2001;1: 749–58.

Tawa R, Ono T, Kurishita A, Okada S, Hirose S, Changes of DNA methylation level during pre- and postnatal periods in mice. Differentiation 1990;45: 44–8.

Tees RC, The influences of rearing environment and neonatal choline dietary supplementation on spatial learning and memory in adult rats. Behav Brain Res 1999a;105: 173–88.

Tees RC, The influences of sex, rearing environment, and neonatal choline dietary supplementation on spatial and nonspatial learning and memory in adult rats. Dev Psychobiol 1999b;35: 328–42.

Tees RC, Mohammadi E, The effects of neonatal choline dietary supplementation on adult spatial and configural learning and memory in rats. Dev Psychobiol 1999;35: 226–40.

Thomas JD, La Fiette MH, Quinn VR, Riley EP, Neonatal choline supplementation ameliorates the effects of prenatal alcohol exposure on a discrimination learning task in rats. Neurotoxicol Teratol 2000;22: 703–11.

Thomas JD, Biane JS, O'Bryan KA, O'Neill TM, Dominguez HD, Choline supplementation following third-trimester-equivalent alcohol exposure attenuates behavioral alterations in rats. Behav Neurosci 2007;121: 120–30.

Trasler JM, Trasler DG, Bestor TH, Li E, Ghibu F, DNA methyltransferase in normal and Dnmtn/Dnmtn mouse embryos. Dev Dyn 1996;206: 239–47.

Trichopoulos D, Hypothesis: does breast cancer originate in utero? Lancet 1990;335: 939–40.

Tucker KL, Methylated cytosine and the brain: a new base for neuroscience. Neuron 2001;30: 649–52.

Wainfan E, Dizik M, Stender M, Christman JK, Rapid appearance of hypomethylated DNA in livers of rats fed cancer- promoting, methyl-deficient diets. Cancer Res 1989;49: 4094–7.

Ward BC, Agarwal S, Wang K, Berger-Sweeney J, Kolodny NH, Longitudinal brain MRI study in a mouse model of Rett Syndrome and the effects of choline. Neurobiol Dis 2008;31: 110–19.

Ward BC, Kolodny NH, Nag N, Berger-Sweeney JE, Neurochemical changes in a mouse model of Rett syndrome: changes over time and in response to perinatal choline nutritional supplementation. J Neurochem 2009;108: 361–71.

Weih F, Nitsch D, Reik A, Schutz G, Becker PB, Analysis of CpG methylation and genomic footprinting at the tyrosine aminotransferase gene: DNA methylation alone is not sufficient to prevent protein binding in vivo. EMBO J 1991;10: 2559–67.

Williams CL, Meck WH, Heyer D, Loy R, Hypertrophy of basal forebrain neurons and enhanced visuospatial memory in perinatally choline-supplemented rats. Brain Res 1998;794: 225–38.

Wilson MJ, Shivapurkar N, Poirier LA, Hypomethylation of hepatic nuclear DNA in rats fed with a carcinogenic methyl-deficient diet. Biochem J 1984;218: 987–90.

Wilson VL, Smith RA, Ma S, Cutler RG, Genomic 5-methyldeoxycytidine decreases with age. J Biol Chem 1987;262: 9948–51.

Wong-Goodrich SJ, Mellott TJ, Glenn MJ, Blusztajn JK, Williams CL, Prenatal choline supplementation attenuates neuropathological response to status epilepticus in the adult rat hippocampus. Neurobiol Dis 2008a;30: 255–69.

Wong-Goodrich SJ, Glenn MJ, Mellott TJ, Blusztajn JK, Meck WH, Williams CL, Spatial memory and hippocampal plasticity are differentially sensitive to the availability of choline in adulthood as a function of choline supply in utero. Brain Res 2008b;1237: 153–66.

Xu X, Gammon MD, Zeisel SH, Lee YL, Wetmur JG, Teitelbaum SL, Bradshaw PT, Neugut AI, Santella RM, Chen J, Choline metabolism and risk of breast cancer in a population-based study. FASEB J 2008;22: 2045–52.

Yang Y, Liu Z, Cermak JM, Tandon P, Sarkisian MR, Stafstrom CF, Neill JC, Blusztajn JK, Holmes GL, Protective effects of prenatal choline supplementation on seizure-induced memory impairment. J Neurosci 2000;20: RC109.

Yossifoff M, Kisliouk T, Meiri N, Dynamic changes in DNA methylation during thermal control establishment affect CREB binding to the brain-derived neurotrophic factor promoter. Eur J Neurosci 2008;28: 2267–77.

Zeisel SH, Char D, Sheard NF, Choline, phosphatidylcholine and sphingomyelin in human and bovine milk and infant formulas. J Nutr 1986;116: 50–8.

Zeisel SH, Da Costa K-A, Franklin PD, Alexander EA, Lamont JT, Sheard NF, Beiser A, Choline, an essential nutrient for humans. FASEB J 1991;5: 2093–8.

Zhu XN, Mar MH, Song JN, Zeisel SH, Deletion of the *Pemt* gene increases progenitor cell mitosis, DNA and protein methylation and decreases calretinin expression in embryonic day 17 mouse hippocampus. Dev Brain Res 2004;149: 121–9.

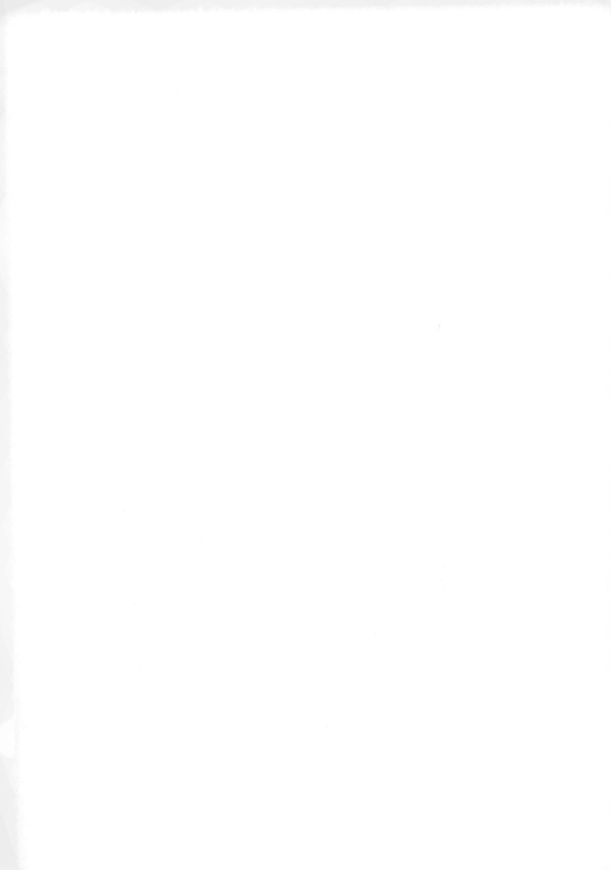

15 Omega-3 polyunsaturated fatty acids (fish oil)

15.1 Omega-3 polyunsaturated fatty acids in human nutrition

Philip C. Calder

15.1.1 Structure, naming and metabolic relations of ω-3 fatty acids

Omega-3 (ω-3 or *n*-3) is a structural descriptor for a family of polyunsaturated fatty acids (PUFAs). The term ω-3 denotes the position of double bond that is closest to the methyl terminus of the acyl chain: in all ω-3 fatty acids this double bond is on carbon 3, counting the methyl carbon as carbon 1 (►Fig. 15.1). As with all fatty acids, ω-3 fatty acids have systematic and common names (►Tab. 15.1); they are also referred to by a shorthand nomenclature that denotes the number of carbon atoms in the chain, the number of double bonds, and the position of the first double bond relative to the methyl carbon (►Tab. 15.1). The simplest ω-3 fatty acid is α-linolenic acid (18:3ω-3). α-Linolenic acid is synthesised from linoleic acid (18:2ω-6) by desaturation, catalysed by delta-15 desaturase (confusingly the desaturase enzymes are named according the first carbon carrying the newly inserted double bond and counting the carboxyl carbon as carbon number one). Animals, including humans, do not possess the delta-15 desaturase enzyme and so cannot synthesise α-linolenic acid. Thus α-linolenic acid is a classically essential fatty acid, along with linoleic acid. Plants possess delta-15 desaturase and so are able to synthesise α-linolenic acid. Although animals cannot synthesise α-linolenic acid, they can metabolise it by further desaturation and elongation; desaturation occurs at carbon atoms below carbon number 9 (counting from the carboxyl carbon) and mainly occurs in the liver. α-Linolenic acid can be converted to stearidonic acid (18:4ω-3) by delta-6 desaturase and then stearidonic acid can be elongated to eicosatetraenoic acid (20:4ω-3) (►Fig. 15.2). This fatty acid can be further desaturated by delta-5 desaturase to yield eicosapentaenoic acid [20:5ω-3; known as eicosapentaenoic acid (EPA)] (►Fig. 15.2). Conversion of α-linolenic acid to EPA is in competition with the conversion of linoleic acid to arachidonic acid (20:4ω-6) because the same enzymes are used. Delta-6 desaturase reaction is rate limiting in this pathway. Although the preferred substrate for delta-6 desaturase is α-linolenic acid, because linoleic acid is much more prevalent in most human diets than α-linolenic acid, metabolism of ω-6 fatty acids is quantitatively the more important. The activities of delta-6 and delta-5 desaturases are regulated by nutritional status, hormones and by feedback inhibition by end products.

A pathway for further conversion of EPA to docosahexaenoic acid [22:6ω-3; known as docosahexaenoic acid (DHA)] exists (►Fig. 15.2): this pathway involves addition of two carbons to form docosapentaenoic acid [22:5ω-3; known as docosapentaenoic acid (DPA)], addition of two further carbons to produce 24:5ω-3, desaturation at the delta-6 position to form 24:6ω-3, translocation of 24:6ω-3 from the endoplasmic reticulum to peroxisomes where two carbons are removed by limited β-oxidation to

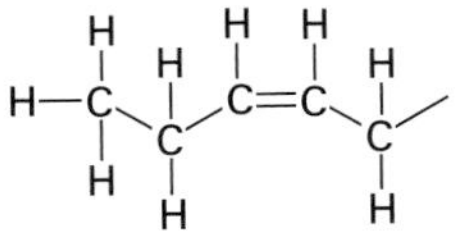

Fig. 15.1: Generic structure of ω-3 fatty acids.

Tab. 15.1: The ω-3 polyunsaturated fatty acid family.

Systematic name	Common name	Shorthand nomenclature
All-*cis*-9,12,15-Octadecatrienoic acid	α-Linolenic acid	18:3ω-3
All-*cis*-6,9,12,15-Octadecatetraenoic acid	Stearidonic acid	18:4ω-3
All-*cis*-8,11,14,17-Eicosatetraenoic acid	Eicosatetraenoic acid	20:4ω-3
All-*cis*-5,8,11,14,17-Eicosapentaenoic acid	Eicosapentaenoic acid	20:5ω-3
All-*cis*-7,10,13,16,19-Docosapentaenoic acid	Docosapentaenoic acid; also Clupanodonic acid	22:5ω-3
All-*cis*-4,7,10,13,16,19-Docosahexaenoic acid	Docosahexaenoic acid	22:6ω-3

yield DHA (▶Fig. 15.3). It is unclear whether the same enzyme is responsible for the initial, rate-limiting desaturation at the delta-6 position of α-linolenic acid and for the synthesis of 24:6ω-3, although enzyme preparations with both activities have been reported. It seems probable that the complex series of fatty acid translocation and β-oxidation steps could act as loci of metabolic control facilitating regulation of DHA synthesis independent from the up-stream activity of the pathway. Short-term studies with isotopically-labelled α-linolenic acid and long-term studies using significantly increased intakes of α-linolenic acid have demonstrated that the conversion to EPA, DPA and DHA is generally poor in humans, with very limited conversion all the way to DHA being observed (Arterburn et al., 2006; Burdge and Calder, 2006).

EPA and DPA can also be synthesised from DHA by retro-conversion owing to limited peroxisomal β-oxidation. EPA, DPA and DHA are referred to as very long chain ω-3 PUFAs.

15.1.2 Dietary sources and typical intakes of ω-3 fatty acids

15.1.2.1 α-Linolenic acid from plant sources

Green leaves contain a significant proportion (typically over 50%) of their fatty acids as α-linolenic acid; however, because green leaves are not rich sources of fat, these are not major dietary sources of fatty acids including α-linolenic acid. Several seeds and seed oils and some nuts contain significant amounts of α-linolenic acid. Linseeds (flaxseeds) and their oil typically contain 45–55% of fatty acids as α-linolenic acid, whereas soybean oil typically contains 5–10% of fatty acids as α-linolenic acid. Rapeseed oil and walnuts also contain α-linolenic acid. Corn oil, sunflower oil and safflower oil are rich

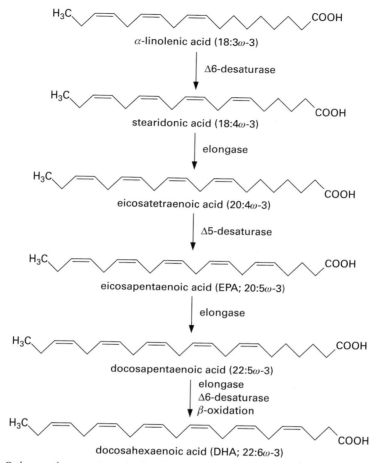

Fig. 15.2: Pathway of conversion of α-linolenic acid to longer chain, more unsaturated ω-3 fatty acids.

in linoleic acid but contain very little α-linolenic acid. Typical intakes of α-linolenic acid among western adults are 0.5–2 g/day (British Nutrition Foundation, 1999; Burdge and Calder, 2006). The main PUFA in most western diets is the ω-6 fatty acid linoleic acid which is typically consumed in 5–20-fold greater amounts than α-linolenic acid (British Nutrition Foundation, 1999; Burdge and Calder, 2006).

15.1.2.2 EPA, DPA and DHA from seafood

Seafoods are a source of the longer chain, more unsaturated ω-3 PUFAs. Fish can be classified into lean fish that store lipid in the liver (e.g., cod) or 'fatty' (oily) fish that store lipid in the flesh (e.g., mackerel, herring, salmon, tuna, sardines). Compared with other foodstuffs, fish and other seafood are good sources of the very long chain ω-3 fatty acids EPA, DPA and DHA (British Nutrition Foundation, 1999). However, different types of fish contain different amounts of these fatty acids and different ratios of

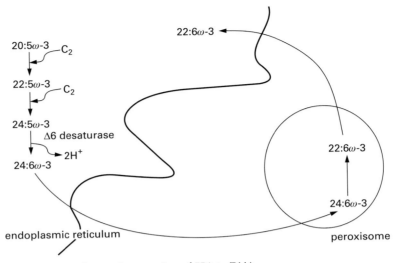

Fig. 15.3: Detail of the pathway of conversion of EPA to DHA.

EPA to DHA (►Tab. 15.2). This is partly dependent upon the metabolic characteristics of the fish and also upon their diet, water temperature, season, etc. Nevertheless, it is clear that a single lean fish meal (e.g., one serving of cod) could provide approximately 0.2–0.3 g very long chain ω-3 fatty acids, whereas a single oily fish meal (e.g., one serving of salmon or mackerel) could provide 1.5–3.0 g of these fatty acids (►Tab. 15.2).

Tab. 15.2: Typical very long chain ω-3 fatty acid contents of seafood.

Seafood	20:5ω-3	22:5ω-3	22:6ω-3	Total long chain ω-3 PUFA per portion
	g/100 g food			g
Cod	0.08	0.01	0.16	0.30
Haddock	0.05	0.01	0.10	0.19
Plaice	0.16	0.04	0.10	0.39
Herring	0.51	0.11	0.69	1.56
Mackerel	0.71	0.12	1.10	3.09
Kippers	1.15	0.10	1.34	3.37
Salmon	0.50	0.40	1.30	2.20
Trout	0.23	0.09	0.83	2.65
Canned crab	0.47	0.08	0.45	0.85
Prawns	0.06	trace	0.04	0.06
Mussels	0.41	0.02	0.16	0.24

The latest estimate for fish consumption among adults in the UK is approximately 100 g lean fish and approximately 50 g oily fish per week (SACN/COT, 2004); similar (and in some countries even lower) intakes are expected in other northern and in eastern European, North American and Australasian countries. Lean fish intake is higher than this in southern European countries and lean and oily fish intake is higher than this in Japan. Average (mean) intakes of very long chain ω-3 fatty acids among adults in the UK, in other northern and in eastern European, North American and Australasian countries are approximately 0.15–0.25 g/day (SACN/COT, 2004). However, the distribution of intakes is bimodal owing to the presence of oily fish consumers and non-consumers and a fairly recent estimate of very long chain ω-3 fatty acid intake among Australian adults gave a median intake of approximately 0.03 g/day, compared with a mean intake of approximately 0.19 mg/day (Meyer et al., 2003). Intakes would be rather higher in those populations, such as the Japanese, who consume oily fish in greater amounts and with greater regularity than seen in Europe, North America and Australasia.

15.1.2.3 Fish oils

The oil obtained from oily fish flesh or lean fish livers (e.g., cod liver) is termed 'fish oil' and it has the distinctive characteristic of being rich in very long chain ω-3 fatty acids. EPA and DHA comprise approximately 30% of the fatty acids in a typical preparation of fish oil, which means that a 1 g fish oil capsule can provide approximately 0.3 g of EPA plus DHA. However, the amount of ω-3 fatty acids that can vary between fish and fish oils, and so can the relative proportions of the individual very long chain ω-3 PUFAs (EPA, DPA and DHA); for example, cod liver oil is richer in EPA than DHA whereas tuna oil is richer in DHA than EPA. Fish liver oils contain significant amounts of fat soluble vitamins, especially vitamins A and D. Encapsulated oil preparations that contain ω-3 fatty acids in higher amounts than found in standard fish oils are available. In fish oil capsules the fatty acids are usually present in the form of triacylglycerols, although ω-3 fatty acids are also available in the phospholipid form (e.g., as krill oil) and as ethyl esters (e.g., in the highly concentrated pharmaceutical preparation Omacor also known as Lovazza in North America). Clearly capsules could make a significant contribution to very long chain ω-3 fatty acid intake. For example, an individual who consumes little or no fish could increase their daily very long chain ω-3 fatty acid intake 5-fold (or more) by taking a single standard fish oil capsule per day.

15.1.2.4 Algal oils

Certain algal oils that are particularly rich in DHA which could comprise as much as 45% of total fatty acids. These oils might be useful where provision of DHA, but not EPA, is particularly desired, for example, in infant formulas.

15.1.2.5 Functional foods as sources of very long chain ω-3 PUFAs

Over the past few years there have been significant moves towards the enrichment of foods with EPA and DHA. Two routes to such enrichment have developed. The first is the addition of fish oil to products such as spreads, yoghurts or milk. The second is feeding of farm animals with ω-3 fatty acids. This results in enrichment of the meat, milk (in the case of cows, sheep or goats) and eggs (in the case of chickens) with EPA and DHA. One attraction of enrichment of foods such as meat, spreads, eggs, yoghurts, dairy products, etc., is that consumers do not have to change their dietary habits to increase their EPA and DHA intake (Givens, 2005). By contrast, the level of enrichment that can be achieved is limited either by metabolic processes in the animals (in the case of the animal feeding approach) or food technology, processing and storage considerations. Thus, the level of enrichment currently achieved can provide at best a few hundred milligrams of EPA and DHA per day obtained from a combination of several enriched foods. Thus, a non-fish eating person could increase their EPA and DHA intake by consuming such enriched foods. However, it is important to consider the amounts of less healthy components such as total fat, saturated fat, and sugar that need to be eaten from an ω-3 PUFA enriched product for that product to deliver a particular amount of EPA plus DHA, which might be only a few tens of milligrams per serving.

15.1.3 Increased intake of very long chain ω-3 fatty acids alters the fatty acid composition of plasma, cells and tissues in humans

Different plasma lipid pools, cells and tissues have different, characteristic, fatty acid compositions. These compositions are influenced by the availability of different fatty acids but also by the metabolic characteristics of the particular pool, cell or tissue. Modification of fatty acid profiles has been widely reported after supplementation of the diet with fish oil capsules; studies report that such supplementation results in appearance of EPA and DHA in plasma lipids, platelets, erythrocytes, leukocytes, colonic tissue, cardiac tissue and most probably in many other cell and tissue types. The incorporation of EPA and DHA from fish oil capsules is partly of the expense of ω-6 PUFAs, such as arachidonic acid, and occurs in a dose-response fashion. For example, studies using a range of EPA+DHA intakes from 1 to 6 g/day report near linear relations between EPA and DHA intake and the EPA and DHA contents of plasma phospholipids (Blonk et al., 1990; Harris et al., 1991; Marsen et al., 1992) and of platelet phospholipids (Sanders and Roshanai, 1983). In other studies incorporation of EPA and DHA into blood neutrophils (Healy et al., 2000) and of EPA into plasma phospholipids and blood mononuclear cells (Rees et al., 2006) occurred in a linear dose-response manner (▶Fig. 15.4). In an elegant study combining dose response and time course over 12 months in older male subjects, Katan et al. (1997) reported the fatty acid compositions of serum cholesteryl esters, erythrocytes and adipose tissue. This study confirmed that EPA and DHA are incorporated into circulating lipid pools and into erythrocytes when their intakes are increased. It also demonstrated EPA and DHA incorporation into adipose tissue, a storage pool, when their intakes are increased. However, this study also clearly showed that incorporation into different pools occurs at different rates and to differing extents (i.e., with different efficiencies) and might not be related to intake in a strictly linear fashion, at least over the intakes studied. The study of Katan et al. (1997) showed that near-maximal incorporation of EPA and DHA into serum cholesteryl esters occurs within 30 days of beginning supplementation, whereas maximal incorporation into erythrocytes does not occur until sometime between 56 and 182 days. Yaqoob et al. (2000) reported the time-dependent incorporation of EPA and DHA into blood mononuclear cells; incorporation of both fatty acids was near-maximal after 4 weeks

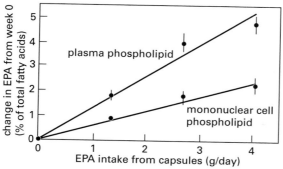

Fig. 15.4: Dose-dependent incorporation of eicosapentaenoic acid into human plasma phospholipids and blood mononuclear cells. Healthy young males supplemented their diet with differing amounts of an EPA-rich oil for a period of 12 weeks. Plasma and blood mononuclear cell phospholipids were isolated and their fatty acid composition determined by gas chromatography. Data are mean ± SEM from 23 or 24 subjects per group and are expressed as a change in EPA from week 0 (study entry). Data are from Rees et al. (2006).

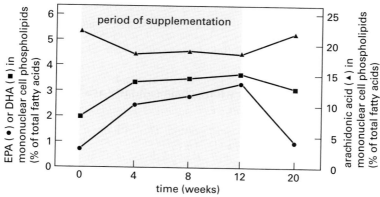

Fig. 15.5: Time course of changes in eicosapentaenoic, docosahexaenoic and arachidonic acid contents of human blood mononuclear cells in subjects consuming fish oil. Healthy subjects supplemented their diet with fish oil capsules providing 2.1 g EPA plus 1.1 g DHA per day for a period of 12 weeks (indicated by the grey area). Blood mononuclear cell phospholipids were isolated at 0, 4, 8, 12 and 20 weeks and their fatty acid composition determined by gas chromatography. Data are the mean from eight subjects and are from Yaqoob et al. (2000) (error bars are omitted for clarity).

of supplementation (▶Fig. 15.5). Upon cessation of supplementation EPA in mononuclear cells returned to starting levels within 8 weeks, whereas the cells appeared to retain DHA. The same observations of loss of EPA and selective retention of DHA upon cessation of fish oil supplementation have been made for erthrocytes (Popp-Snijders et al., 1986) and platelets (von Schacky et al., 1985). Thus, a significant body of literature reports that EPA and DHA are incorporated into blood, cell and tissue lipids when their intake is increased.

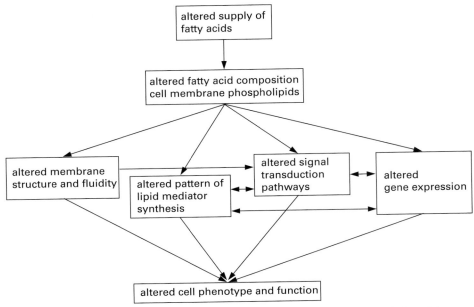

Fig. 15.6: General scheme of the interacting mechanisms whereby very long chain ω-3 fatty acids might influence cell function.

15.1.4 Mechanisms by which very long chain ω-3 fatty acids can influence cell function

Increased cell and tissue ω-3 fatty acid content can influence cell function through a variety of mechanisms as shown in ▶Fig. 15.6.

15.1.4.1 Alterations in membrane structure and function

Increased very long chain ω-3 PUFA content of membrane phospholipids can lead to modifications of the physical properties of the membrane such as membrane order (fluidity) and raft structure (rafts are membrane microdomains with a particular lipid and fatty acid make-up and which play a role as platforms for receptor action and for the initiation of intracellular signalling pathways) which, in turn, influence the activity of membrane proteins including receptors, transporters, ion channels, and signalling enzymes (Yaqoob, 2009).

15.1.4.2 Effects on cell signalling pathways

Very long chain ω-3 PUFAs can affect cell signalling pathways, either through modifying the expression, activity or avidity of membrane receptors or modifying intracellular signal transduction mechanisms (Miles and Calder, 1998). As a result of these effects, transcription factor activation is altered and gene expression modified. Transcription factors reported to be modified by the presence of very long chain ω-3 PUFAs include nuclear factor κ B, peroxisome proliferator activated receptor-α and -γ, and the sterol regulatory element binding proteins (Jump, 2002, 2008; Clarke, 2004; Lapillonne et al., 2004; Deckelbaum et al., 2006). Thus, very long chain ω-3 PUFAs can alter patterns of gene expression.

15.1.4.3 Effects on lipid mediators

Eicosanoids produced from the ω-6 PUFA arachidonic acid, including various prostaglandins, thromboxanes and leukotrienes, have well-established roles in the regulation of inflammation, immunity, platelet aggregation, smooth muscle contraction and renal function (Nicolaou and Kafatos, 2004). Excess or inappropriate production of these eicosanoids is associated with disease processes. For example, cysteinyl-leukotrienes play an important role in asthma. A range of drugs of varying specificity are used clinically to suppress the production of eicosanoids from arachidonic acid. Very long chain ω-3 PUFAs decrease the production of arachidonic acid derived eicosanoids and so can impact on the actions regulated by those mediators (Calder, 2008a). Furthermore, EPA is a substrate for the synthesis of alternative eicosanoids which are typically less potent than those produced from arachidonic acid (Calder, 2008a). Relatively recently a new family of lipid mediators, termed resolvins, synthesised from both EPA (E-series resolvins) and DHA (D-series resolvins) have been described. These mediators have been demonstrated in cell culture and animal feeding studies to be potently anti-inflammatory, inflammation resolving and immunomodulatory (Serhan et al., 2000a,b). Protectin D1, produced from DHA, appears to have an important role in protecting tissue, including neuronal tissue, from excessive damage in a variety of experimental situations (Serhan et al., 2002).

15.1.5 An increased intake of very long chain ω-3 fatty acids is beneficial to health

Through the mechanisms of action outlined above and the resulting modifications of cell and tissue function, very long chain ω-3 fatty acids exert physiological actions. These are summarised in ►Tab. 15.3 where they are linked to certain health or clinical benefits. Several risk factors for cardiovascular disease are modified in a beneficial way by increased intake of very long chain ω-3 fatty acids: these include blood pressure (Geleijnse et al., 2002), platelet reactivity and thrombosis (British Nutrition Foundation, 1992), plasma triglyceride concentrations (Harris, 1996), vascular function (Nestel et al., 2002), cardiac arrhythmias (von Schacky, 2008), heart rate variability (von Schacky, 2008), and inflammation (Calder, 2006). As a result increased very long chain ω-3 fatty acid intake is associated with a reduced risk of cardiovascular morbidity and mortality (Calder, 2004). Indeed supplementation studies with very long chain ω-3 fatty acids have demonstrated reduced mortality (Anonymous, 1999; Bucher et al., 2002; Marchioli et al., 2002; Studer et al., 2005; Yokoyama et al., 2007). Several other, non-cardiovascular, actions of these fatty acids have also been documented (►Tab. 15.3), suggesting that increased intake of these fatty acids could be of benefit in protecting from or treating many conditions. For example, they have been used successfully in rheumatoid arthritis (Calder, 2008b) and, in some studies, in inflammatory bowel diseases

Tab. 15.3: Summary of the physiological roles and potential clinical benefits of very long chain ω-3 fatty acids.

Physiological role of very long chain ω-3 fatty acids	Potential clinical benefit	Target
Regulation of blood pressure	Decreased blood pressure	Hypertension; CVD
Regulation of platelet function	Decreased likelihood of thrombosis	Thrombosis; CVD
Regulation of blood coagulation	Decreased likelihood of thrombosis	Thrombosis; CVD
Regulation of plasma triglyceride concentrations	Decreased plasma triglyceride concentrations	Hypertriglyceridaemia; CVD
Regulation of vascular function	Improved vascular reactivity	CVD
Regulation of cardiac rhythm	Decreased arrhythmias	CVD
Regulation of heart rate	Increased heart rate variability	CVD
Regulation of inflammation	Decreased inflammation	Inflammatory diseases (arthritis, inflammatory bowel diseases, psoriasis, lupus, asthma, cystic fibrosis, dermatitis, neurodegeneration …); CVD
Regulation of immune function	Improved immune function	Compromised immunity
Regulation of fatty acid and triglyceride metabolism	Decreased triglyceride synthesis and storage	Weight gain; weight loss; obesity
Regulation of bone turnover	Maintained bone mass	Osteoporosis
Regulation of insulin sensitivity	Improved insulin sensitivity	Type-2 diabetes
Regulation of tumour cell growth	Decreased tumour cell growth and survival	Some cancers
Regulation of visual signalling (via rhodopsin)	Optimised visual signalling	Poor infant visual development (especially pre-term)
Structural component of brain and central nervous system	Optimised brain development: cognitive and learning processes	Poor infant and childhood cognitive processes and learning

CVD, cardiovascular disease.

(Calder, 2008c), and might be useful in other inflammatory conditions (Calder, 2006). DHA has an important structural role in the eye and brain, and its supply early in life when these tissues are developing is known to be of vital importance in terms of optimizing visual and neurological development (SanGiovanni et al., 2000a,b). Recent studies have highlighted the potential for very long chain ω-3 fatty acids to contribute to enhanced mental development (Helland et al., 2003) and improved childhood learning and behaviour (Richardson, 2004) and to reduce the burden of psychiatric illnesses in adults (Freeman et al., 2006), although these remain controversial areas of possible action which require more robust scientific support. There could also be a role for very long chain ω-3 PUFAs, DHA in particular, in preventing neurodegenerative disease of ageing (Solfrizzi et al., 2010) and the production of protectins, especially protectin D1 (formerly called neuroprotectin D1), appears to be crucial for this effect (Lukiw et al., 2005). The effects of very long chain ω-3 PUFAs on health outcomes are likely to be dose-dependent, but clear dose-response data have not been identified in most cases.

15.1.6 Dietary recommendations for very long chain ω-3 fatty acids

The recognition of the benefits of very long chain ω-3 fatty acids has resulted in a series of recommendations to increase the intake of fish and more specifically of very long chain ω-3 fatty acids by various government, non-government and professional bodies. Typical recommendations to maintain general good health are an intake of at least two fish meals per week including at least one of oily fish (SACN/COT, 2004). Such recommendations are based mainly upon the epidemiological evidence for decreased cardiovascular morbidity and mortality with increased consumption of fish and upon supplementation studies using fish oils investigating impact on cardiovascular risk factors (British Nutrition Foundation, 1999; Calder, 2004; SACN/COT, 2004). In terms of the very long chain ω-3 fatty acids, recommendations that have been made include a minimal intake of 0.2–0.65 g/day for general good health (de Deckere et al., 1998; Simopolous et al., 1999; SACN/COT, 2004), 1.5 g/day for general good health (British Nutrition Foundation, 1999), 1 g/day for secondary prevention of myocardial infarction (Kris-Etheryon et al., 2002; JBS2, 2005; Van der Werf et al., 2008), and 2–4 g/day for blood triglyceride lowering (Kris-Etherton et al., 2002). In those individuals not regularly consuming oily fish, the intake of these fatty acids is likely to be <0.2 g/day and perhaps even much lower than this (Meyer et al., 2003). Strategies to increase intake of very long chain ω-3 PUFAs include eating oily fish, consuming fish oil capsules or liquid, and eating foods specifically enriched in these fatty acids.

15.1.7 Health effects of α-linolenic acid

The foregoing discussion has centred upon the very long chain ω-3 PUFAs for which there is much evidence for human health benefit and an increasing understanding of the multiple mechanisms involved, and for which several recommendations for increased intake have been made. The major plant ω-3 PUFA, α-linolenic acid, is an essential fatty acid and might have human health benefits either in its own right or by acting as a precursor for synthesis of the longer chain more unsaturated derivatives using the pathway shown in ▶Fig. 15.2. These possibilities have been reviewed in some detail fairly recently (Arterburn et al., 2006; Burdge and Calder, 2006). Studies in humans using acute ingestion of stable isotopically-labelled α-linolenic acid have demonstrated some conversion to EPA and to DPA, but much more limited conversion to DHA, although this might be greater in young adult women than in men (Burdge and Wootton, 2002; Burdge et al., 2002), possibly because of up-regulation of the delta-6 desaturase by female sex hormones. Little is known about the extent of α-linolenic acid conversion to EPA and DHA in infancy and childhood, in the elderly or during pregnancy and lactation, times when synthesis of very long chain ω-3 PUFAs might be important or desirable. Several studies have examined the effect of chronic (i.e., weeks to months) consumption of increased amounts of α-linolenic acid. These studies confirm that increasing α-linolenic acid intake increases the EPA (and DPA) content of plasma lipids, platelets, leukocytes and erythrocytes but that DHA content does not increase (Arterburn et al., 2006; Burdge and Calder, 2006); clearly these findings are in agreement with the stable isotope studies. Such studies with α-linolenic acid have demonstrated some effects on cardiovascular risk factors and on inflammatory markers, but where these are reported they are typically weaker than the effects achieved from increasing consumption of EPA+DHA, and might be owing to the increased appearance of EPA (Caughey et al., 1996; Zhao et al., 2004).

15.1.8 Conclusions

Current intakes of very long chain ω-3 fatty acids EPA and DHA are low in most individuals living in western countries. A good natural source of these fatty acids is seafood, especially oily fish. Fish oil capsules contain these fatty acids too, with a standard 1 g capsule providing approximately 0.3 g of EPA plus DHA; more concentrated forms are also available in capsules. Very long chain ω-3 fatty acids are readily incorporated from capsules into transport (blood lipids), functional (cell and tissue) and storage (adipose) pools in humans. This incorporation is dose-dependent and follows a kinetic pattern that is characteristic for each pool. Incorporation is most rapid into blood lipids, followed by platelets and white cells, followed by erythrocytes. At sufficient levels of incorporation into cells, EPA and DHA influence the physical nature of cell membranes and membrane protein-mediated responses, lipid mediator generation, cell signalling and gene expression in many different cell types. Through these mechanisms EPA and DHA influence cell and tissue physiology and the way cells and tissues respond to external signals. In most cases the effects seen are compatible with improvements in disease biomarker profiles or in health-related outcomes. An important aspect of this is the requirement for very long chain ω-3 fatty acids, especially DHA, in early growth and development of the brain and visual system, meaning that adequate provision to the foetus and to the newborn infant is essential. As a result of their effects on cell and tissue physiology, very long chain ω-3 fatty acids play a role in achieving optimal health and in protection against disease. Long chain ω-3 fatty acids not only protect against cardiovascular morbidity but also against mortality. In some situations, e.g., rheumatoid arthritis, they could be beneficial as therapeutic agents although a high intake is required. On the basis of the recognised health improvements brought about by long chain ω-3 fatty acids, recommendations have been made to increase their intake. This can be achieved through increased consumption of oily fish or fish oil capsules. The plant ω-3 fatty acid, α-linolenic acid, can be converted to EPA but in humans conversion to DHA appears to be poor. Effects of α-linolenic acid on human health-related outcomes appear to be owing to conversion to the EPA.

References

Anonymous, Dietary supplementation with n-3 polyunsaturated fatty acids and vitamin E after myocardial infarction: results of the GISSI-Prevenzione trial. Lancet 1999;354: 447–55.

Arterburn LM, Hall EB, Oken H, Distribution, interconversion, and dose response of n-3 fatty acids in humans. Am J Clin Nutr 2006;83: 1467S–76S.

Blonk MC, Bilo HJ, Popp-Snijders C, Mulder C, Donker AJ, Dose-response effects of fish oil supplementation in healthy volunteers. Am J Clin Nutr 1990;52: 120–7.

British Nutrition Foundation, Unsaturated fatty acids: nutritional and physiological significance. London: Chapman & Hall; 1992.

British Nutrition Foundation, Briefing paper: n-3 fatty acids and health. London: British Nutrition Foundation; 1999.

Bucher HC, Hengstler P, Schindler C, Meier G, N-3 polyunsaturated fatty acids in coronary heart disease: a meta-analysis of randomized controlled trials. Am J Med 2002;112: 298–304.

Burdge GC, Calder PC, Dietary α-linolenic acid and health-related outcomes: a metabolic perspective. Nutr Res Rev 2006;19: 26–52.

Burdge GC, Wootton SA, Conversion of α-linolenic acid to eicosapentaenoic, docosapentaenoic and docosahexaenoic acids in young women. Br J Nutr 2002;88: 411–20.

Burdge GC, Jones AE, Wootton SA, Eicosapentaenoic and docosapentaenoic acids are the principal products of α-linolenic acid metabolism in young men. Br J Nutr 2002;88: 355–63.

Calder PC, N-3 fatty acids and cardiovascular disease: evidence explained and mechanisms explored. Clin Sci 2004;107: 1–11.

Calder PC, N-3 polyunsaturated fatty acids, inflammation, and inflammatory diseases. Am J Clin Nutr 2006;83: 1505S–19S.

Calder PC, The relationship between the fatty acid composition of immune cells and their function. Prost Leuk Essent Fatty Acids 2008a;79: 101–8.

Calder PC, PUFA, inflammatory processes and rheumatoid arthritis. Proc Nutr Soc 2008b;67: 409–18.

Calder PC, Polyunsaturated fatty acids, inflammatory processes and inflammatory bowel diseases. Mol Nutr Food Res 2008c;52: 885–97.

Caughey GE, Mantzioris E, Gibson RA, Cleland LG, James J, The effect on human tumor necrosis factor α and interleukin 1β production of diets enriched in n-3 fatty acids from vegetable oil or fish oil. Am J Clin Nutr 1996;63: 116–22.

Clarke SD, The multi-dimensional regulation of gene expression by fatty acids: polyunsaturated fats as nutrient sensors. Curr Opin Lipidol 2004;15:13–8.

Deckelbaum RJ, Worgall TS, Seo T, N-3 fatty acids and gene expression. Am J Clin Nutr 2006;83: 1520S–5S.

de Deckere EA, Korver O, Verschuren PM, Katan MB, Health aspects of fish and n-3 polyunsaturated fatty acids from plant and marine origin. Eur J Clin Nutr 1998;52: 749–53.

Freeman MP, Hibbeln JR, Wisner KL, Davis JM, Mischoulon D, Peet M, Keck Jr PE, Marangell LB, Richardson AJ, Lake J, Stoll AL, Omega-3 fatty acids: evidence basis for treatment and future research in psychiatry. J Clin Psychiatry 2006;67: 1954–67.

Geleijnse JM, Giltay EJ, Grobbee DE, Donders ART, Kok FJ, Blood pressure response to fish oil supplementation: meta-regression analysis of randomized trials. J Hypertens 2002;20: 1493–9.

Givens DI, The role of animal nutrition in improving the nutritive value of animal-derived foods in relation to chronic disease. Proc Nutr Soc 2005;64: 395–402.

Harris WS, N-3 fatty acids and lipoproteins: comparison of results from human and animal studies. Lipids 1996;31: 243–52.

Harris WS, Windsor SL, Dujovne CA, Effects of four doses of n-3 fatty acids given to hyperlipidemic patients for six months. J Am Coll Nutr 1991;10: 220–7.

Healy DA, Wallace FA, Miles EA, Calder PC, Newsholme P, The effect of low to moderate amounts of dietary fish oil on neutrophil lipid composition and function. Lipids 2000;35: 763–8.

Helland IB, Smith L, Saarem K, Saugstad OD, Drevon CA, Maternal supplementation with very-long-chain n-3 fatty acids during pregnancy and lactation augments children's IQ at 4 years of age. Pediatrics 2003;111: e39–44.

JBS2, Joint British Societies' Guidelines on prevention of cardiovascular disease in clinical practice. British Cardiac Society. British Hypertension Society. Diabetes UK. HEART UK. Primary Care Cardiovascular Society. Stroke Association. Heart 2005;91(Supp. 5): v1–v52.

Jump DB, Dietary polyunsaturated fatty acids and regulation of gene transcription. Curr Opin Lipidol 2002;13: 155–64.

Jump DB, N-3 polyunsaturated fatty acid regulation of hepatic gene transcription. Curr Opin Lipidol 2008;19: 242–7.

Katan MB, Deslypere JP, van Birgelen APJM, Penders M, Zegwaars M, Kinetics of the incorporation of dietary fatty acids into serum cholesteryl esters, erythrocyte membranes and adipose tissue: an 18 month controlled study. J Lipid Res 1997;38: 2012–22.

Kris-Etherton PM, Harris WS, Appel LJ, American Heart Association Nutrition Committee, Fish consumption, fish oil, omega-3 fatty acids, and cardiovascular disease. Circulation 2002;106: 2747–57.

Lapillonne A, Clarke SD, Heird WC, Polyunsaturated fatty acids and gene expression. Curr Opin Clin Nutr Metab Care 2004;7: 151–6.

Lukiw WJ, Cui JG, Marcheselli VL, Bodker M, Botkjaer A, Gotlinger K, Serhan CN, Bazan NG, A role for docosahexaenoic acid-derived neuroprotectin D1 in neural cell survival and Alzheimer disease. J Clin Invest 2005;115: 2774–83.

Marchioli R, Barzi F, Bomba E, Chieffo C, Di Gregorio D, Di Mascio R, Franzosi MG, Geraci E, Levantesi G, Maggioni AP, Mantini L, Marfisi RM, Mastrogiuseppe G, Mininni N, Nicolosi GI, Santini M, Schweiger C, Tavazzi L, Tognoni G, Tucci C, Valagussa F, Early protection against sudden death by n-3 polyunsaturated fatty acids after myocardial infarction – time-course analysis of the results of the Gruppo Italiano per lo Studio della Sopravvivenza nell'Infarto Miocardico (GISSI)-Prevenzione. Circulation 2002;105: 1897–903.

Marsen TA, Pollok M, Oette K, Baldamus CA, Pharmacokinetics of omega-3 fatty acids during ingestion of fish oil preparations. Prost Leuk Essent Fatty Acids 1992;46: 191–6.

Meyer BJ, Mann NJ, Lewis JL, Milligan GC, Sinclair AJ, Howe PR, Dietary intakes and food sources of omega-6 and omega-3 polyunsaturated fatty acids. Lipids 2003;38: 391–8.

Miles EA, Calder PC, Modulation of immune function by dietary fatty acids. Proc Nutr Soc 1998;57: 277–92.

Nestel P, Shige H, Pomeroy S, Cehun M, Abbey M, Raederstorff D, The n-3 fatty acids eicosapentaenoic acid and docosahexaenoic acid increase systemic arterial compliance in humans. Am J Clin Nutr 2002;76: 326–30.

Nicolaou A, Kafatos G, Bioactive lipids. Bridgewater: The Oily Press; 2004.

Popp-Snijders C, Schouten JA, van Blitterswijk WJ, van der Veen EA, Changes in membrane lipid composition of human erythrocytes after dietary supplementation of (n-3) fatty acids: maintenance of membrane fluidity. Biochim Biophys Acta 1986;854: 31–7.

Rees D, Miles EA, Banerjee T, Wells SJ, Roynette CE, Wahle KWJW, Calder PC, Dose-related effects of eicosapentaenoic acid on innate immune function in healthy humans: a comparison of young and older men. Am J Clin Nutr 2006;83: 331–42.

Richardson AJ, Clinical trials of fatty acid treatment in ADHD, dyslexia, dyspraxia and the autistic spectrum. Prost Leuk Essent Fatty Acids 2004;70: 383–90.

SACN/COT, Scientific Advisory Committee on Nutrition/Committee on Toxicity. Advice on fish consumption: benefits and risks. London: TSO; 2004.

Sanders TAB, Roshanai F, The influence of different types of ω3 polyunsaturated fatty acids on blood lipids and platelet function in healthy volunteers. Clin Sci 1983;64: 91–9.

SanGiovanni JP, Berkey CS, Dwyer JT, Colditz GA, Dietary essential fatty acids, long-chain polyunsaturated fatty acids, and visual resolution acuity in healthy fullterm infants: a systematic review. Early Hum Dev 2000a;57: 165–88.

SanGiovanni JP, Parra-Cabrera S, Colditz GA, Berkey CS, Dwyer JT, Meta-analysis of dietary essential fatty acids and long-chain polyunsaturated fatty acids as they relate to visual resolution acuity in healthy preterm infants. Pediatrics 2000b;105: 1292–8.

Serhan CN, Clish CB, Brannon J, Colgan SP, Chiang N, Gronert K, Novel functional sets of lipid-derived mediators with antinflammatory actions generated from omega-3 fatty acids via cyclooxygenase 2-nonsteroidal antiinflammatory drugs and transcellular processing. J Exp Med 2000a;192: 1197–204.

Serhan CN, Clish CB, Brannon J, Colgan SP, Gronert K, Chiang N, Anti-inflammatory lipid signals generated from dietary n-3 fatty acids via cyclooxygenase-2 and transcellular processing: a novel mechanism for NSAID and n-3 PUFA therapeutic actions. J Physiol Pharmacol 2000b;4: 643–54.

Serhan CN, Hong S, Gronert K, Colgan SP, Devchand PR, Mirick G, Moussignac R-L, Resolvins: a family of bioactive products of omega-3 fatty acid transformation circuits initiated by aspirin treatment that counter pro-inflammation signals. J Exp Med 2002;196: 1025–37.

Simopolous AP, Leaf A, Salem N, Essentiality and recommended dietary intakes for omega-6 and omega-3 fatty acids. Ann Nutr Metab 1999;43: 127–30.

Solfrizzi V, Frisardi V, Capurso C, D'Introno A, Colacicco AM, Vendemiale G, Capurso A, Panza F, Dietary fatty acids in dementia and predementia syndromes: epidemiological evidence and possible underlying mechanisms. Ageing Res Rev 2010;9: 184–99.

Studer M, Briel M, Leimenstoll B, Glass TR, Bucher HC, Effect of different antilipidemic agents and diets on mortality: a systematic review. Arch Intern Med 2005;165: 725–30.

Van de Werf F, Bax J, Betriu A, Blomstom-Lundqvist C, Crea F, Falk V, Filippatos G, Fox K, Huber K, Kastrati A, Rosengren A, Steg PS, Tubaro M, Verheugt F, Wedinger F, Weis M, Management of acute myocardial infarction in patients presenting with persistent ST-segment elevation. Eur Heart J 2008;29: 2909–45.

von Schacky C, Omega-3 fatty acids: antiarrhythmic, proarrhythmic or both? Curr Opin Clin Nutr Metab Care 2008;11: 94–9.

von Schacky C, Fischer S, Weber PC, Long term effects of dietary marine ω-3 fatty acids upon plasma and cellular lipids, platelet function, and eicosanoid formation in humans. J Clin Invest 1985;76: 1626–31.

Yaqoob P, The nutritional significance of lipid rafts. Annu Rev Nutr 2009;29: 257–82.

Yaqoob P, Pala HS, Cortina-Borja M, Newsholme EA, Calder PC, Encapsulated fish oil enriched in α-tocopherol alters plasma phospholipid and mononuclear cell fatty acid compositions but not mononuclear cell functions. Eur J Clin Invest 2000;30: 260–74.

Yokoyama M, Origasa H, Matsuzaki M, Matsuzawa Y, Saito Y, Ishikawa Y, Oikawa S, Sasaki J, Hishida H, Itakura H, Kita T, Kitabatake A, Nakaya N, Sakata T, Shimada K, Shirato K, Japan EPA lipid intervention study (JELIS) Investigators, Effects of eicosapentaenoic acid on major coronary events in hypercholesterolaemic patients (JELIS): a randomised open-label, blinded endpoint analysis. Lancet 2007;369: 1090–8.

Zhao G, Etherton TD, Martin KR, West SG, Gillies PJ, Kris-Etherton PM, Dietary alpha-linolenic acid reduces inflammatory and lipid cardiovascular risk factors in hypercholesterolemic men and women. J Nutr 2004;134: 2991–7.

15.2 Omega-3-polyunsaturated fatty acids in pregnancy and childhood

Claudia Glaser; Mario Klingler; Berthold Koletzko

15.2.1 Introduction

Genetic inheritance and environmental conditions influence short- or long-term health outcomes and the intellectual development of children (Caspi et al., 2007). The long chain polyunsaturated fatty acids (LC-PUFA) arachidonic acid (AA), docosahexaenoic acid (DHA) and eicosapentaenoic acid (EPA) play a crucial role during growth and development in early life. AA is a member of the omega-6 fatty acid family, DHA and EPA of the omega-3 fatty acid family. An optimal supply of these LC-PUFA during pregnancy and early infancy is important for visual, cognitive and motor development (Beblo et al., 2007; Hibbeln et al., 2007; Koletzko et al., 2007a). The polyunsaturated fatty acid (PUFA) status in humans is also associated with mental health, psychiatric disorders (Muskiet and Kemperman, 2006), cardiovascular diseases and mortality (Leaf, 2006), and immunologic and inflammatory responses (Trak-Fellermeier et al., 2004; Kompauer et al., 2005).

Evidence exists that breastfed children develop higher intelligence quotient (IQ) scores than formula-fed children, which is possibly related to higher amounts of AA and DHA in human milk then in cow's milk or most infant formulas (Caspi et al., 2007). The preferred DHA transport across the placenta could indicate the importance of this fatty acid during late fetal development (Koletzko et al., 2007b). In summary, an optimal LC-PUFA supply during pregnancy, lactation and childhood is crucial for the developing child. However, the development of recommendations for an adequate PUFA intake raises several questions, such as:

- Does the metabolic turnover influence the tissue availability of PUFA?
- What impact has the dietary PUFA intake on maternal, fetal, and infantile PUFA status?
- How are PUFA transported from maternal to fetal circulation?
- How are PUFA related to visual, cognitive and mental development?
- Which roles do genetic variants of the *fatty acid desaturase* (*FADS*) gene cluster play in PUFA metabolism?

This chapter reviews the role of omega-3 LC-PUFA during pregnancy, infancy and childhood. An overview of the metabolism of LC-PUFA, nutritional requirements, and the placental fatty acid transfer will be given. The influence on visual and cognitive development will be discussed in more detail. Finally, a summary of the latest dietary recommendation for adequate PUFA intakes during pregnancy, lactation, infancy and childhood will be provided.

15.2.2 PUFA classification and tissue availability

Fatty acids are monocarboxylic acids composed of a hydrocarbon chain with a methyl group at one end and a carboxyl group at the other end. The carboxyl group is reactive and can be converted into different derivates. Linked to glycerol or cholesterol, fatty acids can form triacylglycerols, phospholipids and cholesterol esters. Fatty acids are differentiated according the hydrocarbon chain, which varies in length and degree of saturation. Commonly, natural fatty acids have straight chains of an even number of four to 28 carbon atoms. Fatty acids with no double bonds in the hydrocarbon chain are referred to as saturated fatty acids. Unsaturated fatty acids contain at least one double bond. They are further divided into monounsaturated fatty acids with one double bond and PUFA with at least two double bonds. PUFA with 20 or more carbon atoms are referred to as LC-PUFA. PUFA can be classified as omega-9, omega-6 and omega-3 fatty acids, depending on whether the last double bond (measured from the carboxyl group) is located at the ninth, sixth, or third carbon atom from the methyl end of the chain.

Oleic acid, linoleic acid (LA) and alpha-linolenic acid (ALA) are the parent fatty acids of omega-9, omega-6 and omega-3 PUFA families, respectively. Saturated fatty acids can be converted into monounsaturated fatty acids by desaturation and further on, desaturation is possible on the carboxyl side of the 9-double bond. However, insertion of double bonds at position 12 and 15 is possible only in plants, not in mammals. Thus, PUFA with these double bond positions cannot be synthesized endogenously in mammals, they must be provided in the diet and are therefore essential for life. Currently, two essential fatty acids are recognized; LA and ALA. These two PUFA cannot be converted into each other, but they can be metabolized to longer chain and higher unsaturated omega-6 and omega-3 fatty acids, respectively. Therefore, in addition to dietary intake, LC-PUFA can also be derived from endogenous synthesis.

15.2.3 Metabolism of PUFAs

There are three main families of unsaturated fatty acids, the omega-9, omega-6 and omega-3 series, which are formed by a series of alternate desaturations and elongations starting from the parent fatty acids, oleic acid (18:1n-9), LA (18:2n-6) and ALA (18:3n-3), respectively. All three metabolic pathways share the same enzymes for desaturation and elongation.

Oleic acid derives from the diet, but also can be synthesized endogenously via elongation of palmitic acid (16:0) to stearic acid (18:0), which is further desaturated by the action of stearoyl-CoA desaturase (delta-9 desaturase) to oleic acid. Oleic acid is desaturated (delta-6 desaturase), elongated and further desaturated (delta-5 desaturase) to the major end-product mead acid (20:3n-9). The desaturase enzymes bind preferably ALA and LA. Thus, only during essential fatty acid deficiency enhanced conversion of oleic acid to mead acid will take place.

In ▶Fig. 15.7 the metabolic conversion of LA and ALA is shown. The main product of the omega-6 family is AA (20:4n-6). In the first step LA is desaturated to gamma-linolenic acid by insertion of an additional double bond catalyzed by the enzyme delta-6 desaturase. The next step of this pathway is a chain elongation with dihomo-gamma-linolenic acid as its product. In addition to this common pathway, Park et al. (2009a) demonstrated an alternative pathway in mammals for dihomo-gamma-linolenic synthesis by delta-8 desaturation of omega-6 eicosadienoic acid (20:2n-6), which is the elongation product of LA. Delta-5 desaturation of dihomo-gamma-linolenic acid leads to AA. Further elongation and desaturation processes are possible.

An analogous pathway exists for the omega-3 family (▶Fig. 15.7). ALA can be converted by delta-6 desaturation to stearidonic acid (18:4n-3), which can be further elongated to

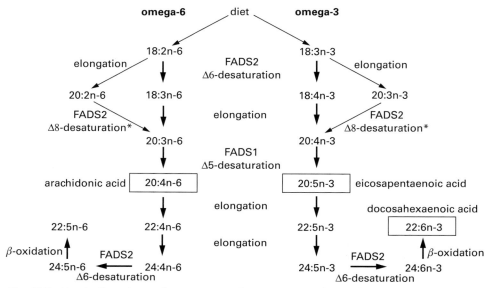

Fig. 15.7: Metabolic pathways for omega-6 and omega-3 long chain polyunsaturated fatty acid synthesis by enzymatic desaturation and chain elongation in humans, *alternative pathway (Park et al., 2009a)

eicosatetraenoic acid (20:4n-3). For eicosatetraenoic acid Park et al. (2009a) reported also an alternative pathway in mammals via elongation of ALA to omega-3 eicosatrienoic acid (20:3n-3) followed by a delta-8 desaturation of this PUFA to eicosatetraenoic acid. EPA (20:5n-3) is the delta-5 desaturation product of eicosatetraenoic acid. The end product of the omega-3 family is DHA (22:6n-3). Previously, it was assumed that in the conversion of EPA into DHA a delta-4 desaturation is involved. However, there is no evidence for the existence of a delta-4 desaturase in mammals. Sprecher (1999) considered a pathway in which DHA is synthesized by two chain elongations of EPA, followed by a delta-6 desaturation and a partial β-oxidation.

All desaturation and elongation steps take place in the endoplasmic reticulum, where as for the last step, the partial β-oxidation, a compartmental translocation to peroxisomes is required (Sprecher, 1999). The conversion rate of omega-3 docosapentaenoic acid (22:5n-3) to DHA has been shown to be low in humans (Burdge, 2004), which could be explained by a low activity of delta-6 desaturases and the compartmental transloca-tion. Conversion of ALA to EPA and DHA is greater in women than in men, which was assumed to be owing to estrogen effects (Burdge, 2006). However, the overall synthesis rate of omega-3 LC-PUFA is limited.

A majority of human tissues produce delta-5 and delta-6 desaturases. The highest levels are found in liver, but also adipose tissue (Sjogren et al., 2008), brain, heart and lung contain significant levels. Minor amounts of both desaturases have been shown in placenta, skeletal muscle, kidney, pancreas and pregnant uterus (Cho et al., 1999a,b). In rats, both desaturases are present in the mammary gland. It could be possible that also the human mammary gland participates in the synthesis of LC-PUFAs, which subsequently can be incorporated into human milk (Rodriguez-Cruz et al., 2006). This assumption needs to be confirmed.

For the mammalian delta-6 desaturase, studies identified until now five substrates (18:2n-6, 24:4n-6, 18:3n-3, 24:5n-3, and 16:0) and showed further a delta-8 desaturase activity of this enzyme on 20:2n-6 and 20:3n-3. Delta-5 desaturase seems to have a higher substrate specificity, because only two substrates, namely 20:3n-6 and 20:4n-3, are known for these enzymes (Park et al., 2009b). The desaturases are thought to be rate limiting in the metabolic pathways of all three PUFA families.

15.2.4 Dietary sources of PUFA

PUFAs comprise up to 20% of dietary fat in typical western diets. LA is the most abundant PUFA in the diet and contributes together with ALA more than 95% of dietary PUFA intake (Calder, 2008). High quantities of LA are found in many vegetable oils (e.g., corn, soybean and sunflower oil) and in products made from such oils (e.g., margarines). Dietary sources of ALA are green plant tissues, some common oils (e.g., flaxseed and rapeseed oil) and nuts. Consumption of LA and ALA in western diets exceeds minimal requirements necessary to prevent essential fatty acid deficiency. In western countries, popularity of cooking oils and margarines increased over the past 40 years, causing an increased LA intake. By contrast, intake of ALA changed rather slightly over this time. This imbalance has changed the ratio of omega-6 to omega-3 PUFA in the diet, which increased markedly and is today estimated at 1:5 to 1:20 in western countries.

Dietary intake of LC-PUFA is significantly lower compared with intakes of LA and ALA. Intakes of AA range typically between 50 and 500 mg/day. Significant quantities of AA can be found in, e.g., meat, eggs and offal. The main dietary sources of the omega-3 LC-PUFA EPA and DHA are fish and other seafood, particularly fatty sea fish (e.g., herring, mackerel, salmon and tuna) is rich in these fatty acids (▶Tab. 15.4). Approximately 1.5–3.5 g of omega-3 LC-PUFA can be provided by one oily fish meal,

Tab. 15.4: EPA and DHA quantities in selected fish (100 g, raw) (USDA, 2009).

Fish	EPA (g)	DHA (g)
Herring, Atlantic	0.71	0.86
Mackerel, Atlantic	0.90	1.40
Salmon		
Atlantic, farmed	0.86	1.10
Atlantic, wild	0.32	1.12
Chinook	1.01	0.94
Coho, farmed	0.36	0.82
Coho, wild	0.43	0.66
Tuna		
Bluefin	0.28	0.89
Skipjack	0.07	0.19
Yellowfin	0.04	0.18

whereas the absence of oily fish consumption leads to a very low omega-3 LC-PUFA intake of less than 100 mg/day.

15.2.5 Genetically determined variation in PUFA metabolism

The genes *FADS1* and *FADS2* encode for the delta-5 and delta-6 desaturases, respectively. Together with a third desaturase, *FADS3*, they build a gene cluster located on the human chromosome 11q12-q13.1 (Marquardt et al., 2000; Nakamura and Nara, 2004). *FADS1* and *FADS2* have a head-to-head orientation, and *FADS2* and *FADS3* have a tail-to-tail orientation. The human *FADS* gene cluster comprises 91.9 kb (Marquardt et al., 2000; Nakamura and Nara, 2004). Approximately 500 single nucleotide polymorphisms (SNPs) are annotated in the NCBI database (dbSNP build 130) for this region. The gene products of *FADS1* and *FADS2* have well known functions (see section 15.2.3), whereas no function has emerged for *FADS3* so far. Park et al. (2009b) identified several alternative splice forms of *FADS3* and hypothesized that *FADS3* has a tissue- or PUFA-specific role in LC-PUFA synthesis.

Genetic variants in the *FADS1 FADS2* gene cluster are associated with blood phospholipid fatty acid levels, as shown in several studies in adults (Glaser et al., 2010). Schaeffer et al. (2006) found that carriers of the minor alleles of 11 selected SNPs (rs174544, rs174553, rs174556, rs174561, rs3834458, rs968567, rs99780, rs174570, rs2072114, rs174583 and rs174589) located in the *FADS1 FADS2* gene cluster had enhanced serum phospholipid fatty acid levels of 18:2n-6, 20:2n-6, 20:3n-6 and 18:3n-3 and decreased levels of 18:3n-6, 20:4n-6, 22:4n-6, 20:5n-3 and 22:5n-3. For DHA, they found no significant association with genetic variants. Further studies confirmed these findings in other populations and reported additionally associations of genetic variants with adipose tissue (Baylin et al., 2007), breast milk (Xie and Innis, 2008) and erythrocyte fatty acid levels (Malerba et al., 2008; Rzehak et al., 2009). The highest proportion of genetically explained variation was shown for AA with 28%, whereas for DHA the primary determinant seems to be dietary supply (Schaeffer et al., 2006).

Further evidence for the importance of *FADS* gene cluster polymorphisms in PUFA metabolism is provided by genome-wide association studies of complex lipid traits, in which *FADS* polymorphisms are among the most significant hits. Gieger et al. (2008) showed that the SNP rs174548, located on the *FADS1* gene, is highly associated with several glycerophospholipid concentrations. Carriers of the minor allele had the lowest levels of glycerophospholipid species containing PUFA with four or more double bonds, whereas those with three or less double bonds showed positive associations with the genotype. Tanaka et al. (2009) reported strongest evidence for the association of plasma PUFA concentrations with SNPs located in a region on chromosome 11. AA levels showed the most significant association with SNP rs174537, located near *FADS1*. Carriers of only minor alleles had lower AA levels compared with homozygous carriers of the major allele. Based on the shown influence of genetic variations on endogenous LC-PUFA production, it is suggested that at similar dietary PUFA intakes, biological and health effects might differ.

Caspi et al. (2007) studied the association between breastfeeding and later IQ development in two independent birth cohorts. They found that breastfeeding had a significant effect on cognitive development in both cohorts. Genetic polymorphism in the *FADS2* gene had no significant effect in the two total study populations, but further analyses revealed that rs174575 polymorphisms interacted with breastfeeding in predicting the IQ. In both cohorts, breastfed children carrying the C allele had a marked IQ advantage over children not breastfed. In GG homozygotes breastfeeding had no influence on the IQ. Caspi et al. (2007) ruled out potential confounding of the gene-environment interaction (gene-exposure correlation, intrauterine growth differences, social class differences and maternal cognitive ability). These observations raise the hypothesis that in subpopulations of infants with genetically determined metabolic conversion activity of LC-PUFA synthesis, breastfeeding might have beneficial effects on later cognitive achievements. This question needs further exploration.

A further study by Moltó-Puigmartí et al. (2010) investigated whether *FADS* gene variants modify the association between maternal fish and fish-oil intake and DHA levels in plasma and human milk. DHA levels increased in plasma phospholipids with increasing fish and fish-oil intake, whereas DHA levels in human milk increased only in lactating women carrying the major allele. Possibly, incorporation of DHA into human milk is limited in women homozygous for the minor allele (Moltó-Puigmartí et al., 2010). Further studies are required to confirm these findings and evaluate whether higher amounts of fatty fish intake or omega-3 LC-PUFA supplementation, as the reported maximum of three portions fatty fish per week, can overcome the limited incorporation into human milk of lactating women homozygous for the minor allele. However, the observed gene-diet interaction could indicate that lactating women homozygous for the minor allele have less advantage of fatty fish or fish-oil intake than women carrying the major allele. These findings together with the observations of Caspi et al. suggest the assumption that the DHA status and the cognitive development of a breastfed child are dependent not only on dietary supply but also on the genotype of the child and the mother.

In conclusion, *FADS* gene variants play an important role in PUFA metabolism and influence PUFA tissue availability. Thus, in relation to *FADS* variants, population subgroups might have different requirements of dietary PUFA intakes to achieve comparable biological effects.

15.2.6 Nutritional requirements and dietary uptake of LC-PUFA during pregnancy

Optimal pregnancy outcomes depend on adequate nutrient intakes to meet maternal and fetal needs during gestation (Wu et al., 2004). ▶Tab. 15.5 contains a summary of recommendations, taken from Dietary Reference Intakes and expert consultations (Kaiser and Allen, 2008; EFSA, 2010).

The energy requirement increases during the course of pregnancy, primarily owing to maternal and fetal tissue accretion and maintenance (Picciano, 2003). The energy demand depends on the maternal body mass index, age, physiologic needs and the rate of weight gain. The additional protein requirement reflects maternal requirements to sustain the nitrogen balance and the protein deposition during pregnancy (Abu-Saad and Fraser, 2010). In Europe, pregnant women can easily meet their enhanced energy and protein needs, with the exception of special subgroups such as women with eating disorders or gastrointestinal diseases (D-A-CH, 2000). However, the pregnancy-associated increase of some micronutrients and omega-3 fatty acids is far higher than the increase in energy (Picciano, 2003). The recommended energy increase during pregnancy is up

Tab. 15.5: Comparison of recommended daily energy and nutrient intakes of adults and pregnant women (19–50 years).

Energy/nutrients	Adults	Pregnant woman	Nutrients	Adults	Pregnant woman
Energy	2nd trimester	+340 kcal/day	Biotin (µg)[b]	30	30
	3rd trimester	+450 kcal/day	Vitamin A (µg)[a]	30	30
			Vitamin D (µg)[b]	5	5
Protein (g)[a]	46	71	Vitamin E (mg)[a]	15	15
DHA+EPA (mg)[c]	250	+100–200 mg DHA	Vitamin K (µg)[b]	90	90
Vitamin C (mg)[a]	75	85	Calcium (mg)[b]	1000	1000
Thiamin (mg)[a]	1.1	1.4	Phosphorus (mg)[b]	700	700
Riboflavin (mg)[a]	1.1	1.4	Magnesium (mg)[a]	310	350
Niacin (ng)[a]	14	18	Iron (mg)[a]	18	27
Vitamin B6 (mg)[a]	1.3	1.9	Zinc (mg)[a]	8	11
Folate (µg)[a]	400	600	Iodine (µg)[a]	150	220
Vitamin B12 (µg)[a]	2.4	2.6	Selenium (µg)[a]	55	60
Pantothenate (mg)[b]	5	6	Fluoride (mg)[b]	3	3

[a] Recommended Dietary Allowance (RDA), average daily dietary intake level that is sufficient to meet the nutrient requirements of almost all (97–98%) individuals in a life stage and gender group based on Estimated Average Requirements (EAR).

[b] Adequate Intake (AI), the value used instead of RDA, if adequate scientific evidence is not available to calculate EAR (Picciano, 2003).

[c] AI, recommended by EFSA (EFSA, 2010).

to approximately 25%, whereas for protein, some vitamins and minerals an increase of approximately 50% is proposed (see ▶Tab. 15.5). The recommendation for omega-3 LC-PUFA intakes during pregnancy relates to DHA only. The European Food Safety Authority (EFSA) suggests an additional uptake of 100–200 mg DHA per day (EFSA, 2010). This is a 40–80% increase of omega-3 LC-PUFA during pregnancy.

Fish and seafood play an important part of a balanced diet during pregnancy. It is a valuable source of omega-3, protein, minerals, vitamin B12, iodine, and is low in saturated fat. Low fish consumption (omega-3) was found to be a strong risk factor for preterm delivery, low birth weight and detrimental effects for child development (Olsen and Secher, 2002; Hibbeln et al., 2007). There are concerns that high fish consumption increases the uptake of methylmercury, which might potentially harm the fetal developing nervous system (Oken and Bellinger, 2008). Recommendations given for fish consumption during pregnancy take into account both the benefits of fish as well as the potential effects of mercury exposure. It is agreed that pregnant women should avoid fish with high mercury levels such as shark, king mackerel, swordfish and tilefish (Ernährung DGf, 2002; USDHHS, 2004; NF Authority, 2009). However, evidence increases that both the mother and the fetus benefit from greater maternal fish consumption, if the woman chooses seafood with low methylmercury levels (Oken and Bellinger, 2008).

15.2.7 Fatty acid transfer across the placenta

The placenta is a barrier between the maternal and fetal circulation. It is composed of endothelium lining fetal vessel walls, connective tissue in the villious stroma, the cytothrophoblast and the syncytiotrophoblast facing intervillious spaces. During the course of pregnancy cytothrophoblast cells merge with syncytiotrophoblast cells, thus the placental barrier consists of three thin layers only (Firth and Leach, 1996) (see ▶Fig. 15.8).

Placental LC-PUFA uptake occurs through simple diffusion (flip-flop) or a saturable, protein-mediated transport mechanism (Kamp et al., 2003). Transporter protein-mediated processes are selective for LC-PUFA, which is crucial for the supply of those fatty acids to the unborn child. Desaturase enzymes, which facilitate the generation of LC-PUFA from their precursors are located in the placenta in minor amounts only (Cho et al., 1999a,b). Moreover, the fetus has limited ability to synthesize DHA and AA owing to the low desaturase activity in the liver. Thus, fetal needs of LC-PUFA in the prenatal period cannot be met by placental or endogenous synthesis (de Groot et al., 2004). Based on this, the fetus depends on the maternal LC-PUFA supply via the placenta (Larque et al., 2002).

The LC-PUFA composition provided to the fetus depends on the maternal dietary fatty acid uptake, but the placenta might be able to modulate its own fatty acid supply by expression of leptin. It is hypothesized that placenta-derived leptin regulates the maternal energy expenditure by mobilizing fatty acid stores from adipose tissue (Sagawa et al., 2002). Placental leptin is also transferred to the fetus to presumably regulate fetal development and growth (Hoggard et al., 1997).

Numerous studies reported higher LC-PUFA contents in cord plasma than in maternal plasma lipids at the time of delivery, whereas EFA are lower in infants than in maternal plasma lipids (Berghaus et al., 2000). In addition, placental tissue preferentially

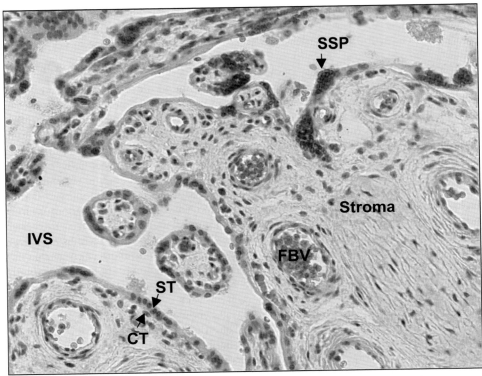

Fig. 15.8: Full-term placental tissue stained with Mayer's haemalum (original magnification 400). From maternal to fetal side: IVS, intervillious space; SSP, syncytium sprout; ST, syncytiotrophoblast; CT, cytotrophoblast; FBV, stroma, fetal blood vessel.

incorporates DHA relative to LA, oleic acid and palmitic acid (Larque et al., 2003). These observations are indicators that the placental fatty acid transfer is selective for individual fatty acids, such as DHA or AA.

The placental transfer of non-esterified fatty acids (NEFA) is a complex process involving membrane-binding proteins and cytoplasmic transport proteins (see ▶Fig. 15.9). The placental fatty acid uptake is facilitated through the plasma membrane fatty acid binding protein (FABP$_{pm}$/GOT2), the fatty acid translocase (FAT/CD36), fatty acid transport proteins (FATP), and fatty acid binding proteins (FABP) (Mantzioris et al., 1994). However, the role of proteins involved in the placental fatty acid uptake and metabolism remains unclear. It is proposed that a complex interaction of these proteins regulates the enrichment of LC-PUFA in the fetal circulation (Koletzko et al., 2007b).

Fatty acids cross the syncytiotrophoblast membranes as NEFA only, which derive mainly from a mixture of triacylglycerols and NEFA of the maternal circulation. The maternal triacylglycerols are primarily transported in lipoproteins, i.e., chylomicrons and very low-density lipoproteins, which can be hydrolyzed by lipoprotein lipases. Although fatty acids bond to phospholipids, albumin or apoprotein receptors represent a source of fatty acid; the lipoprotein lipase activity appears to be of crucial importance for fetal supply (Benassayag et al., 1997; Innis and Elias, 2003).

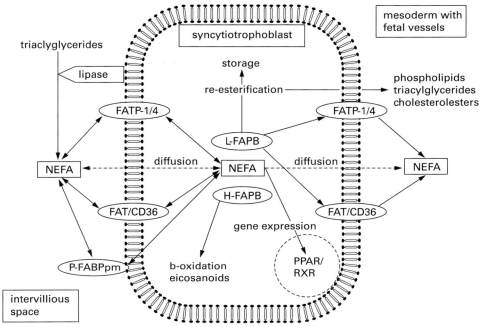

Fig. 15.9: Fatty acid transfer across the placenta. The interaction of fatty acid transport and binding proteins facilitate the fatty acid transfer of NEFA across the placenta. NEFA are also involved in energy generation, eicosanoid synthesis and gene expression. NEFA, non-esterified fatty acid; FATP, fatty acid transport protein; FAT, fatty acid translocase; FABP, fatty acid binding protein; P-FABP$_{pm}$, placental plasma membrane fatty acid binding protein; L-FABP, liver fatty acid binding protein; H-FABP, heart fatty acid binding protein; PPAR, peroxisome proliferator activated receptor; RXR, retinoid X receptor.

In the syncytiotrophoblast, fatty acid are re-esterified into different lipid fractions of the placenta or cross the tissue in either direction bound to cytosolic proteins (Kuhn and Crawford, 1986). Different FABP are involved in the fatty acid transfer to the fetal circulation, the heart-FABP (H-FABP) and liver-FABP (L-FABP). FABP have a higher affinity and binding capacity for DHA and AA compared with LA and ALA, facilitating the preferential transfer of LC-PUFA to the fetal circulation relative to EFA (Rothwell and Elphick, 1982; Kaminsky et al., 1991; Matorras et al., 1999). NEFA are also used for energy generation, eicosanoid synthesis and activation of nuclear transcription factors (PPAR/RXR).

Lipid transport across the placenta depends on a NEFA concentration gradient between maternal and fetal circulation. This gradient increases steadily during pregnancy and drives the materno-fetal fatty acid transport (Hanebutt et al., 2008). Fetal blood flow to the placenta also increases with the course of pregnancy in coincidence with the exponential increase in fetal fat deposition (Sutton et al., 1990).

A better understanding of the placental LC-PUFA transfer is of importance to improve fetal DHA status in uncomplicated and complicated pregnancies. Disorders such as gestational diabetes mellitus (GDM) and intrauterine growth restriction (IUGR) are associated with a poor AA and DHA status of the fetus (Wijendran et al., 2000; Cetin et al., 2002). In women with GDM the placental release of LC-PUFA to the fetal circulation is impaired (Bitsanis et al., 2006), whereas placental insufficiency and fetal abnormalities in lipid metabolism are characteristic for IUGR (Lane et al., 2003; Llanos et al., 2005). GDM can cause negative long-term effects such as an increased susceptibility to develop obesity or diabetes; IUGR might be related to developmental delays (Ong and Dunger, 2002; Brandt et al., 2003). The additional uptake of LC-PUFA during normal pregnancies improves the DHA and AA status of the mother, the placenta and the fetus (Decsi et al., 2005). For the future, targeted LC-PUFA supplementation aiming to improve outcomes of complicated pregnancies is a major challenge.

15.2.8 Role of LC-PUFA during cognitive and visual development

The supply and metabolism of LC-PUFA during pregnancy is important for fetal growth, tissue development and early development of the nervous system (Larque et al., 2002). LC-PUFA are incorporated in practically all tissues; they are the prevalent fatty acids in the mammalian brain, neuronal tissues and visual elements of the retina (Wijendran et al., 2002; Innis, 2008). LC-PUFA are structural components of cell membranes influencing membrane permeability, receptor functions and membrane-associated enzyme activities (Hamosh and Salem, 1998). However, unlike DHA and AA, EPA is not stored in significant quantities in the brain or retina.

In humans, a major portion of LC-PUFA are accumulated in the brain during late intrauterine and early postnatal growth (Neuringer et al., 1988; Innis, 2000). Prenatal DHA accretions also take place in fetal liver and adipose tissue, probably used to facilitate postnatal brain growth (Fewtrell, 2006). Available estimates suggest that on average 67 mg of omega-3 fatty acids are daily accumulated in fetal tissue during the last trimester of gestation (Clandinin et al., 1981). DHA is the predominant structural fatty acid in the developed brain, mostly distributed in the cerebral cortex, synaptic membranes, mitochondria and photoreceptors of the retina (Haag, 2003). At birth, approximately 70% of the total brain size is already developed (Clandinin et al., 1994).

The accumulation of fetal brain DHA and AA derived from dietary preformed LC-PUFA is far more efficient than from dietary EFA precursors and their endogenous desaturation and elongation (Koletzko et al., 2007b). In term newborn baboons approximately half of postnatal brain AA accretion is delivered from dietary preformed AA (Wijendran et al., 2002). It is suggested that the developing human brain depends on dietary DHA to a higher degree than AA, assuming that the endogenous metabolic regulation of AA is more effective (Makrides et al., 1994). In addition, differences are shown for the implementation rate of fetal plasma fatty acids into the brain of baboons; DHA implementation is eight to 20 times higher than ALA (Su et al., 2001).

Biochemical characteristics of brain DHA are linked to lipid-bound DHA in membranes and unesterified DHA in the cytosol. Membrane-bound DHA plays a role in signal transduction, neurotransmission and direct interaction with membrane proteins. Cytosolic DHA appears to be involved in regulating gene expression and ion channel activities, and its metabolites in neuroprotective processes (Innis, 2007).

It is assumed that the time of prenatal and postnatal DHA accrual in the brain is crucial to avoid negative long-term effects for the brain. Follow-up studies with children and adolescents born preterm support this assumption (McNamara and Carlson, 2006).

It has been shown that this children are at risk of incomplete brain DHA accumulation (Makrides et al., 2010). Furthermore, premature infants tend to show a higher incidence for attention-deficit hyperactivity disorders (ADHD), learning disabilities, motor and language impairments and poor social functioning (McNamara and Carlson, 2006). By contrast, DHA supplementation during the first months of life has the potential to improve visual attention processes in premature babies (Werkman and Carlson, 1996). This suggests that prenatal DHA accumulation plays a crucial role in the maturation of brain regions related to attention (McNamara and Carlson, 2006; Makrides et al., 2009).

DHA is abundant in the retina, mostly accumulated in the fragile photoreceptor outer-segment membranes (Neuringer et al., 1988). The DHA content comprises, on average, 30–65% of total fatty acids, which is higher than in any other neural sub-cellular components.

The long-term effect of DHA deficiencies in the retina of infants born preterm is not fully understood yet. Premature infants without major neuromotor disabilities might be affected by subtle visual impairments, such as contrast sensitivity or color vision defects (Dowdeswell et al., 1995). These impairments were not observed in young adolescents born preterm assessed by ophthalmological testing (O'Reilly et al., 2009). Other parameters or physiological processes might compensate the effect of low DHA levels on vision later in life. However, higher DHA levels might improve the visual acuity in early life. This might improve the recognition of the environment at an earlier age and directly influence the mental development.

15.2.9 Effect of additional omega-3 LC-PUFA intakes during pregnancy on early preterm birth and early infancy

The pregnant woman needs to increase the energy and substrate uptake to support the rapid fetal growth during the last trimester of pregnancy. However, the average uptake of omega-3 LC-PUFA, particularly DHA, is low in European mothers (Hornstra, 2000), which could have detrimental effects on the pregnancy outcome.

Increased uptakes of DHA (500 mg) during the second half of pregnancy lead to significantly higher phospholipid DHA levels in maternal and fetal plasma and in the placenta (Klingler et al., 2006; Krauss-Etschmann et al., 2007). This shows that an additional omega-3 LC-PUFA intake during pregnancy improves maternal and fetal DHA status, which could counteract the DHA storage depletion of the mother during the last trimester.

Enhanced DHA uptakes can increase the duration of gestation in low-risk pregnancies (Makrides et al., 2006; Szajewska et al., 2006). It is suggested that effects of omega-3 LC-PUFA on gestation duration might meet a saturation point, above which no further effect can be detected. Supplementation with oils providing LC-PUFA in low-risk pregnancies resulted in a 31% reduced risk of early preterm delivery before 34 weeks of gestation. In high-risk pregnancies the DHA supplementation reduced the risk by about 60% for preterm delivery before 34 weeks of gestation (Szajewska et al., 2006; Horvath et al., 2007). In this context it is discussed that LC-PUFA supplementation functions as an adjuvant to treat preterm labor (Olsen, 2004; Knudsen et al., 2006).

Meta-analyses of randomized clinical trials indicate that a maternal intake of fish or omega-3 supplements during pregnancy has also positive effects on birth weight and head circumference (Olsen, 2004; Decsi and Koletzko, 2005; Makrides et al., 2006; Szajewska et al., 2006). However, differences were small and not significant.

Visual acuity tests or electroretinography have been used to measure the visual development of term infants whose mothers were supplemented with DHA during pregnancy. Significant differences were either not found or showed benefits only at 4 months, but not at 6 months of age (Malcolm et al., 2003a,b; Judge et al., 2007). By contrast, newborns with cord plasma DHA levels greater than 4.3% showed a better visual acuity at 6 months of age compared with infants with lower DHA levels (Jacobson et al., 2008). Observational studies focusing on the seafood intake during pregnancy reported associations between high maternal omega-3 intakes with higher stereo-acuity (Jensen, 2006). However, the benefit of maternal DHA supplementation during pregnancy on visual development remains controversial. A major problem are procedures used to measure visual acuity as they vary in sensitivity or subjectivity (Neuringer and Jeffrey, 2003). Other factors, such as inconsistent habitual and supplemental DHA intakes, DHA source and postnatal DHA availability in human milk or formula might influence the DHA status of the mother and the child, and therefore the interpretation of the studies observations (Birch et al., 2010).

The maternal DHA status at birth might be linked to infantile cognitive function during early life. Cognitive ability is considered to relate to the average look duration in early infancy; shorter peak look duration is interpreted as an indicator of faster information processing. Infants born to mothers with higher DHA levels showed shorter look durations at an age of 4 months compared with infants, whose mothers had lower DHA levels. In this context, shorter duration looking at a young age correlates with higher scores of the Bayley Scale of Mental Development at 18 months of age (Colombo et al., 2004). Similar test outcomes were shown for infants at an age of 11 months, who had increased umbilical cord DHA levels at birth (Jacobson et al., 2008).

In relation to fish consumption a low intake was associated with sub-optimal outcomes in fine motor skills, social developmental scores and a low verbal intelligence at an age of 8 years (Hibbeln et al., 2007). Children at an age of 2.5 years attained higher scores for hand-eye coordination after their mothers received a relatively high dosage of DHA and EPA during pregnancy (Dunstan et al., 2008). Maternal intake of cod liver oil, which contains high levels of DHA, was significantly related to increased IQ scores of children at an age of 4 years compared with children whose mothers were supplemented with lower DHA levels (Helland et al., 2003). However, these differences were not observed in the same cohort at an age of 7 years (Helland et al., 2008). This is in contrast to the birth outcome of non-supplemented pregnant mothers. A correlation of cord blood DHA levels and IQ scores at an age of 4 years was not found (Bakker et al., 2003), but a significant positive relation between DHA levels and motor function at an age of 7 years (Bakker et al., 2009).

These results indicate that long-term benefits of omega-3 LC-PUFA supplementation during pregnancy are difficult to interpret. Factors such as diet, drugs, social stimulation and diseases might have an impact on the outcome of cognitive or functional tests (Helland et al., 2008). It was also shown that relatively large DHA doses are required to detect differences in cognitive ability (Dunstan et al., 2008).

The moderate DHA supplementation during pregnancy is considered to be safe. Studies including LC-PUFA supplementation with up to 20-fold higher DHA dosages as recommended by the EFSA for pregnant women did not describe adverse effects (Dunstan et al., 2008; EFSA, 2010). Other parameters such as placental apoptosis and proliferation or water-soluble and lipid-soluble antioxidants were not affected by DHA supplementation during pregnancy (Klingler et al., 2006; Franke et al., 2010).

15.2.10 Omega-3 fatty acid supply during early infancy

The optimal food for term infants is human milk. The fat content of human milk is relatively constant at 3.5–4 weight %. The dominant LC-PUFA in human milk are DHA and AA, with concentrations several-fold higher than the other LC-PUFA (Brenna and Lapillonne, 2009). PUFA contents are dependent on maternal diet and to a smaller extent on other factors such as certain diseases, gestational age and time postpartum (Jensen, 1999). The level of DHA in human milk is more variable on a worldwide basis than the level of AA. Population means of DHA in human milk range between 0.06 and 1.4 weight % of total fatty acids, whereas AA levels range between 0.24 and 1.0 weight % of total fatty acids (Brenna et al., 2007). The mean ratio of DHA to AA varies widely in regional human milk. The highest amounts are found in coastal populations with higher marine food consumption. Lactating women supplemented with DHA have an increase in milk DHA levels (Fidler et al., 2000; Jensen et al., 2005). Gibson et al. (1997) reported a dose-dependent relation between maternal DHA consumption and DHA levels in human milk, but human milk DHA levels above 0.8% of total fatty acids did little to increase the plasma or red blood cell DHA content of the study infants.

In different studies, infants have been fed formulas with various concentrations and relative ratios of ALA and linoleic acid, to match the LC-PUFA status of breastfed infants. Infants fed formulae with a high ALA/LA ratio showed slightly enhanced DHA levels compared with infants fed lower ratios. However, DHA levels achieved did not reach those found in breastfed infants, but AA levels are suppressed at high ALA/LA ratios (Makrides et al., 2000). In several studies, DHA levels in plasma and erythrocytes have been investigated in infants fed human milk, unfortified formulas and formulas fortified with LC-PUFA (Birch et al., 1998). Only by the addition of DHA and AA to formula, blood levels of both fatty acids can be matched with those of breastfed infants. Provision of omega-3 LC-PUFA without AA in infant formula might negatively affect growth in these infants, because blood AA levels might be reduced in preterm and term infants (Lapillonne et al., 2000a,b; Lapillonne and Carlson, 2001; Udell et al., 2005).

Autopsies from infants who had received breast milk, known to contain DHA, showed significantly higher concentrations of DHA in the cerebral cortex than did infants fed with formulas containing no DHA (Farquharson et al., 1992; Udell et al., 2005). Infants are born with a poorly developed visual system. During the first year of life, vision develops rapidly (Koletzko et al., 2008); therefore, several studies have investigated the effect of DHA and AA on visual development in infants (Fleith and Clandinin, 2005; Koletzko et al., 2008; Brenna and Lapillonne, 2009). Based on 13 randomized controlled studies, the EFSA delivered a scientific opinion on DHA and AA and visual development. They concluded that there is scientific evidence that DHA contributes to the visual development of infants, whereas the role of AA could not be established. For term infants fed formula from 0 to 12 months of age and for breastfed infants after weaning up to 12 months, a formula containing at least 0.3% of total fatty acids has been considered to be positively associated with visual function at 12 months (European Food Safety Authority, 2009a).

The EFSA provided also a scientific opinion on DHA and AA and brain development. They found some evidence for a short-term effect of DHA and AA supplementation on brain development in non-breastfed children but assessed the data available as inconsistent. They considered that currently available data do not provide evidence for an effect of DHA and AA on brain development beyond the supplementation period or beyond the first year of life (European Food Safety Authority, 2009b).

In a study investigating the association of DHA and AA supplementation of infant formula on blood pressure at the age of 6 years, infants fed supplemented formula had significantly lower mean blood pressure and diastolic blood pressure compared with infants given unfortified formula (Forsyth et al., 2003). These findings suggests that early dietary intake of LC-PUFA might have lasting effects on reduced blood pressure and cardiovascular risk, as blood pressure tends to track from infancy into adulthood (Koletzko et al., 2008). Further studies indicate that early LC-PUFA provision might also modulate immune response (Field et al., 2000, 2008).

15.2.11 Effect of additional omega-3 LC-PUFA intakes during childhood

The average uptake of omega-3 LC-PUFA during childhood depends on the availability and access to seafood. The DHA intake of children in a non-marine environment averages 35–50 mg. This is much lower than the DHA content of human milk or infant formulas (Ryan et al., 2010).

There is some evidence that high fish intake or fish oil supplementation improves cognitive abilities in children and young adolescence. Recently, a study demonstrated for the first time a direct link between DHA supplementation and brain function (McNamara et al., 2010). Different levels of DHA (400 versus 1200 mg/day) or placebo were supplied over 8 weeks to children aged between 8 and 10 years. Functional magnetic resonance imaging was used to investigate cortical activation during a continuous performance task. At 8 weeks, the children in the high DHA group had a significantly greater change from baseline in activation of the left dorsolateral prefrontal cortex while performing the sustained task. However, this was not observed in the low DHA group or placebo group. The results suggest that high doses of DHA enhance the functional cortical activity in a brain region, which is related to sustained attention and executive function (McNamara et al., 2010).

A Swedish epidemiological study found a positive correlation between fish consumption of 15-year-old males and their IQ scores at an age of 18 years. Participants were divided in groups depending on fish consumption of more than once per week versus less than once per week. Males with the higher fish consumption performed better in combined intelligence, verbal and visuospatial performance tests, independent of their educational level (Aberg et al., 2009).

Others studies which supplied children with a mix of omega-3 and -6 LC-PUFA found positive correlations of improved short-term and working memory, spelling test performance or ability to recognize words.

It has to be mentioned that some intervention studies could not identify relations between additional DHA uptakes and cognitive improvements during childhood (Kennedy et al., 2009). Other intervention studies could not distinguish between supplements provided and achieved benefits (Osendarp et al., 2007; Muthayya et al., 2009). Therefore it is suggested that study design, DHA concentration of the supplement or study diet and the intervention duration needs to be considered carefully to prove the effects of DHA supplementation during childhood (Ryan et al., 2010).

Omega-3 LC-PUFA play an important role in the treatment of children with phenylketonuria (PKU). The characteristic of this metabolism disorder is the inability to utilize the essential amino acid phenylalanine. Untreated PKU patients tend to develop hyperactivity, aggressiveness, negative mood swings and motor and attention disturbances (Yannicelli and Ryan, 1995). A phenylalanine-free diet is recommended to improve the physical manifestations of PKU patients. However, the proposed diet excludes animal-derived proteins, thus the DHA intake is insignificant. This is reflected in children who follow a phenylalanine-free diet. They exhibit noticeable lower DHA levels in plasma and red blood cell phospholipids (Giovannini et al., 1995). In this context, the intellectual development of treated PKU patients might be influenced by their low DHA status. In comparison with their unaffected siblings, the IQ of treated PKU children is slightly lower, independent of their phenylalanine levels (Burgard et al., 1996). The treatment of PKU children with DHA in combination with AA or EPA significantly improved their performance during visual evoked potential testing (Agostoni et al., 2000; Beblo et al., 2001). The same cohort showed improvements in body coordination and fine motor skills (Beblo et al., 2007; Koletzko et al., 2009). These are strong indicators that the LC-PUFA treatment of PKU children is required to normalize their neural function.

Currently, the effect of LC-PUFA treatment on ADHD was reviewed (Raz and Gabis, 2009; Transler et al., 2010). The authors concluded that the supplementation with individual omega-6 or omega-3 LC-PUFA had no effect on the improvement of ADHD in children. However, the combination of DHA, EPA and gamma-linolenic acid significantly reduced the symptoms of ADHD (Transler et al., 2010). Further effects of this treatment were the improvement in reading and spelling, teacher-rated attention, parent-rated conduct and reduction in the proportion of children showing oppositional defiant behavior (Transler et al., 2010). However, evidence is too minimal at this time for definitive conclusions. Further research needs to focus on individual genetic differences, fatty acid markers, brain imaging methods and systematic observations of behavior.

15.2.12 Summary of recommendations for LC-PUFA intake

Several national and international organizations provide dietary guidelines for adequate intakes of EPA and DHA for adults and infants. Recommendations for adults range from one to two portions of oily fish per week or approximately 500 mg EPA + DHA per day, mainly based on considerations of cardiovascular health (Kris-Etherton et al., 2009; Koletzko et al., 2010).

For pregnant and lactating women recommendations take optimal pregnancy outcomes and possible beneficial effects of EPA and DHA on fetal and infant development into account. According to evidence-based consensus recommendations, developed with support from the European Commission (Koletzko et al., 2007a), pregnant and lactating women should aim to achieve an average daily intake of at least 200 mg DHA. The EFSA (2010) recommends a daily intake of 100–200 mg DHA in pregnancy and lactation in addition to the daily intake of 250 mg EPA + DHA which is recommended for adults. The consumption of one to two portions of oily sea fish per week provides these suggested amounts of DHA. Fish can contribute significantly to the dietary exposure of contaminants. Particularly large predatory fish, which are at the top of the food chain, can contain higher levels of environmental contaminants such as methylmercury, dioxins and polychlorinated biphenyls (European Food Safety Authority, 2007a,b; Koletzko et al., 2007a). The EFSA advises to avoid intake of large amounts of predatory fish. However, the EFSA estimates the risk to exceed the tolerable intake of environmental contaminants by eating one to two portions of oily sea fish per week as very low. Higher intakes of up to 3.3 g omega-3 LC-PUFA per day should not provoke significant adverse effects, as confirmed by randomized trials. There is evidence to suggest that the intake of preformed DHA is more effective in respect to DHA deposition in fetal brain than the intake of the precursor ALA (Koletzko et al., 2007a).

The consensus group found no evidence for the need of an additional dietary AA intake for women of childbearing age, if they have an adequate dietary intake of linoleic acid. Furthermore, they suggest the performance of a screening for dietary inadequacies during pregnancy, particularly during the first trimester, and the offering of an individual counseling if inadequate dietary habits are detected (Koletzko et al., 2007a).

The recommendations and guidelines for perinatal practice supported by the World Association of Perinatal Medicine, the Early Nutrition Academy and the Child Health Foundation (Koletzko et al., 2008) strongly endorse breastfeeding as the preferred method of feeding healthy infants. Breastfeeding women should aim to achieve a balanced diet including a regular supply of DHA. According to the available evidence the recommendations and guidelines for perinatal practice supports the addition of at least 0.2–0.5 % of fatty acids as DHA to infant formula to achieve a benefit on functional endpoints. Infant formula contents of EPA should not exceed levels of DHA, and added AA levels should be at least those of added DHA (Koletzko et al., 2008). The EFSA (2010) recommends an adequate daily intake of 100 mg DHA for infants aged 7–24 months and the FAO/WHO (1993) a daily intake of 20 mg DHA per kg body weight for infants aged 0–2 years to ensure optimal growth and development.

For children above 2 years there are no agreed recommendations for the dietary intake of EPA and/or DHA. In July 2007, a workshop was organized to evaluate whether there are sufficient scientific data for issuing evidence-based guidelines on EPA and DHA intake in children aged 2–12 years (Koletzko et al., 2010). In this workshop, dietary intake recommendations for children could not be established, because available data on the association of dietary EPA and DHA intakes in children with growth, development and health are insufficient. However, there is no reason why children should not consume at least one to two portions of fish per week, as recommended for adults (Koletzko et al., 2010).

In conclusion, scientific data emphasize the importance of a balanced diet in every stage of life. The optimal supply of LC-PUFA is crucial for visual and cognitive development of the fetus, neonate and infant. Dietary intake of omega-3 fatty acids, particularly of DHA, during pregnancy and lactation is associated with positive pregnancy outcomes such as prolonged gestation length, minimized risk of preterm delivery and optimal fetal growth. However, evidence is too minimal at this time to conclude that omega-3 supplementation is beneficial for physical, mental and functional outcomes in children. Further studies need to focus on functional roles of LC-PUFA in pregnancy and early childhood to provide dietary recommendations for mothers and their children.

References

Aberg MA, Aberg N, Brisman J, Sundberg R, Winkvist A, et al., Fish intake of Swedish male adolescents is a predictor of cognitive performance. Acta Paediatr 2009;98: 555–60.

Abu-Saad K, Fraser D, Maternal nutrition and birth outcomes. Epidemiol Rev 2010;32: 5–25.

Agostoni C, Massetto N, Biasucci G, Rottoli A, Bonvissuto M, et al., Effects of long-chain polyunsaturated fatty acid supplementation on fatty acid status and visual function in treated children with hyperphenylalaninemia. J Pediatr 2000;137: 504–9.

Bakker EC, Ghys AJ, Kester AD, Vles JS, Dubas JS, et al., Long-chain polyunsaturated fatty acids at birth and cognitive function at 7 y of age. Eur J Clin Nutr 2003;57: 89–95.

Bakker EC, Hornstra G, Blanco CE, Vles JS, Relationship between long-chain polyunsaturated fatty acids at birth and motor function at 7 years of age. Eur J Clin Nutr 2009;63: 499–504.

Baylin A, Ruiz-Narvaez E, Kraft P, Campos H, alpha-Linolenic acid, delta6-desaturase gene polymorphism, and the risk of nonfatal myocardial infarction. Am J Clin Nutr 2007;85: 554–60.

Beblo S, Reinhardt H, Muntau AC, Mueller-Felber W, Roscher AA, et al., Fish oil supplementation improves visual evoked potentials in children with phenylketonuria. Neurology 2001;57: 1488–91.

Beblo S, Reinhardt H, Demmelmair H, Muntau AC, Koletzko B, Effect of fish oil supplementation on fatty acid status, coordination, and fine motor skills in children with phenylketonuria. J Pediatr 2007;150: 479–84.

Benassayag C, Mignot TM, Haourigui M, Civel C, Hassid J, et al., High polyunsaturated fatty acid, thromboxane A2, and alpha-fetoprotein concentrations at the human feto-maternal interface. J Lipid Res 1997;38: 276–86.

Berghaus TM, Demmelmair H, Koletzko B, Essential fatty acids and their long-chain polyunsaturated metabolites in maternal and cord plasma triglycerides during late gestation. Biol Neonate 2000;77: 96–100.

Birch EE, Hoffman DR, Uauy R, Birch DG, Prestidge C, Visual acuity and the essentiality of docosahexaenoic acid and arachidonic acid in the diet of term infants. Pediatr Res 1998;44: 201–9.

Birch EE, Carlson SE, Hoffman DR, Fitzgerald-Gustafson KM, Fu VL, et al., The DIAMOND (DHA Intake And Measurement Of Neural Development) Study: a double-masked, randomized controlled clinical trial of the maturation of infant visual acuity as a function of the dietary level of docosahexaenoic acid. Am J Clin Nutr 2010;91: 848–59.

Bitsanis D, Ghebremeskel K, Moodley T, Crawford MA, Djahanbakhch O, Gestational diabetes mellitus enhances arachidonic and docosahexaenoic acids in placental phospholipids. Lipids 2006;41: 341–6.

Brandt I, Sticker EJ, Lentze MJ, Catch-up growth of head circumference of very low birth weight, small for gestational age preterm infants and mental development to adulthood. J Pediatr 2003;142: 463–8.

Brenna JT, Lapillonne A, Background paper on fat and fatty acid requirements during pregnancy and lactation. Ann Nutr Metab 2009;55: 97–122.

Brenna JT, Varamini B, Jensen RG, Diersen-Schade DA, Boettcher JA, et al., Docosahexaenoic and arachidonic acid concentrations in human breast milk worldwide. Am J Clin Nutr 2007;85: 1457–64.

Burdge G, Alpha-linolenic acid metabolism in men and women: nutritional and biological implications. Curr Opin Clin Nutr Metab Care 2004;7: 137–44.

Burdge GC, Metabolism of alpha-linolenic acid in humans. Prostaglandins Leukot Essent Fatty Acids 2006;75: 161–8.

Burgard P, Schmidt E, Rupp A, Schneider W, Bremer HJ, Intellectual development of the patients of the German Collaborative Study of children treated for phenylketonuria. Eur J Pediatr 1996;155(Suppl 1): S33–8.

Calder PC, Polyunsaturated fatty acids, inflammatory processes and inflammatory bowel diseases. Mol Nutr Food Res 2008;52: 885–97.

Caspi A, Williams B, Kim-Cohen J, Craig IW, Milne BJ, et al., Moderation of breastfeeding effects on the IQ by genetic variation in fatty acid metabolism. Proc Natl Acad Sci USA 2007;104: 18860–5.

Cetin I, Giovannini N, Alvino G, Agostoni C, Riva E, et al., Intrauterine growth restriction is associated with changes in polyunsaturated fatty acid fetal-maternal relationships. Pediatr Res 2002;52: 750–5.

Cho HP, Nakamura M, Clarke SD, Cloning, expression, and fatty acid regulation of the human delta-5 desaturase. J Biol Chem 1999a;274: 37335–9.

Cho HP, Nakamura MT, Clarke SD, Cloning, expression, and nutritional regulation of the mammalian delta-6 desaturase. J Biol Chem 1999b;274: 471–7.

Clandinin MT, Chappell JE, Heim T, Swyer PR, Chance GW, Fatty acid utilization in perinatal de novo synthesis of tissues. Early Hum Dev 1981;5: 355–66.

Clandinin MT, Jumpsen J, Suh M, Relationship between fatty acid accretion, membrane composition, and biologic functions. J Pediatr 1994;125: S25–32.

Colombo J, Kannass KN, Shaddy DJ, Kundurthi S, Maikranz JM, et al., Maternal DHA and the development of attention in infancy and toddlerhood. Child Dev 2004;75: 1254–67.

D-A-CH, Deutsche Gesellschaft für Ernährung (DGE) ÖGfEÖ, Schweizerische Gesellschaft für Ernährungsforschung (SGE), Schweizerische Vereinigung für Ernährung (SVE). Referenzwerte für Ernährungsforschung, Frankfurt am Main: Umschau Braus Verlag, 2000.

Decsi T, Koletzko B, N-3 fatty acids and pregnancy outcomes. Curr Opin Clin Nutr Metab Care 2005;8: 161–6.

Decsi T, Campoy C, Koletzko B, Effect of N-3 polyunsaturated fatty acid supplementation in pregnancy: the Nuheal trial. Adv Exp Med Biol 2005;569: 109–13.

de Groot RH, Hornstra G, van Houwelingen AC, Roumen F, Effect of alpha-linolenic acid supplementation during pregnancy on maternal and neonatal polyunsaturated fatty acid status and pregnancy outcome. Am J Clin Nutr 2004;79: 251–60.

Dowdeswell HJ, Slater AM, Broomhall J, Tripp J, Visual deficits in children born at less than 32 weeks' gestation with and without major ocular pathology and cerebral damage. Br J Ophthalmol 1995;79: 447–52.

Dunstan JA, Simmer K, Dixon G, Prescott SL, Cognitive assessment of children at age 2(1/2) years after maternal fish oil supplementation in pregnancy: a randomised controlled trial. Arch Dis Child Fetal Neonatal Ed 2008;93: F45–50.

EFSA Panel on Dietic Products Nutrition, and Allergies (NDA), Scientific Opinion on Dietary Reference Values for fats, including saturated fatty acids, polyunsaturated fatty acids, monoun-saturated fatty acids, trans fatty acids, and cholesterol. EFSA J 2010;8:1461.

Ernährung DGf, Roher Fisch und Schwangerschaft. Beratungspraxis 07, 2002.

European Food Safety Authority. Opinion of the Scientific Panel on Contaminants in the Food Chain on a request from the European Parliament related to the safety of assessment of wild and farmed fish (Question No EFSA-Q-2004-022, adopted on 22 June 2005). EFSA J 2007a;236: 1–118.

European Food Safety Authority. Opinion of the Scientific Panel on Contaminants in the Food Chain on a request from the Commission related to mercury and methylmercury in food (Request No EFSA-Q-2003-030, adopted on 24 February 2004). EFSA J 2007b;34: 1–14.

European Food Safety Authority. Scientific Opinion of the Panel on Dietetic Products, Nutrition and Allergies on a request from Mead Johnson Nutrionals on DHA and ARA and visual development. EFSA J 2009a;941: 1–14.

European Food Safety Authority. Scientific Opinion of the Panel on Dietetic Products, Nutrition and Allergies on a request from Mead Johnson & Company on DHA and ARA and brain develop-ment. EFSA J 2009b;941: 1–14.

Farquharson J, Cockburn F, Patrick WA, Jamieson EC, Logan RW, Infant cerebral cortex phospho-lipid fatty-acid composition and diet. Lancet 1992;340: 810–3.

Fewtrell MS, Long-chain polyunsaturated fatty acids in early life: effects on multiple health outcomes. A critical review of current status, gaps and knowledge. Nestle Nutr Workshop Ser Pediatr Program 2006;57: 203–214; discussion 215–221.

Fidler N, Sauerwald T, Pohl A, Demmelmair H, Koletzko B, Docosahexaenoic acid transfer into human milk after dietary supplementation: a randomized clinical trial. J Lipid Res 2000;41: 1376–83.

Field CJ, Thomson CA, Van Aerde JE, Parrott A, Euler A, et al., Lower proportion of CD45R0+ cells and deficient interleukin-10 production by formula-fed infants, compared with human-fed, is corrected with supplementation of long-chain polyunsaturated fatty acids. J Pediatr Gastroen-terol Nutr 2000;31: 291–9.

Field CJ, Van Aerde JE, Robinson LE, Clandinin MT, Effect of providing a formula supplement-ed with long-chain polyunsaturated fatty acids on immunity in full-term neonates. Br J Nutr 2008;99: 91–9.

Firth JA, Leach L, Not trophoblast alone: a review of the contribution of the fetal microvasculature to transplacental exchange. Placenta 1996;17: 89–96.

Fleith M, Clandinin MT, Dietary PUFA for preterm and term infants: review of clinical studies. Crit Rev Food Sci Nutr 2005;45: 205–29.

Food and Agriculture Organization of the UN and WHO, Fats and oils in human nutrition. FAO Food and Nutrition Paper no. 57. Rome: FAO; 1994.

Forsyth JS, Willatts P, Agostoni C, Bissenden J, Casaer P, et al., Long chain polyunsaturated fatty acid supplementation in infant formula and blood pressure in later childhood: follow up of a randomised controlled trial. Br Med J 2003;326: 953.

Franke C, Demmelmair H, Decsi T, Campoy C, Cruz M, et al., Influence of fish oil or folate supple-mentation on the time course of plasma redox markers during pregnancy. Br J Nutr 2010;103: 1648–56.

Gibson RA, Neumann MA, Makrides M, Effect of increasing breast milk docosahexaenoic acid on plasma and erythrocyte phospholipid fatty acids and neural indices of exclusively breast fed infants. Eur J Clin Nutr 1997;51: 578–84.

Gieger C, Geistlinger L, Altmaier E, Hrabe de Angelis M, Kronenberg F, et al., Genetics meets metabolomics: a genome-wide association study of metabolite profiles in human serum. PLoS Genet 2008;4: e1000282.

Giovannini M, Biasucci G, Agostoni C, Luotti D, Riva E, Lipid status and fatty acid metabolism in phenylketonuria. J Inherit Metab Dis 1995;18: 265–72.

Glaser C, Heinrich J, Koletzko B, Role of FADS1 and FADS2 polymorphisms in polyunsaturated fatty acid metabolism. Metabolism 2010;59: 993–9.

Haag M, Essential fatty acids and the brain. Can J Psychiatry 2003;48: 195–203.

Hamosh M, Salem N Jr, Long-chain polyunsaturated fatty acids. Biol Neonate 1998;74: 106–20.

Hanebutt FL, Demmelmair H, Schiessl B, Larque E, Koletzko B, Long-chain polyunsaturated fatty acid (LC-PUFA) transfer across the placenta. Clin Nutr 2008;27: 685–93.

Helland IB, Smith L, Saarem K, Saugstad OD, Drevon CA, Maternal supplementation with very-long-chain n-3 fatty acids during pregnancy and lactation augments children's IQ at 4 years of age. Pediatrics 2003;111: e39–44.

Helland IB, Smith L, Blomen B, Saarem K, Saugstad OD, et al., Effect of supplementing pregnant and lactating mothers with n-3 very-long-chain fatty acids on children's IQ and body mass index at 7 years of age. Pediatrics 2008;122: e472–9.

Hibbeln JR, Davis JM, Steer C, Emmett P, Rogers I, et al., Maternal seafood consumption in preg-nancy and neurodevelopmental outcomes in childhood (ALSPAC study): an observational cohort study. Lancet 2007;369: 578–85.

Hoggard N, Hunter L, Duncan JS, Williams LM, Trayhurn P, et al., Leptin and leptin receptor mRNA and protein expression in the murine fetus and placenta. Proc Natl Acad Sci USA 1997;94: 11073–8.

Hornstra G, Essential fatty acids in mothers and their neonates. Am J Clin Nutr 2000;71: 1262S–9S.

Horvath A, Koletzko B, Szajewska H, Effect of supplementation of women in high-risk pregnancies with long-chain polyunsaturated fatty acids on pregnancy outcomes and growth measures at birth: a meta-analysis of randomized controlled trials. Br J Nutr 2007;98: 253–9.

Innis SM, The role of dietary n-6 and n-3 fatty acids in the developing brain. Dev Neurosci 2000;22: 474–80.

Innis SM, Dietary (n-3) fatty acids and brain development. J Nutr 2007;137: 855–9.

Innis SM, Dietary omega 3 fatty acids and the developing brain. Brain Res 2008;1237: 35–43.

Innis SM, Elias SL, Intakes of essential n-6 and n-3 polyunsaturated fatty acids among pregnant Canadian women. Am J Clin Nutr 2003;77: 473–8.

Jacobson JL, Jacobson SW, Muckle G, Kaplan-Estrin M, Ayotte P, et al., Beneficial effects of a polyunsaturated fatty acid on infant development: evidence from the inuit of arctic Quebec. J Pediatr 2008;152: 356–64.

Jensen CL, Effects of n-3 fatty acids during pregnancy and lactation. Am J Clin Nutr 2006;83: 1452S–7S.

Jensen CL, Voigt RG, Prager TC, Zou YL, Fraley JK, et al., Effects of maternal docosahexaenoic acid intake on visual function and neurodevelopment in breastfed term infants. Am J Clin Nutr 2005;82: 125–32.

Jensen RG, Lipids in human milk. Lipids 1999;34: 1243–71.

Judge MP, Harel O, Lammi-Keefe CJ, A docosahexaenoic acid-functional food during pregnancy benefits infant visual acuity at four but not six months of age. Lipids 2007;42: 117–22.

Kaiser L, Allen LH, Position of the American Dietetic Association: nutrition and lifestyle for a healthy pregnancy outcome. J Am Diet Assoc 2008;108: 553–61.

Kaminsky S, Sibley CP, Maresh M, Thomas CR, D'Souza SW, The effects of diabetes on placental lipase activity in the rat and human. Pediatr Res 1991;30: 541–3.

Kamp F, Guo W, Souto R, Pilch PF, Corkey BE, et al., Rapid flip-flop of oleic acid across the plasma membrane of adipocytes. J Biol Chem 2003;278: 7988–95.

Kennedy DO, Jackson PA, Elliott JM, Scholey AB, Robertson BC, et al., Cognitive and mood effects of 8 weeks' supplementation with 400 mg or 1000 mg of the omega-3 essential fatty acid docosahexaenoic acid (DHA) in healthy children aged 10–12 years. Nutr Neurosci 2009;12: 48–56.

Klingler M, Blaschitz A, Campoy C, Cano A, Molloy AM, et al., The effect of docosahexaenoic acid and folic acid supplementation on placental apoptosis and proliferation. Br J Nutr 2006;96: 182–90.

Knudsen VK, Hansen HS, Osterdal ML, Mikkelsen TB, Mu H, et al., Fish oil in various doses or flax oil in pregnancy and timing of spontaneous delivery: a randomised controlled trial. Br J Obstet Gynaecol 2006;113: 536–43.

Koletzko B, Cetin I, Brenna JT, Grp P, Dietary fat intakes for pregnant and lactating women. Br J Nutr 2007a;98: 873–7.

Koletzko B, Larque E, Demmelmair H, Placental transfer of long-chain polyunsaturated fatty acids (LC-PUFA). J Perinat Med 2007b;35(Suppl 1): S5–11.

Koletzko B, Lien E, Agostoni C, Bohles H, Campoy C, et al., The roles of long-chain polyunsaturated fatty acids in pregnancy, lactation and infancy: review of current knowledge and consensus recommendations. J Perinat Med 2008;36: 5–14.

Koletzko B, Beblo S, Demmelmair H, Hanebutt FL, Omega-3 LC-PUFA supply and neurological outcomes in children with phenylketonuria (PKU). J Pediatr Gastroenterol Nutr 2009;48(Suppl 1): S2–7.

Koletzko B, Uauy R, Palou A, Kok F, Hornstra G, et al., Dietary intake of eicosapentaenoic acid (EPA) and docosahexaenoic acid (DHA) in children – a workshop report. Br J Nutr 2010;103: 923–8.

Kompauer I, Demmelmair H, Koletzko B, Bolte G, Linseisen J, et al., Association of fatty acids in serum phospholipids with hay fever, specific and total immunoglobulin E. Br J Nutr 2005;93: 529–35.

Krauss-Etschmann S, Shadid R, Campoy C, Hoster E, Demmelmair H, et al., Effects of fish-oil and folate supplementation of pregnant women on maternal and fetal plasma concentrations of docosahexaenoic acid and eicosapentaenoic acid: a European randomized multicenter trial. Am J Clin Nutr 2007;85: 1392–400.

Kris-Etherton PM, Grieger JA, Etherton TD, Dietary reference intakes for DHA and EPA. Prostaglandins Leukot Essent Fatty Acids 2009;81: 99–104.

Kuhn DC, Crawford M, Placental essential fatty acid transport and prostaglandin synthesis. Prog Lipid Res 1986;25: 345–53.

Lane RH, Maclennan NK, Daood MJ, Hsu JL, Janke SM, et al., IUGR alters postnatal rat skeletal muscle peroxisome proliferator-activated receptor-gamma coactivator-1 gene expression in a fiber specific manner. Pediatr Res 2003;53: 994–1000.

Lapillonne A, Carlson SE, Polyunsaturated fatty acids and infant growth. Lipids 2001;36: 901–11.

Lapillonne A, Brossard N, Claris O, Reygrobellet B, Salle BL, Erythrocyte fatty acid composition in term infants fed human milk or a formula enriched with a low eicosapentanoic acid fish oil for 4 months. Eur J Pediatr 2000a;159: 49–53.

Lapillonne A, Picaud JC, Chirouze V, Goudable J, Reygrobellet B, et al., The use of low-EPA fish oil for long-chain polyunsaturated fatty acid supplementation of preterm infants. Pediatr Res 2000b;48: 835–41.

Larque E, Demmelmair H, Berger B, Hasbargen U, Koletzko B, In vivo investigation of the placental transfer of (13)C-labeled fatty acids in humans. J Lipid Res 2003;44: 49–55.

Leaf A, Prevention of sudden cardiac death by n-3 polyunsaturated fatty acids. Fundam Clin Pharmacol 2006;20: 525–38.

Llanos A, Lin Y, Mena P, Salem N Jr, Uauy R, Infants with intrauterine growth restriction have impaired formation of docosahexaenoic acid in early neonatal life: a stable isotope study. Pediatr Res 2005;58: 735–40.

Makrides M, Neumann MA, Byard RW, Simmer K, Gibson RA, Fatty acid composition of brain, retina, and erythrocytes in breast- and formula-fed infants. Am J Clin Nutr 1994;60: 189–94.

Makrides M, Neumann MA, Jeffrey B, Lien EL, Gibson RA, A randomized trial of different ratios of linoleic to alpha-linolenic acid in the diet of term infants: effects on visual function and growth. Am J Clin Nutr 2000;71: 120–9.

Makrides M, Duley L, Olsen SF, Marine oil, and other prostaglandin precursor, supplementation for pregnancy uncomplicated by pre-eclampsia or intrauterine growth restriction. Cochrane Database Syst Rev 2006;3: CD003402.

Makrides M, Gibson RA, McPhee AJ, Collins CT, Davis PG, et al., Neurodevelopmental outcomes of preterm infants fed high-dose docosahexaenoic acid: a randomized controlled trial. J Am Med Assoc 2009;301: 175–82.

Makrides M, Smithers LG, Gibson RA, Role of long-chain polyunsaturated fatty acids in neurodevelopment and growth. Nestle Nutr Workshop Ser Pediatr Program 2010;65: 123–36.

Malcolm CA, Hamilton R, McCulloch DL, Montgomery C, Weaver LT, Scotopic electroretinogram in term infants born of mothers supplemented with docosahexaenoic acid during pregnancy. Invest Ophthalmol Vis Sci 2003a;44: 3685–91.

Malcolm CA, McCulloch DL, Montgomery C, Shepherd A, Weaver LT, Maternal docosahexaenoic acid supplementation during pregnancy and visual evoked potential development in term infants: a double blind, prospective, randomised trial. Arch Dis Child Fetal Neonatal Ed 2003b;88: F383–90.

Malerba G, Schaeffer L, Xumerle L, Klopp N, Trabetti E, et al., SNPs of the FADS gene cluster are associated with polyunsaturated fatty acids in a cohort of patients with cardiovascular disease. Lipids 2008;43: 289–99.

Mantzioris E, James MJ, Gibson RA, Cleland LG, Dietary substitution with an alpha-linolenic acid-rich vegetable oil increases eicosapentaenoic acid concentrations in tissues. Am J Clin Nutr 1994;59: 1304–9.

Marquardt A, Stohr H, White K, Weber BH, cDNA cloning, genomic structure, and chromosomal localization of three members of the human fatty acid desaturase family. Genomics 2000;66: 175–83.

Matorras R, Perteagudo L, Sanjurjo P, Ruiz JI, Intake of long chain w3 polyunsaturated fatty acids during pregnancy and the influence of levels in the mother on newborn levels. Eur J Obstet Gynecol Reprod Biol 1999;83: 179–84.

McNamara RK, Carlson SE, Role of omega-3 fatty acids in brain development and function: potential implications for the pathogenesis and prevention of psychopathology. Prostaglandins Leukot Essent Fatty Acids 2006;75: 329–49.

McNamara RK, Able J, Jandacek R, Rider T, Tso P, et al., Docosahexaenoic acid supplementation increases prefrontal cortex activation during sustained attention in healthy boys: a placebo-controlled, dose-ranging, functional magnetic resonance imaging study. Am J Clin Nutr 2010;91: 1060–7.

Moltó-Puigmartí C, Plat J, Mensink RP, Muller A, Jansen E, et al., FADS1 FADS2 gene variants modify the association between fish intake and the docosahexaenoic acid proportions in human milk. Am J Clin Nutr 2010;91: 1368–76.

Muskiet FA, Kemperman RF, Folate and long-chain polyunsaturated fatty acids in psychiatric disease. J Nutr Biochem 2006;17: 717–27.

Muthayya S, Eilander A, Transler C, Thomas T, van der Knaap HC, et al., Effect of fortification with multiple micronutrients and n-3 fatty acids on growth and cognitive performance in Indian schoolchildren: the CHAMPION (Children's Health and Mental Performance Influenced by Optimal Nutrition) Study. Am J Clin Nutr 2009;89: 1766–75.

Nakamura MT, Nara TY, Structure, function, and dietary regulation of delta6, delta5, and delta9 desaturases. Annu Rev Nutr 2004;24: 345–76.

Neuringer M, Jeffrey BG, Visual development: neural basis and new assessment methods. J Pediatr 2003;143: 87–95.

Neuringer M, Anderson GJ, Connor WE, The essentiality of n-3 fatty acids for the development and function of the retina and brain. Annu Rev Nutr 1988;8: 517–41.

North South Wales Food Authority Food safety during pregnancy. 2009.

Oken E, Bellinger DC, Fish consumption, methylmercury and child neurodevelopment. Curr Opin Pediatr 2008;20: 178–83.

Olsen SF, Is supplementation with marine omega-3 fatty acids during pregnancy a useful tool in the prevention of preterm birth? Clin Obstet Gynecol 2004;47: 768–74; discussion 881–2.

Olsen SF, Secher NJ, Low consumption of seafood in early pregnancy as a risk factor for preterm delivery: prospective cohort study. Br Med J 2002;324: 447.

Ong KK, Dunger DB, Perinatal growth failure: the road to obesity, insulin resistance and cardiovascular disease in adults. Best Pract Res Clin Endocrinol Metab 2002;16: 191–207.

O'Reilly M, Vollmer B, Vargha-Khadem F, Neville B, Connelly A, Wyatt J, Timms C, de Haan M, Ophthalmological, cognitive, electrophysiological and MRI assessment of visual processing in preterm children without major neuromotor impairment. Dev Sci 2009; DOI: 10.1111/j.1467-7689.2009.00925.x [E-pub ahead of print].

Osendarp SJ, Baghurst KI, Bryan J, Calvaresi E, Hughes D, et al., Effect of a 12-mo micronutrient intervention on learning and memory in well-nourished and marginally nourished school-aged children: 2 parallel, randomized, placebo-controlled studies in Australia and Indonesia. Am J Clin Nutr 2007;86: 1082–93.

Park WJ, Kothapalli KS, Lawrence P, Tyburczy C, Brenna JT, An alternate pathway to long-chain polyunsaturates: the FADS2 gene product Delta8-desaturates 20:2n-6 and 20:3n-3. J Lipid Res 2009a;50: 1195–202.

Park WJ, Kothapalli KS, Reardon HT, Kim LY, Brenna JT, Novel fatty acid desaturase 3 (FADS3) transcripts generated by alternative splicing. Gene 2009b;446: 28–34.

Picciano MF, Pregnancy and lactation: physiological adjustments, nutritional requirements and the role of dietary supplements. J Nutr 2003;133: 1997S–2002S.

Raz R, Gabis L, Essential fatty acids and attention-deficit-hyperactivity disorder: a systematic review. Dev Med Child Neurol 2009;51: 580–92.

Rodriguez-Cruz M, Tovar AR, Palacios-Gonzalez B, Del Prado M, Torres N, Synthesis of long-chain polyunsaturated fatty acids in lactating mammary gland: role of Delta5 and Delta6 desaturases, SREBP-1, PPARalpha, and PGC-1. J Lipid Res 2006;47: 553–60.

Rothwell JE, Elphick MC, Lipoprotein lipase activity in human and guinea-pig placenta. J Dev Physiol 1982;4: 153–9.

Ryan AS, Astwood JD, Gautier S, Kuratko CN, Nelson EB, et al., Effects of long-chain polyunsaturated fatty acid supplementation on neurodevelopment in childhood: a review of human studies. Prostaglandins Leukot Essent Fatty Acids 2010;82: 305–14.

Rzehak P, Heinrich J, Klopp N, Schaeffer L, Hoff S, et al., Evidence for an association between genetic variants of the fatty acid desaturase 1 fatty acid desaturase 2 (FADS1 FADS2) gene cluster and the fatty acid composition of erythrocyte membranes. Br J Nutr 2009;101: 20–6.

Sagawa N, Yura S, Itoh H, Kakui K, Takemura M, et al., Possible role of placental leptin in pregnancy: a review. Endocrine 2002;19: 65–71.

Schaeffer L, Gohlke H, Muller M, Heid IM, Palmer LJ, et al., Common genetic variants of the FADS1 FADS2 gene cluster and their reconstructed haplotypes are associated with the fatty acid composition in phospholipids. Hum Mol Genet 2006;15: 1745–56.

Sjogren P, Sierra-Johnson J, Gertow K, Rosell M, Vessby B, et al., Fatty acid desaturases in human adipose tissue: relationships between gene expression, desaturation indexes and insulin resistance. Diabetologia 2008;51: 328–35.

Sprecher H, An update on the pathways of polyunsaturated fatty acid metabolism. Curr Opin Clin Nutr Metab Care 1999;2: 135–8.

Su HM, Huang MC, Saad NM, Nathanielsz PW, Brenna JT, Fetal baboons convert 18:3n-3 to 22:6n-3 in vivo. A stable isotope tracer study. J Lipid Res 2001;42: 581–6.

Sutton MS, Theard MA, Bhatia SJ, Plappert T, Saltzman DH, et al., Changes in placental blood flow in the normal human fetus with gestational age. Pediatr Res 1990;28: 383–7.

Szajewska H, Horvath A, Koletzko B, Effect of n-3 long-chain polyunsaturated fatty acid supplementation of women with low-risk pregnancies on pregnancy outcomes and growth measures at birth: a meta-analysis of randomized controlled trials. Am J Clin Nutr 2006;83: 1337–44.

Tanaka T, Shen J, Abecasis GR, Kisialiou A, Ordovas JM, et al., Genome-wide association study of plasma polyunsaturated fatty acids in the InCHIANTI Study. PLoS Genet 2009;5: e1000338.

Trak-Fellermeier MA, Brasche S, Winkler G, Koletzko B, Heinrich J, Food and fatty acid intake and atopic disease in adults. Eur Respir J 2004;23: 575–82.

Transler C, Eilander A, Mitchell S, van de Meer N, The impact of polyunsaturated fatty acids in reducing child attention deficit and hyperactivity disorders. J Atten Disord 2010; [E-pub ahead of print].

US Department of Agriculture ARS, USDA National Nutrient Database for Standard Reference, Release 22. USDA; 2009.

US Department of Health and Human Services, US Environmental Protection Agency, What you need to know about mercury in fish and shellfish. 2004.

Udell T, Gibson RA, Makrides M, PUFA Study Group, The effect of alpha-linolenic acid and linoleic acid on the growth and development of formula-fed infants: A systematic review and meta-analysis of randomized controlled trials. Lipids 2005;40: 1–11.

Werkman SH, Carlson SE, A randomized trial of visual attention of preterm infants fed docosa-hexaenoic acid until nine months. Lipids 1996;31: 91–7.

Wijendran V, Bendel RB, Couch SC, Philipson EH, Cheruku S, et al., Fetal erythrocyte phospho-lipid polyunsaturated fatty acids are altered in pregnancy complicated with gestational diabetes mellitus. Lipids 2000;35: 927–31.

Wijendran V, Huang MC, Diau GY, Boehm G, Nathanielsz PW, et al., Efficacy of dietary arachi-donic acid provided as triglyceride or phospholipid as substrates for brain arachidonic acid accretion in baboon neonates. Pediatr Res 2002;51: 265–72.

Wu G, Bazer FW, Cudd TA, Meininger CJ, Spencer TE, Maternal nutrition and fetal development. J Nutr 2004;134: 2169–72.

Xie L, Innis SM, Genetic variants of the FADS1 FADS2 gene cluster are associated with altered (n-6) and (n-3) essential fatty acids in plasma and erythrocyte phospholipids in women during pregnancy and in breast milk during lactation. J Nutr 2008;138: 2222–8.

Yannicelli S, Ryan A, Improvements in behaviour and physical manifestations in previously untreated adults with phenylketonuria using a phenylalanine-restricted diet: a national survey. J Inherit Metab Dis 1995;18: 131–4.

15.3 Omega-3 polyunsaturated fatty acids and cardiovascular disease

Natalie D. Riediger

15.3.1 Introduction

Omega-3 fatty acids and their role in health have been investigated for over 50 years (Kromann and Green, 1980). Much of the early work on omega-3 fatty acids has been focused on fish-derived omega-3 fatty acids, which include the long-chain eicosapen-taenoic acid (C20:5 n-3; EPA) and docosahexaenoic acid (C22:6 n-3; DHA). Significant sources of long chain omega-3 fatty acids are mostly limited to marine sources such as salmon, mackerel and sardines (Gebauer et al., 2006). The inverse relation between omega-3 fatty acid intake and cardiovascular risk has been known for some time. Early studies indicated Canadian Inuit had a low rate of cardiovascular disease despite high total fat intake, which was attributed to the high fatty fish intake of this northern popu-lation (Kromann and Green, 1980). Over the past decade increased health research surrounding the short chain omega-3 fatty acid, alpha-linolenic acid (C18:3 n-3; ALA), has occurred. The main reasons are that ALA could be an effective alternative to the long-chain omega-3 fatty acids, which might be limited by seafood allergy, organo-leptic properties, vegetarianism and safety for some owing to high levels of mercury in food sources (Gebauer et al., 2006). Natural sources of ALA are mostly plant-based, including flaxseed, canola oil, soybean oil and walnuts (Gebauer et al., 2006). Recently, several functional foods containing omega-3 fatty acids (either as ALA or EPA/DHA) have been created, such as omega-3 enriched eggs, milk, yogurt, spreads and others.

Public nutrition recommendations include omega-3 fatty acids and fish intake, not only because omega-3 fatty acids are essential, but also to obtain the additional cardio-vascular and other health-related benefits. It must be noted that ALA can be converted to EPA and DHA endogenously, therefore only ALA is considered an essential fatty acid. However, the conversion of ALA to EPA and/or DHA is limited (Gerster, 1998), particularly to DHA. The pathway for the conversion of ALA to EPA and DHA has been described elsewhere (Sprecher, 2002) and is not necessary for the understanding of omega-3 fatty acids in the context of this chapter. The Dietary Reference Intakes (DRIs), used in both the USA and Canada, indicate a Recommended Dietary Allowance for omega-3 fatty acids of 1.6 g/day for adult males and 1.1 g/day for adult females; the type of omega-3 fatty acid is not distinguished (National Academy of Sciences, 2002). Furthermore, the American Heart Association Nutrition Committee and Canada's Food Guide recommends consuming at least two servings of fish per week, with an emphasis on oily fish (Lichtenstein et al., 2006). Recommendations from other countries have been summarized by Gebauer et al. (2006). Separate DRI recommendations for EPA and DHA are in the process of being established; the literature supports a DRI of 500 mg/day for EPA and DHA (Harris et al., 2009).

Despite these recommendations, omega-3 fatty acid intake at the population level is considered inadequate. According to a longitudinal trial with over 12 000 male participants, the average intake of long-chain omega-3 fatty acids was approximately 175 mg/day, with 20% reporting no intake (Dolecek and Granditis, 1991). The Japanese population, which typically has had a high omega-3 fatty acid intake, has also reduced their omega-3 fatty acid intake, because of their influence by western culture (Sugano and Hirahara, 2000). In addition, populations with increased needs for omega-3 fatty acid intake, i.e., pregnant women and infants, are also reported to have low consumption (Innis and Elias, 2003).

Cardiovascular disease is the leading cause of death in developing countries. Its pathogenesis is multi-factorial; plasma lipid profile, inflammatory state, hypertension, atherosclerosis and arrhythmia all influence the development and outcomes of cardiovascular disease and could be influenced by omega-3 fatty acid intake. This chapter will review epidemiological and clinical evidence surrounding omega-3 fatty acids, both long-chain (EPA and DHA) and short-chain (ALA), and cardiovascular disease. Mechanisms of omega-3 fatty acids and their cardiovascular benefits are outside the scope of this chapter and will not be discussed in detail. The long chain omega-3 fatty acids, EPA and DHA, and their sources will be discussed separately from research involving ALA because of their differences in sources and efficacy regarding reducing cardiovascular risk.

15.3.2 Dietary intake of omega-3 fatty acids and epidemiological evidence

Epidemiological evidence of associations between EPA and DHA and reduced cardiovascular risk has provided the rationale for many clinical studies conducted in this area. The Physicians' Health Study revealed that fish intake (excluding fish oil supplement use) was associated with reduced risk of sudden cardiac death, but not myocardial infarction, after adjusting for relevant risk factors, even though fish intake was also associated with history of hypertension and high cholesterol (Albert et al., 1998). Conversely, another prospective cohort study, the Chicago Western Electric Study, reported an inverse association between fish intake and both myocardial infarction and all coronary heart disease, but not sudden cardiac death (Daviglus et al., 1997). These studies as well as many other major epidemiological and clinical studies on fish oil were conducted in male populations; Hu et al. (2002) was the first to report this inverse association between fish and coronary heart disease death among women as part of the Nurses' Follow-up Study. This association remained significant after adjusting for age and other relevant cardiovascular risk factors. Other epidemiological studies also support a role of reduced cardiovascular risk with EPA/DHA intake (Mozaffarian et al., 2005).

Population studies including ALA intake and cardiovascular risk have also been conducted. High ALA intake significantly reduced risk of non-fatal myocardial infarction among men with little or no EPA/DHA intake but not among men with high EPA/DHA intake (Mozaffarian et al., 2005); furthermore, ALA intake was not associated with reduced risk of non-fatal myocardial infarction or total coronary heart disease among approximately 45 000 male health professionals (Mozaffarian et al., 2005). In the Nurse's Health Study, intake of ALA was inversely associated with fatal ischemic heart disease but not non-fatal myocardial infarction, other non-sudden fatal cardiac events or non-fatal myocardial infarction (Hu et al., 1999; Albert et al., 2005). Among men at cardiovascular risk followed for 6–8 years, both EPA/DHA and ALA intake, assessed from 24-h recall, were significantly and inversely associated with all cause mortality, coronary heart disease, and all other cardiovascular disease deaths (Dolecek, 1992). By contrast, Oomen et al. (2001) did not report a significant relation between ALA intake and any measure of cardiovascular disease. A meta-analysis of observational studies and clinical trials revealed a reduced risk of fatal coronary heart disease in those with higher ALA intakes, although the risk of prostate cancer was significantly increased (Brouwer et al., 2004).

15.3.3 Plasma lipids

Cardiovascular benefits from omega-3 fatty acids could be mediated through beneficial modifications in plasma lipid profile, particularly plasma triglyceride (TG). For example, supplementation with 4 g/day of EPA reduced plasma concentrations of TG by 23% in mildly hyperlipidemic subjects (Mori et al., 2000), and by 12% in healthy subjects (Grimsgaard et al., 1997). Supplementation with as little as 1 g/day of DHA alone or in combination with EPA (1252 mg total) in hypertriglyceridemic subjects resulted in similar reductions in plasma TG levels (21.8%) (Schwellenbach et al., 2006). In addition, Kris-Etherton et al. (2003) reported that supplementation with 2–4 g/day of EPA+DHA can lower plasma TG levels by approximately 25–30% in hypertriglyceridemic patients. It should be noted that other clinical trials (Yamamoto et al., 1995; Sanders et al., 2006) did not report significant TG-lowering effects. The TG-lowering effects of omega-3 fatty acids might be related to baseline values because reduction in plasma TG seems to be greater among participants with higher baseline values.

Elevated low density lipoprotein cholesterol (LDL-C) and apoB levels have been observed with DHA supplementation (Kestin et al., 1990; Goyens and Mensink, 2006). However, long-chain omega-3 fatty acids have been shown to increase LDL particle size (Mori et al., 2000; Contacos et al., 1993). Contacos et al. (1993), observed a 1 nm increase in the diameter of LDL particles after consumption of 3 g/day fish oil for 6 weeks. Kelley et al. (2007) also observed a significant 21% reduction in the number of small, dense LDL particles and a 0.6 nm increase in LDL particle size in hypertriglyceridemic men receiving 3 g/day DHA. The increase in LDL particle size could explain the increased LDL-C levels observed in some clinical trials (Kestin et al., 1990; Sanders et al., 2006). Therefore, apoB levels should also be measured when LDL is assessed. Overall, influences of EPA/DHA on LDL-C appear inconsistent whereas changes in particle size seem to be key. The influence of EPA/DHA on plasma high-density lipoprotein cholesterol

(HDL-C) is inconsistent. Some studies have shown increases, although small, in HDL-C as a result of long-chain omega-3 fatty acid intake in humans (Calabresi et al., 2004; Breslow, 2006).

The effect of ALA on plasma lipids is not as consistent, nor as strong as EPA/DHA, particularly in regards to plasma TG. Among hypercholesterolemic participants 30–70 years old receiving an average of 6.3 g of ALA/day compared with 1 g/day in the control group in the form of margarine for 2 years, did not have significantly different levels of total cholesterol, TG, HDL-C, LDL-C, blood pressure or BMI (Bemelmans et al., 2002). Daily supplementation of just over 10 g/day of ALA for 6 weeks among males between 18–35 years old also did not significantly alter any plasma lipids compared with baseline or compared with linoleic acid (Pang et al., 1998). Several studies have also noted no significant difference in changes in plasma lipids with ALA supplementation compared with EPA/DHA, with the exception of TG (Finnegan et al., 2003ab; Egert et al., 2007). However, among male dyslipidemic participants, linseed oil supplementation with 8 g/day ALA for 3 months significantly reduced HDL cholesterol compared with baseline (Rallidis et al., 2003).

15.3.4 Blood pressure

EPA/DHA could also play a role in the regulation of blood pressure (Mozaffarian et al., 2007). A meta-analysis of 36 trials with fish oil supplementation showed a weighted reduction of 2.09 mmHg and 1.63 mmHg for systolic and diastolic blood pressure, respectively (Geleijnse et al., 2002). Several factors including the dose of fish oil, concurrent use of medications, an inadequate sample size, population type, choice of placebo oil, and inadequate statistical power might be the reasons for a lack of anti-hypertensive effects of EPA/DHA observed in other studies (Wing et al., 1990; Kelley et al., 2007). Evidence is accumulating that ALA might also have anti-hypertensive effects (Takeuchi et al., 2007; Sioen et al., 2009). The mechanism by which omega-3 fatty acid might exert its anti-hypertensive effects is not completely understood and probably involves several mechanisms including improving endothelial function by way of the series 3 eicosanoids or nitric oxide and by also reducing atherosclerosis. The potential mechanisms have been reviewed in more detail by Abeywardena and Head (2001).

15.3.5 Inflammatory factors

The effect of long chain omega-3 fatty acids that applies to several adverse health conditions including cardiovascular disease is their anti-inflammatory activities. Improvements in production or gene-expression (by either an increase or decrease) of specific cytokines in response to dietary EPA/DHA including interleukin-1β(IL-1β), interleukin-6 (IL-6), tumor necrosis factor-α(TNF-α), and adiponectin have been reported (Endres et al., 1989; Caughey et al., 1996; James et al., 2000; Duda et al., 2009). However, results have not been consistent. Neither purified EPA nor DHA given at 4 g/day for 6 weeks to subjects with type 2 diabetes significantly decreased IL-6 or C-reactive protein (CRP) levels, but both fatty acids reduced the levels of TNF-α by 25% (Mori et al., 2003). Conversely, dietary DHA supplementation in healthy subjects reduced exercise-induced inflammation by decreasing CRP and IL-6 (Philips et al., 2003). ALA has also been shown to decrease inflammation although not as consistently and by as great a margin. Among male dyslipidemic participants, linseed oil supplementation with 8 g/day ALA for 3 months significantly reduced CRP, serum amyloid A and IL-6 (Rallidis et al., 2003). The effect of both types of omega-3 fatty acid on other cytokines and the role these markers play in the development of cardiovascular disease has yet to be fully investigated.

15.3.6 Atherosclerosis

Some of the above mentioned anti-inflammatory effects of omega-3 fatty acids could suggest prevention of atherosclerosis. Therefore, a reduction in atherosclerosis might be secondary to other influences of omega-3 fatty acids. An epidemiological study by Hino et al. (2004) showed an inverse association between long-chain omega-3 fatty acid intake and carotid intima-media thickness, a marker of atherosclerosis, using ultrasonography. Patients with previously diagnosed coronary heart disease receiving 1.5 g/day of omega-3 fatty acids (ALA, EPA and DHA together) for 2 years showed a greater degree of regression of atherosclerosis and less progression compared with participants receiving placebo (Von Schacky et al., 1999). In addition, Thies et al. (2003) have shown that long-chain omega-3 fatty acid intake enhances plaque stability. However, despite some positive results, two large randomized controlled clinical trials failed to show that omega-3 fatty acids prevent restenosis following angioplasty (Leaf et al., 1994; Johansen et al., 1999). Some of the anti-atherosclerotic associations of dietary omega-3 fatty acids that have been reported (Hino et al., 2004) could be owing to their beneficial impacts on platelet activities. In light of this, a 35% decline in platelet-monocyte aggregates was reported after supplementing diets of 14 healthy subjects with 500 g/week of fish oil for 4 weeks (Din et al., 2008). Others have also reported a reduction in platelet aggregation and platelet count following long-chain omega-3 fatty acid intake (Mori et al., 1997). By contrast, ALA alone has not been shown to reduce atherosclerosis or platelet aggregation. In this regard, among Japanese elderly subjects increasing ALA by 3 g/day by switching from soybean oil to perilla oil did not reduce platelet aggregation or plasma fibrinogen (Ezaki et al., 1999). Lastly, there have not been any studies conducted on primary prevention of atherosclerosis with omega-3 fatty acid supplementation. One important barrier is the extensive follow-up time needed to assess atherosclerotic lesions in patients without any previous cardiovascular disease or hyperlipidemia.

15.3.7 Arrhythmia

Many of the beneficial effects on cardiovascular outcomes are thought to be related to the incorporation of DHA and EPA into cardiac cell membranes and their consequent antiarrhythmic effect (Kang and Leaf, 1995). Mozaffarian et al. (2006) has observed slower heart rates, reduced atrioventricular conduction, and lower risk of prolonged ventricular repolarization in participants with higher fish consumption compared with those with the lowest fish intake. Improvement in vagal control by fish consumption could partially explain improved endothelial function and reduced resting heart rate after fish oil supplements in a randomized study with healthy men and women (Shah et al., 2007). Additionally, consuming 3 g/day of encapsulated fish oil for 6 weeks reduced inducible ventricular tachycardia and risk of sudden cardiac death among patients with coronary artery disease (Metcalf et al., 2008). Generally, observational studies support the theory of reduced risk of

Tab 15.6: Summary of major clinical randomized controlled trials on omega-3 fatty acids, both long- and short chain, and cardiovascular risk.

Reference	Subjects (n)[a]	Dose (g)	Duration	Outcomes
Egert et al. (2009)	Normolipidemic non-obese men (27) and women (48)	4.4 g/day ALA; 2.2 g/day EPA; 2.3 g/day DHA	6 weeks	– Serum total and LDL cholesterol did not significantly change in any group – Serum TG significantly decreased in the EPA group ($p < 0.001$), DHA group ($p < 0.001$), and ALA group ($p < 0.05$) – Serum HDL was significantly increased in the DHA group ($p < 0.001$), but not EPA or ALA groups
Finnegan et al. (2003a,b)	Moderately hyperlipidemic adults (25–72 years) (150)	4.5 g/day ALA; 9.5 g/day ALA; 0.8 g/day EPA+DHA; 1.7 g/day EPA+DHA; control: low omega-3	6 months	– Change in plasma TG from baseline to 6 months (reduction) was significantly greater in the 1.7 g EPA+DHA group than the change in the 9.5 g ALA group – Although changes in TC, LDL, HDL, apoB, glucose and insulin compared with baseline were noted for some groups, there was no significant difference in percent difference between any groups – LDL oxidation was significantly reduced after 2 and 6 months in the 1.7 g EPA+DHA group compared with baseline and control, moderate and high ALA groups – No significant difference in coagulation or fibrinolytic factors between groups
Egert et al. (2007)	Healthy male (17) and female (44) students	6.0 g/day ALA; 2.8 g/day EPA; 2.9 g/day DHA	3 weeks	– Serum VLDL, LDL and HDL did not significantly change in any group – Serum TG did not change in the EPA or DHA group but significantly ($p < 0.05$) increased in the ALA group – Results of several tests regarding LDL oxidation were conflicting, DHA appeared to promote oxidation whereas ALA did not
Kestin et al. (1990)	Normotensive and mildly hypercholesterolemic men (33)	14 g/day linoleic acid; 9 g/day ALA; 3.4 g/day EPA+DHA	6 weeks	– EPA/DHA group had significant decrease in plasma VLDL, TG and systolic blood pressure and increase in LDL compared with baseline – Linoleic acid and ALA groups had significant reductions in total cholesterol

(Continued)

Tab 15.6 (*Continued*)

Reference	Subjects (*n*)[a]	Dose (g)	Duration	Outcomes
Wensing et al. (1999)	Healthy adults less than 35 years old (12) and 60 years and older (38)	Oleic acid control group; 6.8 g ALA/day; 1.05 g EPA+0.55 g DHA/day	6 weeks	– None of the diets significantly affected collagen-induced platelet aggregation or plasma thromboxane B2 – *Ex vivo* platelet aggregation was significantly prolonged in the EPA/DHA group compared with oleic acid ($p = 0.004$) or ALA ($p = 0.006$) groups – Effects of ALA were not age-dependent
Goyens and Mensink (2006)	Elderly aged 60–78 years (37)	Oleic acid control group; 6.8 g ALA/day; 1.05 g EPA+0.55 g DHA/day	6 weeks	– Total cholesterol and HDL were not significantly different between the groups – Compared with the ALA group, the EPA/DHA diet significantly increased LDL ($p < 0.05$) and increased apoB compared with both ALA ($p = 0.005$) and oleic acid ($p < 0.005$) groups – Serum TG was non-significantly reduced in the EPA/DHA group compared with both ALA and oleic acid groups – Tissue factor pathway inhibitor, which reduces platelet aggregation, was significantly increased in the EPA/DHA group compared with the ALA group – There was no significant difference in markers of endothelial function between the dietary groups

ALA, alpha-linolenic acid; DHA, docosahexaenoic acid; EPA, eicosapentaenoic acid; HDL, high-density lipoprotein; LDL, low-density lipoprotein; TC, total cholesterol; TG, triglycerides; VLDL, very low-density lipoprotein.

arrhythmia as a result of fish intake because of the inverse association between fish intake and sudden cardiac death (which are mostly accounted for by arrhythmia), but not myocardial infarction (Albert et al., 1998). However, there is also evidence against an antiarrhythmic effect of fish oil from the epidemiological Rotterdam Study (Brouwer et al., 2006) and a clinical trial among patients with implantable defibrillators (Raitt et al., 2005).

Little clinical research of dietary ALA on arrhythmia has been completed and the research reported is inconsistent. Among men, ALA content in platelets, which approximates ALA dietary intake, was not associated with heart rate variability (a precursor to arrhythmia) (Christensen et al., 2000); however, ALA measured in adipose tissue was associated with reduced risk of arrhythmia according to heart rate variability among women with suspected coronary artery disease (Christensen et al., 2005). However, ALA tissue content might not be the best marker for measurement because the conversion of ALA to DHA in heart tissue is what is hypothesized to be part of the mechanism for the antiarrhythmic effect of omega-3 fatty acids. More research is needed to confirm the existence and extent of a possible antiarrhythmic effect of ALA.

15.3.8 Randomized controlled trials

Many randomized controlled trials have been discussed throughout this chapter as they pertain to a respective cardiovascular risk factor. Overall, many trials with EPA/DHA and ALA supplements can be regarded as successful. Some important aspects of success of a trial by reducing cardiovascular risk include dose, type of omega-3 fatty acid (EPA vs DHA vs ALA), duration of treatment, inclusion criteria and variability of participants. Overall, clinical trials consistently show a greater reduction in cardiovascular risk in participants consuming EPA and/or DHA compared with ALA. This is attributed to the fact that the mechanism of some of the beneficial effects of ALA requires that ALA be converted to EPA and DHA, of which the conversion is limited. A summary of major clinical trials comparing cardiovascular risk factors following both EPA/DHA and ALA supplementation is outlined in ▶Tab. 15.6.

15.3.9 Conclusions

Dietary omega-3 fatty acids appear to be beneficial in regards to cardiovascular health by improving plasma lipid profile, reducing inflammation, reducing hypertension, preventing arrhythmia, and potentially slowing atherosclerosis. Research continues to support a more potent effect of EPA and DHA on reducing cardiovascular risk compared with that of ALA. ALA might only have cardiovascular benefit in those consuming little EPA/DHA. Overall however, the influence of omega-3 fatty acids on cardiovascular risk appears to be modest. Omega-3 fatty acid intake is low among western populations. Therefore, strategies to increase omega-3 fatty acid intake should be implemented, with specific emphasis on populations with low intake and on sources of long-chain omega-3 fatty acids to achieve the greatest cardiovascular benefits.

References

Abeywardena MY, Head RJ, Longchain n-3 polyunsaturated fatty acids and blood vessel function. Cardiovasc Res 2001;52: 361–71.

Albert CM, Hennekens CH, O'Donnell CJ, Ajani UA, Carey VJ, Willett WC, Ruskin JN, Manson JE, Fish consumption and risk of sudden cardiac death. J Am Med Assoc 1998;279: 23–8.

Albert CM, Oh K, Whang W, Manson JE, Chae CU, Stampfer MJ, Willett WC, Hu FB, Dietary alpha-linolenic acid intake and risk of sudden cardiac death and coronary heart disease. Circulation 2005;112: 3232–8.

Bemelmans WJ, Broer J, Feskens EJ, Smit AJ, Muskiet FA, Lefrandt JD, Bom VJ, May JF, Meyboom-de Jong B, Effect of an increased intake of alpha-linolenic acid and group nutritional education on cardiovascular risk factors: the Mediterranean Alpha-linolenic Enriched Groningen Dietary Intervention (MARGARIN) study. Am J Clin Nutr 2002;75: 221–7.

Breslow JL, n-3 fatty acids and cardiovascular disease. Am J Clin Nutr 2006;83(Suppl): 1477S–82S.

Brouwer IA, Katan MB, Zock PL, Dietary alpha-linolenic acid is associated with reduced risk of fatal coronary heart disease, but increased prostate cancer risk: meta-analysis. J Nutr 2004;134: 919–22.

Brouwer IA, Heeringa J, Geleijnse JM, Zock PL, Witteman JC, Intake of very long-chain n-3 fatty acids from fish and incidence of atrial fibrillation. The Rotterdam Study. Am Heart J 2006;151: 857–62.

Calabresi L, Villa N, Canavesi M, Sirtori CR, James RW, Bernini F, Franceschini G, An omega-3 polyunsaturated fatty acid concentrate increases plasma high-density lipoprotein 2 cholesterol and paraoxonase levels in patients with familial combined hyperlipidemia. Metabolism 2004;53: 153–8.

Caughey GE, Mantzioris E, Gibson RA, Cleland LG, James MJ, The effect on human tumor necrosis factor α and interleukin1 β production of diets enriched in n-3 fatty acids from vegetable oil or fish oil. Am J Clin Nutr 1996;63: 116–22.

Christensen JH, Christensen MS, Toft E, Dyerberg J, Schmidt EB, Alpha-linolenic acid and heart rate variability. Nutr Metab Cardiovasc Dis 2000;10: 57–61.

Christensen JH, Schmidt EB, Molenberg D, Toft E, Alpha-linolenic acid and heart rate variability in women examined for coronary artery disease. Nutr Metab Cardiovasc Dis 2005;15: 345–51.

Contacos C, Barter PJ, Sullivan DR, Effect of pravastatin and omega-3 fatty acids on plasma lipids and lipoproteins in patients with combined hyperlipidemia. Arterioscler Thromb 1993;13: 1755–62.

Daviglus ML, Stamler J, Orencia AJ, Dyer AR, Liu K, Greenland P, Walsh MK, Morris D, Shekelle RB, Fish consumption and the 30-year risk of fatal myocardial infarction. N Engl J Med 1997;336: 1046–53.

Din JN, Harding SA, Valerio CJ, Sarma J, Lyall K, Riemersma RA, Newby DE, Flapan AD, Dietary intervention with oil rich fish reduces platelet-monocyte aggregation in man. Atherosclerosis 2008;197: 290–6.

Dolecek TA, Epidemiological evidence of relationships between dietary polyunsaturated fatty acids and mortality in the Multiple Risk Factor Intervention Trial. Proc Soc Exp Biol Med 1992;200: 177–82.

Dolecek TA, Granditis G, Dietary polyunsaturated fatty acids and mortality in the multiple risk factor intervention trial (MRFIT). World Rev Nutr Diet 1991;66: 205–16.

Duda MK, O'Shea KM, Tintinu A, Xu W, Khairallah RJ, Barrows BR, Chess DJ, Azimzade AM, Harris WS, Sharov VG, Sabbah HN, Stanley WC, Fish oil, but not flaxseed oil, decreases inflammation and prevents pressure overload-induced cardiac dysfunction. Cardiovasc Res 2009;81: 319–27.

Egert S, Somoza V, Kannenberg F, Fobker M, Krome K, Erbersdobler HF, Wahrburg U, Influence of three rapeseed oil-rich diets, fortified with alpha-linolenic acid, eicosapentaenoic acid or docosahexaenoic acid on the composition and oxidizability of low-density lipoproteins: results of a controlled study in healthy volunteers. Eur J Clin Nutr 2007;61: 314–25.

Egert S, Kannenberg F, Somoza V, Erbersdobler HF, Wahrburg U, Dietary alpha-linolenic acid, EPA, and DHA have differential effects on LDL fatty acid composition but similar effects on serum lipid profiles in normolipidemic humans. J Nutr 2009;139: 861–8.

Endres S, Ghorbani R, Kelley VE, Georgilis K, Lonnemann G, van der Meer JW, Cannon JG, Rogers TS, Klempner MS, Weber PC, Schaefer EJ, Wolff SM, Dinarello CA, The effect of dietary supplementation with n-3 polyunsaturated fatty acids on the synthesis of interleukin-1 and tumor necrosis factor by mononuclear cells. N Engl J Med 1989;320: 265–71.

Ezaki O, Takahashi M, Shigematsu T, Shimamura K, Kimura J, Ezaki H, Gotoh T, Long-term effects of dietary alpha-linolenic acid from perilla oil on serum fatty acids composition and on the risk factors of coronary heart disease in Japanese elderly subjects. J Nutr Sci Vitaminol (Tokyo) 1999;45: 759–72.

Finnegan YE, Howarth D, Minihane AM, Kew S, Miller GJ, Calder PC, Williams CM, Plant and marine derived (n-3) polyunsaturated fatty acids do not affect blood coagulation and fibrinolytic factors in moderately hyperlipidemic humans. J Nutr 2003a;133: 2210–3.

Finnegan YE, Minihane AM, Leigh-Firbank EC, Kew S, Meijer GW, Muggli R, Calder PC, Williams CM, Plant- and marine-derived n-3 polyunsaturated fatty acids have differential effects on fasting and postprandial blood lipid concentrations and on the susceptibility of LDL to oxidative modification in moderately hyperlipidemic subjects. Am J Clin Nutr 2003b;77: 783–95.

Gebauer SK, Psota TL, Harris WS, Kris-Etherton PM, n-3 fatty acid dietary recommendations and food sources to achieve essentiality and cardiovascular benefits. Am J Clin Nutr 2006;83: 1526S–35S.

Geleijnse JM, Giltay EJ, Grobbee DE, Donders AR, Kok FJ, Blood pressure response to fish oil supplementation: meta-regression analysis of randomized trial. J Hypertens 2002;20: 1493–9.

Gerster H, Can adults adequately convert alpha-linolenic acid (18:3n-3) to eicosapentaenoic acid (20:5n-3) and docosahexaenoic acid (22:6n-3)? Int J Vitam Nutr Res 1998;68: 159–73.

Goyens PL, Mensink RP, Effects of alpha-linolenic acid versus those of EPA/DHA on cardiovascular risk markers in healthy elderly subjects. Eur J Clin Nutr 2006;60: 978–84.

Grimsgaard S, Bonaa KH, Hansen JB, Norday A, Highly purified eicosapentaenoic acid and docosahexaenoic acid in humans have similar triacylglycerol-lowering effects but divergent effects on serum fatty acids. Am J Clin Nutr 1997;66: 649–59.

Harris WS, Mozaffarian D, Lefevre M, Toner CD, Colombo J, Cunnane SC, Holden JM, Klurfeld DM, Morris MC, Whelan J, Towards establishing dietary reference intakes for eicosapentaenoic and docosahexaenoic acids. J Nutr 2009;139: 804S–19S.

Hino A, Adachi H, Toyomasu K, Yoshida N, Enomoto M, Hiratsuka A, Hirai Y, Satoh A, Imaizumi T, Very long chain n-3 fatty acids intake and carotid atherosclerosis: an epidemiological study evaluated by ultrasonography. Atherosclerosis 2004;176: 145–9.

Hu FB, Stampfer MJ, Manson JE, Rimm EB, Wolk A, Colditz GA, Hennekens CH, Willett WC, Dietary intake of alpha-linolenic acid and risk of fatal ischemic heart disease among women. Am J Clin Nutr 1999;69: 890–7.

Hu FB, Bronner L, Willett WC, Stampfer MJ, Rexrode KM, Albert CM, Hunter D, Manson JE, Fish and omega-3 fatty acid intake and risk of coronary heart disease in women. J Am Med Assoc 2002;287: 1815–21.

Innis SM, Elias SL, Intakes of essential n-6 and n-3 polyunsaturated fatty acids among pregnant Canadian women. Am J Clin Nutr 2003;77: 473–8.

James MJ, Gibson RA, Cleland LG, Dietary polyunsaturated fatty acids and inflammatory mediator production. Am J Clin Nutr 2000;71(Suppl): 343S–8S.

Johansen O, Brekke M, Sejeflot L, Abdelnoor M, Arnesen H, n-3 fatty acids do not prevent restenosis after coronary angioplasty: results from the CART study. Coronary Angioplasty Restenosis Trial. J Am Coll Cardiol 1999;33: 1619–26.

Kang JX, Leaf A, Prevention and termination of the β-adrenergic agonist-induced arrhythmias by free polyunsaturated fatty acids in neonatal rat cardiac myocytes. Biochem Biophys Res Commun 1995;208: 629–36.

Kelley DS, Siegel D, Vemuri M, Mackey BE, Docosahexaenoic acid supplementation improves fasting and postprandial lipid profiles in hypertriglyceridemic men. Am J Clin Nutr 2007;86: 324–33.

Kestin M, Clifton P, Belling GB, Nestel PJ, N-3 fatty acids of marine origin lower systolic blood pressure and triglycerides but raise LDL cholesterol compared with n-3 and n-6 fatty acids from plants. Am J Clin Nutr 1990;51: 1028–34.

Kris-Etherton PM, Harris WS, Appel LJ, Fish consumption, fish oil, omega-3 fatty acids, and cardiovascular disease. Arterioscler Thromb Vasc Biol 2003;23: 20–30.

Kromann N, Green A, Epidemiological studies in the Upernavik district, Greenland. Incidence of some chronic diseases 1950–1974. Acta Med Scand 1980;208: 401–406.

Leaf A, Jorgensen MB, Jacobs AK, Cote G, Schoenfeld DA, Scheer J, Weiner BH, Slack JD, Kellett MA, Raizner AE, Do fish oils prevent restenosis after coronary angioplasty? Circulation 1994;90: 2248–57.

Lichtenstein AH, Appel LJ, Brands M, Carnethon M, Daniels S, Franch HA, Franklin B, Kris-Etherton P, Harris WS, Howard B, Karanja N, Lefevre M, Rudel L, Sacks F, Van Horn L, Winston M, Wylie-Rosett J, Diet and lifestyle recommendations Revision 2006: a scientific statement from the American Heart Association Nutrition Committee. Circulation 2006;114: 82–96.

Metcalf RG, Sanders P, James MJ, Cleland LG, Young GD, Effect of dietary n-3 polyunsaturated fatty acids on the inducibility of ventricular tachycardia in patients with ischemic cardiomyopathy. Am J Cardiol 2008;101: 758–61.

Mori TA, Beilin LJ, Burke V, Morris J, Ritchie J, Interactions between dietary fat, fish, and fish oils and their effects on platelet function in men at risk of cardiovascular disease. Arterioscler Thromb Vasc Biol 1997;17: 279–86.

Mori TA, Burke V, Puddey IB, Watts GF, O'Neal DN, Best JD, Beilin LJ, Purified eicosapentaenoic and docosahexaenoic acids have differential effects on serum lipids and lipoproteins, LDL particle size, glucose, and insulin in mildly hyperlipidemic men. Am J Clin Nutr 2000;71: 1085–94.

Mori TA, Woodman RJ, Burke V, Puddey IB, Croftt KD, Beilin LJ, Effect of eicosapentaenoic acid and docosahexaenoic acid on oxidative stress and inflammatory markers, in treated-hypertensive Type 2 diabetic subjects. Free Rad Biol Med 2003;35: 772–81.

Mozaffarian D, Fish, n-3 fatty acids, and cardiovascular haemodynamics. J Cardiovasc Med (Hagerstown) 2007; 8: S23–6.

Mozaffarian D, Ascherio A, Hu FB, Stampfer MJ, Willett WC, Siscovick DS, Rimm EB, Interplay between different polyunsaturated fatty acids and risk of coronary heart disease in men. Circulation 2005;111: 157–64.

Mozaffarian D, Prineas RJ, Stein PK, Siscovick DS, Dietary fish and n-3 fatty acid intake and electrocardiographic parameters in humans. J Am Coll Cardiol 2006; 48: 478–84.

National Academy of Sciences, Institute of Medicine. Food and Nutrition Board. Dietary Reference Intakes for energy, carbohydrate, fiber, fat, fatty acids, cholesterol, protein, and amino acids (2002/2005). Accessed March 27, 2009 from http://www.iom.edu/Object.File/Master/7/300/Webtablemacro.pdf

Oomen CM, Ocké MC, Feskens EJ, Kok FJ, Kromhout D, alpha-linolenic acid intake is not beneficially associated with 10-y risk of coronary artery disease incidence: the Zutphen Elderly Study. Am J Clin Nutr 2001;74: 457–63.

Pang D, Allman-Farinelli MA, Wong T, Barnes R, Kingham KM, Replacement of linoleic acid with alpha-linolenic acid does not alter blood lipids in normolipidaemic men. Br J Nutr 1998;80: 163–7.

Philips T, Childs AC, Dreon DM, Phinney S, Leeuwenburgh C, A dietary supplement attenuates IL-6 and CRP after eccentric exercise in untrained males. Med Sports Exerc 2003;35: 2032–7.

Raitt MH, Connor WE, Morris C, Kron J, Halperin B, Chugh SS, McClelland J, Cook J, MacMurdy K, Swenson R, Connor SL, Gerhard G, Kraemer DF, Oseran D, Marchant C, Calhoun D, Shnider R, McAnulty J, Fish oil supplementation and risk of ventricular tachycardia and ventricular fibrillation in patients with implantable defibrillators: a randomized controlled trial. J Am Med Assoc 2005;293: 2884–91.

Rallidis LS, Paschos G, Liakos GK, Vellissaridou AH, Anastasiadis G, Zampelas A, Dietary alpha-linolenic acid decreases C-reactive protein, serum amyloid A and interleukin-6 in dyslipidaemic patients. Atherosclerosis 2003;167: 237–42.

Sanders TA, Gleason K, Griffin B, Miller GJ, Influence of an algal triacylglycerol containing docosahexaenoic acid (22:6n-3) and docosapentaenoic acid (22:5n-6) on cardiovascular risk factors in healthy men and women. Br J Nutr 2006;95: 525–31.

Schwellenbach LJ, Olson KL, McConnell KJ, Stolcpart RS, Nash JD, Merenich JA, The triglyceride-lowering effects of a modest dose of docosahexaenoic acid alone versus in combination with low dose eicosapentaenoic acid alone versus in combination with low dose eicosapentaenoic acid in patients with coronary artery disease and elevated triglycerides. J Am Coll Nutr 2006;25: 480–5.

Shah AP, Ichiuji AM, Han JK, Traina M, El-Bialy A, Meymandi SK, Wachsner RY, Cardiovascular and endothelial effects of fish oil supplementation in healthy volunteers. J Cardiovasc Pharmacol Ther 2007;12: 213–9.

Sioen I, Hacquebard M, Hick G, Maindiaux V, Larondelle Y, Carpentier YA, De Henauw S, Effect of ALA-enriched food supply on cardiovascular risk factors in males. Lipids 2009;44: 603–11.

Sprecher H, The roles of anabolic and catabolic reactions in the synthesis and recycling of polyunsaturated fatty acids. Prostaglandins Leukot Essent Fatty Acids 2002;67: 79–83.

Sugano M, Hirahara F, Polyunsaturated fatty acids in the food chain in Japan. Am J Clin Nutr 2000;71(Suppl): 189S–96S.

Takeuchi H, Sakurai C, Noda R, Sekine S, Murano Y, Wanaka K, Kasai M, Watanabe S, Aoyama T, Kondo K, Antihypertensive effect and safety of dietary alpha-linolenic acid in subjects with high-normal blood pressure and mild hypertension. J Oleo Sci 2007;56: 347–60.

Thies F, Garry JM, Yaqoob P, Rerkasem K, Williams J, Shearman CP, Gallagher PJ, Calder PC, Grimble RF, Association of n-3 polyunsaturated fatty acids with stability of atherosclerotic plaques: a randomised controlled trial. Lancet 2003;361: 477–85.

Von Schacky C, Angerer P, Kothny W, Theisen K, Mudra H, The effect of dietary omega-3 fatty acids on coronary atherosclerosis. A randomized, double-blind, placebo-controlled trial. Ann Intern Med 1999;130: 554–62.

Wensing AG, Mensink RP, Hornstra G, Effects of dietary n-3 polyunsaturated fatty acids from plant and marine origin on platelet aggregation in healthy elderly subjects. Br J Nutr 1999;82: 183–91.

Wing LM, Nestel PJ, Chalmers JP, Rouse I, West MJ, Bune AJ, Tonkin AL, Russell AE, Lack of effect of fish oil supplementation on blood pressure in treated hypertensives. J Hypertens 1990;34: 943–9.

Yamamoto H, Yoshimura H, Noma M, Suzuki S, Kai H, Tajimi T, Sugihara M, Kikuchi Y, Improvement of coronary vasomotion with eicosapentaenoic acid does not inhibit acetylcholine-induced coronary vasospasm in patients with variant angina. Jap Circ J 1995;59: 608–16.

15.4 The effects of omega-3 polyunsaturated fatty acids against cancer

Simona Serini; Idanna Innocenti; Elisabetta Piccioni; Gabriella Calviello

15.4.1 Introduction

The modifications which have taken place in dietary habits over the centuries have deeply changed the ratio of omega-3 (ω-3) to omega-6 (ω-6) polyunsaturated fatty acids (PUFAs) present in the diet (Simopoulos, 2006). Among western populations this change, which has taken place progressively since prehistoric times, has become dramatic over the past two centuries. That has been attributed to the progressive enrichment of the western diet with vegetable oils containing high levels of ω-6 PUFAs, accompanied by the concomitant decreased consumption of fish, rich in ω-3 PUFAs. All these variations in the diet could be related initially to changed socio-economic conditions, such as the industrialization and concentration of population in urban areas (Simopoulos, 2006), and, more recently, to the health recommendations that, by 1970s, had advised the public to avoid the consumption of animal fat because of its high content in deleterious saturated fatty acids and cholesterol (Kritchevsky, 2004). This might have led to dramatic effects on our health, because a low dietary ω-3/ω-6 PUFA ratio has been hypothesized (Simopoulos, 2006) to contribute to the promotion of many chronic diseases including cancer, which are occurring at an increasing rate among western populations. The development of some types of cancer, such as colon, breast and prostate cancer seems particularly related to the amount and type of fat ingested. For this reason considerable effort has been expended in searching whether any inverse association could exist between the increased intake of ω-3 PUFAs and the risk of these cancers. Plenty of results obtained by studying both animal models of cancer or cancer cells cultured *in vitro* concur to suggest a potential remarkable role for these dietary fatty acids as anticancer agents (Calviello et al., 2006). Several mechanistic studies have been performed with the aim of understanding which modifications in cellular functions and molecular pathways induced by these fatty acids could protect the cells from the deregulated growth which leads to cancer. In spite of all the encouraging results obtained, the picture deriving from the human studies, however, does not appear completely clear. The present chapter will deal with the antineoplastic effects of the long-chain ω-3 PUFAs, eicosapentaenoic acid (EPA) and docosahexaenoic acid (DHA), because they are the more widely ω-3 PUFAs studied and because there is large agreement on the efficacy of their antineoplastic action, at least according to the results of the experimental studies. Moreover, only mammary, prostate and colon cancers will be discussed, being, among the most frequent cancers, the most susceptible to the influence of dietary fat.

15.4.2 Epidemiological studies

Plenty of epidemiological studies have been conducted to evaluate the association existing between fish oil or ω-3 PUFA intake and mammary, prostate and colon cancer incidence and mortality. Generally, ample debate exists in this field owing to the conflicting results obtained.

The ecological studies generally have provided strong support to the hypothesis of a role for ω-3 PUFAs as powerful anticancer agents. Different ecological studies have reported an increased risk of breast, colon and prostate cancer among populations previously used to have a fat intake mainly of fish origin and then, in the past century, progressively shifted towards western fish-poor diets (Nielsen and Hansen, 1980; Karmali et al., 1987a; Lanier et al., 2001). Inverse association between incidence and mortality for breast cancer and intake of ω-3 PUFAs has also been supported by ecological cross-national studies performed in different countries (Guo et al., 1994; Hebert and Rosen, 1996). A beneficial effect of fish or fish oil intake has been also reported by two ecological studies which evaluated the mortality rate from colorectal cancer (Caygill and Hill, 1995; Caygill et al., 1996). In agreement, one large ecological study (Hebert et al., 1998) found an inverse association between fish intake and prostate cancer mortality.

These results are very close to those reported by another study conducted on six different Japanese populations that found an inverse relation between the serum level of ω-3 PUFAs and the risk of prostate cancer mortality (Kobayashi et al., 1999). Moreover, observations performed more than 10 years ago on Inuits, a population known for its fish-based diet, reported a risk of prostate cancer much lower than that exhibited by western populations, strongly suggesting that their ω-3 PUFA-rich diet could represent an important protective factor against this type of cancer (Prener et al., 1996). However, contrasting results were reported by a recent large ecological study (Colli and Colli, 2006) which analyzed the data relative to prostate cancer mortality obtained in more than 70 countries. In this study the intake of fish, together with other food categories, had been registered more than 10 years earlier, and no relations have been found with the prostate cancer mortality observed a decade later. In agreement, no relations were observed also in a recent cross-national study (Crowe et al., 2008b).

As far as the epidemiological observational studies are concerned, several of them, mainly having a case-control or a prospective cohort design, have clearly supported consistent inverse association between the increased intake of ω-3 PUFAs (as dietary supplements or fish servings) and the three types of cancers. However, an even larger number of studies have failed to show clear beneficial effects. This discrepancy could be related to many factors which might have influenced the outcomes of this type of studies such as: the method of evaluation of ω-3 PUFA intake (questionnaires or measure of biomarkers); the type of fish species (lean or fat) consumed by the population; the possible carcinogens which could be present in the fish tissues (owing to the fish cooking or to contaminants present in the sea waters of origin); the level of fish intake in the population under study (if it is lower or higher than that of other populations in different studies); etc. All the possible drawbacks have been recently analyzed in detail elsewhere (Calviello et al., 2006; Kimura, 2010). For example, as emphasized recently by Terry and colleagues (Terry et al., 2003; Terry and Mink, 2010), among the studies which evaluated the association between the consumption of fish and the risk for breast cancer, a scarce or null inverse association was found in those conducted in countries with low per-capita intake of fish. By contrast, some small studies implemented in countries with high per-capita fish intake reported interesting inverse associations. As already underlined, it should be noted that the amount of fish ingested is highly variable among countries, and that those subjects classified as 'high fish consumers' in one country might be considered 'low consumers' in another one. For instance, it has been calculated that the energy derived from fish fat is very low (0.2–0.3% of total energy) in western countries, whereas in Japan it is much higher (1.7%) (Sasaki et al., 1993). In the same manner, other than the amount of fish ingested also the features of the fish (i.e., if it is a fat or a lean fish) should been considered in these epidemiological studies. Interestingly, however, some of these studies on breast cancer found that the beneficial effect of fish intake could be better observed in premenopausal women, particularly those with estrogen receptor-negative breast cancer (Hislop et al., 1986, 1988). Inconsistent results have been obtained also when the risk for breast cancer has been studied in relation to the intake of EPA and DHA or to the EPA and DHA levels in serum, erythrocyte membranes or adipose tissues (Zhu et al., 1995; Chajès et al., 1999; Goodstine et al., 2003; Kuriki et al., 2007; Terry and Mink, 2010). Nevertheless, the increasing use of these biomarkers should be regarded as a notable advance for the epidemiological studies, and in particular the measure of adipose tissue EPA and DHA content, which allows a more objective identification of the long-term consumers of dietary ω-3 PUFAs. More agreement has been reached by those studies which investigated the possible inverse relation between the risk of breast cancer and the values of the dietary ω-3/ω-6 PUFA ratio (Terry and Mink, 2010). For this reason, it has been suggested that the increase in ω-3/ω-6 PUFA dietary ratio could beneficially affect the incidence of breast cancer more than the increase in the level of ω-3 PUFAs not accompanied by a concomitant decrease in ω-6 PUFAs (Bagga et al., 2002; Maillard et al., 2002; Simonsen et al., 1998; Kuriki et al., 2007; Terry and Mink, 2010).

The case-control studies performed to investigate the influence of dietary ω-3 PUFAs on colon cancer risk were based only on fish intake. Some showed an inverse significant association with colon cancer (Iscovich et al., 1992; Fernanadez et al., 1999; Kimura et al., 2007), whereas others failed to observe any association (Macquart-Moulin et al., 1986; Lee et al., 1989; Peters et al., 1992; Kimura, 2010). However, it is notable that, when observed and significant, the benefit of fish intake could be much improved by increasing the servings of fish from less than one to two per week to three to four per week (Franceschi et al., 1997; Fernandez et al., 1999; Yang et al., 2003). Interestingly, one of these case-control studies identified distal colon cancer as the more susceptible to the beneficial action of ω-3 PUFAs among the cancers of the large intestine (Kimura et al., 2007). Just a few cohort studies have found significant relations between higher fish consumption and reduced risk of colon cancer. Among these, it is particularly interesting the recent large European Prospective Investigation into Cancer and Nutrition study (EPIC) study, a large cohort study conducted in ten European countries, which underlined the decreased risk for colon cancer in those countries consuming more than 80 g fish per day as compared with those whose intake was less than 10 g fish per day (Norat et al., 2005). However, many of the prospective cohort studies performed so far have not supported the hypothesis of a decreased colon cancer risk with higher fish intake (for a review, see Kimura, 2010). In general, the results of the epidemiological studies on colon cancer give no more than strong suggestions of a decreased cancer risk with higher intake of fish or long chain ω-3 PUFAs.

Also, the numerous cohort and case-control studies aimed to establish the possible inverse association between fish or ω-3 PUFA intake and the risk of prostate cancer have so far failed to produce consistent results, as discussed in detail by Astorg in his exhaustive recent reviews on this topic (Astorg, 2004, 2010). As underlined by him, only a few of all these studies found a decreased risk of prostate cancer with higher intakes. However, encouraging strong associations were observed for metastatic or fatal prostate cancer in subjects consuming high levels of fish or EPA and DHA (Augustsson et al., 2003; Chavarro et al., 2008; Pham et al., 2009). Several studies have analyzed the association between the risk for prostate cancer and the level of several biomarkers, such as ω-3 PUFA levels in blood, erythrocytes, lipid component of serum and prostatic tissues, but mixed results have been obtained so far (for a review, see Astorg, 2010). Analyzing the most recent and largest among these studies, whereas two of them did not found any association (Park et al., 2009) or inverse associations for increased blood EPA and DHA level (Chavarro et al., 2007) and prostate cancer, the European EPIC study (Crowe et al., 2008a) demonstrated a significant positive association with the highest blood level of EPA and DHA. However, when the same population was analyzed not for the blood levels but for the intake of EPA and DHA no associations were observed (Crowe et al., 2008b). Particularly significant is, however, the finding reported by two recently published case control studies (Hedelin et al., 2007; Fradet et al., 2009) according to which some COX-2 polymorphisms could play a crucial role in the preventive effect of fish or ω-3 PUFA intake against prostate cancer. This suggests that the future direction for the epidemiological research in this field and for all types of cancers should be more aimed at the identification of sub-populations possessing specific genetic features which could result favorably sensitive to an increase in fish or ω-3 PUFAs in the diet. Moreover, more attention should also be paid in evaluating the different populations under study, when possible, not only on the basis of their ω-3 PUFA, EPA or DHA intake, which is often hard to calculate precisely. To avoid some of the possible pitfalls of these studies, it would be of great help if more objective biomarkers (ω-3 PUFA levels in serum lipids, red cell membranes or tissues) will be used, as it has been already done in many of the most recent studies. Finally, even though not strictly related to the main aim of this chapter, we have to briefly mention the number of epidemiological studies conducted to clarify whether the dietary intake of α-linolenic acid (ALA, C18:3 ω-3), a ω-3 PUFA with a carbon chain shorter than that of EPA and DHA, and whose dietary sources are mainly vegetables (particularly seed oils), could have a procarcinogenic effect on prostate. Several studies had initially found an increased risk of advanced prostate cancer associated with a high intake of ALA, which, however, was not confirmed by more recent studies (for more details on this point see, Astorg, 2010).

15.4.3 Experimental studies on animals and cultured cells

15.4.3.1 ω-3 PUFA-induced inhibition of tumor growth *in vivo*: animal studies

Three different types of animal models have been used to investigate the antitumor activity of ω-3 PUFAs and to study the molecular mechanisms involved: chemically-induced carcinogenesis in rat, transplanted tumor cells and genetic models of cancer induction.

It was observed that the treatment with fish oils inhibited the growth and incidence of mammary tumors in rats subject to the carcinogenic treatment with N-methyl-N-nitrosourea (NMU) (Jurkowski and Cave, 1985) or 12-dimethylbenz[a]anthracene (DMBA) (Braden and Carroll, 1986). Fish oil treatment in rats was shown to inhibit also the *in vivo* growth of the rat mammary tumor R3230AC (Karmali et al., 1984). Accordingly, the growth of MDA-MB-435 human cells injected in nude mice was strongly inhibited in mice supplemented with EPA and DHA (Rose et al., 1995). It was also demonstrated the ω-3 PUFA treatment inhibited also the metastatic ability of these human cells injected in nude mice (Rose and Connolly, 1993, 1996; Rose et al., 1995). The (MMTV)-HER-2/neu transgenic mouse model has been also used to assess the beneficial effect of ω-3 PUFA dietary treatments on breast cancer growth. These transgenic mice are highly suited to this purpose because they spontaneously develop breast cancer (Guy et al., 1992). It has also been shown that diets enriched with ω-3 PUFAs were able to increase the latency of tumor development as well as to decrease the multiplicity of the tumors which arise in these transgenic mice (Yee et al., 2005; Luijten et al., 2007).

Diets enriched with fish oils have also been shown to reduce the incidence and multiplicity of colon tumors induced by carcinogens such as azoxymethane (AOM) (Minoura et al., 1988; Reddy and Sugie, 1988; Deschner et al., 1990; Takahashi et al., 1994) and 1,2-dimethyl-hydrazine (DMH) (Lindner, 1991; Paulsen et al., 1998; Latham et al., 1999). Also EPA (Minoura et al., 1988) or DHA (Takahashi et al., 1994; Takahashi et al., 1997a,b) given separately to animals subject to colon chemical carcinogenesis showed the same efficiency as fish oils. In agreement, purified EPA or DHA administered to syngeneic mice implanted with the murine MAC16 or CC26 adenocarcinoma colon cells were able to inhibit both weight loss and tumor growth rate (Beck et al., 1991; Hudson et al., 1993; Iigo et al., 1997). The inhibition of metastatic foci formation was also observed when dietary ω-3 PUFAs or EPA alone were supplemented to rats injected with rat colon cancer cells (Iwamoto et al., 1998; Gutt et al., 2007). Furthermore, it has been reported that ω-3 PUFAs can inhibit the growth of human colon cancer cell lines injected in nude mice (Sakaguchi et al., 1990a,b; Boudreau et al., 2001; Kato et al., 2002, 2007; Calviello et al., 2004; Tsuzuki et al., 2004). Very useful in this respect is the transgenic animal model in which the mouse carries the *fat-1* gene from *Caenorhabditis elegans*. The *fat-1* gene encodes for the ω-3 desaturase from *C. elegans*, allowing the endogenous synthesis of ω-3 PUFAs also in mammalian cells (Kang et al., 2004). In the *fat-1* mice the suppression of AOM-induced colon carcinogenesis was observed (Nowak et al., 2007; Jia et al., 2008). Also the APC min/+mouse model, a genetic model of familial adenomatous polyposis, has been used for the same purpose. In this case the supplementation with fish oil reduced significantly the multiplicity and diameter of the tumors that usually arise in the small intestine of these mice (Paulsen et al., 1997).

In agreement with what was observed for breast and colon, diets enriched with ω-3 PUFAs markedly inhibited also the growth of human prostate cancer cell lines transplanted in athymic nude mice (Karmali, 1987b; Rose and Cohen, 1988). Also noteworthy is the study (Lu et al., 2008) performed recently by transfecting the *fat-1* gene into PC3 and DU145 human prostate cancer cells, and implanting the transfected cells in immunodeficient mice. The cells showed markedly reduced *in vivo* growth, clearly indicating the growth-inhibitory role exerted by increased levels of ω-3 PUFAs in cancer cells. The *PTEN* knockout mice is a transgenic mouse model that has been used (Berquin et al., 2007) to demonstrate the efficacy of a diet with an increased ω-3 PUFA/ω-6 PUFA ratio in inhibiting the growth of prostate cancer, a tumor which carries very frequently alterations in the PTEN tumor suppressor gene (Wang et al., 2003). Interestingly, in the same work the authors observed a reduced growth of prostate tumors also in the hybrid mice (*PTEN*-knockout plus *fat-1*) carrying the additional *fat-1* genetic manipulation, which endogenously was able to furnish their tissues with high levels of ω-3 PUFAs (Berquin 2007).

15.4.3.2 ω-3 PUFA inhibition of cancer cell growth *in vitro*: mechanisms of action

The *in vitro* studies, in addition to having clearly shown that the antitumor action of the long chain ω-3 PUFAs is based on their antiproliferative and pro-apoptotic effects, have also allowed to identify a series of possible mechanisms involved. In particular, they have made clear that the induction of apoptosis is crucial for the inhibition of cancer cell growth exerted by ω-3 PUFAs (Mengeaud et al., 1992; Calviello et al., 2005; Schley et al., 2005; Shaikh, 2008; Sun et al., 2008; Tanaka et al., 2008). Particularly, DHA seems to elicit the maximal pro-apoptotic effect (Calviello et al., 2006). Many of the molecular alterations induced by the ω-3 PUFAs in the cancer cells have been considered involved in their effects on cancer growth and apoptosis. Among these alterations, the increased cell lipid peroxidation induced by these fatty acids and the consequent induction of oxidative stress and oxidative adducts are the most often invoked mechanisms to explain the inhibitory effect of ω-3 PUFAs on breast, colon and prostate cancer cell growth *in vitro* (Latham et al., 2001; Baumgartner et al., 2004; Mahéo et al., 2005; van Beelen et al., 2007; Wang, et al., 2007; Pan et al., 2009).

A series of studies performed *in vitro* on these types of cancer cells have also shown that one of the main effects of ω-3 PUFA treatment is to decrease the intracellular levels of arachidonic acid (AA) and its oxygenated metabolites (Noguchi et al., 1995; Calviello et al., 2004; Swamy et al., 2004; Vang and Ziboh, 2005; Kolar et al., 2007). It is generally believed that these are key alterations which can contribute to the antitumoral action of ω-3 PUFAs, because some of the metabolites derived from the activity of cyclo-oxygenases (COX) and lipoxygenases (LOX) on AA exert strong pro-inflammatory and pro-carcinogen activities (Needleman et al., 1979; Gosh and Meyers, 1997; O'Flaherty et al., 2002; Fukuda et al., 2003). Moreover, EPA could function as a substrate for both COX and LOX enzymes, but the EPA-derived metabolites are biologically less active than those derived from AA, and might also antagonize their effects (Needleman et al., 1979; Yang et al., 2004).

Another possible mechanism through which long chain ω-3 PUFAs might act as soon as they become esterified in membrane phospholipids is their ability to alter many crucial properties of membranes such as acyl-chain order, fluidity and permeability (Stillwell and Wassall, 2003). This, as hypothesized by Stillwell and Wassall (2003), might be owed to the high degree of conformational flexibility that the multiple double bonds confer to the long-chain PUFA molecules, particularly to DHA, which makes them able to modify membranes and modulate their enzyme, carrier and receptor activities. The modifications induced could be particularly important at the level of those lipid microdomains in plasma membranes called lipid rafts or caveolae (London, 2002). After a ω-3 PUFA treatment, these fatty acids are incorporated in plasma membrane phospholipids changing raft lipid composition and functions (Webb et al., 2000; Ma et al., 2004; Chapkin et al., 2008). It was observed that dietary treatment of mice with ω-3 PUFAs was able to alter caveolae fatty acyl content and to reduce the levels of cholesterol and caveolin (Ma et al., 2004). Similarly, it has been reported that ω-3 PUFA treatment alters raft lipid composition modifying the EGF receptor expression in lipid rafts of human breast cancer cells cultured *in vitro* (Schley et al., 2007).

Finally, the alterations induced by ω-3 PUFAs in the expression of many molecular factors crucial in the regulation of breast, colon and prostate cancer cell growth are also thought to be involved in the tumor-inhibitory action of these fatty acids. The detailed description of them is not the purpose of this chapter, and numerous exhaustive reviews have been published on this topic (Larsson et al., 2004; Calviello et al., 2006, 2007b; Berquin et al., 2008). For this reason just a brief account of these molecular factors regulated by ω-3 PUFAs will be given here. First, among them, we can include several transcription factors, as well as some of their molecular components, such as the peroxisome proliferator-activated receptors (PPARs), β-catenin, hypoxia inducible factor 1-α (HIF-1α), nuclear sterol regulatory element-binding protein 1 (nSREBP1) and nuclear factor-κB (NF-κB) isoforms (Collett et al., 2001; Narayanan et al., 2001, 2004; Lee and Hwang, 2002; Edwards et al., 2004, 2008; Sun et al., 2005, 2008; Schønberg et al., 2006; Calviello et al., 2007a; Allred et al., 2008). Moreover, protein kinases and other key regulators of signal transduction should be mentioned here, such as different isozymes of protein kinase C (PKC), as well as PI3 kinase, p38,

ERK1/2, AKT/protein kinase B, and Ras (Moore et al., 2001; Calviello et al., 2004; Cha et al., 2005; Engelbrecht et al., 2008; Toit-Kohn et al., 2009). Cellular enzymes have been also reported to exert a crucial role in the ω-3 PUFA antitumoral action. Among them we can include the metabolic enzymes inducible nitric oxide synthase (iNOS), ornithine decarboxylase (ODC), and COX-2 (Chung et al., 2001; Narayanan et al., 2003; Calviello et al., 2004; Swamy et al., 2004), as well as matrix metalloproteinases (MMPs) (Calviello et al., 2007a). Finally, the list might include also those factors whose expression and activity is influenced by ω-3 PUFAs and which act as regulators of cell cycle progression, apoptosis, endoplasmic reticulum (ER) stress response, metastasis and angiogenesis. Among them there are: p21, cyclin D1 and E, (Narayanan et al., 2001; Danbara et al., 2004; Tsujita-Kyutoku et al., 2004), several caspases, Bcl-2 family of proteins, c-myc, the anti-apoptotic protein myeloid cell leukemia sequence-1 (Mcl-1), syndecan-1 (Narayanan et al., 2001; Chiu et al., 2004; Tsujita-Kyutoku et al., 2004; Calviello et al., 2005, 2007b; Hofmanová et al., 2005; Sun et al., 2008), eukaryotic initiation factor 2-α (eIF2α) (Jakobsen et al., 2008), survivin, vascular endothelial growth factor (VEGF), HIF-1α (Calviello et al., 2004, 2007a) and the chemokine receptor CXCR4 (Altenburg and Siddiqui, 2009).

15.4.4 Human trials

The strong body of evidence from epidemiological and experimental studies which suggest a protective role for ω-3 PUFAs against certain types of cancer such as colon, breast and prostate cancer have encouraged the implementation of human intervention trials. In this chapter we will analyze only the trials which evaluate the effects of increased intakes of fish or of supplementations of fish oils, EPA or DHA.

Different intervention trials are currently exploring the possible anti-neoplastic effect of ω-3 PUFAs against breast cancer (http://clinicaltrials.gov/ct2/results?term=breast+omega-3, October 09, 2009). One of them is analyzing the effect of ω-3 PUFA supplementations in preventing breast cancer in women at high risk of developing it (NCT00114296, October 09, 2009). The study is evaluating mammographic breast density, as well as cell atypia, cell proliferation and expression of estrogen-related proteins (using breast cells from ductal lavage specimens). Moreover, in this trial the alteration in the levels of circulating hormones and growth factors related to the incidence of breast cancer, as well as plasma lipid peroxidation markers are being also investigated. Another trial (NCT00627276, October 12, 2009) is a multicenter randomized phase II one, which is studying the effects of ω-3 capsule supplementations for 8 weeks in women with newly diagnosed ductal carcinoma *in situ* and/or atypical ductal hyperplasia. Among other parameters considered in this study it is very interesting the analysis of genetic markers for breast cancer risk and progression evaluated by microarray analysis on blood samples, as well as the analysis of the changes in fatty acid content evaluated in red blood cells and nipple aspirate. Finally, there is a very recently started study (March 2009) analyzing the possible synergistic chemopreventive effect of a combination of ω-3 fatty acids with a low dose of the antiestrogen Raloxifene (NCT00723398, October 12, 2009). The hypothesis from which this study originates is based on the positive findings of a large array of experimental studies, performed both *in vivo* and *in vitro*, which have clearly shown the potential for ω-3 PUFAs to reinforce the action of anti-neoplastic drugs (for a review, see Calviello et al., 2009).

As far as colon cancer is concerned, the first human interventional trials were performed in our laboratory during the early 1990s (Anti et al., 1992, 1994) by supplementing subjects at high risk for sporadic polyposis of colon for periods of 2 weeks or 2–3 months with EPA and DHA (7.8 g EPA+DHA/day or 2.5 g EPA+DHA/day, respectively). The abnormal pattern of proliferation of the rectal mucosal cells present in these patients and considered a marker of colon cancer risk, reverted to normal following the dietary supplementation, even after the shorter treatment. A further double-blind, crossover trial was conducted on healthy volunteers supplemented with fish oil (4.4 g ω-3 PUFAs/day) or corn oil for 4 weeks, and also in this case an antiproliferative effect of ω-3 PUFAs was observed (Bartram et al., 1993). A protective effect of a supplementation with high levels of ω-3 PUFAs (9 g/day) for 3 and 6 months to patients that had been resected for colon carcinoma or adenomatous polyps was also reported (Huang et al., 1996). Subsequently, it was also observed that a dietary switch towards increased levels of dietary ω-3 PUFAs and decreased levels of ω-6 PUFAs and fat in general for 2 years in the same type of patients increased the percentage of apoptotic cells in biopsies from sigmoid colon mucosa (Cheng et al., 2003). However, the recently published outcomes of FISHGASTRO, a multicenter randomized controlled trial, were not in agreement with those of the previous trials because it was observed that the increase in the consumption of either oil-rich or lean fish to two portions weekly over 6 months did not markedly change either the apoptotic and mitotic rates in the colonic mucosa (Pot et al., 2009). Moreover, published outcomes are not yet available for two recently completed trials (NCT00432913 and NCT00510692, http://clinicaltrials.gov/ct2/results?term=colon+omega-3, October 12, 2009) performed supplementing purified EPA to patients with a history of colonic adenoma or familial polyposis. They are much anticipated, because, in contrast to the previous trial, in these cases it is not the effect of a modified diet to be evaluated but the administration of a purified ω-3 PUFA (EPA). However, in our opinion, also the supplementation of purified DHA should be studied, because most of the experimental studies have shown that the strongest pro-apoptotic effect both *in vitro* and *in vivo* is elicited mainly by DHA (Calviello et al., 2007b).

As far as prostate cancer is concerned, a small short-term (3 months) intervention trial was performed treating men with untreated prostate cancer with a low-fat diet supplemented with fish oil. It was shown that the supplementation significantly increased the ω-3/ω-6 PUFA ratio in both plasma and gluteal adipose tissue and reduced the expression of COX-2 in prostate biopsies (Aronson et al., 2001). This is worth noting, because the overexpression of COX-2 has been observed in prostate cancer tissues (Gupta et al., 2000). Moreover, there are different ongoing intervention trials investigating the effects of a dietary supplementation with ω-3 PUFAs on patients showing precancerous condition or malignant prostate cancer (http://clinicaltrials.gov/ct2/results?term=prostate+omega-3, October 09, 2009). Depending on the design of the trial, the ω-3 PUFA supplements are furnished either alone (NCT00458549, October 9, 2009) or in combination with a diet enriched with a series of food components (tomatoes, grape juice, pomegranate juice, tomato, green tea, black tea, soy, selenium, NCT00433797, October 12, 2009). In other cases ω-3 PUFA supplements are given alone or together with green tea extracts at high content in cathechins (NCT00253643, October 13, 2009), lycopene (NCT00402285, October 13, 2009), or together with a low-fat diet enriched in vitamin E (NCT00798876, October 14, 2009). As soon as all the results will be available, we will be able to know the effect of such treatments on different markers which are being evaluated, such as the prostate tissue expression of insulin growth factor-1 (IGF-1), insulin growth factor binding proteins (IGFBPs), sterol regulatory element binding protein (SREBP), as well as the phosphorylation of eIF2α in prostate tissue and the tumor differentiation grade, evaluated by the Gleason score. The possible alterations of biomarkers of oxidative stress, antioxidant status, oxidative damage, inflammation, proliferation and apoptosis following the action of ω-3 PUFAs are being also investigated. Moreover, gene expression in prostate tissue from patients is being evaluated also using the DNA microarray technique, which could enlarge substantially our knowledge.

15.4.5 Conclusions

We can conclude that the study of the potential beneficial role of dietary ω-PUFAs against cancer represents a subject of intense debate in the literature. As far as long chain ω-3 PUFAs are concerned, positive results have been reported for different types of cancers, through experimental studies on animals or cultured cancer cells, by using both ω-PUFAs alone or in combination with other anti-neoplastic agents. These experimental studies have recently enabled remarkable advances in the comprehension of the possible mechanisms involved in the anticancer action of these fatty acids. Among the epidemiological studies the ecological surveys performed in different countries have generally confirmed the experimental laboratory studies. In agreement, a negative association between the dietary intake of these fatty acids and the risk of colon, breast and prostate cancer has been reported also by other epidemiological observational studies, mainly having a case-control or prospective cohort design. However, several of these studies have also failed to report any beneficial effect. This discrepancy could be related to many drawbacks which might affect this type of studies, as well as to the possibility that the occurrence of the beneficial effects of these fatty acids might be influenced by the genetic background of the patient. Moreover, at least for the hormone-related cancers, also the hormonal state of the patients under study (i.e., premenopausal or postmenopausal state) could play a role in determining the outcomes. Furthermore, so far, the number of published human interventional trials is too exiguous to clarify the potential of these fatty acids as preventive agents for cancer, even though different human interventional trials are already ongoing, particularly for prostate cancer, and their results are strongly awaited from the scientific community. In general, however, in our opinion more effort should be devoted designing new observational and analytical human studies to ascertain the actual potential role of these dietary compounds against cancer. Additional experimental studies are also required to further explore the molecular mechanisms underlying their beneficial antineoplastic effects.

References

Allred CD, Talbert DR, Southard RC, Wang X, Kilgore MW, PPARgamma1 as a molecular target of eicosapentaenoic acid in human colon cancer (HT-29) cells. J Nutr 2008;138: 250–6.

Altenburg JD, Siddiqui RA, Omega-3 polyunsaturated fatty acids down-modulate CXCR4 expression and function in MDA-MB-231 breast cancer cells. Mol Cancer Res 2009;7: 1013–20.

Anti M, Armelao F, Marra G, Percesepe A, Bartoli GM, Palozza P, et al., Effects of different doses of fish oil on rectal cell proliferation in patients with sporadic colonic adenomas. Gastroenterology 1994;107: 1709–18.

Anti M, Marra G, Armelao F, Bartoli GM, Ficarelli R, Percesepe A, et al., Effect of omega-3 fatty acids on rectal mucosal cell proliferation in subjects at risk for colon cancer. Gastroenterology 1992;103: 883–91.

Aronson WJ, Glaspy JA, Reddy ST, Reese D, Heber D, Bagga D, Modulation of omega-3/omega-6 polyunsaturated ratios with dietary fish oils in men with prostate cancer. Urology 2001;58: 283–8.

Astorg P, Dietary n-6 and n-3 polyunsaturated fatty acids and prostate cancer risk: a review of epidemiological and experimental evidence. Cancer Causes Control 2004;15: 367–86.

Astorg P, ω-3 Polyunsaturated fatty acids and prostate cancer: epidemiological studies. In: Calviello G, Serini S, editors. Dietary omega-3 polyunsaturated fatty acids and cancer. Dordrecht: Springer; 2010. In press.

Augustsson K, Michaud DS, Rimm EB, Leitzmann MF, Stampfer MJ, Willett WC, et al., A prospective study of intake of fish and marine fatty acids and prostate cancer. Cancer Epidemiol Biomarkers Prev 2003;12: 64–7.

Bagga D, Anders KH, Wang HJ, Glaspy JA, Long-chain n-3-to-n-6 polyunsaturated fatty acid ratios in breast adipose tissue from women with and without breast cancer. Nutr Cancer 2002;42: 180–5.

Bartram HP, Gostner A, Scheppach W, Reddy BS, Rao CV, Dusel G, et al., Effects of fish oil on rectal cell proliferation, mucosal fatty acids, and prostaglandin E2 release in healthy subjects. Gastroenterology 1993;105: 1317–22.

Baumgartner M, Sturlan S, Roth E, Wessner B, Bachleitner-Hofmann T, Enhancement of arsenic trioxide-mediated apoptosis using docosahexaenoic acid in arsenic trioxide-resistant solid tumor cells. Int J Cancer 2004;112: 707–12.

Beck SA, Smith KL, Tisdale MJ, Anticachectic and antitumor effect of eicosapentaenoic acid and its effect on protein turnover. Cancer Res 1991;51: 6089–93.

Berquin IM, Edwards IJ, Chen YQ, Multi-targeted therapy of cancer by omega-3 fatty acids. Cancer Lett 2008;269: 363–77.

Berquin IM, Min Y, Wu R, Wu J, Perry D, Cline JM, et al., Modulation of prostate cancer genetic risk by omega-3 and omega-6 fatty acids. J Clin Invest 2007;117: 1866–75.

Boudreau MD, Sohn KH, Rhee SH, Lee SW, Hunt JD, Hwang DH, Suppression of tumor cell growth both in nude mice and in culture by n-3 polyunsaturated fatty acids: mediation through cyclooxygenase-independent pathways. Cancer Res 2001;61: 1386–91.

Braden LM, Carroll KK, Dietary polyunsaturated fat in relation to mammary carcinogenesis in rats. Lipids 1986;21: 285–8.

Calviello G, Di Nicuolo F, Gragnoli S, Piccioni E, Serini S, Maggiano N, et al., n-3 PUFAs reduce VEGF expression in human colon cancer cells modulating the COX-2/PGE2 induced ERK-1 and -2 and HIF-1alpha induction pathway. Carcinogenesis 2004;25: 2303–10.

Calviello G, Di Nicuolo F, Serini S, Piccioni E, Boninsegna A, Maggiano N, et al., Docosahexaenoic acid enhances the susceptibility of human colorectal cancer cells to 5-fluorouracil. Cancer Chemother Pharmacol 2005;55: 12–20.

Calviello G, Serini S, Palozza P, n-3 Polyunsaturated fatty acids as signal transduction modulators and therapeutic agents in cancer. Curr Signal Transd Ther 2006;1: 255–71.

Calviello G, Resci F, Serini S, Piccioni E, Toesca A, Boninsegna A, et al., Docosahexaenoic acid induces proteasome-dependent degradation of beta-catenin, down-regulation of survivin and apoptosis in human colorectal cancer cells not expressing COX-2. Carcinogenesis 2007a;28: 1202–9.

Calviello G, Serini S, Piccioni E, n-3 polyunsaturated fatty acids and the prevention of colorectal cancer: molecular mechanisms involved. Curr Med Chem 2007b;14: 3059–69.

Calviello G, Serini S, Piccioni E, Pessina G, Antineoplastic effects of n-3 polyunsaturated fatty acids in combination with drugs and radiotherapy: preventive and therapeutic strategies. Nutr Cancer 2009;61: 287–301.

Caygill CP, Hill MJ, Fish, n-3 fatty acids and human colorectal and breast cancer mortality. Eur J Cancer Prev 1995;4: 329–32.

Caygill CP, Charlett A, Hill MJ, Fat, fish, fish oil and cancer. Br J Cancer 1996;74: 159–64.

Cha MC, Lin A, Meckling KA, Low dose docosahexaenoic acid protects normal colonic epithelial cells from araC toxicity. BMC Pharmacol 2005;5: 7.

Chajès V, Hultén K, Van Kappel AL, Winkvist A, Kaaks R, Hallmans G, et al., Fatty-acid composition in serum phospholipids and risk of breast cancer: an incident case-control study in Sweden. Int J Cancer 1999;83: 585–90.

Chapkin RS, Wang N, Fan YY, Lupton JR, Prior IA, Docosahexaenoic acid alters the size and distribution of cell surface microdomains. Biochim Biophys Acta 2008;1778: 466–71.

Chavarro JE, Stampfer MJ, Li H, Campos H, Kurth T, Ma J, A prospective study of polyunsaturated fatty acid levels in blood and prostate cancer risk. Cancer Epidemiol Biomarkers Prev 2007;16: 1364–70.

Chavarro JE, Stampfer MJ, Hall MN, Sesso HD, Ma J, A 22-y prospective study of fish intake in relation to prostate cancer incidence and mortality. Am J Clin Nutr 2008;88: 1297–303.

Cheng J, Ogawa K, Kuriki K, Yokoyama Y, Kamiya T, Seno K, et al., Increased intake of n-3 polyunsaturated fatty acids elevates the level of apoptosis in the normal sigmoid colon of patients polypectomized for adenomas/tumors. Cancer Lett 2003;193: 17–24.

Chiu LC, Wong EY, Ooi VE, Docosahexaenoic acid from a cultured microalga inhibits cell growth and induces apoptosis by upregulating Bax/Bcl-2 ratio in human breast carcinoma MCF-7 cells. Ann N Y Acad Sci 2004;1030: 361–8.

Chung BH, Mitchell SH, Zhang JS, Young CY, Effects of docosahexaenoic acid and eicosapentaenoic acid on androgen-mediated cell growth and gene expression in LNCaP prostate cancer cells. Carcinogenesis 2001;22: 1201–6.

Collett ED, Davidson LA, Fan YY, Lupton JR, Chapkin RS, n-6 and n-3 polyunsaturated fatty acids differentially modulate oncogenic Ras activation in colonocytes. Am J Physiol Cell Physiol 2001;280: C1066–75.

Colli JL, Colli A, International comparisons of prostate cancer mortality rates with dietary practices and sunlight levels. Urol Oncol 2006;24: 184–94.

Crowe FL, Allen NE, Appleby PN, Overvad K, Aardestrup IV, Johnsen NF, Fatty acid composition of plasma phospholipids and risk of prostate cancer in a case-control analysis nested within the European Prospective Investigation into Cancer and Nutrition. Am J Clin Nutr 2008a;88: 1353–63.

Crowe FL, Key TJ, Appleby PN, Travis RC, Overvad K, Jakobsen MU, et al., Dietary fat intake and risk of prostate cancer in the European Prospective Investigation into Cancer and Nutrition. Am J Clin Nutr 2008b;87: 1405–13.

Danbara N, Yuri T, Tsujita-Kyutoku M, Sato M, Senzaki H, Takada H, et al., Conjugated docosahexaenoic acid is a potent inducer of cell cycle arrest and apoptosis and inhibits growth of colo 201 human colon cancer cells. Nutr Cancer 2004;50: 71–9.

Deschner EE, Lytle JS, Wong G, Ruperto JF, Newmark HL, The effect of dietary omega-3 fatty acids (fish oil) on azoxymethanol-induced focal areas of dysplasia and colon tumor incidence. Cancer 1990;66: 2350–6.

Edwards IJ, Berquin IM, Sun H, O'Flaherty JT, Daniel LW, Thomas MJ, et al., Differential effects of delivery of omega-3 fatty acids to human cancer cells by low-density lipoproteins versus albumin. Clin Cancer Res 2004;10: 8275–83.

Edwards IJ, Sun H, Hu Y, Berquin IM, O'Flaherty JT, Cline JM, et al., In vivo and in vitro regulation of syndecan 1 in prostate cells by N-3 polyunsaturated fatty acids. J Biol Chem 2008;283: 18441–49.

Engelbrecht AM, Toit-Kohn JL, Ellis B, Thomas M, Nell T, Smith R, Differential induction of apoptosis and inhibition of the PI3-kinase pathway by saturated, monounsaturated and polyunsaturated fatty acids in a colon cancer cell model. Apoptosis 2008;13: 1368–77.

Fernandez E, Chatenoud L, La Vecchia C, Negri E, Franceschi S, Fish consumption and cancer risk. Am J Clin Nutr 1999;70: 85–90.

Fradet V, Cheng I, Casey G, Witte JS, Dietary omega-3 fatty acids, cyclooxygenase-2 genetic variation, and aggressive prostate cancer risk. Clin Cancer Res 2009;15: 2559–66.

Franceschi S, Favero A, La Vecchia C, Negri E, Conti E, Montella M, et al., Food groups and risk of colorectal cancer in Italy. Int J Cancer 1997;72: 56–61.

Fukuda R, Kelly B, Semenza GL, Vascular endothelial growth factor gene expression in colon cancer cells exposed to prostaglandin E2 is mediated by hypoxia-inducible factor 1. Cancer Res 2003;63: 2330–4.

Goodstine SL, Zheng T, Holford TR, Ward BA, Carter D, Owens PH, et al., Dietary (n-3)/(n-6) fatty acid ratio: possible relationship to premenopausal but not postmenopausal breast cancer risk in U.S. women. J Nutr 2003;133: 1409–14.

Guo WD, Chow WH, Zheng W, Li JY, Blot WJ, Diet, serum markers and breast cancer mortality in China. Jpn J Cancer Res 1994;85: 572–7.

Gupta S, Srivastava M, Ahmad N, Bostwick DG, Mukhtar H, Over-expression of cyclooxygenase in human prostate adenocarcinoma. Prostate 2000;42: 73–8.

Gutt CN, Brinkmann L, Mehrabi A, Fonouni H, Müller-Stich BP, Vetter G, et al., Dietary omega-3-polyunsaturated fatty acids prevent the development of metastases of colon carcinoma in rat liver. Eur J Nutr 2007;46: 279–85.

Guy CT, Webster MA, Schaller M, Parsons TJ, Cardiff RD, Muller WJ, Expression of the neu proto-oncogene in the mammary epithelium of transgenic mice induces metastatic disease. Proc Natl Acad Sci USA 1992;89: 10578–82.

Hebert JR, Rosen A, Nutritional, socioeconomic, and reproductive factors in relation to female breast cancer mortality: findings from a cross-national study. Cancer Detect Prev 1996;20: 234–44.

Hebert JR, Hurley TG, Olendzki BC, Teas J, Ma Y, Hampl JS, Nutritional and socioeconomic factors in relation to prostate cancer mortality: a cross-national study. J Natl Cancer Inst 1998;90: 1637–47.

Hedelin M, Chang ET, Wiklund F, Bellocco R, Klint A, Adolfsson J, et al., Association of frequent consumption of fatty fish with prostate cancer risk is modified by COX-2 polymorphism. Int J Cancer 2007;120: 398–405.

Hislop TG, Coldman AJ, Elwood JM, Brauer G, Kan L, Childhood and recent eating patterns and risk of breast cancer. Cancer Detect Prev 1986;9: 47–58.

Hislop TG, Kan L, Coldman AJ, Band PR, Brauer G, Influence of estrogen receptor status on dietary risk factors for breast cancer. Can Med Assoc J 1988;138: 424–30.

Hofmanová J, Vaculová A, Lojek A, Kozubík A, Interaction of polyunsaturated fatty acids and sodium butyrate during apoptosis in HT-29 human colon adenocarcinoma cells. Eur J Nutr 2005;44: 40–51.

Huang YC, Jessup JM, Forse RA, Flickner S, Pleskow D, Anastopoulos HT, et al., n-3 fatty acids decrease colonic epithelial cell proliferation in high-risk bowel mucosa. Lipids 1996;31: S313–7.

Hudson EA, Beck SA, Tisdale MJ, Kinetics of the inhibition of tumour growth in mice by eicosapentaenoic acid-reversal by linoleic acid. Biochem Pharmacol 1993;45: 2189–94.

Iigo M, Nakagawa T, Ishikawa C, Iwahori Y, Asamoto M, Yazawa K, et al., Inhibitory effects of docosahexaenoic acid on colon carcinoma 26 metastasis to the lung. Br J Cancer 1997;75: 650–5.

Iscovich JM, L'Abbe KA., Castelleto R, Calzona A, Bernedo A, Chopita NA, et al., Colon cancer in Argentina. I: Risk from intake of dietary items. Int J Cancer 1992;51: 851–7.

Iwamoto S, Senzaki H, Kiyozuka Y, Ogura E, Takada H, Hioki K, et al., Effects of fatty acids on liver metastasis of ACL-15 rat colon cancer cells. Nutr Cancer 1998;31: 143–50.

Jakobsen CH, Størvold GL, Bremseth H, Follestad T, Sand K, Mack M, et al., DHA induces ER stress and growth arrest in human colon cancer cells: associations with cholesterol and calcium homeostasis. J Lipid Res 2008;49: 2089–100.

Jia Q, Lupton JR, Smith R, Weeks BR, Callaway E, Davidson LA, et al., Reduced colitis-associated colon cancer in Fat-1 (n-3 fatty acid desaturase) transgenic mice. Cancer Res 2008;68: 3985–91.

Jurkowski JJ, Cave WT Jr, Dietary effects of menhaden oil on the growth and membrane lipid composition of rat mammary tumors. J Natl Cancer Inst 1985;74: 1145–50.

Kang JX, Wang J, Wu L, Kang ZB, Transgenic mice: fat-1 mice convert n-6 to n-3 fatty acids. Nature 2004;427: 504.

Karmali RA, Marsh J, Fuchs C, Effect of omega-3 fatty acids on growth of a rat mammary tumor. J Natl Cancer Inst 1984;73: 457–61.

Karmali RA, Reichel P, Cohen LA, Terano T, Hirai A, Tamura Y, et al., Omega-3 fatty acids and cancer: a review. In: Lands WE, editor. Proceedings of the AOCS short course on polyunsaturated fatty acids and eicosanoids, Mississippi, May 13–19, 1987. Champaign, IL: American Oil Chemists' Society; 1987a. pp. 222–32.

Karmali RA, Reichel P, Cohen LA, Terano T, Hirai A, Tamura Y, et al., The effects of dietary omega-3 fatty acids on the DU-145 transplantable human prostatic tumor. Anticancer Res 1987b;7: 1173–9.

Kato T, Hancock RL, Mohammadpour H, McGregor B, Manalo P, Khaiboullina S, et al., Influence of omega-3 fatty acids on the growth of human colon carcinoma in nude mice. Cancer Lett 2002;187: 169–77.

Kato T, Kolenic N, Pardini RS, Docosahexaenoic acid (DHA), a primary tumor suppressive omega-3 fatty acid, inhibits growth of colorectal cancer independent of p53 mutational status. Nutr Cancer 2007;58: 178–87.

Kimura Y, ω-3 PUFAs and colon cancer: epidemiological studies. In: Calviello G, Serini S, editors. Dietary omega-3 polyunsaturated fatty acids and cancer. Dordrecht: Springer; 2010. In press.

Kimura Y, Kono S, Toyomura K, Nagano J, Mizoue T, Moore MA, et al., Meat, fish and fat intake in relation to subsite-specific risk of colorectal cancer: The Fukuoka Colorectal Cancer Study. Cancer Sci 2007;98: 590–7.

Kobayashi M, Sasaki S, Hamada GS, Tsugane S, Serum n-3 fatty acids, fish consumption and cancer mortality in six Japanese populations in Japan and Brazil. Jpn J Cancer Res 1999;90: 914–21.

Kolar SS, Barhoumi R, Lupton JR, Chapkin RS, Docosahexaenoic acid and butyrate synergistically induce colonocyte apoptosis by enhancing mitochondrial Ca2+ accumulation. Cancer Res 2007;67: 5561–8.

Kritchevsky SB, A review of scientific research and recommendations regarding eggs. J Am Coll Nutr 2004;23: 596S–600S.

Kuriki K, Hirose K, Wakai K, Matsuo K, Ito H, Suzuki T, et al., Breast cancer risk and erythrocyte compositions of n-3 highly unsaturated fatty acids in Japanese. Int J Cancer 2007;121: 377–85.

Lanier AP, Kelly JJ, Holck P, Smith B, McEvoy T, Sandidge J, Cancer incidence in Alaska Natives thirty-year report 1969–1998. Alaska Med 2001;43: 87–115.

Larsson SC, Kumlin M, Ingelman-Sundberg M, Wolk A, Dietary long-chain n-3 fatty acids for the prevention of cancer: a review of potential mechanisms. Am J Clin Nutr 2004;79: 935–45.

Latham P, Lund EK, Brown JC, Johnson IT, Effects of cellular redox balance on induction of apoptosis by eicosapentaenoic acid in HT29 colorectal adenocarcinoma cells and rat colon in vivo. Gut 2001;49: 97–105.

Latham P, Lund EK, Johnson IT, Dietary n-3 PUFA increases the apoptotic response to 1,2-dimethylhydrazine, reduces mitosis and suppresses the induction of carcinogenesis in the rat colon. Carcinogenesis 1999;20: 645–50.

Lee HP, Gourley L, Duffy SW, Esteve J, Lee J, Day NE, Colorectal cancer and diet in an Asian population – a case-control study among Singapore Chinese. Int J Cancer 1989;43: 1007–16.

Lee JY, Hwang DH, Docosahexaenoic acid suppresses the activity of peroxisome proliferator-activated receptors in a colon tumor cell line. Biochem Biophys Res Commun 2002;298: 667–74.

Lindner MA, A fish oil diet inhibits colon cancer in mice. Nutr Cancer 1991;15: 1–11.

London E, Insights into lipid raft structure and formation from experiments in model membranes. Curr Opin Struct Biol 2002;12: 480–6.

Lu Y, Nie D, Witt WT, Chen Q, Shen M, Xie H, et al., Expression of the fat-1 gene diminishes prostate cancer growth in vivo through enhancing apoptosis and inhibiting GSK-3 beta phosphorylation. Mol Cancer Ther 2008;7: 3203–11.

Luijten M, Verhoef A, Dormans JA, Beems RB, Cremers HW, Nagelkerke NJ, et al., Modulation of mammary tumor development in Tg.NK (MMTV/c-neu) mice by dietary fatty acids and life stage-specific exposure to phytoestrogens. Reprod Toxicol 2007;23: 407–13.

Ma DW, Seo J, Davidson LA, Callaway ES, Fan YY, Lupton JR, et al., n-3 PUFA alter caveolae lipid composition and resident protein localization in mouse colon. FASEB J 2004;18: 1040–2.

Macquart-Moulin G, Riboli E, Cornee J, Charnay B, Berthezene P, Day N, Case-control study on colorectal cancer and diet in Marseilles. Int J Cancer 1986;38: 183–91.

Mahéo K, Vibet S, Steghens JP, Dartigeas C, Lehman M, Bougnoux P, et al., Differential sensitization of cancer cells to doxorubicin by DHA: a role for lipoperoxidation. Free Radic Biol Med 2005;39: 742–51.

Maillard V, Bougnoux P, Ferrari P, Jourdan ML, Pinault M, Lavillonnière F, et al., N-3 and N-6 fatty acids in breast adipose tissue and relative risk of breast cancer in a case-control study in Tours, France. Int J Cancer 2002;98: 78–83.

Mengeaud V, Nano JL, Fournel S, Rampal P, Effects of eicosapentaenoic acid, gamma-linolenic acid and prostaglandin E1 on three human colon carcinoma cell lines. Prostaglandins Leukot Essent Fatty Acids 1992;47: 313–9.

Minoura T, Takata T, Sakaguchi M, Takada H, Yamamura M, Hioki K, et al., Effect of dietary eicosapentaenoic acid on azoxymethane-induced colon carcinogenesis in rats. Cancer Res 1988;48: 4790–4.

Moore NG, Wang-Johanning F, Chang PL, Johanning GL, Omega-3 fatty acids decrease protein kinase expression in human breast cancer cells. Breast Cancer Res Treat 2001;67: 279–83.

Narayanan BA, Narayanan NK, Reddy BS, Docosahexaenoic acid regulated genes and transcription factors inducing apoptosis in human colon cancer cells. Int J Oncol 2001;19: 1255–62.

Narayanan BA, Narayanan NK, Simi B, Reddy BS, Modulation of inducible nitric oxide synthase and related proinflammatory genes by the omega-3 fatty acid docosahexaenoic acid in human colon cancer cells. Cancer Res 2003;63: 972–9.

Narayanan BA, Narayanan NK, Desai D, Pittman B, Reddy BS, Effects of a combination of docosahexaenoic acid and 1,4-phenylene bis(methylene) selenocyanate on cyclooxygenase 2, inducible nitric oxide synthase and beta-catenin pathways in colon cancer cells. Carcinogenesis 2004;25: 2443–9.

Needleman P, Raz A, Minkes MS, Ferrendelli JA, Sprecher H, Triene prostaglandins: prostacyclin and thromboxane biosynthesis and unique biological properties. Proc Natl Acad Sci USA 1979;76: 944–8.

Nielsen NH, Hansen JP, Breast cancer in Greenland–selected epidemiological, clinical, and histological features. J Cancer Res Clin Oncol 1980;98: 287–99.

Noguchi M, Earashi M, Minami M, Kinoshita K, Miyazaki I, Effects of eicosapentaenoic and docosahexaenoic acid on cell growth and prostaglandin E and leukotriene B production by a human breast cancer cell line (MDA-MB-231). Oncology 1995;52: 458–64.

Norat T, Bingham S, Ferrari P, Slimani N, Jenab M, Mazuir M, et al., Meat, fish, and colorectal cancer risk: the European Prospective Investigation into cancer and nutrition. J Natl Cancer Inst 2005;97: 906–16.

Nowak J, Weylandt KH, Habbel P, Wang J, Dignass A, Glickman JN, et al., Colitis-associated colon tumorigenesis is suppressed in transgenic mice rich in endogenous n-3 fatty acids. Carcinogenesis 2007;28: 1991–5.

O'Flaherty JT, Rogers LC, Chadwell BA, Owen JS, Rao A, Cramer SD, et al., 5(S)-Hydroxy-6,8,11,14-E,Z,Z,Z-eicosatetraenoate stimulates PC3 cell signaling and growth by a receptor-dependent mechanism. Cancer Res 2002;62: 6817–9.

Pan J, Keffer J, Emami A, Ma X, Lan R, Goldman R, et al., Acrolein-derived DNA adduct formation in human colon cancer cells: its role in apoptosis induction by docosahexaenoic acid. Chem Res Toxicol 2009;22: 798–806.

Park SY, Wilkens LR, Henning SM, Le Marchand L, Gao K, Goodman MT, et al., Circulating fatty acids and prostate cancer risk in a nested case-control study: the Multiethnic Cohort. Cancer Causes Control 2009;20: 211–23.

Paulsen JE, Elvsaas IK, Steffensen IL, Alexander J, A fish oil derived concentrate enriched in eicosapentaenoic and docosahexaenoic acid as ethyl ester suppresses the formation and growth of intestinal polyps in the Min mouse. Carcinogenesis 1997;18: 1905–10.

Paulsen JE, Stamm T, Alexander J, A fish oil-derived concentrate enriched in eicosapentaenoic and docosahexaenoic acid as ethyl esters inhibits the formation and growth of aberrant crypt foci in rat colon. Pharmacol Toxicol 1998;82: 28–33.

Peters RK, Pike MC, Garabrant D and Mack TM, Diet and colon cancer in Los Angeles County, California. Cancer Causes Control 1992;3: 457–73.

Pham TM, Fujino Y, Kubo T, Ide R, Tokui N, Mizoue T, et al., Fish intake and the risk of fatal prostate cancer: findings from a cohort study in Japan. Public Health Nutr 2009;12: 609–13.

Pot GK, Majsak-Newman G, Geelen A, Harvey LJ, Nagengast FM, Witteman BJM, et al., Fish consumption and markers of colorectal cancer risk: a multicenter randomized controlled trial. Am J Clin Nutr 2009;90: 354–61.

Prener A, Storm HH, Nielsen NH, Cancer of the male genital tract in Circumpolar Inuit. Acta Oncol 1996;35: 589–93.

Reddy BS, Sugie S, Effect of different levels of omega-3 and omega-6 fatty acids on azoxymethane-induced colon carcinogenesis in F344 rats. Cancer Res 1988;48: 6642–7.

Rose DP, Cohen LA, Effects of dietary menhaden oil and retinyl acetate on the growth of DU 145 human prostatic adenocarcinoma cells transplanted into athymic nude mice. Carcinogenesis 1988;9: 603–5.

Rose DP, Connolly JM, Effects of dietary omega-3 fatty acids on human breast cancer growth and metastases in nude mice. J Natl Cancer Inst 1993;85: 1743–7.

Rose DP, Connolly JM, Rayburn J, Coleman M, Influence of diets containing eicosapentaenoic or docosahexaenoic acid on growth and metastasis of breast cancer cells in nude mice. J Natl Cancer Inst 1995;87: 587–92.

Rose DP, Connolly JM, Coleman M, Effect of omega-3 fatty acids on the progression of metastases after the surgical excision of human breast cancer cell solid tumors growing in nude mice. Clin Cancer Res 1996;2: 1751–6.

Sakaguchi M, Imray C, Davis A, Rowley S, Jones C, Lawson N, et al., Effects of dietary N-3 and saturated fats on growth rates of the human colonic cancer cell lines SW-620 and LS 174T in vivo in relation to tissue and plasma lipids. Anticancer Res 1990a;10: 1763–8.

Sakaguchi M, Rowley S, Kane N, Imray C, Davies A, Jones C, et al., Reduced tumour growth of the human colonic cancer cell lines COLO-320 and HT-29 in vivo by dietary n-3 lipids. Br J Cancer 1990b;62: 742–7.

Sasaki S, Horacsek M and Kesteloot H, An ecological study of the relationship between dietary fat intake and breast cancer mortality. Prev Med 1993;22: 187–202.

Schley PD, Jijon HB, Robinson LE, Field CJ, Mechanisms of omega-3 fatty acid-induced growth inhibition in MDA-MB-231 human breast cancer cells. Breast Cancer Res Treat 2005;92: 187–95.

Schley PD, Brindley DN, Field CJ, (n-3) PUFA alter raft lipid composition and decrease epidermal growth factor receptor levels in lipid rafts of human breast cancer cells. J Nutr 2007;137: 548–53.

Schønberg SA, Lundemo AG, Fladvad T, Holmgren K, Bremseth H, Nilsen A, et al., Closely related colon cancer cell lines display different sensitivity to polyunsaturated fatty acids, accumulate different lipid classes and downregulate sterol regulatory element-binding protein 1. FEBS J 2006;273: 2749–65.

Shaikh IA, Brown I, Schofield AC, Wahle KW, Heys SD, Docosahexaenoic acid enhances the efficacy of docetaxel in prostate cancer cells by modulation of apoptosis: the role of genes associated with the NF-kappaB pathway. Prostate 2008;68: 1635–46.

Simonsen N, van't Veer P, Strain JJ, Martin-Moreno JM, Huttunen JK, Navajas JF, et al., Adipose tissue omega-3 and omega-6 fatty acid content and breast cancer in the EURAMIC study. European Community Multicenter Study on Antioxidants, Myocardial Infarction, and Breast Cancer. Am J Epidemiol 1998;147: 342–52.

Simopoulos AP, Evolutionary aspects of diet, the omega-6/omega-3 ratio and genetic variation: nutritional implications for chronic diseases. Biomed Pharmacother 2006;60: 502–7.

Stillwell W, Wassall SR, Docosahexaenoic acid: membrane properties of a unique fatty acid. Chem Phys Lipids 2003;126: 1–27.

Sun H, Berquin IM, Edwards IJ, Omega-3 polyunsaturated fatty acids regulate syndecan-1 expression in human breast cancer cells. Cancer Res 2005;65: 4442–7.

Sun H, Berquin IM, Owens RT, O'Flaherty JT, Edwards IJ, Peroxisome proliferator-activated receptor gamma-mediated up-regulation of syndecan-1 by n-3 fatty acids promotes apoptosis of human breast cancer cells. Cancer Res 2008;68: 2912–9.

Swamy MV, Cooma I, Patlolla JM, Simi B, Reddy BS, Rao CV, Modulation of cyclooxygenase-2 activities by the combined action of celecoxib and docosahexaenoic acid: novel strategies for colon cancer prevention and treatment. Mol Cancer Ther 2004;3: 215–21.

Takahashi M, Minamoto T, Yamashita N, Kato T, Yazawa K, Esumi H, Effect of docosahexaenoic acid on azoxymethane-induced colon carcinogenesis in rats. Cancer Lett 1994;83: 177–84.

Takahashi M, Fukutake M, Isoi T, Fukuda K, Sato H, Yazawa K, et al., Suppression of azoxymethane-induced rat colon carcinoma development by a fish oil component, docosahexaenoic acid (DHA). Carcinogenesis 1997a;18: 1337–42.

Takahashi M, Totsuka Y, Masuda M, Fukuda K, Oguri A, Yazawa K, et al., Reduction in formation of 2-amino-1-methyl-6-phenylimidazo[4,5-b]pyridine (PhIP)-induced aberrant crypt foci in the rat colon by docosahexaenoic acid(DHA). Carcinogenesis 1997b;18: 1937–41.

Tanaka Y, Goto K, Matsumoto Y, Ueoka R, Remarkably high inhibitory effects of docosahexaenoic acid incorporated into hybrid liposomes on the growth of tumor cells along with apoptosis. Int J Pharm 2008;359: 264–71.

Terry PD, Mink PJ, ω-3 Polyunsaturated fatty acids and breast cancer: epidemiological studies. In: Calviello G, Serini S, editors. Dietary omega-3 polyunsaturated fatty acids and cancer. Dordrecht: Springer; 2010. In press.

Terry PD, Rohan TE, Wolk A, Intakes of fish and marine fatty acids and the risks of cancers of the breast and prostate and of other hormone-related cancers: a review of the epidemiologic evidence. Am J Clin Nutr 2003 77: 532–43.

Toit-Kohn JL, Louw L, Engelbrecht AM, Docosahexaenoic acid induces apoptosis in colorectal carcinoma cells by modulating the PI3 kinase and p38 MAPK pathways. J Nutr Biochem 2009;20: 106–14.

Tsujita-Kyutoku M, Yuri T, Danbara N, Senzaki H, Kiyozuka Y, Uehara N, et al., Conjugated docosahexaenoic acid suppresses KPL-1 human breast cancer cell growth in vitro and in vivo: potential mechanisms of action. Breast Cancer Res 2004;6: R291–9.

Tsuzuki T, Igarashi M, Miyazawa T, Conjugated eicosapentaenoic acid (EPA) inhibits transplanted tumor growth via membrane lipid peroxidation in nude mice. J Nutr 2004;134: 1162–6.

van Beelen VA, Roeleveld J, Mooibroek H, Sijtsma L, Bino RJ, Bosch D, et al., A comparative study on the effect of algal and fish oil on viability and cell proliferation of Caco-2 cells. Food Chem Toxicol 2007;45: 716–24.

Vang K, Ziboh VA, 15-lipoxygenase metabolites of gamma-linolenic acid/eicosapentaenoic acid suppress growth and arachidonic acid metabolism in human prostatic adenocarcinoma cells: possible implications of dietary fatty acids. Prostaglandins Leukot Essent Fatty Acids 2005;72: 363–72.

Wang S, Gao J, Lei Q, Rozengurt N, Pritchard C, Jiao J, et al., Prostate-specific deletion of the murine Pten tumor suppressor gene leads to metastatic prostate cancer. Cancer Cell 2003;4: 209–21.

Wang Z, Butt K, Wang L, Liu H, The effect of seal oil on paclitaxel induced cytotoxicity and apoptosis in breast carcinoma MCF-7 and MDA-MB-231 cell lines. Nutr Cancer 2007;58: 230–8.

Webb Y, Hermida-Matsumoto L, Resh MD, Inhibition of protein palmitoylation, raft localization, and T cell signaling by 2-bromopalmitate and polyunsaturated fatty acids. J Biol Chem 2000;275: 261–70.

Yang CX, Takezaki T, Hirose K, Inoue M, Huang XE, Tajima K, Fish consumption and colorectal cancer: a case-reference study in Japan. Eur J Cancer Prev 2003;12: 109–15.

Yang P, Chan D, Felix E, Cartwright C, Menter DG, Madden T, et al., Formation and antiproliferative effect of prostaglandin E(3) from eicosapentaenoic acid in human lung cancer cells. J Lipid Res 2004;45: 1030–9.

Yee LD, Young DC, Rosol TJ, Vanbuskirk AM, Clinton SK, Dietary (n-3) polyunsaturated fatty acids inhibit HER-2/neu-induced breast cancer in mice independently of the PPARgamma ligand rosiglitazone. J Nutr 2005;135: 983–8.

Zhu ZR, Agren J, Männistö S, Pietinen P, Eskelinen M, Syrjänen K, et al., Fatty acid composition of breast adipose tissue in breast cancer patients and in patients with benign breast disease. Nutr Cancer 1995;24: 151–60.

Curriculum Vitae

(1/7.3/7.5)

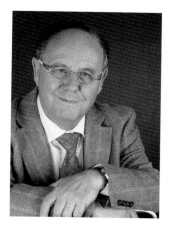

Wolfgang Herrmann

Wolfgang Herrmann is Professor emeritus in the Faculty of Medicine at the Saarland University (Germany). He is the former director of the department of Clinical Chemistry and Laboratory Medicine of the Saarland University. He obtained his academic degrees from the University of Leipzig (Germany) and the University of Regensburg (Germany). He is member of the Editorial Board of the Journal Clinical Chemistry and Laboratory Medicine and member of the Scientific Advisory Board of the journal Clinical Laboratory. He has more than 250 publications and has organized several International Congresses on Hyperhomocysteinemia.

kchwher@uniklinik-saarland.de

(1/7.3/7.5)

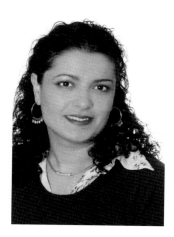

Rima Obeid

Rima Obeid is a Junior-Professor at the Saarland University, Department of Clinical Chemistry, Faculty of Medicine (Germany). She has obtained her academic degrees from the University of Damascus (Syria) and the Saarland University (Germany). She is currently leading a research group and focuses on the role of one-carbon metabolism in human diseases. She has more than 50 publications and has been awarded by the Alexander von Humboldt Foundation.

rima.obeid@uniklinik-saarland.de

(2.1)

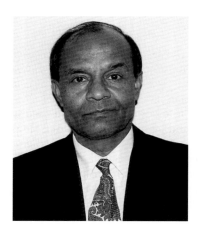

Arun B. Barua

After several years as Lecturer at the Department of Chemistry, Gauhati University in Guwahati, India Arun B. Barua acted as visiting Professor at the Department of Biochemistry and Biophysics, Iowa State University, Ames, IA, USA from 1980 to 1983. Then he began to work permanently at the same department as scientist.

Since 2000 he has been working as an Adjunct Professor at the Department of Biochemistry, Biophysics and Molecular Biology, Iowa State University, Ames until his retirement in 2004. He is an expert in the field of vitamin A metabolism and carotenoid metabolism.

abbarua@gmail.com

(2.1)

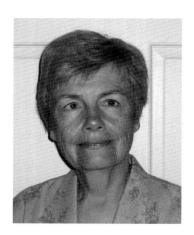

Maria Stacewicz-Sapuntzakis

Dr. Maria Stacewicz-Sapuntzakis graduated from University of Warsaw, Poland, with M.S. degree in Biology. She earned her PhD from the University of Massachusetts, Amherst, MA, USA in Plant Sciences and worked there as a postdoctoral research associate in Biochemistry on vitamin A and carotenoid metabolism. From 1983 till 2008 she was a researcher at the University of Illinois at Chicago, Department of Human Nutrition, investigating fat-soluble vitamin and carotenoid metabolism, oxidative stress parameters and the correlation of diet with health status.

(2.1)

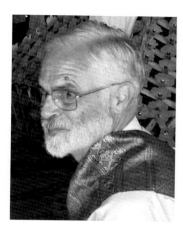

Harold Furr

Dr. Harold Furr holds a BA in Chemistry, and MNS and PhD degrees in Nutritional Biochemistry. He was engaged in research in vitamin A and carotenoids at Iowa State University and held a faculty position at the University of Connecticut before becoming Technical Director at Craft Technologies. He has also been a Visiting Associate Professor at the Institute of Nutrition of Mahidol University in Thailand. He currently holds a part-time position in the Department of Nutritional Sciences of the University of Wisconsin in Madison, Wisconsin.

hfurr581@yahoo.com

(2.2)

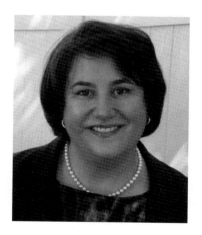

Jenny Libien

Jenny Libien, MD PhD, is Assistant Professor of Pathology and Neurology at the State University of New York – Downstate Medical Center in Brooklyn, New York. She is a neuropathologist and a neuroscientist studying retinoid and glutamate signaling pathways during learning and memory formation and in neurological disorders.

Jenny.Libien@downstate.edu

(3.1)

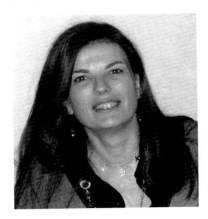

Elena Beltramo

Elena Beltramo is Researcher in Diabetic Retinopathy at the University of Turin (Italy), Deptartment of Internal Medicine.

Her main scientific interests are the study of the mechanisms responsible for the development of diabetic microvascular disease and the protective role of thiamine against high glucose-induced damage.

elena.beltramo@unito.it

(3.2/6.5)

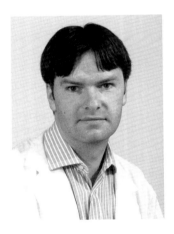

Michael Linnebank

Michael Linnebank is a senior physician at the Department of Neurology of the University Hospital Zurich and since 2008 team leader at the Neuroscience Center Zurich. In 2009, he became head of the neurological day hospital and associate head of the Neurological Outpatients Department.

His main research interests are the homocysteine metabolism and the vitamins involved as well as their effect on metabolic and structural integrity of the central nervous system.

michael.linnebank@usz.ch

(4)

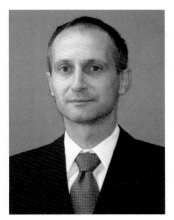

Peter Swaan

Dr. Peter Swaan is Professor of Pharmaceutical Sciences and Director of the Center for Nanomedicine and Cellular Delivery at the University of Maryland School of Pharmacy in Baltimore, MD. He has published over 80 original research articles focusing on all aspects of transport proteins in drug targeting and delivery, pharmacokinetics and pharmacodynamics. His major contributions to this research area involve the application of transporters as targets for prodrugs. Furthemore, Dr. Swaan has pioneered the use of computational techniques to determining structural requirements of membrane transporters which has paved the way for the discovery of novel substrates and inhibitors. He holds several US patents and serves as Editor-in-Chief for the journal Pharmaceutical Research.

pswaan@rx.umaryland.edu

(5)

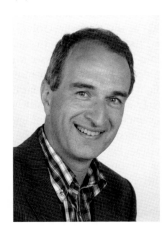

Martin den Heijer

Martin den Heijer is associate professor at the department of Endocrinology and at the department of Biostatistics, Epidemiology and HTA of the Radboud University Nijmegen Medical Centre. His research focus is on homocysteine and B-vitamins especially in relation to vascular disease and venous thrombosis.

M.denHeijer@endo.umcn.nl

(6.1)

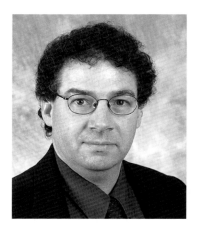

Patrick Stover

Patrick Stover is Professor and Director of the Division of Nutritional Sciences at Cornell University. He graduated from Saint Joseph's University with a BS degree in Chemistry and received a PhD degree in Biochemistry and Molecular Biophysics from the Medical College of Virginia. He performed his postdoctoral studies in Nutritional Sciences at the University of California at Berkeley.

pjs13@cornell.edu

(6.2)

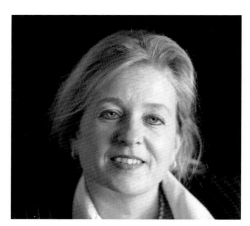

Régine P.M. Steegers-Theunissen

Régine P.M. Steegers-Theunissen fully qualified as M.D. (1986) and acquired her PhD thesis (1993) at the Catholic University in Nijmegen, The Netherlands. In July 2005 she became associate professor in Reproductive Epidemiology at the Erasmus University Medical Center in Rotterdam, The Netherlands. From January 2010 she is professor in Periconception Epidemiology at the Erasmus University Medical Center.

The research line Periconception Epidemiology aims to unravel (epi)genetic mechanisms underlying the influence of periconception health, i.e., gene-environment interactions, of parents-to-be on reproductive performance (congenital malformations) and health in later life. Implementation of the research findings takes place in special preconception clinics developed to provide standardized nutrition and lifestyle screening and intervention programmes.

r.steegers@erasmusmc.nl

(6.2)

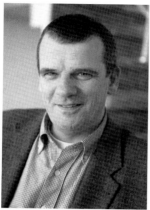

Joop S.E. Laven

Dr. Joop S.E. Laven is a fully registered clinician in Obstetrics and Gynaecology and was initially trained at the university of Utrecht, The Netherlands. After Medical school he completed his Ph.D. thesis on clinical and experimental aspects of varicocele at Utrecht University in 1991. In 1997 he became board certified in OBGYN (FRCOG) and moved to the Erasmus Medical Center in Rotterdam. He is a member of ESHRE, ASRM, Endocrine Society and the Royal Dutch College of Obstetrics and Gynaecology. Recently he became the president of the Dutch Society of Reproductive Medicine.

For many years he had a particular interest in the management of polycystic ovary syndrome covering the full spectrum from the effects of the syndrome during adolescence and adult life on the menstrual cycle, fertility, body weight and cosmetic aspects. More recently the research focussed on more fundamental effects that PCOS may have on quality of life and long-term health risks as well as the genetic basis of the disease.

Clinical work focuses on women's health in particular reproductive endocrinology and menopause as well as on infertility treatment and ART and pregnancy outcome in infertile couples especially women with PCOS. He is the person Responsible for the Rotterdam Erasmus MC Reproductive Medicine Unit, which performs approximately 2400 IVF cycles per year. Works as a full time clinician and is currently acting head of the Division of Reproductive Medicine of the department of OBGYN at Erasmus MC in Rotterdam.

(6.2)

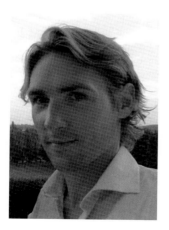

John Twigt

In September 2005 John Twigt started his medical education at the Erasmus Medical Centre in Rotterdam, the Netherlands. Concomitantly he enrolled in the MSc Clinical Research program in 2007. Since 2009 he is affiliated to the department of Obstetrics and Gynecology of the Erasmus MC as a PhD-student. Here, his research focuses on the influence of food and lifestyle factors on fertility treatment, most notably the influence and underlying mechanisms of folic acid supplement use.

(6.3)

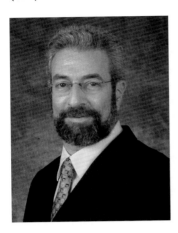

Richard H. Finnell

Dr. Richard H. Finnell earned his B.S. in anthropology at the University of Oregon in 1975, an M.Sc. in medical genetics at the University of British Columbia and his Ph.D. in medical genetics in 1980 from the University of Oregon Health Sciences Center. Over a 30 year academic career, Dr. Finnell has achieved international recognition for his research on the interaction between specific genes and environmental toxicants and nutritional factors, as they influence embryonic development.

rfinnell@ibt.tmc.edu

(6.4)

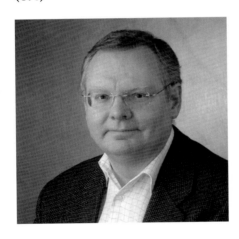

Torbjörn K. Nilsson

Torbjörn K. Nilsson received his MD from Umeå University in 1982 and a PhD in Clinical Chemistry the same year. From 1999 he has held a position as Consultant in the Dept of Laboratory Medicine at Örebro University Hospital and from 2001 as Professor of Biomedicine at the School of Health and Medicine, Örebro University.

torbjorn.nilsson@orebroll.se

(6.4)

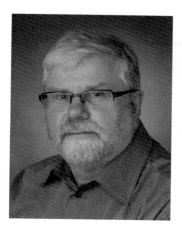

Nils-Olof Hagnelius

Nils-Olof Hagnelius received his MD from Umeå University in 1984, and from 1995 holds a position as Consultant at the Dept of Geriatric Medicine, Örebro University Hospital. In 2009 he received a PhD in Medicine at the School of Health and Medicine, Örebro University.

nils-olof.hagnelius@oru.se

(6.6)

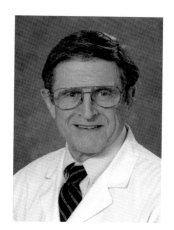

Charles H. Halsted

Dr. Halsted was trained in internal medicine, nutrition, and gastroenterology. He is currently Professor Emeritus of Internal Medicine and Nutritional Sciences at the University of California Davis, USA. His previous appointments include Editor in Chief of the American Journal of Clinical Nutrition. His research career has focused on aspects of the intestinal absorption and metabolism of folate and the relation of abnormal methionine metabolism to alcoholic liver disease. School of Medicine before joining Oregon State University in 1997.

chhalsted@ucdavis.edu

(6.7)

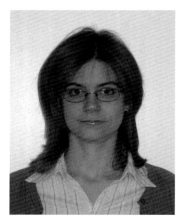

Karen Christensen

Karen Christensen received her Ph.D. from the Department of Biochemistry of McGill University under the supervision of Dr. R.E. MacKenzie. She is currently a post-doctoral fellow in Dr. Rima Rozen's laboratory at the Montreal Children's Hospital Research Institute where she is the recipient of a Thelma Adams Research Fellowship.

(6.7)

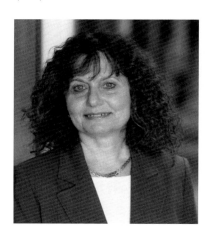

Rima Rozen

Professor Rima Rozen is Interim Vice-Principal (Research and International Relations) at McGill University and a James McGill Professor in the Human Genetics, Pediatrics and Biology Departments. Recognized for her research in the genetics-nutrition field, she has published close to 200 publications, received several awards for her research, and continues to direct her laboratory at the McGill-Montreal Children's Hospital.

rima.rozen@mcgill.ca

(7.1)

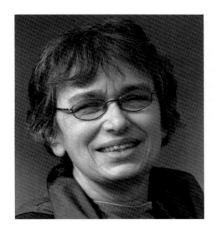

Ebba Nexo

Ebba Nexo is a professor and a consultant of clinical biochemistry. Her main interests are within vitamins and growth factors and she currently supervises projects within both areas. She has served on numerous national and international boards and has amongst others chaired the Danish Medical Research Council, been a co-chair for the board of the Danish Independent Research Councils and a board member of both the EURO-HORCS and ESF.

e.nexo@dadlnet.dk

(7.2)

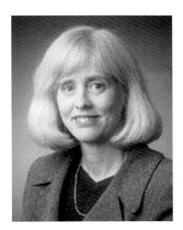

Sally P. Stabler

Sally P. Stabler, M.D. is a Professor of Medicine and Co-Division Chief of Hematology at the University of Colorado School of Medicine. She has studied the clinical and metabolic defects in cobalamin and folate deficiency for almost 3 decades. She has published many manuscripts and reviews on methods of diagnosis of cobalamin deficiency and the prevalence and clinical spectrum of vitamin deficiency.

Sally.Stabler@ucdenver.edu

(7.4)

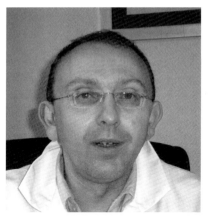

Emmanuel Andrés

Emmanuel Andrés is working as a clinical specialist in the Department of Internal Medicine, Diabetes and Metabolic diseases, University Hospital in Strasbourg (Hôpitaux Universitaires – CHRU de Strasbourg), France, since 1997.

He is currently Professor of Internal Medicine, School of Medicine, University of Strasbourg, France, since 2002. He has received the Robert and Jacqueline Zittoun's Price 2004, Fondation de France, for his research on anemia, metabolism of cobalamin and folate and is Member of the EHA Scientific Working Group on Granulocyte and Monocyte disorders, since 2008 and Member of the french national comity of pharmacovigilance, since 2007.

Emmanuel.andres@chru-strasbourg.fr

(8.2)

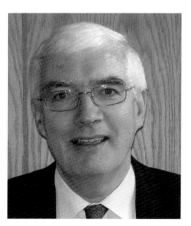

Robert Clarke

Dr. Robert Clarke joined the Clinical Trial Service Unit (CTSU) and Epidemiological Studies Unit at the University of Oxford in 1991. He is currently a Reader in Epidemiology and Public Health Medicine at CTSU and Honorary Consultant in Public Health Medicine at Oxford City Primary Care Trust. In collaboration with others of CTSU, his work has focussed on the generation of reliable evidence for avoidance of death and disability using large-scale observational epidemiological studies and randomised trials. His specific research interests include assessment of the importance of cardiovascular risk factors (blood lipids, blood pressure, and tobacco) and novel risk factors (homocysteine, Lp(a), CRP and genetic variants). This expertise includes use of genetic epidemiology of cardiovascular disease to understand disease mechanisms and define therapeutic targets. In addition, his work on clinical trials of vitamins and fatty acids has helped to define public health policy on nutrition for disease prevention.

robert.clarke@ctsu.ox.ac.uk

(8.3)

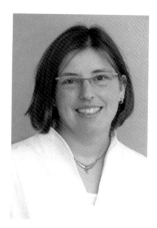

Jutta Dierkes

After academic training including her PhD in human nutrition at the University Bonn, she was a post-doc at Unilever Research in Vlaardingen, the Netherlands. She continued her research then at the Institute of Clinical Chemistry at the Medical Faculty of Magdeburg University, where she studied the effects of vitamin supplementation in patients with end-stage renal disease. Recently, she joined the University of Bergen, Norway, as a professor for clinical nutrition.

jutta.dierkes@landw.uni-halle.de

(8.3)

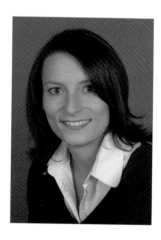

Judith Heinz

After studying nutritional science she conducted her PhD thesis at the Institute of Clinical Chemistry of the University Hospital of Magdeburg (Germany). A randomized, controlled multi-centre trial with B-vitamins in patients with ESRD was the major part of her PhD. In this trial, the effect of B vitamins on the risk of cardiovascular disease and total mortality in patients with end-stage renal disease was investigated. Early in 2009, she started to work at the University Cancer Center, University Hospital Hamburg-Eppendorf (Germany) in the field of cancer epidemiology.

(9.1)

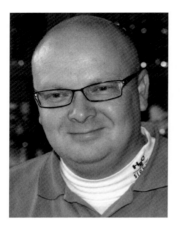

Jens Lykkesfeldt

Jens Lykkesfeldt holds a MSc (chem.), a PhD (biochem.) and a DSc (med.). He worked as Assistant Professor in pharmacology (1992–1995, U. of Copenhagen), visiting scientist (1996–1998; U. of California, Berkeley), Assoc. Professor in pharmacology (1998–2006; U. of Copenhagen), and Professor in biotechnology (2007–2008). Since 2009, he has been Professor and Chair in pharmacology and toxicology at the Faculty of Life Sciences, U. of Copenhagen. Dr. Lykkesfeldt and his group study the effects of redox imbalance in animals and humans and have for many years been particularly interested in vitamin C.

jopl@life.ku.dk

(9.1)

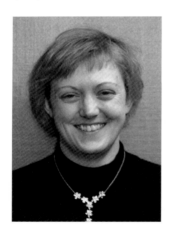

Pernille Tveden-Nyborg

Pernille Tveden-Nyborg holds a DVM and a PhD (vet. med.). In 2007, she became Assistant Professor in pharmacology at the Faculty of Life Sciences, University of Copenhagen. Dr. Tveden-Nyborg is particularly interested in the effects of vitamin C deficiency on the brain.

(9.1)

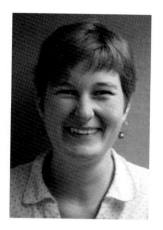

Henriette Frikke-Schmidt

Henriette Frikke-Schmidt holds a MSc in Human Biology. She is currently finishing her Ph.D thesis on the effects of vitamin C deficiency on endothelial function employing both in vitro and in vivo models.

(9.2)

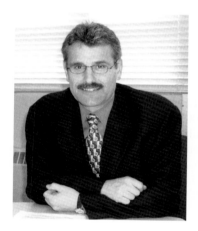

Balz Frei

Dr. Balz Frei is a Distinguished Professor of Biochemistry and Biophysics, and Director and Endowed Chair of the Linus Pauling Institute at Oregon State University in Corvallis, Oregon, USA. Dr. Frei holds a Ph.D. degree in biochemistry from the Swiss Federal Institute of Technology in Zürich, Switzerland; completed a postdoctoral fellowship at the University of California, Berkeley; and served on the faculties of Harvard School of Public Health and Boston University School of Medicine before joining Oregon State University in 1997.

balz.frei@oregonstate.edu

(10.1/10.2)

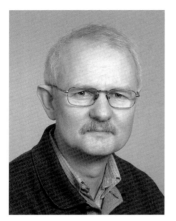

Armin Zittermann

Professor Zittermann is head of study center at the Department of Cardio-Thoracic Surgery, Heart Center North Rhine-Westphalia, Germany, and University Lecturer at the Department of Nutrition and Food Sciences, Bonn, Germany. His main research covers human vitamin D status, including prevalence and consequences of vitamin D insufficiency/deficiency in different population groups. He also investigates immunological aspects of heart transplantation. Moreover, he has a longstanding interest in nutritional aspects of osteoporosis, and cardiovascular diseases and their relation to the interaction of environmental factors and biomedical risk factors. His work spans nutrition, epidemiology, physiology, and biochemical methods, including the basis for causal inference.

azittermann@hdz-nrw.de

(10.3/10.6)

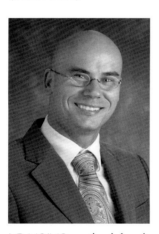

Markus Herrmann

Associate Professor Dr. Markus Herrmann studied medicine at the Universities of Regensburg and Wuerzburg in Germany. After graduation in 2000 he did one year of internship at the Department of Dermatology at the Technical University of Munich. In 2001 he started training as a clinical pathologist at the University of Saarland (Germany). In 2007 he completed his training and subsequently received a grant from the prestigous Akademie der Naturforscher, Leopoldina for a 2-year postdoctoral fellowship at the ANZAC Research Institute in Sydney (Australia). At the ANZAC Institute he studied molecular mechanisms of glucocorticoid induced osteoporosis and developed a new LC-MS/MS method for the detection of 25-OH vitamin D. At present he works as a chemical pathologist at Laverty Pathology and holds an Associate Professor position at the University of Sydney (Australia). Prof. Herrmann is a leading researcher in the FIELD of osteoporosis.

markusherr@aol.com

(10.4)

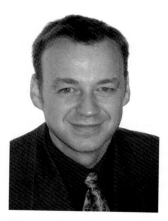

Jörg Reichrath

Jörg Reichrath is Professor for Dermatology and Deputy Director of the Clinic for Dermatology, Allergology and Venerology at the Saarland University Hospital in Homburg/Saar, Germany. Main research interests include photobiology, dermato-endocrinology and dermato-oncology. He is a member of numerous national and international scientific organisations, including the German Dermatological Society (DDG), the Deutsche Krebsgesellschaft (DKG), the German Dermatologic Co-operative Oncology Group (DeCOG), and the European Society of Dermatological Research (ESDR). He has been awarded numerous prices including the Arnold-Rikli-price 2006. Jörg Reichrath received his academic degrees (Dr. med., venia legendi) from the Saarland University, Germany.

Joerg.Reichrath@uniklinikum-saarland.de

(10.5)

Robert Scragg

Dr. Scragg is an Associate Professor in Epidemiology at the School of Population Health at the University of Auckland, New Zealand, where he has worked since 1984. He is a graduate of Adelaide Medical School and trained in epidemiology in the late 1970s at the CSIRO Division of Human Nutrition, Adelaide, South Australia, where he published the hypothesis that sun light and vitamin D may protect against cardiovascular disease.

r.scragg@auckland.ac.nz

(11.1)

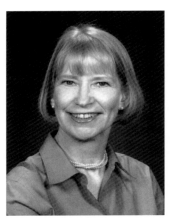

Maret Traber

Dr. Maret Traber is a Principal Investigator in the Linus Pauling Institute, and Professor in the Department of Nutrition and Exercise Sciences at Oregon State University, Corvallis, Oregon, USA. She received both undergraduate and doctoral degrees in Nutrition Science from the University of California at Berkeley. Dr. Traber is considered one of the world's leading experts on vitamin E. Her research efforts are focused on human vitamin E kinetics and the factors that modulate human vitamin E requirements, especially bioavailability and metabolism. She currently serves on the editorial boards of the American Journal of Clinical Nutrition and Free Radical Biology and Medicine. In 2000, Dr. Traber served on the National Academy of Science's, Institute of Medicine Panel on Dietary Antioxidants and Related Compounds that established the dietary requirements for the antioxidant vitamins C and E, selenium and carotenoids.

maret.traber@oregonstate.edu

(11.2)

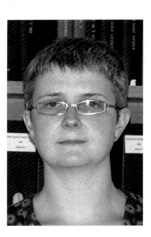

Jayne Woodside

Jayne Woodside is a Reader in Clinical Biochemistry at Queen's University Belfast, Northern Ireland. Her research is focused on how diet and lifestyle factors may affect chronic disease risk, combining both observational epidemiology and intervention study approaches.

(11.2)

Ian S. Young

Ian S. Young is Professor of Medicine at Queen's University Belfast, Northern Ireland. His main research interests are in lipid metabolism, nutrition and cardiovascular risk, with a particular focus on the role of antioxidants in health and disease.

I.Young@qub.ac.uk

(11.3)

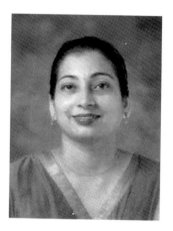

Kanwaljit Chopra

Dr. Kanwaljit Chopra is working as Associate Professor of Pharmacology at University Institute of Pharmaceutical Sciences, Panjab University, Chandigarh, India. Dr Chopra has more than 16 years of research and teaching experience. Dr Chopra's research interests are focused on "Reverse Pharmacology" with emphasis on diabetes and neuropharmacology. Dr Chopra has been a recipient of various prestigious recognitions as AICTE Career Award for Young Pharmacy Teacher, Achari Prize and Chandra Kanta Dandiya Award.

dr_chopra_k@yahoo.com

(11.3)

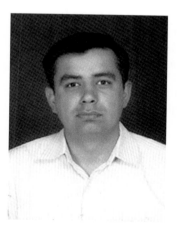

Anurag Kuhad

Mr Anurag Kuhad is serving as Assistant Professor of Pharmacology at University Institute of Pharmaceutical Sciences, Panjab University, Chandigarh, India. He has more than 6 years of research experience (industrial as well as academic) and 3 years of teaching experience. His research area is diabetes and related complications. Mr Kuhad has been selected twice for "Young Investigator Award" at International Conference on Polyphenols and Health 2007 and 2009.

(11.3)

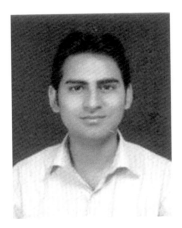

Vinod Tiwari

Mr. Vinod Tiwari is pursuing his PhD under the guidance of Dr. (Ms) Kanwaljit Chopra, Associate Professor of Pharmacology at University Institute of Pharmaceutical Sciences, Panjab University, Chandigarh. His research work is focused on exploring the role of oxidative-nitrosative stress mediated neuroinflammatory cascade in chronic alcohol-induced cognitive deficits, neuropathy and fetal alcohol spectrum disorders.

(11.4)

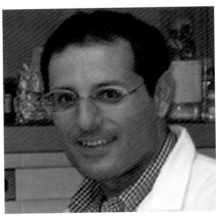

Domenico Praticò

Dr. Praticò received his M.D. from the University of Rome "La Sapienza", School of Medicine where he also completed the residency program in Internal Medicine.

After receiving a European Research Award fellowship, he spent two years of post-doctoral training at the University of Dublin as a fellow in the Center for Cardiovascular Science. In 1994, he joined the Center for Experimental Therapeutics at the University of Pennsylvania as Research Associate, where he was promoted to Assistant Professor of Pharmacology. In 2007, he moved to Temple University in Philadelphia as an Associate Professor of Pharmacology.

His main research interest is oxidative biology with a particular focus on bioactive lipids, their metabolic pathways, and their role as biological mediators of cellular and molecular events in the pathogenesis of human diseases.

praticod@temple.edu

(13)

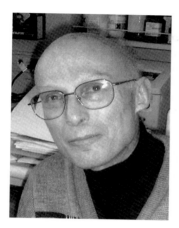

Michael Lever

Michael Lever graduated PhD from Massey University, New Zealand and is a scientist in Canterbury Health Laboratories, the laboratory services of the teaching hospital in Christchurch, New Zealand. His academic affiliations are with the Christchurch School of Medicine and Health Sciences (University of Otago) and the University of Canterbury.

michael.lever@otago.ac.nz

(14.1)

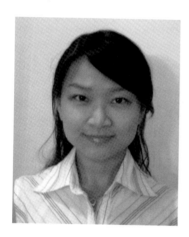

Ya-Wen Teng

Ya-Wen Teng is a Ph.D. candidate in the laboratory of Dr. Zeisel at the Department of Nutrition in the Gillings School of Global Public Health at the University of North Carolina at Chapel Hill. She earned her bachelor of science in Nutrition from UNC-Chapel Hill in 2002 with highest honors. She is a member of the American Society for Nutrition, and was the recipient of the McNeil Nutritionals Predoctoral Fellowship at 2009.

yteng@email.unc.edu

(14.1)

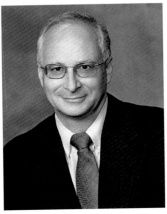

Steven H. Zeisel

Dr. Steven Zeisel is the Kenan Distinguished University Professor in the Department of Nutrition in the Gillings School of Global Public Health at the University of North Carolina at Chapel Hill. He is also the Director of the UNC's Nutrition Research Institute at the newly formed North Carolina Research Campus in Kannapolis, North Carolina. Dr. Zeisel earned his M.D. from Harvard Medical School in 1975, was a resident in pediatrics at Yale University from 1975-1977, and earned his Ph.D. in nutrition at the Massachusetts Institute of Technology in 1980. He served as chair of the Department of Nutrition at the University of North Carolina at Chapel Hill from 1990–2005. He is currently a member of the American Society for Nutrition, the American Society for Parenteral and Enteral Nutrition, the American College of Nutrition and the Society for Pediatric Research, among others.

Dr. Zeisel is a member of the World Cancer Research Fund's Expert Panel on "Food, Nutrition and the Prevention of Cancer: a global perspective." He serves as the principal investigator on multiple federally funded research projects that focus on human requirements for choline and the effects of this nutrient on brain development.

steven_zeisel@unc.edu

(15.1)

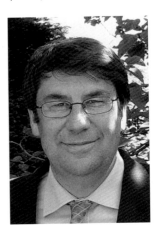

Philip Calder

Philip Calder is Professor of Nutritional Immunology at the University of Southampton, UK. He has been studying the influence of dietary fatty acids on aspects of cell function and human health, in particular in relation to cardiovascular disease, inflammation and immunity, since 1987. He has received several awards and served on a number of committees. He is currently President of the International Society for the Study of Fatty Acids and Lipids (ISSFAL).

(15.2)

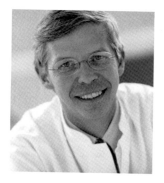

Berthold Koletzko

Berthold Koletzko is Professor of Paediatrics at the Ludwig-Maximilians-University of Munich, Division of Metabolic Diseases and Nutrition, Dr. von Hauner Children's Hospital. He acts as a scientific expert for the Federal Government, the European Parliament, the European Commission, the Food and Agriculture Organization of the United Nations (FAO) and the United Nations University.

office.koletzko@med.uni-muenchen.de

(15.3)

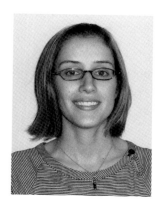

Natalie Riediger

Natalie Riediger completed a B.Sc. and M.Sc. in the Department of Human Nutritional Sciences at the University of Manitoba, Canada. Her M.Sc. work involved investigating the effects of dietary oils low in n-6:n-3 fatty acids, including fish- and flaxseed oil, on cardiovascular risk. Natalie is currently in the PhD program in the Department of Community Health Sciences at the University of Manitoba, where she continues her work on omega-3 fatty acids in addition to other population health research.

umriedin@cc.umanitoba.ca

(15.4)

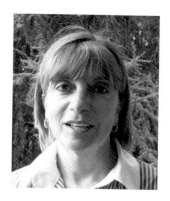

Gabriella Calviello

Gabriella Calviello is currently Associate Professor at the Institute of General Pathology, School of Medicine Catholic University, Rome, Italy, where she has taught General Pathology since 1984. Her main area of research includes the antitumoral and anti-inflammatory effects of n-3 PUFAs.

g.calviello@rm.unicatt.it

Index